GLOBAL HEALTH
Diseases, Programs, Systems, and Policies
THIRD EDITION

Edited by

Michael H. Merson, MD
Wolfgang Joklik Professor of Global Health
Director, Duke Global Health Institute
Duke University
Durham, North Carolina

Robert E. Black, MD, MPH
Edgar Berman Professor and Chair
Department of International Health
Director, Institute for International Programs
Bloomberg School of Public Health
Johns Hopkins University
Baltimore, Maryland

Anne J. Mills, MA, DHSA, PhD
Professor of Health Economics and Policy
Head, Faculty of Public Health and Policy
London School of Hygiene & Tropical Medicine
London, UK

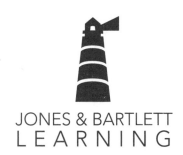

JONES & BARTLETT
LEARNING

World Headquarters

Jones & Bartlett Learning
5 Wall Street
Burlington, MA 01803
978-443-5000
info@jblearning.com
www.jblearning.com

Jones & Bartlett Learning
Canada
6339 Ormindale Way
Mississauga, Ontario L5V 1J2
Canada

Jones & Bartlett Learning
International
Barb House, Barb Mews
London W6 7PA
United Kingdom

Jones & Bartlett Learning books and products are available through most bookstores and online booksellers. To contact Jones & Bartlett Learning directly, call 800-832-0034, fax 978-443-8000, or visit our website, www.jblearning.com.

Substantial discounts on bulk quantities of Jones & Bartlett Learning publications are available to corporations, professional associations, and other qualified organizations. For details and specific discount information, contact the special sales department at Jones & Bartlett Learning via the above contact information or send an email to specialsales@jblearning.com.

This publication is designed to provide accurate and authoritative information in regard to the Subject Matter covered. It is sold with the understanding that the publisher is not engaged in rendering legal, accounting, or other professional service. If legal advice or other expert assistance is required, the service of a competent professional person should be sought.

Production Credits

Publisher: Michael Brown
Editorial Assistant: Teresa Reilly
Editorial Assistant: Chloe Falivene
Associate Production Editor: Kate Stein
Associate Production Editor: Cindie Bryan
Associate Marketing Manager: Jody Sullivan

Manufacturing and Inventory Control
  Supervisor: Amy Bacus
Composition: Achorn International, Inc.
Cover Design: Scott Moden
Cover Image: © argus/ShutterStock, Inc.
Printing and Binding: Courier Kendallville
Cover Printing: Courier Kendallville

Some images in this book feature models. These models do not necessarily endorse, represent, or participate in the activities represented in the images.

Library of Congress Cataloging-in-Publication Data

Global health: diseases, programs, systems and policies / [edited by] Michael H. Merson, Robert E. Black, Anne J. Mills. — 3rd ed.
   p. ; cm.
   Rev. ed. of: International public health. 2nd ed. c2006.
   Includes bibliographical references and index.
   ISBN-13: 978-0-7637-8559-8 (hardcover)
   ISBN-10: 0-7637-8559-8 (hardcover)
   1. World health. 2. Public health—International cooperation.   I. Merson, Michael H.
II. Black, Robert E.   III. Mills, Anne J.   IV. International public health.
   [DNLM: 1. Public Health. 2. World Health. 3. International Cooperation
4. Public Health Administration.   WA 530.1
   RA441.I578 2012
   362.1–dc22

2011000579

6048

Printed in the United States of America
15 14 13 12 11   10 9 8 7 6 5 4 3 2 1

Contents

Chapter 7   Chronic Diseases and Risks   *Derek Yach, George A. Mensah, Corinna Hawkes, JoAnne E. Epping-Jordan, and Krisela Steyn*   **345**

Chapter 8   Unintentional Injuries and Violence   *Robyn Norton, Adnan A. Hyder, and Alexander Butchart*   **407**

Chapter 9   Global Mental Health   *Vikram Patel, Alan J. Flisher, and Alex Cohen*   **445**

About the Authors

Michael H. Merson, MD is the Wolfgang Joklik Professor of Global Health at Duke University and the founding Director of the Duke Global Health Institute and Vice Chancellor for Duke–National University of Singapore Affairs. He has held leadership positions at the Centers for Disease Control and Prevention and the International Center for Diarrheal Diseases Research, Bangladesh, served as Director of the World Health Organization's Diarrheal and Acute Respiratory Control Programs and Global Program on AIDS, and was the first Dean of Public Health at Yale University. Dr. Merson's research and writings have been primarily on the etiology of diarrheal diseases in low- and middle-income countries and on HIV prevention and policy. He has served as an advisor to UNAIDS, the World Bank, and a number of other international organizations and advisory bodies; is an elected member of the U.S. Institute of Medicine; and has received two honorary degrees and the U.S. Surgeon General's Exemplary Service Medal.

Robert E. Black, MD, MPH is the Edgar Berman Professor and Chair of the Department of International Health and Director of the Institute for International Programs of the Johns Hopkins University Bloomberg School of Public Health in Baltimore, Maryland. As a member of the U.S. Institute of Medicine and advisory bodies of the World Health Organization, the International Vaccine Institute, and other international organizations, he assists with the development of programs and policies intended to improve child health and nutrition. Dr. Black currently chairs the WHO/UNICEF Child Health Epidemiology Reference Group and the Child Health and Nutrition Research Initiative. He has more than 500 scientific journal publications derived from his international research. Dr. Black received the Programme for Global Paediatric Research Award for Outstanding Contributions to Global Child Health in 2010, the Prince Mahidol Award in Public Health in 2010, and the Canada Gairdner Global Health Award in 2011.

Anne J. Mills, MA, DHSA, PhD is Professor of Health Economics and Policy at the London School of Hygiene and Tropical Medicine and Head of its Faculty of Public Health and Policy. She has nearly 40 years of experience with the health systems of low- and middle-income countries, and has researched and published widely in the fields of health economics and health systems. Dr. Mills has also had extensive involvement in supporting capacity development in health economics in universities and research institutes. She has advised multilateral, bilateral, and government agencies on numerous occasions; was a member of WHO's Commission on Macroeconomics and Health; and co-chaired Working Group 1 of the 2009 High Level Taskforce on Innovative International Financing for Health Systems. She has been awarded a CBE, is an elected member of the U.S. Institute of Medicine and Fellow of the U.K. Academy of Medical Sciences, and received the Prince Mahidol Award in Medicine in 2009.

Acknowledgments

We would like to acknowledge the technical and editorial assistance of Aisha Jafri and Caroline Hope Griffith.

Contributors

Stuart Anderson, MA, PhD, FRPharmS, FHEA
Associate Dean of Studies
London School of Hygiene & Tropical Medicine
London, U.K.

David E. Bloom, MA, PhD
Clarence James Gamble Professor of Economics
    and Demography
Chair, Department of Global Health and Population
Harvard School of Public Health
Boston, MA

Jennifer Bryce, EdD, MEd
Senior Scientist
Department of International Health
Johns Hopkins Bloomberg School of Public Health
Baltimore, MD

Kent Buse, MSc, PhD
Senior Policy Advisor
UNAIDS
London, U.K.

Alexander Butchart, MA, PhD
Department of Violence and Injury Prevention
    and Disability
World Health Organization
Geneva, Switzerland

Benjamin Caballero, MD, MSc, PhD
Program in Human Nutrition
Johns Hopkins Bloomberg School of Public Health
Baltimore, MD

David Canning, PhD
Professor of Economics and International Health
Department of Global Health and Population
Harvard School of Public Health
Boston, MA

Alex Cohen, MA, PhD
Assistant Professor
Department of Social Medicine
Harvard Medical School
Boston, MA

Charles Collins, PhD, MSoc Sc.
Nuffield Centre for International Health
    and Development
University of Leeds
Leeds, U.K.

Emma Doohan
Project Manager
Centre for Public Health Excellence
National Institute for Health and Clinical Excellence
London, U.K.

JoAnne Epping-Jordan, PhD
Health Consultant
Seattle, WA

William H. Foege, MD, MPH
Senior Fellow
Global Health Program
Bill and Melinda Gates Foundation
Emeritus Presidential Distinguished Professor of
    International Health
Rollins School of Public Health
Emory University
Vashon, WA

**Alan John Flisher, MB ChB, PhD, MSc, MMed, MPhil,
    FCPsych (SA), DCH (*deceased*)**
Professor and Head, Division of Child and
    Adolescent Psychiatry
University of Cape Town and Red Cross War Memorial
Children's Hospital
Cape Town, South Africa

Aubree Gordon, MPH, PhD
Assistant Researcher
School of Public Health
University of California, Berkeley
Berkeley, CA

Andrew Green, MA, PhD
Professor of International Health Planning
Nuffield Centre for International Health and Development
Leeds Institute for Health Sciences, University of Leeds
Leeds, U.K.

Javier Guzman, MD, MSc
Director of Research
Policy Cures
London, U.K.

Kara Hanson, SD
Department of Global Health and Development
London School of Hygiene & Tropical Medicine
London, U.K.

Andrew Harmer, MSc, PhD
Research Fellow
Department of Global Health and Development
London School of Hygiene & Tropical Medicine
London, U.K.

Corinna Hawkes, PhD
Consulting Services
Food and Nutrition Policy
France

Adnan A. Hyder, MD, PhD, MPH
Associate Professor, Department of International Health
Director, International Injury Research Unit
Deputy Director, Health Systems Program
Core Faculty Berman Institute of Bioethics Institute
Johns Hopkins Bloomberg School of Public Health
Baltimore, MD

Dean T. Jamison, MS, PhD
Professor, Global Health
Adjunct Professor, Health Services
Institute for Health Metrics and Evaluation
Department of Global Health
University of Washington
Seattle, WA

Benjamin Johns, MPA, MA
Department of International Health
Johns Hopkins Bloomberg School of Public Health
Baltimore, MD

Adam Kamradt-Scott, BN, MAIS, PhD
Research Fellow
Department of Global Health and Development
London School of Hygiene & Tropical Medicine
London, U.K.

Michael P. Kelly, PhD, FFPH, Hon FRCP
Director
Centre for Public Health Excellence
National Institute for Health and Clinical Excellence
London, U.K.

Tord Kjellstrom, MD, MEng, PhD
Visiting Fellow, Professor
National Centre for Epidemiology and Population Health
Australian National University
Canberra, Australia
Honorary Professor
UCL (London, U.K.), University of Tromso (Norway),
   Umea University (Sweden), Wellington School of
   Medicine (New Zealand)

Kelley Lee, BA MPA, MA, DPhil, FFPH
Professor
Department of Global Health and Development
London School of Hygiene & Tropical Medicine
London, U.K.
Professor
Faculty of Health Sciences
Simon Fraser University
British Columbia, Canada

Anthony J. McMichael, PhD
National Centre for Epidemiology and Population Health
Australian National University
Canberra, Australia

Jane Menken, MS, PhD
Professor, Department of Sociology
Director, Institute of Behavioral Science
University of Colorado at Boulder
Boulder, CO

George A. Mensah, MD
Vice President, Global Nutrition Policy
PepsiCo
Purchase, NY

Tolib Mirzoev, MD, MA, PGCertLTHE, PhD
Lecturer in International Health Systems
Nuffield Centre for International Health and Development
Leeds Institute of Health Sciences, University of Leeds
Leeds, U.K.

Mary Moran, MBBS, Grad Dip FAT, FRSM
Director
Policy Cures
Sydney, Australia

Richard H. Morrow, MD, MPH, FACP
Professor
Department of International Health, Health
   Systems Program
Johns Hopkins Bloomberg School of Public Health
Baltimore, MD

Robyn Norton, PhD, MPH, MA
Principal Director
The George Institute for Global Health
Professor, Public Health
Associate Dean (Global Health)
Sydney Medical School
University of Sydney
Sydney, Australia

Benjamin Palafox, MSc
Research Fellow, Pharmaceutical Policy and Economics
Department of Global Health and Development
London School of Hygiene & Tropical Medicine
London, U.K.

Vikram Patel, MSc, MRCPsych, PhD, FMedSci
Professor of International Mental Health
Wellcome Trust Senior Research Fellow in
   Clinical Science
Centre for Global Mental Health
London School of Hygiene & Tropical Medicine
London, U.K.

Prasanthi Puvanachandra, MB BChir, MPH
Associate
International Injury Research Unit
Johns Hopkins Bloomberg School of Public Health
Baltimore, MD

M. Omar Rahman, MD, MPH, DSc
Vice Chancellor (In Charge)
Independent University
Bangladesh

M. Kent Ranson, MD, MPH, Phd
Technical Officer
Alliance for Health Policy and Systems Research
World Health Organization
Geneva, Switzerland

Arthur L. Reingold, MD
Professor of Epidemiology and Associate Dean
    for Research
Division of Epidemiology
School of Public Health
University of California, Berkeley
Berkeley, CA

Jennifer Prah Ruger, PhD
Associate Professor
Yale Schools of Public Health and Medicine
Professor (Adjunct) of Law
Yale Law School
New Haven, CT

Susan C. Scrimshaw, PhD
President
The Sage Colleges
Troy, NY

Rima Shretta, BPharm, MPH
Principal Program Associate for Malaria
Center for Pharmaceutical Management
Management Sciences for Health
Arlington, VA

Sudhvir Singh
Department of Epidemiology and Biostatistics
School of Population Health
The University of Auckland
Auckland, New Zealand

Kirk R. Smith, MPH, PhD
Professor of Global Environmental Health
University of California, Berkeley
Berkeley, CA

Christine P. Stewart, MPH, PhD
Assistant Professor
Department of Nutrition
Assistant Nutritionist in Agricultural Experiment Station
University of California, Davis
Davis, CA

Krisela Steyn, MSc, NED, MD
Department of Medicine
Faculty of Health Sciences
University of Cape Town
Cape Town, South Africa

Michael J. Toole, BMedSc, MBBS, DTM&H
Head, Centre for International Health
Burnet Institute
Professor, School of Public Health
Monash University
Melbourne, Australia

Cesar G. Victora, MD, PhD
Emeritus Professor of Epidemiology
Federal University of Pelotas in Brazil
Pelotas, Brazil

Ronald J. Waldman, MD
Director, Program on Forced Migration and Health
Professor of Clinical Public Health
Mailman School of Public Health
Columbia University
New York, NY

Damian Walker, PhD
Senior Program Officer, Global Health
Bill and Melinda Gates Foundation
Seattle, WA

Gill Walt, PhD
Emeritus Professor of International Health Policy
Department of Global Health and Development
London School of Hygiene & Tropical Medicine
London, U.K.

Keith P. West, Jr., DrPH, MPH
George G. Graham Professor of Infant and
    Child Nutrition
Department of International Health
Johns Hopkins Bloomberg School of Public Health
Baltimore, MD

Tana Wuliji, PhD, BPharm
Director
Global Develoop
Washington, DC

Derek Yach, MBChB, MPH
Senior Vice President
Global Health Policy
PepsiCo
Purchase, NY

Foreword

WILLIAM H. FOEGE

The change in this book's title, from *International Public Health: Diseases, Programs, Systems, and Policies* to *Global Health: Diseases, Programs, Systems, and Policies*, is a big change. Why a big change? It was possible in the past to see international health as something physically removed—the object of our endeavors. The term "international" suggested a dichotomy between "national" and the rest of the world. In truth, every place on earth is both local and global. The change in title to "global" suggests a unity to health where we are all in this together and where everything affects everything else. It was never possible to adequately protect the health of citizens in one country without being involved with health everywhere, and the title change acknowledges that fact.

In the Foreword for the last edition, published in 2006, I presented a summary of the field from Sumerian times, through the Colonial period, and then on to missionary medicine, military interests, and the modern era since World War II. The second half of the twentieth century was remarkable for the development of global agencies, such as the World Health Organization, UNICEF, the World Bank, and UNDP; large nongovernmental agencies (NGOs) such as CARE and Save the Children; small NGOs by the thousands; bilateral health programs; and the improvement in resources available because of foundations such as the Rockefeller Foundation and the Bill and Melinda Gates Foundation. At the same time that this activity was happening, there was also an evolution in focus from tropical diseases to the health problems of poor countries.

Despite all of the enthusiasm that welcomed the last edition of this book, it is now clear that the past five years have been the most eventful in the history of global health. Suddenly the academic world has changed. In the past, except at a handful of schools, global health—if taught at all—was taught because a single person or a small group had a special interest in the subject. Rarely was it an institutional priority. Today, however, the United States has between 150 and 200 global health programs in institutions of higher learning in both undergraduate and graduate departments. In some universities, this subject has become a school-wide priority, not limited to the health schools. Students in medical schools and schools of public health eagerly seek out courses and experiences in global health. In fact, in some schools of public health, global health is the greatest magnet for new students. It is as if the thirst for knowledge and experience in this field is almost unquenchable.

New tools could narrow what has been a widening gap between the health of poor countries and rich countries. The second anticancer vaccine, directed at the human papillomavirus, holds promise to reduce the toll of cervical cancer in resource-poor areas. The Rotovirus vaccine could save many children in poor countries. A malaria vaccine is in human trials, and a variety of tuberculosis vaccines are now undergoing human trials. This wave of development seems to be a harbinger of what the future holds.

A revolution in support from pharmaceutical companies, accelerated by the gift of Mectizan by Merck for river blindness, has introduced a robust new chapter in global health. Coalitions unimagined in the past are so commonplace that they receive scant notice. A partnership between Merck, the Harvard School of Public Health AIDS Initiative, the Gates Foundation, and the government of Botswana has reduced the HIV-positivity rate of newborns in Botswana from 40% to 4% in a decade. The Jimmy Carter Center has demonstrated the power of involving the political leaders of countries, as it has worked toward reducing river blindness, filariasis, and Guinea worm. The reality of global health today exceeds the dreams of global health practitioners of the past.

Creativity is harnessing new technologies to old problems. For example, the chronic problem of adulterated drugs in Africa might be solved by a scratch-off area on each vial that reveals numbers. A phone number reached by cell phone, followed by the numbers on the vial, would provide immediate feedback regarding the authenticity of that vial. Global health workers have always had a reputation as problem solvers, but now they can tie that ability to technology that ably helps solve problems for many others as well.

Students entering the global health field will have the ability to far surpass the efforts of their predecessors. Now is an absolutely exciting time to engage in the effort to narrow the health gap between poor and rich countries.

But make no mistake: poverty is still the great barrier. It is the major social determinant of health status and is dose related—that is, health status deteriorates with every reduction in financial status. Global health workers will need to be as creative in countering poverty as they are in countering microorganisms. Keeping people healthy is a start toward keeping them productive. Just as coalitions have become standard between corporations, foundations, governments, and NGOs in improving health, so global health workers must now extend their efforts to coalitions that attack poverty. This effort means countering the many other social forces impeding health, through microcredit, employment, education, and opportunities of all kinds.

Drs. Merson, Black, and Mills have once again brought a comprehensive textbook that helps us make sense of an enlarging and confusing field. It is an enormously valuable guide for students, teachers, and practitioners that helps to map out the journeys of those who will change the future.

Introduction

MICHAEL H. MERSON, ROBERT E. BLACK, AND ANNE J. MILLS

The three of us are privileged to serve as faculty at universities that provide education to hundreds of graduate and undergraduate students who are motivated to learn about global health issues and challenges. Many of these students plan to or have already begun careers in global health research, policy, practice, teaching, or administration. This textbook is written for these students around the world, as well as for those who teach and mentor them. In this Introduction, we define global health, provide a brief history of the field, and summarize its many challenges. We then explain how we put this third edition together and how we think it can best be used.

Why Global Health?

Those of you who are familiar with this textbook will have likely realized at first glance that we have changed part of its title from *International Public Health* to *Global Health*. This change reflects the fact that, since the previous edition was published, we have witnessed a major surge in interest in global health, both as a concept and as an area of academic study. Essentially, global health has replaced international health both in concept and reality (Koplan et al., 2009).

International public health, as we defined the term in the previous editions, focuses on the application of the principles of public health to health problems and challenges that affect low- and middle-income countries and to the complex array of global and local forces that influence them. Global health maintains this focus, but places much greater emphasis on health issues that concern many countries or that are affected greatly by transnational determinants, such as climate change or urbanization. This greater emphasis on the scope, in addition to the location, of health problems opens up the opportunity to address cross-border issues as well as domestic health disparities in high-income countries.

Moreover, while international public health primarily applies the principles of public health, there is now agreement that success and progress in improving health around the world requires a multidisciplinary and interdisciplinary approach that includes, yet extends beyond, public health. Professionals from many disciplines and academic fields possess the skills and knowledge needed to understand the various determinants of health and develop strategies that will address these determinants, thereby sharing goals to improve the health of populations. These disciplines and professional fields include social and behavioral sciences (including sociology, economics, psychology, anthropology, political science, and international relations), biomedical and environmental sciences, engineering, business and management, public policy, law, history, and divinity. Furthermore, while efforts to reduce health disparities should focus on prevention, inequalities in treatment, care, and curative strategies must also be addressed when developing solutions to global health challenges, further emphasizing the need for a multidisciplinary approach.

In addition, while social justice—an essential element of public health—should continue to be a central pillar of health, the approach to achieving health equity and finding solutions to reducing health disparities must now much more strongly emphasize global cooperation. Rather than following a model that transfers ideas and resources from high-income countries, organizations, or funding agencies to low-income settings, it is imperative to pursue "a real partnership, a pooling of experience and knowledge, and a two-way flow between developed and developing countries" when implementing health interventions or programs (Koplan et al., 2009).

For all of these reasons, we have embraced the concept of global health and incorporated it in the title of this textbook. Today, there is a greater awareness that we live in an increasingly connected world, and the way in which we view health is no exception. The challenges to reduce health disparities are considerable, and the tenets of global health provide a unique insight and strategic approach to addressing them.

Given this evolution in our thinking, there has been an understandable interest in defining global health. In 1997, the U.S. Institute of Medicine (IOM) released a report that broadly defined global health as "health problems, issues, and concerns that transcend national boundaries, may be influenced by circumstances or experiences in other countries, and are best addressed by cooperative actions and solutions." More than 10 years later, IOM amended its definition, describing global health "not just as a state but also as the *goal of improving health for all people by reducing avoidable disease, disabilities, and deaths* [emphasis added]"(Committee on the U.S. Commitment to Global Health, 2009).

We prefer the definition of global health that was adopted by the Consortium of Universities for Global Health (CUGH). CUGH was recently formed to promote, facilitate, and enhance the growth of global health as an academic field of study. It has defined global health as follows:

> [A]n area for study, research, and practice that places a priority on improving health and achieving equity in health for all people worldwide. Global health emphasizes transnational health issues, determinants, and solutions; involves many disciplines within and beyond the health sciences and promotes interdisci-

plinary collaboration; and is a synthesis of population-based prevention with individual-level clinical care. (Koplan et al., 2009)

When providing this definition, an effort was made to explain the differences between public health, international health, and global health. While these terms certainly share areas of overlap, this comparison helps to draw out global health's distinctive qualities, some to which we have referred previously (Exhibit I-1).

A Brief History of Global Health

Tracing the roots of global health brings us to the history of international public health. This history encompasses the origins of public health and can be viewed as a history of how populations experience health and illness; how social, economic, and political systems create the possibilities for healthy or unhealthy lives; how societies create the preconditions for the production and transmission of disease; and how people, both as individuals and as social groups, attempt to promote their own health or avoid illness

Exhibit I-1	Global Health, International Health, and Public Health	
Global Health	**International Health**	**Public Health**
Focuses on issues that directly or indirectly impact health but can transcend national boundaries.	Focuses on health issues of countries *other* than one's own, especially those of low- and middle-income countries.	Focuses on issues that impact the health of the *population* of a particular community or nation.
Development and implementation of solutions often require global cooperation.	Development and implementation of solutions usually involve binational cooperation.	Development and implementation of solutions usually do not involve global cooperation.
Embraces both prevention in populations and clinical care of individuals.	Embraces both prevention in populations and clinical care of individuals.	Mainly focused on prevention programs for populations.
Health equity among nations and for all people is a major objective.	Seeks to help people of other nations.	Health equity within a nation or community is a major objective.
Highly interdisciplinary and multidisciplinary within and beyond health sciences.	Embraces but has not emphasized multidisciplinarity.	Encourages multidisciplinary approaches, particularly within health sciences and with social sciences.

(Rosen & Morman, 1993). A number of authors have documented this history (Arnold, 1988; Basch, 1999; Leff & Leff, 1958; Rosen & Morman, 1993; Winslow & Hallock, 1933). A brief history is presented here primarily to provide a perspective for the challenges that face us today (Exhibit I-2).

The Origins of Public Health

It is difficult to select a date for the origins of the field of public health. Some would begin with Hippocrates, whose book *Airs, Waters, and Places*, published around 400 BC, was the first systematic effort to present the causal relationships between environmental factors and disease and to offer a theoretical basis for an understanding of endemic and epidemic diseases. Others would cite the introduction of public sanitation and an organized water supply system by the Romans in the first century AD. Many would select the bubonic plague (or Black Death) pandemic of the fourteenth century, which began in Central Asia; was carried on ships to Constantinople, Genoa, and other European ports; and then spread inland, killing 25 million persons in Europe alone. In response to this devastating infectious disease, the Great Council of the city of Ragusa (now Dubrovnik, Croatia) followed a contagion theory, which recommended the separation of healthy and sick populations, and issued a document stating that outsiders entering the city must spend 30 days in the restricted location of nearby islands (Stuard and NetLibrary, 1992). The length of time for this isolation period, dubbed *trentino*, was eventually increased from 30 to 40 days, introducing the concept of the modern quarantine (Gensini et al., 2004).

The Middle Ages was also the period when many cities in Europe, particularly through the formation of guilds, took an active part in founding hospitals and other institutions to provide medical care and social assistance. It was also a time when many European countries expanded their horizons abroad, exploring and colonizing new lands. The travelers brought some diseases with them (e.g., influenza, measles, smallpox), and those who settled in these colonial outposts were forced to confront diseases that had never been seen in Europe (such as syphilis, dysentery, malaria, and sleeping sickness). European explorers also brought new pathogens from one part of Africa to another and from one area of the globe to another

---

Exhibit I-2	The History of Global Health: A Summary

400 BC: Hippocrates presents the causal relationship between environment and disease.

First century AD: Romans introduce public sanitation and organize a water supply system.

Fourteenth century: The "Black Death" (bubonic plague) leads to quarantine and *cordon sanitaire*.

Middle Ages: Colonial expansion spreads infectious diseases around the world.

1750–1850: The Industrial Revolution results in extensive health and social improvements in cities in Europe and the United States.

1850–1910: Knowledge about the causes and transmission of communicable diseases is greatly expanded.

1910–1945: Reductions in child mortality occur. Schools of public health and international foundations and intergovernmental agencies interested in public health are established.

1945–1990: The World Bank and other UN agencies are created. WHO eradicates smallpox. The HIV/AIDS pandemic begins. The Alma Ata Conference gives emphasis to primary health care. UNICEF leads efforts to ensure universal childhood immunization. Greater attention is given to chronic diseases.

1990–2000: Priority is given to health-sector reform, the impact of and responses to globalization, cost-effectiveness, and public–private partnerships in health.

2000–2010: Priority is given to equity, social determinants of health, health and development, use of innovative information and communications technologies, achievement of the Millennium Development Goals (MDGs), and response to influenza.

(e.g., from Africa to North America through the slave trade). On long voyages, however, the greatest enemy of the sailor was often scurvy—at least until 1875, when the British government issued its famous order that all men-of-war should carry a supply of lemon juice.

The Age of Enlightenment (1750–1830) was a pivotal period in the evolution of public health. It was a time of social action in relation to health, as reflected by the new interest taken in the health problems of specific population groups. During this period, rapid advances in technology led to the development of factories. In England and elsewhere, this industrialization was paralleled by expansion of the coal mines. The Industrial Revolution had arrived. During this period, the populations of the cities of England and other industrialized nations grew enormously, creating many unsanitary conditions that caused outbreaks of cholera and other epidemic diseases, which ultimately resulted in high rates of child mortality. Near the end of this period, significant efforts were made to address these problems. Improvements were made in urban water supplies and sewerage systems, municipal hospitals arose throughout cities in Europe and the east coast of the United States, laws were enacted limiting children's ability to work, and data on deaths and births began to be systematically collected in many places.

As industrialization continued, it became obvious that more efforts to protect the health of the public were needed. These changes occurred first in England, which is regarded as the first modern industrial country, through the efforts of Edwin Chadwick. Beginning in 1832, he headed up the royal Poor Law Commission, which undertook an extensive survey of health and sanitation conditions throughout the country. The work of this commission led in 1848 to the Public Health Act, which created a General Board of Health that was empowered to appoint local boards of health and medical officers of health to deal effectively with public health problems. The impact of these developments was felt throughout Europe and especially in the United States, where it stimulated creation of health departments in many cities and states.

Cholera, which in the first half of the nineteenth century spread in waves from South Asia to the Middle East and then to Europe and the United States, did the most to stimulate the formal internationalization of public health. The policy of establishing a *cordon sanitaire*—an action applied by many European nations in an effort to control the disease— had become a major influence on trade, necessitating an international agreement. In 1851, the First International Sanitary Conference was convened in Paris to discuss the role of quarantine in the control of cholera as well as of plague and yellow fever, which were causing epidemics throughout Europe. Although no real agreement was reached, the conference laid the foundations for international cooperation in health.

The latter part of the nineteenth century was distinguished by the enormous growth of knowledge in the area of microbiology, as exemplified by Louis Pasteur's proof of the germ theory of disease, Robert Koch's discovery of the tubercle bacillus, and Walter Reed's demonstration of the role of the mosquito in transmitting yellow fever. Between 1880 and 1910, the etiological cause and means of transmission of many communicable diseases were discovered in laboratories in North America and Europe. The development of this knowledge base was paralleled by related discoveries in the sciences of physiology, metabolism, endocrinology, and nutrition. Dramatic decreases soon were seen in child and adult mortality through improvements in social and economic conditions, discovery of vaccines, and implementation of programs in health education. The way was now clear for the development of public health administration based on a scientific understanding of the elements involved in the transmission of communicable diseases.

The first two decades of the twentieth century witnessed the establishment of three formal intergovernmental public health bodies: the International Sanitary Bureau to serve nations in the western hemisphere (in 1904); l'Office Internationale d'Hygiene Publique in Paris, which was concerned with prevention and control of the main quarantinable diseases (in 1909); and the League of Nations Health Office (LNHO) in Geneva, which provided assistance to member states on technical matters related to health (in 1920). In 1926, LNHO commenced publication of *Weekly Epidemiological Record*, which evolved into a weekly publication of the World Health Organization (WHO). LNHO also established many scientific and technical commissions, issued reports on the status of many infectious and chronic diseases, and sent its staff around the world to assist national governments in dealing with their health problems.

In North America and countries in Europe, the explosion of scientific knowledge in the latter part of the nineteenth century and the belief that social problems could be solved stimulated medical schools, such as Johns Hopkins University, to establish schools of public health. In France, public subscriptions helped to fund the Institut Pasteur (in honor of Louis Pasteur) in Paris, which subsequently developed a network of institutes throughout the francophone world that produced sera and vaccines and conducted research on a wide variety of tropical diseases. Another significant development during this period was the founding of the Rockefeller Foundation (in 1909) and its International Health Commission (in 1913). During its 38 years of operation, the commission cooperated with many governments in campaigns against endemic diseases such as hookworm, malaria, and yellow fever. The Rockefeller Foundation also provided essential financial support to help establish medical schools in China, Thailand, and elsewhere, and later supported international health programs in a number of American and European schools of medicine and public health. All of these developments were paralleled by the development and strengthening of competencies in public health among the militaries of the United States and the countries of Europe, stimulated in great part by the buildup to and realities of World War I. Following the war, there was increasing recognition that much ill health in the colonial world was not easily solvable with medical interventions and was intractably linked to malnutrition and poverty.

Some historians would date the beginning of international public health to the end of World War II. The end of European colonialism, the need to reconstruct the economies of the United States and the countries of Western Europe, and the rapid emergence of newly independent countries in Africa and Asia led to the creation of many new intergovernmental organizations. The United Nations Monetary and Financial Conference, held in Bretton Woods, New Hampshire, and attended by representatives from 43 countries, resulted in the establishment of the International Bank for Reconstruction and Development (more commonly known as the World Bank) and the International Monetary Fund. The former initially lent money to countries only at prevailing market interest rates, but beginning in 1960 also provided loans to poorer countries at much lower interest rates and with far better terms through its International Development Association. It was not until the early 1980s that the World Bank began to accelerate greatly its provision of loans to countries for programs in health and education. By the end of the decade, however, these loans were the greatest source of foreign assistance to low- and middle-income countries (Ruger, 2005).

In the decade after World War II, many other United Nations organizations (e.g., the United Nations Children's Fund, or UNICEF) and specialized agencies (such as WHO) were formed to assist countries in strengthening their health and other social sectors. In addition, most of the wealthier industrialized countries established agencies or bureaus that funded bilateral projects in specific low- and middle-income countries. For the former major colonial powers, such assistance was most often provided to their former colonies.

Many of the international health efforts in the 1960s and 1970s were dedicated to the control of specific diseases. A global effort to control malaria was hampered by a number of operational and technical difficulties, including the vector's increasing resistance to insecticides and the parasite's resistance to available antimalarial drugs. In contrast, the campaign to eradicate smallpox, led by WHO, successfully eliminated the disease in 1981 and stimulated the establishment of the Expanded Program on Immunization, which focused on the delivery of effective vaccines to infants. Also, during the 1970s, two large international research programs were initiated under the co-sponsorship of various United Nations agencies: the Special Program for Research on Human Reproduction (focusing on development and testing of new contraceptive technologies) and the Tropical Disease Research Program (providing support for the development of better means of diagnosis, treatment, and prevention of six tropical diseases, including malaria). Greater attention also was gradually given to chronic diseases, such as cardiovascular and cerebrovascular diseases and cancer.

In 1978, WHO organized a conference in Alma Ata in the former Soviet Union that gave priority to the delivery of primary healthcare services and the goal of "health for all by the year 2000." Rather than focusing solely on control of specific diseases, this conference called for international efforts to strengthen the capacities of low- and middle-income countries to extend their health services to populations with poor access to prevention and care. The concerns of tropical medicine, which were concentrated on the infectious diseases of warm climates, were replaced by an emphasis on the provision of health services to reduce morbidity and premature mortality in resource-poor settings (De Cock et al., 1995). Given the limited financial and managerial capacities of many governments, increased attention was paid to the role of nongovernmental organizations (NGOs) in providing these services. As a result, many mission hospitals, particularly in sub-Saharan Africa, expanded their activities in their local communities, the number of local NGOs began to increase, and a number of international NGOs (e.g., Save the Children, Oxfam, Médecins sans Frontières) greatly expanded their services, often with support of bilateral agencies. Disease-specific efforts—most notably UNICEF's Child Survival Program, with its acronym GOBI (growth charts, oral rehydration, breastfeeding, immunization) and its goal of universal childhood immunization by 1990—were seen by many as programs that both focused on specific health problems and provided an excellent means of strengthening health systems.

The emergence of what is sometimes called "the new public health" was heralded by the Ottawa Charter of 1986, which was meant to provide a plan of action to achieve the "health for all" targets set forth at Alma Ata. The Ottawa Charter pioneered the definition of health as a resource for development, not merely a desirable outcome of development. The prerequisites for health that were outlined in the charter were diverse and included peace, shelter, education, food, income, a stable ecosystem, sustainable resources, social justice, and equity. The charter emphasized the importance of structural factors that affect health on a societal level, rather than focusing only on the risk behaviors of individuals. It called on the worldwide health community to address health disparities by engaging and enabling people to take charge of their health at community and policy-making levels. This shift from a "risk behavior" focus to one of "risk environment" continues to resonate in contemporary public health practice and research.

The one new and unexpected development in the 1980s was the arrival of the HIV/AIDS pandemic. By the time a simple laboratory test to detect HIV was discovered in 1985, more than 2 million persons in sub-Saharan Africa had been infected. In 1987, WHO formed the Global Program on AIDS, which within 2 years became the largest international public health effort ever established, with an annual budget of $90 million and 500 staff working in Geneva, Switzerland, and in more than 80 low- and middle-income countries and regions. In 1995, with some 20 million persons (mostly living in these lower-income countries) infected with HIV, and with the understanding that the pandemic could be brought under control only through a multisectoral effort, the program was transformed into a joint effort of UN agencies known as UNAIDS.

The Origins of Global Health

The end of the Cold War ushered in dramatic changes that stimulated the development of the new concept of global health. Major shifts in political and economic ideologies led to a reconsideration of the role of governments, including how they should finance and deliver public services. Much greater attention was given to focusing government's role more narrowly and to making greater use of civil society and the private sector. Indeed, global health as it relates to

health systems in the last decade of the twentieth century and the first decade of the twenty-first century can be characterized by its emphasis on health-sector reform, cost-effectiveness as an important principle in the choice of interventions, and public–private partnerships in health, paralleled by a rapid expansion of information and communications technologies.

Although rising incomes have long been known to improve health status, during the past decade increased attention has also been paid to the importance of a healthy population for achieving economic development. Participation of sectors other than the health sector is now viewed as essential for achieving a healthy population. More and more countries, experiencing the demographic transition from societies in which most persons are young to societies with rapidly increasing numbers of middle-aged and older adults, have had to provide preventive and care services that address health problems of both the poor and the wealthy simultaneously. Witness the fact that India and China now have high rates of cardiovascular disease, stroke, and diabetes. Not surprisingly, issues regarding equity in the availability of drugs and vaccines and in access to other technological advances have drawn greater attention. Healthy populations are also now viewed as essential for domestic security.

The first decade of the twenty-first century witnessed the addition of new multifaceted and complex issues to the list of global health challenges—among them, human migration and displacement, bioterrorism, pandemic flu, and disaster preparedness. It is within this context that the United Nations General Assembly adopted the Millennium Declaration in September 2000 as a set of guiding principles and key objectives for international cooperation. The declaration underscored the need to address inequities that have been created or worsened by globalization and to form new international linkages to achieve and protect peace, disarmament, poverty eradication, gender equality, a healthy environment, human rights, and good governance. The goals dealing specifically with development and poverty eradication have become known as the Millennium Development Goals (MDGs); three of them pertain primarily to health (shown in bold in Exhibit I-3). All 191 member states of the UN have pledged to meet the MDGs by 2015.

In the five years since the previous edition of this book was published, there have been a number of noteworthy successes in global health. Notably, significant progress has been made in achieving two of the health-related MDG goals. First, mortality among children younger than age five dropped from 12.4

Exhibit I-3	Millennium Development Goals

- Halve extreme poverty and hunger
- Achieve universal primary education
- Promote gender equality and empower women
- **Reduce under-5 mortality by two-thirds**
- **Reduce maternal mortality by three-fourths**
- **Reverse the spread of HIV/AIDS, malaria, tuberculosis, and other major diseases**
- Ensure environmental sustainability
- Develop a global partnership for development, with targets for aid, trade, and debt relief

million deaths in 1990 to 8.1 million deaths in 2009 (WHO, 2011b). Second, some progress has been made in improving maternal health outcomes, as evidenced by the nearly 20% increase between 1980 and 2008 in the proportion of women in low- and middle-income countries who received skilled assistance during delivery (WHO & UNICEF, 2010) and a decrease from 526,300 global maternal deaths in 1980 to 342,900 maternal deaths worldwide in 2008 (Hogan et al., 2010). It is estimated that approximately 289 million insecticide treated nets were delivered to sub-Saharan Africa by the end of 2010, enough to cover 76% of the 765 million persons at risk of malaria (WHO, 2010). The number of people who become infected annually with HIV appears to have peaked at 3.5 million in 1996 and then declined to 2.6 million in 2009, while the number of deaths due to AIDS appears to have peaked at 2.2 million in 2005 and then dropped to 1.8 million in 2009 (United Nations, 2009; WHO, 2011b).

The recent successes in fighting malaria and HIV are attributable in great part to the expansion of access to treatment, financed primarily by the Global Fund to Fight AIDS, Tuberculosis and Malaria and the President's Emergency Fund for AIDS Relief (PEPFAR), the latter now being part of the U.S. government's Global Health Initiative. Both these initiatives were outcomes of the UN's Special Session on HIV/AIDS, convened in June 2001, and its adoption of a Declaration of Commitment on HIV/AIDS. Moreover, the Global Fund's performance-based funding and decision-making processes have made important contributions to the practice of aid, particularly in encouraging management for results, participation of civil society, mutual accountability, and wide-based country and local ownership. The recent involvement of the G8 countries in setting aid

targets in global health and development has also been instrumental in ensuring donor country support to address health problems in lower-income countries (Kurokawa et al., 2009).

Current Challenges in Global Health

We have witnessed major improvements in the health of populations over the past century, with the pace of change increasing rapidly in low- and middle-income countries since the Bretton Woods Conference. Global health—and, more broadly, an improved understanding of how social, behavioral, economic, and environmental factors influence the health of populations—has contributed to these improvements to an extent far greater than expanded access to medical care. Nevertheless, these improvements have not been universal and the challenges of global health have never been greater. For example:

- Despite recent progress, millions of children younger than the age of five whose lives could be saved through access to simple, affordable interventions continue to die each year (UNICEF, 2008).

- Hundreds of thousands of women die annually from complications of pregnancy and childbirth. For each of these deaths, at least 20 other women suffer pregnancy-related health problems that can be permanently disabling and have social consequences (WHO & UNICEF, 2010).

- More than 9.5 million people die each year due to infectious diseases—nearly all of whom live in low- and middle-income countries (WHO, 2008).

- Diarrhea, dysentery, and typhoid are the most prevalent water-related diseases, accounting for more than 90% of deaths and one-third of all outpatient consultations preventable by a safe water supply. Diarrheal disease kills 1.34 million children every year, and it is both preventable and treatable (Black et al., 2010; Disease Control Priorities Project, 2007).

- Noncommunicable diseases (NCDs)—primarily cardiovascular diseases (CVD), cancers, diabetes and chronic lung diseases—are the leading causes of death worldwide and accounted for more than 63% of all global deaths in 2008. 80% of global deaths from CVD and diabetes happen in low- and middle-income countries.

- The number of deaths from NCDs is expected to increase globally by 15% between 2010 and 2020; a 20% increase is projected in Africa, the Eastern Mediterranean, and South-East Asia (WHO, 2011a).
- While sub-Saharan Africa has 11% of the world's population and 24% of the global burden of disease, it has only 3% of the world's health workers (WHO, 2006).

There is a broad consensus that poverty is the most important underlying cause of preventable death, disease, and disability. Unfortunately, more people live in poverty today than did so 20 years ago. Literacy, access to housing, safe water, sanitation, food supplies, and urbanization are determinants of health status that interact with poverty.

In 2008, the world began facing a new economic crisis. Sharply falling economic growth, declines in trade with low- and middle-income countries, and a downturn in foreign aid flows led to a number of outcomes, including larger numbers of people going hungry, living in extreme poverty, and facing unemployment (United Nations, 2009). The economic recovery now under way likely has created a momentum that will result in a reduction of the overall poverty rate by 15% by 2015, giving reason to believe that that the poverty reduction MDG target can still be met (United Nations, 2010). The most rapid economic growth and the sharpest declines in poverty are occurring in Eastern Asia.

Numerous dynamic challenges face global health practitioners in the twenty-first century. Infectious diseases—once thought to have been vanquished as major killers—have emerged or reemerged around the world as top threats to health and well-being. Some of these are variations of familiar, well-understood microbial agents (e.g., multidrug-resistant tuberculosis), whereas others have traveled from endemic regions to previously unaffected areas (e.g., West Nile virus), and still others have newly emerged (e.g., the coronavirus responsible for severe acute respiratory syndrome [SARS] and the H1N1 influenza pathogen) or are threatening on the horizon (e.g., avian influenza). The underlying causes for many emerging infectious diseases can be traced to human-initiated social and environmental changes, including climatic and ecosystem disturbances, trends in food and meat consumption and production, close proximity of humans and animals in household settings, and unsafe medical practices (Kuiken et al., 2003).

Noncommunicable or chronic diseases were once considered a problem afflicting only high-income nations that had achieved long life expectancies. Today, however, millions of people in low- and middle-income countries suffer from chronic conditions such as obesity, cardiovascular disease, hypertension, and diabetes (Abegunde et al., 2007; WHO, 2011a; Yach et al., 2005). Globalizing forces that have imported Western lifestyle habits, such as tobacco use and increased consumption of processed foods, have fueled these disease trends. Mental illness, and depressive disorders in particular, remain a largely ignored and major source of death and disability worldwide (Prince et al., 2007).

The importance of improving the performance of health systems so as to achieve reductions in mortality and morbidity has become widely accepted, especially the need to address the global health workforce crisis (WHO, 2006). WHO has identified six building blocks of health systems, recognizing that to fight poverty, foster development, and maintain and improve the health of people around the world, the need to strengthen health systems is critical. One means for expanding access to health services has been the use of mobile phone technology; it has been estimated that subscriptions to such services per 100 people reached the 50% mark in 2009 (United Nations, 2010). Mobile phone initiatives are now aimed at improving healthcare services in many countries, as they are increasingly being used for disaster management, reminders for people to get vaccinations, and social marketing. This technology, and others like it, will surely play a pivotal role in the future of global health.

The resources required to achieve the MDGs were initially spelled out by a WHO Commission on Macroeconomics and Health (WHO, 2001) and have subsequently been refined (Sachs & McArthur, 2005). Meeting them will require new forms of international and intersectoral cooperation between UN agencies with an established health role, other international bodies such as the World Trade Organization, regional bodies such as the European Union, bilateral agencies, NGOs, foundations, and the private sector, including pharmaceutical companies. Partners also must include the new philanthropists in global health—people such as Bill and Melinda Gates, George Soros, and Ted Turner—who bring not only significant amounts of funds into the global system but also a new, more informal and personal style of operations. Ensuring the ideal formation and effective functioning of this global health system will itself be an enormous challenge for the next decade of global health.

Use and Content of This Textbook

This textbook has been prepared with these challenges foremost in mind. Its focus is on diseases, programs, health systems, and health policies in low- and middle-income countries, making reference to and using examples from the United States, Western Europe, and other high-income countries as appropriate.[1] Individual chapters present information on health problems and issues that transcend national boundaries and are of concern to many countries.

Our intent has been, first and foremost, to provide a textbook for graduate students from various disciplines and professions who are studying global health. Given its broad range of content, the book as a whole may serve as the main source for an introductory graduate course on global health. Experience with the previous editions has shown that the textbook also can be used as a reference text for undergraduate courses in global health. Alternatively, some chapters (or parts of chapters) can be used in graduate or undergraduate courses dedicated to more specific subjects and topics. Ideally, students who use the textbook in this way will be stimulated to explore other chapters once they have read the assigned material. Moreover, the textbook can serve as a useful reference for those already working in the field of global health in government agencies, as well as those employed by health and development agencies, NGOs, or the private sector.

Because of the many dynamic areas and subjects we wanted to cover, we chose to prepare an edited textbook. We selected content experts for each chapter rather than presuming to have the expertise to write the entire book ourselves. We recognize that an edited textbook has its shortcomings, such as some inconsistency in style and presentation and occasional overlap in chapter content. We have done our best to limit these disadvantages, and hope the reader will agree that those that remain are a small price to pay for fulfilling our goal of providing the reader with the highest-quality content.

Another consequence of the dynamic nature of global health is the occasional difficulty in providing the most up-to-date epidemiologic information on all causes of mortality and morbidity. To assist the reader in obtaining this information, we have provided salient references in various chapters, including Internet resources.

The book that you hold in your hands is the third edition of this textbook. In planning its preparation, we sought advice on how to improve it from many of those who prepared chapters in the first two editions, as well as from faculty in various countries who were using the textbook in their courses. The textbook has 18 chapters, three of which are new and are added in response to input from these reviewers.

The first three chapters set the background. Chapter 1 reviews the importance of using quantitative indicators for decision making in health. It presents the latest developments in the measurement of health status and the global burden of disease, including the increasing use of composite measures of health that combine the effects of disease-specific morbidity and mortality on populations. It then reviews current estimates and future trends in selected countries and regions, as well as the global burden of disease.

Chapter 2 examines the social, cultural, and behavioral parameters that are essential to understanding public health efforts. It does so by describing key concepts in the field of anthropology, particularly as they relate to health belief systems, and by presenting theories of health behavior that are relevant to behavior change and examples of specific national and community programs in various areas of health. The importance of combining qualitative and quantitative methodologies in measuring and assessing health status and programs is emphasized.

The newly added Chapter 3 presents the social determinants of health. It considers this area from a historical perspective, presents contemporary examples of patterns of health inequity arising as a consequence of social determinants, illustrates policy implications of the existence of health gradients, and reviews models and theories that explain how some determinants affect health outcomes. The deliberations of the recent Commission on the Social Determinants of Health serve as a key basis for this chapter.

The next three chapters are devoted to the three greatest public health challenges traditionally faced by low-income countries: reproductive health, infectious diseases, and nutrition. Reproductive health has long been addressed primarily through family planning programs directly intended to reduce fertility. Chapter 4 presents more current views of reproductive health that broaden this concept to include empowerment of women in making decisions about their health and fertility. It provides information on population growth and demographic changes around the world, reviews how women control their fertility, and indexes the

---

[1] A classification of countries can be found on the World Bank's website: http://www.worldbank.org/data/countryclass/country class.html.

effects of various social and biological determinants of fertility. It then examines the impact of family planning services and programs on the reduction of fertility and unwanted pregnancies and on the health of children and women.

Collectively, infectious diseases have historically been the most important causes of premature mortality and morbidity in low- and middle-income countries. Chapter 5 presents the descriptive epidemiologic features and available prevention and control strategies for the communicable diseases that are of greatest public health significance in these countries today. These diseases include the vaccine-preventable diseases; diarrhea and acute respiratory infections in children; tuberculosis, malaria, and other parasitic diseases; HIV/AIDS and other sexually transmitted diseases; and the emerging infectious diseases and new disease threats, including avian flu and H1N1. Examples of successful programs using one or more of the available control approaches—prevention of exposure, immunization, drug prophylaxis, and treatment—are described, as are the challenges and obstacles that confront low- and middle-income countries in successfully controlling these diseases.

Nutritional concerns in low- and middle-income countries are diverse, ranging from deprivation and hunger to consequent deficiencies in health, survival, and quality of life in some regions. Chapter 6 focuses on several spheres of nutrition that are of utmost concern in these countries, including undernutrition and its components of protein malnutrition and micronutrient deficiencies (particularly vitamin A, zinc, iron, and iodine) at various stages of life; food insecurity; the interaction of nutrition and infections; the role of breastfeeding and complementary feeding in ensuring healthy children; and the nutrition transition observed in more affluent segments of populations in rapidly developing countries (an issue that is addressed more fully in Chapter 7's exploration of chronic diseases). Chapter 6 also discusses the cost-effectiveness of nutritional interventions.

The book's next four chapters address public health priorities that have been historically associated with higher-income countries but are gaining importance in resource-poor countries as they become more developed economically and their populations live longer and progress through the demographic transition. These issues are chronic diseases, injury, mental health, and environmental health.

Chronic diseases—frequently called noncommunicable or degenerative diseases—are generally characterized by a long latency period, prolonged course of illness, noncontagious origin, functional impairment or disability, and incurability. Chapter 7 provides an overview of chronic diseases in low- and middle-income countries, with particular attention given to cardiovascular diseases (mainly coronary artery disease and stroke), obesity, common cancers, chronic respiratory diseases, and diabetes. The descriptive epidemiology and economic implication of these diseases, the behavioral risk factors that serve as their determinants, and the main approaches, programs, and policy responses required to adequately prevent and manage these diseases at national and global levels are presented.

The subject of injuries is covered in a separate chapter (Chapter 8), reflecting the greater importance and recognition accorded to this problem. The discussion includes both unintentional injuries (ones for which there is no evidence of predetermined intent, such as road accidents and occupational injuries) and intentional injuries or violence that is planned or intended (including injuries related to self-directed, interpersonal, and collective violence). The chapter provides an overview of the global burden of injuries, outlines the causes of and risk factors for them, describes evidence-based interventions that can successfully reduce their impact, and considers the opportunities and challenges that can move forward an injury prevention agenda at the global level.

It is only recently that mental health has received attention commensurate with its great importance to the disability and disease burden in low- and middle-income countries. Chapter 9 charts the historical development of public mental health; considers various concepts and classifications of mental disorders, taking into account the influence of cultural factors in the development of psychiatric classifications; and reviews what is known about the epidemiology and etiology of the more common disorders, including anxiety and mood disorders, psychotic disorders, substance abuse disorders, epilepsy, developmental disabilities, and dementia. Lastly, the chapter reviews mental health policies, human resources for mental health care, and the evidence for the prevention and treatment of major mental disorders.

Chapter 10 provides a comprehensive review of environmental health issues and problems in low- and middle-income countries. It begins by summarizing the conceptual and methodological issues that constitute the important area of risk assessment and monitoring, and then reviews the profiles of environmental health hazards within the household (e.g., water and sanitation), in the workplace (e.g., on farms, in mines, and in factories), in the community (e.g., outdoor air pollution), and at regional and global levels.

The coverage of regional and global threats includes such controversial topics as climate change, ozone depletion, and biodiversity. The chapter concludes with a discussion of the issues and projects that bear on the future of environmental health research and policy.

Chapter 11 focuses on the global health challenges that characterize complex emergencies. These conflicts occur within and across state boundaries, have political antecedents, are protracted in duration, and are embedded in existing social, political, economic, and cultural structures and cleavages. At the end of 2008, there were an estimated 27 million internally displaced persons and more than 14 million refugees seeking asylum across international borders, the vast majority of whom were fleeing conflict zones. Chapter 11 considers the causes of complex emergencies (particularly the political causes) and their impact on populations and health systems, and reviews the technical interventions that can limit their adverse effects on the health of populations. Attention is drawn to the importance of an effective and efficient early response in influencing the long-term survival of populations and health systems and the nature of any postconflict society that is established. The chapter also reviews the impact of natural disasters.

The next two chapters are concerned with the development and implementation of effective health systems, which have a crucial influence on the ability of countries to address their disease burden and improve the health of their populations. Chapter 12 focuses on the design of health systems considered largely from an economic perspective. It provides a conceptual map of the health system along with its key elements; addresses the fundamental and often controversial question as to the role of the state; and considers the key functions of any health system, which include regulation, human resources for health, financing, pay-for-performance approaches, and provision. It concludes by reviewing current trends in health system reform. Four country examples are used throughout the chapter to illustrate key differences in health systems across the world.

As multipurpose and multidisciplinary endeavors, health systems require coordination among numerous individuals and units. Thus they require effective and efficient management. Chapter 13 is dedicated to this topic, which is defined as the process of making decisions as to how resources will be generated, developed, and used in pursuit of particular organizational objectives. It details the important aspects of the political, social, and economic context in which a management process must operate;

discusses the organizational structures under which healthcare systems may be organized, including the role of the private sector; examines the critical process of planning and priority setting; looks at issues in the management of resources, focusing on finance, resource allocation, staffing, transport, and information; and concludes by discussing some cross-cutting themes, such as management style, accountability, and sustainability.

Chapter 14 is a new chapter that is dedicated to the topic of pharmaceuticals, a key part of any health system. It focuses on access, availability (both upstream issues and country-level distribution and management systems), and affordability of pharmaceuticals and their safe and effective use. It also discusses the pharmaceutical system architecture and reflects on coordination and priority setting in a complex global environment.

Health and health systems interrelate with a nation's economy in two main ways. The first, as noted earlier, comprises the bidirectional relationships between health status and national income and development. For example, health affects income through its impact on labor productivity, saving rates, and age structure, while a higher income improves health by increasing the capacity to produce food and have adequate housing and education, and through incentives for fertility limitation. The second concerns linkages between healthcare delivery institutions, health financing (including insurance) policies, and economic outcomes. Chapter 15 reviews information available on both of these challenging and closely related topics, which are critical to government policy makers seeking the best ways to improve the quality of life of their populations, particularly in those countries that carry the heaviest burden of disease and poverty.

Chapter 16, another new chapter, covers the important area of evaluation science and addresses the rationale for and the design of summative impact evaluations of programs being scaled up and delivered to large populations and aimed at delivering several biological and behavioral interventions together. To describe the planning, design, and execution of program evaluations and data analyses, the authors use three evaluations as examples: an integrated management of childhood illness program, an accelerated child survival development initiative, and a voucher scheme for insecticide-treated bed nets.

Chapter 17 presents the current state of affairs regarding global cooperation in international public health. It begins by explaining the reasons why countries seek this cooperation, the processes by which it occurs, the institutions and actors involved, and the global health initiatives that have been implemented and evaluated. The chapter reviews the important shift that has taken place in the overall framework of international cooperation, from one characterized by vertical relationships between states and international and intergovernmental organizations, to one of horizontal, cooperative participation resulting in partnerships and alliances among nation states, UN agencies, the private sector, and NGOs. This shift has great significance for the formation of future international public health policies and programs and for approaches to global governance in the area of global health.

Chapter 18 provides an overview of how globalization is affecting global health in the twenty-first century. It begins by seeking to define the term "globalization" and its key causes (or drivers), then explores how the many changes engendered by globalization are having positive and negative impacts on human societies. A discussion of the links between globalization and shifting patterns of infectious and chronic diseases follows. Next, the chapter explores the impact of globalization on healthcare financing and service provision, using as examples the migration of health workers and the global spread of health-sector reforms. It discusses global health diplomacy and concludes by suggesting ways in which the global health community can promote and protect health in the era of globalization.

Many case studies can be found in exhibits scattered throughout the text. They provide concrete examples and illustrations of key points and concepts covered in each chapter. At the conclusion of each chapter is a list of questions that can help course instructors stimulate classroom discussions about important issues covered in the chapter.

The editors recognize that this book could include separate chapters on many other topics—maternal and child health, health and human rights, and implementation or delivery science, to name but a few. We have opted instead to provide in-depth information on the core subjects that were selected, although we did our best to cover some aspects of all of these subjects in one or more chapters.

In many ways, global health stands today at an important crossroads. Its greatest challenge is to confront global forces, while at the same time promoting local, evidence-based, cost-effective programs that deal with both disease-specific problems and more general issues, such as poverty and gender inequality. Global health–related research is essential to gain a better understanding of the determinants of illness and of innovative approaches to prevention and care and to find means of improving the efficiency and coverage of health systems. Whether as practitioners, policy makers, or researchers, global health professionals can make an enormous difference by being well trained and highly sensitive to the beliefs, culture, and value systems of the populations with whom they collaborate or serve. We hope this textbook will aid in this process.

• • • **References**

Abegunde, D. O., Mathers, C. D., Adam, T., Ortegon, M. & Strong, K. (2007). The burden and costs of chronic diseases in low-income and middle-income countries. *Lancet, 370*(9603), 1929–1938.

Arnold, D. (1988). *Introduction: Disease, medicine, and empire. Imperial medicine and indigenous societies*. Manchester, UK/New York: Manchester University Press/St. Martin's Press: 1–26.

Basch, P. F. (1999). *Textbook of international health*. New York: Oxford University Press.

Black, R. E., Cousens, S., Johnson, H. L., Lawn, J. E., Rudan, I., Bassani, D. G., et al. (2010). Global, regional, and national causes of child mortality in 2008: A systematic analysis. *Lancet, 375*(9730), 1969–1987.

Commission on Macroeconomics and Health. (2001). *Macroeconomics and Health: Investing in Health for Economic Development*. Geneva, Switzerland: World Health Organization.

Committee on the U.S. Commitment to Global Health. (2009). *The U.S. commitment to global health: Recommendations for the new administration*. Washington, DC: Institute of Medicine.

De Cock, K. M., Lucas, S. B., Mabey, D. & Parry, E. (1995). Tropical medicine for the 21st century. *British Medical Journal, 311*(7009), 860–862.

Disease Control Priorities Project. (2007). *Water, sanitation, and hygiene: Simple, effective solutions save lives*. Washington, DC: Author.

Gensini, G. F., Yacoub, M. H. & Conti, A. A. (2004). The concept of quarantine in history: From plague to SARS. *Journal of Infection, 49*(4), 257–261.

Hogan, M., Foreman, K., Naghavi, M., Ahn, S. Y., Wang, M., Makela, S. M, et al. (2010). Maternal mortality for 181 countries, 1980–2008: A systematic analysis of progress towards Millennium Development Goal 5. *Lancet 375*(9726), 1609–1623.

Institute of Medicine. (1997). *America's vital interest in global health*. Washington, DC: Author.

Koplan, J. P., Bond, T. C., Merson, M. H., Reddy, K. S., Rodriguez, M. H., Sewankambo, N. K., et al. (2009). Towards a common definition of global health. *Lancet, 373*(9679), 1993–1995.

Kuiken, T., Fouchier, R., Rimmelzwaan, G. & Osterhaus, A. (2003). Emerging viral infections in a rapidly changing world. *Current Opinion in Biotechnology, 14*(6)4, 641–646.

Kurokawa, K., Banno, Y., Hara, S. & Kondo, J. (2009). Italian G8 summit: A critical juncture for global health. *Lancet, 373*(9663), 526–527.

Leff, S. & Leff, V. (1958). *From witchcraft to world health*. New York: Macmillan.

Prince, M., Patel, V., Saxena, S., Maj, M., Maselko, J., Phillips, M. R., et al. (2007). No health without mental health. *Lancet, 370*(9590), 859–877.

Rosen, G. & Morman, E. T. (1993). *A history of public health*. Baltimore, MD: Johns Hopkins University Press.

Ruger, J. P. (2005). The changing role of the World Bank in global health. *American Journal of Public Health, 95*(1), 60–70.

Sachs, J. D. & McArthur, J. W. (2005). The Millennium Project: A plan for meeting the Millennium Development Goals. *Lancet, 365*(9456), 347–353.

Stuard, S. M. & NetLibrary. (1992). *A state of deference: Ragusa/Dubrovnik in the medieval centuries*. Philadelphia: University of Pennsylvania Press.

UNICEF. (2008). *The state of the world's children 2009*. New York: United Nations Children's Fund.

United Nations (UN). (2009). *The Millennium Development Goals report 2009*. New York: Author.

United Nations (UN). (2010). *The Millennium Development Goals report 2010*. New York: Author.

Winslow, C.-E. A. & Hallock, G. T. (1933). *Health through the ages*. New York: Metropolitan Life Insurance Company.

World Health Organization (WHO). (2006). *The world health report 2006: Working together for health*. Geneva, Switzerland: Author.

World Health Organization (WHO). (2008). *The global burden of disease: 2004 update*. Geneva, Switzerland: Author.

World Health Organization (WHO) & UNICEF. (2010). *Countdown to 2015 decade report (2000–2010) with country profiles: Taking stock of maternal, newborn, and child survival*. Washington, DC: Author.

World Health Organization (WHO). (2010). *World Malaria report 2010*. Geneva, Switzerland: Author.

World Health Organization (WHO). (2011a). *Global status report on noncommunicable diseases 2010*. Geneva, Switzerland: Author.

World Health Organization (WHO). (2011b). *World Health Statistics 2011*. Geneva, Switzerland: Author.

Yach, D., Leeder, S. R., Bell, J. & Kistnasamy, B. (2005). Global chronic diseases. *Science*, 307(5708), 317.

CHAPTER 1

Measures of Health and Disease in Populations

ADNAN A. HYDER, PRASANTHI PUVANACHANDRA, AND RICHARD H. MORROW

In its 1948 charter, the World Health Organization (WHO) defined health as "a state of complete physical, mental and social well-being and not merely the absence of disease or infirmity." Although this is an important ideological conceptualization, for most practical purposes, objectives of health programs are more readily defined in terms of prevention or treatment of disease.

Disease has been defined in many ways and for a variety of reasons; distinctions may be made between disease, sickness, and illness. For purposes of defining and measuring disease burden, a general definition will be used in this book: *Disease* is anything that a person experiences that causes, literally, "dis-ease"; that is, anything that leads to discomfort, pain, distress, disability of any kind, or death constitutes disease. It may be due to any cause, including injuries or psychiatric conditions.

It is also important to be able to diagnose and classify specific diseases to the extent that such classification aids in determining which health intervention programs would be most useful. Thus defining disease, understanding the pathogenesis of the disease process, and knowing which underlying risk factors lead to this process are critical for understanding and classifying causes so as to determine the most effective prevention and treatment strategies for reducing the effects of a disease or risk factor. Just as the purpose of diagnosis of a disease in an individual patient is to provide the right treatment, so the major purpose of working through a burden of disease analysis in a population is to provide the basis for the most effective mix of health and social program interventions.

Recent developments in the measurement of population health status and disease burden include the increasing use of summary, composite measures of health that combine the mortality and morbidity effects of diseases into a single indicator; the availability of results of Global Burden of Disease (GBD) studies, which make use of such summary indicators; and developments in the measurement of disability and risk factors. The more traditional approaches to measuring health are widely available in other public health textbooks and will be used for illustrative and comparative purposes here.

This chapter is divided into five sections. The first section explains the reasons for and approaches to measuring disease burden in populations, describes the need for using quantitative indicators, highlights the importance of using data for decision making in health, and lists a variety of major health indicators in widespread use. The second section critically reviews methods for developing and using composite measures that combine the mortality and morbidity from diseases in populations at national and regional levels. It explores the potential utility of these measures and discusses their limitations and implications. The third section demonstrates the application of these methods for measurement of health status and assessment of global health trends. It reviews current estimates and forecasts trends in selected countries and regions, as well as examines the global burden of disease. The fourth section reviews important underlying risk factors of disease and discusses recent efforts to measure the prevalence of major risk factors and to determine their contributions to regional and global disease burdens. The final section provides conclusions for the chapter.

Reasons for and Approaches to Measuring Health and Disease

Rationale

The many reasons for obtaining health-related information all hinge on the need for data to guide efforts toward reducing the consequences of disease and enhancing the benefits of good health. These include the need to identify which interventions will have the greatest beneficial effect, to identify emerging trends and anticipate future needs, to assist in determining priorities for expenditures, to provide information for education to the public, and to help in setting health research agendas. The primary information requirement is for understanding and assessing the health status of a population and its changes over time. In recent years, practitioners have emphasized the importance of making evidence-based decisions in health care. There is little reason to doubt that evidence is better than intuition, but realizing its full benefits depends upon recognizing and acting upon the evidence (Figure 1-1). This chapter examines evidence—the facts of health and disease—and demonstrates how to assemble this evidence so that it can assist in better decision making concerning health and welfare.

A well-documented example of the relationship between decision making and data can be seen in a health systems project in Tanzania (Exhibit 1-1). This case illustrates how able people with good intentions had been making decisions routinely, only to find that using established methods to collect evidence on the burden of disease changed the nature and effectiveness of their own decisions. A major reason for the effective use of the evidence was that it was collected locally and put forward in a form helpful to decision makers.

Measuring Health and Disease

The relative importance (burden) of different diseases in a population depends on their frequency (incidence or prevalence), severity (the mortality and extent of serious morbidity), consequences (health, social, economic), and the specific people affected (gender, age, social and economic position).

Counting Disease

The first task in measuring disease in a population is to count its occurrence. Counting disease frequency can be done in several ways, and it is important to understand what these different methods of counting

actually mean. The most useful way depends on the nature of the disease and the purpose for which it is being counted. There are three commonly used measures of disease occurrence: cumulative incidence, incidence density, and prevalence.

Cumulative incidence, or *incidence proportion*, is the number or proportion of new cases of disease that occur in a population at risk for developing the disease during a specified period of time. For this measure to have meaning, three components are necessary: a definition of the onset of the event, a defined population, and a particular period of time. The critical point is new cases of disease—the disease must develop in a person who did not have the disease previously. The numerator is the number of new cases of disease (the event), and the denominator is the number of people at risk for developing the disease. Everyone included in the denominator must have the potential to become part of the group that is counted in the numerator. For example, to calculate the incidence of prostate cancer, the denominator must include only men, because women are not at risk for prostate cancer. The third component is the period of time. Any time unit can be used as long as all those counted in the denominator are followed for a period comparable with those who are counted as new cases in the numerator. The most common time denominator is one year.

Incidence density, which is often simply called *incidence rate*, is the occurrence of new cases of disease per unit of person-time. This metric directly incorporates time into the denominator and is generally the most useful measure of disease frequency, often expressed as new events per person-year or per 1,000 person-years. Incidence is a measure of events (in this case, the transition from a nondiseased to a diseased state) and can be considered a measure of risk. This risk can be looked at in any population group, defined by age, sex, place, time, sociodemographic characteristics, occupation, or exposure to a toxin or any other suspected causal factor.

Prevalence is a measure of present status rather than of newly occurring disease. It measures the proportion of people who have defined disease at a specific point of time. Thus it is a composite measure made up of two factors—the incidence of the disease that has occurred in the past and its continuation to the present or to some specified point in time. That is, prevalence equals the incidence rate of the disease multiplied by the average duration of the disease. For most chronic diseases, prevalence rates are more commonly available than are incidence rates.

Exhibit 1-1	Using Evidence to Improve a Health System: An Example from Africa

The **Tanzania Essential Health Interventions Project** (TEHIP), a joint venture of the Tanzanian health ministry and the International Development Research Centre (IDRC), starting in 1996 was conducted in two rural districts—Morogoro and Rufiji—with a combined population of approximately 700,000. The annual health spending in Tanzania was about $8 per capita. In Morogoro and Rufiji, TEHIP added resources on the condition that they must be spent rationally; in other words, the amount of money spent on interventions should reflect the burden of disease. TEHIP conducted burden of disease analysis for the two districts and established a demographic surveillance system. The organization found that the amount the local health authorities spent on addressing each disease bore little relation to the actual burden of disease. Although childhood problems (e.g., pneumonia, diarrhea, malnutrition, measles) constituted 28% of the disease burden, only 13% of the budget was devoted to addressing them. Other conditions, meanwhile, attracted more than their fair share of resources. For example, 22% of the budget was targeted to tuberculosis, even though it accounted for less than 4% of years of life lost.

TEHIP promoted the use of burden of disease analysis, district accounts, and other mapping tools for more rational decision making in the districts. It also brought management tools and community voice techniques to the district teams. The district teams decided to spend more on neglected diseases for which cost-effective treatments or preventive measures were available. The extra $1 per capita was enough to allow the district health authorities to align their spending to reflect the real disease burden. For example, sexually transmitted diseases received 3% of the budget prior to TEHIP's intervention; that percentage changed to 9.5% after the realignment. Malaria accounted for 30% of the years of life lost because of death and debilitating illness; the budget for malaria prevention and treatment programs increased from 5% of total spending in 1996 to 25% in 1998.

The results of TEHIP were documented as changes in health outcomes. In Rufiji, for example, infant mortality fell by 40% in 5 years. In fact, just between 1999 and 2000, infant mortality fell from 100 deaths per 1,000 live births to 72 deaths per 1,000 live births, while the proportion of children dying before their fifth birthdays dropped by 14%, from 140 per 1,000 to 120 per 1,000. The success of TEHIP and its approach led to replication and further innovation in not only Tanzania but also many other low- and middle-income countries.

Although this is a dramatic example of how data can be used to recognize and correct misplaced health resource expenditures, it should be emphasized that health system expenditures should be equitably distributed based on which intervention programs maximize healthy life gains, not according to disease problems per se.

For additional information on the TEHIP success story, visit the following websites: http://www.odi.org.uk/Rapid/Tools/Case_studies/TEHIP.html and http://www.idrc.ca/tehip.

Severity of Disease

To understand the burden of disease in a population, it is important to consider not only the frequency of the disease but also its severity, as indicated by the morbidity and premature mortality that it causes. *Premature mortality* is defined as death before the expected age of death had the disease not occurred. *Morbidity* is a statement of the extent of disability that a person suffers as a consequence of the disease over time and can be measured by a number of indicators, as discussed later in this chapter.

Mortality

Traditionally, mortality has been the most important indicator of the health status of a population. John Graunt developed the first known systematic collection of data on mortality with the *Bills of Mortality*

in the early 1600s in London. He described the age pattern of deaths, categorized them by cause as understood at the time, and demonstrated variations from place to place and from year to year. Mortality rates according to age, sex, place, and cause continue to be central information about a population's health status and a crucial input for understanding and measuring the burden of disease. Considerable literature exists on the use of mortality to indicate health status and its application to national and subnational levels (Murray & Chen, 1992).

The fact of death by age, sex, and place is required by law in most countries through death registration, and in many countries the cause of death through death certification is required as well. Both provide essential information about the health status of a population. Nevertheless, in many low-income countries the fact of death, let alone its cause, is still not reliably available.

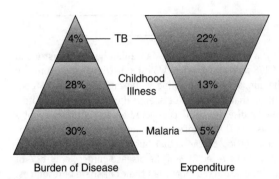

Figure 1-1 Using evidence to improve a health system: an example from Africa.

In high-income countries, vital statistics (i.e., the registration of births and deaths by age, sex, and place) are routinely collected and highly reliable. In most middle-income countries, their reliability and completeness have been steadily improving and often are fairly satisfactory. In many low-income countries, however, the collection of vital statistics remains grossly incomplete. An analysis of death registration in the course of the Global Burden of Disease study showed that vital registration data together with sample registration systems still do not cover 100% of global mortality. Survey data and indirect demographic techniques are needed to provide information on levels of child and adult mortality to provide a complete picture of global mortality (Murray et al., 2001). Nevertheless, even in low-income countries, increasing use of survey methods is delivering useful estimates of the mortality rates for the population younger than age five years and other populations.

Obtaining information about cause of death remains difficult even in many middle-income countries; most information depends on special surveys or studies of select populations. Verbal autopsies (VAs) have been used increasingly for judging the likely cause of death, especially for children younger than age five. This method comprises structured questions administered by trained interviewers with family members after a death; the information is then reviewed by physicians (or computers) to assign a cause of death using algorithms. VAs are quite useful for assessing some causes of death such as neonatal tetanus and severe diarrhea, but their sensitivity and specificity may be limited for diseases whose symptoms are variable and nonspecific, such as malaria (Anker et al., 1999; Thatte et al., 2009).

Age-specific mortality profiles are a prerequisite for a burden of disease analysis. Although extensive work has been done to document and analyze child mortality in low- and middle-income countries, less

has been done for adult mortality (Hill, 2003). Developing countries have higher rates of age-specific adult mortality than do high-income nations (Lopez et al., 2002; Murray & Chen, 1992). Indeed, mortality rates are higher for both women and men at every age when compared with the high-income world. In Africa, the enormous increase in deaths of young and middle-aged women and men from acquired immune deficiency syndrome (AIDS) has had a profound impact on mortality and survival (Exhibit 1-2).

Traditional indicators of mortality have been the standard for assessing population health status. Infant mortality rates (IMR; deaths of live-born infants before 12 months of age per 1,000 live births) and child mortality (deaths of children younger than 5 years of age) are considered sensitive indicators of the overall health of nations. The United Nations Children's Fund (UNICEF) publishes an annual global report that includes a ranking of nations based on these indicators (United Nations Children's Fund, 2009). These indicators have the added advantage of having been studied for their relationships with other indicators of the social and economic development of nations. For example, a clear relation exists between the gross national product (GNP) per capita, an indicator of national wealth, and child mortality. In general, the higher the level of economic development, the lower the rate of child mortality. However, there are exceptions, and they need to be examined carefully. For example, Sri Lanka and the Indian state of Kerala are both low-income regions that have low child mortality rates. These examples demonstrate that the relationship between mortality and poverty is complex and needs in-depth investigation.

There continue to be major deficiencies in cause-specific mortality data in low- and most middle-income countries. In keeping with demographic and epidemiologic transitions (see Exhibit 1-3, later in this chapter), the pattern of cause-specific mortality changes at different levels of total mortality, with a general trend of decreasing infectious and parasitic disease cause-specific mortality with declining total mortality. Indeed, mortality from these communicable causes is a major reason for the difference between high- and low-mortality populations (Murray & Chen, 1992).

The cause of death certification system based on WHO's International *Classification of Diseases* (ICD) has been used widely in many countries for many years (WHO, 1992). Despite the existence of this standardized process for categorizing deaths, variations in the reliability of these data occur because of variations in the training and expertise of the people who are coding causes of death, as well as the supervision

Exhibit 1-2	Trends of the HIV/AIDS Epidemic

Acquired immune deficiency syndrome (AIDS) is the leading infectious cause of adult death in the world. Untreated disease caused by the human immunodeficiency virus (HIV) has a case fatality rate that approaches 100% (WHO, 2003). Unknown 30 years ago, this disease has already killed more than 25 million people, and an estimated 31 to 36 million others are living with HIV/AIDS (UNAIDS, 2008, 2009). The most heavily burdened continent is Africa, home to two-thirds of the world's people living with HIV/AIDS. The prevalence of this disease is rising most rapidly in eastern Europe and Central Asia (e.g., Estonia, Latvia, Ukraine, and the Russian Federation) and in other parts of Asia (Indonesia, Pakistan, and Vietnam) (See Table 1-1) (UNAIDS, 2008, 2009).

Of the leading causes of disease burden among men and women of all ages, HIV/AIDS is the fifth cause, accounting for 4% of the global burden of disease. In terms of mortality, it is the sixth leading cause of death among people of all ages, accounting for 3.5% of all deaths (WHO, 2004). Nearly 72% of the two million global deaths from HIV/AIDS have occurred in sub-Saharan Africa (See Figure 1-2) (UNAIDS, 2009).

Table 1-1	Global Summary of HIV and AIDS Epidemic		
Number of people living with HIV	**Total**	**33.4 million**	**(31.1–35.8 million)**
	Adults	31.3 million	(29.2–33.7 million)
	Women	15.7 million	(14.2–17.2 million)
	Children	2.1 million	(1.2–2.9 million)
Number newly infected with HIV	**Total**	**2.7 million**	**(2.4–3.0 million)**
	Adults	2.3 million	(2.0–2.5 million)
	Children	430,000	(240,000–610,000)
AIDS deaths in 2008	**Total**	**2.0 million**	**(1.7–2.4 million)**
	Adults	1.7 million	(1.4–2.1 million)
	Children	280,000	(150,000–410,000)

Source: UNAIDS, 2009.

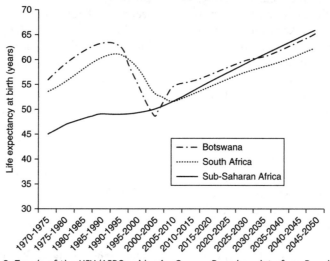

Life Expectancy in Sub-Saharan Africa and Selected Countries, 1970-2050

Figure 1-2 Trends of the HIV/AIDS epidemic. *Source:* Based on data from Population Division of the Department of Economic and Social Affairs of the United Nations Secretariat, *World Population Prospects: The 2008 Revision,* http://esa.un.org/unpp.

and feedback provided. There have been steady improvements in many countries, however, and these kinds of data provide some of the best information available on major causes of mortality.

Mortality can be expressed in two important quantitative measures: (1) *mortality rate* (MR) and (2) *case fatality ratio* (CFR). The MR, a form of incidence rate, is expressed as the number of deaths in a defined population in a defined time period. The numerator can be total deaths, age- or sex-specific deaths, or cause-specific deaths; the denominator is the number of persons at risk of dying in the stated category as defined earlier for incidence. Demographers use the notation XqY for the probability of dying in the Y years following age X at the then prevailing age-specific mortality rates for the population. Thus $5q0$ is the probability of death of newborns by age five (see Table 1-1), and $30q15$ is the probability of death in young adults from age 15 to 45. The CFR is the proportion of those persons with a given disease who die of that disease (at any time, unless specified). The MR is equal to the CFR multiplied by the incidence rate of the disease in the population.

The distinction between the proportion of deaths attributable to a cause (number of deaths due to the cause divided by total number of deaths in a given population in a given time period) as compared to the probability of death from the cause (disease-specific MR) is important to understand. For example, the probability of death (and disability) from noncommunicable causes (indeed, from virtually all causes) is higher in low- and middle-income regions than in the high-income world. However, the proportion of deaths and disability attributable to these chronic causes is smaller in poor countries than in wealthier countries because of the much larger toll taken by infectious and nutritional causes. With increasing economic development, the risk of death and disability from chronic disease does not increase; rather, the proportion of deaths attributable to chronic disease increases as the proportion of deaths attributable to communicable and nutritional disease declines.

Demographic and Epidemiologic Transitions

The demographic transition describes the changes in birth and death rates that historically have accompanied the shift from a traditional society to a modern society; it is detailed in Chapter 3. With modernization, sharp declines in mortality have been followed by a reduction in fertility, albeit one that commonly lags behind the change in the death rate by years or decades. The term *transition* refers to the shift away from a stable population in which very high birth rates are balanced by very high death rates to a stable population in which low birth rates are balanced with low death rates. In between these extremes, as a society undergoes modernization, there is a lag between falling mortality, especially in the under-five age group, and the drop in birth rates that leads to explosive population growth. Thereafter birth rates fall and a new stage is reached in which birth and death rates are low and balance resumes. The result is a striking change in the age structure of the population, with a decreased proportion of children and an aging population. These changes in the population age distributions are reflected in the shift from a wide-based pyramid, reflecting larger numbers in the younger age groups, to a structure with a narrow base, nearly rectangular configuration, and nearly equal percentages in each age group (see Exhibit 1-3).

In 1971, Omran described the underlying reasons for the demographic transition and used the term *epidemiologic transition* to explain the changing causal factors of disease that accounted for the dramatic drop in under-five mortality, which was largely due to reduction in malnutrition and communicable diseases. Although high rates of maternal mortality are characteristic of the low- and middle-income world, reductions of maternal mortality occur in a different time frame from those of under-five mortality. Reductions in maternal mortality require a better-developed infrastructure, including ready availability of surgical and blood transfusion capacity plus improved communication and transportation systems. Thus drops in maternal mortality occur much further along the road toward economic development, and changes occur only after shifts in the child mortality have been seen (see Chapter 3).

Major changes in the patterns and causes of injury are also likely to occur with modernization. For example, road traffic injuries tend to increase as countries go through the stage of development in which there is a great increase in vehicles and in the speeds at which they are operated before improved roads and law enforcement are in place (Crooper & Kopits, 2003). There may also be important shifts in the nature of violence and the people toward whom it is directed, related to crime patterns, civil unrest, ethnic conflicts, and intrafamily tensions (WHO, 2002b). The profound impact of the HIV/AIDS epidemic was discussed earlier in Exhibit 1-2.

Other Health-Related Metrics

In addition to basic measures of mortality, morbidity, and life expectation that are central for population health status assessment, a variety of important

Exhibit 1-3	**The Demographic Transition**

The graphs that follow show the shape of the age structure of the population on the left and the percentage of total deaths attributable to each age group on the right. The age structure for both England and Wales and for Latin America and the Caribbean shifted from a broad base and narrow top to a fairly uniform rectangular shape. At the same time there was a marked shift in the percentage of deaths by age, from children younger than age five to the elderly.

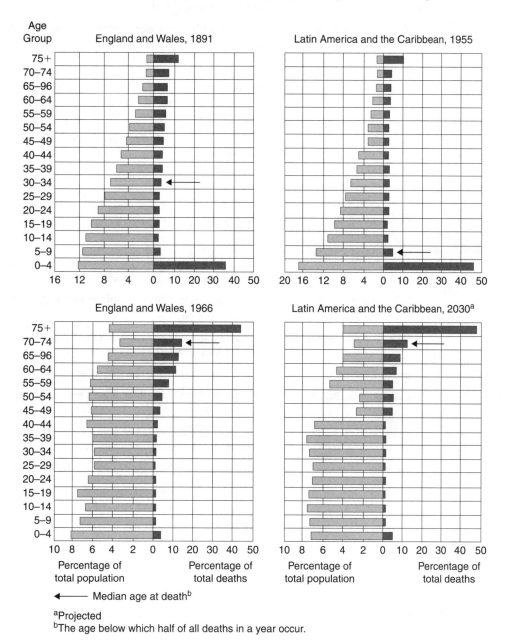

^aProjected
^bThe age below which half of all deaths in a year occur.

Table 1-2	Health-Related Metrics	
Type	**Indicator**	**Definition/Interpretation**
Demographic indicators: reproductive health (see Chapter 4)	Maternal death	Death of a woman while pregnant or up to 42 days post delivery from any cause except accident
	Maternal mortality ratio	Maternal deaths per number of pregnancies (maternal deaths per 100,000 live births)
	Maternal mortality rate	Maternal deaths per number of women of reproductive age (maternal deaths per 100,000 women age 15–49)
	Lifetime risk of maternal mortality	
	Total fertility rate	Average number of children a woman would bear if she lived to the end of her reproductive period
	Life expectation at birth	Average number of years a newborn would live if his or her life were lived under the mortality conditions for the place and year in question
Anthropometric indicators: nutrition (see Chapter 6)	Weight for age	Underweight
	Height for age	Stunting
	Weight for height	Wasting
	Mid-upper arm circumference	Wasting
Mortality (death) indicators	Mortality rate	Number of deaths in a specified time period/number of persons at risk of dying during that period
	Infant mortality rate	Number of deaths of live born infants before 12 months of age per 1,000 live births
	Under-five mortality rate	Number of deaths of children younger than age 5 per 1,000 live births averaged over the last 5 years
	5q0	Probability of death of a newborn by age 5
	Neonatal mortality rate	Number of deaths of live-born infants before 28 days of age per 1,000 live births
	Perinatal mortality rate	Number of fetal deaths (28 or more weeks of gestation) + post natal deaths (first week) per 1,000 live births
Disease frequency	Endemic	Usual occurrence of a given disease in a defined population
	Epidemic	Occurrence of a given disease in a defined population clearly in excess relative to its usual occurrence
	Pandemic	A worldwide epidemic involving large numbers

health-related indicators are useful for specific purposes. Many are discussed more fully in other chapters of this book; they are summarized in Table 1-2. Those related to the Millennium Development Goals (MDGs) are discussed in Exhibit 1-4.

Morbidity and Disability

Measures of mortality have been the principal indicators of population health status for generations. Their relative ease of observation, availability of data, and history of use make mortality information useful for assessing and monitoring the health status of populations. However, the key limitation with mortality-based indicators is that they "note the dead and ignore the living" (Kaplan, 1990). Measurements of morbidity, by comparison, are more problematic because there is not a clearly defined endpoint such as death provides. In addition, several components of disability need to be assessed, and there may be a substantial subjective aspect to grading the extent or severity of a condition.

Exhibit 1-4	Millennium Development Goals

In 2001, UN member states adopted eight Millennium Development Goals (MDGs) to spur social and economic development in the world's poorest countries:

- Goal 1: Eradicate extreme poverty and hunger
- Goal 2: Achieve universal primary education
- Goal 3: Promote gender equality and empower women
- Goal 4: Reduce child mortality
- Goal 5: Improve maternal health
- Goal 6: Combat HIV/AIDS, malaria, and other diseases
- Goal 7: Ensure environmental sustainability
- Goal 8: Develop a global partnership for development

The 8 MDGs were divided into 21 quantifiable targets that are measured by 60 indicators. Of the 21 targets, eight are directly related to health. Of the 60 indicators, 22 are directly to health. The health-related indicators include a variety of indicator types: incidence rates, prevalence "rates," mortality rates, mortality ratios, birth rates, and proportion of target populations receiving an intervention. For examples, the following is a list of MDG indicators:

Target 1c: Reduce by half the proportion of people who suffer from hunger

- 1.8 Prevalence of underweight children younger than five years of age
- 1.9 Proportion of population below minimum level of dietary energy consumption

Target 4a: Reduce by two-thirds the mortality rate among children younger than five

- 4.1 Under-five mortality rate
- 4.2 Infant mortality rate
- 4.3 Proportion of one-year-old children immunized against measles

Target 5a: Reduce by three-fourths the maternal mortality ratio

- 5.1 Maternal mortality ratio
- 5.2 Proportion of births attended by skilled health personnel

Target 5b: Achieve, by 2015, universal access to reproductive health

- 5.3 Contraceptive prevalence rate
- 5.4 Adolescent birth rate
- 5.5 Antenatal care coverage (at least one visit and at least four visits)
- 5.6 Unmet need for family planning

Target 6a: Halt and begin to reverse the spread of HIV/AIDS

- 6.1 HIV prevalence among population aged 15–24 years
- 6.2 Condom use at last high-risk sex
- 6.3 Proportion of population aged 15–24 years with correct knowledge of HIV/AIDS
- 6.4 Ratio of school attendance of orphans to school attendance of non-orphans aged 10–14

Target 6b: Achieve, by 2010, universal access to treatment for HIV/AIDS for all who need it

- 6.5 Proportion of population with advanced HIV with access to antiretroviral drugs

Target 6c: Halt and begin to reverse the incidence of malaria and other major diseases

- 6.6 Incidence and death rates associated with malaria
- 6.7 Proportion of children younger than five sleeping under insecticide-treated bed nets
- 6.8 Proportion of children younger than five with fever who are treated with appropriate antimalarial drugs
- 6.9 Incidence, prevalence, and death rates associated with tuberculosis
- 6.10 Proportion of tuberculosis cases detected and cured under directly observed treatment short course

Target 7c: Reduce by half the proportion of people without sustainable access to safe drinking water and basic sanitation

- 7.8 Proportion of population using an improved drinking water source
- 7.9 Proportion of population using an improved sanitation facility

The *International Classification of Impairments, Disabilities, and Handicaps* (ICIDH) was developed in the 1970s to classify nonfatal health outcomes as an extension of WHO's ICD system (WHO, 1980). It was developed to more fully describe the impact of a given disease on an individual and society, and to account for that disease's heterogeneity of its clinical expression and evolution in different individuals and societies. ICIDH categories included *impairment* (loss or abnormality of psychological, physiological, or anatomical structure or function), *disability* (restriction or lack of ability to perform an activity considered normal), and *handicap* (disadvantage from a disability or impairment for a given individual based on the inability to fulfill a normal role as defined by age, sex, or sociocultural factors). These distinctions clarified more than just processes and helped define the contribution of medical services, rehabilitation facilities, and social welfare to the reduction of disability.

In 2002, WHO built on the ICIDH to develop the *International Classification of Functioning, Disability and Health*, commonly known as ICF (WHO, 2002a), in which health-related domains are classified from the perspectives of the body, of the individual, and of society by means of two lists: a list of body functions and structures, and a list of domains of activity and participation. Because an individual's functioning and disability occurs within a context, the ICF also includes a list of environmental factors that provide a description of that context. The ICF has become WHO's framework for measuring health and disability at both individual and population levels. The ICF was officially endorsed by all 191 WHO member states in the Fifty-Fourth World Health Assembly on May 22, 2001 (resolution WHA 54.21). Unlike its predecessor, which was endorsed for field trial purposes only, the ICF was endorsed for use in member states as the international standard to describe and measure health and disability.

Using such classifications, indicators for disability, such as *impairment-free*, *disability-free*, and *handicap-free*, life expectancies have been developed. These, in turn, have been used to estimate health-adjusted life expectancies using severity and preference weights for time spent in states of less than perfect health.

Hospital inpatient discharge records—when they are based on good clinical evidence and coded by staff well trained in coding procedures—can provide high-quality data on the major causes of morbidity serious enough to require hospitalization. They also can provide good cause-of-death data for hospitalized persons, and some sense of the outcome status of those with serious conditions. Hospital data are generally improving in quality, especially in middle-income countries and in selected sentinel, usually tertiary care, teaching hospitals in low-income countries. Such information is inevitably biased because of the highly skewed distribution of those using such hospitals, but in many situations it is possible to have a good understanding of those biases and make appropriate adjustments to draw useful conclusions.

Generally, outpatient records in most of the world are highly deficient in terms of diagnosis; indeed, they often identify only the patient's chief complaint and the treatment dispensed. The main value of most such records is limited to establishing the fact of using a facility. There are usually strong biases in terms of those patients who use outpatient facilities because of access factors (distance and cost of use), nature and severity of the disease problem, and opportunity for using alternate services.

Visits to healthcare facilities, functional disability (a measure of activity that is less than the norm), and time spent away from work (absenteeism, work days lost) have been used to assess the magnitude of morbidity from various conditions. A commonly used approach to evaluating morbidity in a population has been the assessment of the impact on social roles or functional performance, such as days missed from work or spent in bed (Kaplan, 1990). A considerable body of literature focuses on the wide variety of instruments used to measure such functional capacity, especially in the clinical medical literature, that is not directly useful for population-based morbidity assessment.

Data about morbidity are often based on self-perceived assessments, and are frequently gleaned from survey-based interview information. The perception of morbidity and its reporting, the observation of morbidity and its impact, and other factors are responsible for the wide variations between reported and measured prevalence of conditions (Murray & Chen, 1992). This has resulted in an underestimation of the presence and impact of morbidity in both low- and middle-income as compared with high-income nations. This situation also underscores the variation in morbidity data, which are often interpreted as indicating that wealthy individuals and low-mortality populations report higher rates of morbidity (Lopez et al., 2006).

Measurement of individual preferences for different health states to determine relative severity of disability has been done by a variety of methods (Kaplan, 1990; Murray et al., 2002; Torrence, 1986). Factors that influence the assessment of such preferences include the type of respondent, the type of instrument used to measure the response, and the time from entry into the disabled state. Individuals who are in a particular state, healthy individuals, healthcare providers, caretakers, and family members have all been interviewed in studies. Adaptation, conditioning, development of special skills, and vocational training can all change the response of individuals over time within a particular health state, thereby affecting the value of that state to the individual. As a consequence, the valuation is time dependent—for example, the value placed on a year of life by a paraplegic soon after entering that health state would be different from that obtained after several years of adjustment to that state (Murray & Lopez, 1994.)

Instruments used to extract such preferences involve visual and interview techniques (Lopez et al., 2006; Torrence, 1986). Two alternative scenarios are often presented to the subject and the point of indifference sought (as in standard gamble techniques). Despite much work in this area, there is no consensus or accepted standard method for such elicitation.

Measurement of health-related quality of life has also been discussed in the medical literature for decades. *Health-related quality of life* refers to how well an individual functions in daily life and his or her perception of well-being. Various domains of quality have been defined, such as health perception, functional status, and opportunity, and several instruments have been developed to evaluate them. Both disease-specific and general instruments exist, with such tools abounding in fields dealing with chronic disabled states such as psychiatry, neurology, and counseling. These scales are often dependent on self-reported information, although some incorporate observational data as well. However, there have been concerns about their reliability and validity. These measures are not discussed further in this book, because they have been primarily used in clinical assessments of individuals and do not directly relate to measures of population health.

Measuring Disability

If all the various forms of disability—physical, functional, mental, and social—are to be compared with mortality, they must be measured in an equivalent manner for use in health assessments. To do so, measurement of disability must quantify the duration and severity (extent) of this complex phenomenon. A defined process is needed that rates the severity of disability as compared with mortality, measures the duration of time spent in a disabled state, and converts various forms of disability into a common scale. General measures of disability without regard to cause (often carried out by special surveys) are useful to determine the proportion of the population that is disabled and unable to carry out normal activities, but are not much help for quantifying the extent of disability.

In general, three components of disability need to be assessed. The first component is the *case disability ratio* (CDR)—the proportion of those diagnosed with the disease who have disability. For most diseases that are diagnosed clinically, the CDR will be 1.00 because, by the definition of disease given earlier, patients will have signs or symptoms. In contrast, when the diagnosis is based on, for example, infection rather than disease (such as tuberculosis) or on a genetic marker rather than the physical manifestation (such as sickle cell trait), the CDR is likely to be less than 1.00.

The second component of disability is its *extent or severity*—how incapacitated the person is as a result of the disease. The extent of disability is expressed on a scale, usually from 0 (indicating no disability) to 1.00 (equivalent to death). The assessment of severity can be quite subjective, particularly because so many different types and dimensions of disability exist. A number of methods have been introduced in an effort to achieve comparability and obtain consistency (Murray et al., 2002). For example, severity of disability scales have been developed by group consensus using community surveys (Kaplan, 1990), a mixture of community and expert groups (Ghana Health Assessment Team, 1981), experts only (World Bank, 1993), and population surveys (Murray et al., 2002). These scales usually compare perfect health states to death on a scale of 0 to 1 (Table 1-3).

In the Global Burden of Disease 1990 study, the disability severity estimates were based on expert opinion. Twenty-two indicator conditions were selected and used to construct seven disability classes (see Table 1-3). Outcomes from all other health conditions were categorized within these seven classes (with special categories for treated and untreated groups). Generally, for most conditions a reasonable degree of consensus can be reached within broad categories (e.g., 25% disabled as compared with 50%), but efforts to reach much finer distinctions have proved equivocal. The need to seek out more refined scales for purposes of health program decisions ought to be a national or local decision.

The third component of disability is its *duration*. The duration is generally counted from onset until

Table 1-3	Examples of Disability Classification Systems	
Ghana Health Assessment Team, 1981		
Class	**Severity**	**Equivalent to (Maximum)**
1	0	Normal health
2	0.01–0.25	Loss of one limb function
3	0.26–0.50	Loss of two limbs function
4	0.51–0.75	Loss of three limbs function
5	0.76–0.99	Loss of four limbs function
6	1	Equivalent to death
Global Burden of Disease Study, 1990		
Disability Class	**Severity Weight**	**Indicator Conditions**
1	0.00–0.02	Vitiligo, height, weight
2	0.02–0.12	Acute watery diarrhea, sore throat, severe anemia
3	0.12–0.24	Radius fracture, infertility, erectile dysfunction, rheumatoid arthritis, angina
4	0.24–0.36	Below-knee amputation, deafness
5	0.04–0.50	Rectovaginal fistula, major mental retardation, Down syndrome
6	0.50–0.70	Major depression, blindness, paraplegia
7	0.70–1.00	Psychosis, dementia, migraine, quadriplegia

cure, recovery, or death. Sometimes there is continuing permanent disability after the acute phase is completed; in such a scenario, the duration would be the remaining life expectation from the time of onset of disease.

Data for Decisions

In the collection and assessment of information, the level of precision required should be guided by the purpose of collecting the information and depend on the decisions to be taken. Even rough estimates may be helpful; though disconcerting to some, the time and cost of further precision need to be justified by its potential impact on decision making. Low- and middle-income countries, with their scarce resources, need timely and appropriate information to plan and implement health interventions that maximize the health of their populations. Methods, indicators, and assessments of disease must support and contribute to this primary purpose of health systems.

Decisions concerning deployment of interventions against diseases and underlying risk factors ideally should be taken such that maximum healthy life per resource expenditure is obtained in an equitable, fair, and just fashion. The ultimate reason for obtaining health data is to have the information to guide such decision making.

Summary Measures of Population Health

This section focuses on the major approaches used for developing composite measures of population health status that summarize mortality and morbidity occurring in a population through the use of a single number. It discusses the rationale for composite measures, reviews the origins of each major approach, examines methodological differences among these approaches, makes explicit the value choices that each entails, and outlines the advantages and limitations of each.

Rationale for Composite Measures

Rationing of healthcare resources is a fact of life everywhere; choices about the best use of funds for health must be made (Hyder et al., 1998; World Bank, 1993). The global scarcity of resources for health care is a challenge for every country, rich and poor (Evans et al., 1981; World Bank, 1993), but the realities in low-

and middle-income countries make the issue of choice that much starker. It is even more important for poor countries to choose carefully how to optimize health expenditures so as to obtain the most health in the most equitable fashion from these expenditures. Important tools under development to assist in making better choices for health spending are based on measures of the effectiveness of health interventions in improving health status in relation to their cost.

In most sectors, decisions on resource allocation are based on perceived value for money. The health sector, however, has had no coherent basis for determining the comparative value of different health outcomes (from different health programs). To make decisions about whether to put money into programs that reduce mortality in children, as compared with those programs that reduce disabling conditions in adults, a common denominator is needed. In recent decades, work has been carried out to develop composite indicators combining morbidity and mortality into a single measure that may serve as a common denominator for comparing different health outcomes. A common unit of measure for these different health outcomes is time lost from healthy life.

The most important reason for attempting to capture the complex mix of incommensurable consequences resulting from disease within a single number is the need to weigh the benefits of health interventions against their costs. Costs of health programs are expressed in a unidimensional measure, such as U.S. dollars; therefore, the benefits to be achieved from their expenditure should be expressed in the same manner. Healthy lifetime is a unidimensional measure that can be used to compress health benefits and losses into a single time dimension. An explicit, objective, quantitative approach should enable better budgetary decisions and permit resource allocation in the health sector to be undertaken in a more effective and equitable fashion.

Note that a composite indicator is simply a tool to be used to assist decision makers in resource allocation. Like any tool, it can be misused. Conclusions that are reached on the basis of these indicators must be carefully examined. Not only do problems arise in trying to put so many dimensions together, which inevitably may lead to distortions, but serious issues emerge concerning the reliability and validity of the information on which these indicators are based. Thus all the problems associated with determining causes of death, counting the number of cases of disease, and assessing the extent of disability from a condition will lead to uncertainties when these factors are added and multiplied together. The development of a single indicator consisting of a specific number implies deceptive substantiality about something that may actually be composed of fragile data. Continuing vigilance in how these data are obtained, compiled, and used is critical, and those responsible for using the tool must have a clear technical understanding of what is behind the numbers and which underlying assumptions and limitations are associated with these approaches. Despite all of these caveats, alternative approaches to improved decision making leave even more to be desired.

Uses of Composite Indicators

Measures of health status that combine mortality and morbidity facilitate comparisons both within and across populations. They can be used to estimate the quantitative health benefits from interventions and serve as tools to assist in the allocation of resources. The development of such measures entails two major processes: the measurement of healthy life, including losses of time from premature mortality and disability; and the valuing of life, which incorporates issues of duration, age, extent of future life, productivity, dependency, and equity (Morrow & Bryant, 1995).

The purpose of developing such measures and the need for refining them become clear if the following objectives are to be achieved:

- The use of such methods at the country level for evaluating the impact of diseases
- Their use in the allocation of resources within the health sector
- The generation of more relevant and useful data for policy makers

Understanding Summary Measures

Precursors of composite indicators have been discussed in the literature for decades and generally were developed to assist prioritization of health issues. Usually these metrics were based on the measurement of losses of time, losses of productive time, income forgone, or other costs incurred as a result of diseases. The earlier indicators generally focused on economic losses and estimated time loss due to disease and converted these losses into a dollar value. Thus these measures are more economic measures than disease-burden measures.

Two types of composite summary measures have been developed: *health gap measures* (healthy life lost), such as healthy life years (HeaLY) and disability-adjusted life years (DALY), and *health expectancies*, such as disability-free life expectancy (DFLE) and

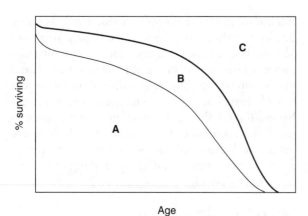

Figure 1-4 Survivorship curve of a hypothetical population showing the areas of health expectancies.
Source: C.J.L. Murray et al. Summary Measures of Population Health (Geneva, Switzerland, WHO, 1999).

health-adjusted life expectancy (HALE). Both types use healthy lifetime lost through disability and death as a common measure of the impact of mortality and nonfatal health outcomes. These two types of measures are complementary and can be studied using survivorship curves, as discussed by Murray and Lopez (Figure 1-4).

In Figure 1-4, the bold line is the survivorship curve based on a standard hypothetical life table population that demonstrates the proportion (*y*-axis) of an initial birth cohort that remains alive at any age (*x*-axis). The area A + B is the total life expectancy at birth of this cohort. A part of this life is spent in full health (area A); the thin line is the survivor curve of those persons in full health. Thus area A represents time lived in full health, whereas area B is time lived in suboptimal health (with disability). Area C represents time lost due to mortality. The area of the complete rectangle (A + B + C) represents the ideal survivorship curve—the theoretical maximum of healthy life for a cohort who lived in full health until a maximum age when all died.

Health expectancies are summary measures that estimate expectancy of life in a defined state of health. Examples include DFLE, active life expectancy, and HALE. These indicators extend the concept of life expectancy to expectations of various states of health, not just of life per se. Health expectancies assign lower weights to life lived in less than full health on a scale of 0 to 1, in which full health is rated 1. In Figure 1-4, health expectancy is given by the following equation:

$$\text{Health expectancy} = A + f(B)$$

where *f* is some function that assigns weights to years lived in suboptimal health.

Health gaps are summary measures that estimate the difference between actual population health and some specified norm or goal. In Figure 1-4, that difference is indicated by area C (loss due to mortality) plus some function of area B—that is, survivorship with disability:

$$\text{Health gap (healthy life lost)} = C + g(B)$$

where *g* is some function that assigns weights to health states lived during time B. Weights range between 0, meaning no disability (full health), and 1, meaning complete disability (equivalent to death). Note that this measure is equivalent to healthy life lost based on the natural history of disease in a population as discussed in the section "Healthy Life Year" later in this chapter.

Although some believe that health expectancies such as the HALE indicator are more readily understood (because they are conceptual extensions of the widely used life expectancy measure), health gap measures have important advantages for the purposes of health policy, planning, and resource allocation decisions. Both HeaLYs and DALYs are developed on the basis of disability and death attributable to a specific disease in an individual person. In their construction, great care is taken to ensure that there is categorical attribution using the ICD classification of disease so that each event (death or disability) is mutually exclusive and collectively exhaustive. With these measures, therefore, summing deaths and disabilities from each disease provides the total amount of death and disability for the population (a property termed *additive decomposition*). Health gap measures have this property, whereas health expectancies do not.

Composite Indicators

A number of composite summary indicators for burden of disease assessment have been developed. We will focus on four of these indicators: three of the health gap type (the healthy life year, the disability-adjusted life year, and the quality-adjusted life year) and one of the health expectancy type (HALE). In addition to measures of morbidity and mortality per se, these composite indicators may incorporate certain social value choices either explicitly or implicitly: the choice of life expectancy tables, valuing future life as compared with present life, valuing life lived at different ages, valuing social or economic productivity, and valuing equity in relation to cost-effectiveness.

These social value choices are discussed later in this chapter (see the section "Valuing Life: Social Value Issues"), but because some social value choices are integral to the calculations of some composite indicators, they are briefly mentioned in this section.

Healthy Life Year

The healthy life year (HeaLY) is a composite measure that combines the amount of healthy life lost due to morbidity with that lost due to death—that is, loss of life expected had the disease not occurred (Hyder et al., 1998). We discuss the healthy life year first because it is conceptually straightforward, serves as a prototype for other health gap indicators, and was the first of the composite measures to be used as a tool in national health planning (Ghana Health Assessment Team, 1981). The HeaLY approach is a direct derivative of the work done in Ghana that incorporates several additional features.

The measure of loss from death is based on the years of life that would have been lived had the disease not occurred. The information needed in addition to the incidence rate and case fatality ratio is the age of disease onset, the age of death, and the expectation of life at these ages. All of this information is objective in nature and potentially available in every country. The main issue centers on the choice for life expectation (see also the section "Expectation of Life" later in this chapter). The original Ghana work was based on expectation-of-life tables specific to Ghana. In later work, considerations of global equity and comparability across countries made it preferable to use the best possible life expectation—that of the female population in Japan.

Measuring the loss of healthy life from disability is more challenging than measuring that from death, and many approaches have been used (Murray & Lopez, 1994.) To incorporate loss from disability in a composite measure, such a loss must have comparable dimensions to that for life lost due to death. The HeaLY includes three components for disability: case disability ratio (comparable to the case fatality ratio), extent of disability, and duration of disability. The CDR and duration of disability can be determined objectively, but assessment of the extent of disability, which ranges from 0 (no disability) to 1 (equivalent to death), has a substantial subjective element (Morrow & Bryant, 1995).

The healthy life approach focuses on knowledge of the pathogenesis and natural history of disease (Last, 2000) as the conceptual framework for assessing morbidity and mortality and for interpreting the effects of various interventions (Figure 1-5). For the purpose of estimating healthy life lost or gained, disease is defined as stated earlier in this chapter: anything that an individual (or population) experiences that causes, literally, "dis-ease"—anything that leads to discomfort, pain, distress, disability of any kind, or death, including injuries and psychiatric disabilities. With some exceptions, those persons with infection or some biological characteristic (such as sickle-cell trait) are considered healthy unless they have specific identifiable symptoms or signs. Preclinical or subclinical disease is not generally counted. However, the diagnostic criteria for some conditions such as hypertension, HIV infection, or onchocerciasis (diagnosed by skin snip) include individuals without signs or symptoms. Such criteria (e.g., indicators of infection, high blood pressure, or genetic markers) are appropriate when they serve as the basis for intervention programs. Interventions may also be directed at reducing identifiable risk factors, such as tobacco smoking or risky sexual behavior. To the extent that risk reduction can be translated into disease reduction, the approach to measuring the benefits and costs of a risk reduction intervention program remains the same as that for disease reduction.

The onset of disease usually will be dated from the start of symptoms or signs, as determined by the individual afflicted, a family member, or a medical practitioner, or as the result of a lab test. Several different patterns of disease evolution are possible, of course. Figure 1-6 illustrates healthy life lost from disability and premature death due to typical cases of cirrhosis, polio, and multiple sclerosis, respectively, in terms of onset, extent and duration of disability, and termination. The conclusion of the disease process depends on the natural history of the disease as modified by possible interventions. The possible outcomes include clinical recovery (the complete disappearance of clinical signs and symptoms), progression to another disease state (such as chronic hepatitis progressing to cirrhosis), and death. The last outcome includes death directly caused by the disease as well as death indirectly brought on by the disease as a result of disability.

The definitions of variables and formulas to calculate HeaLYs are provided later in this section and summarized in Table 1-4. Each disease will have a distribution of ages at which onset or death may occur, but for most diseases the average age will provide a satisfactory approximation for a population. In view of the limitations of data, this is the starting assumption for the application of the HeaLY method in developing countries. Nevertheless, as with other

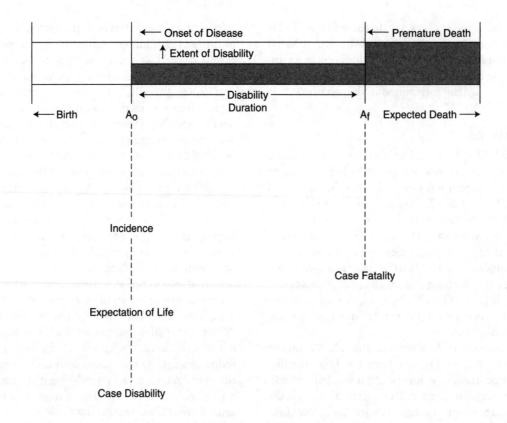

Note: A_o = average age at onset; A_f = average age at death; ■ = healthy life lost.

Figure 1-5 The HeaLY Model: Loss of Healthy Life from Disability and Death.

choices in this method, if sensitivity testing indicates that the average age is not satisfactory, then estimates may be based on age distributions. Similarly, if the natural history of a disease or response to interventions is different in different age groups, then the disease can be specifically classified by age (e.g., neonatal tetanus as compared with adult tetanus, and childhood pneumonia as compared with adult pneumonia).

In recurrent diseases or diseases with multiple episodes (e.g., diarrhea), age at onset denotes the average age at first episode. For some diseases, such as malaria, which is characterized by recurrent episodes, and schistosomiasis, in which reinfection occurs at frequent intervals, it may be useful to view them as single lifetime diseases. For example, malaria in Africa may be considered for each individual as a single, lifelong disease with chronic, usually asymptomatic, parasitemia but with intermittent severe clinical attacks (which result in high mortality in late infancy and early childhood while immunity is being acquired), followed by recurring, nonfatal clinical episodes after age 10.

The expectation of life in HeaLYs is based on normative expectations of what should occur under usual circumstances. Women in Japan, who have the highest global expectation of life, approximate this norm with an expectation of life at birth of 82.5 years for females (model life table west, level 26) (Coale & Demeney, 1983; Coale & Guo, 1989).

The definition of disease ("dis-ease") makes the value of the case disability ratio 1 by default for most disease states because all cases are disabled (to varying degrees and duration) if those persons have been labeled as diseased. For some conditions (e.g., sickle cell trait or HIV positivity) and risk factors, however, cases may not be considered diseased by definition, but the condition nonetheless needs to be assessed.

The duration of disability can be either temporary or permanent (lifelong). If the disability is temporary, then D_t is the duration of that disability until recovery (see Table 1-4). If the disability is permanent and the disease does not affect life expectation, then D_t is the expectation of life at age of onset of disease [$D_t = E(A_o)$]. If the disability is permanent and the disease

Healthy Life Lost (Cirrhosis)

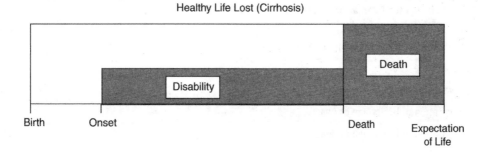

Healthy Life Lost (Polio)

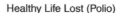
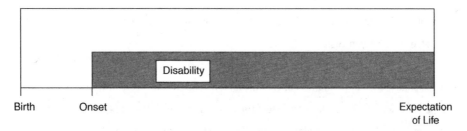

Healthy Life Lost (Multiple Sclerosis)

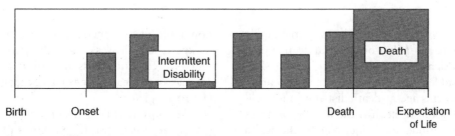

Figure 1-6 Different Patterns of Healthy Life Lost.
Source: Hyder A, Rollant G, Morrow RH. Measuring the Burden of Disease: healthy life-years.
AM J Public Health, Feb. 1998; 88: 196–202. Figure 1 p. 197.

does reduce life expectation, then D_t is the expectation of life at age of onset reduced by the difference between ages of fatality and onset $[D_t = E(A_o) - (A_f - A_o)]$.

A disability severity scale needs to be used to estimate extent (severity) of the disability (see Table 1-4).

The healthy life years lost from death and from disability are added and expressed as the total years of life lost per 1,000 population per year. The loss is attributed to the year in which disease onset occurs and includes the stream of life lost from disability and death at any time after onset, even if these events happen many years later. This method offers a

prospective view of the event (disease onset) and its natural history (or as modified by interventions) over time.

The health status of a population can be considered as the amount of healthy life it achieves as a proportion of the total amount that the people could achieve under optimal conditions. A cohort of 1,000 newborns with an expectation of life of 82.5 years has the potential of 82,500 years of healthy life, for example. In a steady state, a random sample of 1,000 people from a population made up of successive such cohorts has the potential of 41,250 years of healthy life (Hyder et al., 1998; Morrow & Bryant, 1995). Each year this population would experience events

Table 1-4	Variables for Estimating Healthy Life Years (HeaLY)	
Symbol	**Explanation**	**Expression**
I	Incidence rate per 1,000 population per year	/1,000/year
A_o	Average age at onset.	years
A_f	Average age at death.	years
$E(A_o)$	Expectation of life at age of onset.	years
$E(A_f)$	Expectation of life at age of death.	years
CFR	Case fatality ratio: proportion of those developing the disease who die from the disease	0.00–1.00
CDR	Case disability ratio: proportion of those developing the disease who have disability from the disease.	0.00–1.00
D_e	Extent of disability (from none to complete disability equivalent to death)	0.00–1.00
D_t	Duration of disability in years.	years
	Disability can be either permanent or temporary.	
	• If temporary, then D_t = duration of that disability(i.e., until recovery or death)	
	• If permanent and disease does not affect life expectation, then $D_t = E(A_o)$	
	• If permanent and the disease does reduce life expectation, then $D_t = A_f - A_o$	
HeaLY	Healthy life years lost per 1,000 population per year: $I \times \{[CFR \times \{E(A_o) - [A_f - A_o]\}] + [CDR \times D_e \times D_t]\}$	HeaLYs per 1,000 per year

leading to 1,000 years of healthy life lost attributable to mortality, with a distribution of age at death equivalent to that which leads to a life expectation of 82.5. Any disease that leads to disability or to death earlier than that set by this age-at-death distribution would increase the amount of healthy life lost beyond this minimum. This formulation is equivalent to the health gap, as indicated in Figure 1-4. Discounting future life or adding productivity, dependency, or age weighting would modify these denominator numbers.

HeaLYs measure the gap or loss between the current situation in a country as compared to that of an ideal or standard population. In recent work, researchers have used a standard based on the life expectation approximated in Japan. Thus, if exactly the same method were used to estimate the HeaLY losses for females in Japan, they would amount to 0 per 1,000 people for loss due to mortality; only those losses due to disability would be counted. Because the population under study is the ideal (standard), assuming stability of the population with constancy of mortality rates and no disability, there would be no gap to measure. This does not mean that the population is not having a loss of healthy life, but simply that such loss is the minimum as defined by the structure of the population and the expecta-

tion of life, as described previously. Any country that is experiencing losses greater than this minimum, either as a result of excess mortality or disability, will have a gap that can be measured; that gap is what the HeaLYs register.

An important benefit of the HeaLY formulation is that the effects of different kinds of interventions can be readily explored to determine their expected gains in terms of healthy life. Interventions may usefully be divided into two broad categories: those that prevent the initiation of the disease process and those that treat a disease process already under way. Some interventions fall into both categories. The primary effect of preventive strategies is to reduce the incidence of new cases of disease. The main effect of treatment strategies is to interfere with the natural history of the disease process, thereby reducing the case fatality and/or case disability ratios or extending life by providing a later age at death for conditions such as diabetes and AIDS. The HeaLY spreadsheet (available upon request from the authors at ahyder@jhsph.edu) incorporates these concerns; it also includes options for considering the proportion of the population that will be covered by an intervention and allows for different levels of coverage for different segments of the population for each intervention.

Disability-Adjusted Life Year

The disability-adjusted life year (DALY) is a health gap population summary measure that combines time lost due to disability with that lost due to death (life that would have been expected had the disease not occurred), in a manner similar to the healthy life year measure. It first appeared in the World Development Report of 1993 (World Bank, 1993) and has become the most widely used composite measure of population health (Jamison et al., 2006; Lopez et al., 2002; Murray & Lopez, 1994,1999; Murray et al., 2002).

DALYs are calculated as two separate components for the measurement of life lost due to disease, and they may also directly include three social value choices. The two components are (1) years of life lost (YLL), referring to the loss of healthy life from death, and (2) years of life lived with disability (YLD), referring to the loss of healthy life from disability. Thus

$$DALY = YLL + YLD$$

The social value choices that may be included in DALYs are (1) life expectation values, (2) discount rates for future life, and (3) weighting for life lived at different ages, as discussed later.

The calculation for YLL in a population uses the age distribution of all deaths by cause in one year multiplied by life expectation at each age to estimate the loss of life for each disease that would have been expected if not for that disease. The expectation of life is obtained from a model life table based on best achievable low levels of mortality, such as those found in Japan (Coale & Guo, 1989); thus the DALY, as does the HeaLY, directly incorporates this social value choice.

For disability, the DALY uses estimates of incidence, duration, and severity to calculate the time lived with disability (YLD) for each disease. The YLD component equals the number of incident cases in the period multiplied by the average duration of disease multiplied by a weight factor for the degree of severity (extent) of the disease. A description of the severity scale used in one version of DALY was given earlier in this chapter, in the section on measurement of disability (see Table 1-4).

The second social value choice directly incorporated in the original version of DALY is the discount rate of 3% per annum. This social time preference has been used for most estimates; recently, DALY results discounted at 0% have also become available.

The third social value choice concerns weighting life lived at different ages. DALYs are age weighted according to an arbitrary exponential curve designed to give the most value to life lived as a young adult (Hyder et al., 1998; World Bank, 1993). Weighting by age was the most controversial component of the DALYs when they appeared and caused great dissent from other health professionals (see the section "Valuing Life Lived at Different Ages" later in this chapter). Recent DALY listings from GBD studies also include results with no age weighting (all years equally valued). It has been argued that age weighting of DALYs does not affect final results, but this depends on the purpose for making the estimates and has been challenged (Anand & Ranaan-Eliya, 1996; Barendregt et al., 1996; Barker & Green, 1996; Hyder et al., 1998).

An important difference between the HeaLY and DALY is the fact that the starting point for the HeaLY is the onset of disease; the loss of healthy life is based on the natural history of the disease (as modified by interventions), illustrated in Figures 1-4 and 1-5. This is true for the YLD component of the DALY, but the YLL is based on mortality in the current year. In a steady state, there is no difference. When incidence is changing, however—such as with HIV in many parts of the globe—the DALY approach can greatly understate the true situation (Hyder & Morrow, 1999).

The calculation for DALYs can be expressed in the form of an integral that was first published in the World Bank literature (Murray & Lopez, 1994). This single equation incorporating all technical and value choices has the advantage of standardization to ensure comparability of the multiple calculations undertaken in the GBD studies, and it has certainly greatly facilitated the actual computations. Nevertheless, for national and local priority setting, it may be preferable to use an indicator constructed such that the social value choices can be adjusted to suit the national and local preferences (Bobadilla, 1998; Hyder et al., 1998; Morrow & Bryant, 1995). Recent DALY formulations allow for this possibility; indeed, it is useful to think of DALYs as a family of related measures using terminology specifying the formulation as follows: DALYs (r, K) uses a discount rate of r and age weighting indexed to K. Other parameters can be added in a similar fashion (Jamison et al., 2006).

HeaLYs and DALYs are both "health gap" measures and can be considered the same family of measures. In fact, DALYS exactly equal HeaLYs when the following conditions are met: (1) the condition in question is in steady state or equilibrium (that is the incidence, CFR, and disability variables remain constant during the time intervals under consideration); (2) age weighting is not applied ($K = 0$); and (3) the same measures of disability (weights) are used.

Quality-Adjusted Life Year

The quality-adjusted life year (QALY) was introduced in 1976 to provide a guiding principle for selecting among alternative tertiary healthcare interventions (Zeckhauser & Shephard, 1976). The idea was to develop a single measure of quality of life that would enable investigators to compare expected outcomes from different interventions—a measure that valued possible health states both for their quality of life and for their duration.

The central notion behind the QALY is that a year of life spent in one health state may be preferred to a year spent in another health state. This generic measure sums time spent in different health states using weights on a scale of 0.00 (dead) to 1.00 (perfectly healthy) for each health state; it is the arithmetic product of duration of life and a measure of quality of life (health state weight). For example, five years of perfect health = 5 QALYs; 2 years in a state measured as 0.5 of perfect health followed by five years of perfect health = 4 QALYs.

The QALY was originally developed as a differentiating indicator for individual choices among tertiary healthcare procedures, not as a measure of disease burden in a population. It was used to assess individual preferences for different health outcomes from alternative interventions (Morrow & Bryant, 1995). The QALY, too, comprises a large family of measures. Since its introduction, a wide variety of QALY measures have been developed, along with a voluminous literature on alternative methods incorporating a range of disability domains and a diversity of methods to assign weights to generate QALYs (Kaplan, 1990; Nord, 1993). The most widely used measure is the EQ-5D (European Quality of Life with Five Domains and three levels of quality for each domain; www.euroqol.org).

Perhaps the most important use of QALYs has been as a common denominator to measure utility in cost-utility analysis (and effectiveness in cost-effectiveness analysis) to assist in resource allocation among alternative health interventions by ranking interventions in terms of cost per QALY (Kaplan, 1990; Nord, 1992; Torrence, 1986). An early and widely publicized attempt to make the best use of healthcare resources by maximizing QALYs per dollar expended was the well-intentioned but rather unfortunate effort in Oregon in the early 1990s (Exhibit 1-5).

In the United Kingdom, as part of its 1997 National Health Service (NHS) reforms, the National Institute for Clinical Excellence (NICE; www.nice.org.uk) was created to advise public health officials about the effectiveness and cost-effectiveness of various health interventions. In an explicit attempt to introduce economic considerations in addition to medical judgments for the allocation of resources, NICE has produced a large collection of studies on the cost per QALY produced by the interventions it appraises. Some of these appraisals have been the source of considerable controversy. If a treatment is considered cost-effective for a group of patients, NICE will recommend its use throughout the NHS; if not, it will recommend against its use in the NHS. The hope is that use of these cost-effectiveness studies as an aid to decisions will increase the total healthcare benefits gained from the money spent by the NHS.

The QALY as originally used is essentially equivalent to the YLD of the DALY; in fact, it would be exactly the same as the YLD when the following conditions are met: (1) there is no discounting ($r = 0$); (2) there is no age weighting ($K = 0$); and (3) the same disability weights are used. More recently (as used in some cost-effectiveness studies) QALYs have incorporated life expectation as well.

The Health-Adjusted Life Expectancies

Several types of health expectancies exist in the literature. During the 1990s, *disability-free life expectancy* (DFLE) and related measures were calculated for many countries (Mathers et al., 2001; Robine, 1994). However, these measures incorporate a dichotomous weighting scheme in which time spent in any health state categorized as disabled is assigned, arbitrarily, a weight of zero (equivalent to death). Thus DFLE is not sensitive to differences in the severity distribution of disability in populations. In contrast, the *disability-adjusted life expectancy* (DALE) adds up expectation of life for different health states with adjustment for severity weights. In 2001, WHO replaced the DALE terminology with *health-adjusted life expectancy* (HALE); the latter term will be used throughout the remainder of this book.

The HALE is a composite summary measure of population health status that belongs to the family of health expectancies; it summarizes the expected number of years to be lived in what might be termed the equivalent of "full health." Some consider the HALE measure to provide the best available summary measure for measuring the overall level of health for populations (Mathers et al., 2001). WHO has used it as the measure of the average level of health of the populations of member states for annual reporting on population health (WHO, 2000).

Health expectancy indices combine the mortality experience of a population with the disability expe-

---

Exhibit 1-5	Oregon: Application of the QALY for Allocation of Resources

An early and well-known attempt to apply the QALY approach for allocation of health resources occurred in the state of Oregon (Blumstein, 1997). In 1988, Oregon faced a budgetary shortfall for its Medicaid program and coverage for organ transplants was denied. In an effort to prioritize its health services, Oregon undertook a bold attempt to explicitly ration health services. A coalition including consumers, healthcare providers, insurers, business, and labor representatives launched a broad and courageous healthcare reform. It began with a series of "experiments" in which the decision-making process was based on a cost-effectiveness approach using quality of well-being (QWB—essentially a QALY) for comparing the outcomes of treatment options among people.

The initial list, published in 1990, consisted of 1,600 condition/treatment pairs drawn up as follows:

Cost-effectiveness ratio = cost of services / (health gain × duration)

Cost of services = charges for treatment including all services and drugs

Quality of well-being (QWB) = sum of QWB weight (W) × each QWB state × probability that symptoms of that QWB state would occur

Health gain = QWB with treatment − QWB without treatment

From the beginning, there was great opposition to the very notion of rationing; consequent denial of services to those who had conditions that did not make the list contributed to the rancor. There were also unfortunate technical blunders in the generation of the first list. For example, treatment for thumb sucking was ranked higher than hospitalization for starvation, and treatment for crooked teeth higher than early treatment for Hodgkin's disease. Such inconsistencies, together with objections raised by groups advocating for the disabled, gave rise to alternative approaches for establishing rankings.

Although enormous public effort went into the reform and much was accomplished, the explicit cost-effectiveness approach with QALYs as the outcome measure was dropped (Blumstein, 1997; Eddy, 1991; Morrow & Bryant, 1995; Nord, 1993).

---

rience. The HALE is calculated using the prevalence of disability at each age so as to divide the years of life expected at each age (according to a life table cohort) into years with and without disability. Mortality is captured by using a life table method, while the disability component is expressed by additions of prevalence of various disabilities within the life table. This indicator allows an assessment of the proportion of life spent in disabled states. When compared with the total expectation of life, it translates into a measure of the total disability burden in a population. Comparison of the various methods and specific indicators is available in the literature (Robine, 1994). Alternative methods are given in WHO's *National Burden of Disease Studies* manual (Mathers et al., 2001).

As originally designed, the HALE does not relate to specific diseases but rather to the average extent of disability among that proportion of each age group that is disabled. The lack of correlation between a condition or disease entity and the measure makes it less valuable for resource allocation and cost-effectiveness calculations. It is possible to convert health gap measures for specific diseases or interventions and risk factors into HALEs, but it is not clear what would be gained from this exercise.

Although the HALE is conceptually interesting and is now being calculated and included regularly in the WHO annual reports, it is not clear what additional information the HALE provides beyond the standard life expectancy data. At a national level, the amount of healthy life lost due to disability very closely parallels, and is closely proportional to, that lost due to death. As a result, the relative ranking of countries by HALEs is virtually identical to the ranking based on life expectation at birth.

Summary

Table 1-5 summarizes these four summary measures in terms of origins, purposes, level of use, sources of data, and disciplinary background of originators.

Valuing Life: Social Value Issues

The very idea of valuing some lives more than others is jarring, yet these notions are regularly reflected in our actions. The value of life is often implicit in the way resource allocation decisions are made; therefore, as much as possible such decisions should be explicit, open, and transparent. Many thoughtful people have serious reservations about assigning a single number to such a complex multidimensional phenomenon as

Table 1-5	Comparisons of Composite Summary Measures of Population Health			
	Healthy Life Years	**Disability-Adjusted Life Years**	**Quality-Adjusted Life Years**	**Health-Adjusted Life Expectancy**
Origin	Ghana Ministry of Health, 1981	World Bank Development Report, 1993	North America, 1976	World Health Organization Report, 2000
Purpose	Assist in resource allocation decisions	Compare disease burdens in many different populations	Assess individual preferences for various outcomes from complex interventions	Compare national disease burdens
Level of use	National and district level decisions	Broad policy decisions	Personal decisions	Global comparisons
Data	National and local data from multiple sources; expert review	Global data and expert opinion	Tertiary hospital data and personal interviews	Global data and expert opinion
Original discipline base	Epidemiologists, clinicians, national planners	Economists, statisticians	Economists, clinicians	Demographers, economists, statisticians
Social values that may be incorporated	Future life discounted	Age weighting, future life discounted	Generally not included	Not relevant

health. But what is the alternative for use as a measure of utility or effectiveness in economic analyses? Outcome measures must be expressed as a unidimensional measure to be comparable to unidimensional monetary expenditure units for costs. (However, decisions about allocation should not be made on a mechanical basis; other factors, including the effect on equity, may need to be considered in decisions in addition to the goal of maximizing healthy life per unit expenditure.)

To construct composite measures of population health, important social value choices must be made. Choices about which expectation for life should be used and about valuing life lived at different ages, valuing future life as compared with the present, valuing life in terms of economic and social productivity, and valuing equity in relation to efficiency—all raise major ethical concerns.

Expectation of Life

Years of life lost due to death and to chronic disability are based on life expected had the disease not occurred. To estimate the expectation of life in a population, a choice must be made between using a local, national, or model life table. This choice should be determined by the purpose of the study.

For assisting in national and local decision making, it may be more suitable to use national life tables based on the mortality and fertility of the population in question than to use model life tables. Conversely, a model life table might be selected to reflect the best health state possible in the world, such as the west model. This selection allows a fair comparison with other countries. For example, from a global perspective it would be unfair to use national life tables to compare gains that could be achieved from a particular intervention in Ghana with those in the United Kingdom, even if both costs and lives saved were the same in each country. The reason is that those lives saved in Ghana would have a lower life expectancy than those in the United Kingdom, resulting in less healthy life saved for the same expenditure. From the global viewpoint in this example, the priority would be to fund the intervention in the United Kingdom because it would produce more healthy life per expenditure than for Ghana.

Model life tables in common use are the United Nations model life tables and the Coale and Demeney (Coale & Guo, 1989) life tables, which were used in the HeaLY and GBD studies (Hyder et al.,1998; Lopez et al., 2006). The West model life table does not refer to any geographical entity but is considered to represent a mortality pattern typical of the most technologically advanced countries. Level 26 has a female life expectancy at birth of 82.5 years, as actually experienced by women in Japan; therefore, it represents a level that could be achievable elsewhere.

Valuing Life Lived at Different Ages

Age weighting refers to the valuing of a year of life according to the age at which it is lived. This practice immediately raises questions about the basis for valuing human life. Does a day of one person's life have the same value as a day of anyone else's life? Does the value vary with age, economic productivity, or social status? Should life itself be valued separately from what is done with that life?

The Ghana Health Assessment Team (1981) judged that all human life was intrinsically valuable and that a given duration of any life was equal in value to that of any other life. The valuing of a year of life equally, irrespective of age, has been considered egalitarian (Busschbach et al., 1993; Morrow & Bryant, 1995). This choice was incorporated into the development of the HeaLY approach: A year of life lived at any age is equally valued.

The original DALY formulation assigned an exponential function to provide a value chosen so that life lived as a dependent (e.g., infants, children, the elderly) is given less value than life lived during the productive years. With this approach, the intrinsic value of life increases from zero at birth to a maximum at age 25 and declines thereafter, so that a day of life of a 50-year-old is worth about 25% less than that of a 25-year-old. Paradoxically, the age weighting used in the original DALY formulation leads to higher valuation of life lived before age 15 than does the HeaLY formulation, in which life lived at all ages has equal value (Barendregt et al., 1996; Hyder et al., 1998). Current formulations of the DALY leave age weighting as an option, and such weighting is not used with the HALE.

Age-related valuing has been justified by studies showing that individuals value their own life lived at different ages differently. Such values have been reported in the literature, and studies have reported that they are consistent across respondents of different ages (Busschbach et al., 1993). Murray and Lopez (1994) report studies from many countries that reveal a preference for saving younger lives as compared with older ones. Nevertheless, it is not clear how much of the differential valuing of life at different ages is related to an underlying appreciation that economic and social productivity varies at different ages. If it is decided that healthy life should be valued according to economic and social productivity, then an alternative to age weighting might be to explicitly add a productivity factor or subtract for the societal costs of dependents, such as education (see the section "Valuing Life for Its Economic and Social Productivity").

Valuing Future Life Compared with Present Life: Discounting

Discounting is the process for determining the present value of future events. Social time preference takes into account the phenomenon that people value events at present more highly than those in the future (independent of inflation and of uncertainty). For investments in other sectors, time preference is normally taken into account by discounting future returns and costs by some appropriate discount rate. Thus the discount rate can be considered the inverse of an interest rate. The main issue concerning discounting in relation to summary measures is whether discounting life itself is appropriate. There seems little problem about the usefulness of discounting the future value of what is produced by healthy life, but should the life itself be discounted (Morrow & Bryant, 1995)?

Discounting has been applied in the health sector because both the losses from a disease and the benefits from a health intervention often occur in the future. An intervention today may not produce immediate benefits (such as in immunization), or it may result in benefits being sustained over a long time (such as in supplementary nutrition). The costs for these activities must be borne now, but the benefits are realized in the future and are less valuable than if they could occur now. This is equivalent to investing money now so as to obtain more in the future. A healthy life year now has greater intrinsic value to an individual or community than one in the future (Gold et al., 1996; Weinstein et al., 1996).

The rate at which society is supposed to discount has been termed the social discount rate (SDR), a numeric reflection of societal values regarding intertemporal allocation of current resources. There is no consensus about the most appropriate choice of a discount rate in health, but most agree that it should be lower than that used in the private commercial sector. The WDR in 1993 and the GBD studies used a discount rate of 3% per year; in lieu of other information, this rate has come to be used in most international health cost-effectiveness studies. Nevertheless, the impact of using a range of discount rates, including zero, should be explored with each study.

Valuing Life for Its Economic and Social Productivity

Whether and how to value economic and social productivity for purposes of healthcare decision making is highly contentious; to a large extent, the age weighting incorporated in the original DALY formulation was considered by many to be a proxy for productivity. The consensus now seems to be that any such valuations should be considered separately, made explicit, and very much dependent on the purpose of the valuations.

In general, productivity may be attributed to adults aged 15 to 64, and those in these age groups could be given a higher value. Persons younger than age 15 and older than age 65 may be considered as dependents and given a lower value. Many variations for differential valuing are possible, including type of employment. People at different socioeconomic levels in a society are expected to have different capacities for productivity—yet, to value life according to income levels or social class would not seem fair and generally would not be acceptable. In poor countries, the value of marginal wages for subsistence agriculture is negligible, but the value of the workers' lives certainly is not.

A fundamental question is whether to consider adding a productivity component to the summary measure. Health issues do not readily conform to the requirements of market economics; information is inadequate, and misinformation is rife on the part of the providers as well as the public. Externalities from good health are generally large. Demand for costly services is largely determined by the healthcare providers rather than by the consumers. Competitive market forces have not worked well for those in greatest need. In the private sector, demand for services is clearly related to productivity and willingness (and ability) to pay. If left to market forces alone, inequitable distribution would be inevitable.

Economic arguments have been put forward for valuing life according to productivity, but counterclaims have been made that human life cannot and should not be expressed in economic terms for decision-making purposes. Nevertheless, efforts to avoid such expression result in implicit valuation of life. Barnum (1987) has argued for adding productivity to the valuing of human life, stating that it has been ignored in health policy, is readily quantifiable, and does not ignore the welfare of children because the whole population is dependent on adult productivity for quality and sustenance. Such economic appraisal of human life is often based on the net transfer of resources from the "producers" to the "consumers" and the consequent interdependence of people.

In relation to this issue, in the *Report of the Commission on Macroeconomics and Health* (WHO, 2001), a DALY was stated to be worth at least an average annual income per head. Although the basis for such a valuation was not adequately justified, the basic notion seems right. More work on explicit valuations of human life and what it produces are needed, and

will certainly affect health-related cost-effectiveness decisions.

Valuing Equity in Relation to Efficiency

A child born in Malawi or Uganda will likely live only half as long as one born in Sweden or Singapore; one in three babies born in Niger or Sierra Leone will not live to see his or her fifth birthday. These inequalities are unfair and harmful and, therefore, qualify as inequities. In terms of social justice, equity has to do with a fair distribution of benefits from social and economic development. However, the term *equity* is used in different conceptual senses: equal access to health services for all (opportunity equality), equal resources expended for each individual (supply equality), equal resources expended on each case of a particular condition (equality of resource use to meet biological need), equal healthy life gained per dollar expended (cost-effectiveness), care according to willingness to pay (economic-demand equality), care according to biological or socioeconomic need, and equal health states for all.

Decisions based on cost-effectiveness (e.g., cost per healthy life year), therefore, may not accord well with concerns about equity. These calculations are generally indifferent to equity; they are designed to steer interventions to what is efficient, whatever the differential need may be. To meet the requirements of equity, health system planners need to go beyond ensuring equality of access to health care and require a balance so that health system responses are in accord with equity as well as efficiency.

Provided that health information is available according to socioeconomic and vulnerable groups, use of these summary indicators as tools for equity by calculating healthy life per dollar to be gained by all socioeconomic and vulnerable groups could readily be undertaken. It would be straightforward to assess the impact of specific health decisions to ensure that they enhance equity. Summary measures such as HeaLYs and DALYs can be used to guide allocation of resources to ensure equitable distribution of those resources so as to reach those most in need. Cost-effectiveness by itself does not provide adequate guidance; equity should be an associated criterion to govern the distribution of societal benefits.

Data for Composite Measures
Types of Data

The data needs for estimating the burden of disease in a region or country are extensive, and obtaining even reasonable estimates in low- and middle-income countries has been a source of concern (Anand & Ranaan-Eliya, 1996; Barker & Green, 1996; Bobadilla, 1998; Murray et al., 2002). Brief descriptions of the types of data required follow; available data need to be carefully reviewed and optimally utilized.

Demographic Data. Population data are integral to burden of disease estimations and are needed both as denominators and for consistency checks. In a national setting, a recent census is useful for providing population counts by age, sex, and geographic location. Particularly helpful, when there is inadequate death registration, is to have a one-year post-census follow-up on a sample of enumeration areas so as to obtain robust age, sex, and place mortality. The age and sex distribution of the population is critical, and often is a major factor that determines the nature of the disease burden. A good vital registration system is a key asset that will provide both birth and death numbers. Underreporting, age misreporting, and other biases in data may have to be addressed (using standard demographic methods) prior to use of these data in burden of disease estimation.

Mortality. Mortality data are required for any burden of disease analysis. Specifically, age, sex, and place mortality rates greatly assist the analysis by defining the contribution of mortality to the pattern of disease burden. They also serve as an essential framework that constrains estimates obtained from a variety of special studies that fill important information gaps but may be incomplete or biased in the populations covered. Reporting errors, such as underreporting of deaths and reporting of age at death, need to be carefully examined. In particular, information has to be evaluated for deficiencies in the under-five group and older age groups. For the youngest ages, the probabilities of deaths in the first year (1q0) and in the next four years (4q1) provide better estimates of the risk of death than do overall mortality rates. Methods such as the Brass method for indirect estimates of mortality provide useful ways to assess age-specific mortality data for potential errors (Hill, 2001).

For burden of disease studies, cause of death data are required for all ages, but reliable cause of death records are rarely available in low- and middle-income countries, especially for deaths that do not occur in healthcare facilities. Even if available, the classification system used may be outdated rather than ICD based, and the reliability of coding may vary by the type and location of the hospital. Young-adult deaths may be better recorded than deaths of infants and the elderly. Especially in low-income countries, it can be helpful to cross-check death records with other

information, using postmortem interviews and hospital registers to assist in defining causes of death or to extrapolate from other data or other regions to assist in the estimates.

Morbidity. Meaningful data on disability are even more difficult to find and interpret than mortality data. Often morbidity information is institution based or restricted to one or two sources, such as hospital inpatient and clinic outpatient records. The representativeness of small studies and the range and types of morbidity covered in any survey need careful evaluation. National disability surveys or regional studies conducted for the evaluation of disabled people may be available; such research is useful in providing some estimate of the prevalence of serious disabilities and their age and sex distribution. However, linkage between disability and disease is often not available, and attributing one type of disability to specific causes is difficult. For example, because many conditions can lead to blindness—for example, diabetes, hypertension, injuries, trachoma, and cataracts—the attribution of proportions of blindness in a population to its cause can be problematic. Information on the duration of disability may be found in specialized studies and the experience of institutions. The severity of disability will have to be rated on a scale; the various methods used in the literature were described earlier in this chapter.

Variables

The types of data just described need to be processed in the form of specific disease-based estimates. The key variables are defined in Table 1-4.

The incidence rate (usually expressed per 1,000 general population per year) is central to the natural history of disease concept. Although incidence is a basic epidemiologic indicator, it is usually not found in routine data collection systems. Special studies, prospective surveys, or calculations based on the prevalence (which is more commonly available than the incidence) and knowledge of the average duration of the disease can be helpful in developing this measure.

The case fatality rate is the proportion of those developing the disease who die from it at any time. It is expressed as a decimal value between 0 (for nonfatal conditions) and 1 (for universally lethal conditions such as AIDS). The case disability ratio (analogous to the CFR) is the proportion of those diagnosed with a disease who have signs or symptoms, and is usually 1 (as discussed earlier).

Age is required in various formats. Age at onset is when disease onset occurs in a population; age at fatality denotes the age at death as a result of the disease.

The expectation of life at age of onset is the years of life expected at that age had the disease not occurred. Similarly, expectation of life at fatality is the years of life expected at that age had the death not occurred.

Checking Data

Data used for generation of indicators need to be evaluated for validity, reliability, and consistency, using defined qualitative and quantitative criteria. Large population-based studies may be given preference over smaller sample-based work if both are available and the quality of their data is comparable. Better conclusions may be possible by cross-checking different sources of data. Community-based studies, which may be representative of the population but have limited diagnostic validity, may be compared with hospital-based work, in which diagnosis may be valid but would come from a biased population sample. The following subsections profile simple types of checks for data quality.

Comparison of Total Numbers. Cross-checks should be done to compare total numbers. It is essential to check that the number of deaths in a year in a region is the same as the sum of all deaths from all causes in the same region. Similarly, program-based data can be compared with data from other sources to ensure better estimates of causes of death. The comparison of totals allows one to work within a frame of mortality and avoids double counting of one death. However, it does not assist in the distribution of deaths within that frame.

Relationship Between Variables. Checks based on the epidemiologic relationship between parameters refer to the application of simple, yet vital, relationships such as the following:

- Prevalence (point) = incidence × average duration of disease
- Cause-specific mortality rate = incidence × case fatality rate

These checks allow estimates from different sources to be compared for internal consistency. Such relationships can also be used to derive one of the estimates in the equations when the others are known.

Sensitivity Analysis. Sensitivity analysis is a useful tool to determine whether data that are more precise are required for the purposes of a particular decision. A one-way sensitivity analysis (Petiti, 1994) evaluates the effect of manipulating one variable at a time on the dependent variable. If the outcome is sensitive to one or more variables, their precision is more important in the estimation.

Disease Groups: Classification

Murray and Chen (1992) introduced a disease group system based on the WHO ICD classification system. Group I includes conditions characteristic of low-income countries: communicable diseases, maternal and prenatal conditions, and nutritional deficiencies. These conditions decline at rates faster than overall mortality rates as socioeconomic conditions improve; thus group I contributes to a relatively small percentage of deaths in the high-income world. Group II, which consists of noncommunicable and chronic diseases, accounts for most loss of healthy life in the high-income countries and proportionately increases with the epidemiologic transition in low- and middle-income countries (see Exhibit 1-3). Group III consists of injuries, both intentional and unintentional (including violence).

The distribution of the disease burden among these three groups is one indicator of the type of disease burden and the level of epidemiologic transition in a country. It is important to distinguish between the proportions of deaths attributed to these groups, as opposed to the risk of dying from the conditions in these groups. For example, the proportion of deaths attributable to group II causes increases from high- to low-mortality countries (or to an older age structure of the population); however, the risk of death from group II conditions is higher in high-mortality countries.

Implementing a Burden of Disease Study

Knowing how to conduct a burden of disease analysis is important for all countries. Generic steps for a national burden of disease study include the following:

- Assess demographic information, including a census with age, sex, geographic (urban/rural), and selected socioeconomic status information, and vital statistics with births and deaths.
- Collect cause-of-death information for all deaths in a year by age, sex, geographic location, and socioeconomic status as possible, according to the WHO ICD system.
- Define disability by cause/disease, and develop a severity scale using expert and community input.
- Collate information by disease from all sources and assess reliability/validity, using expert

opinion when needed to define variables for a spreadsheet.

- Decide whether social value preferences such as age weighting, discounting, economic and social productivity, and expectation of life will be used and what their values will be.

- Estimate healthy life lost for each disease condition and by disease groups.

- Perform sensitivity analyses to check the robustness of results relative to critical variables and assumptions.

- Consider other variations, including assessment of losses by risk factors; regional, age, and sex breakdowns; and future projections.

- Review the policy implications on overall mortality and morbidity in the country and by cause; feed data into cost-effectiveness analysis and further research.

- Include other modifications as appropriate to the country setting.

To use summary measures to assist in health planning and resource allocation decisions, additional steps include the following:

- Estimate the effectiveness (gains of healthy life) of each intervention under consideration in terms of expected coverage and reductions in incidence and/or case fatality or case disability ratios.

- Work out the costs of the proposed interventions.

- Develop cost-effectiveness ratios to plan which combination of interventions targeted to which groups will provide a maximum return of healthy life per expenditure for the funds allocated to health.

- Review expected gains of healthy life according to age, sex, geographic area, and socioeconomic and vulnerable groups to ensure that all are better off (or at least none are worse off) and adjust as necessary.

Another very important consideration in this process is time. The conduct and analysis of such studies must be timely to assure its appropriate use by policy makers and useful for resource allocation decisions. The precision and comprehensive nature of the study must be balanced by the need for timely results.

The steps described previously may be carried out simultaneously or in some sequence, depending on the specific national situation. Modifications will likely be needed depending on the availability of data (Exhibit 1-6). An actual study requires careful planning on the part of those responsible for its conduct and may include many additional steps that are beyond the scope of this chapter. Even so, these generic steps summarize the essentials of applying the burden of disease methods to a country. Increasingly countries are obtaining, refining, and using these data on an ongoing fashion.

Comparisons and Trends in Disease Burden

This section reviews a number of country-based burden of disease studies so as to compare and assess trends in disease burden from place to place and over time.

Comparative Disease Burden Assessments

Comparing the burden of disease across populations, time, and place is an important aspect of national burden of disease studies. This subsection uses examples from burden of disease studies to illustrate how disaggregated data can help in understanding the distribution of ill health in a country.

The Andhra Pradesh Burden of Disease Study, 2001

The regional distribution (urban/rural, state, district) of the disease burden is important to explore in a national burden of disease study. Andhra Pradesh, a state in India, was the focus of one of the most meticulous burden of disease studies conducted between 1994 and 2001. It had a population of 76 million in 2001, 27% of whom lived in urban areas (20.8 million people); a 1:3 ratio of urban-to-rural disease burden in terms of DALYs lost was identified (Mahapatra, 2001). The burden of disease rates were 19% higher in rural areas than in urban areas, as measured by DALYs lost per 1,000 population (Figure 1-8).

The Burden of Disease and Injury in New Zealand, 1996

Age and ethnicity are key characteristics of a population that require a disaggregation of the burden of disease. The national burden of disease study of New Zealand (1996 population = 3.6 million) provides a clear example of how the DALYs lost in 1996 were predominant among the older age group (65 years and older), even though this group represented only

Exhibit 1-6	The Burden of Disease in Pakistan, 1990

Pakistan is a developing country in South Asia, whose population numbered 112 million in 1990. A study was undertaken to estimate the burden of disease in Pakistan in 1990 and to calculate the loss of healthy life from a spectrum of common conditions. Nearly 200 data sources were evaluated, including national surveys, population-based studies, sentinel survey systems, and disease-specific studies.

Overall, 456 discounted HeaLYs per 1,000 people were lost due to new cases of diseases in 1990. Diarrhea and pneumonia in children caused the greatest loss of healthy life. Sixty-three percent of healthy life was lost from mortality, while 37 percent was lost due to disability. Hypertension and injuries were the leading causes of healthy life lost from disability. Nearly half the healthy life was lost in the under-five age group, demonstrating the great burden on Pakistani infants and children.

Although communicable diseases dominated the burden of disease in Pakistan in 1990, noncommunicable diseases also took a heavy toll. Figure 1-7 and Table 1-6 review the top conditions responsible for loss of healthy life, and the proportion of loss from noncommunicable conditions can only be expected to increase. Injuries also need to be recognized as a major public health problem in the country. According to these estimates, Pakistan had a lower overall burden of disease than most countries in sub-Saharan Africa in 1990, but a burden higher than most countries in Latin America.

Table 1-6	Loss of Healthy Life in Pakistan: Top 10 Conditions for 1990		
	Premature Mortality Only Rank	**Disability Only**	**Healthy Life Years Lost**
Rank	**Disease**	**Disease**	**Disease**
1	Diarrhea	Hypertension	Diarrhea
2	Childhood pneumonia	Injuries	Childhood pneumonia
3	Tuberculosis	Eye diseases	Tuberculosis
4	Rheumatic heart disease	Malnutrition	Birth diseases
5	Chronic liver disease	Birth diseases	Injuries
6	Congenital malformations	Congenital malformations	Hypertension
7	Birth diseases	Dental diseases	Congenital malformations
8	Ischemic heart disease	Ischemic heart disease	Chronic liver disease
9	Child septicemia	Adult female anemia	Ischemic heart disease
10	Other respiratory diseases	Mental retardation	Rheumatic heart disease

Source: Hyder & Morrow, 2000.

Distribution of Disease Burden in Pakistan, 1990

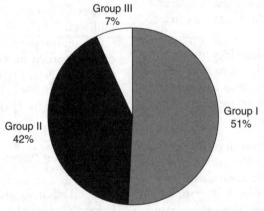

Figure 1-7 The Burden of Disease in Pakistan, 1990.
Source: (Hyder et al, 2000).

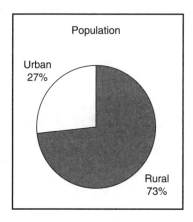

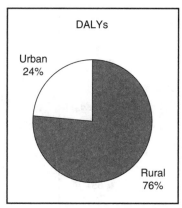

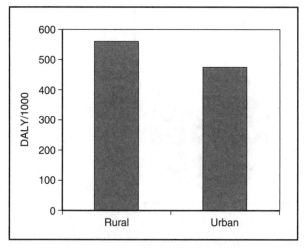

Figure 1-8 Burden of disease in Andhra Pradesh, 2001, by region.
Source: Based on Mahapatra, P. (2001). "Estimating National Burden of Disease: The Burden of Disease in Andhra Pradesh 1990s." Hyberdad: Institute of Health Systems.

Note: Total DALYs lost in Andhra Pradesh = 5 million.

12% of the population (New Zealand Ministry of Health, 2001). The identification of 15% of the burden of disease in the indigenous Maori population, who represent only 9.7% of the total New Zealand population, was an important equity finding (Figure 1-9).

Burden of Disease in Chile, 1993

A disaggregated burden analysis by gender can also be seen in the work done in Chile in 1993, where at that time 49.6% of the population was male. The study found that 56% of the DALYs lost were attributable to males (Figure 1-10). The distribution of the burden by major disease groups—I (communicable, infectious), II (chronic, non-communicable), and III (injuries, violence)—showed the dominance of chronic conditions in the burden (Concha, 1996).

Burden of Disease Estimates for South Africa, 2000

HIV/AIDS is ravaging Africa; thus the impact of HIV/AIDS on the burden of disease in African coun-

tries can be significant. In South Africa, 30% of the 15 million DALYs lost in 2000 were attributed to HIV/AIDS (Figure 1-11) (Burden of Disease Research Unit, 2003); for a population of 45 million, this means 0.33 DALY is lost per capita. Such data are important for national decision making.

The Burden of Disease and Injury in Australia, 1996

The distribution of disease burden by socioeconomic variables is important for poverty and equity analysis. The national burden of disease analysis in Australia for 1996 presented results based on socioeconomic status (defined by the social and economic characteristics of the living area), disaggregated by gender, for both mortality (YLL) and disability (YDL) (Figure 1-12) (Mathers et al., 1999). These results show the high disability losses for women and for the poor. Such explorations of intranational distributions of disease burden are useful in studying the disproportionate effects of ill health on the poor and women.

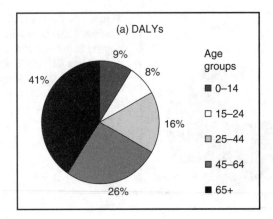

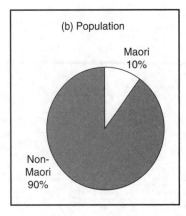

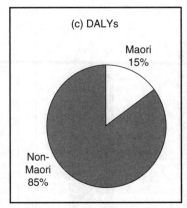

Note: Total DALYs lost in New Zealand for 1996 = 500,000.

Figure 1-9 Burden of disease in New Zealand, 1996, by age (a) and ethnicity (b).
Source: Based on data from New Zealand Ministry of Health. (2001). "Burden of Disease and Injury in New Zealand."

Burden of Disease and National Income

WHO has categorized its member states by income levels into high-, middle-, and low-income nations. The population of the world in 2004 totaled slightly more than 6.4 billion people, with 85% residing in low- and middle-income nations (Figure 1-13). As may be expected, more than 90% of the global burden is found in low- and middle-income nations, reflecting the double challenge faced by the majority of people in the world: They are poor and they are unhealthy. This relationship between ill health and poverty has long been recognized as complex and has been the object of much research and inquiry.

Burden of Disease by Disease Groups

Another way to disaggregate data is to explore the disease burden based on three disease groups: group I (communicable, infectious, maternal, and perinatal), group II (noncommunicable, chronic), and group III (injuries and violence). There is great variation in the portions allocated to these groups; for example, group I conditions may be responsible for anywhere from 12% to 70% of the burden of disease. When the countries are stratified by GNP per capita as a measure of development, an important trend can be seen from historical data (Table 1-7): As income rises, the proportion of the burden attributable to group I conditions decreases, while the share attributable to group II conditions increases. This effect is progressive, although countries such Turkmenistan (a middle-income country) still retain a high group I burden. This finding is consistent with the theory of epidemiological transition, which predicts a change in a country's disease profile with economic development.

Global Assessments of Disease Burden

Information regarding health and disease for all countries of the world can be collated to provide a picture of global health status. In addition, global health assessments may be completed as a separate

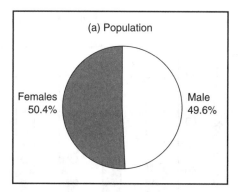

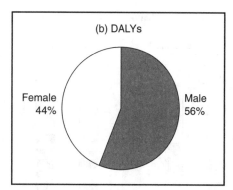

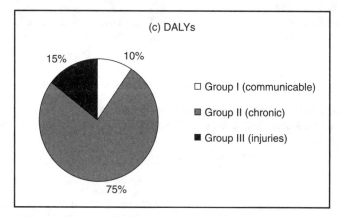

Note: Total DALYs lost in Chile for 1993 = 2 million.

Figure 1-10 Burden of disease in Chile, 1993, by gender (a) (b) and disease groups (c).
Source: Based on data from Concha, M. (1993). "Burden of Disease in Chile."

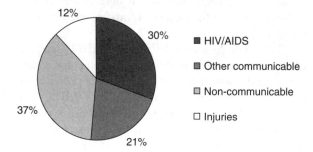

Note: Total DALYs lost in South Africa for 2000 = 15 million.

Figure 1-11 Burden of disease in South Africa, 2000, by disease groups.
Source: Based on data from Burden of Disease Research Unit. (2003). "Initial Burden of Disease Estimates for South Africa, 2000." South Africa: South African Medical Research Council.

activity, and such data can then be disaggregated into regional information. Global assessments serve to highlight major challenges facing the world community, and trends in such assessments indicate progress, if any, in improving the health of people worldwide. Such information is critical to the work of organizations such as WHO and UNICEF in their efforts to combat ill health and disease worldwide. This section highlights results of global exercises for assessment of the disease burden, recent evaluations, and projections for the future.

The Global Burden of Disease

The Global Burden of Disease (GBD) 2000 study constructed estimates of mortality, disability, and DALYs by cause for regions of the world. Demographic estimates of deaths in 2000 by age and sex form the basis of this work. Subsequently, WHO undertook an update of the GBD study to produce reliable estimates of mortality and morbidity for all regions of the world for 2004. The results were based on a variety of sources, including vital registrations systems, special studies, surveys, and expert opinion. This section reviews the 2004 GDB data.

Mortality. Globally, in 2004, an estimated 58.8 million deaths occurred, 53% of whom were males. Ischemic heart disease, cerebrovascular disease, and lower respiratory infections were the top three causes

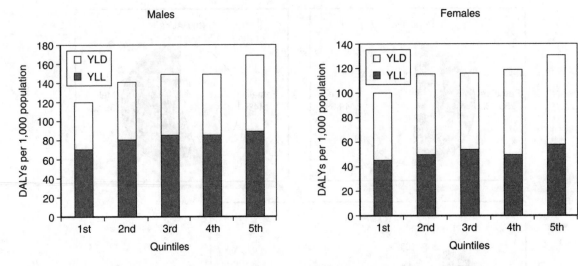

Note: The first quintile corresponds to the highest socioeconomic group, and the fifth quintile to the lowest. Each quintile contains approximately 20% of the total Australian population. Total DALYs lost in Australia for 1996 = 2.5 million.

Figure 1-12 Burden of disease in Australia, 1996, by socioeconomic status and gender.
Source: Based on data from Mathers, C., Vos, T. & Stevenson, C. (1999). "The Burden of Disease and Injury in Australia." Australian Institute of Health and Welfare.

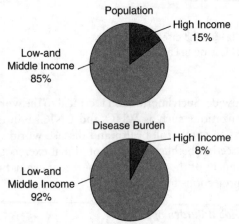

Figure 1-13 Global Burden of Disease, 2004, by Income Level of Countries.
Source: Based on data from World Health Organization. (2004).

of death, while 10 causes accounted for 50% of deaths worldwide. One death in 10 was from injuries, with road traffic accidents included in the top 10 causes of deaths. Approximately 10.4 million deaths occur in children younger than 5 years of age globally, with more than 50% of these fatalities being caused by just four communicable diseases. Of those under-five deaths, 75% occurred in the African and Southeast Asia regions. While the effect is less pronounced in the adult population, the proportion of deaths in the 15-

to 59-year age range remains skewed toward low- and middle-income countries. Mortality in the African region is 40% higher than the next-highest-mortality region and is four times higher than in high-income countries. Thus an inordinate share of the mortality burden at the beginning of this decade was found in low- and middle-income countries, even among adults.

Table 1-8 shows the differences in the 10 leading causes of deaths for 2004 for the high-income countries and the low-income countries. The presence of perinatal conditions, tuberculosis, HIV/AIDS, and malaria in the low-income world is indicative of the high impact of these conditions on premature mortality. These conditions are absent from the top 10 causes in the high-income countries, reflecting the success in combating these infectious conditions in the modern era. It is important to note that noncommunicable diseases such as ischemic heart disease were already prominent causes of premature deaths in the low- and middle-income world in 2000 and remain among the top five causes of death in 2004.

Disability. The GBD study 2004 update also provides an evaluation of the contribution of conditions to disability in the world. Leading causes of disability in 2004 worldwide are shown in Table 1-9. Neuropsychiatric and behavioral conditions dominate the causes of disability, accounting for four of the top 10 conditions. However, a diverse spectrum of

Table 1-7	Historical Distribution of Disease Burden Within Countries		
Disease Burden in Disease Categories (of 100%)			
Country	Group I	Group II	Group III
Low-Income Nations (GNP per capita: $635 or less)*			
Andhra Pradesh	54	30	16
Guinea	70	23	7
Lower Medium-Income Nations (GNP per capita: $636–$2,555)			
Colombia	22	39	39
Jamaica	16	60	24
Turkmenistan	51	45	4
Uzbekistan	46	40	14
Upper Medium-Income Nations ($2,556–$7,911)			
Mauritius	16	74	10
Mexico	32	48	20
Uruguay	12	73	15

Note: Disease classification system: Group I: communicable, infectious, maternal, and perinatal; Group II: noncommunicable and chronic; Group III: injuries and accidents.

Source: World Bank, 1993.

*GNP per capita from World Bank (1993).

often ignored, effects of these conditions are obvious once disability is counted in these estimates of disease burden.

Disease Burden. Based on the estimation of deaths and disability presented in the preceding subsection, the global disease burden for 2004 was estimated using DALYs. Leading causes of the global burden in 2004 (Table 1-10) indicate how those conditions affect the low-middle income world. The top 10 list is a mixture of the unfinished agenda of communicable and perinatal conditions, noncommunicable diseases, and road traffic injuries. This situation highlights the challenge facing the global health community as it simultaneously continues to fight infectious diseases, seeks to improve the response to chronic conditions, and prepares to meet the increasing impact of injuries.

Age and Disease Distributions. Figure 1-14 illustrates the distribution of the global burden in 2004 by disease groups and demonstrates the growing relative impact of chronic diseases (group II) over infectious conditions (group I). Figure 1-15 provides comparable figures for loss of healthy life in sub-Saharan Africa, the Middle Eastern Crescent, Latin America, and the Caribbean. Note that communicable diseases still represent a considerable portion of the disease burden in 2004, especially in sub-Saharan Africa due to HIV/AIDS.

As the figures demonstrate, various subregions within middle- and low-income countries are at different stages of epidemiological transition. The influx of chronic diseases has added another layer of problems in some areas, while the burden of communicable

conditions, such as hearing loss, cataracts, and osteoarthritis, also appear on the list. A unique contribution of the GBD work has been its placement of nonfatal health outcomes in the center of international health policy in recent years. The important, and yet

Table 1-8	Leading Causes of Deaths in High-Income and Low-Income Countries, 2004			
High-Income Countries		**Low-Income Countries**		
Rank	Cause	Rank	Cause	
1	Ischemic heart disease	1	Lower respiratory infections	
2	Cerebrovascular disease	2	Ischemic heart disease	
3	Trachea, bronchus, and lung cancers	3	Diarrheal diseases	
4	Lower respiratory infections	4	HIV/AIDS	
5	Chronic obstructive pulmonary disease	5	Cerebrovascular disease	
6	Alzheimer's and other dementias	6	Chronic obstructive pulmonary disease	
7	Colon and rectum cancers	7	Tuberculosis	
8	Diabetes mellitus	8	Neonatal conditions	
9	Breast cancer	9	Malaria	
10	Stomach cancer	10	Prematurity and low birth weight	

Source: Based on data from WHO, 2008.

Table 1-9	Leading Causes of Disability Losses Globally, 2004
Rank	**Cause**
1	Unipolar major depression
2	Refractive errors
3	Hearing loss, adult onset
4	Other unintentional injuries
5	Alcohol use disorders
6	Cataracts
7	Schizophrenia
8	Osteoarthritis
9	Bipolar disorder
10	Iron-deficiency anemia

Note: Disability losses are defined by years of life lived with disability (YLDs).
Source: Based on data from WHO, 2008.

Table 1-10	Leading Causes of Global Burden of Disease, 2004
Rank	**Cause**
1	Lower respiratory infections
2	Diarrheal diseases
3	Unipolar depressive disorders
4	Ischemic heart disease
5	HIV/AIDS
6	Cerebrovascular disease
7	Prematurity and low birth weight
8	Birth asphyxia and birth trauma
9	Road traffic accidents
10	Neonatal infections and other

Source: Based on data from WHO, 2008.

diseases has not yet been eradicated. This "double burden" poses a major challenge for the health systems in these nations. In addition, the scarcity of resources in many of these countries makes the situation even more critical, and it becomes imperative to define interventions that are cost-effective and able to reduce the burden of disease.

Other Ways Burden Can Be Measured

Mortality and morbidity alone have been used for decades for international comparisons of disease burden. Mortality among children younger than five years is considered a sensitive indicator of overall health of nations, but especially for the health of women and children. UNICEF publishes an annual *State of the World's Children* report that includes a ranking of nations based on this indicator (Table 1-11).

Gross national income (GNI) per capita is an indicator of national wealth, and the relationship between these variables usually follows an expected sequence, such that the country with the lowest GNI per capita has the worst indicators of health. However, as Table 1-11 indicates, even countries that have relatively higher per capita income can have poor indicators of health service accessibility (e.g., coverage of tetanus toxoid vaccination for pregnant women) and health impact (e.g., prevalence of anemia in pregnant women). For example, the per capita GNI for Bhutan is higher than that for Mongolia, yet Bhutan ranks lower than Mongolia in child mortality and life expectancy. Such examples demonstrate that

the relationship between health and poverty is complex and needs in-depth investigation. When seeking to improve the health of nations, both absolute poverty and the disparities within societies serve as impediments to empowerment of the poor and needy, especially women and children.

Projections

Forecasts of disease burden have been attempted with the intent of providing some basis for health planning. Making such projections is a challenging task that requires further data manipulations and the use of assumptions. These assumptions must predict changes

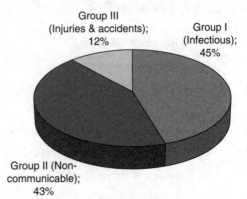

Figure 1-14 Global Burden of Disease 2004 by Disease Groups.
Source: Based on data from WHO. The global burden of disease: 2004 update. Geneva: World Health Organization, 2008.

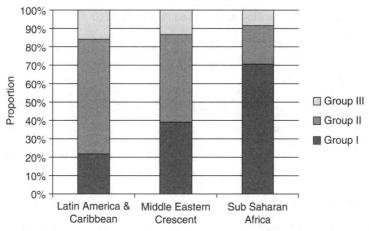

Figure 1-15 Proportion of Disease Burden by Disease Groups in Selected Regions, 2004. *Source*: Based on data from WHO. The global burden of disease: 2004 update. Geneva: World Health Organization, 2008.

in disease prevalence and incidence over time, the effects of interventions, and other factors. As a result, all projections are estimates with substantial variations that are highly dependent on the data used to derive them.

The GBD study updated for 2004 projects the global burden to the year 2030. These estimates are based on projected changes in life expectancy, age structure of the global community, disease profiles based on current states, and other relevant parameters (WHO, 2008). In addition, the projections are guided by forecasts for income per capita, human capital, and smoking intensity. The results of this exercise reveal the leading causes of projected global burden of disease for 2030, as summarized in Table 1-12.

The domination of chronic diseases on this list is obvious, although respiratory conditions still appear to be important. Injuries from road traffic crashes are predicted to become the third leading cause of the global disease burden in the future. In addition, the lower ranking of HIV on the list reflects the assumption that interventions for this condition will succeed in reducing the burden in the intervening decades. This may or may not hold true, and other assumptions may be used to create a different scenario for the future.

The growing importance of noncommunicable diseases is a global phenomenon, and these conditions' impact on low- and middle-income countries and regions needs to be assessed. However, unlike

Table 1-11	Health Status Indicators and National Income for Selected Low- and Middle-Income Countries				
Country	Ranking by Child Mortality (<5 years)	Life Expectation (years)	Stunted Children <5 years (%)	Coverage of Tetanus Vaccination Among Pregnant Women (%)	GNI per Capita (U.S. dollars)
Niger	2	46	40	36	170
Sierra Leone	1	34	34	60	140
Angola	3	40	45	62	660
Afghanistan	4	43	52	34	250
Mongolia	64	64	25	—	440
Pakistan	44	61	37	56	410
Bhutan	50	63	40	70	590
Nicaragua	82	69	20	95	370
Peru	86	70	25	57	2,050
Guatemala	74	67	46	38	1,750

Source: UNICEF, 2004.

Table 1-12	Leading Causes of Disease Burden, 2004 and Projected, 2030		
2004		**2030**	
Rank	**Cause**	**Rank**	**Cause**
1	Lower respiratory infections	1	Unipolar depressive disorders
2	Diarrheal diseases	2	Ischemic heart disease
3	Unipolar depressive disorders	3	Road traffic accidents
4	Ischemic heart disease	4	Cerebrovascular disease
5	HIV/AIDS	5	Chronic obstructive pulmonary disease
6	Cerebrovascular disease	6	Lower respiratory infections
7	Prematurity and low birth weight	7	Hearing loss, adult onset
8	Birth asphyxia and birth trauma	8	Refractive errors
9	Road traffic accidents	9	HIV/AIDS
10	Neonatal infections and other	10	Diabetes mellitus

Source: Based on data from WHO, 2008.

the projected disease burden for the world, there is a persistent burden of respiratory infections and diarrheal diseases in these regions. The situation in the low- and middle-income world is one where the "triple burden" of persistent communicable diseases, prevalent non-communicable conditions, and increasing injuries will call for an appropriate response from public health officials.

Burden of Disease Attributed to Risk Factors

An analysis of risk factors that underlie many important disease conditions can be useful for assisting policy decisions concerning interventions directed toward health promotion and disease reduction. Smoking, alcohol, hypertension, and malnutrition are risk factors for a variety of diseases, for example, and specific interventions have been developed that may reduce their prevalence. Risk factors include an array of human behaviors, nutritional deficiencies and excesses, substance abuse, and certain characteristics such as hypertension. Some factors are both an outcome and a risk factor (hypertension), some are challenging to measure (violence), and yet others (smoking and alcohol) lead to many disease outcomes. The linkage between an identified risk factor and the set of associated disease outcomes may be difficult to

directly quantify, and the portion of specific disease prevalence attributable to any one factor may be problematic.

Relationships such as those shown in Figure 1-16 require careful assessment to determine the proportion of heart disease to be attributed to hypertension in relation to other interacting causal factors. The best way to determine the portion of disease that may be ascribed to hypertension is through randomized trials with careful assessment of disease outcomes over time: Results from studies that control hypertension have shown a reduction of death and disability from not only cardiac disease, but also from cerebrovascular and renal diseases.

Because the most important purpose of risk factor analysis is to assist in decision making about the allocation of resources, the link between the risk factor and the potential intervention to reduce the risk should be clear. The effectiveness of interventions against risk factors ultimately should be judged by their ability to reduce the amount of healthy life lost attributed to the diseases that the risk factor affects. For the evaluation of an intervention that reduces

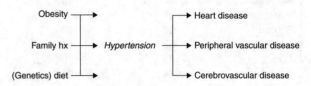

Figure 1-16 Flowchart.

hypertension, for example, the healthy life losses from the entire range of diseases that hypertension influences are therefore required.

Although understanding the underlying factors that lead to disease and the complex interrelations in the web of causation has long been a major focus of epidemiology (http://www.springerlink.com/content/n3mcyxyce7vqn66b/), most analyses of the relationships of risk factors to specific diseases have been done in the context of individual risk factors in limited settings and with wide variations in the criteria for risk assessment. As a consequence, comparisons of risk factors as determinants of disease on a population health level are problematic. The Comparative Risk Assessment (CRA) project of the GBD 2000 study carried out a systematic evaluation of 22 selected risk factors relative to global and regional burdens of disease using a specific model for analysis (Murray et al., 2001); it was updated in 2009 (WHO Global Health Risks) with data for 2004 (Mathers, 2009).

The Burden of Selected Major Risk Factors

The model used in CRA for causal attribution of health outcomes was based on counterfactual analysis that would result in the lowest population risk (Ezzati et al., 2002). Within this analysis, the contribution of one or a group of risk factors to disease or mortality was estimated by comparing the current or future disease burden with the levels that would be expected under an alternative hypothetical scenario. This involved an evaluation of the effect a risk factor has on the disease and its consequences, by setting the risk factor to its minimum while keeping all other factors constant. This method has the advantage of showing the potential gains by risk reduction from all levels of suboptimal exposure in a consistent way across risk factors (Ezzati et al., 2002).

The WHO Global Health Risks (2009) described 24 risk factors that are responsible for 44% of global deaths and 34% of DALYs. As shown in Figure 1-17(a), the five leading risks for mortality globally are high blood pressure (responsible for 13% of deaths globally), tobacco use (9%), high blood glucose (6%), physical inactivity (6%), and overweight and obesity (5%). These five factors especially increase risks for heart disease and cancer and have major consequences for countries across all income groups. In contrast, as Figure 1-17(b) shows, the main risks for burden of disease (DALYs) globally are underweight (6% of global DALYs), unsafe sex (5%), alcohol use (5%), and unsafe water, sanitation, and hygiene (4%); underweight, unsafe sex, and unsafe water, sanitation, and hygiene

all contribute to infectious disease and overwhelmingly affect low-income countries. Alcohol abuse is largely a problem for men, but those mainly affected vary greatly by geographic region: This factor has its greatest impact on men in Africa, in middle-income countries in Latin America, and in a few high-income countries (e.g., Russia).

Eight risk factors—alcohol use, tobacco use, high blood pressure, high body mass index, high cholesterol, high blood glucose, low fruit and vegetable intake, and physical inactivity—account for more than 75% of ischemic heart disease (the leading cause of death worldwide) and 61% of total cardiovascular deaths. Although these major risk factors are associated with high-income countries, in fact more than 84% of the total global burden of disease that they cause occurs in low- and middle-income countries. Reducing exposure to these eight risk factors would increase global life expectancy by almost five years.

Globally, micronutrient deficiencies (including deficiencies of vitamin A, iron, and zinc), suboptimal breastfeeding, and preventable environmental risks account for more than four million deaths (nearly 40% of the 10.4 million under-five children who died in 1994); these deaths are readily preventable. In 1994, 82% of these deaths occurred in Africa and Southeast Asia.

Depression is the leading cause of years lost due to disability; rates of this disease are 50% higher in women than in men. Conversely, men aged 15 to 60 have a much higher risk of dying than do women of the same ages. The main causes of death that result in this differential are injury, particularly from violence and armed conflict, and heart disease.

Some risk factors may have few effects on the total global burden of disease, yet be very important locally within certain populations and regions. For example, iodine deficiency affects certain low- and middle-income countries and results in substantial disability in those populations.

The reasons for the demographic and epidemiologic transitions discussed earlier in this chapter and in Chapter 3 are largely related to shifts in these major risk factors as a result of changing social, economic and political trends and their complex interactions. Low-income countries continue to struggle against the high burdens of infectious diseases, malnutrition (including undernutrition and micronutrient deficiencies), and maternal and child health problems; at the same time, they must deal with the additional burdens of high levels of noncommunicable disease and injuries. The 2009 WHO Global Health Risks report estimates that had the risks analyzed in the report not existed, global life expectancy

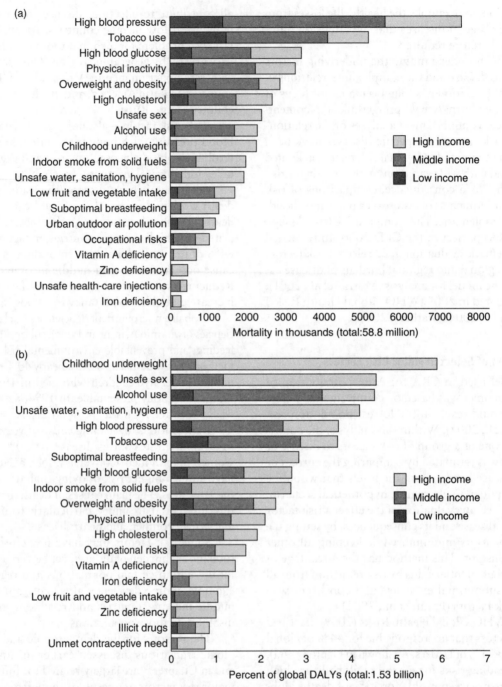

Figure 1-17 Mortality (a) and DALYs (b) due to 19 leading risk factors by country income level, 2004. *Source*: WHO Global Health Risks, 2009, Figures 6 and 7.

would be 10 years longer. This finding largely confirms the hopes first expressed in the 2000 Report to WHO by the Commission on Health and Macroeconomics (Commission on Macroeconomics and Health, 2001) and detailed with the MDGs (United Nations Millennium Declaration, 2000)—namely, that major improvements in the health status

of those in low- and middle-income countries can be achieved:

For example, reducing the burden of disease is possible since many cost-effective interventions are known, and prevention strategies can be transferred between similar countries.

Conclusion

The health of populations is the fundamental concern of global public health. The first step in the pursuit of population health improvement is the measurement of health and disease. Measurement is required to establish the magnitude of disease problems, define causal factors, explore potential solutions, and determine the impact of interventions. Measuring the impact of diseases on populations in terms of mortality and morbidity and their consequences is essential for planning effective ways to reduce the burden of illness and for setting priorities.

The burden of disease in populations has been gauged in many ways. Examples include measures of mortality, such as infant mortality rates; demographic measures, such as expectation of life at birth; and measures of morbidity, such as days away from work. However, for purposes of comparison among populations and for assisting in health planning and resource allocation, a common denominator combining these factors is needed. Summary measures of population health based on the amount of healthy life lost from disability and from death have been developed to serve that purpose.

Composite indicators (such as HeaLYs and DALYs) use duration of time (years, weeks, days) to measure the loss of healthy life from disease and the gain from interventions. These metrics are evolving into important tools for assisting health-related decision making. Nevertheless, to avoid misuse of such indicators, it is critical for those using them to understand the underlying assumptions and limitations and to meet the rather formidable data requirements. These summary measures also could be used to examine the burden of disease among subpopulations defined by socio-cultural-economic attributes and especially on vulnerable groups. Thus they could be used for ensuring that health-related decisions consider equity as well as cost-effective criteria.

Trends in disease burden provide important clues about the success of ongoing health programs and the need for development of new interventions. At the same time, they reflect non-health-related factors that are important to the production or maintenance of health in populations. Intercountry and inter-regional comparisons allow for measuring progress among nations; they can highlight inequalities in health status and examine these disparities in relation to social, economic, educational, and other factors.

Health systems across the world are greatly affected by ongoing changes in disease profiles and population dynamics. These systems must develop the capacity to respond to such changes effectively within the resources of each nation. Decisions must be based on evidence about the patterns of diseases, their risk factors, and the effectiveness of alternative interventions. Timely collection and analysis of appropriate, high-quality data to support such evidence are a prerequisite for improving equitable global health development.

● ● ● Discussion Questions

1. How can data help achieve the main purpose of a health system in any country? Give examples.

2. What are the essential elements of a burden of disease assessment, and which types of data are the most challenging to obtain in a low-income country?

3. What are the relative strengths and weaknesses of summary measures such as HeaLYs and DALYs compared to more traditional indicators of disease burden such as infant or maternal mortality?

4. In your country or city, what would be the most appropriate set of indicators to assess the impact of chronic diseases on the population? Why?

● ● ● **References**

Anand, S., & Ranaan-Eliya. (1996). *Disability adjusted life years: A critical review.* Working Paper No. 95-06. Harvard Center for Population and Development Studies.

Anker, M., Black, R. E., Coldham, C., Kalter, C. D., Quigley, M. A., Ross, D., et al. (1999). *A standard verbal autopsy method for investigating causes of death in infants and children.* WHO/CDS/CSR/ISR/99.4.

Barendregt, J. J., Bonneux, L., & Van Der Maas, P. J. (1996). DALYs: The age weights on balance. *Bulletin of the World Health Organization, 74,* 439–443.

Barker, C., & Green, A. (1996). Opening the debate on DALYs. *Health Policy and Planning, 11*(2), 179–183.

Barnum, H. (1987). Evaluating healthy days of life gained from health projects. *Social Science and Medicine, 24,* 833–841.

Blumstein, J. (1997). The Oregon experiment: The role of cost–benefit analysis in the allocation of Medicaid funds. *Social Science and Medicine, 45,* 545–554.

Bobadilla, J. L. (1998). *Searching for essential health services in low and middle income countries.* Washington, DC: Inter American Development Bank.

Burden of Disease Research Unit. (2003). *Initial burden of disease estimates for South Africa, 2000.* South Africa: South African Medical Research Council. Retrieved from http://www.mrc.ac.za/bod/bod.htm

Busschbach, J. J. V., Hesing, D. J., & de Charro, F. T. (1993). The utility of health at different stages of life: A qualitative approach. *Social Science and Medicine, 37*(2), 153–158.

Coale, A. J., & Demeney, P. (1983). *Regional model life tables and stable populations.* New York: Academic Press.

Coale, A. J., & Guo, G. (1989). Revised regional model life tables at very low levels of mortality. *Population Index, 55,* 613–643.

Commission on Macroeconomics and Health. (2001). *Macroeconomics and health: Investing in health for economic development.* Geneva, Switzerland: World Health Organization.

Concha M, Aguilera X (1996). *Burden of disease in Chile.* Santiago (Chile): Government of Chile Ministry of Health (MINSAL); 1996.

Crooper, M., & Kopits, E. (2003). *Traffic fatalities and economic growth.* World Bank Policy Research Working Paper 3035. Washington, DC: World Bank.

Eddy, D. (1991). Oregon's methods: Did cost-effectiveness analysis fail? *Journal of the American Medical Association, 266,* 2135–2141.

Evans, J.R., Hall, K.L., & Warford, J. (1981). Health care in the developing world: Problems of scarcity and choice. *New England Journal of Medicine, 305, 1117–1127.*

Ezzati, M., Lopez, A., Vander Hoorn, S., Rodgers, A., Murray, C. J. L., & Comparative Risk Assessment Collaborative Group. (2002). Selected major risk factors and global and regional burden of disease. *Lancet, 360*(9343), 1347–1360.

Ghana Health Assessment Team. (1981). A quantitative method for assessing the health impact of different diseases in less developed countries. *International Journal of Epidemiology, 10,* 73–80.

Gold, M. R., Siegel, J. E., Russel, L. B., & Weinstein, M. C. (Eds.). (1996). *Cost- effectiveness in health and medicine.* New York: Oxford University Press.

Hill, K. (2001). Demographic techniques: Indirect estimation. In *International Encyclopedia of Social and Behavioral Sciences* (p. 3461). Oxford, UK: Elsevier Science.

Hill, K. (2003). Adult mortality in the developing world: What we know and how we know it. *Training Workshop on HIV/AIDS and Adult Mortality in Developing Countries.* New York: United Nations Secretariat.

Hyder, A., & Morrow, R. (1999). Steady state assumptions in DALYs: Effect on estimates of HIV impact. *Journal of Epidemiology and Community Health, 53,* 43–45.

Hyder, A. A., & Morrow, R. H. (2000). Applying burden of disease methods in developing countries: A case study from Pakistan. *American Journal of Public Health, 90*(8), 1235–1247.

Hyder, A. A., Rotllant, G., & Morrow, R. H. (1998). Measuring the burden of disease: Healthy life years. *American Journal of Public Health, 88,* 196–202.

Jamison, D.T., Brenan, J.G., Measham, A.R., Alleyne, G., Claeson, M., Evans. D.B., et al. (2006). Disease Control Priorities in Developing Countries. New York: Oxford University Press.

Kaplan, R.M. (1990). The general health policy model: An integrated approach. In B. Spilker (Ed.), *Quality of life assessment in clinical trials* (p. 156). New York: Raven Press.

Last, J. M. (Ed.). (2000). *A dictionary of epidemiology* (4th ed.). New York: Oxford University Press.

Lopez, A., Ahmad, O., Guillot, M., Inoue, M., Fergusson, B., Salomon, J., Murray, C. J. L., & Hill, K. (2002). *World mortality in 2000: Life tables for 191 countries.* Geneva, Switzerland: World Health Organization.

Lopez, A, Mathers, C, Ezzati, M, Jamison, D., & Murray, C. (Eds.). (2006). *Global Burden of Disease and Risk Factors.* The World Bank and Oxford University Press, New York.

Mahapatra, P. (2001). *Estimating national burden of disease: The burden of disease in Andhra Pradesh 1990s.* Hyderabad: Institute of Health Systems. Retrieved from http://www.ihsnet.org.in/BurdenOfDisease/APBurdenofDiseaseStudy.htm.

Mathers, C., Stevens, G., & Mascarenhas, M. (2009). *Global health risks: Mortality and burden of disease attributable to selected major risks.* Geneva, Switzerland: World Health Organization. Retrieved from http://www.who.int/healthinfo/global_burden_disease/global_health_risks/en/index.html.

Mathers, C., Vos., T., Lopez, A., Salomon, J., Lozano, R., & Ezzati, M. (Eds.). (2001). National burden of disease studies: A practical guide (Edition 2.0). Geneva, Switzerland: World Health Organization.

Mathers, C., Vos, T., & Stevenson, C. (1999). *The burden of disease and injury in Australia.* Australian Institute of Health and Welfare. Retrieved from http://www.aihw.gov.au/

Morrow, R. H., & Bryant, J. H. (1995). Health policy approaches to measuring and valuing human life: Conceptual and ethical issues. *American Journal of Public Health, 85,* 1356–1360.

Murray, C. J. L., & Chen, L. C. (1992). Understanding morbidity change. *Population and Development Review, 18*(3), 481–503.

Murray, C. J. L., & Lopez, A. D. (1994). *Global comparative assessments in the health sector.* Geneva, Switzerland: World Health Organization.

Murray, C. J. L., & Lopez, A. D. (Eds.). (1996). *Global health statistics 1990.* Geneva, Switzerland: World Health Organization.

Murray, C. J. L., & Lopez, A. D. (1999). On the comparable quantification of health risks: Lessons from the Global Burden of Disease study. *Epidemiology, 10,* 594–605.

Murray, C. J. L., Lopez, A. D., Mathers, C. D., et al. (2001). *The Global Burden of Disease 2000 project: Aims, methods and data sources.* Geneva, Switzerland: Wohrld Health Organization.

Murray, C. J. L., Salomon, J., Mathers, C., & Lopez, A. (2002). *Summary measures of population health: Concepts, ethics, measurement and applications.* Geneva, Switzerland: World Health Organization.

New Zealand Ministry of Health. (2001). Burden of disease and injury in New Zealand. Retrieved from http://www.moh.govt.nz/moh.nsf/

Nord, E. (1992). Methods for quality adjustment of life years. *Social Science and Medicine, 34,* 559–569.

Nord, E. (1993). Unjustified use of the quality of well being scale in priority setting in Oregon. *Health Policy, 24,* 45–53.

Omran, A. (1971). The epidemiologic transition: A theory of the epidemiology of population change. *Milbank Memorial Fund Quarterly, 49*, 509–538.

Petiti, D. B. (1994). *Meta-analysis, decision analysis and cost-effectiveness analysis: Methods for quantitative synthesis in medicine.* New York: Oxford University Press.

Robine, J. M. (1994). *Disability free life expectancy trends in France: 1981–1991: International comparisons.* Chapter 2 In C. Mathers et al. (Eds.), *Advances in health expectancies.* Canberra, Australia: Australian Institute of Health and Welfare.

Thatte, N., Kalter, H. D., Baqui, A. H., Williams, E. M., & Darmstadt, G. L. (2009). Ascertaining causes of neonatal deaths using verbal autopsy: Current methods and challenges. *Journal of Perinatology: Official Journal of the California Perinatal Association, 29*(3), 187–194.

Torrence, G. W. (1986). Measurement of health state utilities for economic appraisal: A review. *Journal of Health Economics, 5*, 1–30.

UNAIDS. (2008). *Report on the global AIDS epidemic 2008.* Geneva, Switzerland: Joint United Nations Programme on HIV/AIDS.

UNAIDS. (2009). *AIDS epidemic update December 2009.* Geneva, Switzerland: Joint United Nations Programme on HIV/AIDS.

United Nations Children's Fund. (2009). *The state of the world's children 2008.* New York: UNICEF.

United Nations Millennium Declaration. (2000, September 18). Resolution adopted by the General Assembly. 55/2.

Weinstein, M. C., Siegel, J. E., Gold, M. R., Kamlet, M. S., & Russell, L. B. (1996). Recommendations of the Panel on Cost-effectiveness in Health and Medicine. *Journal of the American Medical Association, 276*, 1253–1258.

World Bank. (1993). *World development report 1993: Investing in health.* New York: Oxford University Press.

World Health Organization (WHO). (1980). *International classification of impairments, disabilities and handicaps: A manual of classification relating to the consequences of disease.* Geneva, Switzerland: Author.

World Health Organization (WHO). (1992). *International statistical classification of diseases and related health problem (ICD-10): Tenth revision.* Geneva, Switzerland: Author.

World Health Organization (WHO). (2000). *The world health report 2000.* Geneva, Switzerland: Author.

World Health Organization (WHO). (2002a). *World report on violence and health.* Geneva, Switzerland: Author.

World Health Organization (WHO). (2002b). The international classification of functioning, disability and health: Introduction. Retrieved from http://www.who.int/classifications/icf/en/

World Health Organization (WHO). (2003). *The world health report 2003 – Shaping the Future.* Geneva, Switzerland: Author.

World Health Organization (WHO). (2004). *The world health report 2004 – Changing History.* Geneva, Switzerland: Author.

World Health Organization (WHO). (2008). *The global burden of disease: 2004 update.* Geneva, Switzerland: Author.

World Health Organization (WHO). (2009). *Global health risks: Mortality and burden of disease attributable to selected major risks.* Geneva, Switzerland: Author.

Zeckhauser, R., & Shephard, D. (1976). Where now for saving lives? *Law and Contemporary Problems, 40*(b), 5–45.

2

Culture, Behavior, and Health

SUSAN C. SCRIMSHAW

"If you wish to help a community improve its health, you must learn to think like the people of that community. Before asking a group of people to assume new health habits, it is wise to ascertain the existing habits, how these habits are linked to one another, what functions they perform, and what they mean to those who practice them" (Paul, 1955, p. 1).

People around the world have beliefs and behaviors related to health and illness that stem from cultural forces as well as individual experiences and perceptions. A 16-country study of community perceptions of health, illness, and primary health care found that in all 42 communities studied, people used both the Western biomedical system and indigenous practices, including indigenous practitioners. Also, there were discrepancies between which services the governmental agencies said existed in the community and what was really available. Due to positive experiences with alternative healing systems and shortcomings in the Western biomedical system, people relied on both (Nichter, 2008; Scrimshaw, 1992). Experience has shown that when health programs fail to recognize and work with indigenous beliefs and practices, they also fail to reach their goals. Similarly, research to plan and evaluate health programs must take cultural beliefs and behaviors into account if researchers expect to understand why programs are not working, and what to do about it.

This chapter draws on the social sciences—particularly, anthropology, psychology, and sociology—to examine the cultural and behavioral parameters that are essential to understanding international health efforts. In a sense, it is complementary to Chapter 3, which covers social, political, and economic forces that affect health, but does not go deeply into the cultural components of health. This chapter begins with some key concepts from the field of anthropology and the subfield of medical anthropology. It continues with brief descriptions of the various types of health belief systems and healers around the world. Next, some key theories of health behavior and behavioral and cultural change are described and discussed. Issues of health literacy and health communication are then addressed, along with the myriad health promotion strategies available. Methodological issues are presented, followed by a case study of acquired immune deficiency syndrome (AIDS) in Africa, and another case study of the use of rapid assessment methods to guide the introduction of an improved nutritional cereal for infants and children in Ghana. The chapter concludes by summarizing how all of these areas need to be considered in global health efforts.

Basic Concepts from Medical Anthropology

Health and illness are defined, labeled, evaluated, and acted upon in the context of culture. In the eighteenth century, anthropologist Edmund Tyler (1871) defined culture as "that complex whole which includes knowledge, belief, art, morals, law, custom, and any other capabilities acquired by man as a member of society." Since those early days of anthropology, there have been literally hundreds of definitions of culture, but most have the following concepts in common (Board on Neuroscience and Behavioral Health, 2002):

- Shared ideas meanings and values
- Socially learned, not genetically transmitted

- Patterns of behavior that are guided by these shared ideas, meanings, and values
- Often exists at an unconscious level
- Constantly modified through "lived experiences"

The last of these concepts is a relatively new notion. *Lived experiences* comprise the experiences that people (and sometimes groups of people) go through as they live their lives. These experiences modify their culturally influenced beliefs and behaviors (Garro, 2000; Mattingly and Garro, 2000). As a consequence, culture is not static on either the group or individual level; rather, people are constantly changing. This concept helps allow for cultural change as people migrate to a new setting (community, region, or country), as people acquire additional education and experiences, and as conditions change around them (e.g., armed conflicts, economic changes in a country or region, political changes). This is a helpful viewpoint when looking at cultural change on both individual and group levels.

Medical anthropologists observe different cultures and their perspectives on disease and illness. For example, they look at the biological and the ecological aspects of disease, the cultural perspectives, and the ways in which cultures approach prevention and treatment.

To understand the cultural context of health, it is essential to work with several key concepts. First, the concepts of insider and outsider perspectives are useful for examining when we are seeing things from our point of view and when we are trying to understand someone else's view of things. The insider perspective (*emic*, in anthropological terminology) shows the culture as viewed from within. It refers to the meaning that people attach to things from their cultural perspective. For example, the view that worms (ascaris) in children are normal and are caused by eating sweets is a perspective found within some cultures. The outsider perspective (*etic*, in anthropological terminology) refers to the same thing as seen from the outside. Rather than meaning, it conveys a structural approach, or something as seen without understanding its meaning for a given culture. The outsider perspective can also convey an outsider's meaning attached to the same phenomenon. For example, this view might hold that ascaris is contracted through eggs infected by contact with contaminated soil or foods contaminated by contact with that soil; the eggs get into the soil through fecal wastes from infected individuals. The concepts of insider and outsider perspectives allow us to look at health, illness,

and prevention and treatment systems from several perspectives; to analyze the differences between these perspectives; and to develop approaches that will work within a cultural context (Scrimshaw & Hurtado, 1987).

To continue the example, in Guatemalan villages where the previously mentioned insider beliefs about ascaris prevailed, researchers learned that mothers believed that worms are normal and are not a problem unless they become agitated. In their view, worms live in a bag or sac in the stomach and are fine while so confined. Agitated worms get out and appear in the feces or may be coughed up. Mothers also believed that worms are more likely to become agitated during the rainy season because the thunder and lightning frighten them. From an outsider perspective, this relationship makes sense: Sanitation is more likely to break down in the rainy season, so there is more chance of infection and more diarrheal disease, which will reveal the worms.

The dilemma for the health workers was to get the mothers to accept deworming medication for their children, because most of the time worms were perceived as normal. If the health workers tried to tell the mothers that their beliefs were wrong, the mothers would reason that the health workers did not understand illness in a Guatemalan village and would reject their proposal. The compromise was to suggest that the children be dewormed just before the rainy season, so as to avoid the problem of agitated worms. It worked.*

The insider–outsider approach leads to another set of concepts. According to the Western biomedical definition, disease is the outsider perspective—that is, disease is an undesirable deviation from a measurable norm. Deviations in temperature, white blood cell count, red blood cell count, bone density, and many others are, therefore, seen as indicators of disease. Illness, in contrast, means "not feeling well." Thus it is a subjective, insider view. This sets up some immediate dissonances between the two views. It is possible to have an undesirable deviation from a Western biomedical norm and to feel fine. Hypertension, early stages of cancer, human immunodeficiency virus (HIV) infection, and early stages of diabetes are all instances where people may feel well, yet have a disease. Thus healthcare providers must communicate the need for behaviors to "fix" something that people may not realize is wrong.

---

*I am indebted to Elena Hurtado of Guatemala for this example.

It is also possible for someone to feel ill and for the Western biomedical system not to identify a disease. When this occurs, there is a tendency for Western-trained healthcare providers to say that nothing is wrong or that the person has a "psychosomatic" problem. Although both of these statements can be correct, there are several other explanations for this occurrence. One possibility is that Western biomedical science has not yet figured out how to measure a disease or disorder. Several recent examples of this phenomenon include AIDS, generalized anxiety attacks, and chronic fatigue syndrome. All of these were labeled "psychosomatic" at one time, but now are defined by measurable deviations from a biological norm. Similarly, painful menstruation was labeled "subconscious rejection of femininity" in the past, but is now associated with elevated prostaglandin levels and can be helped by administration of a prostaglandin inhibitor.

Another possibility is something that anthropologists have called "culture-bound syndromes" (Hughes, 1990; Simons, 2001; Simons & Hughes, 1985), but that might be better described as "culturally defined syndromes." *Culturally defined syndromes* are an insider way of describing and attributing a set of symptoms. They often refer to symptoms of a mental or psychological problem, but a physiological disease may also exist, posing a challenge to the health practitioner.

For example, Rubel and colleagues (1984) found that an illness called *susto* ("fright") in Mexico corresponded with symptoms of tuberculosis in adults. If people were told there was no such thing as susto and that they, in fact, had tuberculosis, they rejected the diagnosis and the treatment on the grounds that the doctors obviously knew nothing about susto. This situation was complicated by the fact that tuberculosis was viewed as serious and stigmatizing. The solution was to discuss the symptoms with people and mention that Western biomedicine has a treatment for those symptoms (Rubel et al., 1984). Susto may also be used to describe other sets of symptoms—for example, those of diarrheal disease in children (Scrimshaw & Hurtado, 1988). Other examples of culture-bound syndromes include evil eye (Latin America, the Mediterranean), zar (the Middle East and North Africa), brain fag or brain fog (West Africa), amok (running amok) or *mata elap* (Indonesia, Malaysia, and the Philippines), *latah* (Malaysia and Indonesia), *p'a leng* (wind illness) (China), and *ataque de nervios* (Puerto Rico) (Guarnaccia et al., 2010; Simons & Hughes, 1985).

With culturally defined syndromes, it is essential for an outsider to ask about the symptoms associated with the illness and to proceed with diagnosis and treatment on the basis of those symptoms. This is good practice in any event, because people often make a distinction between the cause of a disease or illness and its symptoms. Even if the perceived cause is inconsistent with the Western biomedical system, a disease can be diagnosed and treated based on the symptoms without challenging people's beliefs about the cause. When people's beliefs about the cause are denied, they may reject prevention or treatment measures entirely (Nichter, 2008).

The term *Western biomedical system* is used throughout this chapter because a term like *modern medicine* would deny the fact that there are other medical systems, such as Chinese and Ayurvedic medicine, that have modern forms. *Indigenous medical system* is used to refer to an insider—"within the culture"—system. Thus the Western biomedical system is an indigenous medical system in some countries, but it still may exist side by side with other indigenous systems, even in the United States and western Europe. In most of the world, the Western biomedical system now coexists with, and often dominates, local or indigenous systems. Because of this multiplicity of systems, and because of class differences, physicians and policy makers in a country may not accept or even be aware of the extent to which indigenous systems exist and their importance (Cameron, 2010). Also, many countries contain multiple cultures and languages. The cross-cultural principles discussed in this chapter may be just as important to work within a country as to work in multiple countries or cultures.

Another key concept from medical anthropology is that of ethnocentrism. *Ethnocentric* refers to seeing your own culture as "best." Ethnocentrism is a natural tendency, because the survival and perpetuation of a culture depend on teaching its children to accept the culture and on its members feeling that it is a good thing. In the context of cross-cultural understanding, ethnocentrism poses a barrier if people approach a culture with the attitude that it is inferior. In anthropology, *cultural relativism* refers to the idea that each culture has developed its own ways of solving the problems of how to live together; how to obtain the essentials of life, such as food and shelter; how to explain phenomena; and so on. No one way is viewed as "better" or "worse"; they are just different.

This understanding works well for classic anthropology but is a challenge when global health is considered. What if a behavior is "wrong" from an epidemiologic perspective? How does one distinguish between a "dangerous" behavior (e.g., using an

HIV-contaminated needle, swimming in a river with snails known to carry schistosomiasis, ingesting a powder with lead in it as part of a healing ritual) and behaviors that are merely different and, therefore, seem odd? For example, Bolivian peasants traditionally used very fine clay in a drink believed to be good for digestion and stomach ailments. Health workers succeeded in discouraging this practice in some communities because "eating dirt" seemed like a bad thing. The health workers then found themselves faced with increased caries and other symptoms of calcium deficiency in these same communities. Analysis revealed that the clay was a key source of calcium for these communities. It turns out that Western biomedicine also uses clay—but we color it pink or give it a mint flavor and put it in a bottle with a fancy label.

Thus there is a delicate balance between being judgmental without good reason and introducing behavior change because there is real harm from existing behaviors. In general, it is best to leave harmless practices alone and focus on understanding and changing harmful behaviors. This task is more difficult than it might seem, because the concept of cultural relativism also applies to perceptions of quality of life. A culture in which people believe in reincarnation may approach death with more equanimity, and may not adopt drastic procedures which only briefly prolong life. In some cultures, loss of a body organ is viewed as impeding the ability to go to an afterlife or the next life, and such surgery may be refused. Thus it is important in global public health for cultural outsiders to be cautious about making statements about what is good for someone elses.

The concept of holism is also useful in looking at health and disease cross-culturally. *Holism* is an approach used by anthropologists that looks at the broad context of whatever phenomenon is being studied. Holism involves staying alert for unexpected influences, because you never know what may have a bearing on the program you are trying to implement. For public health, this consideration is crucial because diverse factors may influence health and health behavior (Nichter, 2008).

One classic example of this situation is the detective work that went into discovering the etiology of the New Guinea degenerative nerve disease, kuru. Epidemiologists could not figure out how people contracted the disease, which appeared to have a long incubation period and to occur more frequently in women and children than in men. Many hypotheses were advanced, including inheritance (genetic), infection (bacterial, parasitic), and psychosomatic explanations.

By the early 1960s, the most widely accepted of the prevailing hypotheses was that kuru was genetically transmitted. Nevertheless, this proposal did not explain the sex differences in infection rates in adults but not in children, nor how such a lethal gene could persist. Working with Gadjusek of the National Institutes of Health (NIH), cultural anthropologists Glasse and Lindenbaum used in-depth ethnographic interviews to establish that kuru was relatively new to that region of New Guinea, as was the practice of cannibalism. Women and children were more likely to engage in the ritual consumption of the brains of dead relatives as a way of paying tribute to them, which was culturally less acceptable for men. Also, this tissue was cooked, but women, who did the cooking, and children, who were around during cooking, were more likely to eat it when it was partially cooked and, therefore, still infectious. Lindenbaum and Glasse suggested the disease was transmitted by cannibalism. To confirm their hypothesis, Gadjusek's team inoculated chimpanzees with brain material from women who had died of kuru; the animals subsequently developed the disease. The disease was found to be a slow virus, transmitted through the ingestion of brain tissue. Since then, the practice of cannibalism has declined and the disease has now virtually disappeared (Gadjusek, Gibbs, & Alpers, 1967; Lindenbaum, 1971).

In recent years, increasing attention has focused on another area that intersects with culture in people's ability to understand and access health care—the concept of health literacy. *Health literacy* is defined as "the degree to which individuals have the capacity to obtain, process, and understand basic health information and services needed to make appropriate health decisions" (Ratzan & Parker, 2000). Health literacy has been most thoroughly explored in the United States, and until recently was seen more as a literacy issue than a cultural issue. A 2004 Institute of Medicine report notes the importance of considering cultural issues such as many of those discussed in this chapter, and of taking a more global look at the problem and needed interventions (Committee on Health Literacy, 2004).

In looking at culture and health literacy, several categories for misunderstandings between provider and patient emerge.

First, there is a difference between medical terminology and lay terminology, which can occur in any language or culture. What is "diastolic" or a "bronchodilator"? What are HDL and LDL? What are T cells?

Second, individual and cultural differences surround concepts. What does it mean to maintain a "moderate" weight? To an anxious teen who wants to become a model, moderate weight might mean something clinically dangerously low (from the outsider, health practitioner perspective). To some women from Latin America or the Middle East, moderate weight will be heavier than U.S. norms, whereas a U.S. woman who fears she weighs too much might be viewed as dangerously thin in those cultures.

Third, meanings may differ. While working with prenatal care programs in Mexico, my team struggled with communicating the concept of risk in pregnancy as we developed materials to help women identify symptoms that meant that they should seek care. It turned out that the direct translation of "risk" into Spanish, or *riesgo,* did not carry the same meaning. When we explained the concept to women, they said, "Oh, you mean *peligro." Peligro* translates directly as "danger."

Finally, language issues may affect understanding. While researchers were investigating seizure disorders in adolescents from three cultures, it became clear that the word "trauma" has two different meanings. It can mean psychological shock, or it can mean physical trauma, such as a blow to the head. The exact same word *trauma* is used in Spanish, with the same two potential meanings. When neurologists talked with epileptic patients and their parents from Latino cultures, the neurologists used the word "trauma" as a cause of seizures to mean a blow to the head. The Latino parents heard the psychological meaning and thought their child had been traumatized psychologically by some fright or shock.

It is particularly important to note that health literacy is as much the problem of the healthcare provider and health communication staff as it is of a patient or the people in a community. If medical "jargon" is used, no amount of education short of experience in medicine or nursing will help someone understand. Terms such as "oncology," "nephrology," and "gastroenterology" have meaning for the medical world, but not for patients. Healthcare providers outside the United States often have a better understanding of this issue than their U.S. counterparts.

A concept related to health literacy is that of cultural competence. *Cultural competence* in health care describes "the ability of systems to provide care to patients with diverse values, beliefs and behaviors, including tailoring delivery to meet patients' social, cultural, and linguistic needs" (Betancourt et al., 2002). Thus cultural competency must include understanding and appreciation of health beliefs and behaviors in their cultural contexts and respectful strategies to negotiate optimal health in the context of these beliefs and behaviors. To achieve this goal, we must understand our own biases.

Cultures vary in their definitions of health and of illness. A condition that is endemic in a population may be seen as normal and may not be defined as illness. Ascaris in young children has already been mentioned as a perceived "normal" condition in many populations. Similarly, malaria is seen as normal in some parts of Africa, because everyone has it or has had it. In Egypt, where schistosomiasis was common and affected the blood vessels around the bladder, blood in the urine was referred to as "male menstruation" and was seen as normal. These definitions may also vary by age and by gender. In most cultures, symptoms such as fever in children are seen as more serious than the same symptoms in adults. Men may deny symptoms more than women in some cultures, but women may do the same in others. Often, adult denial of symptoms is due to the need to continue working.

Sociologist Talcott Parsons (1948) first discussed the concept of the sick role, wherein an individual must "agree" to be considered ill and to take actions (or allow others to take actions) to define the state of his or her health, discover a remedy, and do what is necessary to become well. Individuals who adopt the sick role neglect their usual duties, may indulge in dependent behaviors, and seek treatment to get well. By adopting the sick role, they are viewed as having "permission" to be exempted from usual obligations, but they are also under an obligation to try to restore health. The process of seeking to remain healthy or to restore health is discussed in more detail later in this chapter.

Belief Systems

Exhibit 2-1 depicts types of insider cultural explanations of disease causation. Based on the literature, it attempts to be as comprehensive as possible for cultures around the world. The exhibit consists of generalizations about culture-specific health beliefs and behaviors; these generalizations cannot, however, be assumed to apply to every individual from a given culture. We can learn about the hot/cold balance system of Latinos, Asians, and Middle Easterners, explained in the next section, but the details of the system will vary from country to country, from village to village, and from individual to individual. When someone walks in the door of a clinic, you cannot know whether he or she as an individual adheres to the beliefs described for his or her culture and what shape the individual's belief system takes. This makes the task of the culturally proficient healthcare provider both easier and harder. It means a practitioner working with a Mexican population does not have to

Exhibit 2-1	Types of Insider Cultural Explanations of Disease Causation

Body Balances
Temperature: Hot, cold
Energy
Blood: Loss of blood; properties of blood reflect imbalance; pollution from menstrual blood
Dislocation: Fallen fontanel
Organs: Swollen stomach; heart; uterus; liver; umbilicus; others
Incompatibility of horoscopes

Emotional
Fright
Sorrow
Envy
Stress

Weather
Winds
Change of weather
Seasonal disbalance

Vectors or Organisms
Worms
Flies
Parasites
Germs

Supernatural
Bewitching
Demons
Spirit possession
Evil eye
Offending God or gods
Soul loss

Food
Properties: Hot, cold, heavy (rich), light
Spoiled foods
Dirty foods
Sweets
Raw foods
Combining the "wrong" foods (incompatible foods)
Mud

Sexual
Sex with forbidden person
Overindulgence in sex

Heredity

Old Age

memorize which foods are hot and which are cold in Mexico, but the practitioner does need to know that the hot/cold belief system is important in Mexican culture and be able to be understanding and responsive when people bring up the topic.

The beliefs held by cultures around the world are classified into various categories, which are discussed here. The categories are used for diagnosis and treatment and for explaining the etiology or origin of the illness. Often, multiple categories are used. For example, emotions may be seen as causing a "hot" illness.

Body Balances

Within body balances (opposites) belief systems, the concepts of "hot" and "cold" are among the most pervasive around the world. The hot/cold balance is particularly important in Asian, Latin American, and Mediterranean cultures. Hot and cold beliefs are part of what is referred to as "humoral medicine," which is thought to have derived from Greek, Arabic, and East Indian pre-Christian traditions (Foster, 1953; Logan, 1972; Weller, 1983). The concept of opposites (e.g., hot and cold, wet and dry) also may have developed independently in other cultures (Rubel &

Haas, 1990). For example, in the Chinese medical tradition, hot is referred to as *yin* and cold as *yang* (Topley, 1976).

In the hot and cold belief system, a healthy body is seen as in balance between the two extremes. Illness may be brought on by violating the balance, such as washing the hair too soon after childbirth (cold may enter the body, which is still "hot" from the birth), eating hot or heavy foods at night, or breastfeeding while upset (the milk will be hot from the emotions and make the baby ill). "Hot" does not always refer to temperature, however. Often foods such as beef and pork are classified as hot regardless of temperature, whereas fish may be seen as cold regardless of temperature.

When illness has been diagnosed, the system is used to attempt to restore balance. Thus, in Central America, some diarrheas in children are viewed as hot, and protein-rich "hot" foods such as meats are withheld, aggravating the malnutrition that may be present and may be exacerbated by the diarrheal disease (Scrimshaw & Hurtado, 1988). An extensive literature exists on the topic of hot and cold illness classifications and treatments for them advocated by many of the world's cultures.

Energy balance is particularly important in Chinese medicine, where it is referred to as *chi*. When this balance is disturbed, it creates internal problems of homeostasis. Foods (often following the hot/cold theories) and acupuncture are among the strategies used to restore balance (Topley, 1976).

Blood beliefs include the concept that blood is irreplaceable; thus loss of blood—even small amounts—is perceived as a major risk. Adams (1955) describes a nutritional research project in a Guatemalan village where this belief inhibited the researcher's ability to obtain blood samples until the phlebotomists were instructed to draw as little blood as possible. Also, villagers were told that the blood would be examined to see if it was "sick" or "well" (another belief about blood) and they would be informed and given medicines if it were sick, which in fact did occur.

Menstrual blood is regarded as dangerous, especially to men, in many cultures, and elaborate precautions are taken to avoid contamination with it (Buckley & Gottlieb, 1988). As seen in the Guatemalan example, blood may have many properties that both diagnose and explain illness. Bad blood is seen as causing scabies in south India (Beals, 1976, p. 189). Haitians have a particularly elaborate blood belief system, which includes concepts such as *mauvais sang* (literally, "bad blood," when blood rises in the body and is dirty), *saisissement* (rapid heartbeat and cool blood, due to trauma), and *faiblesses* (too little blood). Blood qualities may also be seen as "opposites," such as clean–unclean, sweet–normal, bitter–normal, high–normal, heavy–weak, clotted–thin, and quiet–turbulent (C. Scott, personal communication, 1976). It is easy to see how these concepts could be used in a current program to prevent HIV infection in a Haitian community, because the culture already has ways of describing problems with blood.

Dislocation of body parts may occur with organs, but also with a physical aspect, such as the fontanel or "soft spot" in a baby's head where the bones have not yet come together in the first year or so to allow for growth. From the outsider perspective, a depression in this spot can be indicative of dehydration, often due to diarrheal disease. From the insider perspective, it is referred to as a cause of the disease (*caida de mollera*) in Mexico and Central America.

Many cultures associate illness with problems in specific organs. Good and Good (1981) talk about the importance of the heart for both Chinese and Iranian cultures. They discuss a case in which problems with

cardiac medication were wrongly diagnosed for a Chinese woman who kept complaining about pain in her heart. In fact, she was referring to her grief over the loss of her son. The Hmong people of Laos link many problems to the liver, referring to "ugly liver," "difficult liver," "broken liver," "short liver," "murmuring liver," and "rotten liver." These terms are said to refer to mental and emotional problems, and so are idiomatic rather than literal (O 'Connor, 1995, p. 92; Thao, 1986).

Topley (1976) mentions incompatibility of horoscopes between mother and child in Chinese explanations for some children's illnesses.

Emotional Illnesses

Illnesses of emotional origin are important in many cultures. Sorrow (as in the case of the Chinese woman mentioned previously), envy, fright, and stress are often seen as causing illnesses. In a Bolivian village in 1965, for example, a young girl's smallpox infection was attributed to her sorrow over the death of her father.

Envy can cause illness because people with envy could cast the "evil eye" on someone they envy, even unwittingly, or the envious person can become ill from the emotion (Reichel-Dolmatoff & Reichel-Dolmatoff, 1961). Fright, called susto in Latin America, has already been mentioned. In addition to the case of tuberculosis in adults discussed previously, susto is a common explanation for illness in children. It is also mentioned in Chinese culture (Topley, 1976).

Weather

Everything from the change of seasons to unusual variations within seasons (too warm, too cold, too wet, too dry) can be blamed for causing illness. Winds, such as the Santa Ana in California or the Scirocco in the North African desert, are also implicated as sources of illness in many cultures.

Vectors or Organisms

Vectors or organisms are blamed for illness in some cultures and represent a blend of Western biomedical and indigenous concepts. "Germs" is a catch-all category, as is "parasites." Worms are seen as causing diarrhea, whereas flies are seen as causing illness and, sometimes, as carrying germs.

The Supernatural

The supernatural is another frequently viewed source of illness, especially in Africa and Asia, though this belief system is certainly not confined to those regions.

In fact, the evil eye is a widespread concept—someone deliberately or unwittingly brings on illness by looking at someone with envy, malice, or too hot a gaze. In cultures where most people have dark eyes, strangers with light eyes may be seen as dangerous. In Latin America, a light-eyed person who admires a child can risk bringing evil eye to that child, but can counter it by touching the child. In other cultures, touching the child can be unlucky, so it is important to learn about local customs. Frequently, amulets and other protective devices, such as small eyes of glass, red hats, and a red string around the wrist, are worn to prevent evil eye. These objects can be viewed as an opportunity to discuss preventive health measures, because they are an indication that people are thinking about prevention.

Bewitching is deliberate malice, done either by the individual who wishes someone ill (literally) or by a practitioner at someone else's request. Bewitching can be countered by another practitioner or by specific measures taken by an individual. In some regions of Africa, epidemics are blamed on "too many witches," and people disperse to get away from them, thereby reducing the critical population density that had previously sustained the epidemic (Alland, 1970).

Belief in soul loss is widespread throughout the world. Soul loss can be caused by sources such as fright, bewitching, evil eye, and demons. It can occur in adults and children. Soul loss is serious and can lead to death. It must be treated through rituals to retrieve the soul. In Bolivia, for example, a village priest complained that his attempt to visit a sick child was thwarted when the family would not allow him to enter the house. The family later reported that an indigenous healer was performing a curing ritual at the time, and the soul was flying around the house as they were trying to persuade it to reenter the child. Opening the door to the priest would have allowed the soul to escape. In the Western biomedical system, the child's symptoms would be attributed to severe malnutrition.

Spirit possession is also a worldwide belief, and one that is found especially frequently in African and Asian cultures. One of the best-known accounts of this phenomenon is *A Spirit Catches You and You Fall Down* (Fadiman, 1997), a moving story of seizure disorders in a Hmong community and the misunderstandings between the family and physicians. In another example, from South India, Beals (1976) mentions spirit possession in a daughter-in-law whose symptoms included refusing to work and speaking insultingly to her mother-in-law. He suggests that spirit possession is a "culturally sanctioned means of

psychological release for oppressed daughters-in-law" (p. 188). Freed and Freed (1967) discuss similar cases in other regions of India. In Tanzania, malaria in children is sometimes blamed on possession by a bird spirit (Kamat, 2008). In Haiti, spirit possession is seen as a mark of favor by the spirits and is actively sought out. One of the drawbacks, however, is that the possessing spirits object to the presence of foreign objects in the body; as a consequence, some women do not want to use intrauterine devices as a means of birth control.

Demons are viewed as causing illness in Chinese culture, while offending God or gods is a problem in other cultures (Topley, 1976). In South India, epidemic diseases such as chickenpox and cholera (and, formerly, smallpox) are believed to be caused by disease goddesses. These goddesses bring the diseases to punish communities that become sinful (Beals, 1976, p. 187). The concept of punishment from God is seen in a case study from Mexico, where onchocerciasis (river blindness), which is caused by a parasite transmitted by the bite of a fly that lives near streams, is often thought to be due to sins committed either by the victim or by relatives of the victim. These transgressions against God are punished by God closing the victim's eyes (Gwaltney, 1970).

Food

In many cultures, food is perceived as being able to cause illness through its role in the hot and cold belief system; through spoiled foods, dirty foods, or raw foods; and by combining the wrong foods. Sweets are implicated as a cause of worms in children, and children who eat mud or dirt may become ill. Foods may also cause problems if eaten at the wrong time of day, such as "heavy" foods at night. An extensive literature describes food beliefs and practices worldwide, which has important implications for public health practice.

Sexual Illnesses

In Ecuador in the early 1970s, children's illnesses were sometimes blamed on affairs between one of the child's parents and a *compadre* or *comadre*—one of the child's godparents (Scrimshaw, 1974). Such a relationship was viewed as incestuous and dangerous to the child. In India, sex is sometimes viewed as weakening to the man, so overindulgence is considered a cause of weakness. To return to the concept of blood beliefs, it is thought that 30 drops of blood are needed to make one drop of semen, so blood loss weakens a man.

Heredity and Old Age

Heredity is sometimes blamed for illness, early death, or some types of death. Similarly, old age may be the simple explanation given for illness or death.

Illness in Various Forms

Exhibit 2-2 illustrates the way in which some of these beliefs are used to explain a particular illness—in this case, diarrheal disease in Central America. It is typical of the way in which an illness may be seen as having different forms, or manifestations, with different etiologies. It is also typical of the way in which several different explanations may be put forth for one set of symptoms.

In this case, Exhibit 2-2 and Figure 2-1 (the diagram of treatments) were key in expanding the orientation of the Central American diarrheal disease program. The program had intended to focus the distribution of oral rehydration solutions (ORS) in the clinics, but the insider perception was that a child should be taken to the clinic only for the worst form of diarrhea, dysentery. Instead, the most common treatment for diarrhea consisted of fluids in the form of herbal teas or sodas with medicines added. Often, storekeepers and pharmacists were consulted. It made sense to provide the ORS at stores and pharmacies as well as at clinics, so that all diarrheas were more likely to be treated (Scrimshaw & Hurtado, 1988).

In a related situation, Kendall, Foote, and Martorell (1983) found that, when the government of Honduras did not include indigenous or "folk" terminology for diarrheal disease in their mass-media messages regarding oral rehydration, people did not use ORS for diarrheas attributed to indigenously defined causes.

Healers

Exhibit 2-3 lists types of healers, which range from indigenous practitioners to Western biomedical providers. Pluralistic healers are those who mix the two traditions, although some Western biomedical healers and those from other medical systems may also mix traditions in their practices.

As with explanations of disease, the types of healers listed here are found in different combinations in different cultures. There is always more than one type of healer available to a community, even if members have to travel to seek care. The 16-country study of health-seeking behavior described earlier found that in all communities, people used more than one healing tradition, and usually more than one type of healer (Scrimshaw, 1992). The process of diagnosing illness and seeking a cure has been referred to as "patterns of resort," a descriptor that is now favored over the older term "hierarchy of resort" (Scrimshaw & Hurtado, 1987). People may zigzag from one practitioner to another, crossing from type to type of healer, and not always starting with the simplest and cheapest, but with the one they can best afford and who they feel will be most effective, given the severity of the problem. Even middle- and upper-class individuals, who can afford Western biomedical care, may use other types of practitioners and practices.

Indigenous practitioners are usually members of the culture and follow traditional practices. Today they often mix elements of Western biomedicine and other traditional systems. In many instances, they are "called" to their profession through dreams, omens, or an illness, which usually can be cured only by their agreement to become a practitioner. Most learn through apprenticeship to other healers, although some are taught by dreams. Often they will take courses in Western practices in programs such as those developed to train Chinese "barefoot doctors" or community-based health promoters. In some instances, they must conceal their role as traditional healer from those running the training programs. The incorporation of some Western biomedical knowledge and skills often enhances a practitioner's prestige in the community.

Some indigenous practitioners charge for their services, but many do not, accepting gifts instead. In a few traditions (including some Chinese cultures), practitioners are paid as long as family members are well, but they are not paid for illness treatment. The duty of the practitioner in those cases is to keep people well, which argues for the acceptability of prevention programs in those cultures.

For the most part, indigenous practitioners do "good," meaning healing. Some can do both good and ill (e.g., shamans, sorcerers, and witches in many cultures). A few practice only evil or negative rituals (e.g., some shamans, sorcerers, and witches). Their work must then be countered by someone who does "good" magic. The power of belief is such that if individuals believe they have been bewitched, they may need a counteractive ritual, even if the Western biomedical system detects and treats a specific disease. In Guayaquil, Ecuador, one woman believed that she had been *maleada* (cursed) by a woman who was jealous of her, and that this curse was making her and her children ill. A *curandera* (curer) was brought in to do a *limpia* (ritual cleansing) of the house and family to remove the curse (Scrimshaw, 1974).

Exhibit 2-2	Taxonomy of Diarrhea

CAUSE			SYMPTOMS All types have watery and frequent stools	TREATMENT
Mother's Milk	Physical activity	Hot		Not breastfeeding when hot
	Hot foods			Mother changes diet
	Pregnancy			Breastfeeding stops
	Anger	Emotional	Very dangerous	Home, drugstore, Injectionist, witch, spiritist
	Sadness			
	Fright			
Food	Bad food		Flatulence, feeling of fullness	Home, folk curer
	Excess			
	Does *not* eat on time			
	Hot	Quality		
	Cold			
Tooth Eruption			Tooth eruption	None
Fallen Fontanel, Fallen Stomach	Fallen stomach		Green with mucus	Folk curer
	Fallen fontanel		Sunken fontanel; vomiting; green in color	
Evil Eye			Fever	Folk curer
Stomach Worms			Worms	Drugstore, home, folk curer
Cold Enters Stomach	From feet		White in color	Folk curer
	From head			
Dysentery			Blood in stools, "urgency;" color is red or black	Home, drugstore, health post

Source: S. C. M. Scrimshaw and E. Hurtado, *Rapid Assessment Procedures for Nutrition and Primary Health Care: Anthropological Approaches to Improving Program Effectiveness (RAP)* (Los Angeles: UCLA Latin America Center, 1987), p. 26. Reprinted with permission of the Regents of the University of California.

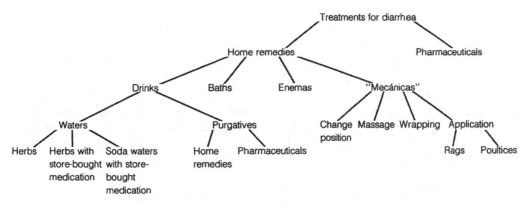

Figure 2-1 Taxonomy of Treatments for Diarrhea. *Source:* S. C. M. Scrimshaw and E. Hurtado, *Rapid Assessment Procedures for Nutrition and Primary Health Care: Anthropological Approaches to Improving Program Effectiveness (RAP)* (Los Angeles: UCLA Latin America Center, 1987), p. 26. Reprinted with permission of the Regents of the University of California.

Exhibit 2-3	Types of Healers

Indigenous	**Western Biomedical**
Midwives	Pharmacists
Shamans	Nurse-midwives
Curers	Nurses
Spiritualists	Nurse practitioners
Witches	Physicians
Sorcerers	Dentists
Priests	Other health professionals
Diviners	
Herbalists	**Other Medical Systems**
Bonesetters	Chinese medical system
Massagers	Practitioners
	Chemists/herbalists
Pluralistic	Acupuncturists
Injectionists	Ayurvedic practitioners
Indigenous health workers	Taoist priests
Western-trained birth	
attendants	
Traditional chemists/	
herbalists	
Storekeepers and vendors	

The importance of the power of belief is not confined only to bewitching. One anthropologist working with a Haitian population discovered that a Haitian burn patient made no progress until she went to a *Houngan* (voodoo priest) on the patient's behalf and had the appropriate healing ritual conducted (J. Halifax-Groff, personal communication, 1976).

In some cultures healers are seen as diagnosticians, while others do the treatment (Alland, 1970).

Other healers may handle both tasks, but refer some kinds of illness to other practitioners. In Haiti, both midwives and voodoo priests refer some cases to the Western biomedical system. Healers who combine healing practices or who combine the ability to do both diagnosis and treatment are viewed as more powerful than other types. Topley (1976, pp. 259–260) discusses this issue in the setting of Hong Kong, noting that Taoist priest healers are particularly respected in that area. They are seen as both priest and doctor and "claim to combine the ethics of Confucianism, the hygiene and meditation of Taoism, and the prayers and self-cultivation of the Buddhist monk."

Pluralistic healers combine Western biomedical and indigenous practices. Injectionists will give an injection of antibiotics, vitamins, or other drugs purchased at pharmacies or stores. Sometimes these injections are suggested by the pharmacist or storekeeper; other times they are self-prescribed. Because antibiotics proved so dramatically effective in curing infections when Western biomedicine was first introduced in many cultures, injections are often seen as conveying greater healing than the same substance taken orally. Thus many antibiotics now available orally and vitamins are injected. In today's environment, this practice increases the risk of contracting HIV or hepatitis if sterile or new needles and syringes are not used.

Traditional chemists and herbalists, as well as storekeepers and vendors (many communities are too small to have a pharmacy), often sell Western biomedical medications, including those that require a prescription in the United States and western Europe. While prescriptions may be "legally" required in many countries, the laws are not always rigorously enforced. This is also true for pharmacies, which are very important—sometimes the most important—sources of diagnosis and treatment in many communities around the world.

For more than 40 years, countries around the world have enlisted and trained indigenous health practitioners to function as part of the national or regional health system. These efforts have ranged from China's "barefoot doctors" to the education of community members in Latin America, Africa, and Asia to provide preventive care and triage. These efforts have nearly disappeared in some areas (e.g., China) and re-emerged in others. For example, in Australia, indigenous people are now involved as indigenous health outreach workers to their communities (2010, healthinfonet@ecu.edu.au). In Nepal, indigenous health workers have been enlisted in programs to address diarrheal disease and acute respiratory infections (Ghimire et al., 2010), and female Ayurvedic doctors are important resources for women's health (Cameron, 2010).

Western biomedical practitioners are an important source of care, but they may also be expensive or difficult to access in remote areas. As mentioned earlier, if an individual believes that an illness is due to a cause explained by the indigenous system and a Western biomedical practitioner denies that cause, the individual may not return to that practitioner but rather seek help elsewhere (Kamat, 2008; Nichter, 2008).

As noted, there are other medical systems with long traditions, systematic ways of training practitioners, and well-established diagnostic and treatment procedures. Until recently Western biomedical practitioners totally rejected both these and indigenous systems, often failing to recognize how many practices and medicines Western biomedicine has derived from other systems (e.g., quinine, digitalis, many anesthetics, aspirin, and estrogen). Elements of these systems that were derided in the past, such as acupuncture, have now found their way into Western biomedical practice and are being "legitimized" by Western research (Baer, 2008).

Theories of Health Behavior and Behavior Change

The fields of sociology, psychology, and anthropology have developed many theories to explain health beliefs and behaviors and behavior change (Schumacher

et al. 2009). Some theories developed by sociologists and psychologists in the United States were developed first for U.S. populations and only later applied internationally. Others were developed with international and multicultural populations in mind from the beginning. Only a few of the many theories of health and illness beliefs and behavior are covered in this section; those included here have been quite influential in general or are applicable for international work in particular.

Health Belief Model

The health belief model suggests that decision making about health behaviors is influenced by four basic premises—perceived susceptibility to the illness, perceived severity of the illness, perceived benefits of the prevention behavior, and perceived barriers to that behavior—as well as other variables, such as sociodemographic factors (Rosenstock et al., 1974). In general, people are seen as weighing perceived susceptibility (how likely they are to get the disease) and perceived severity (how serious the disease is) against their belief in the benefits and effectiveness of the prevention behavior they must undertake and the costs of that behavior in terms of barriers such as time, money, and aggravation. The more serious the disease is believed to be, and the more effective the prevention, the more likely people are to incur the costs of engaging in the prevention behavior.

The health belief model has been extensively studied, critiqued, modified, and expanded to explain people's responses to symptoms and compliance with healthcare regimens for diagnosed illnesses. One concern has been that this model does not work as well for chronic problems or habitual behaviors because people learn to manage their behaviors or the healthcare system. Also, it has been accused of failing to take environmental and social forces into account, which in turn increases the potential for blaming the individual. The difficulty in quantifying the model for research and evaluation purposes is also a problem.

Work by Bandura led to the inclusion of self-efficacy in the model. *Self-efficacy* has been defined as "the conviction that one can successfully execute the behavior required to produce the desired outcome" (Bandura, 1977, 1989). The concept of *locus of control*, or belief in the ability to control one's life, also has been incorporated into this model. In one recent example, a comparison of migrant Yugoslavian and Swedish females with diabetes revealed a stronger locus of control in the Swedish women and more passivity toward self-care in the Yugoslavian women, who also had a lower self-efficacy that the authors attributed to the different political systems in the two countries—collectivism in Yugoslavia versus individualism in Sweden (Hjelm et al., 1999).

The value of the four basic premises of the health belief model has held up well under scrutiny. Perceived barriers have the strongest predictive value of the four dimensions, followed by perceived susceptibility and perceived benefits. Perceived susceptibility is most frequently associated with compliance with health screening exams. Perceived severity of risk has been noted to have a weaker predictive value for protective health behaviors, but is strongly associated with sick-role behaviors.

In *Medical Choice in a Mexican Village,* Young (1981) describes a health decision-making process very similar to that found in the health belief model. In choosing between home remedies, pharmacy or store, and between indigenous healer or doctor, the villagers weigh the perceived severity of the illness, the potential efficacy of the cure to be sought, the cost (money, time, and so on) of the cure, and their own resources to seek treatment and pay the cost as they make their decision. The simplest, least costly treatment is always the first choice, but the severity of illness and efficacy issues may force adoption of a more costly option. Other studies of health-seeking behavior have found similar patterns throughout the world (e.g., Kamat, 2008).

Theory of Reasoned Action

The theory of reasoned action was first proposed by Ajzen and Fishbein (1972) to predict an individual's intention to engage in a behavior in a specific time and place. This theory was intended to explain virtually all behaviors over which people have the ability to exert self-control. Five basic constructs precede the performance of a behavior: behavioral intent; attitudes and beliefs; evaluations of behavioral outcomes; subjective norms; and normative beliefs. Behavioral intent is seen as the immediate predictor of behavior. Factors that influence behavioral choices are mediated through this variable. To maximize the predictive ability of an intention to perform a specific behavior, the measurement of the intent must closely reflect the measurement of the behavior. For example, measurement of the intention to begin to take oral contraceptives must include questions about when a woman plans to visit a clinic and which clinic she plans to attend. The failure to address action, target, context, and time in the measurement of behavioral intention will undermine the predictive value of the model.

In a recent test of this theory in the prediction of condom use intentions in a national sample of young people in England, measures of past behavior were found to be the best predictors of intentions and attenuated the effects of attitude and subjective norms (Sutton et al., 1999).

Diffusion of Health Innovations Model

The diffusion of health innovations model proposes that communication is essential for social change, and that diffusion is the process by which an innovation is communicated through certain channels over time among members of a social system (Rogers, 1983; Rogers & Shoemaker, 1972). An *innovation* is an idea, practice, service, or other object that is perceived as new by an individual or group.

Ideally, the development of a diffusion strategy for a specific health behavior change goal will proceed through six stages:

1. Recognition of a problem or need
2. Conduct of basic and applied research to address the specific problem
3. Development of strategies and materials that will put the innovative concept into a form that will meet the needs of the target population
4. Commercialization of the innovation, which will involve production, marketing, and distribution efforts
5. Diffusion and adoption of the innovation
6. Consequences associated with adoption of the innovation

According to classic diffusion theory, a population targeted by an intervention to promote acceptance of an innovation includes six groups: innovators, early adopters, early majority, late majority, late adopters, and laggards. The rapidity and extent to which health innovations are adopted by a target population are mediated by a number of factors, including relative advantage, compatibility, complexity, communicability, observability, trialability, cost-efficiency, time, commitment, risk and uncertainty, reversibility, modifiability, and emergence.

Relative advantage refers to the extent to which a health innovation is better (faster, cheaper, more beneficial) than an existing behavior or practice. Antibiotics, for example, were quickly accepted in most of the world because they were dramatically faster and more effective than traditional practices.

Compatibility is the degree to which the innovation is congruent with the target population's existing set of practices and values. Polgar and Marshall (1976) point out that injectable contraceptives were acceptable in the village in India where Marshall worked because injections were viewed so positively due to the success of antibiotics.

The degree to which an innovation is easy to incorporate into existing health regimens may also affect rates of diffusion. Iodized salt is easier to use, because salt is already a habit, than taking an iodine pill. Health innovations are also more likely to be adopted quickly and by larger numbers of individuals if the innovation itself can be easily communicated.

The concept of trialability involves the ease of trying out a new behavior. For example, it is easier to try a condom than to be fitted for a diaphragm. Observability refers to role models, such as village leaders volunteering to be the first recipients in a vaccination campaign.

A health innovation is also more likely to be adopted if it is seen as cost-efficient. A famous case study of water boiling in a Peruvian town demonstrated that the cost in time and energy of gathering wood and making a fire to boil the water far outweighed any perceived benefits, so water boiling was seldom adopted (Wellin, 1955). Successful health innovations are likely to be those that do not require expenditure of much additional time, energy, or other resources.

One of the overall messages regarding communicating health education and promotion stated by Rogers (1973) is that mass media and interpersonal communication channels should both be used. Implementing both methods is of particular importance in developing countries, especially in rural communities. Rogers emphasizes that mass media deliver information to a large population and add knowledge to the general knowledge base, but interpersonal contacts are needed to persuade people to adopt new behaviors (thereby using the knowledge function, the persuasion function, and the innovation-decision process). In Rogers's work and other work cited by him, "family planning diffusion is almost entirely via interpersonal channels" (p. 263). Five examples in different countries (including India, Taiwan, and Hong Kong) are presented by Rogers, wherein interpersonal channels were the primary source for family planning information and were the motivating factors to seeking services.

The limitations to mass media in this area include the following issues:

- *Limited exposure.* In low- and middle-income countries, smaller audiences have access to mass media (radio is the most common mass media tool). Low literacy levels are another barrier.

- *Message irrelevancy.* The content of mass-media messages may be of no practical use for many rural and "non-elite" populations. Often instrumental information—"how to" information—is not included in the messages (e.g., where to receive services or the positive and negative consequences of adapting a particular health behavior).

- *Low credibility.* For people to accept and believe the messages being diffused, trustworthiness needs to exist between the sender and the receiver. In many low- and middle-income countries, radio and TV stations are run by a government monopoly and their content may be considered to be government propaganda by the receivers. Radio and TV in Nigeria, Pakistan, and other African and Asian countries, for example, are controlled by the government (Rogers, 1973).

The diffusion of innovations model focuses solely on the processes and determinants of adoption of a new behavior and does not help to understand or explain the maintenance of behavior change. Many health behaviors require permanent or long-term changes. Also, it is important to understand whether a new behavior is being carried out appropriately, consistently, or at all. One salient example involves condom use, which healthcare practitioners demonstrated to a population by unrolling the condom over a banana. Women who became pregnant while they reported using condoms had been faithfully putting them on bananas.

PRECEDE Model

The PRECEDE model of health promotion was first proposed by Green, Kreuter, Deeds, and Partridge in 1980. PRECEDE is an acronym for "predisposing, reinforcing, and enabling causes in educational diagnosis and evaluation." This model focuses on communities, rather than individuals, as the primary units of change. This approach incorporates specific recommendations for evaluating the effectiveness of interventions and provides a highly focused target for the intervention.

The framework of the PRECEDE model outlines progression through seven phases. Phase 1, also known as social diagnosis, relies on the assessment of the general problems of concern that have a negative impact on overall quality of life for members of the target population. Those populations might include patients, healthcare providers, family caregivers, lay health workers, or consumers of health care, for example. During phase 1, emphasis is placed on identification of social problems encountered by the target population. This step provides an important opportunity to involve the community in dealing with the issue. Community participation in and acceptance of programs greatly increase their likelihood of success.

Phase 2 focuses on epidemiologic diagnosis. Activities associated with phase 3 focus on the identification of nonbehavioral (and often nonmodifiable) causes and behavioral causes of the priority health problem. Phase 4 of the model, which is identified as educational diagnosis, consists of activities to identify predisposing, reinforcing, and enabling factors associated with the target health behavior.

In phase 5, intervention planners decide which of the factors will be addressed by various aspects of the intervention. Phase 6, or administrative diagnosis, comprises the development and implementation of the intervention program. Viable intervention strategies suggested by Green and colleagues (1980) include group lectures, individual instruction, mass-media messages, audiovisual aids, programmed learning, educational television, skill development workshops, simulations, role-playing, educational games, peer group discussions, behavior modification, modeling, and community development.

The seventh and final phase focuses on evaluation. This type of analysis begins during each of the preceding six phases, and ranges from simple process evaluation to impact and outcome evaluation.

Transtheoretical Model

Theories around the concept of stages of change have been evolving since the early 1950s. Currently, the most widely accepted stage change model is the transtheoretical model of behavior change developed by Prochaska, DiClemente, and Norcross (1992). This model includes four core constructs: (1) stages of change, (2) decisional balance, (3) self-efficacy, and (4) processes of change. Interventions relying on this model are expected to include all four constructs in the development of strategies to communicate, promote, and maintain behavior change.

The model identifies five stages of change. The first is precontemplation, in which individuals have no intention to take action within the next six months. In the contemplation stage, individuals express an intention to take some action to change a negative health behavior or adopt a positive one within the next six months. The preparation stage refers to the intent to make a change within the next 30 days. The action stage involves the demonstration of an overt behavior change for an interval of less than six months. In the fifth stage, known as maintenance, a person will have sustained a change for at least six months.

Decisional balance is an assessment of the costs and benefits of changing, which will vary with the stage of change.

Self-efficacy is divided into two concepts within the transtheoretical model. First, confidence exists that one can engage in the new behavior. Second, the temptation aspect of self-efficacy refers to factors that can tempt one to engage in unhealthy behaviors across different settings.

The fourth construct of the transtheoretical model deals with the process of change. It includes 10 factors that can influence the progression of individuals from the precontemplation stage to the maintenance stage.

Explanatory Models

Explanatory models were initially proposed by the physician-anthropologist Kleinman (1980, 1986, 1988). They differ from some of the theories described earlier in this section in that they are designed for multicultural settings. They include models such as the meaning-centered approach to staff–patient negotiation described by Good and Good (1981). Although such models focus on individual interactions between physician or other staff and patients, the concepts underlying them—such as Kleinman's negotiation model—have proved useful for research and for behavioral interventions for larger populations. An explanatory model is seen as dynamic, and can change based on individual experiences with health, health information, or with the illness in question (McSweeney et al., 1997).

Exhibit 2-4 adapts and summarizes concepts from Good and Good's (1981) description of the meaning-centered approach. This approach involves mutual interpretations across systems of meaning. The interpretive goal is understanding the patient's perspective. The underlying premise is that disorders vary profoundly in their psychodynamics, cultural influences in interpretation, behavioral expression, severity, and duration. As noted earlier, it is difficult to provide "codes" to culture and symptoms due to factors such as individual variations, groups assimilating or changing, and groups adding beliefs and behaviors from other cultures. For example, belief in *espiritismo* (spiritism) was traditionally strongest among Puerto Rican groups in the United States, but this belief has now been adopted by other cultures of Latin American origin as well. Thus, instead of trying to provide "formulas" for understanding health and illness belief systems for different cultures, the focus with the meaning-centered approach is on the meaning of symptoms. The medical encounter must involve the interpretation of symptoms and other relevant information.

Exhibit 2-4	Meaning-Centered Approach to Clinical Practice

Primary Principles

Groups vary in the specificity of their medical complaints.

Groups vary in their style of medical complaining.

Groups vary in the nature of their anxiety about the meaning of symptoms.

Groups vary in their focus on organ systems.

Groups vary in their response to therapeutic strategies.

Human illness is fundamentally semantic or meaningful (it may have a biological base, but is a human experience).

Corollary

Clinical practice is inherently interpretive.

Actions

Practitioners must

Elicit patients' requests, questions, etc.

Elicit and decode patients' semantic networks

Distinguish disease and illness and develop plans for managing problems.

Elicit explanatory models of patients and families, analyze conflict with biomedical models, and negotiate alternatives

Source: B. J. Good and M. J. D. Good, "The Meaning of Symptoms: A Cultural Hermeneutic Model for Clinical Practice," in I. Eisenberg and A. Kleinman, *The Relevance of Social Science for Medicine* (Dordrecht: Kluwer Academic Publishers, 1981). Adapted and reprinted with kind permission of Kluwer Academic Publishers.

Other Theories

A number of other theories can be useful in looking at culture and behavior. For example, multi-attribute utility theory predicts behavior directly from an individual's evaluation of the consequences or outcomes associated with both performing and not performing a given behavior. Some models, such as social learning theory, have been criticized by anthropologists who argue against the notion that people are like a "black box" into which you can pour information and expect a specific behavior change.

Common Features of Successful Health Communication and Health Promotion Programs

When applied in practice, many of the principles discussed in this chapter help increase the success of health communication and health promotion programs. In particular, understanding and incorporating people's insider cultural values, beliefs, and behav-

iors; a community-based approach with strong community participation; recognition of gender issues (Zamen & Underwood, 2003); peer group education, including use of community-based outreach workers; and multilevel intervention approaches have proved essential to program success.

The Agita Sao Paulo Program provides a case study in using local culture to design both the content and the delivery system for a program to use physical activity to promote health (Matsudo et al., 2002). Just the word *agita* (which means to move the body—to "agitate" in the sense of "stirring," but also to change) is more culturally understood and internalized than a literal translation of "exercise." In addition to representing careful work on culturally acceptable ways of delivering the message, this project provides multiple culturally valued ways to increase physical activity, and "tailors" these options to the age, gender, and lifestyles of community members.

In a very different project, work in three townships in South Africa focused on identifying where AIDS prevention would be most effective from the culturally appropriate, insider perspective (Weir et al., 2003). Among other things, researchers learned that ideal prevention intervention sites varied depending on whether the central business district or the township was the most popular location for initiating new sexual encounters. The type of sex (commercial versus casual) as well as the availability of condoms varied with the site. The age of people engaging in risky behaviors and risk behaviors by gender also varied by site. Again, prevention programs needed to be tailored.

In another HIV/AIDS prevention project, this time in Vietnam, paying attention to culture and religion was essential to program strategies (Rekart, 2002). In Belize, understanding adolescents and making sure the program met their needs in both cultural- and age-appropriate ways was key (Martiniuk et al., 2003). In Nepal, the use of indigenous workers and attention to cultural practices helped lower the incidence and severity of diarrheal and respiratory infections in the districts targeted for interventions (Ghimire et al., 2010). Evaluation of programs addressing family planning and HIV prevention shows that behavior-change communication increases knowledge and interpersonal communication among audience members and motivates positive changes in behavior (Salem et al., 2008).

Another example of focusing on understanding and changing cultural values around unhealthy behaviors is found in the area of smoking cessation. Abdullah and Husten (2004) set forth a framework for public health intervention in this area that addresses multiple levels of society.

The need for the involvement of communities is also clearly demonstrated in the literature. Literally hundreds of references exist on this topic. A recent summary article on this topic outlines many of the broad principles underlying this approach, including community analysis with community participation, action plans designed with community input, and community involvement in implementation. Community involvement may take the form of ongoing oversight and evaluation as well as the more usual modes of community outreach workers (e.g., Thevos et al., 2000), working through community organizations, and getting individuals involved (Bhuyan, 2004). A report from a recent project in Bolivia documents the success of involving community members in everything from mapping the villages to priority setting for the program (Perry et al., 2003). A recent book by the former head of the United Kingdom's National Health Service argues strongly that the quest for global health in the twenty-first century must involve a paradigm shift in which nations, communities, and indigenous peoples around the world have a much greater voice in the design and implementation of health services (Crisp, 2010).

Two projects in Chicago demonstrate the success of the community outreach worker approach. In one case, the project focuses on intravenous drug abusers, helping them to reduce their HIV/AIDS-related risk behaviors and to initiate drug abuse treatment programs. This work simply could not have been accomplished without the efforts of community outreach workers, all of whom are former addicts who know how and when to reach current addicts. Also, the outreach workers come from the predominant cultural/ethnic group in each community (Booth & Wiebel, 1992; Wiebel, 1993; Wiebel et al., 1996). Similarly, the Chicago Project for Violence Prevention involves ex-gang members as outreach workers. Both programs have been adopted internationally as well as in other cities in the United States. A similar focus on peer group education in Botswana led to increased knowledge and prevention behaviors among women at risk for HIV/AIDS infection (Norr et al., 2004).

Methodologies for Understanding Culture and Behavior

Many of the research methodologies developed in the United States do not translate easily, literally, or figuratively to international settings. Differences in linguistic nuances, in the meanings of words and concepts, in what people would reveal to a stranger, and in what they would reveal to someone from their community have all complicated the application of the quantitative methodologies used by sociologists, psychologists, and epidemiologists. The realization of these problems came about gradually, through failed projects and missed interpretations, and especially once AIDS appeared. As a disease whose only prevention is still behavioral, and with which many hidden or taboo behaviors are involved, AIDS highlighted the need for qualitative research and for research conducted by individuals from the cultures being studied.

The field of global public health has now moved from an almost exclusively quantitative orientation to the recognition that a toolbox of methodologies is available. Some of these tools may be more valuable than others for some situations or questions; at other times, a mix of several methodologies may offer the best approach. These methodologies derive from epidemiology, survey research, psychology, anthropology, marketing (including social marketing), and other fields. The biggest disagreement has been over the relative value of quantitative and qualitative methods.

The debate on the scientific value of qualitative versus quantitative research is well summarized by Pelto and Pelto (1978). They define *science* as the "accumulation of systematic and reliable knowledge about an aspect of the universe, carried out by empirical observation and interpreted in terms of the interrelating of concepts referable to empirical observations" (p. 22). The Peltos add that "if the 'personal factor' in anthropology makes it automatically unscientific, then much of medical science, psychology, geography, and significant parts of all disciplines (including chemistry and physics) are unscientific" (p. 23).

In fact, scientific research is not truly objective, but rather is governed by the cultural framework and theoretical orientation of the researcher. One example of this bias is the past tendency of biomedical researchers in the United States to focus on adult men for many health problems that also occur in women (such as heart disease). The earlier example of kuru also demonstrates the limitations of cultural bias.

Qualitative research techniques include the following:

- Observation: Behaviors are observed and recorded.
- Participant observation: The researcher learns by participating in cultural events and practices.

- Interviews: Both open-ended and semistructured queries are possible, usually based on interview guides or checklists.

- Focus groups: A group of people are asked to discuss specific questions and topics.

- Document analysis: Existing documents and prior research are evaluated.

- Systematic data collection: This technique ranges widely, from photography and video taping to asking informants to draw maps' sort cards with pictures, words, or objects; answer questions based on scales; and many more (Bernard, 2006; Pelto & Pelto, 1978; Scrimshaw & Hurtado, 1987).

A key feature of qualitative research is the use of these multiple methods to triangulate, or compare, data so as to ensure accuracy. With these approaches, the researcher does not simply rely on what is said, but can observe what is actually done. Another feature is that the researcher spends enough time in the community to be able to interview, observe, or otherwise evaluate the same individuals or behaviors multiple times, thereby further ensuring the depth and accuracy of the resulting data.

These techniques yield data that are descriptive and exploratory, and that serve to investigate little-understood phenomena, identify or discover important variables, and generate hypotheses for further research. Results are often explanatory, helping researchers to understand the social and cultural forces causing the phenomenon and to identify plausible causal networks. They also present the "voices" of the participants, and introduce context and meaning into the findings. They yield themes, patterns, concepts, and insights related to cultural phenomena. They can be particularly valuable for behaviors that are often hidden, such as sexual risk taking and drug abuse (Dickson-Gomez, 2010; Wiebel, 1993) In evaluations, they help practitioners make judgments about a program, improve its effectiveness, and inform decisions about future programming, as illustrated in the case study on acceptability of an infant cereal found later in this chapter.

The methodological concepts of validity and reliability provide a common foundation for the integration of quantitative and qualitative techniques. *Validity* refers to the accuracy of scientific measurement—"the degree to which scientific observations measure what they purport to measure" (Pelto & Pelto, 1978, p. 33). For example, in Spanish Harlem in New York City, a study using the question "¿Sabe como evitar los hijos?" ("Do you know how to avoid [having] children?") elicited responses on contraceptive methods and was used as the first in a series of questions on family planning. By not using family planning terminology at the outset, the study was able to avoid biasing respondents (Scrimshaw & Pasquariella, 1970). The same phrase in Ecuador, however, produced reactions like "I would never take out [abort] a child!" If the New York questionnaire had been applied in Ecuador without first testing it through semistructured ethnographic interviews, the same words would have produced answers to what was, in fact, a different question (Scrimshaw, 1974). Qualitative methods often provide greater validity than quantitative methods because they rely on multiple data sources, including direct observation of behavior and multiple contacts with people over time. Thus they can be used to increase the validity of survey research.

Reliability refers to replicability—the extent to which scientific observations can be repeated and the same results obtained. In general, this goal is best accomplished through survey research or other quantitative means. Surveys can test hypotheses and examine questions generated through qualitative data. Qualitative methods may help us discover a behavior or learn how to ask questions about it, while quantitative data can tell us how extensive the behavior is in a population and which other variables are associated with it.

Murray (1976) describes just such a discovery during qualitative research in a Haitian community, where a simple question—"Are you pregnant?"—had two meanings. Women could be pregnant with *gros ventre* ("big belly") or could be pregnant and in *perdition*. Perdition meant a state where a woman was pregnant, but the baby was "stuck" in utero and refused to grow. Perdition was attributed to causes such as "cold," spirits, or ancestors. Women may be in perdition for years, and may be separated, divorced, or widowed, but the pregnancy is attributed to her partner when it commenced. Murray subsequently included questions about perdition in a later survey, which revealed that it was apparently a cultural way of making infertility or subfecundity socially acceptable, as many women in perdition fell into these categories.

Surveys are effective tools for collecting data from a large sample, particularly when the distribution of a variable in a population is needed (e.g., the percentage of women who obtain prenatal care) or when rarely occurring events must be assessed (e.g., neonatal deaths). Surveys are also used to record people's answers to questions about their behavior, motivations, perception of an event, and similar topics. Although surveys are carefully designed to collect data in the most objective manner possible, they often suffer inaccuracies based on respondents' perceptions of their own behavior, their differing interpretations of the meaning of the question, or their desire to please the interviewer with their answers. Surveys also can encounter difficulty in uncovering motives (i.e., why individuals behave as they do), and they are not apt to uncover behaviors that may be consciously or unconsciously concealed. In "Truths and Untruths in Village Haiti: An Experiment in Third World Survey Research," Chen and Murray (1976) describe some of these problems.

The traditional anthropological approach involves one person or a small team who remain at the research site for at least a year. This practice is intended to ensure that the findings take into account the changes in people's lifestyles with the changes in seasons, activities, available food, and so on. Also, the anthropologist often needs time to learn a language or dialect and learn enough about the culture to provide a context for questions and observations. More recently, a subset of anthropological tools (ethnographic interview, participant observation, conversation, and observation) plus the market researchers' tool of focus groups have been combined in a rapid anthropological assessment process known as the Rapid Assessment Procedure (RAP) (Scrimshaw et al., 1992; Scrimshaw et al., 1991; Scrimshaw & Hurtado, 1987).

RAP evolved around the same time as Rapid Rural Appraisal was developed by rural sociologists (Chambers, 1992). Both methods made listening to community voices easier for program planners and healthcare providers and became frequently used tools for program development and evaluation. RAP is designed to involve local researchers who already know the language and much of the cultural context. Such procedures have been developed for many topics, including AIDS, women's health, diarrheal disease, seizure disorders, water and health, and childhood obesity prevention. RAP has become a generic concept, and has been modified for many uses. Modified titles include RARE, ERAP, and FES (focused ethnographic study). In the past 20 years, the RAP methodologies have been embraced by community members, researchers, and funders alike and have been broadly used in community participatory research.

The case study on the use of focused ethnographic methods to assess the feasibility of introducing a fortified infant cereal in an African country, which appears in the next section of this chapter, is a good example of the use and value of this approach. With a relatively small number of interviews, researchers were able to establish that the cereal as constituted and packaged would be unlikely to succeed. Minor modifications (i.e., a cereal that did not require cooking and was packaged in small amounts) were recommended to change the product's likely acceptability.

In community participatory research, community members become involved in the design, conduct, and interpretation of research. This approach has been used most often for health intervention and behavior change programs where community acceptance of such interventions and programs is essential for success. It also has been found to increase the validity (accuracy) of the data, as community members are invested in developing programs that work.

A final comment on methodology is that as the social sciences are increasingly combining methodologies and sharing each other's tools, it is also important to share theoretical approaches. Where methodology is concerned, this leads to using multilevel approaches to research, in which environment, biological factors, cognitive issues, societal and cultural context, and political and economic forces all can contribute to the analyses. This should take place at least to the extent that an examination is made of data one step above and one step below the phenomenon being explained (Rubenstein et al., 2000).

An example of a logic framework using this approach can be found in the work of the Centers for Disease Control and Prevention task force that has been developing *Guide to Community Preventative Services*—a series of evidence-based recommendations for community public health practice based on a systematic and critical review of the evidence. Topics considered in the guide include major risk behaviors (e.g., tobacco use, alcohol abuse and misuse, other substance abuse, nutrition, physical activity, healthy sexual behavior), specific illnesses (e.g., cancer, diabetes), and one overarching topic, the sociocultural environment. Figure 2-2 presents the logic framework for this topic. The outcomes of community health (on the right side of the figure) stem from factors in the physical environment and societal resources; outcomes related to equity and social justice issues derive from factors on the left side of the figure. The immediate outcomes, which are listed in the middle of the figure, range from neighborhood living conditions to prevailing community norms to prevention and healthcare (Anderson, Fielding, et al., 2003; Anderson, Scrimshaw, et al., 2003). This approach greatly broadens the context for understanding and addressing the health of individuals and of communities.

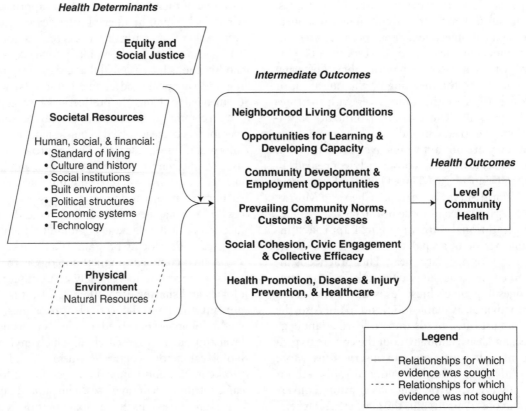

Figure 2-2 The *Guide to Community Preventive Service's* Social Environment and Health Model. *Source:* L. M. Anderson, S. C. Scrimshaw, M. T. Fuillilove, et al., "The Community Guide's Model for Linking the Social Environment to Health," 2003, *American Journal of Preventive Medicine, 24*(35), p. 13. Reprinted with permission.

The CDC Community Guide can be accessed through the following website: www.thecommunity guide.org. That website and related publications listed there provide evidence-based guidelines for improving community health, many of which have global relevance.

Case Study: Use of a Focused Ethnographic Study to Assess the Acceptability of a Fortified Infant Cereal in Africa*

Earlier in this chapter, qualitative methods derived largely from anthropology were described as being important tools for ascertaining cultural facilitators and impediments to behavior changes that lead to improved health. As discussed then, these tools have been adapted for use in rapid assessment. This case study involves a rapid (focused) ethnographic study that was conducted before a new infant cereal was introduced to assess the potential success of this cereal by investigating household and local market behaviors.

Many infants and young children (IYC) in Africa continue to suffer from malnutrition or undernutrition. Where mothers breastfeed exclusively for at least six months, quality foods that complement the nutrients in human milk are important after six months when human milk alone is not adequate to meet nutritional needs.

In one African country, a project was devised to introduce a fortified cereal-based food that could help contribute to improved nutrition for infants and children consuming it. The aim of the focused ethnographic study was to determine whether families would purchase the food if available and, if the product was purchased, who actually consumed it. Why each of these steps did or did not occur was also im-

---

*This case study is based on Pelto, G. H., & Armar-Klemesu, M. (2010). *Focused ethnographic study to assess the potential of a commercial complementary food.* Report prepared for the Global Alliance for Improved Nutrition, Geneva, Switzerland.

portant to assess. The price of the product was pegged at the amount that most urban families, even the poor, could afford to spend per day for a cereal.

It was important to the researchers to make the study framework broad enough to include key variables, so that they could avoid mistakes made by intervention projects that fail to take important cultural, economic, access, and other factors into account. A household perspective was chosen because the purchase and preparation of the cereal would be done at the household level.

Research questions included the following items:

- How much are households currently spending on food for their infants?

- Are their current expenditures providing a nutritionally adequate diet?

- Do households that are spending less than x amount (e.g., cents/day) have the potential to shift their expenditures?

- Which other factors determine household buying and/or preparation of foods for the infant or young child, and would these other factors interfere with making a switch, even if the family could afford it monetarily?

It was also important to take into account the possible foods for infants and young children in this environment: (1) human milk, (2) home-prepared foods that are made for family members and are also given to the infant or young child, (3) home-prepared foods that are made exclusively for the IYC, (4) commercial products that are marketed and purchased for household consumption, (5) commercial products that are marketed and purchased exclusively for the infant or young child, and (6) commercial products that are marketed for household consumption, but are purchased exclusively for the infant or young child.

The focused ethnographic study interviewed key informants—people who had personal knowledge and experience in an area of concern to the project. Four different techniques were used:

1. Free listing exercises. The respondent is asked a question or set of questions that elicit a series of items (objects, events, issues) pertaining to a particular cultural domain. For example, one can ask, "What are all the different places where one can get food for infants or young children?"

2. Open-ended interviewing, with guiding questions. In open-ended questions, the interviewer writes down what the respondent says in response to a question without using precoding. Questions can be broad or narrow—for example, "How do you prepare cereal for your baby?"

3. Rating and ranking exercises. Respondents are asked to rate and rank items such as foods and sources of health care. Methods include handing respondents cards with pictures of objects to be ranked and asking them to arrange these from most to least important, as well as asking them to assign the card to a slot along a continuum. (A similar technique for the latter method is the familiar scale of perceived pain.)

4. Mapping exercises. Respondents create visual maps on which they indicate the locations of specific features of concern for the researcher, such as places to obtain commercial foods.

In this case study, there were two main types of key informant-respondents: (1) women who gave information from the perspective of people who take care of children and (2) people who gave information from the perspective of marketing infant and young child foods. Thirty primary care givers, 10 alternate caregivers, and 12 sellers of these foods were interviewed. The sellers were divided into street venders and keepers of small shops.

The results of the study provided evidence to answer the key question about the potential acceptability of a new fortified cereal for infants and young children. They revealed that fortified cereals are, indeed, used and accepted, and that a relatively high proportion of the food budget for households with infants is spent on these items. Thus the key question about a dietary niche for a fortified cereal was answered affirmatively.

Importantly, the study also uncovered the reality that a food that must be cooked, however briefly, is *unlikely* to be chosen over instant foods that do not require cooking. Busy mothers will spend more money to purchase prepared cooked cereals from street vendor or buy small packets of instant cereal that can be mixed with water rather than cooking a cereal themselves. This was extremely important guidance, as it showed that the cereal planned for introduction would need to be modified so that it would not require cooking if it was to be a success.

Because families were already spending so much for these foods, there was clearly a niche for a lower-cost fortified cereal, but it must be instant and available in small packets to be financially available. The findings of this study were valuable in planning a program to introduce the cereal, providing the guidance healthcare practitioners needed to proceed with an appropriately modified product, and avoid spending time and money on something that will not work.

Case Study: The Slim Disease— HIV/AIDS in Sub-Saharan Africa*

AIDS changed the way in which epidemiologic and behavioral research is conducted and health interventions designed and carried out. This case study illustrates virtually all the topics covered in this chapter.

Epidemiology

As of 2008, 33.4 million adults and children were living with HIV/AIDS worldwide (UNAIDS, 2009). Nearly half (15.7 million) were women, and 2.1 million were children. Of the 33.4 million persons with HIV/AIDS, 22.4 million reside in sub-Saharan Africa, where 1.8 million children younger than age 15 are infected and 1.4 million adults and children younger than 15 died in 2008. An estimated 1.9 million people in this region became infected in 2008, down from 2.1 million people infected in 2004. Infection rates have decreased by 17% in the past eight years, as a result of a combination of aggressive use of antiretroviral therapies and prevention strategies (World Health Organization [WHO], http://www.who.int/hiv/en/, June 2010).

Unlike in the Western world, where AIDS has been largely associated with gay men and injection-drug users, in Africa the most common route of transmission is through heterosexual sex. A husband often infects his wife as a result of his involvement with other partners. A pregnant, HIV-positive woman may transmit the virus to her fetus through the placenta or to her infant through breastfeeding

Generally, AIDS patients in Africa suffer from intestinal infections, skin disease, tuberculosis, herpes zoster, and meningitis. In the industrialized countries, AIDS is associated with Kaposi's sarcoma (a skin cancer), meningitis, and pneumonia.

Why does the same disease spread so differently from one region of the world to another? History, politics, economics, and cultural and social environments influence the course of a disease in a society. In the case of Africa, traditional family, social, and environmental structures were disrupted by European colonization, which imposed changes on the existing culture. Even after countries became independent from Europe, their political, ecological, and economic structures remained disrupted and often unstable. Many of these factors contribute to an environment in which AIDS easily took hold (Akeroyd, 1997; Bond et al., 1997; Hunt, 1989; Madut Jok, 2001). These factors and their association with the AIDS pandemic are described in the following subsections. In addition to illustrating the relationship between cultural norms, prevention and healthcare access, and disease, this case study demonstrates the profound relationship between the general sociocultural, political, physical, and economic environment and health.

Risk of AIDS Associated with Migratory Labor

The integral family structure of the African culture has been broken up by the migratory labor system in eastern, central, and southern Africa. The migratory labor system is historically part of the region's industrial development and colonization by European powers. These large industries, which include mining, railroad work, plantation work, and primary production facilities (e.g., oil refineries) have absorbed a massive labor influx from rural areas. Men typically leave their homes and travel outside their communities to work sites for long periods of time. This system has not only kept families apart, but has also increased the numbers of sex partners—in turn, giving rise to a higher prevalence of sexually transmitted infections (STIs) and later AIDS. In many African cultures, regular sex is believed essential to health. Men in the migratory labor system have sex with prostitutes close to their work sites, become infected, and eventually return home and infect their wives, whose babies may in turn become infected (Hunt, 1989; Salopek, 2000).

War

In 2008, there were 28 major armed conflicts globally, 11 of which occurred in Africa. A country at war typically faces a weakening of its political system, and this situation in Africa has intensified the impact of the AIDS epidemic. Several populations become more vulnerable to HIV/AIDS during wartime, including those affected by food emergencies and scarcity, displaced persons, and refugees. Women are especially at risk. They are six times more likely to contract HIV in refugee camps than populations that reside outside such camps. In addition, women are often victims of rape as a weapon of war by the enemy side. Armed forces and the commercial sex workers soldiers interact with are also affected by the epidemic

---

*This case study was developed by Isabel Martinez, MPH.

(Akeroyd, 1997; Carballo & Siem, 1996; Madut Jok, 2001; UNAIDS, 1999; United Nations, 1999a; Uppsala Conflict Data Program, 2008; Wallensteen & Harbom, 2009).

Gender Roles and Cultural Traditions

The African woman's struggle with the AIDS pandemic has been depicted often in the literature (Akeroyd, 1997; Carballo & Siem, 1996; Hunt, 1989; Messersmith, 1991; Salopek, 2000; UNAIDS, 1999; Watkins, 2004). The risk to women from husbands or partners returning from work in other areas has already been discussed. Another risk—sex work or prostitution by women as a means of survival—is now almost a death sentence in Africa, considering the great risk of contracting HIV/AIDS through such employment. There are many reasons why some African women find the need to engage in sex work, although studies have linked most of these reasons to a political economy context. Sex in exchange for favors, material goods, or money is conducted in all socioeconomic levels, from female entrepreneurs in foreign trade having to use sexual ploys to ensure business to impoverished young women needing money to support themselves and their families (Swidler & Watkins, 2007). Even if women in sex work are knowledgeable about preventing HIV infection through use of condoms, their cost, availability, and resistance of some males to use them raise barriers for the safety of these women and play a part in further transmission of the disease (Akeroyd, 1997; Messersmith, 1991).

Having multiple sexual partners has increasingly been implicated in raising the risk for HIV for both men and women (Helleringer et al., 2009). Called "concurrency," these practices are now a major focus of intervention efforts (Shelton, 2009).

Other cultural factors that place young women at greater risk for HIV infection include a superstition in some areas that having sex with a virgin will cure an HIV-infected man, and the practice of female circumcision. In both of these circumstances, the risk of contracting HIV through sex or infected surgical instruments increases for adolescents (Akeroyd, 1997; Salopek, 2000).

Additional Cultural Beliefs

Secrecy regarding HIV/AIDS is common within regions of the sub-Saharan culture. Denying that AIDS is affecting one's community or that one is infected increases the chances that the virus will be transmitted to other people because preventive actions are not taken (Akeroyd, 1997; Salopek, 2000; UNAIDS,

1999; United Nations, 1999d). Preventive actions go beyond preventing sexual transmission, to include concerns about transmission during treatment of ill individuals and during funeral practices.

In some parts of Africa, AIDS is referred to as the "slim disease" because of the wasting away that occurs as a result of the infections. Because of this belief, men prefer sex with plump women, believing that they are not infected. AIDS is called "white man's disease" in Gabon and "that other thing" in Zimbabwe. HIV and AIDS are a source of shame and denial in these African cultures. AIDS is also considered a punishment for overindulgence of the body. One *sangoma* (faith healer), who has helped revive an ancient Zulu custom of virginity testing of young girls, supported her belief in reviving this custom by saying, "We have adopted too many Western things without thinking, and we lost respect for our bodies. This has allowed things like AIDS to come torture us" (Akeroyd, 1997; Hunt, 1989; Salopek, 2000; UNAIDS, 1999).

Barriers to Prevention or Treatment of HIV/AIDS

Barriers to prevention of HIV/AIDS include lack of financial resources and allocation of funds to projects that might be less crucial than those related to health. For example, a foreign country funded a multimillion-dollar hospital in Zambia, even though the rural clinics where the majority of the population live are often not even stocked with aspirin (Bartholet, 2000; Salopek, 2000).

Changing people's health behavior and addressing cultural beliefs has also been a tough challenge when it comes to prevention efforts. Promoting safe sex and the use of contraception, and abstaining from some cultural rituals can be perceived as changing traditional gender roles for both men and women, and may go against some religious values that are part of the core for some communities. The need to hide or look away from the problem of HIV/AIDS stems from the disgrace attached to the disease, which makes it difficult for people even to discuss it, much less be tested for this infection. The stigma of HIV/AIDS needs to be removed for prevention efforts to be more widely accepted by the African people (Akeroyd, 1997; Bartholet, 2000; *Newsweek*, 2000; Salopek, 2000; UNAIDS, 1999; United Nations, 1999c).

One project in Ghana used both the health belief model and social learning theory to examine the determinants of condom use to prevent HIV infection among youth. The authors of the study found that perceived barriers significantly interacted with perceived susceptibility and self-efficacy. Youth who perceived a high level of susceptibility to HIV infection and a low level of barriers to condom use were almost six times as likely to have used condoms at last intercourse. A high level of perceived self-efficacy and a low level of perceived barriers increased the likelihood of use three times (Adih & Alexander, 1999).

Prevention Efforts by Community and Governmental Agencies and Nongovernmental Organizations

In the 1990s, Uganda and Senegal reduced their HIV infection rates through aggressive public education and condom promotion campaigns, expanded treatment programs for other STIs, mobilization of nongovernmental organizations (NGOs), and reduction of stigma for people with HIV/AIDS. Health officials believe the education efforts surrounding AIDS have contributed to women choosing to remain virgins longer and increased condom use among sex workers and men and women who have casual sex (*Newsweek*, 2000; UNAIDS, 1999; United Nations, 1999a).

The theory of self-efficacy has proved useful in addressing AIDS. For example, one study in South Africa found that knowledge of risk and its prevention was important, but not sufficient to change behavior. The authors stress the need to improve personal autonomy in decision making about sexual behavior and condom use for both men and women through skills development programs that promote self-efficacy (Reddy et al., 1999).

The United Nations and its specialized agencies have created major programs to assist countries and communities in prevention efforts, including joining forces to accelerate the development of experimental vaccines. Academic institutions have also teamed up with local community and church organizations to create prevention projects and help organize the communities to reach more of the public. These efforts have assisted in empowering many volunteers, mostly women, to motivate others in their communities through education and increasing women's negotiation skills for safe sex or condom use (Msiza-Makhubu, 1997; United Nations, 1999d; WHO, 1997).

There is also a growing movement of doctors in Africa working with traditional healers to do outreach and education on AIDS. As discussed earlier, traditional healers have better access to many populations. People seek their help because of tradition and lack of adequate health care (Associated Press, 2000; Green, 1994).

Antiretroviral Therapy

Donor agencies/organizations such as the Global Fund to Fight AIDS, TB and Malaria; the U.S. President's Plan for AIDS Relief; the World Bank; the European Commission; WHO; and the Gates Foundation have aggressively provided testing and antiretroviral (ARV) therapy during the past eight years, and infection rates have come down (UNAIDS, 2004a; WHO, 2004).

Innovative prevention programs such as the introduction of male circumcision in areas where it had not been practiced are helping to reduce infection rates. Male circumcision has been found to help protect against infection, reducing transmission rates by as much as 60% (Bailey & Mehta, 2009; Bailey et al., 2007; Tobian et al., 2009; Westercamp & Bailey, 2007).

Antiretroviral Treatment Challenges

Diminished political and economic support for antiretroviral programs could lead to the interruption of treatment of HIV/AIDS patients, which in turn would provide the HIV virus with the potential to become drug resistant. Other challenges include the shortage in Africa of health professionals, many of whom have left their home countries for better opportunities in higher-income countries. In addition, a lack of treatment literacy poses a huge challenge for effective antiretroviral treatment (UNAIDS, 2004b).

The individual behaviors that place people at risk are part of the larger root causes of the problem in Africa, including colonialism, big industry's design of mass labor migration, poverty, gender inequalities, and war. The ideal prevention and intervention strategies would address health behavior changes as well as economic and community barriers to the provision of social services and treatment options (Akeroyd, 1997; Bond et al., 1997; Tylor, 1871; United Nations, 1999c, 1999d; WHO, 1997).

Conclusion

This chapter has briefly explored cultural and behavioral issues that influence global public health. Anthropology, sociology, and psychology have much greater depth in both method and theory than can be described in this chapter, of course. A rich and extensive literature exists on health beliefs and behaviors, environmental and biological contexts, health systems, and programmatic successes and failures. It is essential to take these factors into account in considering global public health work. In addition, a program must consider structural factors, such as setting, hours, child care, and ambience, as well as factors of content, such as culturally acceptable services, which includes providers who treat patients with respect and understanding.

Research and preventive services regarding health beliefs and behaviors must accept and integrate concepts different from those held by Western biomedicine, by middle- or upper-class healthcare providers, or by healthcare providers from an ethnic or cultural group that is different from their patients. This requirement demands the ability inherent in some of the anthropological methods and approaches discussed earlier—that is, the ability to "get into someone's head" and understand things from an insider perspective. There is nothing like the experience of spending time with people, in their own homes or community, and striving to reach that insider understanding.

Acknowledgments

I would like to thank Carolyn Cline, Rose Grignon, and Lisa Brainard for their assistance in editing and preparing the bibliography, Pamela Ippoliti for her editorial assistance, Susan Levy and John Justino for providing key examples from the intervention literature, and Isabel Martinez and Janel Heinrich for their assistance with the literature search, for helpful comments on the chapter, and, in particular, for preparing and revising the case study on AIDS. I am also grateful to Carole Chrvala for sharing notes on the various intervention theories. In addition, I would like to thank and acknowledge Professor Gretel Pelto and Dr. Margaret Armar-Klemesu for permission to base the case study on the introduction of a fortified infant cereal on one of their recent projects.

• • • Discussion Questions

1. Which prevention strategies for AIDS would you develop if you were the minister of health of a sub-Saharan African country? Which strategies would you use if you were a community leader? Would the strategies used for these two perspectives differ? If so, how? How would you address some of the cultural beliefs or traditions associated with HIV/AIDS mentioned in the case study?

2. If you were entering a community to introduce a health program, who would you talk to? What would you ask? Why?

3. Discuss the concepts of validity and reliability in research as they apply to the use of quantitative and qualitative methods. Next, discuss the same concepts as they apply to community participatory research.

4. What is the hot/cold illness belief system? Why is it important? How would you incorporate it into a maternal and child health program?

5. Many people believe that healers such as midwives and shamans are called to their profession by a greater spiritual power. What significance does this belief have for official health programs around the world? How should they address this belief?

6. If an indigenous practice seems peculiar to you, but does no apparent harm, what should you do?

7. How could you learn what people in a community really believe about health and illness?

8. Based on the theories of behavior change, create your own model by taking what you think is the best content from existing theories. Explain your reasoning.

• • • References

Abdullah, A., & Husten, C. (2004). Promotion of smoking cessation in developing countries: A framework for urgent public health interventions. *Thorax, 59*, 623–630.

Adams, R. N. (1955). A nutritional research program in Guatemala. In B. D. Paul (Ed.), *Health, culture, & community* (pp. 435–458). New York: Russell Sage Foundation.

Adih, W. K., & Alexander, C. S. (1999). Determinants of condom use to prevent HIV infection among youth in Ghana. *Journal of Adolescent Health, 24*(1), 63–72.

Africa matters: Interview with U.S. ambassador to the United Nations, Richard Holbrooke. (2000, January 17). *Newsweek* (U.S. Edition: International).

Ajzen, I., & Fishbein, M. (1972). Attitudes and normative beliefs as factors influencing behavioral intentions. *Journal of Personality and Social Psychology, 21*(1), 1–9.

Akeroyd, A. V. (1997). Sociocultural aspects of AIDS in Africa: Occupational and gender issues. In G. C. Bond, J. Kreniske, I. Susser, & J. Vincent (Eds.), *AIDS in Africa and the Caribbean*, 11–32. Boulder, CO: Westview Press.

Alland, A. (1970). *Adaptation in cultural evolution: An approach to medical anthropology*. New York: Columbia University Press.

Anderson, L. M., Fielding, J. E., Fullilove, M. T., Scrimshaw, S. C., Carande-Kulis, V. G., & Task Force on Community Preventive Services. (2003, April). Methods for conducting systematic reviews of the evidence of effectiveness and economic efficiency of interventions to promote healthy social environments. *American Journal of Preventive Medicine, 24*(3S), 25–31.

Anderson, L. M., Scrimshaw, S. C., Fullilove, M. T., Fielding, J. E., & Task Force on Community Preventive Services. (2003, April). The community guide's model for linking the social environment to health. *American Journal of Preventive Medicine, 24*(3S), 12–20.

Associated Press. (2000, February 8). Conference stress uses for traditional healers in AIDS battle.

InteliHealth. Retrieved from www.intelihealth.com/IH/ihtIH/EMIHc000/333/333/268121.html

Baer, H. (2008). The emergence of integrative medicine in Australia: The growing interest of biomedicine and nursing in complementary medicine in a southern developed society. *Medical Anthropology Quarterly, 22*(1), 52–66.

Bailey, R. C., & Mehta, S. (2009). Circumcision's place in the vicious cycle between HSV-2 and HIV. *Journal of Infectious Diseases, 199*, 923–925.

Bailey, R. C., Moses, S., Parker, C. B., Agot, K., Maclean, I., Krieger, J. N., et al. (2007). Male circumcision for HIV prevention in young men in Kisumu, Kenya: A randomised controlled trial. *Lancet, 369*, 643–656.

Bandura, A. (1977). *Social learning theory*. Englewood Cliffs, NJ: Prentice Hall.

Bandura, A. (1989). Human agency in social cognitive theory. *American Psychologist, 44*, 1175–1184.

Bartholet, J. (2000, January 17). The plague years. *Newsweek, 135*(3).

Beals, A. R. (1976). Strategies of resort to curers in south India. In C. Leslie (Ed.), *Asian medical systems: A comparative study* (pp. 184–200). Berkeley, CA: University of California Press.

Bernard, R. (2006). *Research methods in anthropology: Qualitative and quantitative approaches* (4th ed.). Lanthan, MD: Altamira Press.

Betancourt, J. R., Green, A. R., & Carrillo, J. E. (2002). *Cultural competence in health care: Emerging frameworks and practical approaches*. New York: Commonwealth Fund.

Bhuyan, K. (2004). Health promotion through self-care and community participation: Elements of a proposed programme in the development countries. *BMC Public Health, 4*, 11. Retrieved from http://www.biomedcentral.com/1471-2458/4/11.

Board on Neuroscience and Behavioral Health, Institute of Medicine. (2002), *Committee on Communication for Behavior Change in the 21st Century: Improving the health of diverse populations. Speaking of health: Assessing health commu-*

nication strategies for diverse populations. Washington, DC: National Academy Press.

Bond, G. C., Kreniske, J., Susser, I., & Vincent, J. (1997). The anthropology of AIDS in Africa and the Caribbean. In G. C. Bond, J. Kreniske, I. Susser, & J. Vincent (Eds.), *AIDS in Africa and the Caribbean* (pp. 3–9). Boulder, CO: Westview Press.

Booth, R., & Wiebel, W. (1992). Effectiveness of reducing needle related risk for HIV through indigenous outreach to injection drug users. *American Journal of Addictions, 1,* 227–287.

Buckley, T., & Gottlieb, A. (Eds.). (1988). *Blood magic.* Berkeley, CA: University of California Press.

Cameron, M. (2010). Feminization and marginalization? Women Ayurvedic doctors and modernizing health care in Nepal. *Medical Anthropology Quarterly, 24*(1), 42–63.

Carballo, M., & Siem, H. (1996). Migration, migration policy and AIDS. In M. Knipe & R. Rector (Eds.), *Crossing borders: Migration, ethnicity and AIDS* (pp. 31–48). London: Taylor and Francis.

Chambers, R. (1992). Rapid but relaxed and particularly rural appraisal: Towards applications in health and nutrition. In N. S. Scrimshaw & G. R. Gleason (Eds.), *Rapid assessment procedures: Qualitative methodologies for planning and evaluation of health related programmes* (pp. 295–305). Boston: International Nutrition Foundation for Developing Countries.

Chen, K.-H., & Murray, G. F. (1976). Truths and untruths in village Haiti: An experiment in Third World survey research. In J. F. Marshall & S. Polgar (Eds.), *Culture, natality, and family planning* (pp. 241–262). Chapel Hill, NC: Carolina Population Center.

Committee on Health Literacy, Board on Neuroscience and Behavioral Health. (2004). *Health literacy: A prescription to end confusion.* Ed. by L. Nielsen-Bohlman, A. M. Panzer, & D. Kindig. Washington, DC: National Academies Press.

Crisp, Lord Nigel. (2010). Turning the world upside down: The search for global health in the 21st century. London: Hodder Education.

Dickson-Gomez, J. (2010). Structural factors influencing the patterns of drug selling and use and HIV risk in the San Salvador metropolitan area. *Medical Anthropology Quarterly, 24*(2), 157–181.

Fadiman, A. (1997). *A spirit catches you and you fall down: A Hmong child, her American doctors, and the collision of two cultures.* New York: Farrar, Straus, and Giroux.

Foster, G. M. (1953). Relationships between Spanish and Spanish-American folk medicine. *Journal of American Folklore, 66,* 201–17.

Freed, S. A., & Freed, R. S. (1967). Spirit possession as illness in a north Indian village. In J. Middleton (Ed.), *Magic, witchcraft, and curing* (pp. 295–320). Garden City, NY: Natural History Press.

Gadjusek, D. C., Gibbs, C. J., & Alpers, M. (1967). Transmission and passage of experimental "kuru" to chimpanzees. *Science, 155,* 212–214.

Garro, L. (2000). Remembering what one knows and the construction of the past: A comparison of cultural consensus theory and cultural schema theory. *Ethos, 28,* 275–319.

Ghimire, M., Pradhan, Y. V., & Mahesh, M. K. (2010). Community-based interventions for diarrhoeal diseases and acute respiratory infections in Nepal. *Bulletin of the World Health Organization, 88,* 216–221.

Good, B. J., & Good, M. J. D. (1981). The meaning of symptoms: A cultural hermeneutic model for clinical practice. In L. Eisenberg & A. Kleinman (Eds.), *The relevance of social science for medicine* (pp. 165–196). Dordrecht, Netherlands: Reidel.

Green, E. (1994). *AIDS and STDs in Africa: Bridging the gap between traditional healing and modern medicine.* Boulder, CO: Westview Press.

Green, L., Kreuter, M., Deeds, S., & Partridge, K. (1980). *Health education planning: A diagnostic approach.* Palo Alto, CA: Mayfield.

Guarnaccia, P. J., Lewis-Fernandez, R., Martinez Pincay, I., Shrout, P., Guo, J., Torres, M., et al. (2010, May 1). Ataque de nervios as a marker of social and psychiatric vulnerability: Results from the NLAAS. *International Journal of Social Psychiatry, 56*(3), 298–309.

Gwaltney, J. L. (1970). *The thrice shy.* New York: Columbia University Press.

Helleringer, S., Kohlerb, H., & Kalilani-Phiric, L. (2009). The association of HIV serodiscordance and partnership concurrency in Likoma Island (Malawi). *AIDS, 23,* 1285–1290.

Hjelm, K., Nyberg, P., Isacsson, A., & Apelqvist, J. (1999). Beliefs about health and illness essential for self-care practice: A comparison of migrant Yugoslavian and Swedish diabetic females. *Journal of Advanced Nursing, 30*(5), 1147–1159.

Hughes, C. (1990). Ethnopsychiatry. In T. M. Johnson & C. E. Sargent (Eds.), *Medical anthropology: Contemporary theory and method.* (p. 131). New York: Praeger.

Hunt, C. W. (1989). Migration labor and sexually transmitted diseases: AIDS in Africa. *Journal of Health in Social Science Behavior, 30,* 353–373.

Kamat, V. R. (2008). Dying under the bird's shadow: Narrative representations of *degedege* and child survival among the Zaramo of Tanzania. *Medical Anthropology Quarterly, 22*(1), 67–93.

Kendall, C., Foote, D., & Martorell, R. (1983). Anthropology, communications, and health: The mass media and health practices program in Honduras. *Human Organization, 42,* 353–360.

Kleinman, A. (1980). *Patients and healers in the context of culture.* Berkeley, CA: University of California Press.

Kleinman, A. (1986). *Social origins of distress and disease.* New Haven, CT: Yale University Press.

Kleinman, A. (1988). *The illness narratives.* New York: Basic Books.

Lindenbaum, S. (1971). Sorcery and structure in fore society. *Oceania, 41,* 277–287.

Logan, M. H. (1972). Humoral folk medicine: A potential aid in controlling pellagra in Mexico. *Ethnomedizin, 4,* 397–410.

Madut Jok, J. (2001). *War and slavery in Sudan.* Ethnography of Political Violence Series. Philadelphia: University of Pennsylvania Press.

Martiniuk, A., O'Connor, K., King, W. (2003). A cluster randomized trial of a sex education programme in Belize, Central America. *International Journal of Epidemiology, 32,* 131–136.

Mattingly, Cheryl & Garro, Linda, Eds. (2000) *Narrative and the Cultural Construction of Illness and Healing.* Berkeley, CA: University of California Press.

Matsudo, V., Matsudo, S., Andrade, D., Araujo, T., Andrade, E., de Oliveira, L., et al. (2002). Promotion of physical activity in a developing country: The Agita São Paulo experience. *Public Health Nutrition. 5*(1A), 253–61.

McSweeney, J. C., Allan, J. D., & Mayo, K. (1997). Exploring the use of explanatory models in nursing research and practice. *Image Journal of Nursing Scholarship, 29*(3), 243–248.

Messersmith, L. J. (1991). *The women of good times and Baba's Place: The multi-dimensionality of the lives of commercial sex workers in Bamako, Mali.* PhD dissertation, University of California at Los Angeles.

Msiza-Makhubu, S. B. (1997). *Peer education and support for AIDS prevention among women in South Africa.* PhD dissertation, University of Illinois at Chicago.

Murray, G. F. (1976). Women in perdition: Ritual fertility control in Haiti. In J. F. Marshall & S. Polgar (Eds.), *Culture, natality, and family planning* (pp. 59–78). Chapel Hill, NC: Carolina Population Center.

Nichter, M. (2008). *Global health: Why cultural perceptions, social representations and biopolitics matter.* Tucson, AZ: University of Arizona Press.

Norr, K., Norr, J., McElmurray, B., Tlou, S., & Moeti, M. (2004). Impact of peer group education on HIV prevention among women in Botswana. *Health Care for Women International, 25,* 210–226.

O'Connor, B. (1995). *Healing traditions.* Philadelphia: University of Pennsylvania Press.

Parsons, T. (1948). Illness and the role of the physician. In C. Kluckholm & H. Murray (Eds.), *Personality in nature, society, and culture* (pp. 609–617). New York: Alfred A. Knopf.

Paul, B. D. (Ed.). (1955). *Health, culture, and community.* (p. 1). New York: Russell Sage Foundation.

Pelto, P. J., & Pelto, G. H. (1978). *Anthropological research: The structure of inquiry.* New York: Cambridge University Press.

Perry, H. Shanklin, D., & Schroeder, D. (2003). Impact of a community-based comprehensive primary healthcare programme on infant and child mortality in Bolivia. *Journal of Health, Population, and Nutrition, 21*(4), 383–395.

Polgar, S., & Marshall, J. F. (1976). The search for culturally acceptable fertility regulating methods. In J. F. Marshall & S. Polgar (Eds.), *Culture, natality, and family planning* (pp. 204–218). Chapel Hill, NC: Carolina Population Center.

Prochaska, J., DiClemente, C., & Norcross, J. (1992). In search of how people change: Applications to addictive behaviors. *American Psychologist, 47,* 1102–1104.

Ratzan, S. C., & Parker, R. M. (2000). Introduction. In C. R. Selden, M. Zorn, S. C. Ratzan, & R. M. Parker (Eds.), *National Library of Medicine current bibliographies in medicine: Health literacy.* NLM Pub. No. CBM 2000-1. Bethesda, MD: National Institutes of Health, U.S. Department of Health and Human Services.

Reddy, P., Meyer-Weitz, A., van den Borne, B., & Kok, G. (1999). STD-related knowledge, beliefs and attitudes of Xhosa-speaking patients attending STD primary health-care clinics in South Africa. *International Journal of Sexually Transmitted Diseases and AIDS, 10*(6), 392–400.

Reichel-Dolmatoff, G., & Reichel-Dolmatoff, A. (1961). *The people of Aritama.* London: Routledge and Kegan Paul.

Rekart, M. (2002). Sex in the city: sexual behavior, societal change, and STDs in Saigon. *Sexually Transmitted Infections. 78* (Suppl. I), i47–i54.

Rogers, E. M. (1973). *Communication strategies for family planning.* New York: Free Press.

Rogers, E. M. (1983). *Diffusion of innovations* (3rd ed.). New York: Free Press.

Rogers, E. M., & Shoemaker, F. F. (1972). *Communication of innovations* (2nd ed.). New York: Free Press.

Rosenstock, I., Strecher, V., & Becker, M. (1974). Social learning theory and the health belief model. *Health Education Monograph, 2,* 328–386.

Rubel, A. J., & Haas, M. R. (1990). Ethnomedicine. In T. M. Johnson & C. D. Sargent (Eds.), *Medical anthropology, contemporary theory and method* (pp. 115–131). New York: Praeger.

Rubel, A. J., O'Nell, C. W., & Collado-Ardon, R. (1984). *Susto: A folk illness.* Berkeley, CA: University of California Press.

Rubenstein, R. A., Scrimshaw, S. C., & Morrissey, S. (2000). Classification and process in sociomedical understanding towards a multilevel view of sociomedical methodology. In G. L. Albrecht, R. Fitzpatrick, & S. C. Scrimshaw (Eds.), *The handbook of social studies in health & medicine* (pp. 36–49). London: Sage.

Salem, R. M., Bernstein, J., Sullivan, T. M., & Lande, R. (2008, January). *Communication for better health.* Population Reports, Series J, No. 56, 28 pages. Baltimore, MD: INFO Project, Johns Hopkins Bloomberg School of Public Health.

Salopek, P. (2000, January 10). We die lying to ourselves. Part 2. *Chicago Tribune.*

Schumacher, S. A., Ockene, J. K., & Riekert, K. A. (2009). *The handbook of health behavior change.* New York: Springer.

Scrimshaw, S. C. (1974). *Culture, environment, and family size: A study of urban in-migrants in Guayaquil, Ecuador.* PhD dissertation, Columbia University, New York.

Scrimshaw, S. C. M. (1992). Adaptation of anthropological methodologies to rapid assessment of nutrition and primary health care. In N. S. Scrimshaw & G. R. Gleason (Eds.), *Rapid assessment procedures: Qualitative methodologies for planning and evaluation of health related programmes* (pp. 25–49). Boston: International Nutrition Foundation for Developing Countries.

Scrimshaw, S. C. M., Carballo, M., Carael, M., Ramos, L., & Parker, R. G. (1992). *HIV/AIDS rapid assessment procedures: Rapid anthropological approaches for studying AIDS related beliefs, attitudes and behaviours*. Monograph. Tokyo: United Nations University.

Scrimshaw, S. C. M., Carballo, M., Ramos, L., & Blair, B. A. (1991). The AIDS rapid anthropological assessment procedures: A tool for health education planning and evaluation. *Health Education Quarterly, 18*(1), 111–123.

Scrimshaw, S. C., & Hurtado, E. (1987). *Rapid assessment procedures for nutrition and primary health care: Anthropological approaches to improving program effectiveness (RAP)*. Tokyo: United Nations University.

Scrimshaw, S. C., & Hurtado, E. (1988). Anthropological involvement in the Central American diarrheal disease control project. *Social Science and Medicine, 27*(1), 97–105.

Scrimshaw, S. C., & Pasquariella, B. G. (1970). Obstacles to sterilization in one community. *Family Planning Perspectives, 2*(4), 40–42.

Shelton, J. (2009, August 1). Why multiple sexual partners? *Lancet, 374,* 367–368.

Simons, R. C. (2001, November 1). Introduction to culture-bound syndromes. *Psychiatric Times, 18*(11).

Simons, R. C., & Hughes, C. C. (Eds.). (1985). *The culture-bound syndromes: Folk illnesses of psychiatric and anthropological interest*. Dordrecht, Netherlands: D. Reidel.

Sutton, S., McVey, D., & Glanz, A. (1999). A comparative test of the theory of reasoned action and the theory of planned behavior in the prediction of condom use intentions in a national sample of English young people. *Health Psychology, 18*(1), 72–81.

Swidler, A., & Watkins, S. C. (2007). AIDS and transactional sex in rural Malawi. *Studies in Family Planning, 38*(3), 147–162.

Thao, X. (1986). Hmong perception of illness and traditional ways of healing. In G. L. Hendricks, B. T. Downing, & A. Deinard (Eds.), *The Hmong in transition* (pp. 365–378). New York: Center for Migration Studies of New York & Southeast Asian Refugee Studies Project of the University of Minnesota.

Thevos, A. K., Quick, R. E., & Yanduli, V. (2000). Motivational interviewing enhances the adoption of water disinfection practices in Zambia. *Health Promotion International, 15*(3) 207–214.

Tobian, A., Serwadda, D., Quinn, T., Kigozi, G., Gravitt, P., Laeyendecker, O., et al. (2009, March 26). Male circumcision for the prevention of HSV2 and HPV infections and syphilis. *New England Journal of Medicine, 360*(13), 1298–1309.

Topley, M. (1976). Chinese traditional etiology and methods of cure in Hong Kong. In C. Leslie (Ed.), *Asian medical systems: A comparative study* (pp. 243–265). Berkeley, CA: University of California Press.

Tylor, E. B. (1871). *Primitive culture*. London: J. Murray.

UNAIDS. (1999). *AIDS epidemic update: December 1999*. Geneva, Switzerland: World Health Organization.

UNAIDS. (2004a). *2004 report on the global HIV/AIDS epidemic: 4th global report*. Geneva, Switzerland: Author. Retrieved from http://www.unaids.org/bangkok2004/GAR2004_html/GAR2004_00_en.htm

UNAIDS. (2004b). *AIDS epidemic update: 2004*. Geneva, Switzerland: Author. Retrieved from http://www.unaids.org/wad2004/EPI update2004_html_en/epi04_00_en.htm

UNAIDS. (2009). *AIDS epidemic update December 2009*. Geneva, Switzerland: Joint United Nations Programme on HIV/AIDS.

United Nations. (1999a). *Acting early to prevent AIDS: The case of Senegal*. UNAIDS.

United Nations. (May 6–8, 1999b). HIV/AIDS in Africa: Socio-economic impact and response. Joint conference of African ministers of finance and ministers of economic development and planning, Addis-Ababa, Ethiopia. Retrieved from http://www.unaids.org/publications/graphics/addis/sld001.htm

United Nations. (June 1999c). *Sexual behavioral change for HIV: Where have the theories taken us?* UNAIDS, 199.27E (English original, text by Rachel King).

United Nations, Wellcome Trust Centre for the Epidemiology of Infectious Disease. (1999d). *Trends in HIV incidence and prevalence: Natural course of the epidemic or results of behavioral change?* UNAIDS.

Uppsala Conflict Data Program. (n.d.). UCDP database, Uppsala University. Retrieved July 8, 2010, from www.ucdp.uu.se/database

Wallensteen, P., & Harbom, L. (2009). Armed conflict, 1946–2008. Department of Peace and Conflict Research. *Harbom Journal of Peace Research, 46*(4), 577–587.

Watkins, S. C. (2004, December). Navigating the AIDS epidemic in rural Malawi. *Population and Development Review, 30*(4), 673–705.

Weir, S.S., Pailman, C., Mahalela, X., Coetzee, N., Meidany, F., & Boerma, J.T. (2003). From people to places: focusing AIDS prevention efforts where it matters most. *AIDS, 17*(6), 895–903.

Weller, S. C. (1983). New data on intracultural variability: The hot–cold concept of medicine and illness. *Human Organization, 42,* 249–257.

Wellin, E. (1955). Water boiling in a Peruvian town. Paul (Ed.), Health, culture, & community. (pp. 71–103). New York: Russell Sage Foundation.

Westercamp, N., & Bailey, R. C. (2007). Acceptability of male circumcision for prevention of HIV/AIDS in sub-Saharan Africa: A review. *AIDS and Behavior, 11*(3), 341–355.

Wiebel, W. (1993). *The indigenous leader outreach model: Intervention manual.* DHHS Publication 93-3581.Washington, DC: National Institute on Drug Abuse, National Institutes of Health, U.S. Department of Health and Human Services.

Wiebel, W., Jimenez, A., Johnson, W., Oulette, L., Jovanovic, B., Lampinen, T., et al. (1996). Risk behavior and HIV seroincidence among out of treatment injection drug users: A four-year prospective study. *Journal of Acquired Immune Deficiency Syndromes and Human Retrovirology, 12,* 282–289.

World Health Organization (WHO). (1997). *Women and HIV/AIDS prevention training manual: Peer education program, a global approach.* Collaborating Centre for International Nursing Development in Primary Health Care Research, Geneva, Switzerland: Author.

World Health Organization (WHO). (2004). *Investing in a comprehensive health sector response to HIV/AIDS: Scaling up treatment and accelerating prevention. WHO HIV/AIDS plan.* Geneva, Switzerland: Author. Retrieved from http://www.who.int/entity/3by5/en/HIV_AIDSplan.pdf

Young, C. J. (1981). *Medical choice in a Mexican village.* New Brunswick, NJ: Rutgers University Press.

Zamen, F., & Underwood, C. (2003). *The gender guide for health communication programs.* Baltimore, MD: Population Communications Services, Center for Communications Programs, Johns Hopkins.

3

The Social Determinants of Health

MICHAEL P. KELLY AND EMMA DOOHAN

Introduction

This chapter provides a comprehensive overview of the empirical and theoretical literature that has described how social, economic, political, legal, and material factors—sometimes collectively called the *social determinants of health*—affect health and cause disease. In dealing with specific aspects of these issues, the chapter draws upon examples from low-income, middle-income, and high-income societies.

The Social Determinants of Health

In 2005, the World Health Organization (WHO) established a Commission on the Social Determinants of Health (CSDH), chaired by Michael Marmot, an eminent epidemiologist based in the United Kingdom (Marmot & Friel, 2008). The CSDH, which published its report in 2008, was heralded in a speech by Lee Jong-Wook, Director General of WHO, at the 57th World Health Assembly meeting on May 17, 2004, in Switzerland:

> We have yet to get to grips with the links between health, equity, and development. The underlying theme of my first year as Director-General is equity and social justice. To support our work in this area, I am setting up a new commission to gather evidence on the social and environmental *causes* [emphasis added] of health inequities, and how to overcome them. The aim is to bring together the knowledge of experts, especially those with practical experience of tackling these problems. This can provide guidance for all our programmes.

The principle behind Lee's speech, and the subsequent work of the CSDH, was that not only is disease a biological process in the human body with immediate and proximal causes, like germs and viruses, but that it also has much broader social origins (Irwin et al., 2006). Thus factors such as poverty and wealth, political systems, the types of housing in which people live, sanitary systems and access to clean water, for example, are directly linked to health and disease. This idea was the guiding principle behind the search for evidence that the CSDH undertook to inform its work.

As part of the CSDH study, eight evidence hubs were established. The areas covered by the evidence hubs were early child development (Irwin et al., 2007), employment conditions (Benach et al., 2007), globalization (Labonte et al., 2008), health systems (Gilson et al., 2007), priority public health conditions (Blas & Sivasankara Kurup, 2008), social exclusion (Popay et al., 2008), urban settings (Kjellstrom, 2007), women and gender equity (Sen et al., 2007), and they were supported by a measurement and evidence hub (Kelly et al., 2007). The reports of the hubs provide the most comprehensive evidence base assembled to date on the broad range of issues and factors involved in the social determinants of health.

A huge amount and range of material have been collected through this effort. Figure 3-1 provides the classification developed some years ago to clarify this evidence. This diagram was originally prepared for the WHO by Dahlgren and Whitehead (1993) as a way of capturing all of the potential wider determinants of health—and that it does. This framework is a useful starting point for the discussion in this chapter and for arranging the information collected to support the CSDH's work.

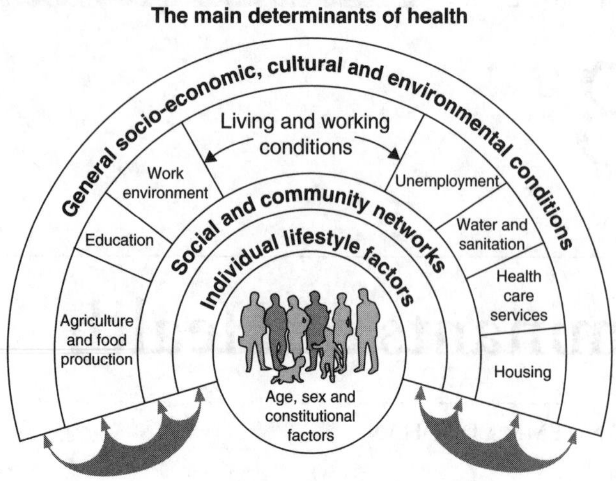

The main determinants of health

Figure 3-1 The Determinants of Health.
Source: Dahlgren, G. and Whitehead, M. (1991), Policies and strategies to promote social equity in health. Stockholm, Sweden Institute for Futures Studies.

The focus of this chapter is not a simple classification of the possible determinants of health, however. Rather, it seeks to explore the underlying causal relationships between the social determinants and health outcomes and their link to health inequity. This is a tricky question scientifically. It is relatively straightforward to imagine how a virus causes a particular disease: The causal pathway from the pathogen to the pathology is biologically familiar and clear. However, while social disadvantage is certainly associated with poor health, precisely how does this linkage work? What is the causal relationship between social, economic, political, and legal factors and disease? What is the relationship between the social determinants and the biological processes in the human body (Boxall & Short, 2006; Galea et al., 2009)? A "black box" metaphor in which somehow the social forces exert an undefined influence is not very precise and, therefore, not much help (Glass & McAtee, 2006).

In his speech to the World Health Assembly, Lee Jook-Wong emphasized his interest in *causes*. The purpose of this chapter is to describe the issues involved and to explore the question of cause. To do so, it develops and uses a conceptual model of the causal pathways from the wider determinants to both individual disease outcomes and population-level patterns of disease (Kelly, 2009, 2010a; Kelly et al., 2009). We return to the issue of cause later in this investigation.

Historical Background: Social Determinants and Health

Whatever the precise causal mechanisms, the social determinants have long been known to produce patterns of disease at the population level. These pat-

terns of disease are not randomly spread across the population, but rather cluster with aspects of social disadvantage (Beaglehole & Bonita, 2008). In the CSDH's final report, the central argument was that social justice, economic systems, and political arrangements are the principal macro determinants of patterns of health and disease within and between societies. This report makes it clear that economic systems, political processes, social structures, and legal arrangements—the macro determinants or social determinants of health—can be as toxic to populations as any viral or bacterial pandemic.

That the broader environment affects health is not a new idea. To both ancient Chinese and ancient Greek medico-philosophical systems, the relationship between disease and the wider social and material environment was a fundamental one. Population-level measures to tackle disease are not new either; in fact, quarantine was practiced as early as 1377 in Marseilles, for example (Etches et al., 2006). Nevertheless, it was not until the nineteenth century that the idea of a relationship between the pattern of disease in the population and the social characteristics of that population was put onto a scientific footing. Both Virchow in Germany (Mackenbach, 2009) and Duncan (Frazer, 1947) in Britain, for example, observed that epidemic prevalence was associated with poor social and economic conditions, with others such as Chadwick, Snow, and Bazalgette making important contributions to this understanding (Webster, 1990).

William Duncan was the first Medical Officer of Health anywhere in Britain. This role meant that he was the physician with responsibility to the local municipality for the health of the public. He was appointed in Liverpool, a port in northern England, which in the nineteenth century was growing quickly as a consequence of the Industrial Revolution and British trade with North America and elsewhere. The city was a focus for immigration from Ireland, Scotland, and the surrounding countryside, as well as a magnet for business, manufacturing, and commerce. Social conditions were extremely bad and the health of the population very poor, with periodic outbreaks of deadly infectious disease sweeping through the city. Duncan gave evidence in Parliament to the Royal Commission on the Health of Towns about what he encountered in Liverpool. In particular, he described the very strong association between patterns of the outbreak of disease and local social conditions (Frazer, 1947).

William Tennant Gairdner was the first Medical Officer of Health in the city of Glasgow, another large port, on the River Clyde in the west of Scotland. In the 1860s, he showed how social, environmental, and economic conditions demonstrated remarkable patterning and argued for the authorities to take seriously the connection between material circumstances and the outbreak of disease (Gairdner, 1862).

These and other public health pioneers described in vivid and sometimes lurid detail the *lifeworlds* of socially disadvantaged people in Victorian Europe. The lethal cocktail of filth, overcrowding, poverty, hunger, drunkenness, and sexual license is graphically and sometimes horrifically described in their reports. These pioneers could not necessarily detect the immediate causal factors—that is, bacteria and viruses—empirically. Nevertheless, they gathered enough other circumstantial evidence to demonstrate the association between poor social conditions and disease.

Their findings shocked Victorian Britain. Comprehensive social and health reforms followed gradually in housing, sanitation, nutrition, and—in due course—education, social welfare, and health care (Briggs, 1959, 1963; Ensor, 1946). The upshot was that over the course of the nineteenth century, the population of Britain became gradually healthier, infant mortality declined, and life expectancy increased. All of these changes took place for the most part in advance of effective medical interventions for treatment of bacterial and viral diseases (McKeown, 1976). These public health medical pioneers, along with the engineers who built the sanitation systems, the reformers who championed the cause of the poor, and the politicians who showed the political will to enact the legislation that made these things possible, are rightly credited with bringing about health improvement on a grand scale (Webster, 1990). These reformers understood the fact that social factors caused disease. They did not know precisely how, but they observed enough to prompt actions that helped to prevent some illnesses, improve infant mortality, virtually eradicate some major infectious diseases, and build a much healthier society. (See Chave, 1958; Checkland & Lamb, 1982; Ferguson, 1948, 1958; Frazer, 1947; Gairdner, 1862; Hamlin, 1995; Mackenbach, 2009; and Webster, 1990 for details especially of the British case.)

It is not surprising, given the degree of biological variation in the population, that we should see differences in health among different individuals. The key point that the Victorian public health or sanitary movement grasped was that some differences in mortality and morbidity are, in principle, preventable. Such prevention is possible because the causes of the patterning of disease arise from the operation of the social determinants, which, as we will see below, are themselves the results of human activities of various kinds, not the results of random biological fluctuation or variation. The cornerstone of the social determinants approach, then, is that the impact of these factors on the lives of people can be ameliorated by various kinds of preventive activity. The desire to act is driven by a view that the patterns of disease that are the result of social factors are unfair and that prevention is a matter of social justice, just as Lee's speech in 2004 noted.

Global Health Inequities

It is helpful to distinguish between health inequity and health inequality when addressing the influence of social determinants of health. The CSDH (2008) defined health *equity* as "the absence of unfair and avoidable or remediable differences in health among social groups" (Solar & Irwin, 2007). This idea is adapted from Whitehead's (1992) definition of health equity. Health inequity is, therefore, considered unfair and avoidable, but potentially amenable to change. Health *inequality* refers simply to differences in health between different individuals; it is seen as primarily the consequence of individual biological differences.

Health inequity is seen as something on which it is possible to act and change because its origins are the consequences—albeit indirectly—of human actions in the first place through the social determinants (Starfield, 2006). Reducing these inequities in health has become a goal of governments across the globe. While differences in wealth or status are accepted—even valued—in some market-driven societies, preventable differences in health status are not. This situation arises because the value placed on health in most societies is unique. The WHO constitution, for example, states that "the enjoyment of the highest attainable standard of health is one of the fundamental rights of every human being" (WHO, 2006a).

Thus a key goal for many governments has been to consider how preventable differences in health might be changed in the future. It is now well accepted from epidemiological research that a macro social approach is likely to bring about the greatest level of improvement in the reduction of health inequities (Putnam & Galea, 2008; Rose, 2008; Woolf et al., 2007).

In contemporary society, the distribution of income, employment, education, and housing is still linked to poor health, just as it was in Victorian times (Braveman, 2003, 2006; Graham, 2000; Starfield, 2007). This is true both within each country and between different countries. As illustrated in Figure 3-2, global patterns of life expectancy vary widely between countries in ways that are associated with different levels of economic development and different forms of social and political organization (Beaglehole & Bonita, 2008).

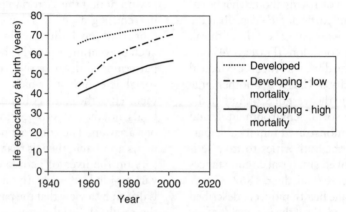

Figure 3-2 Trends in life expectancy at birth 1955–2006.
Source: Beaglehole & Bonita, 2008.

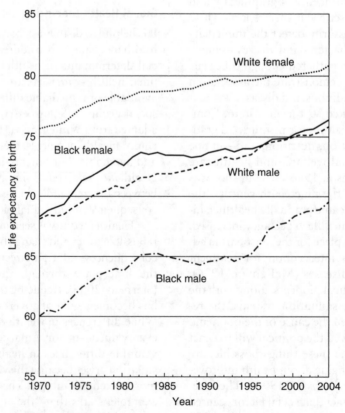

Figure 3-3 Life expectancy at birth by race and sex USA 1970–2004.
Source: CDC Atlanta.

Table 3-1	Infant Mortality in Selected Countries
Place	**Infant Mortality Rate**
Gaza	18.35 deaths per 1,000 live births
Israel	4.22 deaths per 1,000 live births
Tunisia	22.57 deaths per 1,000 live births
Italy	5.51 deaths per 1,000 live births
Portugal	4.78 deaths per 1,000 live births
France	3.33 deaths per 1,000 live births

Source: Central Intelligence Agency, 2009.

ucational levels. Nevertheless, maternal health—to take one example—varies enormously in societies with different political infrastructures. It is as low as 4 maternal deaths per 100,000 live births in Australia and as high as 2,100 maternal deaths per 100,000 births in Sierra Leone, a 500-fold difference (Beaglehole & Bonita, 2008). This enormous disparity reflects the effects of wealth as well as political will (Blas et al., 2008).

Type of Social Determinants

By convention, the term usually used in discussions of public health is *social* determinants—hence the title of the chapter. In fact, this term is slightly misleading, as "social" in this context includes a number of discrete types of factors already alluded to: economic, legal, political, and material factors, as well as social factors that are more narrowly defined (Kelly et al., 2009). Each of these factors is explored in more detail in this section.

Economic Factors

Typically the kinds of economic factors that are most relevant to health include absolute and relative poverty, the size and distribution of the gross domestic product (GDP—a measure of the wealth of a society), the proportion of GDP spent on health care, and the infrastructure of health protection and improvement such as water, sanitation, housing, roads, and education (especially the amount spent on women's education) (see Bunker, 2001; McKeown, 1976; Marmot & Bell, 2009). The market offers incentives and rewards to some and barriers to opportunities to others; markets produce winners and losers. Thus market arrangements and practices in specific

Within nations, very wide, widespread, and persistent differences can be found in the patterns of mortality and morbidity between different social, racial, and ethnic groups; between young and old; and between men and women. Figure 3-3 shows the differences in life expectancy of blacks and whites in the United States, for example.

The differences in the health of the population are not randomly distributed, but rather follow certain predictable patterns. The principal pattern is that various types of economic and social characteristics, such as occupation, housing tenure, and education, are associated with poor health. The patterning of health inequities across the globe within and between societies is associated with systematic inequalities in access to the social, economic, political, and cultural resources necessary to promote health or prevent disease. These resources are generated by the macro legal, political, social, and economic systems. For some people, these systems are health enhancing; for others, they are lethal. Data on infant mortality demonstrate this dichotomy very strikingly (Table 3-1 and Figure 3-4).

The political infrastructure is also a macro determinant, although the precise way its relationship with health works is complex, and the pathway is confounded by other variables such as income and ed-

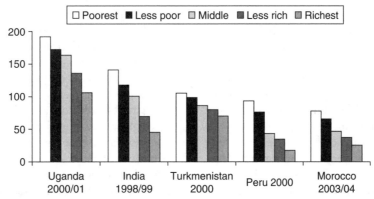

Figure 3-4 Under-5 mortality rate per 1000 live births by level of household wealth. *Source*: Marmot and Friel, 2008.

Table 3-2	Wealth and Health				
Country	Total Expenditure on Health per Capita (International $)	Gross National Income per Capita (PPP International $)	Total Expenditure on Health as a Percentage of GDP (2006)	Life Expectancy at Birth (Male/Female)	Probability of Dying Before Age 5 Years (per 1,000 Live Births)
United States	6,714	44,070	15.3	75/80	8
Switzerland	4,312	40,840	11.3	79/84	5
Canada	3,672	36,280	10	78/83	6
United Kingdom	2,784	33,650	8.4	77/81	6
Chile	697	11,300	5.3	75/81	9
Colombia	626	6,130	7.3	71/78	21
Cuba	363	N/A	7.1	76/80	7
Iraq	124	N/A	3.8	48/67	47
Sudan	61	1,780	3.8	59/61	89

Source: WHO, 2006b.

societies are also relevant. Regulation of market failure and of the labor market in particular is very significant. Economic growth and rates of employment are very important as well. Economic freedom to promote market opportunity and cause damage when people lose their jobs or businesses fail is another potent part of the mix. The extent to which markets are regulated and managed and the degree to which protection is offered against the vicissitudes of the market are fundamental aspects that affect all parts of the society, including health care. As part of the regulatory structure of the economy the taxation system is core including taxes on tobacco and alcohol. The general fiscal structure, especially its regressive or progressive nature, and the amount of value-added tax (VAT) on food and clothing are very important determinants of health, too.

At the most basic level, being poor is very bad for an individual's health. Nevertheless, it does not follow that the populations of rich countries that spend a lot on health care enjoy uniformly good health. Table 3-2 compares the total wealth of different countries (measured by their GDP), their expenditures on health, and various measures of health.

Three particular examples from the table—the United States, Chile, and Cuba—are worth examining in more detail. The total expenditure on health per capita varies enormously among these three countries: The United States spends approximately 10 times more than Chile, and nearly 20 times more than Cuba. Even so, life expectancy at birth is remarkably similar for all three countries. This is a good example of the enormous complexity of the relationship between social factors (in this case, economic factors) and their effect on health outcomes.

In summary, economic factors have direct effects on the livelihoods and life chances of people. They not only set a context for people's lives, but also fundamentally shape and constrain the lifeworlds of every man, woman, and child. As explained in detail later in this chapter, the lifeworld is the bridge between the wider determinants (the social determinants) and disease.

Political and Legal Factors

The political and legal factors that are relevant to health involve the actions of states, governments, corporations, and supranational state formations such as the European Union, as well as the concomitant legislation, taxation, and the rules and regulation used to manage relations within civil society and between civil society and the state (Beaglehole & Bonita, 2008; Blas et al., 2008; Boxall & Short, 2006). The degree to which the state permits democratic engagement, political and economic freedoms, and free speech, and the degree to which the state is itself fragile or secure, corrupt or efficient, set a context that affects health (Espelt et al., 2008).

Types of legislation and its enforcement are important for such things as compulsory wearing of seat belts in cars, bans on smoking in public places or working environments, and prohibition of the sale of cigarettes, tobacco, and alcohol to young people. Laws to protect goods and services of high quality (e.g., certification of physicians and of drugs), the enforcement of these laws, and the efficient use of information are other examples of key legal and political determinants of health. In societies that are totalitarian, authoritarian, or dictatorial, or where the state is not self-regulated by principles of equality before the law, the impacts on the health and well-being of the population can be negative, although some authoritarian states have pursued successful programs of health improvement.

Like the economic factors discussed in the preceding section, these political and legal factors structure individuals' lifeworlds and hence directly affect health. Table 3-3 compares the life expectancy in selected countries with different political systems.

Figure 3-5 depicts smoothed trends in life expectancy at age 20 by educational level in Russia. This figure shows values for persons who have achieved one of three educational levels: elementary (open circles), intermediate (triangles), and university (filled circles). As can be seen, the gap between expected survival of university-educated and elementary-educated men and women actually grew between 1980 and 2000 following the collapse of the political system of the Soviet Union. This is a very interesting finding. Under an authoritarian system, but one with an avowed commitment to equity, the differences in life expectancy between social groups measured by educational levels were relatively small. Following the dramatic political change and the emergence of a new socioeconomic and political system, the differences became much greater. Of course, there is no simple explanation for this finding, but these data do point to the importance of political and economic systems and their links to health, and particularly the link between political commitment and equity (Blas et al., 2008).

Material and Physical Factors

The material and physical elements of relevance to health include all of those potentially noxious substances, microbes, and particles that might be present in macro and micro environments, such as dust, lead,

radon, asbestos, and other things associated with industrial, agricultural, transport, or construction activities or occurring naturally in the environment. These elements may be present in the micro environments of homes or workplaces or in the atmosphere of the wider environment. They include all water-, air-, plant-, insect-, animal-, and human-borne infections. For example, material and physical factors include meteorological, tidal, and geophysical hazards such as radiation, floods, and drought as well as longer-term potential climatic threats and dangers. They include microbiological agents, germs, viruses, bacteria, prions, and other biological phenomena. Moreover, some psychological stressors and mediators such as noise and working conditions fall within this category. Material and physical factors also include transport systems, buildings, homes, and the structural organization of workplaces and schools. Finally, they include the systems of sanitation and provision of clean water and spatial planning (Thomson et al., 2006).

In many ways, these factors constitute the traditional fare of public health. Clear causal pathways through well-defined vectors from agent to host are the basic tools employed for understanding the interaction of the various elements and their effects on individual health. The evidence base here is grounded in the biomedical and epidemiological sciences' explanations of vulnerability, exposure, and risk. Material and physical factors are linked to social factors in that social factors determine degrees of exposure and risk to these environmental phenomena and, therefore, the consequent disease outcomes.

Material and physical factors are mediated in part by the actions of the state and in part by various economic actors such as businesses and labor unions. Some of the hazards in the environment are more amenable to amelioration and control than others—for example, by regulation and management, by immunization and screening, or by other forms of medical intervention. Even here, however, the degree of protection that in principle should apply to everyone varies, with the poor generally being at greater risk. Others factors, such as the forces of tides and climate, are less easily immediately controlled through regulation and legislation or any kind of direct medical intervention, but the consequent risks to the population nevertheless vary by social advantage and disadvantage.

Epidemiology has consistently demonstrated that the levels of risk associated with these material factors and the degree of exposure to them are themselves socially patterned, with the poor and disadvantaged experiencing greater exposure, higher levels of risk, and consequently greater levels of morbidity and

Table 3-3	Life Expectancy at Birth in Selected Countries	
Place	Life Expectancy at Birth: Male (years)	Life Expectancy at Birth: Female (years)
Sweden	78.7	83
Denmark	76.2	81
Cuba	75.9	80.1
Iraq	47.9	67.4
Sierra Leone	38.6	42.3
Zimbabwe	43.9	42.7
Sri Lanka	68.7	76.3

Source: WHO, 2006b.

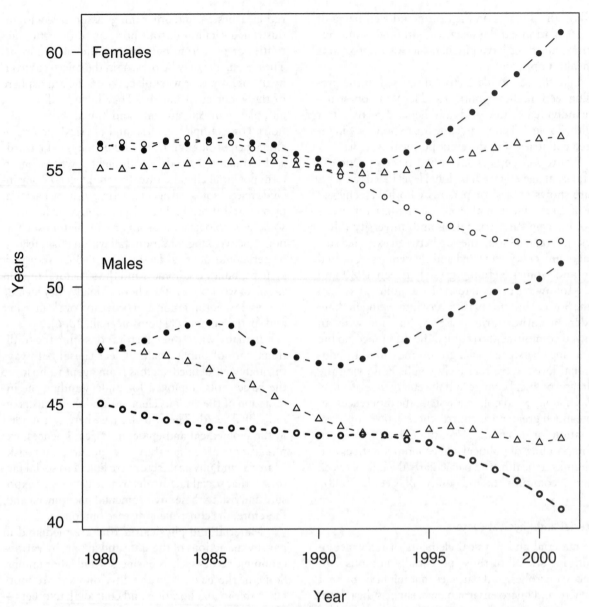

Life Expectancy in Russia at Age 20: Males & Females by Educational Level

Figure 3-5 Expected survival by level of education in the former Soviet Union. *Source*: From Murphy et al., 2006.

mortality. In summary, these individuals' lifeworlds are more risky and hazardous places.

Social Factors

Social factors, as their name suggests, derive from society. *Society*, although a very widely used term, is quite tricky to define scientifically. Society is real, and its effects are as real as those of the environment or the economy. Nevertheless, those effects are more dif-

ficult to see (Kelly, 2009). Society arises spontaneously from the billions of human actions that take place every second of every minute of every day. These individual actions, in turn, produce the patternings of human actions and behaviors that we call "society." The patterns exert influence on the individual actions that gave rise to the patterns in the first place. As such, society impinges on, constrains, and organizes human affairs in ways that, for the most part, are not a *direct* result of intentional human agency or intention (Giddens, 1979, 1982, 1984).

The billions of individual actions produce individual heterogeneity (i.e., individual differences) between people. These differences between different people are easy to see all around us. When one takes a larger view of the many millions of individually different people doing countless human actions, however, regular patterns in human behavior, human institutions, human culture, human economies, and human political systems emerge. It is these patterns we call society. These patterns and regularities appear and reappear generation after generation. They also change and develop generation after generation, even as they continue generation on generation. One of the most important patterns is that of the appearance of heterogeneous social groups in competition with one another for scarce resources and control of their life chances and lifeworlds (Lenski, 1966; Lenski & Lenski, 1971).

Group social difference—in whatever great variety of forms it may take—is a universal characteristic of human social systems. These differences have important consequences, including health consequences, because they determine access to and possession of assets and resources and exposure to vulnerability. Social difference determines access to resources and, therefore, life chances (Weber, 1948). The key dynamic here is the competition between those groups for scarce resources in the civil, political, and economic spheres. Social categories such as those demarcated by class, status groups, ethnic groups, castes and tribes, and age, gender, disability, and religion are the groupings that are the most well known, and in health terms the most important, because each of these categories maps against patterns of disease.

Power relations are of particular interest to public health practitioners. To a very significant degree, the shape of society reflects struggles for power and competition for resources. Sometimes power is played out as violent aggression, sometimes as legally sanctioned oppression and violence, and sometimes as the micro politics of the office or institution. The structures of power and domination, from the most benign to the most malevolent, are intrinsic to the human condition. From the perspective of public health, their effects—especially effects related to the negative experience of power, domination, aggression, and force, as well as the more benevolent forms of social control—have direct impacts on health (Kelly, 2001).

Among the most important social structural consequences of power relations are patterns of inequality and their resulting patterns of health inequity and differences. These disparities arise because the result of competition for scarce resources is unequal access to them, and consequently limits life chances. This unequal distribution creates lifeworlds that are more risky and noxious for some people than for others.

Access to resources is fundamental to the ability to cope with the travails of life. The term "resources," in the sense used here, can refer to money, social support, social capital, skills, psychological resilience, and market position (Cobb, 1976; Taylor et al., 1997). None of these factors are distributed equally or randomly in the population. Rather, they are differentially distributed according to social difference and are the outcome of power struggles. (This idea is explored in more detail later in this chapter.)

The general principle of the approach enshrined in the idea of the social determinants of health is that relationships exists between a variety of economic, political, legal, social, and physical factors and health. However, as noted previously, this observation alone leaves open the question of the causal relationship between social factors and disease—a topic we will explore later in this chapter. First, though, the concept of the health gradient is introduced.

The Health Gradient

Demonstrating Social Patterns of Health

The most well-known social pattern of health demonstrating the operation of the social determinants is called the *health gradient* (Kelly, 2010a). The health gradient describes a pattern that is formed by comparing measures of mortality and morbidity with some measure of social position (Table 3-4). In Great Britain, where the earliest records were collected making this link, the social measure was originally defined as an individual's occupation or the occupation of the head of the household (Graham & Kelly, 2004), a convention also used since in many other developed countries. Occupation has tended to be readily available in official statistics and has proved to be a good proxy for a range of other aspects of life chances, including education, income, housing tenure, and social class.

Data collected by Banks and colleagues (2006) nicely illustrate the gradient. Comparing the United Kingdom and the United States, these researchers found similar patterns of graded health differences measured by income for, among other things,

Table 3-4	Inequalities in Mortality by Socio-Economic Position in 21 European Countries					
Country	Indicator of socio-economic position	Period	Age-group	Rate Ratio[b] Men	Women	Source
Austria	Education[2]	1991–1992	45+	1.43*	1.32*	National census-linked mortality follow-up
Belgium	Education[2]	1991–1995	45+	1.34*	1.29*	National census-linked mortality follow-up
	Housing tenure[1]	1991–1995	60–69	1.44*	1.43*	
Czech Republic	Education[6]	End 1990s	20–64	1.66*	1.09*	Unlinked cross-sectional study
Denmark	Education[1]	1991–1995	60–69	1.28*	1.26*	National census-linked mortality follow-up
	Housing tenure[1]	1991–1995	60–69	1.64*	1.47*	
	Occupation[3]	1981–1990	45–59	1.33*	n.a.	National census-linked mortality follow-up
England/Wales	Education[2]	1991–1996	45+	1.35*	1.22*	National census-linked mortality follow-up
	Housing tenure[1]	1991–1996	60–69	1.65*	1.58*	
	Occupation[3]	1981–1989	45–59	1.61*	n.a.	National census-linked mortality follow-up; representative sample
Estonia	Education[11]	2000	20+	2.38*	2.23*	National cross-sectional study
	Education[6]	1988	20–74	1.50*	1.31*	National cross-sectional study
Finland	Education[2]	1991–1995	45+	1.33*	1.24*	National census-linked mortality follow-up
	Housing tenure[1]	1991–1995	60–69	1.90*	1.73*	
France	Education[1]	1990–1994	60–69	1.31*	1.14	National census-linked mortality follow-up
	Housing tenure[1]	1990–1994	60–69	1.27*	1.25*	
	Occupation[3]	1980–1989	45–59	2.15*	n.a.	National census-linked mortality follow-up; representative sample
Hungary	Education[9]	2002	45–64	1.97*	1.58*	Cross-sectional ecological analysis
	Occupation[10]	1984–1985	45–64	1.61	1.33	National cross-sectional study
Ireland	Occupation[3]	1980–1982	45–59	1.38*	n.a.	National cross-sectional study
Italy	Education[2]	1991–1996	45+	1.22*	1.20*	Urban census-linked mortality follow-up (Turin)
	Housing tenure[1]	1991–1996	60–69	1.37*	1.33*	
	Education[4]	1981–1982	18–54	1.85*	n.a.	National census-linked mortality follow-up
	Occupation[3]	1981–1982	45–59	1.35*	n.a.	National census-linked mortality follow-up
Latvia	Education[7]	1988–1989		1.50	1.20	National cross-sectional study
Lithuania	Education[5]	2001	25+	2.40*	2.90*	Unlinked cross-sectional analysis
Netherlands	Education[23]	1991–1997	25–74	1.92*	128	GLOBE Longitudinal study (Eindhoven)
Norway	Education[2]	1990–1995	45+	1.36*	1.27*	National census-linked mortality follow-up
	Housing tenure[1]	1990–1995	60–69	1.44*	1.36*	
	Occupation[3]	1980–1990	45–59	1.47*	n.a.	National census-linked mortality follow-up
Poland	Education[8]	1988–1989	50–64	2.24	1.78	National cross-sectional study
Portugal	Occupation[3]	1980–1982	45–59	1.36*	n.a.	National cross-sectional study
Slovenia	Education	1991 & 2002	25–64	2.44	2.66	Unlinked cross-sectional study
Spain	Education[2]	1992–1996	45+	1.24*	1.27*	Urban and regional census-linked mortality follow-up (Barcelona & Madrid)
	Occupation[3]	1980–1982	45–59	1.37*	n.a.	National cross-sectional study
Sweden	Occupation[3]	1980–1986	45–59	1.59*	n.a.	National census-linked mortality follow-up
Switzerland	Education[2]	1991–1995	45+	1.33*	1.27*	National census-linked mortality follow-up
	Occupation[3]	1979–1982	45–59	1.37*	n.a.	National cross-sectional study

a Because of differences in data collection and classification, the magnitude of inequalities in health cannot always directly be compared between countries.

b Rate Ratio: ratio of mortality rate in lower socio-economic groups as compared to that in higher socio-economic groups. Asterisk (*) indicates that difference in mortality between socio-economic groups is statistically significant. Notes refer to references given in the back of this report. N.a. indicates 'not available'.

Source: From Mackenbach, 2006.

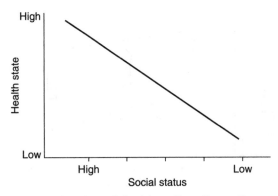

Figure 3-6 The schematic health gradient. *Source*: From Kelly, 2010.

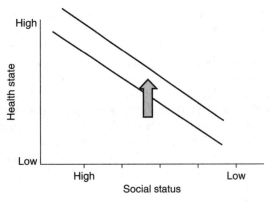

Figure 3-7 The health gradient showing uniform improvement. *Source*: From Kelly, 2010.

self-assessed health, diabetes, heart disease, and lung disease. The gradient is described in many texts, reports, and papers (see, for example, Acheson, 1998; CSDH, 2008; Mackenbach, 2006a; 2006b; Marmot, 2010; Siegrist & Marmot, 2006; Starfield, 2006; Townsend & Davidson, 1982; Wilkinson & Pickett, 2009). The steepness of the gradient and the differences between the top and bottom do vary between societies (Bonnefoy et al., 2007). Even so, a degree of commonality can be found in higher-income societies in that the nature of the gradient tends to be smooth, showing a gradual rise in mortality and morbidity as social position declines (Figure 3-6). That said, the most disadvantaged members of society do carry by far the greater level of risk (Kaplan, 2007). In low- and middle-income countries, the shape of the gradient tends to be less smooth, reflecting different patterns of income distribution and levels of poverty, as data collected by Victora and colleagues (2005) demonstrate.

The measures used to describe health or disease at any point on the gradient represent a value.[1] This value could be, for example, a measure of mortality, the number of cases of cardiovascular disease, or responses to a questionnaire describing self-rated health. Figure 3-6 shows schematically the way that advantage is associated with good health and disadvantage is associated with poor health. It also indicates that the decline in health status is gradual across the social groups. Such measures are helpful in observing changes in health over time for particular groups, because mortality rates may change, the number of cases may rise or fall, and people's feelings about their health may change.

Thinking about the measures *relatively*, however, lies at the heart of the idea of the gradient. This approach allows comparisons to be made between groups and elucidates how these comparisons may change *relative to each other* over time. Thus it becomes possible to think of a particular gradient as being made up of absolute measures of health at a particular point in time. If we imagine a population-level public health intervention that would affect the whole population similarly and improve health in some way, then we would anticipate that the gradient as a whole would be shifted upward uniformly and by the same amount (Figure 3-7). Under such circumstances, the absolute health of everyone in the group would be seen to have improved by the same amount, which might be judged to be a good thing. Nevertheless, if the gradient simply shifts upward at the same rate for all groups, then the *relative* differences between the groups remain unchanged, and in that sense health inequity has not changed.

The health gradient exhibits still more complex behavior because the effect of some public health interventions is to improve the health of the already advantaged more quickly than the less advantaged, or sometimes earlier in the life cycle of an intervention (Victora et al., 2000). As a consequence, although the absolute health of all groups might be improving, the rate at which it is improving will be faster in absolute terms for those persons already in the best health. In this case, the relative differences become greater or worse and the pattern of health inequity becomes relatively worse across society as a whole (Figure 3-8). This outcome is not an inevitability, however; the magnitude of the shift either to widen or lessen inequity needs to be assessed on an empirical basis (Krieger et al., 2008). Indeed, in some countries in recent years the absolute values for the worse off have grown worse anyway (Murphy et al., 2006).

In schematic terms, if the goal of a policy or an intervention is to change the overall pattern of health inequity, a more targeted or directed approach is

---

[1] The text that follows is based on Kelly (2010a).

required that would result in the rate of improvement being faster for those groups whose starting point is worse initially, with the health gradient being altered such that it becomes less steep (Figure 3-9). Achieving this goal, of course, would require a detailed knowledge of what is labeled in Figures 3-6, 3-7, 3-8, and 3-9 on the *x*-axis as *social status*. Social status is a catch-all term that involves a number of distinct dimensions. To make a difference in the way described in Figure 3-9 requires a detailed understanding of these dimensions and the ways in which they relate to one another (Kelly, 2010a).

When analyzing inequality patterns in low- and middle-income countries, it is important to be aware that the health gradients in these countries can have different shapes than those found in higher-income countries (Bonnefoy et al., 2007). This can be a critical factor when selecting a social policy approach intended to reach different populations. The differences in the shape of the gradient are well illustrated by Victora and colleagues' (2005) evaluation of coverage of preventive child-survival interventions in nine low-income countries in Africa, Asia, and Latin America. Figure 3-10 shows the distribution of children according to the number of preventive interventions they received in relation to the socioeconomic group to which they belonged.

Victora and colleagues (2005) identify three inequity patterns: linear, top, and bottom. The *linear inequity* corresponds to the classic gradient situation. Although the steepness of their health gradients varies, Bangladesh, Benin, and Nepal represent this pattern. The *top inequity* pattern corresponds to countries where the great majority of the population does not receive interventions and a disproportion of benefits is concentrated in the higher socioeconomic groups (e.g., Cambodia, Eritrea, Haiti, and Malawi). Finally,

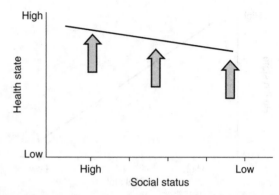

Figure 3-9 Shifting the health gradient through universal and targeted action. *Source:* From Kelly, 2010.

the *bottom inequity* pattern is found where most children do have access to interventions, but there is a clear group that lags behind. Such is the case in Brazil and Nicaragua; in fact, this pattern is a common one in many Latin American countries.

Closing the Equity Gap: A Case Study of the Health Gradient

The next example illustrates the way the health gradient responds to public health interventions and the degree to which the gradient can be a stubborn feature of the patterning of health despite well-intentioned efforts to change it. It also demonstrates the power of the social determinants in the face of attempts to arrest their influence (Bonnefoy et al., 2007).

Early in the 1980s, the infant mortality rate (IMR) in the state of Ceará, in the poor northeastern area of Brazil, was greater than 100 infant deaths per 1,000 live births. Malnutrition was also very common in this region. In 1986, the new state government requested UNICEF support to help improve child health, and a state-wide survey of child health and nutrition was commissioned. More than 4,500 children younger than 3 years of age were surveyed in 8,000 families in 40 different municipalities. Based on the survey's conclusions, new health policies were implemented, including growth monitoring, oral rehydration, breast-feeding promotion, immunization, and vitamin A supplementation—interventions collectively known as GOBI (*g*rowth monitoring, *o*ral rehydration, *b*reast-feeding, and *i*mmunization). Because lack of access to healthcare facilities was a major problem, a large new program for community health workers was established and another program for traditional birth attendants was expanded. Responsibility for health services was decentralized to rural municipalities, which were the areas with the worst health indicators. A

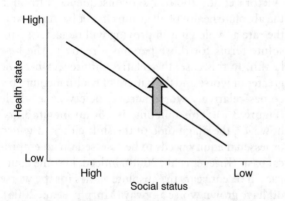

Figure 3-8 The health gradient showing relative health inequalities getting worse. *Source:* From Kelly, 2010.

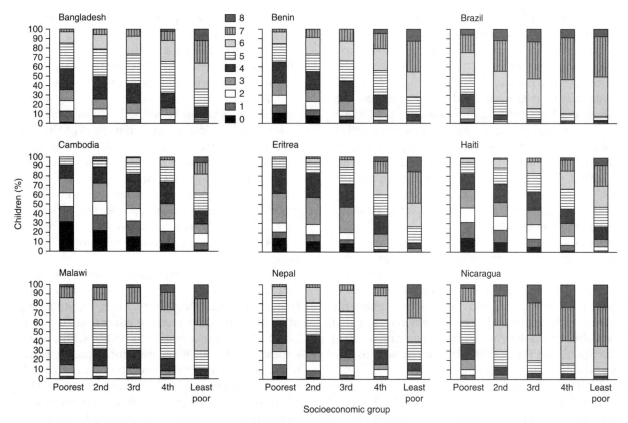

Figure 3-10 Different types of health gradients as represented by percentage of children aged 1–4 according to the number of child survival interventions received, by socioeconomic group and country. *Source*: From Victora et al., 2005.

social mobilization campaign for child health was implemented, which included the use of the media and small radio stations to broadcast educational messages.

Similar surveys were repeated again in 1990 and 1994. After each one was completed, the results were incorporated into health policy. This process was sustained by four consecutive state governors, all of whom gave high priority to improving child health. The experience in Ceará drew international attention, and in 1993 the state received the Maurice Pate Award, the annual UNICEF prize for successful progress toward child health and well-being.

Considerable advances in the population coverage of the four GOBI interventions had been made by 1994. The use of oral rehydration solution had increased to more than 50% in children with diarrhea. Nearly all children had a growth chart, and half had been weighed within the previous three months. Immunization coverage was 90% or higher. Moreover, median breastfeeding duration—a difficult indicator to improve—had apparently increased from 4.0

months to 6.9 months. Disease frequency and mortality outcome indicators for the whole population also showed considerable improvement between 1987 and 1994. The prevalence of low-weight-for-age children younger than age five fell from 13% to 9%, the prevalence of low-height-for-age children decreased from 27% to 18%, and the prevalence of reported episodes of diarrhea in children in the previous two weeks declined from 26% to 14%. Infant mortality was estimated at 39 deaths per 1,000 live births in 1994, a 37% reduction from the estimated 63 deaths per 1,000 births in 1987. Immunization rates improved remarkably in all income groups, with the inequity gap between rich and poor closing as the wealthy reached near-universal coverage. For both growth monitoring and use of oral rehydration solution, the inequity gap was also narrowed. Assessment of breastfeeding duration showed that in 1987 it was longer among the poorest, whereas by 1994 the gap between rich and poor had narrowed in favor of the wealthier—an interesting "trickle up" phenomenon, given that health messages had been primarily directed toward the poorest people.

Despite the progress achieved in improving coverage for public health interventions, the inequity between rich and poor as measured by disease frequency and infant mortality remained largely unchanged between 1987 and 1994. The proportions of children in the extreme categories of family income remained almost the same in both years, showing that income inequalities had persisted and remained largely unchanged. Cases of diarrhea remained approximately 60% higher among the poor.

Thus, in Ceará, despite the implementation of child health interventions for the poorest families, inequities appeared to remain largely unchanged for four health status impact indicators—weight, stunted growth, prevalence of diarrhea, and infant mortality. Despite an overall improvement in health, the inequity ratio between rich and poor stubbornly persisted. An explanation for this phenomenon is that wealthy families had made greater and earlier use of both public-sector and private-sector services to protect their children's health.

The conclusions from Ceará suggest that, even with public health programs targeted at the poorest, it is difficult to close the inequity gap (Victora et al., 2000). This example highlights the stubbornness of the health gradient, and the reality of the gradient as a social fact. It also raises a fundamental question about our ability to describe the social differences between the various social groups accurately enough to target interventions appropriately. In short, how good is our understanding of the factors that make up the x-axis? This is the subject of the next section.

Measuring the Health Gradient

In the previous section, a schematic representation of the gradient was used to illustrate the phenomenon and to demonstrate the overall impact of social determinants. As noted in that discussion, the nature of the x- and y-axes on the graphs needs further elaboration.

The x-Axis of the Health Gradient: Social Variation

The x-axis representing difference in social status is, in fact, composed of a range of measurable elements, comprising an amalgam of different aspects of social difference in the population. It is important to understand the nature of the relationship between these different aspects—that is, how they interact with one another—to develop appropriate responses to the social determinants (Kelly, 2010a).

The starting point is the measures of social difference themselves.[2] The classic core indicators for measuring socioeconomic status on the x-axis are education, occupation, and income (including income defined as expenditure/consumption or wealth/assets). In low- and middle-income countries (LMIC), appropriate data are not always available about occupation. In addition to socioeconomic status, the x-axis represents gender, ethnic group (made up of ethnic, racial, tribal, caste, religious, and national-origin groups), and place of residence (e.g., urban versus rural, northern versus southern regions), as these aspects constitute important dimensions of social difference.

Education is an important measure, albeit one that has multiple levels. Specifically, distinctions may be made between elementary, lower secondary, upper secondary, and tertiary education (based on UNESCO's International Standard Classification of Educations, 1997). When no information on educational levels is available, a substitute measure is the number of years of school attended. In many LMIC, a category of "no education" needs to be included as well. It is also important to distinguish between complete and incomplete educational levels, given their differential impact on health outcomes and health equity. Illiteracy is another necessary indicator making up the x-axis.

Education is highly interactive with other variables such as income, occupation, gender, age, and place of residence. A higher-income family will tend to assure its children a higher level of education, which in turn will affect the child's income once he or she becomes an adult. Gender affects the educational level attained in the first place; it also interacts with income, given that women and men who have attained the same educational level do not usually receive the same income. In contrast, age should be considered as a confounding factor: Younger populations are expected to have more education than older ones because the highest level of education is constantly increasing. This factor reveals the dynamic social nature of education—while its absolute value increases, its relative value decreases such that newer generations require greater education for similar occupations.

---

[2] The next section is based on the work of Bonnefoy et al. (2007). We are grateful to Johan Mackenbach for the classification described here.

There are several ways to classify people by occupation. The main approach in many European countries is the "class structural" approach. Distinctions are made between people who have structurally different positions in the labor market and who, as a result, differ in terms of income, privileges, lifestyles, and characteristics such as voting behavior. The resulting groups of people are usually referred to as "occupational classes" or "social classes."

In many LMIC, however, "occupation" data, as collected in vital statistics or censuses, are not adequate for stratifying populations. First, questions about occupation are not usually asked consistently and hence the data are unreliable. Second, in LMIC the influence of occupation is highly dependent on working conditions: The same occupation might have quite different income levels and health effects depending on whether the person works in the formal sector of the economy or in the informal sector. Third, significant levels of underpaid and nonpaid employment (e.g., unpaid family workers especially in farming) occur in LMIC. Finally, high levels of economic inactivity are typically present; in some cultures, this inactivity may be particularly concentrated in the female population.

The income level of a person can be used in two ways: (1) to indicate the socioeconomic status of the income recipient, with higher personal income indicating a better labor market position, or (2) to indicate access to scarce material resources, where measurement of household equivalent income is more appropriate. Household equivalent income is a measure that takes into account different household compositions. Income level may be measured in different ways—income per se, consumption/expenditure, or wealth/assets. These may be expressed in quintiles or deciles, which classify the population by aggregating households into groups of equal number according to the household equivalent per capita income, expenditure, consumption, or wealth/assets.

This information is also aggregated around the poverty/indigence line, which may be defined in either absolute or relative terms. In most LMIC, poverty is measured in absolute terms—that is, in relation to the level necessary to cover food and nonfood needs. A frequently used metric in high-income countries sets the relative poverty line at 50% of the nation's median income. Dachs and colleagues (2002) has argued that total household expenditure per capita is considered to be "less biased, less prone to seasonal variations, particularly in rural areas, and is considered a better indicator of household economic status overall." Ideally, household expenditure should be cross-referenced with household income to obtain the most accurate understanding of household wealth, but these data are not always available.

The Wealth Index (Rutstein & Johnson, 2004), which was adopted in analyzing the Demographic and Health Surveys, provides an important alternative to standard measures (such as income, education, and occupation) for measuring social inequalities in health in LMIC. This index is calculated using easy-to-collect data on a household's ownership of selected assets, ranging from a fan to televisions, bicycles, or a car; materials used for housing construction such as flooring material; types of drinking water source and sanitation facilities; and other context-specific characteristics related to wealth status.

Gender as an equity stratifier presupposes the need for distinguishing between sexes when collecting and processing data. Because gender is a relational concept, analyzing data by gender means more than simply distinguishing the data between men and women or boys and girls; it means using indicators that allow comparisons between both genders. One such instrument that facilitates such comparisons is the Gender Parity Index (GPI), developed by the United Nations Educational, Scientific and Cultural Organization (UNESCO), which gives the ratio of female-to-male value of a given indicator. In this scheme, a GPI of 1 indicates parity between sexes; a GPI that varies between 0 and 1 indicates a disparity in favor of boys; and a GPI greater than 1 indicates a disparity in favor of girls (UNESCO, 2006). In education, for instance, one could assess literacy in terms of the number of literate women per 1,000 literate men.

Ethnic groups, race, caste, tribe, and religion may also be used to stratify populations so as to reveal inequities in health, particularly but not exclusively in LMIC (Anderson et al., 2006; Montenegro & Stephens, 2006; Ohenjo et al., 2006; Stephens et al., 2006). At first glance, ethnicity might seem a simple issue to identify. Nonetheless, problems of under-representation and differences within and between the groups arise that need to be properly addressed in the data sources. The two main approaches to identifying ethnicity rely on self-identification and language. In some cases, self-identification has problems of under-representation, especially among young people (Economic Commission for Latin America and the Caribbean [ECLAC], 2006). This factor is also potentially unstable in repeated surveys. When language is used as an indicator, as well as identifying the native language, it is also important to assess whether people are monolingual or bilingual, as this is a key issue in determining access to and utilization of health services.

As well as the classic rural–urban distinction, place of residence implies administrative units (villages, municipalities, provinces, regions, or states) and geo-climate areas. Disaggregation is needed not only to identify inequities based on this factor, but also to facilitate decision making at the local level. Recently, geographic software programs have enhanced researchers' ability to carry out spatial analysis. As a consequence, research on the influences of climatic parameters (e.g., rainfall, aridity, farming systems, length of growing season, stability of malaria transmission) and geographic parameters (e.g., population density, urban proximity, coastal proximity, distance to roads) may be able to explain differences in health outcomes (e.g., in child mortality). The use of these diverse geographic variables has the potential to go beyond the traditional urban–rural dichotomy and lead to analysis based on an "urban–rural continuum" (Balk et al., 2003).

The x-axis for the health gradient represents social variation in the population. A reasonably good toolbox of methods is available to researchers to help them do the measuring of this aspect. This is an important first step because in all societies—but especially in complex multicultural ones—the x-axis is made up of many elements and facets (Kelly, 2006a). Public health researchers, however, need to go beyond simple measurement and description, which can prove a much more difficult task. These different elements and facets interact with one another, they overlap, they are mutually reinforcing, and they are dynamic and changing. In contrast, efforts to capture the complexity in a single measure such as occupation, socioeconomic grouping, or income will always be both static and blunt. Little direction is available regarding the best means to target the different parts of the population so as to accelerate the absolute improvements in the health status of the most disadvantaged groups. Further, basic measurement of social variation leaves unanswered the question of which elements are the most important to act upon first to achieve the desired outcomes. It is vitally important to remember that health and disease outcomes are the consequence of the synergies between these stratifiers in the dynamic lifeworlds of ordinary people (Kelly, 2010a). To capture the dynamism of the impact of different factors requires more than simply measuring each one

against a health outcome. The section on the lifeworld later in this chapter offers a solution to this problem.

The *y*-Axis of the Health Gradient: Health Outcomes

The y-axis of the health gradient consists of health outcomes—and, like the x-axis, its definition presents a number of other problems. The measures on the y-axis can also take many forms (Bonnefoy et al., 2007; for a review, see Etches et al., 2006).

In many countries three types of data are available:

- Nationally representative, individual-level data on mortality according to socioeconomic indicators and other social stratifiers
- Nationally representative data from health interviews or multipurpose surveys
- Nationally representative data from routine health records

When nationally representative data are not available, regional or local studies may be used as long as the restriction to specific regions or areas is explicitly recognized, and extrapolation to the country as a whole is done only if representativeness has been confirmed. Another alternative is to use "ecological" studies, in which mortality or morbidity indicators are linked to socioeconomic indicators at the level of small areas, as long as the potential for bias is recognized.

Tabular representation of data is usually the starting point, and health measures should be standardized for age in such a way that comparisons can be made not only between socioeconomic groups, but also between periods and countries (if applicable). It is important to look not only at rates of health problems, but also at the distribution of the population over socioeconomic groups, as the size of the relatively disadvantaged groups will determine the impact of health inequities. To measure the magnitude of health inequities is important, for example, to determine whether it has changed over time or whether it differs between countries.

Table 3-5 outlines the most commonly used summary indices of the magnitude of health inequities. The choice of whether to use absolute or relative measures can affect the assessment of whether a health inequity exists and what its magnitude is. Sometimes a disparity on the relative scale (i.e., the rate ratio of a health outcome between a low- and a high-socioeconomic status group) may not appear to be a disparity on the absolute scale (i.e., the rate difference between the two groups). It is critical that

Table 3-5	Overview of Summary Indices of the Magnitude of Health Inequities		
		Summary Index	
		On the Absolute Occurrence of Health Problems	**On the Relative Occurrence of Health Problems**
Indices That Compare Two Contrasting Groups	**Compare Extreme Groups**	**Rate Difference** Example: the absolute difference in mortality between professionals and unskilled manual workers	**Rate Ratio** Example: the proportional difference in mortality between professionals and unskilled manual workers
	Compare Broad Groups	**Rate Difference** Example: the absolute difference in mortality between non-manual and manual classes	**Rate Ratio** Example: the proportional difference in mortality between non-manual and manual classes
Regression-Based Indices That Take into Account All Groups Separately	**Based on Absolute SES**	**Absolute Effect Index** Example: the absolute increase in health associated with an income increase of $100	**Relative Effect Index** Example: the proportional increase in health associated with an income increase of $100
	Based on Relative SES	**Slope Index of Inequity (SII)** Example: the health difference between the top and bottom of the income hierarchy	**Relative Index of Inequity (RII)** Example: the proportional health difference between the top and bottom of the income hierarchy
Total Impact Indices That Explicitly Take into Account Population Distributions	**The PAR Perspective (Equality by Leveling Up)**	**Population Attributable Risk (PAR)** Example: the total number of cases that would be avoided if everyone had tertiary education	**PAR (%)** Example: the proportion of all cases in the total population that would be avoided if everyone had tertiary education
	The ID Perspective (Equality by Redistribution)	**Index of Dissimilarity (ID)** Example: the total number of cases to be redistributed between groups to obtain the same average rate for all groups	**ID (%)** Example: the proportion of all cases in the total population to be redistributed between groups to obtain the same average rate for all groups

Source: From Kunst et al., 2001

researchers and policy makers are clear about which type of measure they are using.

It is generally best to use, where possible, both relative and absolute measures of health inequities (i.e., both rate ratios and rate differences comparing two contrasting groups) to ensure that inequities are identified. Other, more sophisticated measures can also be used to gain more insight into the patterns of health inequities, such as the Gini coefficient or the concentration index (Alleyne et al., 2002; Schneider et al., 2002a, 2002b).

Vital statistics, censuses, population-based surveys, and health records are the basic elements of the *y*-axis of the health gradient. These documents are found in all countries, although they differ greatly in their coverage, quality, and frequency. Vital registries in the developed world are core instruments providing continuous information on births and deaths by age and sex, as well as causes of death. Birth registries provide diverse health indicators such as birth weight, delivery assistance, teenage fertility, and other health-relevant indicators (e.g., mother's education level).

They also give statistics on live births, which are used to calculate infant mortality rates. Death registries provide useful information on gender, age, education, occupation, and residence. In the case of infants younger than one year old, information on the mother and the father is collected in most countries. Cause-of-death registries enable monitoring of age-specific and age-standardized death rates for total and cause-specific mortality, allowing calculation of specific rates according to social stratifiers such as social class, gender, ethnicity, or place of residence. In the higher-income world, in countries where vital registries are very incomplete, Demographic Surveillance Sites (DSS) can provide these data for specific geographical areas. For example, InDepth, a network of DSS, has exploited such data to explore health equity issues.

Population and housing censuses are a rich source of data, providing useful information on most stratifiers (e.g., age, gender, education, occupation, ethnicity, residence), although by and large they do not gather information on health or income. Because censuses provide information on fertility, mortality, and migration, they are the basis for (1) population projections, which are vital for mortality rate calculations because they provide the rates' denominator, and (2) life tables, which allow life expectancy to be calculated and, therefore, represent a key component of monitoring systems.

Although they are not the preferred way of monitoring mortality, in many LMIC where vital registries' coverage is less than 90% of the total population, censuses are an essential instrument in measuring mortality, especially infant and child mortality (Vapattanawong et al., 2007), and even maternal mortality in some countries (Stanton et al., 2001).

Population-based surveys, including health interview surveys, epidemiological studies, longitudinal studies, and small-area studies, can provide relevant information on health outcomes as well. In many LMIC, such surveys are conducted at regular intervals to examine trends in health; like censuses, they are a useful source when vital registries lack appropriate coverage. A wide range of such surveys exist, the best known of which are the Demographic and Health Surveys (ORC Macro), the Multiple Indicator Cluster Survey (UNICEF), the World Health Surveys (WHO), and the Core Welfare Indicators Questionnaire (World Bank). These surveys provide information on recent illness episodes in relation to access to care, maternal and child health practices, health knowledge, sexual behavior, anthropometric measures, and biological testing for HIV, anemia, and malaria. In many countries, they also serve as the main source of data on

mortality (Korenromp, 2003; Setel et al., 2005; Soleman et al., 2005, 2006). In addition, most countries routinely conduct multipurpose household surveys that contain health modules—for example, living standards measurement surveys, integrated household surveys, and household income, expenditure, and consumption surveys.

Multipurpose household surveys are increasingly being used to monitor health inequities because the data from their health modules (e.g., self-reported health status, out-of-pocket health expenditures, access and utilization of health services) may be analyzed according to diverse equity stratifiers. The added value of such surveys is that they provide data on individuals and populations outside the institutional registries—for example, the population outside the labor force, children who have never enrolled in school or those who have abandoned the formal educational system, and people who do not access health services.

Health records are also important. They encompass a range of routine data sources, such as disease surveillance systems (e.g., notifiable conditions), healthcare utilization registries, health services statistics, and administrative records, which provide information for monitoring health status (e.g., nutritional status) and health outcomes (e.g., morbidity and mortality) based on social determinants. One drawback is that these records provide information only on those individuals who seek health care. Furthermore, in many LMIC these records are often poor and incomplete.

Many high-income countries regularly conduct health interviews or multipurpose surveys to collect population-wide data on health and population stratifiers, particularly socioeconomic indicators. Measurement and classification of these main social and economic indicators is far from straightforward, however—whether in high-income countries or in LMIC.

Implications of the Health Gradient for Policy Makers

The evidence available to policy makers is largely based on an understanding of the social determinants of health rather than the social determinants of health inequities. This distinction is important at a policy level because the actions required to address the social determinants of health are not the same as the actions required to address the social determinants of health inequities (Graham, 2004a, 2004b, 2004c;

Kaplan, 2007). The factors that lead to general health improvement—improvements in the environment, good sanitation and clean water, better nutrition, high levels of immunization, good housing—do not always translate into reduced health inequities, because the determinants of good health at the individual level are not necessarily the same as the determinants of inequities in patterns of health at population level (Graham & Kelly, 2004). As a consequence, policy makers need to distinguish between the causes of health improvement and the causes of health inequities.

The factors that improve overall health have differential effects on the population, with the better off always benefiting disproportionately when universal interventions are applied (Kelly, 2006b). Sometimes there is a "catching up" effect, in which the less well off makes up ground later, but a differential inevitably remains (Antonovsky, 1967; Victora et al., 2000). Perhaps the widening differential does not matter, as everyone is benefiting to some degree, so the differential is not a reason not to carry out general health improvement. It is important, however, not to define universal and targeted approaches as simple opposites. Hybrid policies that contain elements of, for example, universal actions with targeted follow-through will sometimes be the most appropriate choices.

Where equity is the explicit policy focus, two potential policy implications arise: (1) a clear description of the social structure is required (i.e., a clear description of the relevant elements in the x-axis of the health gradient) to target and tailor interventions and to nuance universal interventions appropriately, and (2) there must be a focus on the determinants of the inequities. The causes and the dynamics whereby different groups respond differentially to health initiatives and the ways in which health-damaging effects operate need to be specified in any intervention (NICE, 2007). The "causes of the causes" of inequities, as they are sometimes known, are located in the divisions of labor within and between societies, the lifecourse and lifeworlds of individuals, and the interaction between them (discussed later in this chapter; see also Kelly, 2006a; NICE, 2007).

Although the evidence base is limited in various ways, "equity proofing" provides a solution that, while evidence based, can proceed without waiting on the results of future studies and the introduction of better conceptual apparatus. Equity proofing involves checking what the equity implications and consequences—both intended and, if possible, unanticipated—are likely to be of a particular action, policy, or intervention (Mahoney et al., 2004; Simpson et al., 2005).

Equity proofing[3] is important for the effective implementation of policies and programs that seek to address the social determinants of health and health equity, as well as for the sustainability of the overall approach to improving health equity. Because solutions to tackling health inequities cannot be universally applied to all contexts (e.g., all countries, all sociopolitical contexts, all economic systems), it is important to review proposed policy and program approaches in context. Also, the best intentions in any policy or major program can go astray in the implementation. Therefore any policy or program development process needs to include the opportunity to identify, assess, and address its potential health equity impacts (positive and negative, intended and unintended) so as to maximize the potential health equity outcomes and minimize any potential harm. In summary, it is essential that policies aiming to address the social determinants of health are equity proofed to ensure the gaps in health experience are not inadvertently increased.

The equity proofing approach should be applied not only to policies and programs with an explicit equity objective, but also to policies or major programs without a stated equity focus. This step is particularly important for policies outside the health sector, where policy makers may not have considered any potential health impacts (not to mention health equity impacts) and where such impacts (positive as well as negative) could potentially be significant.

A recommended approach to equity proofing is a health impact assessment (HIA). This structured process assesses the potential health impacts of a proposal (positive and negative, intended and unintended) and makes recommendations for improving the proposal (Quigley et al., 2005; Simpson et al., 2005). An equity-focused HIA provides a systematic approach to consideration of equity in each step of an HIA (Mahoney et al., 2004; Simpson et al., 2005).

Models and Explanations

We now move on to consider the explanations that have been developed for the actions of the social determinants. Various explanations have been advanced to explain the observed relationships between the social determinants and disease outcomes. The precise ways in which the social determinants of health operate is an area of considerable research interest.

---

[3] This discussion follows from the work of Bonnefoy et al. (2007).

Much is known. For example, it is clear that social determinants of health inequities exist because at both population and individual levels, poor health is linked to social and economic disadvantage. Nevertheless, while the general relationship between social factors and health is well established (Marmot & Wilkinson, 1999; Solar & Irwin, 2007), the relationship is not precisely understood in causal terms (Glass & McAtee, 2006; Shaw et al., 1999).

The Commission on the Social Determinants of Health recommends four key research areas should be explored further to more fully elucidate this relationship:

- Global factors and processes that affect health equity

- Structures and processes that differentially affect people's chances to be healthy within a given society

- Health system factors that affect health equity

- Policy interventions to reduce health inequity— that is, how to influence the first three areas effectively, such as by identifying policy and program interventions with the potential to reduce inequities in the determinants of health and health services and opportunities to transfer the findings of research to potential users with maximum effectiveness (Ostlin et al., 2009)

In the absence of such evidence, a number of theories have been developed. Some propose that inadequacy in individual income levels leads to a lack of resources to cope with stressors of life, which in turn produces ill health (Frohlich et al., 2001; Goldberg et al., 2003; Macintyre, 1997). Others have taken a more psychosocial approach, arguing that that discrimination based on a person's place in the social hierarchy causes stress, which then triggers a neuroendocrine response that produces disease (Evans & Stoddart, 2003; Goldberg et al., 2003; Karasek, 1996; Siegrist & Marmot, 2004). Cobb (1976) proposed that protection from stress by social support could protect people in crises from a wide variety of pathological states, ranging from low birth weight to death, arthritis, tuberculosis, depression, and alcoholism. Brown and colleagues (Brown, 1987; Brown et al., 1975) presented a model in which the absence of social support amplified the effects of stressful life events, producing negative effects on mental health. Still others have sought an explanation that considers how social and physical environments interact with biology and focus on the contexts in

which people live and work (Cockerham et al., 1997; Frohlich, 2001; Goldberg et al., 2003; Krieger, 2001). Glass and McAtee (2006) in an important paper develop an explanation in which the complex relationship between social structure and human behavior is articulated, with reference to the lifecourse, risk, and human behavior. (For a review of approaches, see Berkman et al., 2000; Cockerham, 2007; Evans & Stoddart, 2003; Krieger, 2008a, 2008b; Levine et al., 2004; Solar & Irwin, 2007; Starfield, 2006, 2007; Taylor et al., 1997; Warnecke et al., 2008; World Cancer Research Fund/American Institute of Cancer Research, 2009.)

This section puts forward our own causal explanation, which acknowledges the previously mentioned models but develops a distinctive approach based on the theory of the lifeworld. Two causal pathways of interest need to be distinguished from each other as part of this model development: the individual and the social (Galea et al., 2009; Hawe et al., 2009; Kelly, 2009).

The Individual Causal Pathway

The individual pathway manifests within a person's body. In the conventional biomedical arena, if someone becomes unwell because he or she has developed a specific illness, then the biomedical processes at work in the individual human body are described as the cause. Pathological events in the human body have preceding pathogenic causes. These causes can take many forms, ranging from viruses, bacteria, and genes to physical trauma. Modern medicine is concerned with the causation of disease by these various agents, with the amelioration, prevention, or limitation of these pathological outcomes in the human body being the center of attention.

As an example, consider someone who is HIV positive and, therefore, potentially at risk of developing a series of other diseases. In this case, the HIV virus is the biological agent, the vector of transmission might be the sharing of infected drug-injecting paraphernalia among illicit drug users, and the host is the person who becomes HIV positive. Very precise causal pathways can be conceptualized as residing in individual biology—the serology of the individual—and in individual behavior—injecting heroin using a needle that other people have already used for the same purpose.

There are many diseases whose origins may be identified similarly using this type of biomedical explanation. Sometimes those origins are distal. Mesothelioma, for example, is caused by inhalation of asbestos fibers into the lung. In this case, the vector would be exposure to asbestos fibers; the reason for the exposure could be industrial or occupational. The ultimate cause, however, would reside in the job that person did. An even more distal set of causes might also be operating, in that the choice of occupation in the first place would have been driven by opportunity, education, and place of residence and the local presence of ship building or lagging industries using asbestos. For each individual with mesothelioma, an individual causal pathway, unique to that person, exists in which the reasons for the presence of the disease can be plotted.

The same is true of infectious diseases such as measles and mumps: The person who gets measles or mumps will have been exposed to another infected person. It is also true of coronary disease and lung cancer, although in these cases the cause may reside in diet, exercise habits, and smoking. In any event, there will be an individual causal pathway producing a particular pathology in the individual human body.

The conventional public health contribution is to acknowledge and to bring into the causal explanation the more distal factors that will be behavioral, social, or economic in nature (Putnam & Galea, 2008). Having identified the causal pathway, preventive action can follow by finding specific points along the pathway where the process could be blocked or arrested. For example, programs might be developed to reduce exposure to the causative agent. Occupational health and safety in the asbestos industry is concerned, among other things, with enforcing regulation to reduce exposure. To prevent the spread of HIV among injecting-drug users, the solution might be to encourage the use of sterile needles and syringes among illicit drug users. In the case of measles and mumps, protection can be afforded by immunization. For cardiovascular disease, the preventive effort involves detection and early intervention by screening for hypertension or elevated cholesterol levels, or more distally by taking action to prevent people smoking or helping them to quit.

Such efforts are the realm of classic public health, which is conventionally defined as being devoted to either primary prevention (the protection from risk in the first place) or secondary prevention (stopping the progress of disease once it has begun). The interventions require a good understanding of the individual causal pathways. Classic epidemiology has been very successful in identifying such causal pathways. Indeed, some of the most important and historically significant epidemiological studies, which shifted the way in which we think about disease, its cause, and its prevention, were studies of this type. For example, the investigations linking smoking and lung cancer (Doll & Hill, 1952), lack of exercise and heart attack (Morris et al., 1953), and asbestos and lung cancer (Doll, 1955) stand as testimonies to the effectiveness of this individual level approach.

The Social Causal Pathway

It is relatively easy to see how individual actions located in particular social and economic contexts combine with specific pathogens to produce disease at the individual level. Beyond these examples of individual-level explanations, however, we need also to consider the social level of causation (see Putnam & Galea, 2008). The social level focuses on the causes of the *patterning* of health and illness. Virchow, the great European public health pioneer, was one of the earliest proponents of the view that the population level needs explanation as well as the individual level (Mackenbach, 2009). Durkheim (1897/1952), however, was the principal exponent of the idea that the patterning of events in the population was not merely the aggregation of individual events, but rather a social fact in its own right that required a social-level explanation. The patternings of disease and death referred to in the previous sections according to class, wealth, status, ethnicity, and gender are real social things in themselves that require their own causal explanation. Such patterning has causes separate from, although linked to, the causes of individual pathologies.

The idea that the patterns or structures at the social or population level require explanation is a difficult concept to grasp. Surely it is nothing more than the aggregate of the many individual actions of individual people? The answer is complex: Yes, it is the aggregate, but that aggregate has a reality of its own, as distinct from the biological, cellular, and molecular levels. Population health differences are themselves particularly powerful examples of the social level. Population variations in blood pressure, distributions of levels of lipids, population distributions of body mass index, population self-reported health, and, of course, patterns of mortality and morbidity for cancer, cardiovascular disease, obesity, and alcohol consumption are the empirical representations of the social reality that we also know as health inequity.

The patternings of health at population level are not static: They change and evolve, yet at the same time they persist through time. The capacity for some of the same structures of health inequity to be reproduced through every generation provides, in part, for the stability and continuity in social systems. At the same time, it provides for the enduring problem of public health—persistent and recurring patterns of health iniquity—cited by Lee Jook-Wong in the quote at the beginning of this chapter. This statement is not meant to suggest that in a population group with high rates of a particular disease, all members of the group will necessarily become ill; making such assumption is equivalent to committing the ecological fallacy (Subramanian et al., 2009). Individual differences will inevitably arise. Nevertheless, the existence of these individual differences should not obscure the larger picture of distinct patterning that requires examination.

Hawe and colleagues (2009) make a clear distinction between the two levels of causation, arguing that a focus on the individual level has been a significant impediment to understanding the types of effects that might act at population level, particularly with respect to heart health promotion, where a focus on individual psychology blinded researchers to the importance of the dynamics of social systems and heart disease and its patterning as part of that social system. These authors argue that systems are dynamic, ecological, and complex, and they suggest that health and disease is produced through that complexity and dynamism. Within these ecological systems, the context, the nature of relationships, and the distribution of resources need to be captured analytically. This is what we mean here by the social level.

The social level of explanation is about the explanation of the patterns. The question may be approached by thinking about the fact that the patterns recur year after year, generation after generation. An examination of data for nineteenth-century Britain, for example, reveals that certain districts had much higher rates of mortality than others. These same districts are the places very largely where the highest rates of early mortality can be found in contemporary Britain. Some of these districts have undergone massive demographic change, such that the population mix is now quite different, ethnically and culturally, from that found in the nineteenth century. In other districts, the same poor, white, working-class communities remain largely intact. The early deaths have different causes in the present day: In the nineteenth century, most were due to infectious disease; in the twentieth century, most are caused by diseases of lifestyle. Nevertheless, the *social pattern* of early death remains, although, of course, the mortality rate is very much lower now than in the nineteenth century.

The Lifecourse Approach

The *explanation* for the patterning involves describing the links between the social determinants and human biology (Galea et al., 2009; Taylor et al., 1997). The links between the social, population, organization, and environment determinants of health are to be found at the intersections between the lifecourse and the lifeworld (Galea et al., 2009; Glass & McAtee, 2006; Kaplan, 2007; Kelly, 2006a, 2010b; Kelly et al., 2009; Taylor et al., 1997; Warnecke et al., 2008).

The epidemiology and sociology of the lifecourse are very straightforward.[4] Through numerous studies of birth and other cohorts (Kuh et al., 2003) and a consideration of the associations between insults and benefits in utero (Barker & Martyn, 1992) and subsequent patterns in later life (Graham & Power, 2004; Hertzman et al., 2001), it is possible to show that from the moment of conception to the moment of death, the human organism is subject to both positive and negative forces. These accumulate over the course of a lifetime to produce the health state of an individual at any point in time. Sometimes earlier negative impacts will be cancelled out by later benefits; conversely, previously gained benefits may be wiped out by some subsequent negative impact. However, mostly health is a cumulative outcome of factors that impinge on the individual over his or her lifetime.

The lifecourse approach sees health state at any given point in life as a cumulative health profit-and-loss account. It attends to the fact that along life's pathway, there are often critical moments when particular directions are taken that will have short- and long-term costs and benefits (Graham & Power, 2004). Sometimes the pathway choice is largely driven by social circumstances; sometimes it is a real choice. In any event, the choice has consequences. Thus the type of job entered may be entirely driven by local labor markets, decisions to start to smoke by peer pressure, use of a condom during first intercourse (or not) by the state of alcoholic intoxication at the time, and even the decision to add salt to food by cultural habit. Each of these actions has potential short- and long-term health consequences.

It is important to note that the trajectory through the lifecourse is neither uniform nor, strictly speaking, chronological. Most assuredly, the velocity and shape of the lifecourse trajectory of a boy born to white middle-class parents in upstate New York and a girl born in very poor circumstances in Dakar in Bangladesh will be different. The accumulated health benefits and insults and the critical decision points and opportunities available to each will mean they may follow quite different paths.

---

[4] This section is based on Kelly (2010b).

The Lifeworld Approach

The *lifeworld* is the personal experience of the lifecourse (Kelly, 2006a, 2010b). It is a private, psychological, subjective space where conscious cognitive processes operate. It is where thinking takes place and where perceptions of internal and external experience are lodged. The lifeworld is where humans make sense of the social and physical world around them. It is also the place where mind, by mediating external sensory experience, interacts with others external to self (Mead, 1934; Schutz, 1964, 1967, 1970). It is where the world of pain and suffering is experienced, where feelings of disadvantage are noted (Kelly, 1996, 2001, 2006a). It is where the physical world is interpreted as malevolent or benign. In this sense, the lifeworld is also a physical space where interaction takes place—not just symbolic interaction (in the mind), but the real physical interaction between people and the self. It is the place where the insults and benefits of the lifecourse are experienced, mediated, and moderated. (See Exhibit 3-1).

The idea of the power of the lifeworld—of immediate social experience to exert a profound effect on health—has been around a long time. Cobb reviewed the state of the literature in relation to social support in 1976, and Brown and colleagues (1975) proposed a model of mediation of stressors in the lifeworlds about the same time. More recently, a number of researchers have pursued the same idea, albeit not calling it the lifeworld (Berkman et al., 2000; Cockerham, 2007; Evans & Stoddart, 2003; Krieger, 2008a, 2008b; Levine et al., 2004; Solar & Irwin, 2007; Starfield, 2006, 2007; Taylor et al., 1997).

Exhibit 3-1	Jan's Lifeworld and the Way It Affects Her Health

Jan lives in the East End of London. It is a poor part of London, where car manufacturing was once the main industry, employing hundreds of thousands of factory workers. The other main industry was associated with the Port of London, its docks, and their associated trades. The East End was and is a working-class community. It was badly damaged by German bombs in World War II, was rebuilt in the post-war era, and until the 1970s was a thriving working-class community. Then the car plant was scaled down, with production eventually being transferred to Germany in the 1990s. The docks closed finally in the 1980s. The district where Jan lives was once an affluent community, but it is now characterized by joblessness and by inward migration; in recent years, many migrants from the wars in Eastern Europe have flooded the area.

Jan is 30 years of age. She lives on the fourth floor of a tower block of apartments built in the in 1960s. It is in a bad state of repair. Often the elevators are broken, and Jan has to walk up and down the stairs; sometimes she doesn't bother. She does not own her own apartment, but rather rents it from a local housing association that now runs the flats, which were originally built and managed by the local city council.

Jan does not work as she has a young family. She has four children, Kirsty (age 2), Jamie (age 4), Ross (age 5), and Lee (age 7). None of the children were breastfed. Jan's mother and her aunt share the flat with her. Both her father and her uncle, who worked in the car factory, are dead. Jan's father died of lung cancer at the age of 50, and her uncle died following a massive stroke at the age of 60.

Jan was not married to Bill, the father of her children, but lived with him for five years. The couple separated before Kirsty was born. Bill also lives in the same district but seldom visits his family. He was unemployed all the years they were together. Jan threw him out of the home because she found that Bill had been taking money from her purse, which he used to buy alcohol. His drinking had become out of control, with the episodes of drinking frequently being followed by episodes of violence toward his girlfriend. Bill provides no financial support to the family. He is now using drugs and has started injecting heroin. When he does come to Jan's flat, he is frequently drunk or under the influence of drugs and wants money. On a number of occasions, Jan has had to call the police to have Bill removed from the flat.

The apartment is not well cared for. The carpets are worn; the furniture was bought originally very cheaply, and is now grubby and dilapidated. None of the furniture is flame retardant; if a cigarette or match were to fall into the fabric, the chances of it igniting are high. Although smoke detectors are installed in the flat, Jan's aunt removed the batteries because the alarm would go off when she fried chips (potatoes). There is mold inside the flat on some of the walls in the children's bedrooms. The children all have persistent runny noses and coughs. The flat is difficult and expensive to heat using the inbuilt central heating system. This unit is usually turned off; instead, Jan relies on two secondhand oil-burning heaters to keep the flat warm. When these heaters are in use, there is a pervasive smell of petroleum in the apartment.

Jan, her mother, and her aunt are smokers. Jan has smoked since she was 12 years old. Each woman smokes approximately 30 cigarettes every day, and the trio will sometimes go without food to buy tobacco. They get their cigarettes from an ice cream van; while ostensibly selling ice cream, the driver also sells illicit tobacco products that are either smuggled or imported illegally into the country. These illegal cigarettes are cheaper than those sold in legitimate outlets where duty (tax) is payable.

continued

Exhibit 3-1	continued

Jan is obese. She has put on weight since her first pregnancy; before then, she had a normal body mass index (BMI). Jan, her mother, and her aunt drink alcohol when they can afford it. On most weekends, they get drunk together in the flat. Often this behavior occurs when Jan's mother and aunt return from visiting one of the local bars, where they go most Fridays, Saturdays, and Sundays, usually staying from about lunchtime until early evening.

The family eats a diet that is very high in saturated fat, sugar, and salt. They often buy ready-made meals from the local Indian fast-food shop and sometimes from the local Chinese restaurant. They never buy fresh fruit, and the only vegetables they buy are potatoes. They drink sugary soft drinks throughout the day; the women often mix these beverages with the cheap vodka that they buy from the local supermarket.

Jan developed gestational diabetes in her second pregnancy, and she now is borderline diabetic. Her family doctor has advised her of the risks of smoking and her alcohol consumption, and has tried to monitor her diabetic state. Jan is unconvinced that she can do much about her weight. Indeed, she is of the view that doctors and others who focus on her weight do not know what they are talking about: Everyone she knows, except her ex-boyfriend, seems to be the same shape as Jan.

Before she got pregnant, Jan had a job working in a local shop. She stopped working to have her first baby and has not returned to work. She receives a variety of benefits from the state. Although she tries to feed her children a good diet, her understanding of what constitutes a "good diet" is very limited. She knows that the children like chocolate and fizzy drinks, biscuits, crisps, and cakes—and that is what she gives them. The family does not sit down and eat together, as they do not have a table. The children snack during the day. When Jan eats her Indian or Chinese food, she usually does so while sitting and watching the television. The television is on most of the day, and the children are allowed to use the remote control.

The family has neighbors in their block of apartments, but they have little contact with them. The neighbors on one side are an Asian family. Although Jan, her mother, and her aunt are on nodding terms, she has never been inside these neigbors' apartment. They know the children by sight, but not well enough to ask any of the children into the home despite the fact that one of the children is in the same class as Lee at the local primary school.

During the school term, Jan takes Lee and Ross to the local school each morning. She is slightly troubled by their appearance, because some of the other children seem better dressed. Jan has tried to budget better to provide nice clothes for her children. She talks to the other mothers at the school gate, but has not struck up friendships with any of them. Jan took her oldest daughter to the local children's center a few times, and she has tried the local mother-and-toddler group. She found it a great deal of effort and in the end stopped going because it seemed like too much trouble.

Sometimes Jan feels like it is all too much. Some days, especially when her mother and her aunt have gone out, she feels terribly lonely and sits in front of the television crying. She describes her feelings as like staring into a dark black hole. The future seems to hold out little hope that things will change. She worries about the future for her children. She knows that drugs are widely available locally and that many youngsters can be seen locally sitting in the parks drinking alcohol and smoking marijuana. She feels very vulnerable and sometimes has suicidal thoughts. She worries about her health, but feels helpless to do anything much about it. The alcohol helps in the short run, but she knows that after each weekend, she feels worse and often highly anxious after the hangover. Jan often feels a tightening across her chest and pains around her jaw. She is unaware that she is hypertensive.

Applying the Principles of the Lifeworld

Jan and her family are very vulnerable. Jan lives in a narrowly circumscribed, highly threatening lifeworld, with limited contacts with others. Her only confiding relationships with other adults are with her mother and her aunt. She has four children younger than age seven. The children put enormous demands on her, both emotionally and physically. She finds the television very useful as a way of keeping the children occupied, and feeding them chocolate and fizzy drinks serves as a way of keeping them reasonably quiet. Even so, the youngest still wakes at night and wets the bed. When Lee and Ross went to school, they could not read or write, and both have struggled to keep up with their classmates. Jan, her mother, and her aunt do not have any books in the apartment. Sometimes they buy a newspaper, and occasionally a magazine featuring celebrities. The children receive no stimulation other than the television in the home. There is little by way of obvious love and affection. Jan feels detached from much of what else is going on the world.

Four dimensions help people control their lifeworlds—technical skills, interpersonal relationships, intrasubjectivity, and intersubjectivity. Jan is very limited in all of these areas; thus she is very vulnerable psychologically and physically. She barely manages to cope with life most of the time.

Jan is limited by the few skills that she possesses. She is an unskilled worker, and the opportunities for this type of work are limited. In any event, she feels tied to looking after the children. She does not have a bank account. Although she did once have a credit card, she exceeded the limit on spending and it was eventually withdrawn. Jan has little knowledge about a good diet for her or her children, and she has few cooking or food preparation skills. She has no understanding that she has a large number of risk factors for cardiovascular disease, stroke, and cancer. Indeed, she disbelieves some health messages she has heard. Her own reading and writing skills are very limited—she could not have helped her children learn to read and write,

continued

Exhibit 3-1	continued

even if she had wanted to. She cannot use a computer. She does have a mobile cell phone, which she bought when she had use of the credit card. However, she uses it only to play games rather than to communicate with anyone.

Jan's interpersonal skills are also limited. Her dealings with authority in all its forms are characterized by anger and hostility. She feels intimidated by officials from the housing association, the local health visitor, and the social workers who have visited from time to time. She has found over the years that the only way to get any attention is to shout. As a consequence, when she deals with authority, she often gets angry and shouts. She shouts at her children—and they are learning to shout back. Jan's contacts outside the home are limited, and she has few ordinary adult conversations during a day. She has no friends outside the immediate circle of her family.

Her intrasubjective world is where Jan feels vulnerable. She feels anxious most of the time. She is often frightened, especially when her ex-boyfriend comes to the flat. She is often very unhappy, which she deals with by drinking alcohol. The cigarettes help her; indeed, she sometimes thinks that cigarettes are the only things that make life worthwhile. She does not really enjoy all of the Indian and Chinese food she eats, and sometimes the smell of last night's food, the damp, and urine that permeates the flat makes her feel physically sick.

Finally, Jan's sense of what life means or its purpose—the intersubjectivity—is almost all negative. She cannot see much reason for struggling on, except for the sake of her children, who do seem to give her life some purpose. Even so, she wonders what kind of future awaits them. When she looks around at her immediate social and physical environment, it does not seem to offer much by way of hope for the future for them. Her sense of being a valued person is eroding every day.

Jan is clearly very vulnerable to psychological morbidity and is already experiencing symptoms of depression and anxiety. Her alcohol consumption compounds her psychiatric symptoms. Her physical environment is also very risky. Not only does it feel very insecure, but it is badly heated, damp, and moldy, and is producing respiratory symptoms in her children and her. Jan has no opportunity to take exercise, and the children have nowhere to play safely in the open air. Her own behavior and choices contribute to her own poor physical health. Her diet, her lack of exercise, and her smoking have all taken their toll, so that Jan has prediabetes, angina, and hypertension. In fact, both her environment and her emotional state mean that her choices are very limited, and her options to change things on her own account almost completely zero. Jan is the bottom of the pile in terms of future job opportunities.

The life world Jan inhabits is, to a very significant degree, out of her control; that is, it is controlled either directly by others or by the operation of forces of which Jan is only dimly aware. These forces ultimately create the circumstances that proscribe Jan's lifeworld. They include the economy; high-level policies related to housing, the family, and alcohol liberalization; and failure to control the import of illicit tobacco. Global markets have eliminated the local industries that used to provide plentiful opportunities for unskilled manual work, and the new high-tech industries offer nothing for Jan or the many other people living in similar lifeworlds.

Jan's lifeworld is an example of the social determinants writ large.

The origins of the idea of the lifeworld are to be found in the philosophy of the Enlightenment, that period of great scientific advance that took place in the seventeenth and eighteenth centuries in Europe. David Hume (1748/2007), Bishop Berkeley (1713/1996), and Rene Descartes (1997), among others, set out some of the basic ideas underlying the Enlightenment, which were then developed by other philosophers in the twentieth century. Lifeworlds consist of internal representation of external and internal sense experiences (Hume, 1748/2007). External interaction critically depends not only on having an inner sense of self, but also on that self making the assumption that others who come into the lifeworld, and with whom the self interacts, perceive and see the world—and more or less make sense of it—in much the same way that the perceiving self does (Schutz, 1964, 1967). Such an assumption can never be proven. This point has served as a considerable source of anxiety for some philosophers, who have concluded that it is impossible to prove the existence of the external world at all (Berkeley, 1713/1996).

Empirical confirmation that others see and interpret the world in much the same way as the self does comes from two sources. First, both the future and external others' behavior tend to be reasonably predictable. Things on the whole tend to turn out pretty much like the past of which the self has already had experience. In that past, others mostly behaved as if they saw things in the same way as the self. Second, the causal attributions that the self makes tend to be confirmed by the way others see, understand, and explain the reasons for events (Hume, 1748/2007). Lifeworlds tend to consist of unexceptional confirmation that even though we know that things do change, mostly we live in a predictable world; that understanding permits life to flow along without the need for too much philosophical speculation.

Of course, things do change. People's lifeworlds are sometimes subject to seismic shocks—some of which may be predictable, some of which may not. Nevertheless, it is the predictability that is of particular interest here. This predictability resides in the fact that lifeworlds, although subjectively unique, are also shared with others in similar social positions. In essence, lifeworlds have a shared predictability. That sharing is cultural. Coping in the lifeworld is the keynote to understanding vulnerability, both individual and collective.

Shared backgrounds, patterns of socialization, and even the recurrent patterning of social life at the social level mean that large areas of localized lifeworlds are similar but not the same. Thus families, coworkers, and friendship groups—the primary attachments of social life—have the characteristic not of producing exact copies of one another's lifeworlds, but rather lifeworlds where a great deal overlaps. Of course, as people move through space and time, their lifeworlds change and the potential malleability is large. Even so, the coalescence of lifeworlds, the development of shared patterns of meaning and cultural assumptions, produces a predictable patterning of everyday life, of interrelationships between different but overlapping lifeworlds. The patterning of disease at population level is a consequence of this shared nature. Lifeworlds are shared among similar individuals who have like social positions. They experience similar consequences of the social determinants of health, and their patterns of behavior have high degrees of similarity. Consequently, the individual disease pathways acquire a population-level dimension.

The social determinants produce individual-level diseases through the lifeworld. Individual disease pathways manifest themselves and operate via the lifeworld of the individual. Certain individual biological differences between individuals inevitably exist because of differences related to genetics, nutritional status, and previous disease exposure—indeed, the accumulated benefits and insults of unique passages through the life course. There are also differences in the assets that people have at their disposal to help them cope with their lifeworlds. Along with individual biological differences, these variations produce individual health differences.

Lifeworlds are the locus of experience, of pain and suffering, of discrimination and disadvantage. Lifeworlds are the place where the vagaries and the good fortunes of life, as they are visited upon us, take their toll across the lifecourse and have their direct effects. This is why the Commission on the Social Determinants of Health makes the point in its Executive Summary that social injustice is a cause of mortality (Blakely, 2008). Social injustice is experienced in the lifeworld. (See Exhibit 3-2).

Exhibit 3-2	Susana's Lifeworld and the Way It Affects Her Health[5]

Susana lives in Orocuina, in Honduras. She is 23 years old. She is married to Gerardo, who does not have a full-time job but who migrates for the harvests in the northern part of the country periodically. He is 25. The couple has four children, but Susana has recently had another pregnancy that ended in a stillbirth.

The area where Susana lives with her children; her mother, Gracy; and a younger sister, Marta, is very poor. All of the adult women spend time in some agricultural work. In fact, Susana continued working in the fields until the day before she delivered the stillborn child. The family's home is a rough wooden shack. Sanitation takes the form of a septic pit located approximately 100 meters from the home. There is limited running water, but it is of uncertain quality and should be boiled before drinking—something that is not always possible in the home. There is a television, and they have a radio; the electricity supply is unreliable, however.

The climate is tropical, and flies and insects are a constant problem. Malaria-carrying mosquitoes are rare in their area, but are more common in the northern parts of the country, where Gerardo goes to work at harvest time.

Susana's father died in an accident in a lead mine when she was a child. Susana did go to school, but did not complete her primary education. Although she can read and write, she struggles with complex written materials and her understanding of human biology is limited. Despite the fact that she has only ever had sex with her husband, he frequently accuses her of past infidelities and has subjected her to violence and verbal abuse on a regular basis as a consequence.

Life in the rural community is hard, and communication with the nearest urban center, San Lorenzo, is difficult because of the poor state of the roads. There is one local medical center and a birthing center (*clinicas materno-infantiles*) staffed

continued

[5] The authors would like to acknowledge the assistance of Shital Chauhan of Global Brigades, Honduras, Rachel Kelly and Tessa Moore in the preparation of this case study.

Exhibit 3-2	continued

by a trained midwife. Although these facilities are run by the Honduran Ministry of Health, neither has a regular physician in attendance. While Susana visited the centers when she was pregnant, she was not seen by a physician through her pregnancy. When she visits the medical center, Susana usually has to wait about 90 minutes to be seen.

It costs five lempira (Lps 5) to visit the medical center and Lps 100 to visit the birthing center. Tests and medicines cost additional amounts; because there is no pharmacy attached to the medical center, obtaining the medicines requires a three-hour round trip to the nearest pharmacy. Susana's family income is the Honduran average, approximately Lps 500 per month, which translates into less than one U.S. dollar per day. More than 50% of the Honduran population lives below the poverty line.

When her youngest child was born two years ago, Susana had a complex pregnancy and was seen by a physician. She was strongly advised that further pregnancies would be a potential hazard to her health and that she and her husband should use some form of contraception. Gerardo was incensed at this suggestion and refused to use any form of contraception. He became abusive and violent when Susana raised the issue, claiming that if his wife used contraception, it would mean she would be unfaithful to him while he was away working at harvest time. Gerardo has always had a tendency toward violence. Although she does not like being assaulted in this way by her husband, Susana believes that the violence is Gerardo's way of telling her that he loves her and wants her only to be his woman. Susana has heard that while the men are away, some of them are unfaithful to their wives, but she believes that her Gerardo is not like that. She also knows that HIV is a problem in Honduras, and that the greatest bulk of infections come from heterosexual transmission. She would not dare raise this issue with her husband. She tried talking to the local Catholic priest about her fears of getting pregnant again, but he made it clear that in the eyes of the church, using contraception is a sin, and whether she got pregnant is God's will.

The result was, of course, another complex pregnancy. In the last trimester, Susana was frequently unwell and in considerable pain. When her baby was delivered, it was born dead. Since the stillbirth, Susana has felt very sad and has grieved for the lost child. She has cried many times over the death of her baby and feels that no one really understands how she feels. Infant death is not uncommon in Honduras; likewise, the death rate for children younger than the age of five is relatively high (40 per 1,000 live births). Even so, Susana feels the pain of loss intensely and mourns the fact that she was not allowed to have a proper funeral for the child. Gerardo was not sympathetic, and her mother and sister continued with their own preoccupations; also, the other children needed to be fed and looked after, and the work in the fields needed to continue, too.

Aside from her mental distress, Susana feels tired and unwell much of the time and has experienced periodic postpartum bleeding that has not resolved. She is constantly tired, yet sleeps very badly. Her own health is deteriorating as each day goes past.

In Susana's case, we can see very clearly the way that the social determinants of health operate. There are two sets of health outcomes in this scenario—the child who was stillborn and Susana's poor and deteriorating physical and mental health. We can track the individual-level causal chains back to the social determinants: The health of the fetus and the health of the mother are attributable to a set of gynecological complications that the absence of good antenatal care failed to identify and to prevent.

In turn, we might reasonably assume that the mother's health has been rendered at greater risk by a combination of factors, including the physical environment in which she lives, the poor sanitation, the lack of clean water, the nature of the overcrowded conditions in which she and her family live, the lack of a supportive relationship with her husband, and the sheer difficulty of trying to survive in an environment characterized by poverty. Susana lives in a world in which the dangers of infection from a variety of potential sources are ever present, including those arising as a consequence of poor sanitation and the threat of HIV, tuberculosis, and malaria. The climate is favorable to many toxic microorganisms. Medical services are very limited. The rural isolation compounds the issues raised by the general lack of public services associated with living in a country that spends only $197 per person per year on health care, and where only 57 doctors are available per 100,000 population. The political system is unstable, and this instability means that governments find it difficult to invest much time and effort in improving services delivery.

Thus a combination of economics and politics, climate and microbes, conspire to make Susana's lifeworld a very risky place, indeed. She is surrounded by hazards that she has very limited resources to control in any way at all. Her means of control over her lifeworld in the form of technical, interpersonal, intrasubjective, and intersubjective dimensions are very limited.

Technically, the options for Susana are highly limited. She has little more than a basic education. Although she does read and write, she has almost no access to the kinds of written resources that could help her in her situation. She has only a very limited understanding of her own reproductive system and the dangers posed to her as a consequence of not controlling her own fertility. Her husband has very traditional views about the role of women, which prevent both of them from acquiring the skills that could ultimately save her life. Of course, even if the couple had the necessary knowledge, their ability to act on it would be severely curtailed by their lack of access to basic services. Access to the Internet, to the kinds of things that might be available in an urban environment, are nonexistent in rural Honduras.

At the level of the interpersonal dimension, things are tricky, too. Susana has what we might perceive as a very traditional relationship with her husband, but at times Gerardo is abusive and violent. Susana does not like this, but she has tried

continued

| Exhibit 3-2 | continued |

to understand it within the cultural norms and values with which she has grown up. She sees her husband's behavior as just typical of men. She thinks her father behaved much the same way with her mother, and certainly neither her mother nor her sister has ever suggested that Gerardo's behavior is out of the ordinary or in any way unacceptable. Thus, not only does Susana find herself in a set of interpersonal relationships that provide little social and emotional support, but those relationships also reinforce a set of stereotypes abut male and female behavior that merely compounds the difficult situation she is in. The idea that life might be different is not part of the thinking Susana does about her own situation. She knows little of other alternatives; in that sense, her lifeworld is highly restricted.

Emotionally—at the level of her intrasubjectivity—Susana is very vulnerable. She has suffered the loss of her baby. She feels helpless in the face of a pregnancy that she did not want; nevertheless, once she had carried the child for nine months, she felt a strong maternal bond that was severed abruptly at the stillbirth. Susana has not really grieved properly for the child; that is an underlying risk for her, because there are no services standing ready to provide help, and neither her mother, sister, or husband has done anything to help her deal with her grief. Susana herself does not recognize that she has a potential psychiatric problem, as such illnesses are not really part of her understanding of illness and death. She does know that she feels terribly sad, that sometimes everything just seems to be too much, and that she cannot see any hope looking forward.

Susana has very little to help her make sense of it all (the intersubjective dimension). The local culture is highly traditional, and in many ways it offers little to the poor people who spend their life working on the land. Susana thinks that it is some way her fault that the baby died. Traditional religious views do not help her much either: They emphasize the role of God in determining what happens to people, place very strong prohibitions on fertility control, and offer tacit support for the status quo in which men and women occupy distinctive and separate roles, and in which men have more freedom.

Of course, there is a pattern here. Although Susana's personal tragedy and deteriorating health are the story of just one individual, Susana also exemplifies the challenges faced by many millions of women across the globe in low- and middle-income societies. Some fare better than Susana; some do much worse. Indeed, although it is a poor country, Honduras is by no means the poorest country on the planet. The problems attached to the very risky lifeworlds of the poor in agricultural economies may differ in some of the details, but Susana's story depicts a fundamental paradigm of how the social determinants affect health—how the lifeworlds for some people are treacherous and risky, and how many individuals who find themselves in such circumstances have only a very limited ability to change their lives.

Coping Mechanisms: Surviving the Lifeworld

The human lives in a world—a lifeworld—that is intrinsically threatening, dangerous, risky, noxious, and stressful, but with which each person copes (Lazarus, 1969, 1974, 1976, 1980, 1985, 2001; Lazarus & Cohen, 1977; Lazarus & Folkman, 1984a, 1984b; Lazarus & Launier, 1978). The stresses and stimuli are chronic, only interrupted by occasional periods of more or less acutely high levels of even more extremely stressful stimuli. In this regard, humans are all subject to stresses all of the time, because ordinary human life is a life of routine aggravation and difficulty. From time to time, these daily hassles are overlaid by major life events such as illness, death of loved ones, divorce, and war. In this view of things, there are relatively few periods of calm and peace in the human condition. The lifeworlds of most people most of the time are routinely difficult.

Despite the ubiquitous nature of problems, most people get through them, although some individuals deal with these stressors better than others. Some seem to have more assets with which to cope, and coping seems to be intrinsic to maintaining a balance in the lifeworld (Cobb, 1976). There must be some-thing intrinsic to some people's lifeworlds that produces a greater ability to cope. These capabilities are assets, not psychological traits; they are skill-based transactions between persons and their environment.

Four assets, or groups of coping skills, help to clarify the way people survive their own lifeworlds: technical, interpersonal, intrasubjective, and intersubjective. These are the four different types of skills or assets with which we master the lifeworld in varying degrees; they mediate the stressors originating from the social determinants.

The technical level comprises the technical tool-based skills that people use to deal with situations and people, things and the environment. Keeping some sense of control over one's immediate environment is linked to good health (Ellaway et al., 2005); the technical dimension of coping captures this important dimension. Humans have evolved the ability to fashion and to use tools. Tools take many forms, including the use of language to shape thought. Our access to tools and our ability to use those tools skillfully, including in particular occupational and professional configurations, determine our place not only in the labor market, but also in the wider world and within our own lifeworlds. Skills are the basis, in evolutionary terms, of survival; they are the basis of being able to handle and deal with everyday life.

Max Weber (1948), the German sociologist, pointed out that the possession of skills for use in the labor market is a powerful determinant of life chances, by which he meant access to or the means to exert power over others. This statement is still fundamentally true—although extending Weber's ideas to skills to deal with everyday life means that we include not just professional market skills and qualifications, but also the ability to manage encounters with bureaucracy, handle money, and use devices and machines. In today's world, such skills include using the Internet, mobile phone, and automobile, as well as reading, writing, and communicating. These tools allow for mastery of the lifeworld and enhance the ability to negotiate meaning and interaction. They are the principal mediators of life chances in the face of powerful others. In other words, they are fundamental assets: They allow individuals to exercise control over the vagaries of their lives and, in turn, act as mediators against the negative forces that impinge on their lifeworlds.

The second key component of managing the lifeworld—the second asset—is the interpersonal dimension. This component focuses on managing relationships with others. The basis of human society is interaction, which incorporates two elements. The first element is actual physical interaction, either face to face or through an electronic means such as a telephone, that happens in real time. The second element is symbolic interaction. As we physically interact with others, or as we anticipate or reflect upon interacting with others, we rehearse symbolically in our minds what the other person is thinking and will do next in response to what we do and say. We put ourselves figuratively in the shoes of the person with whom we are interacting. This ability to more or less accurately take the role of the other is the core component of what makes interaction work. Our management of relations with others and our ability to interact successfully provides us with a fundamental means of being able to control our lifeworlds.

Life is made up of both routine skirmishes and smooth transactions with bureaucracies, retailers, institutions of all kinds, tradespeople, neighbors, coworkers, relatives, and friends. Most people have the interactive skills to take the rough with the smooth, but a few do not (May & Kelly, 1992). Although some of these interactions may be deeply unsatisfactory, we can at least extricate ourselves from them and move on to other arenas of our lives, where we can escape the hassle and deal with other more satisfactory aspects of our lives. For some people, however, their lifeworld includes chronically difficult ways of interacting with others, be they neighbors, members of the domestic environment, coworkers, community members, or officialdom of various sorts; these interactions are characterized by struggles where the person's claims to be taken seriously as a human being are denied by others who act in ways that seek to exert power over the individual in one way or another. In other words, some individuals spend much more of their time having others define what and who they are, rather being self-directed. At this very micro level, the ability to control the life world may be severely undermined.

The next type of assets is termed intrasubjective, meaning "inside the subject." At the heart of our lifeworld is the emotional or intrasubjective epicenter. This is the world of raw feeling and emotion, of sensibilities and sensitiveness, of fear and hatred, of love and empathy, of all those psychological states of which the human is capable. It is also the cognitive and calculating seat of thinking and feeling. Modern psychology classifies all of these aspects in a variety of ways; likewise, psychoanalytic approaches offer degrees of insight into the origins of these feelings. The task here is not to arbitrate between the various approaches that may be brought to bear to explain these aspects, nor to consider the great philosophical debates from Descartes (1997) and Berkeley (1713/1996) onward, which have sought to reflect on these concerns. Rather, we simply acknowledge that the human is a thinking being who is sensitive to its external environment and stimuli in it, who is capable of manipulating sensations and ideas into highly complex patterns of reasoning and understanding, who is a reasoning, calculating being with a continuous sense of self existing through time and space, and who is a highly volatile emotional creature capable of feelings of great passion and emotion.

Most germane to the question here is the reality that those emotions and feelings can be decidedly painful, and even distressing to the point of psychological morbidity. Some people seem better able to withstand inner turmoil and distress. This capacity might be thought of as encompassing varying degrees of an inner toughness or psychological resilience. The inescapable fact is that the individual feels psychological distress, which is itself linked to somatic changes in the human body. The link between the emotional state of the person and underlying biology is real, although all the precise pathways remain to be fully elucidated. At the heart of the lifeworld for each person is either a relatively robust set of mechanisms that mediate stressors or a relative vulnerability offering at least a partial explanation of the link between the social and the biological mediated via the psyche. This intrasubjective dimension is not the whole story, however: It will apply in some, but probably by no means all, causes of morbidity.

The final asset is intersubjectivity—a term deliberately borrowed from phenomenological philosophy. In that context, intersubjectivity refers to shared meanings between subjects, between human actors. Interaction depends on intersubjectivity. As noted earlier, the basic operating premise on which most human actors work is the assumption that other people see and understand the world in more or less the same way that they do. In real time during shared interactions, meanings are not merely assumed, but tend to emerge and change through processes of negotiation and testing during the interaction. Shared meaning is important because it enables humans to make sense of the world. In other words, as humans, we are constantly engaged in a process, usually at quite a low level, of providing psychologically satisfying accounts of our own actions, the actions of others around us, and other events in the world.

One of the most difficult and shocking things for us to have to deal with is the situation in which the accounts of the world we carefully rehearse and then test in interaction are undermined by the actions of others or by other external events. Reappraisal is called for as we then repair our sense of who and what we are and recalculate our place in the scheme of things. The ability to provide satisfactory accounts lies at the heart of being able to cope with stressors great and small. The inability to do so leads to an overwhelming sense of dread and failure and potentially psychologically terrifying experiences. This dimension is closely linked to the intrasubjective dimension, of course, but is the part that emerges through the social and psychological aspects of the lifeworld. To make things meaningful is a basic element of coping with a hostile environment (Antonovsky, 1985, 1987; Cobb, 1976).

Lifeworlds are also physical. This is what the great Victorian public health pioneers understood. The lifeworld is not just a space where cognitive processes and the experience of stress reside; it is also the place where material circumstances and all the forces of the environment rain down. The point is that the four elements of coping—technical, interpersonal, intrasubjective, and intersubjective—are the basis of resilience and of vulnerability. Where individuals and communities are able to control their lifeworlds, these components offer up some degree of protection. Where they do not have sufficient control over their lifeworlds, individuals and communities are intrinsically vulnerable. Of course, control is never absolute: None of us—no matter how privileged or powerful—ever has complete control of our lifeworld. Relative control makes a huge difference, however, and provides a mechanism that serves as the gateway between the social and the biological.

Conclusion

The social determinants of health are real, and they have real consequences. They are describable and measurable and we know a great deal about them. We also know that their effects have a stubborn and enduring quality that, to a significant degree, has proved not amenable to easy and swift change. The work of the Commission on the Social Determinants of Health is a watershed, but not because it holds all the answers—far from it. Rather, this effort represented the first systematic accumulation of the evidence base across a range of areas of interventions, programs, policies, politics, and economics. To change things requires political will, and the political will to change things most certainly lags behind our ability to describe the problem. Nevertheless, we have very good descriptions of the problem and now, with the evidence accumulated on the social determinants of health, the framework for action. We also have a range of ways of understanding the causal relationships between these factors and health outcomes. These first steps, along with the various hypotheses concerning the way that the determinants link social and biological factors outlined in this chapter, provide the beginnings of a research program that will lead to further accumulation of evidence focusing on effective ways to bring about change.

• • • Discussion Questions

1. What is the difference between health inequity and health inequality?
2. Give some examples of the links between economic factors and health.
3. What is a health gradient?
4. What is the difference between an absolute measure and a relative measure of health state?
5. Why might overall health improvement in the population not lead to a reduction in health inequity?
6. What are the most common measures of social differences?
7. What is the lifecourse and why is important in studies of the social determinants of health?

• • • References

Acheson, D. (1988). *Public health in England: The report of the Committee of Inquiry into the Future Development of the Public Health Function*, Cm 289. London: The Stationery Office.

Alleyne, G. A., Castillo-Salgado, C., Schneider, M. C., Loyola, E., & Vidaurre, M. (2002). Overview of social inequalities in health in the Region of the Americas, using various methodological approaches. *Pan American Journal of Public Health, 12*(6), 388–397.

Anderson, I., Crengle, S., Leialoha-Kamaka, M., Chen, T., Palafox, N., & Jackson-Pulver, L. (2006). Indigenous health in Australia, New Zealand, the Pacific. *Lancet, 367*(9524), 1775–1785. Retrieved from http://www.who.int/social_determinants/ resources/articles/lancet_anderson.pdf

Antonovsky, A. (1967). Social class, life expectancy and overall mortality, *Milbank Memorial Fund Quarterly, 45*, 31–73.

Antonovsky, A. (1985). *Health stress and coping.* San Francisco: Jossey-Bass.

Antonovsky, A. (1987). *Unraveling the mystery of health: How people manage stress and stay well.* San Francisco: Jossey-Bass.

Balk, D., Pullum, T., Storeygard, A., Greenwell, F., & Neuman, M. (2003). *Spatial analysis of childhood mortality in west Africa.* DHS Geographic Studies 1. Calverton, MD: ORC Macro and Center for International Earth Science Information (CIESIN), Columbia University. Retrieved from http://www3.interscience.wiley.com/cgi-bin/ abstract/108565124/ABSTRACT?CRETRY=1& SRETRY=0

Banks, J., Marmot, M., Oldfield, Z., Smith, J.P. (2006). *The SES Health Gradient on Both Sides of the Atlantic.* Cambridge, MA: National Bureau of Economic Research.

Barker, D., & Martyn, C. (1992). The maternal and foetal origins of cardiovascular disease. *British Medical Journal, 304*, 9–11.

Beaglehole, R., & Bonita, R. (2008). Global public health: A scorecard. *Lancet.* doi: 10.1016/S0140-6736(08)61558-5

Benach, J., Muntaner, C., & Santana, V. (2007). *Employment conditions and health inequalities: Final report of the Employment Conditions Knowledge Network of the Commission on Social Determinants of Health.* Geneva, Switzerland: World Health Organization. Retrieved from http://www.who.int/social_determinants/resources/ articles/emconet_who_report.pdf

Berkeley, G. (1713/1996). *Principles of human knowledge and three dialogues.* Edited and with an introduction by H. Robinson. Oxford, UK: Oxford University Press. *Principles of human knowledge* first published 1710; *Three dialogues* first published 1713.

Berkman, L. F., Glass, T., Brissette, I., & Seeman, T. E. (2000). From social integration to health: Durkheim in the new millennium. *Social Science and Medicine, 51*, 843–857.

Blakely, T. (2008). Iconography and Commission on the Social Determinants of Health (and health inequity), *Journal of Epidemiology and Community Health, 62*, 1018–1020.

Blas, E., Gilson, L., Kelly, M. P., Labonte, R., Lapitan, J., Muntaner, C., et al. (2008). Addressing social determinants of health inequities: What can the state and civil society do? *Lancet, 372*, 1684–1689.

Blas, E., & Sivasankara Kurup, A. (2008). *Priority public health conditions: From learning to action on social determinants of health.* Geneva, Switzerland: World Health Organization.

Bonnefoy, J., Morgan, A., Kelly, M. P., Butt, J., Bergman, V., et al. (2007). *Constructing the evidence base on the social determinants of health: A guide. Report to the World Health Organization Commission on the Social Determinants of Health, from Measurement and Evidence Knowledge Network.* Retrieved from http://www.who.int/ social_determinants/knowledge_networks/add_ documents/mekn_final_guide_112007.pdf

Boxall, A-M., & Short, S. (2006). Political economy and population health: Is Australia exceptional? *Australia and New Zealand Health Policy, 3*, 6–10. doi: 10.1186/1743-8462-3-6.

Braveman, P. (2003). Monitoring equity in health and health care: A conceptual framework/ *Journal of Health Population Nutrition, 21*(3), 181–192.

Braveman, P. (2006). Health disparities and health equity: Concepts and measurement. *Annual Review of Public Health, 27*, 167–194.

Briggs, A. (1959). *The age of improvement.* London: Longmans.

Briggs, A. (1963). *Victorian cities.* London: Odhams.

Brown, G. W. (1987). Social factors and disease: The sociological perspective. *British Medical Journal, 294*, 1026–1028.

Brown, G. W., Brolchain, M., & Harris, T. (1975). Social class and psychiatric disturbance among women in an urban population, *Sociology, 9*, 225–254.

Bunker, J. (2001). *Medicine matters after all: Measuring the benefits of medical care, a healthy lifestyle, and a just social environment.* London: Stationery Office/Nuffield Trust.

Centers for Disease Control and Prevention (CDC). (n.d.). Retrieved from http://www.cdc.gov/DataStatistics/

Central Intelligence Agency (CIA). (2009). *The world factbook.* Retrieved from https://www.cia.gov/library/publications/the-world-actbook/rankorder/2091rank.html

Chave, S. W. P. (1958, June 13). John Snow, the Broad Street pump and after. *The Medical Officer, 99*, 347–349.

Checkland, O., & Lamb, M. (Eds.). (1982). *Health care as social history: The Glasgow case.* Aberdeen: Aberdeen University Press.

Cobb, S. (1976). Social support as a moderator of life stress. *Psychosomatic Medicine, 38*, 300–314.

Cockerham, W. C. (2007). *Social causes of health and disease.* Cambridge, UK: Polity.

Cockerham, W. C., Ritten, A., & Abel, T. (1997). Conceptualizing contemporary lifestyles: Moving beyond Weber. *Sociological Quarterly, 38*, 601–622. Retrieved from http://www.blackwell-synergy.com/doi/abs/10.1111/j.1533-8525.1997.tb00480.x

Commission on the Social Determinants of Health (CSDH). (2008). *Closing the gap in a generation: Health equity through action on the social determinants of health.* Geneva, Switzerland: World Health Organization.

Dachs, N. S., Ferrer, M., Florez, C. E., Barros, A. J. D., Narvaez, R., Valdivia, M. (2002). Desigualdades de salud en América Latina y el Caribe: resultados descriptivos y exploratorios basados en la autonoti-ficación de problemas de salud y atención de salud en doce países [Inequalities in health in Latin America and the Caribbean: descriptive and ex-ploratory results of self-reported health problems and health care in twelve countries]. *Pan American Journal of Public Health.11*(5–6), 335–355. Available at: http://www.scielosp.org/scielo.php?script=sci_arttext&pid=S1020-49892002000500009

Dahlgren, G., Whitehead, M. (1991). *Policies and Strategies to Promote Social Equity in Health.* Stockholm, Sweden: Institute for Futures Studies.

Dahlgren, G., & Whitehead, M. (1993). *Tackling inequalities in health: What can we learn from what has been tried?* Working paper prepared for the King's Fund International Seminar on Tackling Inequalities in Health. London: Kings Fund.

Descartes, R. (1997). *Key philosophical writings.* Trans. by E. S. Haldane & G. R. T. Ross' edited and with an introduction by E. Chavez-Arvizo, Ware: Wordsworth.

Doll, R. (1955). Mortality from lung cancer in as-bestos workers. *British Journal of Industrial Medicine, 12*, 81–86.

Doll, R., & Hill, A. B. (1952). Smoking and carci-noma of the lung. *British Medical Journal, 2*, 84–92.

Durkheim, E. (1897/1952). *Suicide: A study in soci-ology.* Trans J. A. Spaulding & G. Simpson. London: Routledge & Kegan Paul.

Economic Commission for Latin America and the Caribbean (ECLAC). (2006). *Social Panorama 2006.* Santiago, Chile: ECLAC. Retrieved from http://www.eclac.cl/cgi-bin/getProd.asp?xml=/publicaciones/xml/4/27484/P27484.xml&xsl=/dds/tpl-i/p9f.xsl&base=/tpl/top-bottom.xslt

Ellaway, A., Macintyre, S., & Bonnefoy, X. (2005). Graffiti, greenery, and obesity in adults: Secondary analysis of European cross sectional survey. *British Medical Journal, 331,* 611–612.

Ensor, R. C. K. (1946). *England 1870–1914.* Oxford, UK: Clarendon Press.

Espelt, A., Borrell, C., Rodriguez, M., Muntaner, C., Pasarin, M. I., Benach, J., et al. (2008). Inequalities in health by social class dimensions in European countries of different political traditions. *International Journal of Epidemiology.* doi: 10.1093/ije/dyn051

Etches, V., Frank, J., Di Ruggerio, E., & Manuel, D. (2006). Measuring population health: A review of indicators. *Annual Review of Public Health, 27,* 29–55.

Evans, R. G., & Stoddart, G. L. (2003). Consuming research, producing policy. *American Journal of Public Health, 93,* 371–379.

Ferguson, T. (1948). The dawn of Scottish social welfare: *A survey from medieval times to 1863.* London: Nelson.

Ferguson, T. (1958). *Scottish social welfare 1864–1914.* Edinburgh: Livingston.

Frazer, W. M. (1947). *Duncan of Liverpool: Being an account of the work of Dr W. H. Duncan, Medical Officer of Health of Liverpool 1847–63.* London: Hamish Hamilton. Republished by Preston: Carnegie in 1997.

Frohlich, K. L., Corin, H., & Potvin, L. (2001). A theoretical proposal for the relationship between context and disease. *Sociology of Health & Illness,* 23(6), 776–797. Retrieved from http://www.ingentaconnect.com/content/bpl/shil/2001/00000023/00000006/art00002;jsessionid=8pesprj7e3q98.alice?format=print

Gairdner, W. T. (1862). *Public health in relation to air and water.* Edinburgh: Edmonston & Douglas.

Galea, S., Riddle, M., & Kaplan, G. A. (2009). Causal thinking and complex system approaches in epidemiology. *International Journal of Epidemiology, 39,* 97–106.

Giddens, A. (1979). Central problems in social theory: Action, structure and contradiction in social analysis. Berkeley, CA: University of California Press.

Giddens, A. (1982). Profiles and critiques in social theory. London: Macmillan.

Giddens, A. (1984). The constitution of society: Outline of the theory of structuration. Berkeley, CA: University of California Press.

Gilson, L., Doherty, J., Loewenson, R., & Francis, V. (2007). *Challenging inequity through health systems: Final report of the Health Systems Knowledge Network of the Commission on Social Determinants of Health.* Geneva, Switzerland: World Health Organization. Retrieved from http://www.who.int/social_determinants/resources/csdh_media/hskn_final_2007_en.pdf

Glass, T. A., & McAtee, M. J. (2006). Behavioral science at the crossroads in public health: Extending horizons, envisioning the future. *Social Science and Medicine, 62,* 1650–1671.

Goldberg, M., Melchior, M., Leclerc, A., & Lert, F. (2003). Épidémiologie et déterminants sociaux des inégalités de santé. *Revue d'épidémiologie et de santé publique, 51,* 381–401. Retrieved from http://cat.inist.fr/?aModele=afficheN&cpsidt=15109036

Graham, H. (Ed.). (2000). *Understanding health inequalities.* Buckingham, UK: Open University Press.

Graham, H. (2004a). Social determinants and their unequal distribution: Clarifying policy understandings. *Milbank Quarterly, 82,* 101–124.

Graham, H. (2004b). Tackling health inequalities in England: Remedying health disadvantages, narrowing gaps or reducing health gradients. *Journal of Social Policy, 35,* 115–131.

Graham, H. (2004c). Intellectual disabilities and socioeconomic inequalities in health: An overview of research. *Journal of Applied Research on Intellectual Disabilities, 18,* 101–111.

Graham, H., & Kelly, M. P. (2004). *Health inequalities: Concepts, frameworks and policy.* London:

Health Development Agency. Retrieved from http://www.nice.org.uk/page.aspx?o=502453

Graham, H., & Power, C. (2004). *Childhood disadvantage and adult health*. London: Health Development Agency. Retrieved from http://www.nice.org.uk/page.aspx?o=502707

Hamlin, C. (1995). Could you starve to death in England in 1839? The Chadwick–Farr controversy and the loss of social in public health. *American Journal of Public Health, 85*, 856–866.

Hertzman, C., Power, C., Mathews, S., & Manor, O. (2001). Using an interactive framework of society and lifecourse to explain self-rated health in early adulthood. *Social Science and Medicine, 53*, 1575–1585.

Hawe, P., Shiell, A., Riley, T. (2009). Theorising interventions as events in systems, *American Journal of Community Psychology, 43*, 267–76.

Hume, D. (1748/2007). *An enquiry concerning human understanding*. Edited and with an introduction by P. Millican. Oxford, UK: Oxford University Press.

Irwin, A., Valentine, N., Brown, C., Loewenson, R., Solar, O., Brown, H., et al. (2006). The Commission on Social Determinants of Health: Tackling the social roots of health inequalities, *PLoS Med, 3*(6), e106.

Irwin, L. G., Siddiqi, A., & Hertzman, C. (2007). *Early child development: A powerful equalizer. Final report of the early child development knowledge network of the Commission on Social Determinants of Health*. Geneva, Switzerland: World Health Organization. Retrieved from http://whqlibdoc.who.int/hq/2007/a91213.pdf

Kaplan, G. (2007). Health inequalities and the welfare state: Perspectives from social epidemiology. *Norsk Epidemiolgi, 17*, 9–20.

Karasek, R. (1996). Job strain and the prevalence and outcome of coronary artery disease. *Circulation, 94*(5), 1140–1141. Retrieved from http://www.circ.ahajournals.org/cgi/content/full/92/3/327

Kelly, M. P. (1996). Negative attributes of self: Radical surgery and the inner and outer lifeworld.

In C. Barnes & G. Mercer (Eds.). *Exploring the divide: Illness and disability*. 74–93. Leeds: Disability Press.

Kelly, M. P. (2001). Disability and community: A sociological approach. In G. Albrecht, K. Seelman, & M. Bury (Eds.), *Handbook of disability studies*. 396–411. London: Sage.

Kelly, M. P. (2006a). Mapping the life world: A future research priority for public health. In A. Killoran, C. Swann, & M. P. Kelly (Eds.), *Public health evidence: Tackling health*. 553–574. Oxford, UK: Oxford University Press.

Kelly, M. P. (2006b). The development of an evidence based approach to tackling health inequalities in England. In. A. Killoran, C. Swann, & M. P. Kelly (Eds.), *Public health evidence: Tackling health inequalities*. 41–62. Oxford, UK: Oxford University Press.

Kelly, M. P. (2009). The individual and the social level in public health. In A. Killoran & M. P. Kelly (Eds.), *Evidence based public health: Effectiveness and efficiency*. 425–435. Oxford, UK: Oxford University Press.

Kelly, M. P. (2010a). The axes of social differentiation and the evidence base on health equity. *Journal of the Royal Society of Medicine, 103*, 266–272. doi: 1258/jrsm.2010.100005

Kelly, M. P. (2010b). A theoretical model of assets: The link between biology and the social structure. In A. Morgan, M. Davies, & E. Ziglio (Eds.), *Health assets in a global context: Theory, methods, action*. 41–58. New York: Springer.

Kelly, M. P., Morgan, A., Bonnefoy, J., Butt, J., & Bergman, V. (2007). *The social determinants of health: Developing an evidence base for political action: Final report of the Measurement and Evidence Knowledge Network of the Commission on Social Determinants of Health*. Geneva, Switzerland: World Health Organization. Retrieved from http://www.who.int/social_determinants/resources/mekn_final_report_102007.pdf

Kelly, M. P., Stewart, E., Morgan, A., Killoran, A., Fischer, A., Threlfall, A., et al. (2009). A conceptual framework for public health: NICE's emerging approach, *Public Health, 123*, e14–e20. doi: 10.1016/j.puhe.2008.10.031

Kjellstrom, T. (2007). *Our cities, our health, our future: Acting on social determinants for health equity in urban settings. Final report of the Urban Settings Knowledge Network of the Commission on Social Determinants of Health*. Geneva, Switzerland: World Health Organization. Retrieved from http://www.who.int/social_determinants/ resources/knus_report_ 16jul07.pdf

Korenromp, E. L., Williams, B. G., Gouws, E., Dye, C., & Snow, R. W. (2003). Measurement of trends in childhood malaria mortality in Africa: An assessment of progress toward targets based on verbal autopsy. *Lancet Infectious Diseases, 3*(6), 349–358. Retrieved from http://www.thelancet.com/journals/ laninf/article/PIIS1473309903006571/fulltext

Krieger N. (2001). Theories for social epidemiology in the 21st century: An ecosocial perspective. *International Journal of Epidemiology, 30*(4), 668–677.

Krieger, N. (2008a). Proximal, distal and the politics of causation: what's level got to do with it? *American Journal of Public Health, 98*, 221–230.

Krieger, N. (2008b). Ladders, pyramids, and champagne: The iconography of health inequities. *Journal of Epidemiology and Community Health, 62*, 1098–1104.

Krieger, N., Rehkopf, D. H., Chen, J. T., Waterman, P. D., & Marcelli, M. (2008). The fall and rise of US inequalities in premature mortality. *PLoS Med, 5*(2), e46. doi: 10.1371/journal.pmed .0050046

Kuh, D., Ben-Shlomo, Y., Lynch, J., Hallqvist, J., & Power, C. (2003). Life course epidemiology. *Journal of Epidemiology and Community Health, 57*, 778–783.

Kunst, A. E., Bos, V, Mackenbach, J. P., & EU Working Group on Socio-economic Inequalities in Health. (2001). *Monitoring socio-economic inequalities in health in the European Union: Guidelines and illustrations*. Rotterdam: Erasmus University. Retrieved from http://ec.europa.eu/ health/ph_projects/1998/monitoring/fp_ monitoring_1998_frep_06_a_en.pdf

Labonte, R., Blouin, C., Chopra, M., Lee, K., Packer, C., Rowson, M., et al. (2008). *Towards health equitable globalisation: Rights, regulation and redistribution. Final report of the Globalization Knowledge Network of the Commission on Social Determinants of Health*. Geneva, Switzerland: World Health Organization. Retrieved from http://www.who.int/social_determinants/resources/ gkn_report_ 06_2007.pdf

Lazarus, R. (1969). *Patterns of adjustment and human effectiveness*. New York: McGraw-Hill.

Lazarus, R. S. (1974). Psychological stress and coping in adaptation and illness. *International Journal of Psychiatry in Medicine, 5*, 321–333.

Lazarus, R. (1976). *Patterns of adjustment* (3rd ed.). New York: McGraw-Hill.

Lazarus, R. (1980). The stress and coping paradigm. In L. A. Bond & J. C. Rosen (Eds.), *Competence and coping during adulthood*. 20–64. Hanover, NH: University Press of New England.

Lazarus, R. S. (1985). The costs and benefits of denial. In A. Monat & R. Lazarus, *Stress and coping: An anthology*. 154–173. New York: Columbia University Press.

Lazarus, R. S. (2001). Relational meaning and discrete emotions. In K. R. Scherer, A. Schorr, & T. Johnstone (Eds.), *Appraisal processes in emotion: Theory, methods, research*. 37–67. Oxford, UK: Oxford University Press.

Lazarus, R. S., & Cohen, J. B. (1977). Environmental stress. In I. Altman & J-F. Wohlwill (Eds.), *Human behavior and the environment: Advances in theory and research*. 2, 81–112. New York: Plenum.

Lazarus, R., & Folkman, S. (1984a). *Stress, appraisal and coping*. New York: Springer.

Lazarus, R., & Folkman, S. (1984b). Coping and adaptation. In W. D. Gentry (Ed.), *Handbook of behavioral medicine*. 283–309. New York: Guilford.

Lazarus, R. S., & Launier, R. (1978). Stress related transactions between person and environment. In L. A. Pervin & M. Lewis (Eds.), *Perspectives in interactional psychology*. 288–320. New York: Plenum.

Lenski, G. E. (1966). *Power and privilege: A theory of social stratification*. London: McGraw-Hill.

Lenski, G., & Lenski, J. (1971). *Human societies: An introduction to macro sociology* (3rd ed.). New York: McGraw-Hill.

Levine, R., What Works Working Group, & Kinder, M. (2004). *Millions saved: Proven successes in global health*. Washington, DC: Center for Global Development.

Macintyre, S. (1997). The Black report and beyond: What are the issues? *Social Science & Medicine, 44*(6), 723–745. Retrieved from http://www.ingentaconnect.com/content/els/02779536/1997/00000044/00000006/art00183

Mackenbach, J. P. (2006a). *Health inequalities: Europe in profile*. European Commission.

Mackenbach, J. P. (2006b). Socioeconomic inequalities in health in Western Europe: From description to explanation to intervention. In J. Siegrist & M. Marmot, *Social inequalities in health: New evidence and policy implications*. 223–246. Oxford, UK: Oxford University Press.

Mackenbach, J. P. (2009). Politics is nothing but medicine at a larger scale: Reflections on public health's biggest idea. *Journal of Epidemiology and Community Health, 63*, 181–184.

Mahoney, M., Simpson, S., Harris, E., Aldrich, R., & Stewart Williams, J. (2004). *Equity-focused health impact assessment framework*. Sydney: Australasian Collaboration for Health Equity Impact Assessment. Retrieved from http://www.hiaconnect.edu.au/files/EFHIA_Framework.pdf

Marmot, M. (2010). *Fair society, healthy lives: Strategic review of health inequalities in England post 2010*. London: UCL. Retrieved from http://www.ucl.ac.uk/gheg/marmotreview/Documents/finalreport

Marmot, M., & Bell, R. (2009). Action on health disparities in the United States: Commission on the Social Determinants of Health. Journal of the American Medical Association, 301, 1169–1171.

Marmot, M., & Friel, S. (2008). Global health equity: Evidence for action on the social determinants of health. *Journal of Epidemiology and Community Health, 62*, 1095–1097.

Marmot, M., & Wilkinson, R. (Eds.). (1999). *Social determinants of health*. Oxford, UK: Oxford University Press.

May, D., & Kelly, M. P. (1992). Understanding paranoia: Towards a social explanation. *Clinical Sociology Review, 10*, 50–69.

McKeown, T. (1976). *The role of medicine: Dream, mirage or nemesis?* London: Nuffield Provincial Hospitals Trust.

Mead, G. H. (1934). *Mind, self and society: From the standpoint of the social behaviorist*. Chicago: Chicago University Press.

Montenegro, R., & Stephens, C. (2006). Indigenous health in Latin America and the Caribbean. *Lancet, 367*(9525), 1859–1869. Retrieved from http://www.who.int/social_determinants/resources/articles/lancet_montenegro.pdf

Morris, J., Heady, J. A., Raffle, P. A. B., & Parks, J. W. (1953). Coronary heart disease and physical activity at work. *Lancet, ii*, 1053–1057, 1111–1120.

Murphy, M., Bobak, M., Nicholson, A., Rose, R., & Marmot, M. (2006). The widening gap in mortality by educational level in the Russian Federation, 1980–2001. *American Journal of Public Health, 96*(7), 1293–1299.

NICE. (2007). *Behaviour change at population, community and individual levels*. London: NICE. NICE Public Health Guidance 6. Retrieved from http://guidance.nice.org.uk/PH006

Ohenjo, N., Willis, R., Jackson, D., Nettleton, C., Good, K., & Mugarura, B. (2006). Health of indigenous people in Africa. *Lancet, 367*(9526), 1937–1946. Retrieved from http://www.who.int/social_determinants/resources/articles/lancet_ohenjo.pdf

Ostlin, P., Schrecker, T., Sadana, R., Bonnefoy, J., Gilson, L., Hertzman, C., et al. (2009). *Priorities for research on equity and health: Implications for global and national priority setting and the role of WHO to take the health equity research agenda forward*. Geneva, Switzerland: World Health Organization. Retrieved from http://www.global healthequity.ca/electronic%20library/Priorities%20for%20research%20on%20equity%20and%20health.pdf

Popay, J., Escorel, S., Hernandez, M., Johnston, H., Mathieson, J., & Rispel, L. (2008). *Understanding and tackling social exclusion: Final report of the Social Exclusion Knowledge Network of the Commission on Social Determinants of Health*. Geneva, Switzerland: World Health Organization. Retrieved September 30, 2008, from http://www.who.int/social_determinants/knowledge_networks/final_reports/sekn_fi nal%20report_042008.pdf

Putnam, S., & Galea, S. (2008). Epidemiology and macro social determinants of health, *Journal of Public Health Policy, 29*, 275–289.

Quigley, R., Cavanagh, S., Harrison, D., Taylor, L., & Pottle, M. (2005). *Clarifying approaches to health needs assessment, health impact assessment, integrated impact assessment, health equity audit, and race equality impact assessment*. London: Health Development Agency. Retrieved from http://www.nice.org.uk/page.aspx?o=505665

Rose, G. (2008). *Rose's strategy of preventive medicine: The complete original text*. Commentary by K-T. Khaw & M. Marmot. Oxford, UK: Oxford University Press.

Rutstein, S., & Johnson, K. (2004). *The DHS wealth index* (DHS Comparative Reports No. 6). Calverton, MD: ORC Macro. Retrieved from http://www.datadyne.org/files/reference/CR6.pdf

Schneider, M. C., Castillo Salgado, C., Bacallao, C., Loyola, E., Mujica, O. J., Vidaurre, M., et al. (2002a). Métodos de medición de las desigualdades de salud. *Revista Panamericana de Salud Publica, 12*(6), 398–414. Retrieved from http://www.scielosp.org/pdf/rpsp/v12n6/a08v12n6.pdf

Schneider, M. C., Castillo Salgado, C., Bacallao, C., Loyola, E., Mujica, O. J., Vidaurre, M., et al. (2002b). Resumen de los indicadores más utilizados para la medición de desigualdades en salud. *Revista Panamericana de Salud Publica, 12*(6), 462–464. Retrieved from http://www.scielosp.org/scielo.php?script=sci_arttext&pid=S1020-49892002001200012

Schutz, A. (1964). *Collected papers: II. Studies in social theory*. The Hague: Martinus Nijhoff.

Schutz, A. (1967). *The phenomenology of the social world*. Trans. b G. Walsh & F. Lehnert. Evanston, IL: Northwestern University Press.

Schutz, A. (1970). *On phenomenology and social relations: Selected writings*. Trans. by H. R. Wagner. Chicago: Chicago University Press.

Sen, G., Östlin, P., & George, A. (2007). *Unequal, unfair, ineffective and inefficient: Gender inequity in health: Why it exists and how we can change it. Final report of the Women and Gender Equity Knowledge Network to the Commission on Social Determinants of Health*. Bangalore: Indian Institute of Management. Retrieved from http://www.who.int/social_determinants/resources/csdh_media/wgekn_final_report_07.pdf

Setel, P. W., Sankoh, O., Rao, C., Velkoff, V. A., Mathers, C., Gonghuan, Y., et al. (2005). Sample registration of vital events with verbal autopsy: A renewed commitment to measuring and monitoring vital statistics. *Bulletin of the World Health Organization, 83*(8), 611–617. Retrieved from http://www.who.int/bulletin/volumes/83/8/setelabstract0805/en/index.html

Shaw, M., Dorling, D., Gordon, D., & Davey Smith, G. (1999). *The widening gap: Health inequalities and policy in Britain*. Bristol, UK: Policy Press.

Siegrist, J., & Marmot, M. (2004). Health inequalities and the psychosocial environment: Two scientific challenges. *Social Science & Medicine, 58*, 1463–1473.

Siegrist, J., & Marmot, M. (2006). *Social inequalities in health: New evidence and policy implications*. Oxford, UK: Oxford University Press.

Simpson, S., Mahoney, M., Harris, E., Aldrich, R., & Williams, S. J. (2005). Equity-focused health impact assessment: A tool to assist policy makers in addressing health inequalities. *Environmental Impact Assessment Review, 25*, 772–782.

Solar, O., & Irwin, A. (2007). *Towards a conceptual framework for analysis and action on the social determinants of health* [draft]. Geneva,

Switzerland: World Health Organization, Commission on Social Determinants of Health.

Soleman, N., Chandramohan, D., & Shibuya, K. (2005). *WHO Technical Consultation on Verbal Autopsy Tools: Final Report. Review of the literature and currently-used verbal autopsy tools.* Geneva, Switzerland: World Health Organization.

Soleman, N., Chandramohan, D., & Shibuya, K. (2006). Verbal autopsy: Current practices and challenges. *Bulletin of the World Health Organization, 84*(3), 239–245. Retrieved from http://www.who.int/bulletin/volumes/84/3/soleman0306abstract/en/index.html

Stanton, C., Hobcraft, J., Hill, K., Nicaise, K., Mapeta, W. T., Munene, F., et al. (2001). Every death counts: Measurement of maternal mortality via a census. *Bulletin of the World Health Organization, 79*, 657–664. Retrieved from http://www.who.int/bulletin/archives/79(7)657.pdf

Starfield, B. (2006). State of the art in research on equity and health. *Journal of Health Politics, Policy and Law, 31*, 11–32.

Starfield, B. (2007). Pathways of influence on equity in health. *Social Science and Medicine, 64*, 1355–1362.

Stephens, C., Porter, J., Nettleton, C., & Willis, R. (2006). Disappearing, displaced, and undervalued: A call to action for Indigenous health worldwide. *Lancet, 367*(9527), 2019–2028. Retrieved from http://www.who.int/social_determinants/resources/articles/lancet_stephens.pdf

Subramanian, S. V., Jones, K., Kaddour, A., & Krieger, N. (2009). Revisiting Robinson: The perils of individualistic and ecologic fallacy. *International Journal of Epidemiology*, 1–19. doi: 10.1093/ije/dyn359

Taylor, S. E., Repetti, R. L., & Seeman, T. (1997). Health psychology: What is an unhealthy environment and how does it get under the skin? *Annual Review of Psychology, 48*, 411–447.

Thomson, H., Atkinson, R., Petticrew, M., Kearns, A. (2006). Do urban regeneration programmes improve public health and reduce health inequalities? A synthesis of the evidence from UK policy and practice, *Journal of Epidemiology and Community health; 60*, 108–115.

Townsend, P., & Davidson, N. (Eds.). (1982). *Inequalities in health: The Black report.* London: Penguin.

United Nations Educational, Scientific and Cultural Organization (UNESCO). (2006). *Education for All global monitoring report 2006: Literacy for life.* Paris: Author. Retrieved from http://unesdoc.unesco.org/images/0014/001416/141639e.pdf

Vapattanawong, P., Hogan, M., Hanvoravongchai, P., Gakidou, E., Vos, T., Lopez, A., et al. (2007). Reductions in child mortality levels and inequalities in Thailand: Analysis of two censuses. *Lancet, 369* (9564), 850–855. Retrieved from http://www.thelancet.com/journals/lancet/article/PIIS0140673607604139/fulltext

Victora, C. G., Fenn, B., Bryce, J., & Kirkwood, B. R. (2005). Co-coverage of preventive interventions and implications for child-survival strategies: Evidence from national surveys. *Lancet, 366*(9495), 1460–1466.

Victora, C. G., Vaughan, J. P., Barros, F. C., Silva, A. C., & Tomasi, E. (2000). Explaining trends in inequalities: Evidence from Brazilian child health studies. *Lancet, 356*, 1093–1098.

Warnecke, R. B., Oh, A., Breen, N., Gehlert, S., Paskett, E., Tucker, K. L., et al. (2008). Approaching health disparities from a population perspectives: The National Institutes of Health Centers for Population Health and Health Disparities. *American Journal of Public Health, 98*, 1608–1615.

Weber, M. (1948). Class, status, party. In H. H. Gerth & C. W. Mills (Eds.), From *Max Weber: Essays in sociology.* 180–194. London: Routledge & Kegan Paul.

Webster, C. (1990). *The Victorian public health legacy: A challenge to the future.* London: Institution of Environmental Health Officers/Public Health Alliance.

Whitehead, M. (1992). Perspectives in health inequity. *International Journal of Health Services, 22*, 429–445.

Wilkinson, R., & Pickett, K. (2009). *The spirit level*. London: Allen Lane.

Woolf, S., Johnson, R. E., Phillips, R. L., & Philipsen, M. (2007). Giving everyone the health of the educated: An examination of whether social change would save more lives than medical advances. *American Journal of Public Health, 97*, 679–683.

World Cancer Research Fund/American Institute for Cancer Research. (2009). *Policy and action for cancer prevention. Food nutrition and physical ac-tivity: A global perspective*. Washington, DC: American Institute of Cancer Research.

World Health Organization (WHO). (2006a). Constitution of the World Health Organisation. Retrieved from http://www.who.int/governance/eb/constitution/en/

World Health Organization (WHO). (2006b). WHO statistical information systems. Retrieved from http://apps.who.int/whosis/database/life_tables/life_tables.cfm

CHAPTER

4

Reproductive Health

M. OMAR RAHMAN AND JANE MENKEN

Reproductive health in low- and middle-income countries has long been addressed primarily through family planning and maternal and child health programs, and through programs to prevent and treat sexually transmitted infections (STIs) and their consequences. HIV/AIDS prevention and treatment is increasingly essential in addressing this area of global health.

Reproductive health is tied to policy concerns about population growth as well as health. In 1994, the United Nations (UN) sponsored the third decennial International Conference on Population and Development (ICPD) in Cairo. The previous two conferences had emphasized family planning and economic development, respectively, as the major focus of population policy—policy that was intended to reduce fertility and, thereby, population growth. The rationale for support of family planning programs included both the right of individuals to control their own fertility and the belief that reduced fertility would lead to reduced population growth, which would have benefits for individuals, nations, and the world. In 1994, for the first time, women's health advocates, including many from nongovernmental organizations (NGOs), played a key role in the ICPD and brought to the fore issues of reproductive health that went beyond family planning. They called for a fundamental redefinition of population policy that focused on the status of women and gave "prominence to reproductive health and the empowerment of women while downplaying the demographic rationale for population policy" (McIntosh & Finkle, 1995, p. 223).

The 1994 ICPD adopted a Programme of Action that included the following definition of reproductive health:

Reproductive health is a state of complete physical, mental and social well-being, and not merely the absence of disease or infirmity, in all matters relating to the reproductive system and its processes. Reproductive health therefore implies that people are able to have a satisfying and safe sex life and that they have the capability to reproduce and the freedom to decide if, when, and how often to do so. Implicit in this last condition are the right of men and women to be informed and to have access to safe, effective, affordable and acceptable methods of family planning of their choice, as well as other methods of their choice for the regulation of fertility which are not against the law, and the right of access to appropriate health-care services that enable women to go safely through pregnancy and childbirth and provide couples with the best chance of having a healthy infant. . . . It also includes sexual health, the purpose of which is the enhancement of life and personal relations, and not merely counseling and care related to reproduction and sexually transmitted diseases (United Nations, 1994).

This vision of reproductive health has, not unexpectedly, proved controversial and has not been achieved to the extent hoped for by its proponents (see, for example, "Conference Adopts Plan," 1999; "Population Control Measures," 1999). Nor have donors met the pledges made at the Cairo conference. The UN estimated in 2003 that the international donor community had contributed far less than the pledges for reproductive health made at Cairo. Of the $6.1 billion promised by 2005, slightly more than $3 billion had been provided through 2003 (Population Reference Bureau, 2004; United Nations Commission on Population and Development, 2004).

A less controversial and more limited version of the vision for reproductive health guided the 1997 U.S. National Academy of Sciences report on reproductive health (Tsui, Wasserheit, & Haaga, 1997):

1. Every sex act should be free of coercion and infection.

2. Every pregnancy should be intended.

3. Every birth should be healthy for both mother and child.

Even so, no country, according to Tsui, Wasserheit, and Haaga (1997), had met these more limited goals by 1997, and the problems were greatest in the low- and middle-income countries.

In 2000, the United Nations Millennium Declaration was adopted as a commitment to "making the right to development a reality for everyone and to freeing the entire human race from want" (United Nations General Assembly, 2000). Eight Millennium Development Goals (MDGs) were established as part of the Roadmap Toward the Implementation of the United Nations Millennium Declaration (United Nations General Assembly, 2001). Goal 5 is to improve maternal health with a specific target of reducing "by three quarters, between 1990 and 2015, the maternal mortality ratio." In mid-2008, the UN found little change in maternal mortality had occurred in sub-Saharan Africa and Southern Asia. Only in countries with moderate to low levels of maternal mortality in 1990 had significant improvement occurred ("Maternal Deaths," 2008; United Nations Statistics Division, 2010a, 2010b; World Health Organization [WHO], 2008b).

This chapter emphasizes both the older and the newer views of family planning and reproductive health. In the section on demographic trends, the focus is on population growth and change and the transitions under way around the world from situations of high fertility and high mortality to those of low fertility and low mortality. The ways in which people control their fertility and indices of the effects of various fertility determinants on overall fertility in a range of countries are then considered. The third section examines family planning programs and their role in the reduction of fertility and unintended pregnancy. The next two sections consider the role of fertility patterns in the health of children and women,

respectively. The final section presents brief recommendations for future research and programs. Because Chapter 5 focuses on STIs, including HIV/AIDS, these crucial aspects of reproductive health are mentioned only briefly here.

Demographic Trends and Fertility Determinants

History of Population Growth

To understand the context of the concerns about population and reproductive health in the world today, it is instructive to review the history of population growth and its associated impacts. Figure 4-1 shows the growth of population and, in particular, the extraordinary changes in growth rates over the past 200 years. World population reached 1 billion just after 1800. By the turn of the twentieth century it had reached 1.6 billion, and before 1930 it had surpassed 2 billion. Thus it took less than 125 years to add the second billion people, an astounding feat given the long sweep of history needed to reach the first billion. World population passed the 3 billion mark in 1960. Each additional billion of people has taken less time to add, so that by the year 2000, population had reached 6.1 billion. Thus population doubled between 1960 and 2000, adding 3 billion people in only 40 years. In the last 10 years, almost 1 billion people have been added, so that world population in 2010 was 6.9 billion (United Nations Population Division, 2009; Figure 4-1).

The majority of this expansion has taken place in the low- and middle-income regions of Asia, Africa, Latin America, and Oceania (Figure 4-2), which accounted for 82% of the world's population in 2010, compared with 71% in 1950. The share of world population in these regions is expected to continue increasing, reaching 86% in the middle of the twenty-first century (United Nations Population Division, 2009).

The encouraging news is that the rate at which the world's population is growing has declined continuously since about 1960 (Figure 4-3), although the absolute *number* of people added in each decade has continued to increase. After 2000 that number is projected to decline. Population growth rates are declining in most low- and middle-income countries, albeit at an uneven pace; that is, some countries and regions are experiencing much more rapid change than others. China is a particularly prominent example; its growth rate was 2.1% in 1960, increased to 2.6% in 1965, but then steadily dropped to less than 1% by

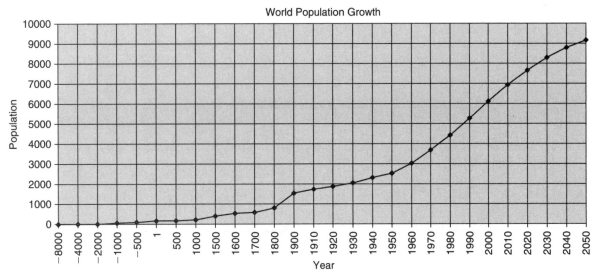

Figure 4-1 The Growth of Population and, in Particular, the Extraordinary Changes of the Past 200 Years. *Source*: Data for the years 8000 to 1900: US Bureau of the Census, Population Division, International Programs Center, (http://www.census.gov/ipc/www/worldhis.html), and for the years 1910-2050: United Nations Population Division, 2009: *World Population Prospects: The 2008 Revision Population Database* (http://esa.un.org/unpp/). Accessed March 26, 2010.

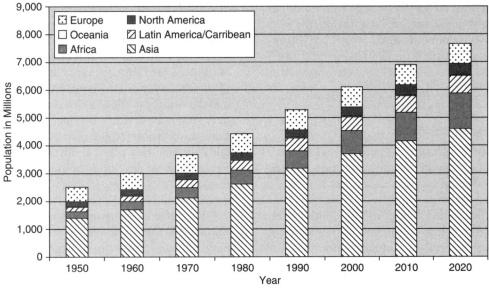

Figure 4-2 Population Size by Continent, 1950–2020 *Source*: Data from United Nations Population Division, 2009: *World Population Prospects: The 2008 Revision Population Database* (http://esa.un.org/unpp/). Accessed March 26, 2010.

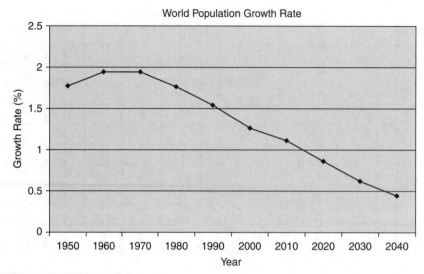

Figure 4-3 World Population Growth Rate: 1950–2040. *Source*: Data from United Nations Population Division, 2009: *World Population Prospects: The 2008 Revision Population Database* (http://esa.un.org/unpp/). Accessed March 26, 2010.

1995. The UN estimates that world population in the middle of the twenty-first century will total between 8 billion and 11 billion people. By that time, the growth rate will be significantly less than 1% but will not yet have achieved the no-growth stable situation.

Because of reduced fertility and increased life expectancy, the 2050 population will have more people older than 60 than children younger than age 15. As of 2010, 11% of all people were older than 60 and 26.9% were younger than 15. Nevertheless, the world population will continue to age, so that 21.9% are expected to be older than 60 in 2050, while only 19.6% are younger than 15 (United Nations Population Division, 2009).

The Demographic Transition

What explains the historic experience of low initial growth, followed by an explosive increase and finally by a steady decline in growth? The classic theory of demographic transition proposed by Notestein (1953) and others postulated that all societies initially start off with high fertility and high mortality levels. At some point in societal development, mortality rates fall due to public health advances, while fertility rates remain high. This combination results in explosive population growth, with birth rates far exceeding death rates, until at some point birth rates also start to decline and a new equilibrium is reached at low fertility and low mortality levels.

Until fairly recently, the classic theory of demographic transition held sway, and all societies were supposed to go through it in a lock-step manner. In the early to mid-1970s, however, an international team of researchers participated in the Princeton University European Fertility Project and carefully examined historical fertility declines in Europe. They came to a somewhat surprising conclusion: The process of demographic transition is quite varied and does not always follow the path suggested by classic theory (Coale & Watkins, 1986). Under that scenario, a certain level of socioeconomic development was required for the initial mortality decline, which was followed, at some later point, by fertility decline. Researchers in the European Fertility Project, however, found that mortality decline took place in different societies at different levels of development and that there was no magic threshold of mortality above which fertility decline would not take place.

The current consensus about demographic transition is that there is no specific sequence in which fertility and mortality decline. They can decline together, or one can decline before the other. Furthermore, no specific thresholds of development are required for either process to start. Moreover, the intervals between a high-fertility and high-mortality regime and a subsequent low-fertility and low-mortality regime are also not fixed and can vary considerably. The experience of the low- and middle-income countries has borne out this new consensus. Demographic transitions have taken place at different rates in different places and with different sequences; a common thread, however, is that the transition has often been

considerably more rapid than those seen in the European or North American historical record.

Population growth rates and fertility and mortality for different parts of the world since the mid-twentieth century are shown in Table 4-1, and for the specific cases of Bangladesh and Kenya, in Exhibit 4-1. Growth rates are given as the percent change in

Table 4-1	Growth Rate, Total Fertility Rate, and Life Expectancy for Regions of the World, by Time Period

Region	1950	1970	1990	2000	2010[a]	2020[a]
World						
Growth rate	1.77	1.94	1.54	1.26	1.11	0.86
TFR	4.92	4.32	3.08	2.67	2.49	2.30
Life expectancy	46.6	58.2	64.0	66.4	68.9	71.1
Low- and Middle-Income Countries						
Growth rate	2.03	2.37	1.82	1.47	1.28	1.00
TFR	6.00	5.18	3.43	2.89	2.62	2.39
Life expectancy	41.0	54.9	61.7	64.4	67.0	69.4
High-Income Countries						
Growth rate	1.21	0.77	0.47	0.36	0.28	0.14
TFR	2.82	2.17	1.67	1.58	1.65	1.67
Life expectancy	66.0	71.3	74.1	75.8	78.0	79.7
Asia						
Growth rate	1.89	2.26	1.63	1.25	1.05	0.75
TFR	5.73	4.76	3.01	2.50	2.26	2.09
Life expectancy	41.2	56.6	64.2	67.6	70.3	72.6
Africa						
Growth rate	2.18	2.65	2.57	2.34	2.20	1.85
TFR	6.63	6.69	5.65	4.91	4.27	3.54
Life expectancy	38.7	46.5	51.6	52.7	56.0	59.5
Latin America & Caribbean						
Growth rate	2.71	2.42	1.73	1.31	0.99	0.73
TFR	5.85	5.01	3.02	2.50	2.09	1.90
Life expectancy	51.3	60.9	68.9	72.1	74.5	76.5
Oceania						
Growth rate	2.15	1.61	1.52	1.48	1.23	1.05
TFR	3.83	3.29	2.49	2.42	2.39	2.25
Life expectancy	60.4	65.8	72.3	75.2	77.3	79.0
Northern America						
Growth rate	1.71	0.94	1.19	0.96	0.91	0.72
TFR	3.33	2.07	1.99	1.99	1.98	1.87
Life expectancy	68.8	71.6	75.9	78.4	77.3	81.1
Europe						
Growth rate	1.00	0.60	0.18	0.08	−0.13	−0.22
TFR	2.65	2.19	1.57	1.43	1.53	1.60
Life expectancy	65.6	70.8	72.6	73.8	76.1	78.1

Note: Growth rate (% per year), TFR, and life expectancy are for the subsequent 5-year period (e.g., 1950–1955). Life expectancy is for both sexes combined.

[a]Figures for 2010 and 2020 are from the medium-variant projection.

Source: Data from United Nations Population Division, *World Population Prospects: The 2004 Revision Population Database* (http://esa.un.org/unpp/). Accessed June 22, 2005.

Exhibit 4-1   **Demographic Change in Kenya and Bangladesh**

Kenya (population = 41 million) and Bangladesh (population = 164 million) will be used as case studies to illustrate demographic change in this chapter for a number of reasons. There are both similarities and differences in their experiences.

First, similar to Bangladesh, Kenya experienced high population growth rates that were the result of continuing high fertility during a period when mortality was declining quite sharply. Thus, in the period 1950–1955, life expectancy was 40.5 years for males and 44.2 years. By 1980–1985, almost 16.5 years had been added to life expectancy for both males and females in Kenya, raising life expectancy there to 57 years for males and 60.7 years for females. In comparison, although life expectancy also rose sharply during the same period for Bangladesh, the increase was notably less than in Kenya (10 years for males and 14 years for females). Because Bangladesh started from a lower base in 1980–1985, life expectancy in Bangladesh was actually significantly (almost 10 years) lower than that in Kenya (male = 48.9 years; female = 50.2 years). As a result of the sharp decline in mortality coupled with continuing high fertility rates (during that period, the total fertility of Kenya exceeded 7 births per woman), population growth rates in Kenya increased from 2.77% per year in 1950–1955 to 3.78% per year in 1980–1985. Similarly, for Bangladesh, due to the sharp drop in mortality and the continued high fertility (TFR remained between 6 and 7), there was also a sharp increase in population growth rates, from 2.11% in 1950–1955 to 2.61% in 1980–1985.

Second, as was the case in Bangladesh, a successful family planning program in Kenya managed to bring about a fertility decline despite relatively little improvement in socioeconomic indicators (Toroitich-Ruto, 2001). Fertility dropped sharply over the next 15 years, from 7.22 births per woman in 1980–1985 to 5.07 births per woman in 1995–2000. Fertility subsequently appears to have plateaued; in 2005–2010, it was estimated at approximately 4.96 births per woman. Both the initial decline and the subsequent plateauing in total fertility rates are similar to the experience of Bangladesh, although TFR in Bangladesh plateaued at a significantly lower level—approximately 3.3 in 1995–2000—and subsequently dropped very slowly to an estimated 2.36 in 2005–2010.

Kenya, like other countries severely affected by AIDS, saw its life expectancy fall in the latter part of the twentieth century, to 51 years for males and 52.3 years for females in 2000, with life expectancy expected to rise thereafter.

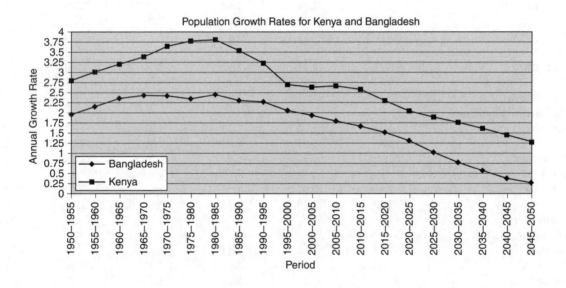

(continued)

Exhibit 4-1 | **Continued**

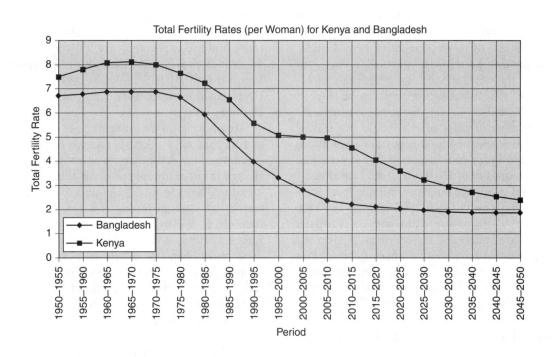

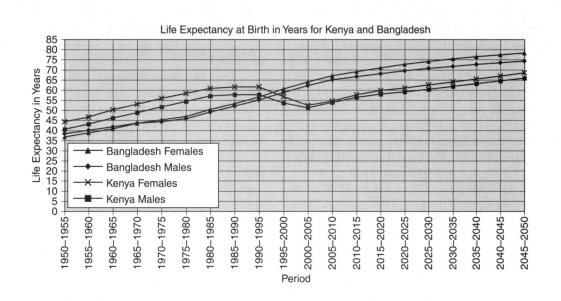

population per year for the five years subsequent to the specified date. When a population stops changing in size, it becomes *stationary* and its growth rate is zero. The total fertility rate (TFR) is the number of children a women would bear, on average, if they lived to the end of the reproductive period under the childbearing pattern of a particular year—for example, if they had, at age 15, the birth rate of 15-year-olds in 1970; at age 16, the birth rate of 16-year-olds in 1970; and so on. Life expectancy at birth is the average number of years people would live if their entire life were spent under the mortality conditions of a particular year—for example, if they experienced the infant mortality of 1970, the death rate at age 1 of 1970, and so on. The numbers resulting from these examples would be the 1970 TFR and the 1970 life expectancy. A TFR of approximately 2.1 is usually referred to as *replacement level* fertility. If, over the long run, women have that number of children on average, the population will become stationary, neither growing nor declining. Women will be contributing to the next generation one child for themselves and one for their partner, and a bit more for girls who were born but did not survive to reproduce.

As shown in Table 4-1, life expectancy has risen continuously over the latter half of the twentieth century. The exceptions (not shown) are in the countries of Africa hardest hit by AIDS, where, by 2000, disease wiped out much if not all earlier gains (see Exhibit 4-1 for the specific case of Kenya). According to the UN, nine countries had adult HIV prevalence of 10% or more in 2009: Swaziland, Botswana, Lesotho, Zimbabwe, South Africa, Namibia, Zambia, Malawi, and Mozambique (UNAIDS Fact Sheets, 2009). The U.S. Census Bureau (2004) estimated that, on average, life expectancy in 2010 will be 30.5 years less in these countries than it would have been in the absence of AIDS. Much of the increase in every country in life expectancy is due to improvements in infant and child survival; by contrast, the HIV-related declines are primarily the result of increased adult mortality.

Total fertility rate had declined by 1970 in all parts of the world with the exception of Africa. That decline was, in low- and middle-income regions, overwhelmed by increases in life expectancy, so that these regions' growth rates—and their population growth—increased. Fertility continued to fall, however, and at sufficient rates to counteract the continuing increased in life expectancy. This fertility transition is serving to bring growth rates down in all low- and middle-income regions today. HIV/AIDS may be contributing to recent declines in fertility in the parts of the

world hardest hit by this disease; a mounting body of evidence indicates that infected women have reduced fecundity (United Nations Population Division, 2002; Lewis, Ronsmans, Ezeh, & Gregson, S. (2004). The changes in population growth rates, total fertility rates, and life expectancy are illustrated in Exhibit 4-1, which provide information for Bangladesh and Kenya from 1950 to 2050 using the medium variant UN population estimates (United Nations Population Division, 2009).

To understand the different types of fertility transitions that have taken place, we need an understanding of the determinants of fertility and fertility change in different contexts. An extensive body of literature has examined the impact of socioeconomic factors on desired family size (see, for example, Bankole & Westoff, 1995; Bulatao & Lee, 1983; Rutstein, 1998). Much of this discussion centers on the costs and benefits of children and the notion that couples desire additional children as long as the benefits are greater than the costs. These benefits and costs are, in turn, determined by a range of factors, some of which are *structural* (e.g., wages, rates of return on investments, opportunity costs), and some of which are attitudinal (i.e., changes in values and expectations). Improvements in the educational status of women, for example, are thought to decrease desired family size because such trends increase the potential wages that women can earn and thus raise the opportunity costs of childbearing and childrearing. Education may, in addition, lead to attitudinal change about quantity–quality tradeoffs in numbers of children—for example, having fewer children so that greater investment in the education of each child is feasible.

Implicit in this theoretical framework is the idea that couples weigh a variety of alternatives, with childbearing being just one of the possible behavioral choices available. Other structural factors affecting fertility rates include trends such as increasing landlessness, which decreases the benefits of the labor provided by children and thereby tends to reduce family sizes. More recent research emphasizes attitudinal change as affecting fertility rate. It posits that values and expectations can change as a result of outside influences. Thus exposure to messages in which small families are treated as a marker for modernity may motivate couples to reduce their desired family sizes even in the absence of any changes in the structural costs and benefits of children.

Although this chapter focuses on low- and middle-income countries, in almost none of which has fertility declined to replacement level, it is worth noting that high-income countries, especially those in Europe, are concerned about their very low fertility rates and population declines. For Europe as a whole, TFR fell to less than 1.9 births per woman before 1980 and has continued to decline. It is expected that the entire continent will have a negative growth rate for 2000–2020 (United Nations Population Division, 2009). Understanding what maintains below-replacement fertility and what causes it to increase is an important issue for high-income countries.

How Do People Control Their Fertility?

In addition to considering *why* people control their fertility, we need to understand *how* people actually do so. It is useful first to consider the *proximate determinants* that lead to variation in fertility in the absence of deliberate family planning (see, for example, Bongaarts, 1978; Bongaarts & Potter, 1983; Menken & Kuhn, 1996; Sheps & Menken, 1973). These proximate determinants can be divided into those that affect the *reproductive span* and those that influence the *intervals between successive births* within that span. As shown in Figure 4-5, the *effective reproductive span* exists within boundaries set by both the *biological span* and the *social reproductive span*. The biological span is the time during which a woman is capable of childbearing because she has the biological capacity to ovulate and to carry a pregnancy to a

live birth. It is usually marked by menarche and menopause, but first ovulation may occur well after menarche and last ovulation precedes menopause.

In no society, however, do women devote their full biological span to reproduction. Were they to do so, according to Bongaarts (1978), women who survive to sterility would bear more than 15 children on average. This figure is well beyond the maximum ever recorded for any population.

Every society has social controls on initiation and cessation of sexual activity. We will refer to entry into sexual activity as *marriage* and cessation as *marriage dissolution*. We use these terms as social markers rather than as representing legal ceremonies and arrangements of the state. Specifically, marriage dissolution can occur through breakup of the relationship or through widowhood. The social reproductive span is, therefore, the interval between initiation and cessation of sexual activity. The effective reproductive span is the overlap of the biological and the social spans. It begins with the later of menarche and marriage and ends with the earliest of sterility, death, and cessation of sexual activity. In many societies, the effective reproductive span is interrupted by time between successive unions or by temporary separation of spouses.

Within the effective reproductive span, the pace of childbearing is determined by the lengths of the successive intervals between births (B_1, B_2, and so on

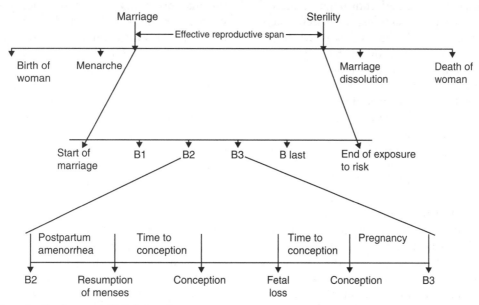

Figure 4-5 Reproductive Span and Birth Intervals.

in Figure 4-5). We will first discuss birth intervals in the absence of deliberate family planning. The birth interval may be divided into several segments:

- The postpartum period after a birth until both ovulation and sexual relations resume
- The time to conception
- Additional time due to fetal loss through spontaneous abortion
- The pregnancy leading to the next live birth

Fertility in the Absence of Contraception and Induced Abortion

The postpartum period ends when both ovulation and intercourse have resumed. It is largely determined by the duration and intensity of breastfeeding and by postpartum taboos against intercourse by a nursing mother. Women who do not breastfeed usually menstruate for the first time approximately two months after giving birth (Salber, Feinleib, & MacMahon, 1966). Frequent, intense breastfeeding, however, can postpone average time of ovulation to more than 20 months (see, for example, Wood, Lai, Johnson, Campbell, & Maslar, 1985). Some populations, particularly in sub-Saharan Africa, have traditionally had taboos against intercourse that can lengthen the postpartum period beyond the resumption of ovulation, but these practices are rare outside this region and their observance is believed to be decreasing.

Breastfeeding not only provides the child with nourishment, but also, depending on the pattern of suckling, can postpone the return of ovulation for many months. It exerts this effect through a maternal response to suckling that suppresses the secretion of gonadotrophins. The classic studies of McNeilly (1996) and his colleagues showed that "if the frequency of suckling is maintained above five times a day and the duration is maintained above 65 minutes a day, amenorrhea will often be the consequence." Others have found that night feeds are particularly important in maintaining amenorrhea (Jones, 1988). Women who fully breastfeed their infants and are amenorrheic are highly unlikely to conceive in the first six months after a birth. Indeed, one multinational study estimated that fewer than 2% would do so (Labbok, Hight-Laukaran, Peterson, Fletcher, von Hertzen, & Van Look, 1997). In addition, demographic studies suggest that the duration of lactational amenorrhea increases with the age of the woman (Wood, 1994). The effects of breastfeeding patterns are so important that they are the major factor in explaining differences in fertility among populations in which no family planning is practiced.

The time to conception depends on the monthly probability of conception in the absence of birth control and can vary among populations, by age, and according to the frequency and pattern of intercourse. The monthly probability of conception, known as *fecundability*, is extremely difficult to measure. Estimates of this probability differ in part because of the methods used to determine that a conception has occurred. If early fetal loss occurs before the woman is aware she is pregnant, then the estimates of conception are biased downward. According to Wood (1994), the best study of early fetal loss was conducted by Wilcox and associates (1988), who followed a group of women aged 20 to 35 and collected blood and urine samples from them regularly. There were 198 pregnancies detected by assays of these samples; 43 pregnancies, or about 22%, were lost before the woman realized she was pregnant and before clinical diagnosis was made.

More traditionally, fecundability has been measured by accepting a woman's report of her pregnancy. This measure of *apparent* fecundability has yielded rates that range from approximately 0.10 to 0.30 for relatively young women (Menken, 1975; Wood, 1994). The waiting time to conception is, on average, the inverse of fecundability; for younger women, this time is 3 to 10 months on average. In many cases, fecundability has been estimated from reported waiting times to conception using a variety of mathematical models (some of which are summarized by Wood, 1994).

Fecundability depends in part on a couple's frequency and pattern of intercourse, which determines the likelihood that coitus will occur during the woman's fertile period. Both those couples wishing to conceive a wanted child and those couples hoping to avoid pregnancy without the use of hormonal or barrier contraceptives depend on knowledge of the woman's cycle to time their sexual activity, thereby changing their probability of conception. Whether ovulation is discerned by changes in cervical mucus or basal body temperature, conception is most likely to occur when intercourse takes place shortly before ovulation (Colombo & Masarotto, 2000).

Fecundability declines with the age of the woman, although there is increasing evidence that the decline does not take place until the late thirties, on average, if patterns of intercourse remain unchanged. Decline with age of the man is quite slow.

Lactation has a fertility-reducing effect even after a woman has resumed menstruation and ovulation (see Wood, 1994). Apparently, continued suckling beyond ovulation reduces fecundability through a response that interferes with the functioning of the corpus luteum. Although fertilization can occur, the corpus luteum may not produce sufficient progesterone to enable the pregnancy to continue (McNeilly, 1996).

HIV also affects fertility. Notably, it reduces conception rates beginning in the earliest asymptomatic stages of infection (Gray et al., 1998; Ross, Van der Paal, Lubega, Mayanja, Shafer, & Whitworth, 2004; United Nations Population Division, 2002).

Spontaneous abortion occurs frequently; the estimated rate, as already described, depends on how early the pregnancy is detected. From the time conceptions are recognizable by virtue of late menses, approximately 24% end in spontaneous abortion (French & Bierman, 1962). Even higher proportions of fertilized ovum do not lead to live births. Wilcox and associates (1988), in the study cited earlier in which urine specimens were collected so that early pregnancy could be detected, found that 31% of the pregnancies ended in fetal loss. Rates of spontaneous abortion increase with the age of the woman (Nybo Andersen, Wohlfahrt, Christens, Olsen, & Melbye, 2000; Wood, 1994) and, more slowly, with the age of the man (Nybo Anderson, Hansen, Andersen, & Davey Smith, 2004; Slama, Werwatz, Boutou, Ducot, Spira, & Hardle, 2003). The time added to the birth interval by a recognized fetal loss is the sum of the time from pregnancy to the next ovulation (usually estimated to be slightly more than 3 months on average, as the vast majority of spontaneous abortions occur very early in pregnancy) plus the time to the next conception. There is little evidence that rates of spontaneous abortion vary to any great extent among populations.

Gestation leading to a live birth does not vary much, usually lasting between 35 and 40 weeks, with few differences noted between population groups (Wood, 1994, p. 207). In some populations with outstanding care of premature infants or increasing maternal risks, gestation may be somewhat shorter on average. In the United States, the percentage of live births reported as preterm (fewer than 37 weeks' gestation) increased from 9.4% in 1981 to 12.1% in 2002, a jump of 29% (Martin, Hamilton, Sutton, Ventura, Menacker, & Munson, 2003). In 2009, the highest rates of preterm births occurred in Africa (11.9%) and North America (10.6%), with Europe (6.2%) having the lowest rate (Beck et al., 2009).

A cross-cutting issue that affects fertility rates is that of infertility and sterility. Especially in parts of Africa, infertility and early sterility are major factors affecting fertility. This effect may take the form of absolute sterility that causes the effective reproductive span to end early, or decreased fecundability or increased risk of spontaneous abortion (see, for example,

Larsen, 2000). In most cases, however, the concern is with early sterility, much of which is believed to be due to sexually transmitted infections.

Thus the main reasons that populations not practicing family planning vary in terms of their fertility rates are differences in the effective reproductive span and the duration of the postpartum amenorrheic period, with variation in time to conception and infertility playing lesser roles.

Deliberate Control of Fertility

People can deliberately reduce their fertility in three ways: (1) by reducing the effective reproductive span through postponement of marriage or interrupted marriage or by sterilization that ends reproductive capacity early; (2) by using contraception, which increases the time to conception; and (3) by induced abortion, which increases the time added to the birth interval by pregnancies that do not lead to a live birth. Family planning programs can both promote the motivation to reduce fertility and provide the means to do so. Many governments encourage or enforce later marriage explicitly through changes in the legal age of marriage and implicitly through programs that foster female education. Family planning programs have traditionally focused on education regarding methods of fertility control, motivation to reduce the number of wanted children, and provision of family planning methods themselves. Such methods include promotion of breastfeeding, both for the health of the infant and to prolong the postpartum period; contraception, which is intended to prolong the time to conception; and, except where there is opposition for religious reasons, abortion, which increases the time added to the birth interval.

Although specific family planning methods are discussed in greater detail in the section on family planning programs later in this chapter, it seems appropriate to consider two important general issues here. First, why do populations in which the desired number of children is low still have high proportions of unintended births? Second, why is reliance on abortion an inefficient approach to family planning?

Contraception, even when highly effective, may not prevent all unintended pregnancies. A simple calculation makes this problem clear. Suppose a woman is using a highly effective method—one that reduces her probability of conceiving to about 1 in 1,000 per month. She begins using this method at age 30 and wants no more children before she reaches menopause at age 45. We can calculate the probability that she has no pregnancy in each of 13 lunar months over the next 15 years, or a total of 195 lunar months. The probability of succeeding (not getting pregnant) is

.999 each month. The probability of not getting pregnant in 195 months is $.999^{.195}$, which equals .38. In other words, this woman has only a 38% chance of avoiding pregnancy for 15 years. Among women like her, 62% will have at least one unintended pregnancy in that time period. For this reason, even women who are very serious users of contraception are at high risk of unintended pregnancy. Family planning program and health planners need to be aware of this high risk when they are developing their programs.

In a population that relies primarily on induced abortion to reduce fertility, if a woman becomes pregnant unintentionally, she may choose to have an abortion. Approximately three months after the abortion, she again begins ovulating and is capable of conceiving. Suppose her time to conception averages 10 months. Then 13 months after the first abortion, she is again pregnant and must have another abortion if she is not to have an unwanted birth. Another 13 months later, an abortion is again performed, and so on. Preventing a birth for 15 years may, therefore, require 15 abortions.

Given this pattern, it is not surprising that many women in Eastern European countries who relied primarily on abortion for birth control reported numbers of abortions in the double digits. Women in the former Soviet Union, for example, are believed to have had six or more abortions on average over the course of their lifetime (David, 1992). While abortion rates in Eastern Europe have declined sharply in the last decade or so with increased access to modern contraception services, they remain the highest in any region in the world (44 women undergoing abortions per 1,000 women of childbearing age; 105 abortions for every 100 births) (Alan Guttmacher Institute, 2009a, 2009b). Abortion, is, however, extremely effective as a backup to effective contraception. A woman who has an abortion and subsequently uses extremely effective contraception is unlikely to have more than one or two unintended pregnancies—but our previous analysis shows that she may, indeed, have these one or two.

For these reasons, it is not surprising that sterilization—the one method that has a failure rate near zero—is so widely selected by women and couples who want no additional children. In the United States in 2002, sterilization of the woman or of the man was the modal method used by women older than age 30 (Mosher, Martinez, Chandra, Abma, & Wilson, 2004). In low- and middle-income countries, 26% of married women relied on sterilization to prevent additional births; 22% of wives and an additional 4% of their husbands had been sterilized (Population Reference Bureau, 2002).

The Effect on Fertility of the Proximate Determinants: *Bongaarts' Indices*

Bongaarts (1978) developed a set of indices to measure the effect on fertility of some of these proximate determinants. They are based on the assumption that there is some maximum potential fertility, TF, for women. This figure is usually estimated to be slightly more than 15 children.

C_i The **index of postpartum infecundity** varies from 0 to 1. It represents the proportion of potential fertility, TF, remaining when the average postpartum period of the population of interest is taken into account. Therefore, $C_i = 1$ if the population does not breastfeed at all. The fertility-reducing effect of postpartum infecundity is $(1 - C_i)$.

C_A The **index of abortion** is the proportion of TF, after postpartum infecundity is first taken into account, remaining when the effect of induced abortion in reducing live births is taken into account. Spontaneous abortions are included in the original estimate of TF, because they are treated as a purely biological occurrence. Few countries have sufficient information available on abortion to make reasonable estimates of C_A, so it usually must be disregarded in application.

C_C The **index of contraception** is the proportion of TF, after the effects of postpartum infecundity and induced abortion are taken into account, remaining after contraceptive use is considered.

C_m The **index of marriage** is the proportion of TF, after the first three factors are considered, remaining when the particular marriage or sexual union pattern is taken into account.

Thus, in the Bongaarts decomposition of the total fertility rate,

$$TFR = TF \leftrightarrow C_i \leftrightarrow C_A \leftrightarrow C_C \leftrightarrow C_m$$

Both C_C and C_m contain adjustments for infertility and sterility. In the first index, the adjustment takes into account infertility and sterility and assumes no use of contraception by infertile and sterile couples. In the second index, a weighting factor is present, in that nonmarriage has a greater effect on fertility reduction when the woman is young (e.g., the effect of nonmarriage is much greater for a 25-year-old than a 42-year-old).

Table 4-2 presents these indices, except for C_A, which is assumed to be 1 because of the lack of data, for a number of populations around 1970 and for several historical populations (Bongaarts & Potter, 1983). The major impact of breastfeeding can be seen

Table 4-2	Estimates of Total Fertility Rate and the Bongaarts's Proximate Determinants Indices*			
Region and Year	**Total Fertility Rate (TFR)**	**Index of Postpartum Infecundity (C_i)**	**Index of Marriage (C_m)**	**Index of Contraception (C_c)**
Low- and Middle-Income Countries				
Bangladesh, 1975	6.34	0.54	0.85	0.90
Colombia, 1976	4.57	0.84	0.58	0.61
Dominican Republic, 1975	5.85	0.61	0.60	1.0
Indonesia, 1976	4.69	0.58	0.71	0.75
Jordan, 1976	7.41	0.80	0.74	0.81
Kenya, 1976	8.02	0.67	0.77	1.0
Korea, 1970	3.97	0.66	0.58	0.68
Lebanon, 1976	4.77	0.78	0.58	0.69
Sri Lanka, 1975	3.53	0.61	0.51	0.74
Syria, 1973	7.00	0.73	0.73	0.86
Thailand, 1975	4.70	0.66	0.63	0.74
Industrialized Countries				
Denmark, 1970	1.78	0.93	0.55	0.23
France, 1972	2.21	0.93	0.52	0.30
Hungary, 1966	1.80	0.93	0.62	0.21
United Kingdom, 1967	2.38	0.93	0.61	0.27
United States, 1967	2.34	0.93	0.63	0.26
Historical Populations				
Bavarian villages, 1700–1850	4.45	0.85	0.37	0.91
Grafenhausen, 1700–1850	4.74	0.67	0.44	1.0
Hutterites	9.50	0.82	0.73	1.0
Quebec, 1700–1730	8.00	0.81	0.63	1.0

Note*: Each index represents the proportion of potential fertility remaining after the particular factor is taken into account in the following order: postpartum infecundity, marriage, and contraceptive use.

Source: Adapted with permission of the Population Council, from John Bongaarts, "The Fertility-Inhibiting Effects of the Intermediate Fertility Variables," *Studies in Family Planning*, 13 (6/7), pp. 182–183.

through the values of the index C_i in countries whose populations used little contraception during the period in question. All of the South and East Asian countries, as well as Kenya, have indices that do not exceed 0.67; thus their potential fertility is reduced by at least one-third by long postpartum periods. In fact, the long breastfeeding periods employed in Bangladesh and Indonesia reduced these countries' fertility rates to only about half of their potential. In Europe, the demographic transition to low levels of fertility was caused, to a great extent, by very late marriage and a relatively high degree of nonmarriage. The index of marriage is far lower, on average, for high-income countries around 1970 than for low- and middle-income countries. Two historical populations shown, however, had indices of marriage less than 0.45, indicating that nonmarriage reduced their potential fertility by at least 55%. By 1970, fertility in all the developed countries shown was reduced by contraceptive use to no more than 30% of its potential level.

Thus, in high-income countries, breastfeeding has little effect on fertility, but nonmarriage and use of contraception reduce the TFR to relatively low levels. In the 1970s, contraceptive use had little impact on fertility in the low- and middle-income countries included in Table 4-2; lower fertility was achieved in some of these countries through long-term breastfeeding (see Exhibit 4-2 for the example of Kenya). Populations that had very high TFRs achieved these rates through a combination of high indices of marriage and breastfeeding and little or no contraception.

Stover's Revision of Bongaarts' Indices

The indices of the effects of the proximate determinants on fertility have been revised a number of times by Bongaarts and others to take advantage of more recent detailed and reliable data and to substitute more realistic assumptions. Stover (1998), for example, dropped the original indices of marriage and contraceptive use; he also attempted to treat infertility and sterility more directly and to deal with sexual activity rather than using the proxy of marriage or stable sexual union incorporated in the earlier version of the indices. He includes, instead, three new indices:

Exhibit 4-2	Proximate Determinants of Fertility in Kenya

The fertility rate in Kenya was estimated to be approximately 8.20 births per woman in 1978. This high fertility was due to the combination of very high rates of marriage for women of reproductive age (C_m = .91) and essentially no fertility control within marriage (C+ = 0.96). Fertility could, however, have been much higher except for prolonged amenorrhea, which is related to the long breastfeeding practiced in this country (C_f = .64). Total fertility, at 8.20 births per woman, was slightly more than half (.56) of what it would have been (TFR = 14.7) if women had not breastfed at all (Toroitich-Ruto, 2001).

The focus of the Kenyan Family Planning Program has been to increase fertility control within marriage by increasing the use of contraception by married women. This emphasis paid off at least initially and resulted in sharp declines in TFR between 1978 and 1989 (from 8.20 births per woman to 6.60 births per woman). Estimates of Bongaarts' proximate determinants of fertility for Kenya in 1989 compared to 1978 support the notion that this sharp decline in TFR was essentially due to a rise in contraceptive prevalence rates. The Bongaarts' estimates show a significantly lower index of contraception (C_c) of approximately 0.80 in 1989 compared to 0.96 in 1978, reflecting the rapid rise in contraceptive prevalence over a period of 12 years (33% in 1989 versus 7% in 1978); a relatively unchanged index for marriage (C_m = 0.86 in 1989 versus 0.91 in 1978), reflecting the continuing high rates of marriage; and a relatively unchanged index of postpartum infecundity (0.66 in 1989 versus 0.64 in 1978), reflecting continued long breastfeeding durations (Toroitich-Ruto, 2001).

Total fertility rates continued to decline relatively rapidly until 1993 (TFR = 5.4) Subsequently, fertility decline stalled. In 2003 (the most recently available data), TFR in Kenya was 4.9, with contraceptive prevalence rates having risen to 41%, up from 33% in 1989 (Macro International, 2010c).

Table 4-3	Estimates of Total Fertility Rate (TFR) and Revised Bongaarts's Proximate Determinants Indices				
Region (Year)	**TFR**	**Index of Sexual Activity (C_x)**	**Index of Postpartum Infecundity (C_i)**	**Index of Infecundity (C_f)**	**Index of Contraceptive Use (C_u)**
Africa					
Burkina Faso, 1993	6.9	.66	.49	.88	.94
Cameroon, 1991	5.8	.69	.57	.81	.84
Ghana, 1993	5.5	.64	.55	.86	.81
Madagascar, 1992	6.1	.71	.61	.83	.89
Namibia, 1992	5.4	.59	.59	.86	.70
Niger, 1992	7.4	.86	.58	.78	1.0
Nigeria, 1990	6.0	.73	.53	.80	.93
Rwanda, 1992	6.2	.60	.56	.85	.86
Senegal, 1993	6.0	.63	.56	.81	.93
Zambia, 1992	6.5	.69	.60	.86	.90
Latin America and the Caribbean					
Brazil, 1991	3.7	.59	.83	.88	.39
Colombia, 1990	2.9	.53	.77	.89	.36
Dominican Republic, 1991	3.3	.54	.81	.88	.41
Paraguay, 1990	4.7	.49	.76	.86	.47
Peru, 1992	3.5	.55	.68	.89	.53

Source: Adapted with permission of the Population Council, from Stover, J. (1998). Revising the proximate determinants of fertility framework: What have we learned in the past 20 years? *Studies in Family Planning, 29*(3), 263.

C_x The **index of sexual activity** depends on the reported proportion of women in the population who are sexually active. Its interpretation is, therefore, the proportion of potential fertility remaining after celibacy is taken into account.

C_f The **index of infecundity** reflects the effect on fertility of infecundity among sexually active women, and is simply $1 - f$, where f is the proportion who report that they believe themselves to be infecund.

C_u The **index of contraceptive use** reflects actual contraceptive use by women who believe themselves to be fecund and who are not experiencing postpartum amenorrhea.

Thus the fertility-reducing effect of the proximate determinants is given by

$$C_x \leftrightarrow C_i \leftrightarrow C_A \leftrightarrow C_u \leftrightarrow C_f$$

where the index of abortion (C_A) is rarely estimated and C_i is the index of postpartum infecundity as previously defined by Bongaarts.

These results show that the two main factors producing lower fertility in Latin America are relatively low participation in sexual activity and relatively high contraceptive use (Table 4-3). By contrast, in most countries of Africa, there is much higher participation in sexual activity and lower use of contraception. Fertility would be even higher were it not for the effects of postpartum infecundity, which reduces fertility by at least 40% in the countries represented here. What is striking is the documentation of the rather large impact on overall fertility (approximately 20%) in some countries due to infertility among sexually active women.

Family Planning Programs

A fundamental rationale for family planning programs is to reduce unintended fertility because of its negative health and welfare consequences and because control of fertility has been recognized as a human right of women and couples. Over the last 50 years, societal changes have included reduced infant mortality, increased urbanization, improved education for women, increased economic opportunities, and the dissemination and adoption of modern ideas about small families. The response by couples in the low- and middle-income countries has been accelerated change in expectations about both the number and the timing of births (Bongaarts, 1983; Freedman, 1987).

In 1997, 155 countries had programs that subsidized the cost of family planning services (Gelbard, Haub, & Kent, 1999). However, in part due to the lack of available, accessible, and effective contraception, the gap between observed and desired fertility grew, leading in turn to an increase in unintended fertility (Bankole & Westoff, 1995; Bulatao, 1998). Out of 211 million pregnancies in 2005, 87 million women become pregnant unintentionally. Due to concerted family planning efforts in the last three decades to increase access to contraceptive services (which worldwide have increased from about 10% in the early 1960s to 59% in 2000), many more women are now able to avoid unintentional pregnancies (WHO, 2005). For example, in Kenya, 35.5% of women expressing a desire to control their fertility were not able to meet this need in 1989. By 2003, this figure had decreased to 24.5% (Exhibit 4-3).

Unintended Fertility

A number of definitional issues complicate the process of estimating unintended fertility and its distribution. In general, data on unintended fertility come from representative population surveys in which women who are pregnant at the time of the survey or who have had at least one birth in the five years prior to the survey are asked whether each of those births (including the outcome of the current pregnancy) was

---

Exhibit 4-3   Desired Family Size and Unmet Need for Contraception in Kenya

One rationale for family planning programs was that couples who wanted to have fewer children were unable to do so either because they lacked knowledge of the means of fertility control or because they lacked access to those means, owing to an absence of supplies or services.

In the case of Kenya, even in the earliest surveys carried out, a high proportion of married women reported that they wanted no more children. At that time, the mean ideal number of children was reported to be 4.4, and 45.5% of women reported they did not want to have another child. The desired TFR (wanted fertility) was 4.5, while the actual TFR was 6.7. Thus there was a big gap between desired fertility and actual fertility despite the inception in late 1970s of a nationwide family planning program. Among the barriers to achieving this low desired fertility were (1) the economic costs of access to services, including the cost of transportation, and supplies; (2) the social costs, including travel by women whose mobility was traditionally constrained; (3) the psychic costs of contraceptive use in a society that offered little social or familial support for low fertility; and (4) the health costs of side effects, whether subjective or objective, from contraceptive use.

These barriers have been overcome to the extent that in 2003, 43% of married women of reproductive age in Kenya were current contraceptive users, compared to 33% in 1989. Also, actual TFR in Kenya declined from 6.7 in 1989 to 4.9 in 2003. However, wanted fertility did not remain at the 1989 level: It fell to 3.6. The need for contraception in 2003 remained unmet for 24.5% of women at risk of pregnancy, down from 35.5% in 1989.

intended, *mistimed* because it came too early but was still within the desired number of births, or *unwanted* in that no more children were desired. Unfortunately, usage of these terms is not completely consistent; some authors include mistimed births as part of their estimates of unwanted births, while others count only those births that exceed the desired family size as unwanted (Brown & Eisenberg, 1995). The major weakness of this approach is that women may be reluctant to classify specific births as unwanted, leading to artificially low estimates of unwanted births.

Measurement of fertility intentions has been criticized because it relies exclusively on mothers' intentions and not the intentions of other family members—most importantly, fathers—to gauge unintended fertility. It has been argued that the intentions of the mother, especially in many low- and middle-income countries, may not accurately reflect the desirability of a birth. Evidence suggests that intergenerational differences in family size goals (i.e., preferences of grandparents versus parents) may be more pronounced than interspousal differences (Caldwell, 1986; Mason & Taj, 1987). Ultimately, the justification for relying on the stated preferences of the mother in determining desired family size and unintended or unwanted births stems from the fact that the mother is the person most responsible for the birth and child care (Tsui et al., 1997).

Demographic and Health Surveys (DHS) have been conducted since 1984 in approximately 75 low- and middle-income countries (www.measuredhs .com/). This research is intended to provide comparable information on a variety of subjects related to health and fertility issues. DHS calculates, for each survey, both the total fertility rate (the number of children a woman would bear were she to live her reproductive life under the fertility conditions just prior to the survey) and the unwanted total fertility rate (the number of those children who would be unwanted) (Westoff, 2001). A birth is counted as unwanted only when the mother states she wanted no more children at the time of the pregnancy.

The results of DHS surveys conducted over the period 2003–2010 in 41 countries are shown in Table 4-4. On average, 18% of total fertility was unwanted, with the percentage varying considerably by region. The lowest and the highest fertility regions (Eastern Europe and sub-Saharan Africa, respectively) had the lowest proportions of unwanted births (the mean percentages were 8% for Eastern Europe and 16% for sub-Saharan Africa). Some countries with high total fertility rates had low proportions unwanted (e.g., Niger). The highest percentages unwanted (one-third

or more) were found in countries with TFRs between 3 and 5. Finally, in low fertility countries where the TFR is less than 4 births per woman, a substantial proportion of those births remain unwanted (Macro International, 2010b).

Note that this and earlier evidence suggest that increases in contraception prevalence rates do not necessarily cause a decline in the proportion of unwanted births and, in fact, may initially be associated with an increase in the proportion of unwanted births (Tsui et al., 1997). This scenario can happen if desired fertility rates drop faster than the compensating rises in contraceptive prevalence rates and if the use of methods of fertility control is so effective that unintended births rarely occur. Thus, when couples have very high fertility desires, it is difficult to exceed those desires, so nearly all children are wanted. As desired fertility falls, use and effective use of contraception and abortion may not increase quickly enough to avoid unwanted births. Finally, at low levels of fertility, women want so few children that there remain many years after the last wanted child during which an unwanted pregnancy and birth can, and frequently do, occur. The differences by education within a country can, in part, be explained by this phenomenon: More-educated women within a society frequently are earlier adopters of contraception and, because they desire few children, a higher proportion of their children are unwanted.

With regard to mistimed births, DHS data from around 1990 suggest that roughly 20% of births in low- and middle-income countries were mistimed—that is, they came too early. There were no apparent regional differences in mistimed births and no clear association between contraceptive prevalence and the proportion of mistimed births. Thus, even in a region such as sub-Saharan Africa, which has a low rate of unwanted fertility, considerable mistimed fertility was still observed. This finding suggests that there is a need for contraception to delay first births and control spacing of subsequent births even when there may be little demand for contraception to control the number of births (Bankole & Westoff, 1995; Rafailimanana & Westoff, 2001).

Consequences of Unintended Pregnancies and Births

Aside from helping individual couples fulfill their desires and expectations, why should we care about unintended pregnancies and births and, moreover, try to reduce them? A compelling public health reason is their negative consequences. Unintended pregnancies

Table 4-4	Total Fertility Rate and Percentage of Births Unwanted, by Mother's Education, in Countries with DHS Surveys Conducted Around 2000							
	No Education		Primary Education		Secondary or Higher Education		Total	
	TFR	Percentage Unwanted	TFR	Percentage Unwanted	TFR	Percentage Unwanted	TFR	Percentage Unwanted
Sub-Saharan Africa								
Benin, 2006	6.4	0.16	5.2	0.15	3.3	0.11	5.6	0.1
Cameroon, 2004	6.3	0.05	5.6	0.09	3.5	0.09	4.8	0.10
Chad, 2004	6.3	0.05	7.4	0.11	4.2	0.07	6.3	0.03
Congo, 2005	6.2	0.05	6.3	0.09	4	0.07	4.8	0.08
Congo Democratic Republic, 2007	7.1	0.11	7.1	0.11	5	0.01	6.3	0.11
Euthopia, 2005	6.1	0.25	5.1	0.31	2	0.25	5.4	0.26
Ghana, 2008	6.0	0.12	4.9	0.14	3.0	0.17	4.0	0.12
Guinea, 2005	6.2	0.01	5.8	0.14	3.3	0.12	5.7	0.1
Kenya, 2003	6.7	0.15	5.5	0.31	3.2	0.28	4.9	0.27
Lesotho, 2004	5.2	0.25	4	0.3	2.9	0.45	3.5	0.29
Liberia, 2007	6	0.08	5.9	0.01	3.3	0.15	5.2	0.11
Madagascar, 2003/2004	6.5	0.11	5.7	0.12	3.4	0.12	5.2	0.12
Malawi, 2004	6.8	0.18	6.2	0.19	3.8	0.16	6.0	0.18
Mali, 2006	7.0	0.09	6.3	0.11	3.8	0.05	6.6	0.09
Namibia, 2006/2007	6.3	0.24	4.5	0.27	3.0	0.20	3.6	0.25
Niger, 2006	7.2	0.03	7.0	0.04	4.8	0.06	7.0	0.03
Nigeria, 2008	7.3	0.07	6.5	0.08	4.2	0.07	5.7	0.07
Rwanda, 2005	6.9	0.23	6.1	0.25	4.3	0.23	6.1	0.25
Senegal, 2005	6.0	0.12	4.8	0.19	2.9	0.14	5.3	0.15
Swaziland, 2006/2007	4.9	0.39	4.5	0.51	3.4	0.41	3.9	0.46
Tanzania, 2004/2005	6.9	0.10	5.6	0.08	3.3	0.09	5.7	0.14
Uganda, 2006	7.7	0.19	7.2	0.25	4.4	0.18	6.7	0.24
Zambia, 2007	8.2	0.13	7.1	0.15	3.9	0.10	6.2	0.16
North Africa/West Asia/Europe								
Armenia, 2005	0	0	3.1	0	1.7	0.06	1.7	0.06
Azerbaijan, 2006	1.8	0.11	2.8	0.18	2	0.1	2	0.1
Egypt, 2005	3.8	0.32	3.4	0.29	2.9	0.21	3.1	0.26
Jordan, 2007	2.6	0.31	3.9	0.31	3.6	0.22	3.6	0.22
Eastern Europe								
Ukraine, 2007	1.8	0	5.1	0	1.2	0.08	1.2	0.08
South & Southeast Asia								
Bangladesh, 2007	3.0	0.37	2.9	0.31	2.5	0.24	2.7	0.30
Cambodia, 2005	4.3	0.21	3.5	0.17	2.6	0.15	3.4	0.18
India, 2005/2006	3.6	0.33	2.6	0.27	2.1	0.19	2.7	0.37
Indonesia, 2007	2.4	0.17	2.8	0.14	2.6	0.15	2.6	0.15
Nepal, 2006	3.9	0.33	2.8	0.32	2.2	0.27	3.1	0.35
Pakistan, 2006/2007	4.8	0.23	4.0	0.27	2.8	0.21	4.1	0.24
Latin America & Caribbean								
Colombia, 2005	4.5	0.44	3.4	0.38	2.1	0.24	2.4	0.29
Dominican Republic, 2007	3.9	0.26	3.0	0.3	2.2	0.14	2.4	0.21
Ecuador, 2004	5.9	0.27	4.1	0.22	2.6	0.15	3.2	0.22
Haiti, 2005/2006	5.9	0.41	4.3	0.37	2.4	0.17	3.9	0.38
Honduras, 2005/2006	4.9	0.33	3.8	0.32	2	0.15	2.7	0.15
Nicaragua, 2006	4.4	0.14	3.2	0.19	2.0	0.15	2.7	0.15
Paraguay, 2004	4.3	0.09	4	0.15	2.4	0.08	2.9	0.10

Source: Macro International, 2010b.

increase the lifetime risk of maternal mortality simply by increasing the number of pregnancies (Alan Guttmacher Institute, 2009a; Koenig, Phillips, Campbell, & D'Souza, 1988). Unintended pregnancies can lead to unsafe abortion, poor infant health, and lower investment in the child.

Abortion

In many cases, unintended pregnancies are terminated by abortions, which are currently the outcome of roughly 20% of all pregnancies. Most abortions, especially those in low- and middle-income countries, continue to be conducted illegally under unhygienic conditions and pose significant health risks to the mother.

The legal status of abortion and, consequently, access to safe abortion services is highly variable. Roughly 40% of women of childbearing age (15 to 44 years) currently live in countries where abortion is highly restrictive (Alan Guttmacher Institute, 2009a; Rahman, Katzive, & Henshaw, 1998). Women in low- and middle-income countries (except for China and India) are much more likely to live under restrictive abortion laws than women in high-income countries. In fact, out of 193 countries, only 52 countries allow abortion on request; in 110 countries, abortion remains illegal even in the face of incest or rape (WHO, 2007b). There has been some positive change in access to legal abortion since 1995, with 19 new countries broadening the grounds under which abortion can be performed.

Despite these differences in legal access, there is little difference in the likelihood of having an abortion. Thus the abortion rate is 29 per 1,000 women of childbearing age (15 to 44 years) in Africa, where abortion is fairly restrictive, compared to 28 per 1,000 women in Europe, where it is very accessible (Alan Guttmacher Institute, 2009b). As a result, women in low- and middle-income countries (excluding China) are more likely to have illegal abortions, and their abortion mortality rate is many times higher than that for women in high-income countries (330 deaths versus 0.2 to 1.2 deaths per 100,000 abortions) (Alan Guttmacher Institute, 1999a, 1999b, 2009a, 2009b).

Henshaw, Singh, and Haas (1999) estimated that approximately 26 million legal abortions and 20 million unsafe (illegal) abortions were performed worldwide in 1995, resulting in a worldwide abortion rate of 35 per 1,000 women aged 15 to 44. In the last decade or so, however, there has been some significant progress on this front. The total number of abortions worldwide decreased from 45.5 million to 41.6 million in 2003, though the total number of unsafe (il-legal) abortions (almost all in low- and middle-income countries) has essentially remained the same, at about 20 million. The overall worldwide abortion rate has come down from 35 per 1,000 women to 29 per 1,000 women largely due to reductions in safe abortions associated most likely with increases in contraceptive use in the high-income world. Most strikingly, in Eastern Europe, which had the highest abortion rates in 1995, abortion rates declined dramatically—from 90 per 1,000 women in 1995 to 44 per 1,000 women in 2003—coincident with a substantial increase in contraceptive use. Western Europe continues to have the lowest abortion rate, which has not changed since 1995 (12 per 1,000) (Alan Guttmacher Institute, 2009a, 2009b).

Even where abortion is legal, access is very limited, there are poor systems of referral, and very often services are of poor quality. For example, despite the fact that manual vacuum extraction is much safer, the most frequently used method for abortion in most countries is dilatation and curettage, which has significant associated morbidity. In recent years, some encouraging signs indicate that use of manual vacuum extraction and medications to end unwanted pregnancies is increasing (Alan Guttmacher Institute, 2009a).

WHO estimates that approximately 20 million unsafe abortions (i.e., those not attended by a trained health professional) are performed each year, resulting in nearly 66,500 deaths in low- and middle-income countries. Globally, unsafe abortion accounts for 13% of maternal deaths (WHO, 2007b). Case fatality rates (deaths per 100,000 unsafe abortion procedures) vary tremendously by region, with the world average being 300 deaths per 100,000 unsafe abortions and ranging from 10 deaths per 100,000 unsafe abortions in the high-income world to 750 deaths per 100,000 unsafe abortions in sub-Saharan Africa. It is worth noting that case fatality rates for unsafe abortions are many times higher than for safe abortions, again with significant regional differences—ranging from 10 times higher in the developed world to 1,000 times higher in sub-Saharan Africa.

Another abortion-related issue is the recent rise in the male-to-female sex ratio at birth in Southeast Asia. Data from a number of countries, including China and Korea, show that the sex ratio at birth in these areas is unusually high compared with the expected ratio of 1.06 male births to each female birth, and is steadily increasing. Rising sex ratios at birth suggest that selective abortion of female fetuses may be increasing (Arnold, Kishor, & Roy, 2002; Larsen, Chung, & Das Gupta, 1998; Westley, 1995). This practice is embedded in the context of strong societal preferences for male children and declining family size desires, which increase the incentives to have both the desired family composition and the desired number of children.

In recent decades, the broader availability of modern technology has provided the means to actualize these preferences. There are basically three ways of determining the sex of a fetus: chorionic villus sampling, amniocentesis, and ultrasound. Ultrasound is the safest and cheapest method, but only works reliably 5 to 6 months into the pregnancy (i.e., the end of the second trimester). It is widely available in rural areas in India, China, and other parts of East Asia. Despite strong legal sanctions against sex-selective abortion, the availability of relatively cheap ultrasound technology has promoted this practice, leading to deleterious consequences for women who undergo late-term, riskier abortions and possibly for children due to the increasing sex imbalance in the population.

Consequences of Unintended Births for Infant Health

Data on the consequences of unintended births for infant health are available for the period before 1990. They show that these births were concentrated in demographically high-risk categories (Tables 4-5, 4-6, and 4-7); that is, the proportion of unintended births was much higher among young mothers and older mothers, among higher-parity mothers, and following a short birth interval (National Research Council, 1989). Why these demographic characteristics are associated with high risks for infant health is discussed in greater detail in the next section. Notably, unwanted births have higher mortality even when the pregnancy fits into otherwise demographically low-risk categories (mothers aged 24 to 29; parity of 2 to 4).

Table 4-5	Percentage Unintended of Most Recent Birth or Current Pregnancy by Mother's Age		
	Mother's Age		
Country (Year)	Younger Than 20 Years	2–4 Years	35 Years or Older
Bolivia, 1993	41.5	53.9	74.0
Colombia, 1986	34.9	48.3	60.5
Egypt, 1988	13.9	41.3	75.0
Kenya, 1993	61.2	55.3	65.4
Nigeria, 1990	13.7	12.5	21.6
Philippines, 1993	37.6	46.4	58.2
Tanzania, 1991	22.7	26.1	31.7
Thailand, 1987	28.3	38.4	47.2

Source: Adapted with permission from Tsui, A. O., Wasserheit, J. N., & Haaga, J. G. (Eds.). (1997). *Reproductive health in developing countries: Expanding dimensions, building solutions.* Washington, DC: National Academies Press. Copyright 1997 by the National Academy of Sciences.

Table 4-6	Percentage Unintended of Most Recent Birth or Current Pregnancy by Birth Order		
	Birth Order		
Country (Year)	1	2–4	5+
Bolivia (1993)	32.7	50.1	78.6
Colombia (1986)	25.0	50.7	68.8
Egypt (1988)	3.8	39.5	67.2
Kenya (1993)	52.1	52.1	66.2
Nigeria (1990)	11.2	9.9	22.7
Philippines (1993)	22.3	47.4	63.6
Tanzania (1991)	18.7	25.0	39.5
Thailand (1987)	20.7	36.3	64.4

Source: Adapted with permission from Tsui, A. O., Wasserheit, J. N., & Haaga, J. G. (Eds.). (1997). *Reproductive health in developing countries: Expanding dimensions, building solutions.* Washington, DC: National Academies Press. Copyright 1997 by the National Academy of Sciences.

Table 4-7	Percentage Unintended of Recent Higher-Order Birth or Current Pregnancy by Interval from Previous Birth to Conception	
	Interval from Previous Birth to Conception	
Country (Year)	Birth Interval <24 months	Birth Interval ≥24 months
Bolivia (1993)	68.4	60.1
Colombia (1986)	67.6	49.2
Egypt (1988)	54.0	50.2
Kenya (1993)	67.2	56.1
Nigeria (1990)	21.1	13.0
Philippines (1993)	62.1	49.3
Tanzania (1991)	33.5	27.5
Thailand (1987)	53.4	36.5

Source: Adapted with permission from Tsui, A. O., Wasserheit, J. N., & Haaga, J. G. (Eds.). (1997). *Reproductive health in developing countries: Expanding dimensions, building solutions.* Washington, DC: National Academies Press. Copyright 1997 by the National Academy of Sciences.

Human Capital Investments

In addition to deleterious health consequences for the mother and the index child, unintended births have spillover and long-term cumulative effects by reducing human capital investments (i.e., allocation of resources for education and health) in the family as a whole. A number of studies in low- and middle-income countries have shown that older children, especially girls, suffer disproportionately in terms of lower educational attainment and health status as family size increases—the latter being a proxy for unwanted births (Bledsoe & Cohen, 1993; Desai, 1995; Frenzen & Hogan, 1982; Lloyd, 1994).

Cross-sectional associations between large family sizes and lower health and educational attainments need to be interpreted cautiously, given that parents who choose to have large families may also choose to invest differently in different children (Knodel, Chamrathrithirong, & Debavalya, 1987). Nevertheless, some evidence, from a family planning quasi-experiment in which villages were assigned different levels of family planning services, suggests that part of the relationship between large family sizes and low human capital investments is causal (Foster & Roy, 1996).

Unmet Need for Contraception

A primary objective of family planning programs has been to reduce unintended births by addressing "the unmet need for contraception." This unmet need is conventionally estimated from representative population-based surveys of currently married women as the sum of the number of currently pregnant women who report that their pregnancy is unintended and the number of currently nonpregnant women who are not using contraception and would not like to have any more children or, at least, none in the next two years (Bankole & Westoff, 1995). On the basis of this definition, the unmet need for contraception (Table 4-8) is estimated to be 12% or less for married women in countries with high contraceptive prevalence rates (e.g., 55% or higher) and ranges up to 40% (Uganda) of women in countries with lower contraceptive prevalence rates.

The definition of "unmet need for contraception" has been criticized as an underestimate of actual need because it excludes both currently married women who are not pregnant and who are using inappropriate (because of health consequences or side effects) methods of contraception and sexually active women who are not currently married and who do not wish to become pregnant, at least in the next two years (Bongaarts, 1991; Dixon-Mueller & Germain, 1992;

Pritchett, 1994a, 1994b). An additional criticism revolves around the issue of ineffective contraception. Large numbers of women currently use traditional methods, which have much higher failure rates than available modern contraceptives. Current estimates of unmet need do not include women who are using traditional (i.e., ineffective) contraceptives methods.

More recent estimates (Ross & Winfrey, 2002) consider unmarried as well as married women. They show that for all low- and middle-income countries, approximately 113.2 million women have an unmet need for contraception (105.2 million married and 8.4 million unmarried). These numbers translate into 17% of married women having an unmet need versus 3% of unmarried women, with women aged 15 to 24 accounting for one-third of the unmet need. Of the 17% total unmet need for contraception, 9% is attributed to the need to space births and 8.1% to the need to limit births. The total number of women whose needs are unmet results from the combination of upward pressure due to population growth and downward pressure due to the success of family planning programs (Ross & Winfrey, 2002).

Family planning programs have played an important role in reducing the unmet need for contraception by making contraception both physically accessible and financially affordable. Since the late 1950s, when the first national family planning programs in low- and middle-income countries were established, there has been a significant increase in the prevalence of contraceptive use. This increase has played an important role in the significant reduction in fertility that has taken place especially over the last three decades in these regions, where the average number of births per couple declined from more than 6 to fewer than 3 in the latter half of the twentieth century.

Program success in improving contraceptive prevalence rates has, however, been somewhat uneven. It has depended on a number of factors, including a receptive social and family environment that accepts fertility control as legitimate behavior, a favorable political and bureaucratic climate, a management structure that pays close attention to both quality and quantity of services, and reliable sources of funding. Furthermore, those programs that have succeeded have invested considerable resources in evaluation, research, and monitoring of their services, and have had the flexibility to adapt to local conditions (Bongaarts, 1997; Bongaarts & Watkins, 1996; Bulatao, 1993, 1998; Freedman, 1987).

A long-standing debate has focused on the relative merits of "demand side" versus "supply side" inter-

Table 4-8	Unmet Need for Contraception and Demand for Family Planning for Married Women in 37 Countries, Based on DHS Survey in 2005–2010			
Country	**Unmet Need**	**Current Use of Contraception**	**Demand for Family Planning**	**Percentage of Total Demand Satisfied**
Sub-Saharan Africa				
Benin, 2006	29.9	17	46.9	36.3
Cameroon, 2004	20.2	26	46.2	56.2
Chad, 2004	20.7	2.8	23.5	11.8
Congo, 2005	16.2	44.3	60.4	73.3
Congo Democratic Republic, 2007	24.4	20.6	45	45.9
Ethiopia, 2005	33.8	14.7	48.7	30.6
Ghana, 2008	35.3	23.5	58.9	40.0
Guinea, 2005	21.2	9.1	30.3	30.0
Lesotho, 2004	31.0	37.3	68.3	54.6
Liberia, 2007	35.6	11.4	47.0	24.3
Madagascar, 2003/2004	23.6	27.1	50.8	53.4
Malawi, 2004	27.6	32.5	61.7	55.2
Mali, 2006	31.2	8.2	39.5	20.9
Namibia, 2006/2007	20.6	55.1	75.6	72.8
Niger, 2006	15.8	11.2	27.1	41.5
Nigeria, 2008	20.2	14.6	34.8	41.9
Rwanda, 2005	37.9	17.4	55.3	31.4
Senegal, 2005	31.6	11.8	43.4	27.2
Swaziland, 2006/2007	24.0	50.6	74.7	67.8
Tanzania, 2004/2005	21.8	26.4	49.5	55.9
Uganda, 2006	40.6	23.7	64.2	36.9
Zambia, 2007	26.5	40.8	67.2	60.6
Zimbabwe, 2005/2006	12.8	60.2	73.7	82.6
North Africa/West Asia/Europe				
Armenia, 2005	13.3	53.1	66.7	80.1
Azerbaijan, 2006	22.7	51.1	73.9	69.4
Egypt, 2005	10.3	59.2	70.4	85.4
Jordan, 2007	11.9	57.1	71.4	83.3
Moldova, 2005	6.7	67.8	75.2	91.1
Asia				
Bangladesh, 2007	16.8	55.8	72.6	76.8
Cambodia, 2005	25.1	40.0	65.1	61.5
India, 2005/2006	12.8	56.3	69.3	81.6
Indonesia, 2007	9.1	61.4	70.6	87.2
Pakistan, 2006/2007	24.9	29.6	54.5	54.3
Latin America and the Caribbean				
Colombia, 2005	5.8	78.2	86.2	93.3
Dominican Republic, 2007	11.4	72.9	84.2	86.5
Haiti, 2005/2006	37.5	32.0	69.5	46.1
Honduras, 2005/2006	16.9	65.2	82.1	79.5

Source: Macro International, 2010b.

ventions to reduce unmet need in contraception (Bongaarts, 1997; Pritchett, 1994a, 1994b). Demand-side proponents argue that improvements in women's socioeconomic status are an essential and necessary prerequisite to the success of family planning programs. Thus educated women with higher status, compared to their less-educated and lower-status peers, are more likely to know about contraception and seek it out to actualize their latent fertility desires. Supply-side proponents, in contrast, posit that family planning programs, when properly managed, can increase access to and availability of contraception, even in the absence of changes in socioeconomic status of women. Thus they can lead to increased contraceptive prevalence rates and initiation of fertility decline.

The experience of many countries shows that the onset of fertility decline[1] is not dependent on any particular threshold in socioeconomic factors such as levels of urbanization, female education, or infant mortality. In fact, fertility decline appears to have started in a wide range of low- and middle-income countries at quite varied levels of socioeconomic status. Bangladesh is frequently cited as the best example of improved contraceptive prevalence rates and dramatic fertility decline in the absence of socioeconomic improvements but in the presence of a well-run, sharply focused family planning program (Cleland, Phillips, Amin, & Kamal, 1994), although the absence of socioeconomic change has recently come under question (Caldwell, Barkat, Caldwell, Pieris, & Caldwell, 1999; Menken, Khan, & Williams, 1999). While there appears to be no magic threshold of socioeconomic development for initiation of fertility decline, the decline occurs more rapidly in countries with greater levels of socioeconomic development (Bongaarts & Watkins, 1996).

The demand side versus supply side debate is basically a false dichotomy. Neither development nor family planning programs are a necessary prerequisite, nor is either sufficient to induce fertility decline on its own (see, for example, Ross & Mauldin, 1996). Rather, these factors work in complementary fashion, with the time scale of their respective impacts being very different. On the one hand, investments in improving women's status and educational attainment certainly have an important impact in reducing unmet need, but it is a long-term impact. On the other hand, family planning programs can increase access to contraception in the short run, thereby enhancing knowledge about its use and availability and addressing many of the negative myths about particular methods of contraception. Appropriately crafted and focused media campaigns, when implemented as part of family planning programs, can also help legitimize contraception as an acceptable and desirable form of behavior. Moreover, it is important to note that access to the means to limit fertility in and of itself helps improve the status of women. Family planning programs work synergistically with improvements in socioeconomic status and are most effective when they are directed at an informed, educated, empowered client base (Freedman, 1987).

In summary, Bongaarts (1997) estimates that approximately 40% of the fertility decline in the last three decades of the twentieth century in low- and middle-income countries (from a TFR of 6 to 3) can be attributed to family planning programs, and approximately 60% to changes in socioeconomic status, particularly for women.

The Challenges Facing Family Planning

Despite significant family planning program success in reducing financial and logistic constraints to contraceptive access, the unmet need for contraception remains high in many countries. Studies by Bongaarts and Bruce (1995) and Casterline and associates (1996) reported that the major barriers to use of contraception appear to be lack of knowledge about contraception availability and use, concerns about the deleterious health consequences of contraception, and opposition from family and community to contraception use.

Given that physical access and financial constraints are not considered to be significant barriers to the use of contraception, the major challenges for family planning revolve around improving the quality of services, particularly in the areas of information exchange and method choice; integration with reproductive health services other than contraception; and last, but not least, financial sustainability.

Information Exchange

In upgrading the quality of family planning services, the major area of concern is information exchange between providers and clients. The fragmentary evidence that exists suggests that inadequate information is often provided about the proper use of contraceptives, alternatives in the event of non-optimal use, contraceptive side effects, and the appropriateness of the chosen method for women who have particular health problems (Winikoff, Elias, & Beattie, 1994). For example, quite a few women who are using oral birth control pills do not know that they can make up for a missed day by taking two pills the next day. Similarly, not enough women know that birth control pills should not be used if a woman is a smoker or has a heart condition (Trottier, Potter, Taylor, & Glover, 1994).

In general, far fewer than 50% of women have meaningful knowledge about contraceptive methods (Bongaarts & Bruce, 1995). This lack of specific knowledge often leads to exaggerated notions of the health risks of contraception (Casterline et al., 1996). It is worth reiterating that contraception is, by and

---

[1] The onset of fertility decline is usually dated from an initial decline of at least 0.7 point in total fertility over a five-year period, following the practice employed by Bulatao & Elwan (1985).

large, very safe, especially when compared to the health risks deriving from an unplanned pregnancy. Ross and Frankenberg (1993) have estimated that the mortality risk of an unplanned, unwanted pregnancy is 20 times the risk of any modern contraceptive method and 10 times the risk of a properly performed abortion. Although the last two decades have witnessed great success in social marketing, whereby most women are aware of the benefits of small families and the existence and availability of contraception, much more needs to be done to educate women about method choice and associated health risks and benefits.

Although concern about information exchange in family planning programs is long-standing, progress in addressing this problem has been uneven. An issue that comes up repeatedly is whether there is a quality–quantity tradeoff. Program managers voice a common complaint that they have their hands full just providing physical access to contraceptives. Many feel they do not have the luxury of providing extensive information about contraception because of the time-intensive nature of this type of activity.

In reality, there is little contradiction or tradeoff between paying attention to quality issues and achieving quantity targets for numbers of users. The two are integrally linked in several ways. First, the key steps needed to improve quality—such as attention to logistics, adequate supervision, motivation of workers at every level, real feedback to managers and supervisors, and accountability for supplies and money—are exactly the same steps needed to improve quantity.

Second, family planning services are inseparable from information provision. In fact, provision of information is one of the key services that a family planning program can offer. Third, attention to quality will improve efficiency and will allow the addition of new users without new costs (Tsui et al., 1997).

Contraceptive Use and Method Choice

Modern contraceptive methods are now so widely available in low- and middle-income countries that approximately one-third of all couples outside of China and more than half of all couples in high-income countries in which the woman is of reproductive age use such methods (Robey, Rutstein, & Morris, 1992). In 1993, the estimated number of contraceptive users in low- and middle-income countries was 436 million. By 2000, this number had grown to 549 million, and it is expected to reach 816 million during the next 25 years according to UN projections (Bongaarts & Johansson, 2002). This rapid growth rate is a result of population increases and a concomitant rise in contraceptive prevalence in low- and middle-income countries, from 55% in 1993 to 60% in 2000, and expected to reach 67% in 2025 due to declines in desired fertility.

Table 4-9 shows the worldwide distribution of contraceptive use according to method using the most recent data (2002). In addition to demonstrating the great variation in use, these data are remarkable in that they show, for much of the world, a high proportion of those couples using contraception are

Table 4-9	Contraception Use, 2000: Percentage of Married Couples[a] in Which the Woman Is of Reproductive Age, by Region					
	Sterilization					
Region	**Female**	**Male**	**Pill**	**IUD**	**Condom**	**Total**
World	21.0	4.0	7.0	15.0	5.0	61.0
Low- and middle-income regions						
Africa	2.0	0.1	7.0	5.0	1.0	26.0
Asia	25.0	4.0	5.0	18.0	4.0	64.0
Latin America and Caribbean	31.0	2.0	13.0	8.0	4.0	70.0
Oceania	12.0	9.0	21.0	2.0	9.0	59.0
Industrialized regions						
Japan	3.0	0.6	0.8	1.5	43.0	56.0
Europe	4.0	2.0	16.0	15.0	10.0	67.0
Northern America	23.0	14.0	15.0	1.0	13.0	76.0
New Zealand	14.0	19.3	20.5	3.3	11.0	74.0

Note: The table is based on the most recent data available as of 2002; pertaining approximately to 2000.

[a]Including, where possible, those in consensual unions.

Source: Population Reference Bureau. (2002). *Family planning worldwide: 2002 data sheet.* Washington, DC: Author. Adapted with permission.

using sterilization—the one method that has almost zero risk of failure. Note that the average for low- to middle-income countries in Asia (64%) is heavily influenced by the very high rate of contraceptive prevalence in China (83%). Without China, the average for all low- and middle-income countries would drop from 55% to only 43% (Bongaarts & Johansson, 2002). Figures based on more recent data do not show major changes in contraceptive method choice except for the case of condom use in Oceania, which has increased significantly—from 9% in 2000 to 17% in 2009 (Macro International, 2010b).

It is much more difficult to judge how much *choice* of method women in low- and middle-income countries have, and how their array of choices has changed in recent years. With the exception of sub-Saharan Africa, where contraceptive prevalence rates are low, significant progress in overall method availability occurred in most countries between 1982 and 1994 (Ross & Mauldin, 1996). In all 22 countries (with the exception of Nigeria) where DHS surveys were conducted between 1990 and 1993, at least half of all women had heard of at least one modern contraceptive method; in 13 of these countries, more than 90% of women knew of at least one contraceptive method (Curtis & Neitzel, 1996).

Table 4-10 shows historical data on contraceptive method mix and alternative projections for the year 2015 (Bongaarts & Johansson, 2002). Although the two projection methodologies have varying estimates for specific methods, female sterilization appears likely to remain the most popular method of choice in 2015, followed by IUDs and pills. An issue of considerable concern is that despite evidence of a spreading HIV epidemic in low- and middle-

income countries, condom use remains low in these projections.

Largely due to a lack of funding and the long lead time required for new methods to gain acceptance, there has been relatively little innovation in contraceptive technology in the last 30 years. Thus, in an era of increasing expectations for contraception, the menu of choices has not expanded greatly. Given the AIDS pandemic, new contraceptive methods that are of high priority are vaginal microbicides, which protect women from STIs, in combination with spermicides, which provide contraceptive protection (Bongaarts & Johansson, 2002; Harrison & Rosenfield, 1996; Tsui et al., 1997).

In some situations, knowledge and use of existing technology have not been widely disseminated. One example is emergency contraception—that is, the prevention of pregnancy through the use of contraceptive methods after unprotected sex—for which appropriate technologies (e.g., a combination of oral contraceptive pills, progestin-only pills, and the copper-T IUD) have long been available but are not used by many women (e.g., victims of coercive sex) who could benefit from them (International Planned Parenthood Foundation, 1995; Trussell, Ellertson, & Stewart, 1996). Although this treatment was discovered in 1966, it was not until 1995 that the International Consortium for Emergency Contraception (ICEC, 2010) was formed to promote and mainstream emergency contraception worldwide. However, progestin-only preparations, commonly known as the "morning after pill," are now available commercially in most countries as a dedicated emergency contraception product under many names worldwide (Trussell & Cleland, 2010).

Table 4-10	Estimates of Contraceptive Method Distribution in 1980 and 1993 and Alternative Projections for 2015, Low- and Middle-Income Countries				
				Futures Group	New Procedure
Method	1980	1993	2015	2015
Female sterilization	24	39	26	37
Male sterilization	13	8	3	5
Pill	13	11	22	17
Injectables	0	4	6	5
IUD	32	26	18	20
Vaginal methods	0	0.3	0.6	0.4
Condom	5	4	10	9
Traditional methods	12	9	14	7
Total	100	100	100	100

Note: The figures for 1993 are proportions of total contraceptive use; the analogous figures for 1993 are proportions of married women using contraceptives. Thus 21% of married couples used female sterilization. As the total number of married couples using contraceptive methods was 55%, this translates into (21/55 = 39%) of total contraceptive use.

Source: Adapted with permission of the Population Council, from Bongaarts, J., & Johansson, E. (2002). Future trends in contraceptive prevalence and method mix in the developing world. *Studies in Family Planning, 33*(1), 24–36.

Political, Social, and Financial Constraints

Although high unmet need is in part a function of specific management deficiencies in family planning programs, it is important to recognize that broader political and societal constraints also play a role. Kenney (1993) has identified policies in a variety of countries that retard access to safe contraception: (1) health and safety regulations that restrict choice of methods or providers (e.g., the failure to approve oral contraceptives for use in Japan for more than nine years; a committee finally recommended their approval after the male impotence-relieving drug Viagra received endorsement within six months [Insurance for Viagra spurs coverage for birth control, 1999]); (2) taxes and barriers to trade that affect importation of contraceptives; (3) regulation of advertising (usually due to concerns about modesty and privacy); and (4) restrictions on private-sector involvement in family planning. In addition, law and policies in many countries restrict or forbid access to abortion.

In any discussion of family planning programs and their performance, the issue of financial sustainability is key. Family planning expenditures in low- and middle income countries as a whole are estimated to be slightly less than $10 billion annually, or roughly $1–2 per person per year in 2000. In the last two decades, most of this expense has been paid for by national governments (50%) and individual households (20%), with international donor assistance accounting for only 30% of the total. If donor assistance for family planning had kept pace with the historical record of 30%, it would have risen from its 1994 level of $1.37 billion to $3.0 billion in 2000. In reality, there was a decline—rather than an increase in funding—over this period. In particular, the share of funding provided by the United States, by far the largest historical donor for family planning programs, has fallen by 30%. In the coming decades, rising demand for contraception and increasing budget constraints will require that programs either mobilize more public resources or increase the cost of family planning services to the individual, so that more users can be accommodated (Bulatao, 1998).

The Broader Effects of Family Planning Programs

Even before the 1994 International Conference on Population and Development (ICPD) in Cairo, concerns were expressed, both by women's groups and by policy makers, about the effects of family planning programs on the lives of individual women. Family planning programs have been criticized as exclusively concerned with reducing population growth. Studies in recent years have broadened research to include consideration of the effects of programs on the quality of life for women. In particular, the Women's Studies Project found that family planning programs provided the following benefits to women:

- "Most women and men are convinced that practicing family planning and having smaller families provide health and economic benefits."

- Family planning offers freedom from fear of unplanned pregnancy and can improve sexual life, partner relations, and family well-being.

- Where jobs are available, family planning users are more likely than non-users to take advantage of work opportunities.

- "Family planning helps women meet their practical needs and is necessary, but not sufficient, to help them meet their strategic needs" (Women's Studies Project, 1999, p. 2).

The Women's Studies Project also found costs to women from such programs:

- "Contraceptive side effects—real or perceived—are a serious concern for many women, more so than providers realize.

- When partners or others are opposed, practicing family planning can increase women's vulnerability.

- When women have smaller families, they may lose the security of traditional roles and face new and sometimes difficult challenges, including the burden of multiple responsibilities at home and work" (Women's Studies Project, 1999, p. 2).

In addition, the Women's Studies Project found that the exclusion of men from most family planning programs affected the ability of women to take advantage of their services, because men play a dominant role in family planning decisions in many regions.

Most family planning programs have emphasized only the positive benefits of family planning; they are now being urged to pay attention to at least some of these broader considerations.

A Broader Definition of Family Planning and Reproductive Health Programs

As discussed earlier, the 1994 ICPD brought about an international reevaluation of the conceptualization of family planning programs. They are now viewed as falling under the larger rubric of more general reproductive health services and interventions, some of which are directly health related, whereas others are related indirectly. It is useful, however, to first consider conventional family planning programs.

Organization and Structure of Family Planning Programs

While nearly all low- and middle-income countries have established an infrastructure to deliver family planning services, their organization varies markedly. One example, Bangladesh, is discussed in Exhibit 4-4.

According to Tsui, Wasserheit, and Haaga (1997), successful performance in the family planning realm is influenced by a focused commitment to achieving program objectives and access to adequate resources. At the national level, strong leadership, clearly formulated policies, explicit goals and objectives, and a clear agenda for meeting those goals can all contribute to the success of programs. In some countries, political commitment is evidenced by placing the family planning program under a national supervisory coun-

cil or by establishing a separate ministry. Programs also need ways of assessing progress toward meeting their objectives. Indicators such as contraceptive prevalence, proportion of unwanted births, maternal morbidity and mortality, pregnancy complications and their management, and actual fertility levels all provide information that, over time, can permit program evaluation. Therefore, one element of successful programs is the definition of result measures to be used and establishment of mechanisms for collecting the needed information. Caution is in order, however. For example, goals that are defined in terms of targets, such as the number of acceptors of particular methods in a given time, may lead workers to exert pressure on clients and reduce their options.

Family planning service programs have focused on a narrow set of goals—reducing unwanted fertility by providing access to the means of fertility control. Several models have been used for the design of programs. In the vertical model, family planning ad-

---

Exhibit 4-4	The Bangladesh Family Planning Program

Family planning in Bangladesh can be traced to the private Family Planning Association created in 1953, before Bangladesh achieved its independence from Pakistan. By 1960, Pakistan had begun public-sector programs, which Bangladesh continued after becoming a nation in 1971. The overall program has grown and changed over the years, but throughout there has been high-level political support and considerable funding from external donors. The Family Planning Association program has emphasized provision of services, outreach activities at the village level, and mass communication through a variety of media.

As part of the early 1960s public-sector programs, family planning services were offered in government health clinics as part of regular health services. A system of using village aides to provide education was established but abandoned after only 18 months for a variety of reasons, including poor training of the aides, complaints that their services were directed only to family planning and not to other health problems, inadequate resources, and poor supervision. It was followed by renewed efforts run by a new Family Planning Board independent of the Ministry of Health.

Bangladesh's family planning efforts in the late 1960s met with little success, primarily because of poor-quality services provided by a program that had been instituted on a large scale, with little pilot testing and poor organization. The program emphasized use of the intrauterine device (IUD), which was met with resistance by many concerned about side effects and problems with its use. It did not help that the program was seen by many as having been imposed on Bangladesh, then East Pakistan, by a government whose political support was declining.

In the aftermath of the country's war for independence, although the health and social sectors of the government were particularly negatively affected, it was felt that family planning was urgently needed. A large and complex program was established. A separate Population Wing was created within the Ministry of Health and Population to run the program. Thus health and family planning services were separated. At the local level, the primary healthcare staffs were predominantly male. In a society where little interaction is permitted between women and men who are not members of their families, male workers cannot provide maternal and child health services except for immunizations. This staffing was a legacy of early programs to combat smallpox, tuberculosis, and malaria; it was ill suited to the new focus. By contrast, local family planning workers were women, although their supervisors were men. These female workers went directly to households and offered family planning counseling and free supplies. They spent some time on maternal and child health, although they were not well trained for this purpose.

Over the years, the Bangladeshi program has continued to be revised and expanded. In all cases, the elements of strong political support, strong financial support, and extensive administrative support have remained.

Source: Cleland, J., Phillips, J. F., Amin, S., & Kamal, G. M. (1994). *The determinants of reproductive change in Bangladesh*. Washington, DC: World Bank. Adapted with permission.

ministration and service delivery are carried out by staff for whom this is their single function. In a second model, a separate family planning administration unit is established, but field staff at each level of the healthcare system can deliver a variety of linked services. In practice, the linkage between family planning and maternal and child health services has been the most common. Under the new broader definition of reproductive health, it is expected that other types of services will be offered, so that the ways in which they are linked, both administratively and in provision of care, will have to be addressed.

No matter which model is followed, the program design involves decisions on which services will be offered and at which level of the healthcare system. Tsui, Wasserheit, and Haaga (1997) illustrate the possibilities as follows:[2]

Level

- Interventions for prevention and management of unintended pregnancies

Community

- Information, education, and communication programs
- Community-based distribution
- Social marketing of condoms and oral pills

Health Post

- Counseling/screening for contraception
- Counseling and referral for menstrual regulation or abortion
- Provision of injectable contraceptives
- IUD insertions
- Counseling and treatment of contraceptive side effects

Health Center

- Menstrual regulation/manual vacuum aspiration abortion
- Performing surgical contraception on set days
- Post-abortion counseling and contraception
- Counseling and treatment of contraceptive side effects

---

[2] Reprinted with permission from Tsui, A.O., Wasserheit, J. N., & Haaga, J. G. (Eds.). (1997). *Reproductive health in developing countries: Expanding dimensions, building solutions. Panel on Reproductive Health, Committee on Population, Commission on Behavioral and Social Sciences, and Education.* Washington, DC: National Academy Press. Copyright 1997 by the National Research Council.

District Hospital

- Surgical contraception
- Abortions through 20 weeks, where indicated
- Post-abortion counseling and contraception

These authors' report concludes that the breadth and scope of the services to be delivered present a formidable challenge in design, execution, administration, and evaluation. Even if this challenge is met, a program can falter if inadequate resources are allocated to meet its needs for trained staff, equipment, and supplies. Additional demands will be placed on whatever system is in place if services related more generally to reproductive health are provided.

Research on design and implementation can help improve family planning and reproductive health programs. Exhibits 4-5 and 4-6 illustrate the approach taken by Bangladesh in this regard.

Additional Reproductive Health Care Services

Some reproductive health services are closely linked to contraception; it is likely that, without much added expense, they can be integrated into conventional family planning programs relatively easily. These services may include pregnancy tests, Pap smears, and screening for sexually transmitted infections. STI screening has been carried out, in many cases, only in the context of separate programs to treat such infections. That type of intervention misses the general population of women who may not realize that they are infected or understand that they may pass their infection to their unborn or nursing children.

HIV/AIDS deserves special mention. In 1999, the United Nations convened a conference to assess the progress made on this front since the 1994 ICPD. Attendees concluded that the earlier conference had greatly underestimated the effects of HIV/AIDS on the populations of the low- and middle-income countries and called for specific programs and targets to reduce the spread of infection ("Conference Adopts Plan," 1999). Directly related to the family planning realm is their call for greater access to methods such as the female and male condoms that can reduce or prevent transmission of the virus. This and other approaches to preventing the spread of HIV/AIDS are discussed in Chapter 5.

Other desirable reproductive health interventions remain within the health realm but will require significant changes in staffing and significantly more financial resources. These services include emergency obstetrics, general women's health services, abortion services where they are not already available, infertility services, and greatly expanded testing and counseling for HIV/AIDS.

| Exhibit 4-5 | Research to Improve the Family Planning Program in Bangladesh |

How well does a family planning program work? Few experiments in applied research have been conducted to determine whether a particular design is more effective in reaching the objectives of the program. The International Centre for Dirarrhoeal Disease Research, Bangladesh (ICDDR,B) has carried out just these kinds of operations research experiments, which have served to improve the ways in which services are delivered within the Bangladeshi family planning program.

An early effort, in 1975, was intended to test the hypothesis that there was latent demand for family planning. ICDDR,B maintains a field station in Matlab, approximately 40 kilometers from the capital, Dhaka. A family planning program was introduced in roughly half of the area in which the center provided services, while people living in the remainder of the area had access only to standard government or private services. Local women, mostly illiterate widows, were hired to visit households approximately every 90 days to offer oral contraception to women. Later, condoms were added to the offerings. The hypothesis was that couples wanted to reduce the fertility but would do so if only they were supplied with the necessary means. Initial acceptance was good; prevalence of use rose in the early stage of the program to almost 20% from its near-zero level prior to the program. But within less than nine months, it had dropped, so that the program area prevalence was only 6 percentage points higher than in the comparison area.

Lessons learned: This type of demand-oriented program was inadequate in a situation where women and couples had little social support for contraceptive use. Rather, a system that addressed the non-economic costs of use—whether social, psychological, or based on health concerns—was essential. In addition, problems arose in complying with a daily pill regimen, and condoms were not popular. Analysis of the experiment through interviews with people in the community also demonstrated the importance of the characteristics of the family planning worker. Women who had little status in the community and who were past the reproductive age themselves did not have sufficient credibility to help others withstand the social costs of use. Improving access was simply not enough.

A subsequent experiment begun in 1978 tested better follow-up for users, an expanded set of method choices, employment of better educated and younger women, and new management strategies. These steps were undertaken to ensure that women received regular visits and that problems were addressed rapidly. A new dual leadership system was introduced, which included both technical (paramedical) and administrative supervision. The interval between visits was reduced to 14 days. Within a year, nearly one-third of women in the study area were contraceptive users, while there was little change in the comparison area. Increases in contraceptive use continued so that by 1990 nearly 60% of women in the targeted area were users, compared to only 25% in the comparison area. Clearly, taking advantage of latent demand for contraception required that the program address the social costs of contraceptive use. It also demonstrated the value of providing service in the home.

In 1983, a new experiment was begun outside of Matlab, to see if the lessons learned there could be applied within the government family planning program and without major additional resources or changes in administration. This pilot project was carried out in two areas. Because of the success of this Extension Project, the government changed the national program to increase the number of female village workers, train them to provide injectable contraception within the home, and upgrade management to provide better support, both technical and supervisory, for local workers. In fact, one of the main lessons learned from these experiments was that careful supervision and support of workers were critical factors for success. Another lesson emphasized the importance of designing a program for local cultural circumstances—in this case, providing basic services in the home.

Since these experiments were conducted, other projects have tested variations of the Extension Project model to see how much it can be altered and still achieve the objectives of increased use of family planning and reduced fertility. The Extension Project (now known as the Operations Research Project) has, since the International Conference on Population and Development, initiated studies of how the family planning program can be expanded to provide a wide array of reproductive and other health services under what is termed the Essential Services Package.

Source: Cleland, J., Phillips, J. F., Amin, S., & Kamal, G. M. (1994). *The determinants of reproductive change in Bangladesh.* Washington, DC: World Bank. Adapted with permission.

Some infertility services are already provided within the context of programs to reduce STIs, as these diseases are a major cause of infertility and premature sterility (see, for example, Tsui et al., 1997). The others, however, are generally lacking. Without considerable expansion of the financial base for family planning and for the expanded reproductive health program, it is unlikely that these services can be provided in many low- and middle-income countries.

Reproductive Health Beyond Direct Health Care

Reproductive health interventions that go beyond the healthcare realm, while clearly valuable, are not linked in any obvious way to conventional family planning services. The ICPD's Cairo agenda focused on improving the status of women. It called for interventions such as income-generating activities for women and female education that affect overall status of women as well as for sex education for youth, both

Exhibit 4-6	**Strategies Used by the Bangladesh Family Planning and Reproductive Health Programs**

According to Cleland et al. (1994), at least four sets of strategies have been implemented:

1. Strategies to improve the coverage and quality of services

   - Clinics, located within 5 miles of most couples, now provide free contraception and treatment of side effects.
   - Sterilization is offered without charge at all subdistrict hospitals and is carried out by well-trained personnel.
   - Related health services for children and women are provided either in the home or in clinics.
   - Community-based distribution of low-cost nonclinical contraceptives is provided through pharmacies and is well publicized through various media.

2. Strategies to improve awareness and motivation:

   - Mass media are used to provide extensive relevant information; family planning and reproductive health are openly discussed in public media.
   - Focused programs (for example, with religious leaders) are carried out to build awareness and consensus.

3. Strategies to foster village-based and household services:

   - Outreach involves female workers who deliver services in the home. These services are now provided by both the government and nongovernmental organizations.
   - This strategy has been questioned in recent years by critics who say the time is past when women should be provided with services that encourage continued seclusion. They argue that the demand for family planning and reproductive health services is now so great that women will travel outside their homes to obtain these services and that this type of modernization is to be encouraged. In addition, issues of cost of maintaining the large cadre of home visitors is encouraging experimentation with less costly alternatives.

4. Strategies to foster community development and demand generation:

   - These strategies have not been carried out within the family planning program itself but are directed toward improving the status of women. They include micro-credit and other programs sponsored by local organizations, such as Grameen Bank and the Bangladesh Rural Advancement Committee, and government strategies to increase education of girls. In fact, education of women has increased substantially in recent years. In many parts of Bangladesh, nearly all children—male and female—receive at least several years of primary schooling.

   As a final note, the Bangladesh effort is characterized by the use of research to help determine the design of programs. Ongoing studies at the International Centre for Diarrhoeal Disease Research, Bangladesh (ICDDR,B) are addressing how the new Essential Services Package (which includes reproductive health, child survivals, and curative care) can best be implemented within existing fixed service provision sites, how to meet the health needs of adolescents, how to improve prevention and management of reproductive tract and sexually transmitted infections (RTI/STI), and how to provide essential obstetric care.

Source: Cleland, J., Phillips, J. F., Amin, S., & Kamal, G. M. (1994). *The determinants of reproductive change in Bangladesh.* Washington, DC: World Bank. Adapted with permission.

male and female, to increase responsible sexual behavior. The 1999 follow-up conference reiterated and intensified these calls ("Conference Adopts Plan," 1999).

Others have called for programs that decrease violence against women. Violence in women's intimate relationships can lead to death through homicide or through driving the woman to suicide. A less drastic outcome is loss of control by women over their sexuality and, therefore, their sexual health.

Another kind of violence against women is female genital mutilation, a practice that has been reported in more than 40 low- and middle-income countries and has followed immigrants from these areas to high-income countries (Tsui et al., 1997). It is estimated that more than 130 million women have been affected globally by female genital mutilation and approximately 3 million girls are at risk for female genital cutting every year (IRIN, 2010). Although any type of genital cutting carries a risk of infection, the implications of genital cutting for long-term reproductive health differ according to the severity of cutting, conditions of delivery, and sociodemographic factors. It is generally accepted that women who have undergone the most severe type of cutting, which includes removal of external genitalia and infibulation (stitching or narrowing of the vaginal opening), have an increased likelihood of delivery complications or obstetric morbidity (Slanger, Snow, & Okonofua, 2002). Even death may occur from excessive bleeding and infection resulting from use of unsterile equipments for performing the procedure by quacks. In some countries, evidence suggests that a growing proportion of these procedures are being carried out by medical personnel (Yoder, Abderrahim, & Zhuzhuni, 2004).

Can These Goals Be Achieved?

All parts of this new "beyond family planning" mandate are worthwhile. Nevertheless, it remains unclear how this expansion, in the absence of clearly designated additional funds to finance it, will affect the ability of family planning programs to reach their objective of promoting safe contraception (Cleland et al., 1994; Finkle & Ness, 1985). In addition, concerns have been raised that the expansion from family planning programs to reproductive health programs without additional funds will not only dilute what traditional family planning does reasonably well but also fail to provide significant improvements in other areas (Bulatao, 1998; Mukaire, Kalikwani, Maggwa, & Kisubi, 1997; Twahir, Maggwa, & Askew, 1996). Exhibit 4-7 discusses these issues in the context of Bangladesh.

In fact, the new agenda comes in an era when many high-income countries are reducing their aid contributions. At the Cairo conference, high-income country donors pledged to provide $5.7 billion per year for family planning, but as of 1999 their contributions totaled only $1.9 billion annually ("Population Control Measures," 1999). Increasing the political

---

Exhibit 4-7	Challenges and Constraints for Family Planning and Fertility Reduction in Bangladesh

In the early 1990s, following the rapid decline in Bangladesh fertility from a TFR of 6.3 in 1975 to 3.4 in 1994, much optimism was voiced that fertility would continue to decline and that replacement-level fertility would be reached by 2005. However, fertility in Bangladesh has plateaued at a TFR of approximately 3 children per woman for the last decade. This lack of change in fertility (a trend also noted in Bangladesh's regional neighbor India) has become a source of major concern, and puzzlement.

The initial dramatic fall in fertility took place within the context of relatively insignificant overt improvements in socioeconomic development, and was largely attributed to "supply-side initiatives"—that is, the impact of an intensive family planning program. In contrast, the last decade has witnessed quite significant improvements in socioeconomic development in Bangladesh, including a rapid rise in educational enrollment for women and increased employment opportunities for women in the fast-growing garment sector. Moreover, the family planning program has continued to enjoy high levels of funding and resources.

Various hypotheses have been put forth to try to explain this lack of progress in diminishing fertility. Advocates of conventional family planning programs suggest that the trend may be due to the change of focus (in the mid-1990s, following the expansion of the family planning agenda to include broad-based reproductive health services—see Exhibit 4-4) from household distribution of contraceptives by a vertical cadre of family planning workers to clinic-based family planning and reproductive health services provided by a unified integrated health and family planning service. They argue that this change has (1) reduced the motivation of the family planning workers, who now have an expanded set of health-related duties they are ill prepared to fulfill, and (2) made contraceptive provision just one of many government-sponsored healthcare activities, none of which have adequate resources committed to their fulfillment. Moreover, they question the optimism that family planning is so well established that women in rural Bangladesh no longer have social constraints vis-à-vis seeking family planning and reproductive health services outside the home.

Those who favor clinic-based services point out that contraception prevalence rates have continued to rise in Bangladesh over the last decade and note that a change of method mix from predominantly oral contraceptives to more long-term methods with lower failure rates requires clinic-based initiatives. In fact, due to the lack of progress in fertility, the government of Bangladesh has just recently switched back from clinic-based services to household distribution.

Demand-side advocates argue that the exclusive focus on fine-tuning family planning programs to bring about fertility reduction is misplaced. They contend that further reductions in fertility require broad-based initiatives to improve socioeconomic development (with a particular focus on improving women's status), which will help to reduce the benefits of additional children and increase their costs. They point to continued desired fertility of 2.5 children per woman—still higher than the replacement level, with quite significant regional variations that can be correlated with differences in women's education and employment, as well as continued son-preference.

The debate about demand-side versus supply-side policy initiatives as the best approach to fertility reduction continues. Most researchers and policy makers feel that both kinds of initiatives are important, but there is growing appreciation that the final stretch of fertility decline to replacement levels may well be a long, hard battle.

will and raising the funding for these new programs and for maintaining existing effective ones is perhaps the greatest challenge for reproductive health in the twenty-first century.

Impact of Reproductive Patterns on the Health of Children

Over the last several decades, an impressive body of evidence has accumulated suggesting that certain kinds of reproductive patterns are injurious to infant and child health (Table 4-11). These risk factors are usually discussed as if they were completely independent. In reality, a number of problematic issues arise with this approach to deleterious reproductive patterns. For example, many of the risk factors are integrally linked with one another and their independent effects are difficult to disentangle. Thus first births and young age of mothers are separately cited as risk factors, but young mothers usually are having their first birth. Similarly, children of high parity come from large families and are likely to have older mothers, yet all three are referred to individually.

Parity and Child Health

First births are known to be more dangerous for the child than subsequent births. The excess risk relative to births of order 2–4 is limited to the first year of life, however—particularly to the neonatal period (the first 28 days of life), when the odds ratio for mortality is 1.7. There appears to be no survival disadvantage after the child reaches his or her first birthday (Hobcraft, 1987; Hobcraft, McDonald, & Rutstein, 1985).

Moreover, the excess risk for first-born children varies considerably across countries. It is not clear whether this risk reflects inadequate physiologic adjustment of first-time mothers to pregnancy (leading to lower intrauterine growth, shorter gestation, lower birth weight, a higher probability of birth trauma, higher risks of pregnancy-induced hypertension, higher prevalence of placental malaria in malaria-endemic areas, and so on) or whether it arises because of the lack of experience of first-time mothers in care seeking and care taking. The latter factor is, of course, amenable to policy prescriptions that encourage first-time mothers to seek prenatal and postnatal care (Haaga, 1989; National Research Council, 1989).

Table 4-11	Mechanisms by Which Reproductive Patterns Affect Child Health
Reproductive Pattern	**Mechanism Through Which Child Health Is Affected**
Firstborn children	First-time mothers have a higher frequency of health problems during pregnancy and childbirth; parents have less experience with child care; poorer intrauterine growth
Higher-order children	Possible cumulative effect of earlier maternal reproductive injury—"maternal depletion" syndrome—leading to poorer intrauterine growth
Large families	Competition for limited resources, with some children, possibly disproportionately girls, losing out; possible spread of infection
Children born to very young mothers	Inadequate development of maternal reproductive system and incomplete maternal growth; young mothers less likely to know about and use prenatal and delivery care or provide good child care
Children born to older mothers	Greater risk of birth trauma; greater risk of genetic abnormalities
Short interbirth intervals	Inadequate maternal recovery time (maternal depletion); competition among similar-aged siblings for limited family resources; early termination of breast-feeding; low birth weight; increased exposure to infection from children of similar ages
Unwantedness	(Conscious or unconscious) neglect; child born into a stressful situation
Maternal death or illness (e.g., chronic infection such as AIDS)	Early termination of breastfeeding; no maternal care; disease may be passed to child
Contraceptive use	Hormonal contraception may interrupt breastfeeding

Source: Adapted with permission from National Research Council. (1989). *Contraception and reproduction: Health consequences for women and children in the developing world.* Washington, DC: National Academies Press. Copyright 1989 by the National Academy of Sciences.

Higher-order births may suffer due to poor maternal health as a result of cumulative exposure to previous pregnancies (Hobcraft et al., 1985; Pebley & Stupp, 1987). Mothers may suffer from inadequate recovery of their energy store after earlier pregnancies (maternal depletion hypothesis) or from the long-term cumulative effects of prior delivery-related injuries. Thus higher-order children (parity of 5 or greater) may be at greater risk of poor intrauterine growth, greater trauma during birth, and, more generally, poorer health than lower-parity (2–4) children. Although these mechanisms are plausible, the empirical evidence for them is inconsistent and suggests that little additional risk can be attributed to higher order-births, once short birth intervals are taken into account (Gubhaju, 1986; Hobcraft et al., 1985; National Research Council, 1989).

In addition to physiologic deficiencies, higher-order children may suffer deleterious consequences of competition for limited family resources. Thus they may get proportionately less food and less attention from their parents. This negative consequence of large families may not be limited solely to higher-order births. If family resources are limited and there is no preference for specific children, all children may suffer as a result of large family sizes. Some evidence suggests that certain children (particularly higher-order girls, and especially those with older sisters) suffer disproportionately from the impact of large family size in specific social settings (Muhuri & Menken, 1997).

Maternal Age

Hobcraft (1987) found that children born to teenage mothers had significantly higher risks of dying than children born to mothers aged 25 to 34 years. This excess mortality risk was 1.2 for the neonatal period, 1.4 for the post-neonatal period, 1.6 for toddlers, and 1.3 for children aged 2 to 5 years. Nevertheless, considerable variability was observed among countries in terms of the excess mortality risk for children born to young mothers.

Plausible explanations reflecting both physiological and social causes have been offered for the health disadvantage of children born to young mothers. Perhaps these children are disadvantaged because maternal reproductive systems are inadequately industrialized (Aitken & Walls, 1986) or because young mothers lack experience and knowledge about prenatal and postnatal care (Geronimus, 1987). Unfortunately, there is little solid empirical evidence from low- and middle-income countries to prove any

of these hypotheses. It has been difficult to study possible competition between fetal growth and maternal development as underlying the excessive mortality of children born to young mothers in low- and middle-income countries. Due to lack of reliable data on gynecological age (i.e., age since menarche—a particularly important concern because of delayed age at menarche in low- and middle-income countries; Foster, Menken, Chowdhury, & Trussell, 1986) or chronological age of mothers younger than 20, Haaga (1989) concluded that there was only weak evidence for this mechanism. Studies that have addressed social causes (i.e., poor knowledge and use of prenatal care) have used socioeconomic status as a crude proxy for use of prenatal care services. In multivariate analyses, this measure fails to help explain the high risk of infants and children born to young mothers.

Children born to older mothers may suffer because of poorer maternal health due to age-related declines in physiologic function and a higher risk of genetic abnormalities (Hansen, 1986). Little proof exists that this is a major risk factor in low- and middle-income countries, however.

Short Birth Intervals

Short birth intervals, both prior and subsequent to the birth of a child, are probably the most consistent reproductive pattern identified as a risk factor for excess child mortality. Hobcraft (1987) reports that the excess mortality risk of children born less than 24 months after the preceding birth compared to those born 24 months or more after the preceding birth is 1.8 in the first year of life, 1.3 for toddlers (ages 1–2), and 1.3 for children aged 2 to 5 years. In terms of subsequent birth intervals, Hobcraft reports that, on average, across 34 countries, children whose birth was followed by a subsequent birth within less than 24 months had 2.2 times the risk of dying than did children for whom the subsequent birth interval was longer. As is the case for other demographic risk factors, considerable variation exists between countries in terms of risks related to short birth intervals.

A number of plausible explanations have been put forth for the relationship between short prior and subsequent birth intervals (less than 24 months) and a child's risk of poor health and increased mortality. First, due to maternal depletion (resulting from inadequate recovery time from the nutritional burdens of breastfeeding and prior pregnancy; Merchant & Martorell, 1988), children born after a short birth interval may suffer poorer intrauterine growth, and possibly have a higher risk of preterm birth. To date, little empirical evidence has been collected that supports this mechanism (Ferraz, Gray, Fleming, & Maria, 1988; National Research Council, 1989; Pebley & DaVanzo, 1988; Winikoff & Sullivan, 1987).

Second, children born before a short birth interval may suffer from premature cessation of breastfeeding (which has been shown to be an important correlate of child survival in low- and middle-income countries; Palloni & Millman, 1986), as the mother shifts her attention to the more recent arrival. Given that studies that have controlled for the length of breastfeeding still show an association between short subsequent birth interval and high infant mortality (Pebley & Stupp, 1987), premature termination of breastfeeding does not entirely explain this effect.

Third, children born in close proximity to each other may suffer from competition for limited family resources of time and food. The evidence for this type of competition is unclear and sometimes contradictory (DaVanzo, Butz, & Habicht, 1983; Palloni, 1985).

Fourth, close birth spacing may increase the likelihood of transmission of infectious diseases such as diarrhea and measles, due to overcrowding and presence of children of similar ages (Aaby, Bukh, Lisse, & Smits, 1984).

Finally, despite adequate controls for observable confounding factors in multivariate analyses, part of the relationship between short birth intervals (either preceding or following the index birth) and increased child mortality may be due to unobserved factors such as short gestational length or parental characteristics. Babies born before or after very short birth intervals are known to be at high risk for short gestational durations, which independently have been shown to increase child mortality dramatically (Miller, 1989; Pebley & Stupp, 1987).

In terms of unobserved parental characteristics, it is possible that women who are likely to have short birth intervals are inherently at higher risk for poorer child health outcomes than their peers who have longer birth intervals. This would lead to a spurious inference that short birth intervals are causally related to higher child mortality (Pebley & Stupp, 1987; Potter, 1988; Rosenzweig & Schultz, 1983).

Unwanted Pregnancy and Birth

As discussed previously, unwanted children have much higher risks of morbidity and mortality. They may suffer from both conscious and unconscious neglect, due to lower allocations of food, parental time and attention, and access to health care. In countries

with a strong son preference (South and Southeast Asia), there is significant evidence for higher mortality for female children relative to their male siblings (Das Gupta, 1987; D'Souza & Chen, 1980; Muhuri & Menken, 1997). Moreover, as discussed earlier, the recent rise in sex-selective abortion in China and Southeast Asia (which has led to a disproportionately high male-to-female sex ratio at birth) is evidence of the high risk of mortality for unwanted female fetuses (Larsen et al., 1998; Tsui et al., 1997). The pattern of gender discrimination is, however, complex and nuanced and may vary by societal setting (Muhuri & Menken, 1997).

Maternal Health

Maternal morbidity and mortality can have profoundly negative effects on child health, leading to high rates of morbidity and mortality. Population-based studies in South and Southeast Asia suggest that more than half of all perinatal deaths (deaths in the first week of a child's life) are associated with poor maternal health and pregnancy and delivery-related complications (Fauveau, Wojtyniak, Mostafa, Sarder, & Chakraborty, 1990; Kusiako, Ronsmans, & Van der Paal, 2000; National Statistics Office [Philippines] & Macro International, 1994). These deleterious consequences may result from a combination of direct delivery-related consequences, such as premature labor, prolonged or obstructed labor, abnormal fetal position (Kusiako et al., 2000); physiologic processes, such as cessation of breastfeeding following maternal morbidity and mortality as well as maternal fetal transmission of a variety of infectious agents, including HIV, toxoplasmosis, cytomegalovirus (CMV), rubella, hepatitis B virus, herpes simplex, syphilis, malaria, and tuberculosis; and emotional impacts and lower levels of caregiving (National Research Council, 1989; Overall, 1987; Turner, Miller, & Moses, 1989; Weinbreck, Loustaud, Denis, Vidal, Mounier, & DeLumley, 1988). This is particularly a major concern in sub-Saharan Africa, where significant numbers of mothers are suffering from HIV and other STIs (National Research Council, 1989; Turner et al., 1989; Weinbreck et al., 1988).

Methodological Concerns

The previously mentioned mechanisms by which specific reproductive patterns affect infant and child health are certainly plausible and suggestive. Nevertheless, it is important to reiterate that the empirical evidence—in terms of the appropriateness of both data and statistical methods—supporting such mechanisms zis variable and needs to be interpreted cautiously. Women have some control over their choices of reproductive patterns (i.e., whether to have children early or late, whether to have shorter or longer birth intervals, whether to have high parity births). Therefore unobservable factors that are associated with both reproductive patterns and child health may be operating, and reverse causality may be a problem. As a consequence, our estimates of the impact of specific reproductive patterns on the risk of poor infant and child health may be overstated.

For example, if women who choose to be young mothers are prone to behavior patterns that devalue prenatal and postnatal care, delaying childbirth for these women will not produce the salutary effects that the earlier discussion suggests. Similarly, unobserved selection biases may operate such that a significant proportion of women who choose to have births at older ages, higher-parity births, and closely spaced births, are intrinsically in better health—most likely because of higher socioeconomic status. If that is the case, then reducing higher-parity births, increasing inter-birth intervals, and reducing births to older women (older than age 35) will not result in the degree of improvement that the current studies suggest.

With regard to reverse causality, one example is the often-cited relationship between the mortality of an index child and a short subsequent birth interval. The inference is that a child is at a higher risk of death if the next-younger sibling arrives after only a short interval, presumably because the pregnancy and the arrival of a newborn cause early cessation of breastfeeding for the older child and a shift of other maternal resources. In reality, it is quite possible that the subsequent birth interval is short because the index child died, or was ill and weaned earlier because of his or her existing health problems. Thus the direction of causation is not from the short subsequent birth interval to the death of the preceding child but

rather in the reverse direction—from the death of the preceding child to a short subsequent birth interval. Although in principle statistical methods can deal with this kind of potential bidirectionality (Rosenzweig & Schultz, 1983; Schultz, 1984), in practice relatively few published studies have employed such sophisticated methods of analysis. In summary, because of these methodological concerns, we should be careful not to over-interpret the evidence linking specific reproductive patterns and poor child health.

Summary of the Impact of Reproductive Patterns on Child Mortality

Despite these caveats about over-interpretation and overestimation, it is instructive to consider the impact of specific deleterious reproductive patterns on infant and child mortality. The National Research Council (1989) has simulated the impact of various reproductive patterns on child mortality rates using data from 18 low- and middle-income countries reported by Hobcraft (1987). The simulations in Table 4-12 refer to death rates that would be observed in individual families with particular reproductive patterns; they assume the mortality risks associated with the specific reproductive pattern are causative.

Table 4-12 shows that children of parity 2 and greater are at much higher risk of mortality if they are born to teenage mothers than if their mothers are aged 20 to 34 years. Moreover, both teenage and nonteenage mothers can significantly reduce the risks of child mortality by adopting better spacing patterns (i.e., birth intervals of 24 months or more). The best-case scenario for children of parity 2 and greater is for those born to mothers between the ages of 20 and 34, whose older sibling has survived, and whose birth interval is 24 months or more. Only 67 of 1,000 such children fail to reach their second birthday. This is less than half the mortality risk of their peers born to

Table 4-12	Estimated Risk of Dying (Deaths per 1,000 Births) Prior to their Second Birthday for Second-and Higher-Order Births to Women with Different Reproductive Patterns	
Age of Mother	**Better Spacing Pattern**	**Poor Spacing Pattern**
Teenaged mothers	92	165
Mothers aged 20 to 34	67	120

Note: Better spacing pattern: birth intervals both proceeding and subsequent to this birth were 24 months or more and the older sibling survived. Poor spacing pattern: birth intervals both preceding and subsequent to this birth were less than 24 months and the older sibling survived.

Source: Data from National Research Council. (1989). *Contraception and reproduction: Health consequences for women and children in the developing world.* Washington, DC: National Academy Press; and Hobcraft, J. N. (1987). *Does family planning save lives?* Paper presented at the International Conference on Better Health for Women and Children Through Family Planning, Nairobi, October 5–9, 1987.

teenage mothers, where their birth intervals are less than 24 months. In the latter situation, 165 of 1,000 such children die before age 2 years.

Other simulations show the deleterious consequences of increasing family size and birth intervals on the probability of a child surviving to his or her fifth birthday. These calculations were carried out under low, moderate, and high baseline child mortality rates (to take into account variation in overall mortality among populations). The baseline child mortality rates represent the probability of a child surviving to his or her fifth birthday for children who have the lowest risk profile—that is, parity 2–3, preceding and subsequent birth intervals of 24 months or more, and the older sibling survived. Thus, in a population with a baseline child mortality rate of 150/1,000, out of 1,000 births of children who were parity 2–3, had long preceding and subsequent birth intervals (24 months or more), and whose older sibling survived, 150 would die before their fifth birthday.

Mortality rates for specific combinations of parities below and above the baseline, of short and long intervals, and of survival of older sibling were estimated by Hobcraft (1987). He then simulated the average number of children per 1,000 births who would die before their fifth birthday. Here we discuss only those cases where the older sibling survived. In terms of family size, small families were much better off than large families. Regardless of the baseline mortality rates or the closeness of birth spacing, the larger the family size, the higher the child mortality rates. In all cases, four-child families experienced fewer than half the deaths per 1,000 births of nine-child families. Similarly, families with long spacing experienced half or less the mortality per 1,000 births of families with consistently short spacing. Clearly, the most beneficial scenario for children is that of well-spaced births and small overall family sizes.

Impact of Reproductive Patterns on the Health of Women

Pregnancy is one of the major health risks for women in low- and middle-income countries. Nearly 536,000 women die worldwide each year due to pregnancy-related causes, and the vast majority (99%) of these deaths occur in low- and middle-income countries (Filippi et al., 2006; Ronsmans & Graham, 2006; WHO, 2007a). Although these numbers are alarming, it is important to recognize that 230 million pregnancies and approximately 118 million births occur annually in the world (WHO, 2007a); thus, by and large, reproduction is relatively safe for women.

Maternal mortality risks are a fraction of infant mortality risks. For example, Bangladesh has both high infant mortality and very high maternal mortality risks, but the latter are roughly a 1/17th of the former. The maternal mortality ratio is approximately 380 deaths per 100,000 births, while the infant mortality rate (which has fallen considerably in the last decade) is approximately 66 deaths per 1,000 births (Macro International, 2010a). Similarly, for Kenya, the maternal morality ratio at 590 deaths per 100,000 births is roughly one-tenth of the infant mortality rate, which is approximately 63 deaths per 1,000 births (NationMaster.com, 2010).

Definitions

In any discussion of maternal mortality, a number of potentially confusing definitional issues arise. The first is the definition of a maternal death. A maternal death is usually defined as a death of a woman while pregnant or up to 42 days post delivery from any cause (except accidents). There has been some discussion as to whether this definition is overly restrictive (i.e., leading to an undercount of maternal deaths) and should be expanded to include female deaths up to 90 days post delivery. In reality, data from a number of well-conducted population-based studies using different post-delivery durations show that the majority of maternal deaths occur within 42 days post-delivery, with approximately 40% occurring within 24 to 48 hours of delivery. Furthermore, extending the definition to up to 90 days would result in only a marginal increase (6%) in the number of deaths classified as related to maternal causes (Egypt Ministry of Health, 1994; Fauveau, Koenig, Chakraborty, & Chowdhury, 1988).

The second issue is the measure of maternal mortality risk that should be used in comparing and contrasting the situations in different populations both geographically and across time. Maternal mortality risks are conventionally described using three measures. It is important to understand and to think of them separately, because they are conceptually distinct.

The first measure is the *maternal mortality ratio*, which is defined as the ratio of the number of maternal deaths to the number of pregnancies. It is an indicator of the risk of death that a woman faces for each pregnancy she undergoes. Although conceptually the denominator for such a risk measure should include all pregnancies, operationally, because of the difficulty of counting miscarriages and induced abortions, the denominator used is live births.

The second measure is the *maternal mortality rate,* which is defined as the number of maternal deaths divided by the number of women of reproductive age (i.e., between ages 15 and 49). This composite measure is the product of the maternal mortality ratio (number of maternal deaths per births) and the birth rate in the reproductive age group (number of births for women between ages 15 and 49).The maternal mortality can be changed by altering the frequency of pregnancies or births in the population without changing the risk of maternal death per pregnancy/birth. Although the maternal mortality ratio and the maternal mortality rate are conceptually distinct, they are often confused in the public health literature, with rates referring to ratios, and vice versa. In this book, these two measures are carefully distinguished.

The third measure is the *lifetime risk of maternal mortality.* Also a composite measure, it takes into account not only the maternal mortality risk per pregnancy, but also factors in the cumulative exposure to pregnancy that an individual woman experiences. The average cumulative exposure to pregnancy is usually taken to be the total fertility rate for the population. It is an estimate of the number of births a woman in a particular society would have over her lifetime if she were to adhere to the current age-specific fertility rates in that population.

The lifetime maternal mortality risk for a woman in one of the low- and middle-income countries in 2005 was estimated to be 1/75 (Population Reference Bureau, 2008; UNFPA, 2004, 2009). This estimate can be interpreted as follows: A woman in the low- and middle-income countries who (1) has the same total number of pregnancies over her lifetime as the current fertility norm (estimated to be 2.7 births) and (2) experiences at each pregnancy the same independent risk of maternal death as the current maternal mortality ratio (approximately 500 maternal deaths per 100,000 births) would have 1 chance in 75 of dying from pregnancy-related causes. This lifetime risk captures both the risk of dying per pregnancy and the cumulative effect of exposure to multiple pregnancies.

Maternal Mortality Risks

A major constraint with respect to investigating the magnitude of maternal mortality risks and its determinants is the lack of available and reliable population-based data. Even in low- and middle-income countries, many of which have high maternal mortality rates and ratios, maternal deaths are relatively rare. For example, in sub-Saharan Africa and South Asia, where maternal mortality ratios of 800 maternal deaths per 100,000 live births have been reported, one would need very large sample sizes to obtain reasonable estimates of maternal mortality risks and their accompany determinants. A sample of 10,000 births (a very large sample by any standards) would be expected to yield only 80 maternal deaths. In contrast, infant mortality rates in these settings are typically 15 times as large, and the same sample would yield 1,050 infant deaths.

To date, relatively few large-scale population-based studies of maternal mortality have been conducted in low- and middle-income countries. The major investigations were carried out in Bangladesh (Alauddin, 1986; National Institute of Population Research and Training, 2003; Chen, Gesche, Ahmed, Chowdhury, & Mosley, 1975; Fauveau et al., 1988; Khan, Jahan, & Begum, 1986; Koenig et al., 1988), Ethiopia (Kwast, Rochat, & Kildane-Mariam, 1986), Egypt (Egypt Ministry of Health, 1994; Fortney, Susanti, Gadalla, Saleh, Feldblum, & Potts, 1985), and Jamaica (Walker, Ashley, McCaw, & Bernard, 1985). Estimates for other countries are derived from model-based assumptions and thus are not as precise.

There are huge disparities in maternal mortality among various regions of the world. The disparity between low-and middle-income countries and high-income countries is much greater for maternal mortality (20 times higher risk of maternal death per pregnancy) than infant mortality (10 times higher risk of infant death per pregnancy). Lifetime risks of maternal mortality vary from 1/75 in low- and middle-income countries to 1/7,300 in high-income countries (Table 4-13).

As is shown in Table 4-13, both the total number of pregnancies per woman and the individual risk of dying per pregnancy are much higher in low- and middle-income countries than in high-income countries. But it is the risk of dying per pregnancy that accounts for the vast majority of the difference in lifetime risk of maternal mortality. Total fertility rates in low- and middle-income countries are, on average, 1½ times as high as in the industrialized countries (2.7 births per woman versus 1.7 births per woman). Maternal mortality ratios are 50 times as high (450 maternal deaths per 100,000 births in low- and middle-income countries versus 9 maternal deaths per 100,000 births in high-income countries). Fourteen countries—Afghanistan, Angola, Burundi, Cameroon, Chad, Democratic Republic of the Congo, Guinea-Bissau, Liberia, Malawi, Niger, Nigeria, Rwanda, Sierra Leone, and Somalia—have maternal mortality

Table 4-13	Total Fertility Rate, Maternal Mortality Ratios, and Lifetime Risks of Maternal Death, by Region, 2005			
Region	Total Fertility Rate (Births per Woman)	Maternal Mortality Ratio (Deaths per 100,000 Live Births)	Maternal Deaths Lifetime Risk	Deaths per Year
World	2.6	400	1 in 92	536,000
Industrialized countries	1.7	9	1 in 7,300	960
Low-and middle-income countries	2.7	450	1 in 75	533,000
Africa	4.8	820	1 in 26	276,000
Asia	2.3	330	1 in 120	241,000
Latin America and the Caribbean	2.3	130	1 in 290	15,000

Source: Population Reference Bureau. (2008). *Family planning worldwide: 2008 data sheet.* Washington, DC: Author. Adapted with permission. Retrieved February 28, 2010, from http://www.prb.org/Datafinder/Geography; and World Health Organization. (2007). *Maternal mortality in 2005: Estimates developed by WHO, UNICEF, UNFPA and the World Bank.* Geneva, Switzerland: Author. Retrieved March 30, 2010, from http://www.who.int/reproductive-health/publications/maternal_mortality_2005/index.html.

ratios of at least 1,000 deaths per 100,000 live births; all of these countries are in sub-Saharan Africa, except for Afghanistan. For most of the poorest countries (most of South Asia and Africa, as opposed to the middle-income countries such as China, Egypt, Indonesia, Jordan, Mexico, Sri Lanka, and Tunisia), there was not much change in the maternal mortality ratios between 1900 and 2000 (United Nations Statistics Division, 2009, 2010a, 2010b; WHO, 2007a).

Direct and Indirect Causes of Maternal Mortality and Morbidity

What are the sources of the mortality risk per pregnancy? The causes of maternal mortality are conventionally divided into direct causes—those that occur only during pregnancy and the immediate postdelivery period—and indirect causes—those derived from conditions that precede, but are aggravated by, pregnancy, such as anemia, diabetes, malaria, tuberculosis, cardiac disease, hepatitis, and increasingly AIDS (Ronsman & Graham, 2006; WHO, 2005).

In low- and middle-income countries, direct causes account for 75% to 80% of maternal mortality and include, in approximate order of importance, hemorrhage (25%), sepsis (15%), hypertensive disorders of pregnancy (eclampsia—12%), complications of unsafe abortion (13%), obstructed or prolonged labor (8%), and other direct causes (8%) (Fauveau et al., 1988; Maine & McGinn, 1999; WHO, 2005, 1993c; WHO & UNICEF, 1996). The vast majority of these maternal deaths can be attributed to just three causes: hemorrhage, sepsis, and eclampsia. Attribution of cause of death is complicated by the fact that in most cases unsafe abortion and obstructed or prolonged labor eventually cause death via the proximate causes of hemorrhage or sepsis. There is variation in the order of importance of these causes in different studies from different parts of the world (Jamison, Mosley, Measham, & Bobadilla, 1993), partly due to real differences in the availability and use of obstetric care and partly due to differences in the quality of reporting. Thus, in countries that have poor access to obstetric care facilities, a relatively large proportion of deaths is attributed to hemorrhage, sepsis, and abortion. Differential reporting—particularly reluctance to attribute maternal deaths to abortion in countries where it is illegal—also artifactually inflates the proportion of deaths attributed to hemorrhage and sepsis. For example, Jamison and associates (1993) estimated that, for the period 1980–1985, these two causes were responsible for 56% of maternal deaths in Indonesia, 40% of such deaths in Egypt, and 18% of these in the United States.

The remaining 20% to 25% of maternal deaths can be attributed to illnesses aggravated by pregnancy (Jamison et al., 1993; WHO, 1993b). For example, anemia hampers a woman's abilities to resist infection and to survive hemorrhage; it may increase the likelihood of her dying in childbirth by a factor of 4 (Chi, Agoestina, & Harbin, 1981). Hepatitis can cause hemorrhage or liver failure in pregnant women (Kwast & Stevens, 1987). Latent infections such as tuberculosis, malaria, or STIs can also be activated or exacerbated during pregnancy and cause potentially severe complications for both mother and child (Jamison et al., 1993).

In keeping with the high rates of maternal mortality in low- and middle-income countries, there are also high rates of maternal morbidity. An estimated 30 to 50 morbidities (temporary and chronic) occur for every maternal death (Safe Motherhood Initiative, 2010). Between 30% and 40% of the approximately 180 million women who are pregnant annually in the world, or roughly 54 million women, report some kind of pregnancy-related morbidity (Koblinsky, Campbell, & Harlow, 1993; WHO, 1993b). Of these women, 10 to 15 million each year develop relatively long-term disabilities deriving from complications from obstetric fistula or prolapse, uterine scarring, severe anemia, pelvic inflammatory disease, reproductive tract infections, and infertility (Filippi et al., 2006; Ronsmans & Graham, 2006; Tsui et al., 1997).

These figures demonstrate significant variability from one country to another (Tsui et al., 1997). For example, Guatemalan women report one in five pregnancies as being complicated (Bailey, Szaszdi, & Scheiber, 1994), women in West Java report one in three pregnancies as being complicated (Alisjahbana, Williams, Dharmayanti, Hermawan, Kwast, & Koblinsky, 1995), and two out of three pregnancies in Ghana had some complications (De Graft-Johnson, 1994). This variability in rates stems at least in part from differences in study design and data quality. To date, relatively few population-based surveys have been carried out. Moreover, much of the maternal morbidity data is based on self-reported symptoms— a data collection technique that has been shown to have relatively low reliability and validity (Stewart & Festin, 1995). A few data sets with reliable information have come from the United States and Canada (Koblinsky et al., 1993; WHO, 1994b) and from specific validation studies (Stewart & Festin, 1995). These data show that annually 12% to 15% of women who are pregnant suffer life-threatening obstetric complications, equivalent to approximately 20 million women in low- and middle-income countries (assuming approximately 150 million women giving birth annually). In contrast to the evidence on acute pregnancy-related morbidity, little is known about the long-term chronic morbidity sequelae of pregnancy-related complications, which may significantly affect women's lives.

Specific Causes of Pregnancy-Related Morbidity and Mortality

This section focuses on some of the more prominent causes of pregnancy-related morbidity and mortality in low- and middle-income countries.

Obstructed and Prolonged Labor

Obstructed or prolonged labor leads to approximately 40,000 maternal deaths annually, with high proportions of survivors suffering from obstetric fistulas and their newborn often suffering from long-term sequelae of anoxia and even death (Kusiako et al., 2000). Predictive risk factors for this outcome are not particularly reliable (Fortney, 1995; Maine, 1991). Monitoring during labor using a partograph is the only effective way to detect such problems (WHO, 1994a).

Obstetric Fistula and Genital Prolapse

Both obstetric fistulas and genital prolapse have severe consequences for the pregnant woman. As a consequence, they represent a major global health problem.

An obstetric fistula is a passage or channel from the vaginal wall to either the rectum (recto-vaginal fistula) or the bladder (vesico-vaginal fistula). It is usually a result of a tear in the vaginal wall during complicated labor. Risk factors for obstetric fistulas include being a young mother, stunted mother, or a mother who has complicated labor and delivers in a nonhospital setting with the help of traditional birth attendants (Lawson, 1992; Tahzib, 1983, 1985). Population-level estimates of obstetric fistulas are hard to come by, but fragmentary reports suggest that it is a significant cause of morbidity for pregnant women in low- and middle-income countries (Lawson, 1992; WHO, 1991). The consequences of fistulas are quite severe, especially for young primipara women. The baby is often stillborn, and the mother is incontinent of urine and/or feces. This condition is a source of enormous personal discomfort, whose consequences are exacerbated by social stigma. In many cases, it leads to divorce and social ostracism—these women are often barred from food preparation or even participating in prayer, due to lack of personal hygiene (Reed, Koblinsky, & Mosley, 2000).

Genital prolapse occurs when the vagina and uterus descend below their normal positions. This condition is usually a result of damage to supporting muscles and ligaments during childbirth and is most often associated with high parity. It is particularly uncomfortable for women who are squatting, which is the normal position for doing many chores in low- and middle-income countries. It can also lead to chronic backache, urinary problems, and pain during sexual intercourse. Subsequent pregnancies have a higher probability of fetal loss and further maternal morbidity.

Although good estimates of these conditions are difficult to obtain, some reliable population studies suggest very high prevalence rates—as much as one-third of all pregnant women (Omran & Standley, 1981; Younis, Khattab, Zurayk, el-Mouelhy, Fadle Amin, &

Farag, 1993). The Giza study (Younis et al., 1993), which clinically validated reported prolapse, found that one-third of women suffered from genital prolapse and also documented a relationship between genital prolapse and risk of reproductive tract infections.

Anemia

Approximately 50% of pregnant women around the world are estimated to be anemic (i.e., to have hemoglobin levels less than 11 g/dL). Dietary iron deficiency is the primary cause of this condition, followed by malaria, other parasitic diseases (schistosomiasis, hookworm), folate deficiency, AIDS, and sickle cell disease (Tsui et al., 1997). In addition to its well-documented effects on pregnancy outcomes—prematurity, stillbirths, and spontaneous abortions (Levin, Pollitt, Galloway, & McGuire, 1993)—anemia, even at fairly mild levels, has been implicated directly as contributing to maternal deaths (Harrison & Rossiter, 1985; United Nations, 1991). In addition, some evidence suggests that anemia predisposes women to higher risks of complications during pregnancy, including urinary tract infections, pyelonephritis, and pre-eclampsia (Kitay & Harbort, 1975). Anemia is also associated with reduced productivity and quality of life for women (Bothwell & Charllton, 1981).

Data on the effectiveness of iron supplementation in reducing the prevalence of iron-deficiency anemia are not encouraging (Sloan, Jordan, & Winikoff, 1992). While a significant part of the failure to reduce anemia is due to inadequate efforts to provide iron supplementation, even in situations where properly conducted supplementation trials have been conducted, these programs do not appear to be very effective in reducing baseline anemia levels (Sood et al., 1975). The relatively poor outcomes may reflect inadequacies of strategies that focus just on pregnant women. Long-term success probably will require the use of a multipronged strategy including iron supplementation schemes, efforts to raise household income, and efforts to reduce workload during pregnancy (Tsui et al., 1997).

Pregnancy-Related Hypertension

Both eclampsia and pre-eclampsia are significant causes of maternal morbidity. Unfortunately, these conditions are difficult to predict and prevent, although routine prenatal blood pressure measurements and urinalysis for proteinuria in the first prenatal visit continue to be recommended for this purpose (Rooney, 1992; Stone, Lockwood, Berkowitz, Alvarez, Lapinski, & Berkowitz, 1994). Women with moderate hypertension and proteinuria require appropriate follow-up. Treatment options and their effectiveness vary, so no

definitive conclusions or recommendations can be made. As a general rule, a combination of bed rest, antihypertensive agents, and anticonvulsant medications (especially magnesium sulfate for frank convulsions) may provide some relief (Eclampsia Trial Collaborative Group, 1995; Rooney, 1992).

Consequences of Pregnancy and Delivery Complications for Infants

Pregnancy- and delivery-related complications have important health consequences not only for mothers but also for infants, particularly in the neonatal period (the first 28 days following birth/delivery), and especially in the early neonatal period (i.e., the first 7 days of birth/delivery) (Kusiako et al., 2000; WHO, 2006; Zupan, 2005). Each year, out of the 10.7 million children who die before their fifth birthday, approximately 3.3 million (31%) are stillborn and 4 million (38%) die during the first 28 days. Developing countries account for more than 98% of both stillbirths and neonatal deaths (WHO, 2005). Of the 4 million neonatal deaths, 75% (3 million deaths) occur in the first 7 days of life (WHO, 2006).

For most low- and middle-income countries, neonatal mortality rates range between 10 and 62 deaths per 1,000 live births, with the median being 33 neonatal deaths per 1,000 live births (Hill & Choi, 2006). Low- and middle-income countries have six times the neonatal mortality rate of high-income countries. The highest neonatal mortality rates are in Central and Western Africa (41/1,000) and the lowest in Latin America and the Caribbean (25/1,000). Early neonatal mortality rates (ENMR—deaths in the first 7 days of life, including stillbirths) average 24 deaths per 1,000 live births, ranging from 9 to 45 deaths per 1,000 live births (Hill & Choi, 2006; WHO, 2006). Most neonatal deaths occur in Asia, which is where most children are born. Within Asia, the most strongly affected region is South Central Asia (e.g., Afghanistan, Bangladesh, India, Nepal and Pakistan), which accounts for more than 40% of global neonatal deaths (WHO, 2006).

In 2005, a total of 4 million neonatal deaths and 7.6 million infant deaths (not including stillbirths) occurred. Thus neonatal deaths accounted for approximately 53% of all infant deaths worldwide. As infant mortality rates drop, the proportion of infant deaths attributed to the neonatal period actually increases, because post-neonatal deaths (those after the first 28 days of life, which are most sensitive to environmental contamination and amenable to public health interventions) are the first to decrease (Black, Morris & Bryce, 2003; Hill & Choi, 2006; WHO, 2006; Zupan, 2005).

Of the estimated 3.3 million stillbirths and 4 million neonatal deaths worldwide, the vast majority are associated with maternal health problems during pregnancy (e.g., preterm birth, maternal infections, severe malformations) and around delivery (e.g., asphyxia or trauma during birth, infections such as tetanus). The contribution of each of these factors varies with the level of neonatal mortality. In areas where neonatal mortality is high, birth trauma and infections play larger roles; in contrast, in areas where neonatal mortality is low, preterm birth and severe malformations predominate (Beck et al., 2009; Fauveau et al., 1990; Hill & Choi, 2006; Zupan, 2005). Most of the adverse outcomes leading to stillbirth and neonatal death are due to poor antenatal care (e.g., non-immunization against tetanus, poor prevention of HIV and other STIs) inadequately treated maternal complications such as eclampsia, poor-quality neonatal care, and harmful traditional practices such as discarding the colostrums, nonsterile umbilical cord cutting, and failure to keep babies warm. Roughly one-third of the 3.3 million stillbirths are due to delivery complications and could largely be prevented by skilled care during delivery and in the first 24 hours post delivery (WHO, 2006; Zupan, 2005).

One of the most important risk factors for neonatal mortality is low birth weight, with babies weighing less than 2,500 grams having 20 to 30 times the mortality risk of babies of normal weight. In addition to increasing the risk of neonatal mortality, low birth weight is associated with a substantial burden of long-term disability (e.g., impaired immune function and greater susceptibility to infection, long-term undernourishment and decreased muscle strength throughout the child's life, inhibited cognitive development, higher incidence of diabetes and heart disease, cerebral palsy, seizures, and severe learning disorders) for babies who survive (Jamison et al., 1993; Tsui et al., 1997; United Nations Children's Fund/WHO, 2004; WHO, 2006; Zupan, 2005). Women who have inadequate nutritional status (including short stature, poor prepregnancy weight, inadequate weight gain during pregnancy, and anemia) or infections during pregnancy are more likely to have low-birth-weight (LBW) babies (United Nations Children's Fund/WHO, 2004;WHO, 1993b; Zupan, 2005).

When assessing outcomes for LBW babies, it is necessary to distinguish between those who are appropriate for their gestational age but are mostly preterm (less than 37 weeks' gestation) and those who are inappropriately small for their gestational age (mostly full term) and have suffered from intrauterine growth retardation (IUGR). In low- and middle-income countries, the majority of LBW babies are full term but suffer from IUGR; in contrast, in the high-income world, most LBW babies are preterm. These distinctions are important, as LBW babies with IUGR have higher morbidity and higher mortality than LBW babies who are appropriately sized given their (preterm) gestational age. The worst-off babies are those who are both preterm and suffer from IUGR (Childinfo, 2009; Qadir & Bhutta, 2009; United Nations Children's Fund/WHO, 2004). In 2000, out of approximately 132 million babies born worldwide, 15.5%— 20.5 million—were LBW (96% in developing countries). The level of LBW in low- and middle-income countries was more than double that in high-income countries (16.5% versus 7%), with the highest rates being found in South Asia (27%). Of these 20.5 million LBW babies, only one-third (7 million) suffered from IUGR and were full term. The remaining two-thirds (14 million) of LBW babies were preterm births who were appropriately sized given their gestational age (De Onis, Blossner, & Villar, 1998; Qadir & Bhutta, 2009; United Nations Children's Fund/WHO, 2004).

Preterm birth is a major risk factor for neonatal mortality and morbidity, accounting for 28% of early neonatal mortality (deaths of infants in the first 7 days of life) other than those deaths related to congenital malformations. It is estimated that 9.6% of all births worldwide in 2005 were preterm, which translates into a total of 12.9 million preterm births. In light of the earlier discussion of LBW and IUGR, it is important to note that most preterm babies are, in fact, appropriately developed for their gestational age and have LBW (i.e., weigh 2,500 g or less) because of premature delivery. In 2005, the majority of these births occurred in Asia (54%) and Africa (31%), with only 7.4% being in Europe and North America. The highest preterm birth rates occurred in Africa and North America (11.9% and 10.6%, respectively), with Europe having the lowest rates (approximately 6.2%) (Beck et al., 2009). A variety of factors are associated with preterm birth, including medical conditions of the mother or the fetus, genetics, environmental exposures, infertility treatments, behavioral and socioeconomic factors, and iatrogenic interventions (Goldenberg, Culhane, Iams, & Romero, 2008).

High-Risk Pregnancies

For the sake of simplicity, the calculations of lifetime risk presented earlier assumed that the risk of maternal death per pregnancy is the same across all women and across successive pregnancies within each woman.

The reality is somewhat more complicated, with some types of pregnancies being riskier than others. Higher-risk conditions include pregnancies of first-time mothers, mothers with multiple previous pregnancies (five or more pregnancies), very young and older mothers, women already in poor health, and pregnancies that are terminated by unsafe abortions (National Research Council, 1989; Tsui et al., 1997). Table 4-14 summarizes the hypothesized mechanisms by which different reproductive patterns affect maternal health.

First pregnancies have a higher risk of maternal mortality than subsequent pregnancies (up to give) both in high-income and low- and middle-income countries. Population-based data from Bangladesh (Koenig et al., 1988), Ethiopia (Kwast, Rochat, & Kidane-Mariam, 1986), and the Gambia (Greenwood et al., 1987) suggest that first pregnancies may be as much as three times riskier than later pregnancies.

The impact of young maternal age on maternal mortality is more difficult to evaluate because relatively few studies have disaggregated the confounding effect of young maternal age and first pregnancy. Among those that have controlled for confounding factors appropriately, the largest study to date looked at maternal mortality among 14,631 first births in rural Bangladesh (Koenig et al., 1988); it showed no age effect. Other smaller studies from the same area

(Chen et al., 1975), Indonesia (Chi et al., 1981), and Jamaica (Walker et al., 1985) have shown a higher mortality risk for mothers younger than age 20 compared to mothers aged 20 to 24. A further problem that makes interpretation of data difficult is that maternal age younger than 20 is not disaggregated into single years of age; in fact, the highest risk may be for young mothers in the 15- to 17-year-old age group (Harrison & Rossiter, 1985).

The major causes of morbidity and mortality for young primigravida women include a high risk of pregnancy-induced hypertension (WHO, 1988), a high frequency of obstructed labor due to the pelvis being too small for the child's head to pass (Aitken & Walls, 1986), and a high incidence of placental malaria (MacGregor, Wilson, & Billewicz, 1983).

A number of studies have shown that women with four or more pregnancies have 1.5 to 3 times the risk of maternal death as women of parities 2 and 3. In general, for any given parity, older women—particularly those beyond age 35—have higher risks of maternal death (Chi et al., 1981; Koenig et al., 1988; Walker et al., 1985). A major cause of maternal morbidity and mortality for older multiparous women is the higher risk of malpresentation (in which the fetus assumes a position other than the usual head-first delivery, as in a breech or transverse lie presentation). Malpresentation of the fetus may occur due to the

Table 4-14	Mechanisms by Which Reproductive Patterns Affect Maternal Health
Reproductive Pattern	**Mechanism Through Which Maternal Health Is Affected**
Number of pregnancies	Each pregnancy carries a risk of morbidity and mortality
High-risk pregnancies	
First-time mothers	Higher risk than pregnancies 2–4 for obstructed labor, pregnancy-induced hypertension, other obstetric complications due to initial adaptation to pregnancy
Higher-order pregnancies	Higher risk for hemorrhage and uterine rupture, due to the cumulative toll of previous pregnancies and reproductive injuries
Pregnancy at very young maternal ages	Higher risk due to physiologically immature reproductive systems and reduced propensity for timely care seeking
Pregnancy at old maternal ages	Body in poorer condition for pregnancy and childbirth
Short interbirth intervals	Inadequate time to rebuild nutritional stores and regain energy levels
Unwanted pregnancies ending in unsafe abortions	Unsafe abortions increase exposure to injury, infection, hemorrhage, and death
Pregnancies for women already in poor health	Aggravated health condition

Source: Adapted with permission from National Research Council. (1989). Contraception and reproduction: Health consequences for women and children in the developing world. Washington, DC: National Academies Press. Copyright 1989 by the National Academy of Sciences.

flaccidity of the uterine wall from repeated stretching from successive pregnancies. It can lead to uterine rupture, hemorrhage associated with rupture, or infections resulting from unsuccessful attempts to deal with malpresentation. Another major cause of morbidity and mortality in older multiparous women is hemorrhage due to placental abnormalities such as placenta previa (where the placenta overlies the cervical opening of the uterus) and placenta abruptio (where the placenta separates prematurely from the uterus prior to delivery of the baby) (Faundes, Fanjul, Henriquez, Mora, & Tognola, 1974).

There has been much talk about the possibility of a maternal depletion syndrome whereby multiple short birth intervals result in women not having enough time to recover their energy and nutritional levels, which in turn may lead to higher risks of maternal mortality (Jelliffe, 1976; Winikoff, 1983). As yet, no convincing evidence validating this hypothesis has been presented (Koenig et al., 1988; National Research Council, 1989; Ronsman & Campbell, 1998). This could be due to the fact that intrinsically healthier women (in this case, women of higher socioeconomic status) may be more likely to have multiple short birth intervals, whereas less healthy women may take longer between subsequent births (Duffy & Menken, 1998).

Pregnancy is more dangerous for women who are already in poor health. It increases the likelihood that a woman will die if she has certain preexisting conditions, such as malaria, hepatitis, anemia, sickle cell disease, rheumatic heart disease (Koblinsky et al., 1993; Morrow, Smetana, Sai, & Edgcomb, 1968; National Research Council, 1989; Tsui et al., 1997; WHO, 1993b).

Finally, unsafe abortions are a significant cause of maternal death in countries where abortion is not legal and regulated. Kwast, Rochat, and Kidane-Mariam (1986) reported that the primary cause of maternal mortality in Addis Ababa, Ethiopia, especially among primigravida, unmarried women is complications from illegal abortions. In Bangladesh, Koenig and colleagues (1988) reported that 18% of all maternal deaths in the Matlab surveillance area were from abortion complications (see the earlier discussion of abortion and its health consequences for women in the family planning program section). More recent data from WHO (2007b) indicate that in low- and middle-income countries, a woman dies from an unsafe abortion every 8 minutes. Approximate one in every four women having unsafe abortions develops significant medical complications, and unsafe abortion causes approximately 13% of all maternal deaths

and approximately 20% of the overall burden of maternal death and long-term sexual and reproductive ill health.

Mechanisms to Reduce Maternal Morbidity and Mortality in Low- and Middle-Income Countries

The fifth Millennium Development Goal (MDG) to reduce maternal mortality by 75% between 1990 and 2015 has made the least progress of all the MDGs (United Nations Statistics Division, 2009). The current maternal mortality decrease, which amounts to less than 1% per year between 1990 and 2005 globally, is far less than the required annual decrease of 5.5% improvement needed to reach the target by 2015 ("Maternal Deaths," 2008; United Nations Statistics Division, 2009, 2010a, 2010b; WHO, 2008b). Weak health systems, continuing high fertility, and poor availability of data to monitor change have further jeopardized progress in the low- and middle-income countries where 99% of maternal deaths occur, and particularly in sub-Saharan Africa (Koblinsky et al., 2006; Ronsman & Graham, 2006; WHO, 2008a). Researchers have suggested that a multisectoral approach will be required to decrease the number of maternal deaths through reduced exposure to pregnancy (i.e., by reducing fertility), optimization of access to emergency obstetric care, and improvement of general health status and treatment of pregnancy- and childbirth-related complications (Barlett et al., 2005, Campbell & Graham, 2006; Dogba & Fournier, 2009; Koblinsky et al., 2006; Paxton, Maine, Freedman, Fry, & Lobis, 2005; WHO, 2005, 2007a).

The major emphasis in the last few decades in low- and middle-income countries in reducing maternal morbidity and mortality has been on decreasing the total number of pregnancies per woman. As documented earlier, the total number of pregnancies per woman has fallen quite sharply in many of these countries; this drop has contributed significantly to the decrease in the lifetime risk of maternal mortality by reducing cumulative exposure. For example, assume a constant maternal mortality ratio of 750 maternal deaths per 100,000 live births. In Kenya, if the total fertility rate had remained at its 1975 level of 8.2 instead of dropping to the 2003 level of 4.9, the lifetime risk of maternal mortality would have been 1/16 instead of 1/32. In addition to the significant drop in TFR, some fairly modest improvement in mortality risk per pregnancy has occurred; the 2003 maternal mortality ratio was 590 deaths per 100,000 births (NationMaster.com, 2010). Taken together, these changes have led to the decrease in the lifetime maternal mortality risk to its current level of 1/34, with most of the improvement in lifetime risk coming from reduction of the overall number of births and, therefore, women's exposure to the risk of maternal mortality.

In addition to the reduction in the TFR in low- and middle-income countries, some progress has been made in reducing the numbers of high-parity births (Table 4-15), births to older women (Table 4-16),

and births following short intervals (i.e., less than 24 months). By 2000, however, as fertility continued to decline in most of these countries, the proportion of births to older women increased again due to postponement of births (United Nations Population Division, 2009). Access to safe abortion has also increased (Alan Guttmacher Institute, 2009a, 2009b; Tsui et al., 1997); unfortunately, the number of unsafe abortions remained more or less steady from 1995 to 2003 at approximately 20 million per year, with 98%

Table 4-15	Change in the Distribution of Birth Order over the Course of Fertility Decline and Percentage Decline in Total Fertility Rates for Selected Countries				
	Percentage of All Births of Order 1		Percentage of All Births of Order 5		
Country	1960s	1970s–1980	1960s	1970s–1980	Percentage Decline in TFR
Singapore	23	44	33	2	65
Hong Kong	25	43	23	4	64
Barbados	22	40	35	10	54
Mauritius	18	36	36	11	52
Costa Rica	18	32	45	17	50
Chile	25	41	31	9	49
Trinidad and Tobago	19	32	37	19	43
Puerto Rico	27	32	27	10	42
Panama	21	29	35	22	42
Malaysia	12	26	41	22	42
Fiji	23	35	36	13	41

Source: Adapted with permission from National Research Council. (1989). *Contraception and reproduction: Health consequences for women and children in the developing world.* Washington, DC: National Academies Press. Copyright 1989 by the National Academy of Sciences.

Table 4-16	Change in the Distribution of Births by Maternal Age in Selected Countries over the Course of Fertility Decline and Percentage Decline in Total Fertility Rates Between 1960 and 1980				
	Percentage of All Births to Women Younger Than Age 20		Percentage of All Births to Women Aged 35 and Older		
Country	1960s	1970s–1980	1960s	1970s–1980	Percentage Decline in TFR
Singapore	8	4	14	5	65
Hong Kong	5	4	20	6	643
Barbados	21	25	15	6	54
Mauritius	13	14	15	7	52
Costa Rica	13	20	18	9	50
Chile	12	17	17	9	49
Trinidad and Tobago	17	19	11	8	43
Puerto Rico	18	18	11	7	42
Panama	18	20	11	9	42
Malaysia	11	7	14	13	42
Fiji	13	11	12	8	41

Source: Adapted with permission from National Research Council. (1989). *Contraception and reproduction: Health consequences for women and children in the developing world.* Washington, DC: National Academies Press. Copyright 1989 by the National Academy of Sciences.

of these procedures occurring in developing countries (Alan Guttmacher Institute, 2009a, 2009b; WHO, 2007b). An often-overlooked benefit of fertility-reduction initiatives is their impact on reducing the frequency of unsafe abortions by providing access to effective contraception for those who want it (Alan Guttmacher Institute, 2009a, 2009b; Bulatao, 1998; National Research Council, 1989; WHO, 2007b).

Despite these positive efforts, a significant burden of maternal mortality persists in low- and middle-income countries. Two reasons explain why this condition remains in spite of the increase in the proportion of pregnancies that are in the demographically low-risk category (i.e., parity 2–4 among mothers aged 24 to 29 with birth intervals of 24 months or more). First, the absolute risk of maternal death is still very high in these settings, even in low-risk pregnancies. Second, some of the factors associated with the highest-risk pregnancies, such as first pregnancies, are unavoidable.

In this regard, it is worth considering the following scenario. Kenya—which has very high risks of maternal mortality per pregnancy—experiences no change in the mortality risk per pregnancy (now 590 maternal deaths per 100,000 live births), but fertility declines to replacement levels (i.e., each woman has just 2.1 births over her lifetime). Under these conditions, the lifetime risk of maternal mortality would still be 1/81—almost 90 times as high as the lifetime maternal mortality risk (1/7,300) of women in high-income countries.

Even this scenario may be overly optimistic. Our calculation does not allow for any heterogeneity in maternal mortality risks across pregnancies. If first pregnancies are intrinsically more dangerous or if healthier women were the ones who had more pregnancies, simply reducing the number of births would not achieve the reduction in maternal mortality estimated previously.

Finally, a number of studies have shown that older women with more surviving sons have significantly lower mortality than their peers with fewer sons (Rahman, 1998; Rahman, Menken, & Foster, 1992). This research suggests that although increased numbers of pregnancies may expose a woman to considerable risk of morbidity and mortality, women in certain social settings (where family support is crucial) are actually better off when they are older if they have had higher fertility. These considerations lead to the conclusion that, to reduce maternal deaths to a significant extent in low- and middle-income countries, an emphasis on reducing overall fertility levels and the frequency of high-risk pregnancies is unlikely to be

sufficient. Instead, the emphasis must be on reducing the mortality risk for each and every pregnancy.

Obstetric Care

As pointed out earlier, the majority of maternal and perinatal mortality and morbidity stems from complications related to the delivery process, which are difficult to predict and avoid prenatally (Maine, 1991; National Statistics Office [Philippines] & Macro International, 1994; Ronsman & Graham, 2006; Thaddeus & Maine, 1994; WHO, 2005). Perhaps the most important benefit of prenatal care is in sensitizing the mother to warning signs of obstetric emergencies and the need to seek appropriate obstetric care when they occur (Tsui et al., 1997).

It is instructive to review briefly what qualifies as the basic acceptable package of obstetric care. WHO uses the following eight criteria to assess the adequacy of obstetric care facilities (Campbell & Graham, 2006; Dogba & Fournier, 2009; Paxton et al., 2005; WHO, 1995):

1. The ability to treat infection, both orally and intravenously

2. The ability to provide intravenous labor-inducing agents such as oxytocin

3. The facilities for the medical treatment of shock, anemia, and hypertensive disorders of pregnancy (provision of parenteral anticonvulsants)

4. The ability to provide manual procedures for removal of the placenta, including vacuum extraction

5. The ability to carry out the removal of retained products of conception and ectopic pregnancy and provide safe abortion services

6. The ability to carry out assisted vaginal delivery and monitor labor

7. The ability to carry out caesarean section along with appropriate facilities for anesthesia

8. The ability to provide blood transfusions

Facilities that can carry out the first six interventions are called basic EmOC (Emergency Obstetric Care) centers; those that can carry out all eight interventions are termed complete EmOC centers (Campbell & Graham, 2006; Paxton et al., 2005).

The historical record in the United States and Europe (Hogberg, Wall, & Brostroin 1986; Loudon, 1991) and the more recent experience of specific low- and middle-income countries such as Sri Lanka show that the implementation of even limited parts of the essential obstetric care package can result in major declines in maternal mortality. The maternal mortality ratio in Sri Lanka dropped dramatically, from 555 maternal deaths per 100,000 births in the mid-1950s to 239 maternal deaths in the 1960s and again to 95 maternal deaths in 1980 (WHO, 1995). These gains were largely due to the expansion of health centers appropriately equipped for essential obstetric care and the increase in births attended by trained personnel.

A 2008 report focusing on maternal health interventions in 68 countries that experience 97% of maternal and child deaths worldwide suggested that several interventions have been proven to improve maternal survival (United Nations Children's Fund, 2008; Bryce et al., 2008; Bhutta et al. 2008). Under the circumstances when complications are not predictable, skilled care at delivery is the key to reduce maternal mortality. For example, a package healthcare service consisting of skilled care by doctors, nurses, and midwives during pregnancy and childbirth, including family planning and emergency medical services, and costing less than $1.50 per person can reduce an estimated 80% of maternal mortality. Increased access to hospital and midwifery care, improved quality of care, and control of infectious diseases have been successfully combined to significantly lower maternal mortality in several low-income countries, including Bangladesh, Nepal, Thailand, Malaysia, Sri Lanka, Egypt, Honduras, and some states of India ("The World Health Report," 2005; WHO, 2005).

For a variety of reasons—including cultural taboos, lack of social mobility, lack of economic resources, lack of logistic resources, and lack of information—women in low- and middle-income countries for the most part do not use appropriate obstetric care services, with the most vulnerable group in this regard being rural, less educated, and poorer women (Govindasamy, Stewart, Rutstein, Boerma, & Sommerfelt, 1993). In 1993, only 37% of births in low- and middle-income countries took place in a health facility (WHO, 1993a). The remaining deliveries (some 55 to 60 million infants) were carried out with the help of traditional birth attendants, family members, or no assistance at all.

In this regard, it is interesting to note that prenatal care services are used significantly more than obstetric care services. In 39 of 43 countries covered by DHS surveys between 1985 and 1994, prenatal care coverage was significantly higher than delivery care from a trained provider (i.e., doctor, nurse, or midwife) (Macro International, 1994). These results need to be viewed with some caution, however, as prenatal care is self-reported and may include very low and episodic use of appropriate services.

There is considerable variation in the DHS-surveyed countries in use of both prenatal and maternal care services. South Asia (with the exception of Sri Lanka) has particularly low rates of use for prenatal care and maternal care services. More recent data show that there has been significant improvement in developing countries in terms of access to both antenatal and skilled care services during delivery, with the latter showing a greater increase in the utilization rate. Approximately 66% of pregnant women in low- and middle-income countries currently receive at least one antenatal care visit, compared to at least four antenatal care visits for most women in high-income countries. There are huge disparities in the distribution of antenatal care, however: In Ethiopia, for example, this figure is only 12%. Moreover, only 62% of pregnant women in low- and middle-income countries currently receive assistance from skilled birth attendants during their deliveries. As in the case of antenatal care, large regional differences in access to these services exist, with utilization rates ranging from 34% in Eastern Africa to 93% in South America ("Maternal Deaths," 2008; United Nations Children's Fund, 2008; WHO, 2008c).

Despite these improvements in access to skilled delivery care, there is currently a 50% deficit worldwide against the estimated demand of 700,000 midwives needed to ensure universal coverage with maternity care. More generally, there is a global shortage of 4.3 million health workers (WHO, 2008c).

Leaving aside the significant gaps in the availability of skilled maternal care/delivery services, even when such services are available they are not used to the degree they should be. The failure to use appropriate maternal/delivery care services can be viewed as resulting from a multipart process, which includes the following factors:

- Deficiencies in identifying life-threatening medical complications that would benefit from obstetric care services

- Constraints that prevent the use of obstetric services even when appropriate conditions for such use are identified (these may include lack of financial resources, transportation difficulties, other logistic problems)

- Obstetric care facilities of such poor quality that they are ineffective in preventing obstetric complications and death, even when pregnant women come to such facilities (Thaddeus & Maine, 1994; Tsui et al., 1997)

Each of these problems is elaborated upon in the following subsections.

Identification of Serious Medical Complications That Will Benefit from Obstetric Care

It is important to reiterate that most women in low- and middle-income countries deliver their babies at home, far away from even rudimentary obstetric care facilities, and assisted for the most part by family members and/or traditional birth attendants. The ability to recognize a potentially life-threatening complication (such as obstructed or prolonged labor, incipient hemorrhage, or other fetal distress), and the corresponding need for specialized obstetric care, depends on appropriate education and sensitization of both family members and traditional birth attendants, with the former being perhaps the more important constituency.

A number of cultural factors affect recognition that obstetric complications can benefit from specific kinds of medical care. When a woman is bleeding, the need for obstetric intervention by trained medical personnel is better recognized. Other complications, however, are generally not viewed as benefiting from specialized obstetric care. In some cultures, complications are seen as determined by fate, with little that can be done to alter the course of events. In Indonesia, for example, malposition of the fetus is seen as the domain of traditional birth attendants, who deal with it with soothing massage whereby pregnant women maintain the inner calm considered necessary for correcting the baby's position (Ambaretnani, Hessler-Radelet, & Carlin, 1993). As a result, referral to obstetric care services is often significantly delayed. In other instances, due to concerns about privacy and modesty, the home is perceived as the more natural and fitting place for birth than any healthcare facility. For the Fulani and Hausa in Nigeria, pregnancy is seen as a shameful period with unpredictable outcome; thus no preparations are made for referral for obstetric services (Public Opinion Polls, 1993; Tsui et al., 1997).

It is clear from these examples that cultural sensitivities need to be taken into account when constructing appropriate educational messages that emphasize the identification of particularly serious obstetric risks and the need to refer these women to health facilities with adequate obstetric care services. A purely technocratic approach, which focuses on modern systems of logic and evidence, may not be very effective in bringing about changes in behavior. Much attention has been focused on training birth attendants, given that they are present in the majority of births in low- and middle-income countries. However, the evidence suggests that focusing on just training birth attendants leads to mixed results in terms of increased referrals for appropriate conditions. In urban/periurban areas, such training appears to be no impact, whereas there is some improvement in rural areas with low prevalence rates of use of maternal care services (Alisjahbana et al., 1995; Bailey, Dominik, Janowitz, & Aaujo, 1991). The consensus from a number of sources is that husbands and possibly other family members (mothers-in-law, mothers, and sisters) are the key people who should be targeted, as they are the final decision makers with regard to whether the woman will go to a modern healthcare facility (Alisjahbana et al., 1995; Bailey et al., 1991; Bower & Perez, 1993; Center for Health Research, Consultation and Education and MotherCare/John Snow, 1991; Howard-Grabman, Seoane, & Davenport, 1994).

Constraints Affecting Use of Obstetric Care Services Once Complications Are Identified

Several concerns affect the decision to use modern obstetric care services once a life-threatening complication is identified and the need for obstetric care is acknowledged. These issues include economic constraints (i.e., not being able to afford the costs of such care, including transportation costs), logistic constraints (taking time off to accompany the patient to often distant care facilities), and quality concerns (attitude and treatment of healthcare providers) (Sundari, 1992; Thaddeus & Maine, 1994).

The economic costs of care include not only the nominal costs charged by the healthcare facility for delivery-related services, but also transportation costs (which are not insubstantial in many rural settings), costs of medications, and costs of housing. In many cultures, family members need to accompany the patient, which adds to transportation and housing costs. In addition to these direct costs, opportunity costs or lost wages for the patient and particularly family members who accompany the patient are key considerations. Relatively few population-based data have been gathered from which to estimate the various components of costs that are incurred for a maternal delivery in a healthcare facility, but some reports suggest that such costs may be a real barrier to the use of obstetric services. For example, data from three countries in Africa (Nigeria, Ghana, and Sierra Leone) show that there were declines in deliveries in seven referral sites from 1983 to 1989, paralleling increases in costs to patients for drugs and services (Prevention of Maternal Mortality Network,

1995). To date, the impact of user fees on the decision to seek out obstetric care for complicated cases (as opposed to normal deliveries) has not been adequately investigated. The existing evidence shows a mixed response to the imposition of user fees, with use of modern medical facilities for obstetric complications being reduced to different degrees in different countries (Ambaretnani et al., 1993; Prevention of Maternal Mortality Network, 1995).

Clearly, much more information needs to be collected to understand the changes in demand and use of obstetric care services with changes in costs of services. Special attention needs to be focused on obtaining data on the nonservice components of obstetric costs (i.e., travel costs, opportunity costs).

Aside from economic costs, transportation constraints are a major factor in the low use of maternal care services. In most low- and middle-income countries, advanced obstetric care (including surgical services with appropriate transfusion capabilities) is available only in a few healthcare facilities, which are often located at a considerable distance from the patient. Transportation facilities are, for the most part, poorly developed and quite expensive. Thus problems need to be anticipated in advance to allow for enough time for the patient to reach the care facility. The degree to which lack of transportation infrastructure is a major constraint on the use of modern obstetric services is not certain; the evidence on this issue is mixed. On the one hand, data from rural Bangladesh suggest that relatively modest investments in transportation can have a significant impact on use of obstetric services, leading to reductions in maternal mortality (Fauveau, Stewart, Khan, & Chakraborty, 1991; Maine, Akalin, Chakraborty, de Francisco, & Strong, 1996). On the other hand, three different experiments that aimed at ensuring transport did not by themselves increase the use of obstetric services (Alisjahbana et al., 1995; Poedje et al., 1993; Prevention of Maternal Mortality Network, 1995).

Transportation concerns assume the patient has to be brought to the care facility. A complementary approach is to bring the provider closer to the patient. Some limited success has been achieved with programs that place certified midwives in health posts closer to the pregnant patient population, but such staffing may be difficult to sustain logistically and financially (Fauveau et al., 1991; Tsui et al., 1997).

Finally, the perception of the welcoming nature of the referral site and its flexibility in accommodating accompanying family members are often ignored, but are particularly important constraints to seeking modern obstetric care. Oftentimes, referral sites are perceived as impersonal and unfriendly and are passed over in favor of care from traditional birth attendants (Bailey et al., 1994; Eades, Brace, Osei, & LaGuardia, 1993).

Quality of the Obstetric Care in the Healthcare Facility

Relatively few systematic data on the quality of healthcare services in obstetric care facilities exist. The rare studies that do exist suggest that the majority of obstetric care facilities in low- and middle-income countries fall far short of minimal acceptable standards of care. Important indicators of quality include waiting time from admission to treatment, trends in numbers and rates of maternal and perinatal deaths, and trends in case fatality rates for all complications including cesarean deliveries (O'Rourke, 1995; Prevention of Maternal Mortality Network, 1995).

Much of this problem can be traced to lack of adequate resources in terms of trained personnel (Dogba & Fournier, 2009), equipment, and bed capacity. For example, a UNICEF survey of three districts in India in 1993 found not only inadequate numbers of beds, but also huge disparities in bed allocation between different levels of the healthcare system. The majority of beds were allocated to referral sites, where a small minority of complicated births were managed. There were also major deficiencies in availability of essential drugs and appropriately trained surgical and anesthesia professionals.

In addition to supply constraints, major deficiencies in the management of services and in provider attitudes are often in evidence in obstetric facilities located in low- and middle-income countries. Triaging is not done systematically, such that very sick patients are often left waiting for much longer than medically desirable, while others with less severe problems are treated before them. Obstetric care is often provided in an ad hoc manner, with no consistent set of case management algorithms being followed. Nursing is often seriously below standard, and basic levels of hygiene are not adhered to, leading to considerable postoperative morbidity and mortality. There is also very little sensitivity to patient concerns, and little effort is expended in explaining complexities of care to patients, leading to widespread patient dissatisfaction (Dogba & Fournier, 2009).

In a nationally representative study of 718 maternal deaths in Egypt in 1992 (Egypt Ministry of Health, 1994), avoidable factors (i.e., those that could have been changed by either the health delivery system or the patient) were assessed by an expert panel. In approximately half of the cases, the primary avoidable factor identified was poor management and diagnoses by healthcare professionals. In the other half of cases, patient factors—particularly delay in seeking medical care or compliance with medical recommendations—were implicated as key issues in the mother's death. Notably, the health professionals most often cited for poor quality of care were not traditional birth attendants or general practitioners, but rather obstetricians with supposedly appropriate training. This sorry state of affairs is significantly related to the lack of consistent management guidelines for complicated obstetric cases.

Similar results have been reported from China (WHO, 1994b), where a study of 1,173 maternal deaths in 1990 implicated deficiencies in the healthcare system as the major contributor (48%), followed by individual and family delays in using health care and transport problems. There appears to be a clear rural/urban divide in this situation, with rural areas having a much higher frequency of problems that are avoidable both from the point of view of the healthcare system and from the point of view of the patient.

Improvements in the quality of care require a number of initiatives to be undertaken simultaneously. Governments must appropriately fund healthcare referral facilities so that they have adequate supplies and equipment and are staffed by adequate numbers of appropriate specialists. There must be a clear chain of referral whereby trained birth attendants refer complicated obstetric cases to higher-level facilities, where specialist care is available. Efforts must be made to follow consistent management protocols that are clearly articulated, and both birth attendants and specialists must be trained to adhere to these protocols (Marshall & Buffington, 1991; Scheiber, Mejia, Koritz, Gonsalez, & Kwast, 1995). In addition, a monitoring system must be established to provide regular audits of both process and outcome indicators such as waiting times and case fatalities, with the results being used in a continuous process of review and upgrading of the healthcare system (Egypt Ministry of Health, 1994).

If even some of these improvements in quality of care are made, they will not only improve outcomes for those women who reach the healthcare facility but also increase the demand for such services by pregnant women (Dogba & Fournier, 2009; Mantz & Okong, 1994; O'Rourke, 1995).

Conclusion

This chapter has outlined the need for reproductive health and family planning to help individual women and men and larger populations reduce fertility and maintain reproductive health. Population growth rates are declining in much of the world because people are reducing their fertility. The primary factors effecting this reduction are early termination of the reproductive period through sterilization, use of contraception to reduce conception rates, and induced abortion. Because of increased desire for smaller families, both unwanted fertility and unmet needs for family planning and reproductive health services exist in most low-and middle-income countries. To meet this challenge, improvements are needed in the quality of family planning services, especially in the areas of information exchange and method choice, interaction of reproductive health services and contraceptive provision, and financial sustainability. Maternity care needs to be significantly expanded so that the adverse sequelae of pregnancy and childbearing can be reduced. While preventive services (including education of both men and women regarding health and sexuality, family planning, and prevention of STIs) need to be increased and targeted to those at greatest risk of adverse outcomes, special attention needs to be paid to increasing access to skilled birth attendants and emergency obstetric care.

At the societal level, programs need to be supported to improve the status of women, whether through education or through changes in laws and culture to reduce violence. Although this may be unfamiliar territory for public health professionals, the consequences for the health of women and children make it essential that this broader perspective become part of global health programs.

An overriding concern regarding continuing—let alone expanded—funding remains. Many high-income countries have reduced their aid contributions; many low- and middle-income countries are undergoing financial and health crises. Part of the agenda for the future must be research to determine cost-effective programs that will address the reproductive health needs of the twenty-first century.

● ● ● **Discussion Questions**

1. Using the proximate determinants framework (originally proposed by Bongaarts and subsequently revised by Stover), discuss the relative impacts of contraception, breastfeeding, abortion, sexual activity, and infecundity on total fertility rates in Latin America versus Africa. What are the policy implications of these findings?

2. Discuss fertility changes using the framework of wanted versus unwanted fertility and the forces that drive each of them. How do you

explain unwanted fertility increasing with increasing contraceptive prevalence? What are the policy approaches that stem from a consideration of this kind of framework?

3. The 1994 Cairo ICPD substantially enlarged the scope of family planning to include a broader conception of women's health and development. Discuss the pros and cons of this expansion in the context of limited financial and logistic resources, particularly in sub-Saharan Africa, with its very heavy HIV/AIDS burden.

4. Discuss the impact of the birth interval length, both prior and subsequent, on the health of children, taking into account methodological concerns about reverse causality. What are the implications for policy?

5. Consider the following statement: "Family planning has only a limited role to play in reducing the risk of maternal mortality." Do you agree with this statement? Elaborate on the policy implications of your analysis.

6. Discuss the reasons why, in the context of low- and middle-income countries, there has been relatively little improvement in maternal mortality and the policy implications that follow from this analysis.

7. Consider the following statement: "Specific health technological inputs are a necessary but not sufficient determinant of significant improvements in reproductive health." Using the example of changes in women's status, discuss the validity of this proposition.

• • • References

Aaby, P., Bukh, J., Lisse, I. M., & Smits, A. J. (1984). Overcrowding and intensive exposure as determinants of measles mortality. *American Journal of Epidemiology, 120*(1), 49–63.

Aitken, I. W., & Walls, B. (1986). Maternal height and cephalopelvic disproportion in Sierra Leone. *Tropical Doctor, 16*(3), 132–134.

Alan Guttmacher Institute. (1999a). *Sharing responsibility: Women, society, and abortion worldwide.* New York: Author.

Alan Guttmacher Institute. (1999b). *Facts in brief: Induced abortion worldwide.* New York: Author.

Alan Guttmacher Institute. (2009a). *Abortion worldwide: A decade of uneven progress.* New York: Author.

Alan Guttmacher Institute. (2009b). Facts on induced abortion worldwide. Retrieved from http://www.guttmacher.org/sections/abortion .php?scope=comparative%20international

Alauddin, M. (1986). Maternal mortality in rural Bangladesh: The Tangail district. *Studies in Family Planning, 17*(I), 13–21.

Alisjahbana, A. C., Williams, C., Dharmayanti, R., Hermawan, D., Kwast, B. E., & Koblinsky, M. (1995). An integrated village maternity service to improve referral patterns in a rural area in West Java. *International Journal of Gynecology and Obstetrics, 48*(suppl), s83–s94.

Ambaretnani, N. P., Hessler-Radelet, C., & Carlin, L. E. (1993). *Qualitative research for the social marketing component of the Perinatal Regionalization Project, Tanjungsari, Java* (MotherCare Working Paper No. 19, prepared for the U.S. Agency for International Development, Project No. 936-5966). Arlington, VA: John Snow, Inc.

Arnold, F., Kishor, S., & Roy, T. K. (2002). Sex-selective abortions in India. *Population and Development Review, 28*(4), 759–785.

Bailey, P. E., Dominik, R. C., Janowitz, B., & Aaujo, L. (1991). Obstetrica e mortalidade perinatal em uma area rural do nordeste Brasileiro. *Boletin de la Oficina Sanitaria Panamericana, 111*(4), 306–318.

Bailey, P. E., Szaszdi, J. A., & Scheiber, B. (1994). *Analysis of the vital events reporting system of the Maternal and Neonatal Health Project: Quetzaltenango, Guatemala* (MotherCare Working Paper No. 3, prepared for the U.S. Agency for International Development, Project No. DPE-5966-Z-00-8083-00). Arlington, VA: John Snow, Inc.

Bankole, A., & Westoff, C. F. (1995). *Childbearing attitudes and intentions* (DHS Comparative Studies No. 17). Calverton, MD: Macro International.

Bartlett, L. A., Mawji, S., Whitehead, S., Crouse, C., Dalil, S., Ionete, D., & Salama, P. (2005). Where giving birth is a forecast of death: Maternal mortality in four districts of Afghanistan, 1999–2002. *Lancet, 365*(9462), 864–870.

Beck, S., Wojdyla, D., Say, L., Betran, A. P., Merialdi, M., Requejo, J. H., et al. (2009). The worldwide incidence of preterm birth: A systemic review of maternal mortality and morbidity. *Bulletin of the World Health Organization,88,* 31–38.

Bhutta, Z. A., Ahmed, T., Black, R. E., Cousens, S., Dewey, K., Glugliani, E., et al. (2008). What works? Interventions for maternal and child undernutrition and survival. *Lancet, 371*(9610), 417–440.

Black, R. E., Morris, S. S., & Bryce, J. (2003). Where and why are 10 million children dying every year? *Lancet, 361*(9376), 2226–2234.

Bledsoe, C. H., & Cohen, B. (Eds.). (1993). *Social dynamics of adolescent fertility in sub-Saharan Africa. Working Group on the Social Dynamics of Adolescent Fertility in Sub-Saharan Africa, Committee on Population, National Research Council.* Washington, DC: National Academies Press.

Bongaarts, J. (1978). A framework for analyzing the proximate determinants of fertility. *Population and Development Review, 4,* 105–132.

Bongaarts, J. (1983). The proximate determinants of natural marital fertility. In R. A. Bulatao & R. D. Lee (Eds.), *Determinants of fertility in developing countries* (Vol. 1, pp. 103–108). New York: Academic Press.

Bongaarts, J. (1991). Do reproductive intentions matter? *Demographic and Health Surveys World Conference, 1,* 223–248.

Bongaarts, J. (1997). The role of family planning programs in contemporary fertility transitions. In G. W. Jones, R. M. Douglas, J. C. Caldwell, & R. M. D'Souza (Eds.), *The continuing demographic transition* (pp. 422–443). New York/Oxford, UK: Oxford University Press.

Bongaarts, J., & Bruce, J. (1995). The causes of unmet need for contraception and the social context of services. *Studies in Family Planning, 26*(2), 57–76.

Bongaarts, J., & Johansson, E. (2002). Future trends in contraceptive prevalence and method mix in the developing world. *Studies in Family Planning, 33*(1), 24–36.

Bongaarts, J., & Potter, R. G. Jr. (1983). *Fertility, biology, and behavior: An analysis of the proximate determinants.* New York: Academic Press.

Bongaarts, J., & Watkins, S. C. (1996). Social interactions and contemporary fertility transitions. *Population and Development Review, 22*(4), 639–682.

Bothwell, T. H., & Charllton, R. (1981). *Iron deficiency in women.* Washington, DC: International Nutrition Anemia Consultative Group.

Bower, B., & Perez, A. (1993). *Final project report: Cochabamba Reproductive Health Project* (MotherCare Project No. 5966-C-00-3038-00). Arlington, VA: John Snow, Inc.

Brown, S. S., & Eisenberg, L. (Eds.). (1995). *The best intentions: Unintended pregnancy and the well-being of children and families. Committee on Unintended Pregnancy, Institute of Medicine.* Washington, DC: National Academies Press.

Bryce, J., Coitinho, D., Darnton-Hill, I., Pelletier, D., & Pinstrup-Anderson, P. for the Maternal and Child Undernutrition Study Group. (2008). "Maternal and child undernutrition: effective action at national level." *Lancet 371*(9611): 510–26.

Bulatao, R. A. (1985). *Fertility and mortality transition: Patterns, projections, and interdependence* (World Bank Staff Working Paper No. 681). Washington D.C.: The World Bank.

Bulatao, R. A. (1993). Effectiveness and evolution in family planning programs. In *International Union for the Scientific Study of Population, International Population Conference* (Vol. 1, pp. 189–200). Liege, Belgium: International Union for the Scientific Study of Population.

Bulatao, R. A. (1998). *The value of family planning programs in developing countries.* Santa Monica, CA: RAND Corporation.

Bulatao, R. A., & Lee, R. (1983). *Determinants of fertility in developing countries: Vol. I. Supply and demand for children.* New York: Academic Press.

Caldwell, J. C. (1986). Routes to low mortality in poor countries. *Population and Development Review, 12*(2), 171–200.

Caldwell, J. C., Barkat, H. B., Caldwell, B., Pieris, I., & Caldwell, P. (1999). The Bangladesh fertility decline: An interpretation. *Population and Development Review, 25*(1), 67–84.

Campbell, O. M. R., & Graham, W. J. (2006). Maternal survival 2: Strategies for reducing maternal mortality: Getting on with what works. *Lancet, 368,* 1284–1299.

Casterline, J., Perez, A. E., & Biddlecom, A. E. (1996). *Factors underlying unmet need for family planning in the Philippines* (Research Division Working Paper No. 84). New York: Population Council.

Center for Health Research, Consultation and Education & MotherCare/John Snow, Inc. (1991). *Qualitative research on knowledge, attitudes, and practices related to women's reproductive health* (MotherCare Working Paper No. 9, prepared for the U.S. Agency for International Development, Project No. 936-5966). Arlington, VA: John Snow, Inc.

Chen, L. C., Gesche, M. C., Ahmed, S., Chowdhury, A. I., & Mosley, W. H. (1975). Maternal mortality in Bangladesh. *Studies in Family Planning, 5*(11), 334–341.

Chi, I.C., Agoestina T, & Harbin J. (1981). Maternal mortality at twelve teaching hospitals in Indonesia: An epidemiologic analysis. *International Journal of Gynecology & Obstetrics, 19,* 259–266.

Childinfo. (2009). Monitoring the situation of children and women. Retrieved from http://www.childinfo.org/low_birthweight.html

Cleland, J., Phillips, J. F., Amin, S., & Kamal, G. M. (1994). *The determinants of reproductive change in Bangladesh*. Washington, DC: World Bank.

Coale, A. J., & Watkins, S. C. (1986). *The decline of fertility in Europe*. Princeton, NJ: Princeton University Press.

Colombo, B., & Masarotto, G. (2000). Daily fecundability: First results from a new data base. *Demographic Research, 3*(Article 5). Retrieved from http//www.demographic-research.org/Volumes/Vol3/5

Conference adopts plan on limiting population. (1999, July 3). *New York Times*.

Curtis, S. L., & Neitzel, K. (1996). *Contraceptive knowledge, use, and sources* (DHS Comparative Studies No. 19). Columbia, MD: Institute for Resource Development.

Das Gupta, M. (1987). Selective discrimination against female children in rural Punjab. *Population and Development Review, 13*(1), 77–100.

DaVanzo, J., Butz, W. P., & Habicht, J. P. (1983). How biological and behavioral influences on mortality in Malaysia vary during the first year of life. *Population Studies, 37*(3), 381–402.

David, H. P. (1992). Abortion in Europe, 1920–91: A public health perspective. *Studies in Family Planning, 23*(1), 1–22.

De Graft-Johnson, J. (1994, May 5–7). *Maternal morbidity in Ghana*. Paper presented at the annual meeting of the Population Association of America, Miami, FL.

De Onis, M., Blosssner, M., & Villar, J. (1998, January). Levels and patterns of intrauterine growth retardation in developing countries. *European Journal of Clinical Nutrition, 52*(suppl 1), S5–S15.

Desai, S. (1995). When are children from large families disadvantaged? Evidence from cross-national analyses. *Population Studies, 49*, 195–210.

Dixon-Mueller, R., & Germain, A. (1992). Stalking the elusive "unmet need" for family planning. *Studies in Family Planning, 23*(5), 330–335.

Dogba, M., & Fournier, P. (2009). Human resources and the quality of emergency obstetric care in developing countries: A systematic review of the literature. *Human Resources for Health, 7*. doi: 10:1186/1478-4491-7-7. Retrieved from http://www.humarn-resources-health-.com/contect/7/1/7

D'Souza, S., & Chen, L. C. (1980). Sex differentials in mortality in rural Bangladesh. *Population and Development Review, 6*(2), 257–270.

Duffy, L., & Menken, J. (1998). *Health, fertility, and socioeconomic status as predictors of survival and later health of women: A twenty-year prospective study in rural Bangladesh* (Working Paper WP-98-11). Boulder, CO: Population Program, Institute of Behavioral Science, University of Colorado.

Eades, C., Brace, C., Osei, L., & LaGuardia, K. (1993). Traditional birth attendants and maternal mortality in Ghana. *Social Science and Medicine, 36*(11), 1503–1507.

Eclampsia Trial Collaborative Group. (1995). Which anticonvulsant for women with eclampsia? Evidence from the Collaborative Eclampsia Trial. *Lancet, 345*, 1455–1463.

Egypt Ministry of Health. (1994). *National maternal mortality study: Egypt, 1992–1993*. Alexandria, Egypt: Ministry of Health, Child Survival Project.

Faundes, A., Fanjul, B., Henriquez, G., Mora, G., & Tognola, C. (1974). Influencia de la edad y de la paridad sobre algunos parametros de morbilidad materna y sobre la morbimortalidad fetal. *Revista Chileña de Obstetrica y Ginecologia, 37*(1), 6–14.

Fauveau, V., Koenig, M., Chakraborty, J., & Chowdhury, A. (1988). Causes of maternal mortality in rural Bangladesh, 1976–1985. *Bulletin of the World Health Organization, 66*(5), 643–651.

Fauveau, V., Stewart, K., Khan, S. A., & Chakraborty, J. (1991). Effect on mortality of community-based maternity-care programme in rural Bangladesh. *Lancet, 338*, 1183–1186.

Fauveau, V., Wojtyniak, B., Mostafa, G., Sarder, A. M., & Chakraborty, J. (1990). Perinatal mortality in Matlab, Bangladesh: A community-based study. *International Journal of Epidemiology, 19,* 606–612.

Ferraz, E. M., Gray, R. H., Fleming, P. L., & Maria, T. M. (1988). Interpregnancy interval and low birthweight: Findings from a case-control study. *American Journal of Epidemiology, 128,* 1111–1116.

Filippi, V., Ronsmans, C., Campbell, O. M. R., Graham, W. J., Mills, A., Borghi, J., et al.(2006). Maternal survival 5: Maternal health in poor countries: The broader context and a call for action. *Lancet, 368,* 1535–1541.

Finkle, J. L., & Ness, G. D. (1985). *Managing delivery systems: Identifying leverage points for improving family planning program performance.* Ann Arbor, MI: Department of Population Planning and International Health, University of Michigan.

Fortney, J. A. (1995). Antenatal risk screening and scoring: A new look. *International Journal of Gynecology and Obstetrics, 2*(suppl), s53–s58.

Fortney, J. A., Susanti, I., Gadalla, S., Saleh, S., Feldblum, P. J., & Potts, M. (1985, November 11–15). *Maternal mortality in Indonesia and Egypt.* Paper presented at the WHO Inter-regional Meeting on Prevention of Maternal Mortality, Geneva, Switzerland.

Foster, A., Menken, J., Chowdhury, A. K. M. A., & Trussell, J. (1986). Female reproductive development: A hazard model analysis. *Social Biology, 33*(3–4), 183–198.

Foster, A., & Roy, N. (1996). *The dynamics of education and fertility: Evidence from a family planning experiment.* Working paper, University of Pennsylvania, Department of Economics.

Freedman, R. (1987). The contribution of social science research to population policy and family planning effectiveness. *Studies in Family Planning, 18*(2), 57–82.

French, F. E., & Bierman, J. M. (1962). Probabilities of fetal mortality. *Public Health Report, 77,* 835–847.

Frenzen, P. D., & Hogan, D. P. (1982). The impact of class, education, and health care on infant mortality in a developing society: The case of rural Thailand. *Demography, 19,* 391–408.

Gelbard, A., Haub, C., & Kent, M. M. (1999). World population beyond six billion. *Population Bulletin, 54*(1), 1–40.

Geronimus, A. T. (1987). On teenage childbearing and neonatal mortality in the United States. *Population and Development Review, 13*(2), 245–279.

Goldenberg, R. L., Culhane, J. F., Iams, J. D., & Romero, R. (2008). Epidemiology and causes of preterm birth. *Lancet, 371,* 75–84. PMID: 18177778. doi:10.1016/S0140-6736(08)60074-4.

Govindasamy, P., Stewart, K., Rutstein, S., Boerma, J., & Sommerfelt, A. (1993). *High-risk births and maternity care* (Demographic and Health Surveys Comparative Studies No. 8). Columbia, MD: Macro International, Inc.

Gray, R. H., Wawer, M. J., Serwadda, D., Sewankambo, N., Li, C., Wabwire-Mangen, F., et al. (1998). Population-based study of fertility in women with HIV-1 infection in Uganda. *Lancet, 351*(9096), 98–103.

Greenwood, A. M., Greenwood, B. M., Bradley, A. K., Williams, K., Shenton, F. C., Tulloch, S., et al. (1987). A prospective survey of the outcome of pregnancy in a rural area in the Gambia. *Bulletin of the World Health Organization, 65*(5), 635–643.

Gubhaju, B. (1986). Effect of birth spacing on infant and child mortality in rural Nepal. *Journal of Biosocial Science, 18*(4), 435–447.

Haaga, J. (1989). Mechanisms for the association of maternal age, parity, and birth spacing with infant health. In A. M. Parnell (Ed.), *Contraceptive use and controlled fertility: Health issues for women and children* (pp. 96–139). Washington, DC: National Academy Press.

Hansen, J. P. (1986). Older maternal age and pregnancy outcome: A review of the literature. *Obstetrical and Gynecological Survey, 41,* 726–742.

Harrison, K. A., & Rossiter, L. A. (1985). Childbearing, health and social priorities: A survey of 22,774 consecutive hospital births in Zaria, Northern Nigeria. *British Journal of Obstetrics and Gynecology, 5*(suppl), 1–119.

Harrison, P. F., & Rosenfield, A. (Eds.). (1996). *Contraceptive research and development: Looking to the future.* Committee on Contraceptive Research and Development, Institute of Medicine. Washington, DC: National Academies Press.

Henshaw, S., K., Singh, S., & Haas, T. (1999). The incidence of abortion worldwide. *Family Planning Perspectives, 25*(suppl), S30–S38.

Hill, K., & Choi, Y. (2006, May 23). Neonatal mortality in the developing world. *Demographic Research, 24*(18), 429–452. Retrieved from http://www.demographic-research.org/ Volumes/ Vol14/18/

Hobcraft, J. N. (1987, October 5–9). *Does family planning save children's lives?* Paper presented at the International Conference on Better Health for Women and Children Through Family Planning, Nairobi.

Hobcraft, J. N., McDonald, J. W., & Rutstein, S. O. (1985). Demographic determinants of infant and child mortality: A comparative analysis. *Population Studies, 39*(3), 363–385.

Hogberg, U., Wall, S., & Brostroin, G. (1986). The impact of early medical technology on maternal mortality in late 19th century Sweden. *International Journal of Gynecology and Obstetrics, 24,* 251–261.

Howard-Grabman, L., Seoane, L. G., & Davenport, C. A. (1994). *The Warmi Project: A participatory approach to improve maternal and neonatal health. An implementor's manual.* Arlington, VA: MotherCare Project, John Snow, Inc.

Insurance for Viagra spurs coverage for birth control. (1999, June 30). *New York Times.*

International Consortium for Emergency Contraception (ICEC). (2010). Background. Retrieved from http://www.cecinfo.org

International Planned Parenthood Foundation. (1995). *Consensus statement on emergency contraception.* London: International Planned Parenthood Federation.

IRIN. (2010). In-depth: Razor's edge: The controversy of female genital mutilation. Retrieved from http://www.irinnews.org/IndepthMain.aspx/ IndepthId=15&ReportId=62462

Jamison, D. T., Mosley, W. H., Measham, A. R., & Bobadilla, J. L. (1993). *Disease control priorities in developing countries.* New York: Oxford University Press.

Jelliffe, D. B. (1976). Maternal nutrition and lactation. In *CIBA Foundation Symposium, Breastfeeding and the mother* (pp. 119–143). Amsterdam: Excerpta Medica.

Jones, R. E. (1988). A biobehavioral model for breastfeeding effects on return to menses postpartum in Javanese women. *Social Biology, 35,* 307–323.

Kenney, G. M. (1993). *Assessing legal and regulatory reform in family planning: Manual on legal and regulatory reform* (OPTIONS Projects Policy Paper No. 1). Washington, DC: Futures Group.

Khan, A. R., Jahan, F. A., & Begum, S. F. (1986). Maternal mortality in rural Bangladesh: The Jamalpur district. *Studies in Family Planning, 17*(1), 7–12.

Kitay, D., & Harbort, R. (1975). Iron and folic acid deficiency in pregnancy. *Clinical Perinatology, 2,* 255–273.

Knodel, J., Chamrathrithirong, A., & Debavalya, N. (1987). Societal change and the demand for chidren. In *Thailand's reproductive revolution: Rapid fertility decline in a third world setting* (pp. 117–142). Madison: University of Wisconsin Press.

Koblinsky, M. A., Campbell, O., & Harlow, S. (1993). Mother and more: A broader perspective on women's health. In M. A. Koblinsky, J. Timyan, & J. Gay (Eds.), *The health of women: A global perspective* (pp. 33–63). Boulder CO: Westview Press.

Koblinsky, M., Matthews, Z., Husssein, J., Mavalankar, D., Mridha, M. K., Anwar, I., et al. (2006). Going to scale with professional skilled care [see comment]. *Lancet, 368,* 1377–1386. Erratum appears in *Lancet, 368* (9554), 2210, December 23, 2006.

Koenig, M. A., Phillips, J., Campbell, O., & D'Souza, S. (1988). Maternal mortality in Matlab,

Bangladesh: 1976–1985. *Studies in Family Planning, 19*(2), 69–80.

Kusiako, T., Ronsmans, C., & Van der Paal, L. (2000). Perinatal mortality attributable to complications of childbirth in Matlab, Bangladesh. *Bulletin of the World Health Organization, 78*(5), 621–627.

Kwast, B. E., Rochat, R. W., & Kidane-Mariam, W. (1986). Maternal mortality in Addis Ababa, Ethiopia. *Studies in Family Planning, 17*(6), 288–301.

Kwast, B. E., & Stevens, J. A. (1987). Viral hepatitis as a major cause of maternal mortality in Addis Ababa, Ethiopia. *International Journal of Gynecology and Obstetrics, 25*, 99–106.

Labbok, M. H., Hight-Laukaran, V., Peterson, A. E., Fletcher, V., von Hertzen, H., & Van Look, P. F. (1997). Multicenter study of the lactational amenorrhea method (LAM): I. Efficacy, duration, and implications for clinical application. *Contraception, 55*(6), 327–336.

Larsen, U. (2000). Primary and secondary infertility in sub-Saharan Africa. *International Journal of Epidemiology, 29*, 285–291.

Larsen, U., Chung, W., & Das Gupta, M. (1998). Fertility and son preference in Korea. *Population Studies, 52*(3), 317–325.

Lawson, J. (1992). Vaginal fistulae. *Journal of the Royal Society of Medicine, 85*, 254–256.

Levin, H., Pollitt, E., Galloway, R., & McGuire, J. (1993). Micronutrient deficiency disorders. In D. Jamison, W. H. Mosley, A. Measham, & J. L. Bobadilla (Eds.), *Disease control priorities in developing countries* (pp. 421–451). New York: Oxford University Press.

Lewis, J. J. C., Ronsmans, C., Ezeh, A., & Gregson, S. (2004). The population impact of HIV on fertility in sub-Saharan Africa. *AIDS, 18*(suppl 2), S35–S43.

Lloyd, C. (1994). Investing in the next generation: The implications of high fertility at the level of the family. In R. Cassen (Ed.), *Population and development: Old debates, new conclusions* (pp. 181–202). New Brunswick, NJ: Transaction Publishers.

Loudon, I. (1991). On maternal and infant mortality 1900–1960. *Social History of Medicine, 4*(1), 29–73.

MacGregor, I. A., Wilson, M. E., & Billewicz, W. Z. (1983). Malaria infection of the placenta in Gambia, West Africa: Its incidence and relationship to stillbirth, birthweight and placental weight. *Transactions of the Royal Society of Tropical Medicine and Hygiene, 77*(2), 232–244.

Macro International, Inc. (1994). Selected statistics from DHS. *Demographic and Health Survey Newsletter, 6*, 2.

Macro International, Inc. (2010a). Bangladesh demographic and health survey, 2007. Retrieved from http://www.measuredhs.com

Macro International, Inc. (2010b). MEASURE DHS STAT compiler. Retrieved from http://www.measuredhs.com

Macro International, Inc. (2010c). Selected statistics from DHS. *Demographic and Health Surveys.* Retrieved from http://www.measuredhs.com

Maine, D. (1991). *Safe motherhood programs: Options and issues.* New York: Columbia University, Center for Population and Family Health, School of Public Health.

Maine, D., Akalin, M. Z., Chakraborty, J., de Francisco, A., & Strong, M. (1996). Why did maternal mortality decline in Matlab? *Studies in Family Planning, 27*, 179–187.

Maine, D., & McGinn, T. (1999). Maternal mortality and morbidity. In M. Goldman & M. Hatch (Eds.), *Women and health* (pp. 395–403). San Diego, CA: Academic Press.

Mantz, M. L., & Okong, P. (1994). *Evaluation report: Uganda life saving skills program for midwives, October–November, 1994* (MotherCare Project No. 5966-C-00-3038-00, prepared for the U.S. Agency for International Development). Arlington, VA: John Snow, Inc.

Marshall, M. A., & Buffington, S. T. (1991). *Lifesaving skills manual for midwives* (2nd ed.). Washington, DC: American College of Nurse-Midwives.

Martin, J. A., Hamilton, B. E., Sutton, P. D., Ventura, S .J., Menacker, F., & Munson, M. L. (2003). Births: Final data for 2002. *National Vital Statistics Reports, 52*(10), 1–114.

Mason, K. O., & Taj, A. M. (1987). Differences between women's and men's reproductive goals in developing countries. *Population and Development Review, 13*(4), 611–638.

Maternal deaths per 100,000 live births, 1990 and 2005. (2008). *Millennium Development Goals report 2008*, (p. 25). Retrieved from http://www.undp .org/publications/MDG_Report_2008_En.pdf

McIntosh, C. A., & Finkle, J. L. (1995). The Cairo Conference on Population and Development: A new paradigm? *Population and Development Review, 21*, 223–260.

McNeilly, A. (1996). Breastfeeding and the suppression of fertility. *Food and Nutrition Bulletin, 17,* 340–345.

Menken, J. (1975). *Estimating fecundability.* Unpublished doctoral dissertation, Princeton University, Princeton, NJ.

Menken, J., Khan, M. N., & Williams, J. (1999, March 27). *The role of female education in the Bangladesh fertility decline.* Paper presented at the annual meeting of the Population Association of America, New York.

Menken, J., & Kuhn, R. (1996). Demographic effects of breastfeeding: Fertility, mortality and population growth. *Food and Nutrition Bulletin, 17,* 349–361.

Merchant, K., & Martorell, R. (1988). Frequent reproductive cycling: Does it lead to nutritional depletion of mothers? *Progress in Food and Nutrition, 12,* 339–369.

Miller, J. E. (1989). Is the relationship between birth intervals and perinatal mortality spurious? Evidence from Hungary and Sweden. *Population Studies, 43*(3), 479–495.

Morrow, R. H. Jr., Smetana, H. F., Sai, F. T., & Edgcomb, J. H. (1968). Unusual features of viral hepatitis in Accra, Ghana. *Annals of Internal Medicine, 68*(6), 1250–1264.

Mosher, W. D., Martinez, G. M., Chandra, A., Abma, J. C., & Wilson, S. J. (2004). *Use of contraception and use of family planning services in the United States: 1982–2002.* Advance Data from Vital and Health Statistics, Number 350. Retrieved from http://www.cdc.gov/nchs/data/ad/ad350.pdf

Muhuri, P., & Menken, J. (1997). Adverse effects of next birth, gender, and family composition on child survival in rural Bangladesh. *Population Studies, 51,* 279–294.

Mukaire, J., Kalikwani, F., Maggwa, B. N., & Kisubi, W. (1997). *Integration of STI and HIV/AIDS services with MCH-FP services: A case study of the Busoga Diocese Family Life Education Program, Uganda.* Nairobi: Operations Research Technical Assistance, Africa Project II, Population Council.

National Institute of Population Research and Training (NIPORT), ORC Macro, Johns Hopkins University and ICDDR,B. 2003. *Bangladesh Maternal Health Services and Maternal Mortality Survey 2001.* Dhaka, Bangladesh and Calverton, Maryland (USA): NIPORT, ORC Macro, Johns Hopkins University, and ICDDR,B.

National Research Council. (1989). *Contraception and reproduction: Health consequences for women and children in the developing world. Committee on Population, Working Group on Healthy Consequences of Contraceptive Use and Controlled Fertility.* Washington DC: National Academy Press.

National Statistics Office (Philippines) & Macro International, Inc. (1994). *Philippines National Safe Motherhood Survey, 1993.* Calverton MD: National Statistics Office and Macro International, Inc.

NationMaster.com. (2010). Retrieved from http://www.nationmaster.com/country/ke-kenya/hea-health

Notestein, F. W. (1953). Economic problems of population change. In *Proceedings of the Eighth International Conference of Agricultural Economics* (pp. 13–31). London: Oxford University Press.

Nybo Andersen, A. M., Hansen, K. D., Andersen, P. K., & Davey Smith, G. (2004). Advanced paternal age and risk of fetal death: A cohort study. *American Journal of Epidemiology, 160*(12), 1214–1222.

Nybo Andersen, A. M., Wohlfahrt, J., Christens, P., Olsen, J., & Melbye, M. (2000). Maternal age and fetal loss: Population based register linkage study. *British Medical Journal, 320*(7251), 1708–1712.

Omran, A. R., & Standley, C. C. (Eds.). (1981). *Further studies on family formation patterns and health: An international collaborative study in Colombia, Egypt, Pakistan, and the Syrian Arab Republic.* Geneva, Switzerland: World Health Organization.

O'Rourke, K. (1995). The effect of hospital staff training on management of obstetrical patients referred by traditional birth attendants. *International Journal of Gynecology and Obstetrics, 48*(suppl), s95–s102.

Overall, J. C. (1987). Viral infections of the fetus and neonate. In R. D. Feigin & J. D. Cherry (Eds.), *Textbook of pediatric infectious diseases* (2nd ed., pp. 966–1007). Philadelphia: WB Saunders.

Palloni, A. (1985). Health conditions in Latin America and policies for mortality changes. In J. Vaillin & A. Lopez (Eds.), *Health policy, social policy, and mortality prospects. Proceedings of a seminar, Paris, February 28–March 4, 1983* (pp. 465–492). Liege: Ordina Editions.

Palloni, A., & Millman, S. (1986). Effects of inter-birth intervals and breastfeeding on infant and early childhood mortality. *Population Studies, 40*(2), 215–236.

Paxton, A., Maine, D., Freedman, L., Fry, D., & Lobis S. (2005). The evidence for emergency obstetric care. *International Journal of Gynaecology & Obstetrics, 88*, 181–193.

Pebley, A. R., & DaVanzo, J. (1988, April). *Maternal depletion and child survival in Guatemala and Malaysia.* Paper presented at the annual meeting of the Population Association of America, New Orleans, LA.

Pebley, A. R., & Stupp, P. W. (1987). Reproductive patterns and child mortality in Guatemala. *Demography, 24*(1), 43–60.

Poedje, R., Setjalilakusuma, L., Abadi, A., Soegianto, B., Rihadi, S., Djaeli, A., et al. (1993). *Final project report: East Java Safe Motherhood Study* (MotherCare Project No. 936-5966, prepared for the U.S. Agency for Interna-tional Development). Arlington, VA: John Snow, Inc.

Population control measures to aid women are stumbling. (1999, April 10). *New York Times.*

Population Reference Bureau. (2002). *Family planning worldwide 2008 data sheet.* Washington DC: Population Reference Bureau.

Population Reference Bureau. (2004). The unfinished agenda: Meeting the need for family planning in less developed countries. *PRB Policy Brief.* Retrieved from http://www.prb.org/Template.cfm?Section=PRB&template=/ContentManagement/ContentDisplay.cfm&ContentID=11948

Population Reference Bureau. (2008). *Family planning worldwide 2008 data sheet.* Washington DC: Population Reference Bureau. Retrieved from http://www.prb.org/Publications/Datasheets/2008/familyplanningworldwide.asp

Potter, J. E. (1988). Does family planning reduce infant mortality? *Population and Development Review, 14*(1), 179–187.

Prevention of Maternal Mortality Network. (1995). Situational analyses of emergency obstetric care: Examples from eleven operations research projects in West Africa. *Social Science and Medicine, 40*(suppl), 657–667.

Pritchett, L. (1994a). Desired fertility and the impact of population policies. *Population and Development Review, 20*(1), 1–55.

Pritchett, L. (1994b). The impact of population policies: Reply. *Population and Development Review, 20*(3), 621–630.

Public Opinion Polls. (1993). *MotherCare Nigeria maternal healthcare project qualitative research* (MotherCare Working Paper No. 17B, prepared for the U.S. Agency for International Development, Project No. 936-5966). Arlington, VA: John Snow, Inc.

Qadir, M., & Bhutta, Z. (2009). Low birth weight in developing countries. In W. Kiess, S. D. Chernausek, & A. C. S. Hokken-Koelega (Eds.), *Small for gestational age, causes and consequences* (pp. 148–162). Pediatric Adolescent Medicine 13. Basel: Karger. doi: 10.1159/000165998.

Rafailimanana, H., & Westoff, C. F. (2001). *Gap between preferred and actual birth intervals in sub-Saharan Africa: Implications for fertility and child health*. Calverton, MD: ORC Macro. Retrieved from http://www.measuredhs.com/pubs/pdf/AS2/AS2.pdf

Rahman, A., Katzive, L., & Henshaw, S. K. (1998). A global review of laws on induced abortion, 1985–1997. *International Family Planning Perspectives, 24*(2), 56–64.

Rahman, O. (1998). Family matters: The impact of kin on elderly mortality in rural Bangladesh. *Population Studies, 53*(2), 227–235.

Rahman, O., Menken, J., & Foster, A. (1992). Older widow mortality in rural Bangladesh. *Social Science and Medicine, 34*(1), 89–96.

Reed, H. E., Koblinsky, M. A., & Mosley, W. H. (Eds.). (2000). *The consequences of maternal morbidity and maternal mortality. Committee on Population, Commission on Behavioral and Social Sciences and Education, National Research Council*. Washington, DC: National Academies Press.

Robey, B. K., Rutstein, S. O., & Morris, L. (1992). *The reproductive revolution: New survey findings* (Population Reports Series M, No. 11). Baltimore: The Johns Hopkins University.

Ronsman, C., & Campbell O. (1998). Short birth intervals don't kill women: Evidence from Matlab, Bangladesh. *Studies in Family Planning, 29*(3), 282–290.

Ronsman, C., & Graham, W. J. (2006). Maternal survival 1: Maternal mortality: Who, when, where, and why. *Lancet, 368*(9542), 1189–1200.

Rooney, C. (1992). *Antenatal care and maternal health: How effective is it? A review of the evidence* (WHO/MSM/92.4). Geneva, Switzerland: World Health Organization.

Rosenzweig, M. R., & Schultz, T. P. (1983). Estimating a household production function: Heterogeneity, the demand for health inputs, and their effects on birth weight. *Journal of Political Economy, 91*(5), 723–746.

Ross, A., Van der Paal, L., Lubega, R., Mayanja, B. N., Shafer, L. A., & Whitworth, J. (2004). HIV-1 disease progression and fertility: The incidence of recognized pregnancy and pregnancy outcome in Uganda. *AIDS, 18*(5), 799–804.

Ross, J., & Frankenberg, E. (1993). *Findings from two decades of family planning research*. New York: Population Council.

Ross, J. A., & Mauldin, W. P. (1996). Family planning programs: Efforts and results, 1972–1994. *Studies in Family Planning, 27*(3), 137–147.

Ross, J. A., & Winfrey, W. L. (2002). Unmet need for contraception in the developing world and the former Soviet Union: An updated estimate. *International Family Planning Perspectives, 28*(3), 138–143.

Rutstein, S. O. (1998). *Change in the desired number of children: A cross-country cohort analysis of levels and correlates of change* (DHS Analytical Report No. 9). Calverton, MD: Macro International, Inc.

Safe Motherhood Initiative. (2010). Retrieved from http://www.safemotherhood.org

Salber, E. J., Feinleib, M., & MacMahon, B. (1966). The duration of postpartum amenorrhea. *American Journal of Epidemiology, 82*, 347–358.

Scheiber, B. A., Mejia, M., Koritz, S., Gonsalez, C., & Kwast, B. (1995). *Medical audit of early neonatal deaths—INCAP: Quetzaltenango Maternal and Neonatal Health Project* (Technical Working Paper No. 1, prepared for the U.S. Agency for International Development, MotherCare Project No. 936-5966). Arlington, VA: John Snow, Inc.

Schultz, T. P. (1984). Studying the impact of household economic and community variables on child mortality. *Population and Development Review, 10*(suppl), 215–235.

Sheps, M. C., & Menken, J. (1973). *Mathematical models of conception and birth*. Chicago: University of Chicago Press.

Slama, R., Werwatz, A., Boutou, O., Ducot, B., Spira, A., & Hardle, W. (2003). Does male age affect the risk of spontaneous abortion? An approach using semiparametric regression. *American Journal of Epidemiology, 157*(9), 815–824.

Slanger, T. E., Snow, R., & Okonofua, F. E. (2002). The impact of female genital cutting on first delivery in southwest Nigeria. *Studies in Family Planning, 33*(2), 173–184.

Sloan, N. L., Jordan, E. A., & Winikoff, B. (1992). *Does iron supplementation make a difference?* (MotherCare Working Paper No. 15, prepared for the U.S. Agency for International Development, MotherCare Project No. 936-5966). Arlington, VA: John Snow, Inc.

Sood, S. K., Ramachandran, K., Mathur, M., Gupta, K., Ramalingaswamy, V., Swarnabai, C., et al. (1975). WHO sponsored collaborative studies on nutritional anemia in India. Part I: The effects of supplemental oral iron administration to pregnant women. *Quarterly Journal of Medicine, 174,* 241–258.

Stewart, M. K., & Festin, M. (1995). Validation study of women's reporting and recall of major obstetric complications treated at the Philippine General Hospital. *International Journal of Gynecology and Obstetrics, 48*(suppl), s53–s66.

Stone, J. L., Lockwood, C. J., Berkowitz, G., Alvarez, M., Lapinski, R., & Berkowitz, R. (1994). Risk factors for severe preeclampsia. *Obstetrics and Gynecology, 83,* 357–361.

Stover, J. (1998). Revising the proximate determinants of fertility framework: What have we learned in the past 20 years? *Studies in Family Planning, 29*(3), 255–267.

Sundari, T. K. (1992). The untold story: How the health care systems in developing countries contribute to maternal mortality. *International Journal of Health Service, 22*(3), 513–528.

Tahzib, F. (1983). Epidemiological determinants of vesicovaginal fistulae. *British Journal of Obstetric Gynaecology, 90,* 387–391.

Tahzib, F. (1985). Vesicovaginal fistula in Nigerian children. *Lancet, 2*(8467), 1291–1293.

Thaddeus, S., & Maine, D. (1994). Too far to walk: Maternal mortality in context. *Social Science and Medicine, 38*(8), 1091–1110.

Toroitich-Ruto, C. (2001). The evolution of the family planning programme and its role in influenc-ing fertility change in Kenya. *Journal of Biosocial Science, 33,* 245–260.

Trottier, D. A., Potter, L. S., Taylor, B., & Glover, L. H. (1994). User characteristics and oral contraceptive compliance in Egypt. *Studies in Family Planning, 25*(4), 284–292.

Trusell, J., & Cleland, K. (2010). The emergency contraceptive. Retrieved from http://ec.princeton .edu/questions/dedicated.html

Trussell, J., Ellertson, C., & Stewart, F. (1996). The effectiveness of the Yuzpe regimen of emergency contraception. *Family Planning Perspectives, 28*(2), 58–87.

Tsui, A. O., Wasserheit, J. N., & Haaga, J. G. (Eds.). (1997). *Reproductive health in developing countries: Expanding dimensions, building solutions. Panel on Reproductive Health, Committee on Population, Commission on Behavioral and Social Sciences and Education, National Research Council.* Washington, DC: National Academies Press.

Turner, C. F., Miller, H. G., & Moses, L. E. (Eds.). (1989). *AIDS, sexual behavior, and intravenous drug use. Committee on AIDS Research and the Behavioral, Social, and Statistical Sciences. Commission on Behavioral and Social Sciences and Education, National Research Council.* Washington, DC: National Academy Press.

Twahir, A., Maggwa, B. N., & Askew, I. (1996). *Integration of STI and HIV/AIDS services with MCH-FP services: A case study of the Mkomani Clinic Society in Mombasa, Kenya, Nairobi.* Operations Research Technical Assistance, Africa Project II, Population Council.

UNAIDS Fact Sheets (2009). AIDSinfo Database, Country Fact Sheets. Retrieved from http://www .unaids.org/en/regionscountries/countries/

UNFPA. (2004). State of the world's population 2004: The Cairo Consensus at Ten: Population, reproductive health, and the global effort to end poverty. Retrieved from http://www.unfpa.org/ swp/ swpmain.htm

UNFPA. (2009). State of the world's population 2009: Facing a changing world: Women,

population and climate. Retrieved from http://www
.unfpa.org/swp/2009/en/overview.shtml

United Nations. (1991). *Controlling iron deficiency*
(Nutrition State-of-the-Art Series, Nutrition Policy
Discussion Paper No. 9). Geneva, Switzerland:
Author.

United Nations. (1994). Programme of action of
the 1994 International Conference on Population
and Development (A/CONF.171/13). Reprinted in
Population and Development Review, 21(1),
187–213 & 21(2), 437–461.

United Nations Children's Fund. (2008).
*Countdown to 2015: Tracking progress in mater-
nal, newborn and child survival: The 2008 report.*
New York: Author. Retrieved from http://www
.countdown2015mnch.org/index.php?option=com_
content&view=article&id=68&itemid=61

United Nations Children's Fund & World Health
Organization (WHO). (2004). *Low birthweight:
Country, regional and global estimates.* New York:
UNICEF.

United Nations Commission on Population and
Development. (2004). Flow of financial resources
for assisting in the implementation of the
Programme of Action of the International
Conference on Population and Development: A 10-
year review. Retrieved from http://daccessdds.un.org/
doc/UNDOC/GEN/N04/206/10/PDF/N0420610
.pdf?OpenElement

United Nations General Assembly. (2000). United
Nations Millennium Declaration (A/RES/55/2).
Retrieved from http://daccessdds.un.org/doc/
UNDOC/GEN/N00/559/51/PDF/N0055951
.pdf?OpenElement

United Nations General Assembly. (2001). Road
map towards the implementation of the United
Nations Millennium Summit: Report of the
Secretary-General (A/56/326). Retrieved from
http://www.un.org/documents/ga/docs/56/a56326
.pdf

United Nations Population Division. (2002).
HIV/AIDS and fertility in sub-Saharan Africa: A re-
view of the research literature (ESA/P/WP.174).
Retrieved from http://www.un.org/esa/population/

publications/fertilitysection/HIVAIDSPaperFertSect
.pdf

United Nations Population Division. (2009). World
population prospects: The 2008 revision population database. Retrieved from http://esa.un.org/
unpp/

United Nations Statistics Division. (2009). MDG
progress chart 2009. Retrieved from http://mdgs.un
.org/unsd/mdg

United Nations Statistics Division. (2010a).
Millennium Development Goals report 2009.
Retrieved from http://unstats.un.org/unsd/
mdg/Resources/Static/Products/Progress2009/MDG
_Report_2

United Nations Statistics Division. (2010b).
Millennium Development Goals indicators: World
and regional trends. Retrieved from http://mdgs.un
.org/unsd/mdg/Host.asp

U.S. Census Bureau. (2004). Global population
profile 2004: The AIDS pandemic in the 21st century. Retrieved from http://www.census.gov/ipc/
prod/wp02/wp02-2.pdf

Walker, G. J., Ashley, D. E., McCaw, A., &
Bernard, G. W. (1985). *Maternal mortality in
Jamaica: A confidential enquiry into all maternal
deaths in Jamaica, 1981–1983* (WHO FHE/
PMM/85.9.10). WHO Inter-regional Meeting on
Prevention of Maternal Mortality, Geneva,
Switzerland.

Weinbreck, P. V., Loustaud, F., Denis, B., Vidal, M.,
Mounier, M., & DeLumley, L. (1988). Postnatal
transmission of HIV infection. *Lancet, 1*, 482.

Westley, S. B. (1995). *Evidence mounts for sex-
selective abortion in Asia* (Asia-Pacific Population
and Policy No. 34). Honolulu, HI: East-West
Population Center.

Westoff, C.F. (2001). *Unmet need at the end of the
century.* Calverton, MD: ORC Macro. Retrieved
from http://www.measuredhs.com/pubs/pdftoc
.cfm?ID=349

Wilcox, A. J., Weinberg, C. R., O'Connor, J. F.,
Baird, D. D., Schlatter, J. P., Canfield, R. E., et al.

(1988). Incidence of early loss of pregnancy. *New England Journal of Medicine, 319,* 189–194.

Winikoff, B. (1983). The effect of birthspacing on child and maternal health. *Studies in Family Planning, 18*(3), 128–143.

Winikoff, B., Elias, C., & Beattie, K. (1994). Special issues of IUD use in resource-poor settings. In C. W. Bardin & D. R. Mishell, Jr. (Eds.), *Proceedings of the Fourth International Conference on IUDs* (pp. 230–238). New York: Population Council.

Winikoff, B., & Sullivan, M. (1987). Assessing the role of family planning in reducing maternal mortality. *Studies in Family Planning, 18*(3), 128–143.

Women's Studies Project. (1999). *The impact of family planning on women's lives.* Research Triangle Park, NC: Family Health International.

Wood, J. W. (1994). *Dynamics of human reproduction: Biology, biometry, demography.* New York: Aldine de Gruyter.

Wood, J. W., Lai, D., Johnson, P. L., Campbell, K. L., & Maslar, I. A. (1985). Lactation and birth spacing in highland New Guinea. *Journal of Biosocial Science, 9*(suppl), 157–173.

World Health Organization (WHO). (1988). Geographic variation in the incidence of hypertension in pregnancy. *American Journal of Obstetrics and Gynecology, 158*(1), 80–83.

World Health Organization (WHO). (1991). *Maternal mortality: A global factbook.* Geneva, Switzerland: Author.

World Health Organization (WHO). (1993a). *Coverage of maternity care: A tabulation of available information* (WHO/FHE/MSM/ 93.7). Geneva, Switzerland: Author.

World Health Organization (WHO). (1993b). *Making maternity care more accessible* (Press release No. 59). Geneva, Switzerland: Author.

World Health Organization (WHO). (1993c). *The global burden of disease. Background paper pre-pared for the World Development Report.* Geneva, Switzerland: Author.

World Health Organization (WHO). (1994a). *Maternal health and Safe Motherhood Programme: Research progress report 1987–1992* (WHO/FHE/ MSM94.18). Geneva, Switzerland: Author.

World Health Organization (WHO). (1994b). *The mother–baby package: Implementing safe mother-hood in countries* (Document FRH/MSM/94.11). Geneva, Switzerland: Author.

World Health Organization (WHO). (1995). Essential or emergency obstetric care. *Safe Motherhood Newsletter, 18*(2), 1–2.

World Health Organization (WHO). (2005). *The world health report 2005: Make every mother and child count.* Geneva, Switzerland: Author. Retrieved from http://www.who.int/whr/2005/en

World Health Organization (WHO). (2006). *Neonatal and perinatal mortality: Country, re-gional and global estimates.* Geneva, Switzerland: Author.

World Health Organization (WHO). (2007a). *Maternal mortality in 2005: Estimates developed by WHO, UNICEF, UNFPA and the World Bank.* Geneva, Switzerland: Author. Retrieved from http://www.who.int/reproductive-health/ publications/maternal_mortality_2005/index.html

World Health Organization (WHO). (2007b). *Unsafe abortion: Global and regional estimates of incidence of unsafe abortion and associated mortal-ity in 2003.* Geneva, Switzerland: Author.

World Health Organization (WHO). (2008a). *Maternal mortality factsheet* (Document WHO/MPS/08.12). Geneva, Switzerland: Author.

World Health Organization (WHO). (2008b). *Millennium Development Goal 5 factsheet* (Document WHO/MPS/08.15). Geneva, Switzerland: Author.

World Health Organization (WHO). (2008c). *Skilled birth attendants factsheet* (Document WHO/MPS/08.11). Geneva, Switzerland: Author.

World Health Organization (WHO) & UNICEF. (1996). *Revised estimates of maternal mortality: A new approach by WHO and UNICEF.* Geneva, Switzerland: Author.

The world health report 2005: Make every mother and child count. (2005). *Lancet, 365*(9463), 977–988.

Yoder, S., Abderrahim, N., & Zhuzhuni, A. (2004). *Female genital cutting in the demographic and health surveys: A critical and comparative analysis.* Calverton, MD: ORC Macro.

Younis, N., Khattab, H., Zurayk, H., el-Mouelhy, M., Fadle Amin, M., & Farag, A. M. (1993). A community study of gynecological and related morbidities in rural Egypt. *Studies in Family Planning, 24*(3), 175–186.

Zupan, J. (2005, May 19). Perinatal mortality in developing countries. *New England Journal of Medicine, 352,* 2047–2048.

5

Infectious Diseases

ARTHUR L. REINGOLD AND AUBREE GORDON

This chapter describes the epidemiological features of the infectious diseases of greatest public health significance in low- and middle-income countries and details available strategies to prevent and control them. Because these diseases cannot be covered in depth in a single chapter, the emphasis here is on their unique epidemiological features and the relevant technological challenges, resource limitations, and cultural barriers that have shaped current approaches to their prevention and control. Conceptually, these approaches include preventing exposure to the infectious agent; making otherwise susceptible individuals or populations immune to the infectious agent; treating infected individuals or populations to prevent illness and transmission of the agent to others; and improving the timeliness and appropriateness of care for symptomatic individuals so as to minimize morbidity and mortality and, in some instances, to reduce the likelihood of transmission to others. Examples of successful programs using one or more of these various conceptual approaches are discussed, as are the challenges and obstacles that confront low- and middle-income countries and their partners as they seek to reduce the burden of disease caused by infectious agents.

Overview

Collectively, infectious diseases have undoubtedly been the single most important contributors to human morbidity and mortality throughout history. Over the past 150 years, the mortality attributable to them has declined substantially in high-income countries, and chronic diseases such as cardiovascular disease, cancer, stroke, chronic obstructive pulmonary disease, and diabetes mellitus have assumed prominence as the leading causes of death in these countries. Although uncertainty exists about the relative importance of various social, economic, environmental, and public health factors in this epidemiologic transition, most of the reductions in mortality attributable to infectious diseases clearly preceded any advances in clinical medicine and public health that plausibly could have had an impact on the infectious diseases of public health significance of the time (e.g., tuberculosis, rheumatic fever, scarlet fever, typhoid fever, and cholera). At present, only pneumonia, influenza, and septicemia rank among the top 10 causes of mortality in the United States.

The global burden of disease and the epidemiologic transition are discussed in detail elsewhere in this book (see Chapter 1). Although current projections suggest that acute infectious diseases will decrease substantially in their absolute and relative importance as causes of death and disability in low- and middle-income countries in the decades to come, today they remain issues of great public health significance. Acute infectious diseases are, collectively, the leading cause of death among children, accounting for more than half of all deaths in low-income countries (see Chapter 1), as well as being important causes of morbidity and mortality in people at all stages of life. In many countries, the HIV/AIDS pandemic has, in recent years, reversed decades of progress in reducing mortality due to acute infectious diseases, with a resulting decrease in life expectancy. Further, it is now well accepted that chronic infection contributes in important—if poorly understood—ways to the pathogenesis of a number of chronic diseases, including cervical cancer (in which human papillomavirus [HPV] plays a role), hepatic cancer and cirrhosis (in which hepatitis B virus [HBV] and probably hepatitis C virus [HCV] play a role), gastric cancer and peptic ulcer disease (in which *Helicobacter pylori* plays a role), and possibly cardiovascular disease (in which *Chlamydia pneumoniae* and perhaps other infectious agents may play roles). Hepatic cancer and cirrhosis due to HBV were the first vaccine-preventable chronic diseases, and it is expected that recently licensed vaccines against HPV will prevent many cases of cervical cancer. Thus, for all the reasons just mentioned, infectious diseases and their prevention and control will remain of major public health importance for low- and middle-income countries for the foreseeable future.

Underlying virtually every infectious disease of public health importance in low- and middle-income countries is the significant role played by poverty and its associated problems. For example, both obvious and more subtle forms of malnutrition and micronutrient deficiencies are associated with an increased risk of severe morbidity and mortality from a wide range of infectious diseases. At the same time, lack of education, poor access to clean drinking water, inability to dispose properly of human waste, household crowding, and lack of access to medical care—all manifestations of poverty—also make substantial contributions to their prevalence.

However, low- and middle-income countries and the people living in them cannot be lumped together into a single group insofar as their risk of various infectious diseases is concerned. Important geographic differences arise in the incidence and public health significance of various infectious diseases, due to differences in climate, the distribution of insect vectors and intermediate hosts, and variations in other environmental, social, and cultural factors. In addition, all low- and middle-income countries are not equally resource poor—they vary enormously in the resources that are available to provide clinical services (e.g., oral rehydration therapy), mount public health programs (e.g., vaccination programs), and reduce environmental sources of infection (e.g., provide clean drinking water and adequate sanitation or control vector populations). Also, all low- and middle-income countries include within them culturally, economically, and sometimes geographically diverse subpopulations with very different needs and resources, particularly with regard to infectious diseases. Given the enormous diversity of low- and middle-income countries and the infectious diseases that confront them, it will be possible in this chapter to discuss these diseases only selectively, using representative examples when appropriate.

Control of Infectious Diseases

The twentieth century saw an ever-increasing number of programs to prevent morbidity and mortality from specific infectious diseases in low- and middle-income countries. Strategies that have been employed include various combinations of vector control (e.g., for malaria, dengue, yellow fever, and onchocerciasis [river blindness]); vaccination (e.g., for smallpox, measles, polio, neonatal tetanus, diphtheria, pertussis, tetanus, hepatitis B, meningococcal meningitis, and yellow fever); mass chemotherapy (e.g., for hookworm, onchocerciasis, dracunculiasis [Guinea worm], and sexually transmitted infections [STIs]); improved sanitation and access to clean water (e.g., for diarrheal diseases); improved care seeking and caregiving (e.g., for diarrheal diseases and acute respiratory infections); and behavior change (e.g., for HIV and other STIs, diarrheal diseases, and dracunculiasis), among others. The successful eradication of smallpox in the late 1970s through a combination of enhanced case finding, containment, and vaccination gave considerable impetus to attempts to control other infectious diseases (Exhibit 5-1).

As the world health community has established goals for reducing morbidity and mortality from other infectious diseases, a variety of terms describing different levels of control have come into use. Organizations such as the World Health Organization (WHO) and its governing body, the World Health Assembly (WHA), have been careful to define their prevention goals vis-à-vis various diseases; these are set forth in appropriate sections of this chapter. A useful set of definitions of such terms was put forward at the Dahlem workshop on the Eradication of Infectious Diseases (Dowdle & Hopkins, 1998):

- *Control:* Reduction of disease incidence, prevalence, morbidity or mortality to a locally acceptable level as a result of deliberate efforts; continued intervention measures are required to maintain the reduction.

- *Elimination of disease:* Reduction to zero of the incidence of a specified disease in a defined geographic area as a result of deliberate efforts; continued intervention measures are required.

- *Elimination of infection:* Reduction to zero of the incidence of infection caused by a specific agent in a defined geographic area as a result of deliberate efforts; continued measures to prevent reestablishment of transmission are required.

| Exhibit 5-1 | Smallpox Eradication |

Most individuals who work in the area of global health consider the eradication of smallpox to have been the single most important contribution of public health efforts in the twentieth century, and possibly the most significant accomplishment in the field of human health in recorded history. Although the ultimate eradication of smallpox through the use of vaccine was foreseen by Edward Jenner and President Thomas Jefferson at the beginning of the nineteenth century, it took more than 150 years for it to become a reality. Eradication of smallpox was possible because of several important features of the disease itself; technological advances in vaccine preparation and administration; development and application of a new approach to using the vaccine selectively rather than in mass campaigns; and a combination of international will and cooperation, strong leadership, and the focused effort of large numbers of health workers in multiple countries.

One feature of smallpox that made it a candidate for eradication was its relatively inefficient transmission from person to person. In addition, individuals with smallpox were generally bedridden before the appearance of the rash—the stage in the illness when person-to-person transmission was most likely to occur. Moreover, subclinical cases did not occur in unvaccinated individuals, and vaccinated individuals who developed mild smallpox did not efficiently transmit the virus. Smallpox was also characterized by a lack of a carrier state and the existence of a single serotype of the virus. Other notable features of the disease included a marked seasonal fluctuation in cases and the lack of a nonhuman reservoir for the virus in nature.

A key advance in vaccine development and delivery that was crucial to smallpox eradication was the development of a heat-stable, freeze-dried vaccine. In addition, two improved methods of delivering the vaccine were introduced—a bifurcated needle that was inexpensive, easy to use, and economical in its use of a small volume of vaccine, and jet injector guns that allowed a team to vaccinate more than 1,000 persons per hour.

Nevertheless, despite the availability of a heat-stable smallpox vaccine and the means of vaccinating large numbers of persons, mass vaccination campaigns intended to render entire populations immune to smallpox were unsuccessful in eradicating the disease, even in countries that achieved vaccine coverage in the range of 80% to 95%. Smallpox virus continued to circulate among the remaining unvaccinated individuals, who were extremely difficult to identify and vaccinate.

A delay in the arrival of sufficient vaccine to mount a mass campaign against smallpox in Nigeria in 1966 led to the development of an alternative approach to preventing the spread of smallpox in an area: energetic case detection followed by isolation of all infected individuals and intense vaccination efforts focused on the area and population immediately surrounding a case. This approach, dubbed a surveillance containment strategy, proved to be remarkably successful in eradicating smallpox once imaginative and locally acceptable approaches to detecting all suspected cases, isolating individuals with smallpox, and vaccinating those around them were implemented. Surveillance containment ultimately replaced mass vaccination campaigns, and global efforts to complete eradication of smallpox relying on this approach gained momentum.

In 1967, as many as 10 to 15 million cases of smallpox occurred in 33 countries with endemic smallpox and 14 other countries with imported cases of smallpox. These countries, which had a total population of more than 1.2 billion persons at the time, included many of the poorest countries in the world and those presenting the greatest logistical barriers to mounting an effective eradication program. As a result of the efforts of dedicated public health workers in these countries and a small cadre of public health professionals from unaffected countries, the last person with smallpox not caused by a laboratory accident had onset of a rash on October 26, 1977, in Somalia. On December 9, 1979, the World Health Organization's Global Commission for the Certification of Smallpox Eradication concluded that "smallpox eradication has been achieved throughout the world," a conclusion accepted by the World Health Assembly in May 1980.

Source: The Eradication of Infectious Diseases: Report of the Dahlem Workshop on the Eradication of Infectious Diseases, W. R. Dowdle and D. R. Hopkins, March 16–22, 1998. Copyright John Wiley & Sons Limited. Reproduced with permission.

- *Eradication:* Permanent reduction to zero of the worldwide incidence of infection caused by a specific agent as a result of deliberate efforts; intervention measures are no longer needed.

- *Extinction:* The specific infectious agent no longer exists in nature or in the laboratory.

In the near term, extinction is possible only for smallpox, although concerns about its use as an agent of bioterrorism have prevented the long-awaited destruction of the last known stocks of the virus. Eradication of other diseases, such as polio, measles, and dracunculiasis, is considered theoretically possible using existing control methods and is being actively pursued. Unfortunately, for most of the infectious diseases responsible for the majority of morbidity and mortality in low- and middle-income countries at the beginning of the twenty-first century, only their control is considered achievable in the foreseeable future (Table 5-1).

Table 5-1	Levels of Control Considered Achievable for Selected Infectious Diseases in the Foreseable Future Using Currently Available Methods			
Extinction	**Eradication**	**Elimination of Infection**	**Elimination of Disease**	**Control**
Smallpox	Polio Measles Dracunculiaisis (Guinea worm)	Onchocerciasis	Rabies Trachoma	Malaria Neonatal tetanus Cholera Tuberculosis Schistosomiasis Diarrheal disease ARIs AIDS STIs Leprosy

Note: ARIs = acute respiratory infections; AIDS = acquired immune deficiency syndrome; STIs = sexually transmitted infections.

Childhood Vaccine-Preventable Diseases: The Expanded Program on Immunization

Overview

Based on the success of the vaccination program mounted to control and then eradicate smallpox, WHO and various partner agencies launched the Expanded Program on Immunization (EPI, or PEV in French) in 1974. At that time it was estimated that fewer than 5% of infants and children in low- and middle-income countries were receiving relatively inexpensive and highly effective vaccines, despite the fact that these vaccines had been licensed and available for a number of years. Many obstacles to vaccinating these children existed, including the lack of demand for vaccines on the part of the community; the small number of sources of vaccines of adequate quality; the lack of the infrastructure needed to purchase, store, and distribute vaccines, some of which were temperature sensitive; a deficiency in the number of trained personnel to administer vaccination programs; and insufficient funds to purchase vaccines and vaccination supplies and equipment. Further, most countries lacked health information and surveillance systems to assess the burden of disease caused by various vaccine-preventable diseases or to evaluate the impact of a vaccination program. Remarkable progress since 1974 in correcting these problems has led to the possible eradication through immunization of polio; dramatic reductions in morbidity and mortality from measles and neonatal tetanus worldwide; and likely, but harder to demonstrate, reductions of a similar magnitude in morbidity and mortality from diphtheria and pertussis.

For the first 20 years or so of its existence, the EPI focused on diseases for which safe, effective, and inexpensive vaccines were available and could be given entirely during the first year of life. These included oral polio vaccine (OPV, a trivalent live vaccine against poliomyelitis); measles vaccine (a live vaccine); a three-component killed vaccine against diphtheria, pertussis, and tetanus (DPT); and bacillus Calmette-Guérin (BCG, a live vaccine against tuberculosis). Vaccination with tetanus toxoid (TT) was included for women of childbearing age to prevent neonatal tetanus in their newborn babies, even though the group being targeted for vaccination was not infants in the first year of life. Subsequently, it has been recommended that vaccine against yellow fever and Japanese B encephalitis be added in countries where these two diseases pose a threat. Vaccines against hepatitis B and *Haemophilus influenzae* b were then included after large quantities of these relatively inexpensive vaccines became available. Newer vaccines, including rotavirus vaccine, pneumococcal conjugate vaccine, and human papillomavirus (HPV) vaccine, have also recently been added. (Table 5-2 provides the current WHO recommendations concerning infant and childhood immunizations.) Hepatitis B, *H. influenzae* b, *Streptococcus pneumoniae*, HPV, yellow fever, and tuberculosis are discussed elsewhere in this chapter, so they will not be considered here.

Poliomyelitis

Etiologic Agent, Clinical Features, and Characteristics of the Currently Available Vaccines

Poliomyelitis (polio) may be caused by any of the three known serotypes (1, 2, and 3) of poliovirus. This virus is efficiently transmitted through the fecal–oral route. Ingestion of the virus leads to asymptomatic or mild, self-limited infection and shedding of the virus from the throat and gastrointestinal tract in

Table 5-2	Recommended Routine Immunizations for Children: Summary of WHO Position Papers*		
Disease/Vaccine	**Age of First Dose**	**Dose in Primary Series**	**Booster Dose**
Recommended for All Children			
BCG	As soon as possible after birth	1	
DTP	6 weeks	3	1–6 years of age
H. influenzae b	6 weeks	3	
Hepatitis B	With DPT1 or as soon as possible after birth	3	
HPV	10–13 years of age	3	
Pneumococcal (conjugate)	6 weeks	3	
Polio (OPV)	6 weeks	3	
Measles	9–15 months	2	
Recommended for Children Residing in Certain Regions			
Japanese B encephalitis	1 year	2 (mouse brain derived)	
Japanese B encephalitis	9–12 months	1 (live attenuated)	
Yellow fever	9–12 months, with measles	1	
Rotavirus	6 weeks	2 (Rotarix)	
Rotavirus	6 weeks	3 (RotaTeq)	

Note: *Not including vaccines recommended only for children in selected high-risk populations.

the vast majority of exposed persons. However, an estimated 1 in 100 to 1 in 850 infected persons develops symptomatic polio, with or without paralysis. Of those who develop paralysis, which primarily affects one or both legs, approximately 10% die acutely, 10% to 15% are left permanently unable to walk, and 10% to 15% are left lame (unable to walk normally).

Treatment for polio is entirely supportive in nature. Before widespread vaccination was undertaken, polio was the leading cause of lameness in low- and middle-income countries, and many of its victims remain a visible sign of the ravages of the disease and will need assistance long after acute cases of polio have been eradicated.

Killed injectable polio vaccine (IPV) and live OPV became available in the 1950s and 1960s, respectively. Both types of vaccines are safe and highly effective, and each has been used successfully to eliminate disease caused by wild-type poliovirus in high-income countries. Although there are extremely rare cases of polio caused by the vaccine strain of the virus when OPV is given, WHO and other supporters of the EPI have always considered OPV to be preferable to IPV for routine use in low- and middle-income countries. Reasons for preferring OPV have included its extremely low cost (approximately $0.02 per dose); its ease of administration; its ability to induce intestinal immunity that inhibits shedding of wild-type poliovirus; and its transmission to household and other close contacts through the fecal–oral route, thereby providing repeated exposures to the vaccine and boosting immunity to polio through such contacts. However, for unclear reasons, the efficacy of OPV in low- and middle-income countries has consistently been found to be lower than that in high-income countries—approximately 85% versus approximately 95% for the primary series (Patriarca, Wright, & John, 1991).

Descriptive Epidemiologic Features and Risk Factors

Before the widespread use of polio vaccine, polio was endemic in virtually all low- and middle-income countries, and most children were asymptomatically infected during the first few years of life. Symptomatic acute polio was similarly seen primarily in infants and young children. Based on surveys of the prevalence of lameness in school-aged children, the annual incidence of symptomatic polio in low- and middle-income countries was estimated to be in the range of 20 to 40 cases per 100,000 total population (LaForce, Lichnevski, Keja, & Henderson, 1980).

As oral polio vaccine came into widespread use and vaccine coverage increased, endemic infections with wild-type poliovirus decreased. However, vaccine coverage levels in the range of 40% to 80%, combined with a vaccine efficacy of approximately 85%, led to an accumulation of susceptible individuals and subsequent outbreaks in many countries with "good" EPI programs (Sutter et al., 1991). In the early 1980s, more than 50,000 cases of polio were being reported annually to WHO (Otten et al., 1992). However, as described in the next subsection, polio has now been eliminated in much of the world as a result of intensified surveillance and immunization efforts and in 2010 remains a problem in only a small number of countries.

Current Approaches to Prevention and Control

In 1988, the WHA set a goal of interrupting polio transmission worldwide by 2000 and certifying that polio had been eradicated by 2005. The polio eradication effort put into place at that time was based on a combination of ongoing routine immunization of infants, annual national immunization days, and house-to-house mop-up campaigns to vaccinate those persons who were missed by these other approaches (Hull, Ward, Hull, Milstien, & de Quadros, 1994). In addition, sensitive surveillance for and laboratory testing of specimens from individuals with acute flaccid paralysis were put into place to help identify cases of polio, thereby allowing targeting of additional vaccination efforts and monitoring of the impact of the eradication program.

The last confirmed case of paralytic polio caused by wild-type poliovirus in the Western Hemisphere was detected in Peru in 1991, and three WHO regions (Americas, western Pacific, and European) had been certified as polio free by 2002 (Centers for Disease Control and Prevention [CDC], 2002). By 2006, indigenous transmission of wild poliovirus type 2 had been interrupted globally, and indigenous transmission of types 1 and 3 had been interrupted in all but four countries (Afghanistan, India, Nigeria, and Pakistan).

Unfortunately, major resurgences of polio in India in 2002 and in northern Nigeria in 2003 and 2004 led to reintroduction of wild polio virus type 1 into more than 20 previously polio-free countries in Africa and Asia. While renewed control efforts had stopped transmission in all but five of these countries by the end of 2007, multiple new importations from India and Nigeria led to additional cases in previously polio-free African countries in 2008 and 2009 (CDC, 2009c). Renewed efforts, including various supplementary immunization activities (e.g., national and subnational immunization days), are now under way as part of the concerted effort to complete polio eradication. In addition, the emergence of circulating, vaccine-derived polio viruses, which consist of genetically unstable OPV strain viruses that revert to the profile of the virulent parent strain, needs to be addressed. This issue will eventually require the worldwide use of only IPV once eradication of wild polio virus is assured (Modlin, 2010).

Measles

Etiologic Agent, Clinical Features, and Vaccine Characteristics

Measles is caused by measles virus. Although some genotypic variation occurs, all measles virus strains are considered to be of a single type. Measles virus is spread via the respiratory route and is transmitted extremely efficiently. It is highly infectious, and in the absence of vaccine-induced immunity, virtually every child can be expected to develop measles if the virus is circulating in the community.

Measles is characterized initially by fever, cough, runny nose, and malaise, making it indistinguishable from many other viral respiratory infections for the first several days, during which the child is highly infectious. A characteristic rash then appears. Although most cases are self-limited, complications commonly include pneumonia, diarrhea, and ear infections. Less common complications include encephalitis and blindness. Measles is not amenable to antibiotic therapy, but treatment with vitamin A can reduce the case fatality ratio (Hussey & Klein, 1990).

Before the measles vaccine came into widespread use, measles was consistently one of the leading causes of death among children worldwide, accounting for an estimated 20% to 30% of such fatalities (Walsh, 1983). Although the estimates of the case fatality ratio for measles have varied from 1% to greater than 30%, depending in part on whether the studies were community or hospital based, it is clear that the most potent predictors of mortality among children with measles are young age; malnutrition, particularly vitamin A deficiency (Markowitz et al., 1989); and HIV infection. Furthermore, measles frequently leaves a child weakened and at increased risk of illness and death from other causes for a year or more after the acute episode.

The measles vaccine consists of a live, attenuated strain of the measles virus. It is safe, inexpensive, and highly effective when given to a child after circulating measles antibody acquired from the mother have disappeared. Because the maternal antibodies tend to disappear somewhat later and exposure to measles virus is substantially less common in high-income countries, the measles vaccine is typically given at 15 months of age in such countries. In low- and middle-income countries, the intensity of exposure to measles and the poorly understood, more rapid decline in maternal antibodies combine to put infants at much greater risk of acquiring measles at a young age, when complications and death are more likely. As a result, measles vaccine is typically given to infants at 9 months of age in low- and middle-income countries.

Descriptive Epidemiologic Features and Risk Factors

In the absence of vaccination, every child in an area where measles virus is circulating would be expected to contract measles. In the early 1980s, an estimated 3 million children died annually of measles and its sequelae. By 2008, however, the number of measles deaths had declined to an estimated 164,000 (CDC, 2009a).

The age at which an unvaccinated child develops measles is a function of when maternal antibodies disappear (generally at 6 to 12 months of age) and the intensity of exposure to measles virus in the community. Thus, in crowded urban areas, most unvaccinated children will develop measles between 6 months and 5 years of age; in contrast, in more sparsely populated, rural areas, such children acquire measles at an older age (Walsh, 1983). Family size, travel patterns, and types and locations of social interactions (e.g., marketplaces) also influence the local epidemiologic features of measles. HIV infection appears to increase the risk of acquiring measles in infancy, presumably by decreasing the level of circulating maternal antibody in the infant.

Current Approaches to Prevention and Control

Like smallpox, measles can, in theory, be completely eradicated because the causative virus does not infect other species or live in the environment. However, because measles is more widespread and much more infectious than smallpox, and because substantial transmission of the virus occurs among infants prior to the age of routine vaccination, eradication of measles will be more difficult to achieve. Thus, rather than establish a goal of measles eradication, the WHA resolved in 1989 to reduce measles-related morbidity by 90% and measles-related mortality by 95% by 1995. As with polio, improved routine immunization of infants and periodic mass vaccination campaigns targeting infants and children from 9 months to 5 (or even up to 14) years of age have been undertaken as complementary strategies.

Based on the significant success achieved in reducing the incidence of measles and even interrupting measles virus transmission over large geographic areas for substantial periods of time, the 1994 Pan American Sanitary Conference made elimination of measles from the Western Hemisphere a goal for the year 2000 (Pan America Health Organization, 1994). As a result of this concerted effort, indigenous measles virus circulation has not been observed in the region of the Americas since 2002, although continuing circulation of the virus elsewhere in the world poses an ongoing threat of measles importations (de Quadros,

Izurieta, Venczel, & Carrasco, 2004). Substantial progress has also been made in reducing morbidity and mortality due to measles in Africa. Through a combination of approaches, including supplemental immunization activities, improved surveillance, and improved case management, measles cases and deaths have been reduced in some African countries by 91% and 84%, respectively, compared with findings in the immediately preceding years (CDC, 2004; CDC, 2009b). Despite these impressive gains, worldwide eradication of measles is unlikely in the immediate future.

Diphtheria

Etiologic Agent, Clinical Features, and Vaccine Characteristics

Diphtheria is caused by the bacterium *Corynebacterium diphtheriae*. It is spread primarily via the respiratory route, although in low- and middle-income countries the organism is also a cause of ulcerative skin lesions and can be transmitted from such lesions. The incidence of diphtheria and the morbidity and mortality attributable to it in such countries are largely unknown, but the disease is not believed to pose a major public health threat.

Diphtheria is a disease of the upper respiratory tract, manifested by fever, sore throat, an inflamed pharynx (and possibly nose and larynx), and a grayish membrane covering the inflamed mucosa. With involvement of the larynx, the airways can be blocked and death can result. The disease is toxin mediated, and use of both antibiotics and diphtheria antitoxin (which is rarely, if ever, available in low- and middle-income countries) is beneficial in its treatment.

The diphtheria component of the DPT vaccine is composed of inactivated diphtheria toxin adsorbed to aluminum salts. Two or more doses of DPT result in protection against diphtheria in 90% to 100% of those vaccinated.

Descriptive Epidemiologic Features and Risk Factors

Although diphtheria is easier to diagnose than pertussis, it is likely underreported in many low- and middle-income countries. Thus the approximately 30,000 cases of diphtheria reported to WHO in 2000 almost certainly do not reflect the actual burden of disease.

Most cases of diphtheria occur in young children, primarily among those living in impoverished, crowded conditions. Lack of vaccination is undoubtedly the most important risk factor for developing or dying from diphtheria.

Current Approaches to Prevention and Control

The current approach to reducing morbidity and mortality from diphtheria is to improve levels of vaccine coverage achieved through ongoing infant immunization programs (i.e., EPI) in various countries. Strategies for improving vaccine coverage include expanding the times when vaccinations are offered in clinics, reducing waiting times, and reducing the number of missed opportunities to vaccinate unvaccinated infants, among other options. Because vaccination does not lead to elimination of carriage of *C. diphtheriae* from the nasopharynx, ongoing control of diphtheria requires achieving and maintaining high levels of vaccine coverage among the target population.

Pertussis

Etiologic Agent, Clinical Features, and Vaccine Characteristics

Pertussis (whooping cough) is caused by the bacterium *Bordetella pertussis*. Like measles, pertussis is spread via the respiratory route and is highly contagious, particularly within a household and in crowded institutional settings. In classic cases of pertussis, nonspecific respiratory tract symptoms are followed by severe and protracted bouts of coughing that typically end with an inspiratory whooping sound. These bouts of coughing can persist for many weeks and be quite debilitating, even when complications such as pneumonia and neurologic damage do not develop. Antibiotic treatment has little or no impact on the natural course of the disease once symptoms have begun, but probably shortens the time during which an individual is infectious.

Pertussis is believed to be the cause of substantial morbidity and mortality in the absence of high levels of coverage with pertussis vaccine, but it is difficult to assess the proportion of respiratory infections and related deaths due to pertussis. In part, this difficulty arises from the fact that many infants with pertussis never have the characteristic whoop seen in older children. Similarly, a growing body of evidence suggests that in high-income countries, and presumably in low- and middle-income countries as well, *B. pertussis* is the cause of many cough illnesses in young adults that are never recognized as pertussis. Finally, the laboratory diagnosis of pertussis has been plagued by the insensitivity, nonspecificity, technical difficulty, and cost of the various diagnostic tests, making research studies difficult and routine surveillance extremely inaccurate.

Pertussis vaccines have, for many years, consisted of killed whole bacteria adsorbed to aluminum salts to make them more immunogenic. In most instances, pertussis vaccine is given to infants and young children as a part of the DPT vaccine. When a full series of three doses is given, the efficacy of the pertussis component of DPT is in the range of 80%. Because whole-cell pertussis vaccine contains many bacterial products, it is the most reactogenic component of DPT and makes the vaccine the most reactogenic of those included in the EPI. Thus pain and tenderness at the injection site, with or without fever, is common after a DPT injection.

More serious but rare complications of whole-cell pertussis vaccine (e.g., encephalopathy) have been at the center of a protracted debate in many high-income countries over its safety. Concern over these rare complications and attendant declines in vaccine acceptance led to the development and licensure of acellular pertussis vaccines that are far less reactogenic and equally efficacious, but also far more expensive than whole-cell pertussis vaccine. Because of this large difference in cost, the EPI continues to use whole-cell pertussis vaccine in virtually all low- and middle-income countries.

Descriptive Epidemiologic Features and Risk Factors

The number of pertussis cases reported to WHO annually in the early 1980s was in the range of 1.5 to 2 million; by 1997, this number had decreased to less than 200,000 (WHO, 1998b). In the mid-1980s, it was estimated that more than 600,000 children died of pertussis annually. By 2008, the estimated annual death toll from pertussis had declined to approximately 195,000. As noted earlier, any estimate of the burden of disease caused by pertussis is likely to underestimate the actual toll due to the difficulty of making the diagnosis.

Limited studies suggest that most cases of pertussis in low- and middle-income countries occur in infancy and early childhood and that the highest case fatality ratio is seen in infants. It is likely that poverty and the resultant crowding increase the risk of pertussis and that malnutrition increases the likelihood of dying among those who develop the disease, although lack of vaccination is undoubtedly the most important risk factor for developing or dying from pertussis at any age.

Current Approaches to Prevention and Control

As is the case for diphtheria, the current approach to reducing morbidity and mortality from pertussis is to improve levels of vaccine coverage through the EPI and strategies for improved vaccine coverage. Because vaccination does not lead to elimination of carriage of *B. pertussis,* ongoing control of pertussis requires high levels of vaccine coverage among the target population.

Tetanus

Etiologic Agent, Clinical Features, and Vaccine Characteristics

Tetanus is caused by the toxin produced by the anaerobic bacterium *Clostridium tetanus*. It is commonly found in the gastrointestinal tract of many domesticated animals (e.g., cows, sheep, and goats). When deposited in the soil, *C. tetanus* cells form spores that are highly resistant to heat and desiccation and remain viable for years or even decades. When these spores are introduced into a wound or other suitable environment, they sporulate and the bacterial cells reproduce, forming and releasing a highly potent neurotoxin as they grow. Symptoms produced by the neurotoxin include painful stiffening and spasms of the muscles, including those of the jaw (hence the common name "lockjaw"), and, particularly in newborn infants, a resultant inability to suck or otherwise feed.

Treatment of tetanus is largely supportive, even in the rare circumstance when tetanus antitoxin is available. It consists largely of giving muscle relaxants and fluids intravenously. Even with such treatment, the case fatality ratio is very high, particularly in infants with neonatal tetanus, of whom 80% to 90% will die.

The vaccine against tetanus, either in a single preparation or in DPT, is a toxoid—an inactivated form of tetanus toxin, adsorbed to aluminum salts. Tetanus toxoid (TT) is extremely safe and produces few reactions. The three doses of DPT given to infants and the two doses of TT given to women of childbearing age or pregnant women through the EPI produce immunity in 90% to 100% of those vaccinated.

Descriptive Epidemiologic Features and Risk Factors

While tetanus in adults is an avoidable and tragic illness, tetanus in newborn infants is a public health problem. Studies in the 1970s and 1980s showed that as many as 60 newborn babies per 1,000 (6%) were developing neonatal tetanus in some low-income countries, primarily due to contamination of the umbilical stump, and that virtually all these babies died (Stanfield & Galazka, 1984). Deaths due to neonatal tetanus accounted for one-fourth to three-fourths of all neonatal deaths and as much as one-fourth of infant mortality in these countries. Neonatal tetanus caused more than 500,000 deaths worldwide in 1993 (WHO, 1994), but that number had declined to an estimated 128,000 by 2004.

Neonatal tetanus is more common in rural areas, particularly those where animal husbandry practices lead to substantial fecal contamination of the soil, and tends to be more common during the rainy season (Schofield, 1986). Nevertheless, the key risk factors for neonatal tetanus clearly relate to the site where a delivery occurs, the level of training of the person assisting with the delivery, the manner in which the umbilical cord is cut, and the way the umbilical stump is treated. Because there is enormous diversity of cultural practices regarding how the cord is cut and what is placed on the umbilical stump (including mud, animal dung, clarified butter, and other nonsterile materials), the rate of and risk factors for neonatal tetanus vary substantially in different regions of the world (Stanfield & Galazka, 1984).

Current Approaches to Prevention and Control

Because the *C. tetanus* spores that cause neonatal tetanus are ubiquitous in soil and can persist there indefinitely, the organism itself cannot be eradicated. Neonatal tetanus, however, can be controlled or eliminated as a public health problem (defined as fewer than 1 case per 1,000 live births in each health district) by ensuring that a high proportion of women giving birth have received two doses of TT or that the delivery and subsequent cord care practices minimize the chance that *C. tetanus* spores will be introduced. Studies such as those conducted in Egypt (Figure 5-1) demonstrate clearly that immunization of women of reproductive age or of pregnant women has a dramatic impact on the risk of neonatal tetanus (CDC, 1996). Other studies suggest that training and equipping birth attendants so they can perform a clean delivery (the "three cleans"—delivery with clean hands, delivery on a clean surface, and use of clean instruments and dressings to cut and dress the umbilical cord) may be somewhat less effective at reducing the risk of neonatal tetanus but has a greater impact on the risk of neonatal mortality from all causes combined. These two approaches can and have been used together. In recent years, the proportion of women giving birth in various geographic regions who have been adequately immunized with TT has increased substantially, but neonatal tetanus remains a problem in many low- and middle-income countries where many deliveries still occur at home.

Obstacles to Prevention and Control

Despite Herculean efforts on the part of WHO, UNICEF, and others, it has been challenging to achieve and maintain high levels of vaccine coverage in many countries, particularly in rural areas of the

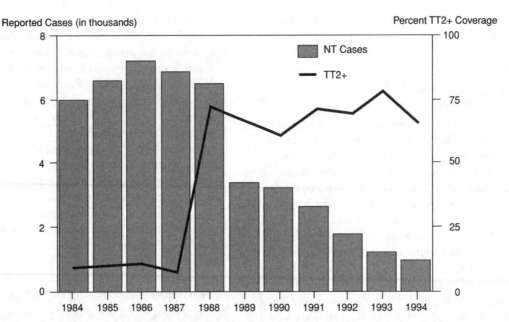

Figure 5-1 Number of Reported Cases of Neonatal Tetanus (NT) and Percentage of Pregnant Women Receiving at Least Two Doses of Tetanus Toxoid (TT2+), by Year, in Egypt, 1984–1994. *Source:* Centers for Disease Control and Prevention, "Progress Toward Elimination of Neonatal Tetanus: Egypt, 1988–1994," 1996, Morbidity and Mortality Weekly Report, 45, pp. 89–92.

low-income countries. By 2008, 151 and 120 countries reported coverages with the third dose of DTP vaccine of 80% and 90%, respectively. Current estimates suggest that worldwide, 24 million children remain unvaccinated, of whom an estimated 2 million die of childhood vaccine-preventable diseases (Senior, 2009).

For a number of years, substantial controversy persisted regarding the relative merits of vertical approaches to vaccinating children (e.g., mass campaigns) and horizontal approaches (i.e., improving access to and use of primary care services that provide routine immunizations). Although the debate over vertical versus horizontal programs continues in some health areas, it has largely been replaced with respect to vaccination of infants and children by a broad consensus that the two approaches can be complementary rather than conflicting. Thus attempts to strengthen routine infant (and pregnant woman) immunization programs in low- and middle-income countries around the world have proceeded in parallel with mass campaigns intended to hasten the eradication of polio and the elimination of measles.

Further reduction or elimination of the childhood vaccine-preventable diseases discussed in this section is contingent on the availability of sustained funding of and technical support for immunization programs, stimulation of increased demand for vaccination on the part of parents and communities, expanded access to immunization services, and effective surveillance for these diseases. At the same time, there is a need to continue to develop, test, and make available new and improved vaccines; to expand local production of existing vaccines in low- and middle-income countries; to ensure the potency and safety of the vaccines produced; and to ensure the availability and proper use (and disposal) of sterile injection equipment. The Global Alliance for Vaccines and Immunizations (GAVI; see Exhibit 5-2), together with the Bill and Melinda Gates Foundation and other partners, is working to ensure the earliest possible incorporation of other vaccines into the EPI. As existing and newly licensed infant and childhood vaccines are added to those recommended by WHO, countries with limited resources will need to establish their own priorities for which vaccines to add.

Based on the model of smallpox eradication, one argument used to support the drive for worldwide polio eradication was that it would be possible to discontinue routine polio vaccination at some point after eradication was achieved. However, outbreaks of polio caused by circulating vaccine-derived polioviruses in Hispaniola, the Philippines,

Exhibit 5-2	The Global Alliance for Vaccines and Immunizations

An estimated 2 million infants and children still die each year from diseases that can be prevented by currently available vaccines. Several million more infants and children die each year from tuberculosis, malaria, and AIDS—infectious diseases for which new vaccines are urgently needed.

Numerous obstacles, many of which are external to the public health and health care delivery systems, make it difficult to achieve and sustain high levels of coverage with existing vaccines in low- and middle-income countries. These obstacles include limited financial resources, insufficient numbers of trained healthcare workers, poor roads and other barriers to reaching remote parts of some countries, civil wars, and natural disasters. Other barriers hinder the development, testing, licensure, and ultimate availability of new vaccines, including the cost of research and testing (and hence the eventual cost of new vaccines, particularly those requiring technological sophistication, such as conjugated vaccines) and liability concerns on the part of potential manufacturers.

Recognizing these problems and wishing to increase the speed with which current and new vaccines reach the world's children, a group of international agencies—including WHO, UNICEF, the World Bank, and others—launched the Global Alliance for Vaccines and Immunizations (GAVI) in 2000. The mission of GAVI is "to fulfill the right of every child to be protected against vaccine-preventable diseases of public health concern." The initial activities of GAVI focused on establishing a children's vaccine fund and on conducting an analysis of those research and development gaps that impede the development and distribution of vaccines. More recently, GAVI has begun working with multilateral and international agencies, vaccine manufacturers, foundations, and low- and middle-income countries to promote the rapid development of new vaccines and greater access to both current and new vaccines. For example, this organization has been instrumental in helping make *H. influenzae* b conjugate vaccine available to millions of children in poor countries and is currently working to speed the introduction of *S. pneumoniae* conjugate vaccines, as well as vaccines against rotavirus and HPV.

and Madagascar, together with the widespread presence of wild-type polio virus in numerous laboratories and vaccine production facilities around the world, have challenged previous notions about the need for ongoing polio vaccination after eradication (Fine, Oblapenko, & Sutter, 2004; Sutter, Cáceres, & Mas Lago, 2004).

The inexplicable and unfortunate increase in all-cause mortality seen in infants (primarily female infants) given experimental high-titer measles vaccine at a young age has clearly set back efforts to develop a more potent measles vaccine (Aaby et al., 1994). Therefore, for the foreseeable future, efforts to eliminate measles will, of necessity, rely on the currently available vaccine. Important unanswered questions relate to how best to use the currently available vaccine and which vaccination strategies or combinations of strategies will be most effective in interrupting transmission of this highly infectious agent, particularly in Africa. Although there is a clear need to sustain high levels of routine immunization against measles at or around 9 months of age, the relative importance of various strategies for increasing population-level immunity, such as periodic mass campaigns and routinely giving a second dose of measles vaccine at some time after the first birthday, remains to be determined. Nevertheless, it is now recognized that giving all children an opportunity to receive a second dose of measles vaccine is an important component of measles elimination strategies. It is, at best, uncertain whether a new measles vaccine that is immunogenic at a younger age (in the face of circulating maternal antibodies) and that is safe can be developed and tested, or whether it is even needed to eliminate measles.

Historically, rubella vaccine has not been included in the EPI package of vaccines, even though it has been available for 30 years. In recent years, there has been growing recognition that congenital rubella syndrome is a problem in low- and middle-income countries, where an estimated 110,000 cases occur annually (Cutts & Vynnycky, 1999). All countries in the Americas now include rubella vaccine in the EPI package, and there is growing interest in using it routinely in Africa and Asia as well (Banatvala & Brown, 2004).

Enteric Infections and Acute Respiratory Infections

Although it might seem odd to discuss enteric infections and acute respiratory infections (ARIs) together in one section, these seemingly disparate conditions have much in common. Each accounts for a substantial amount of childhood morbidity and mortality, as well as for a large proportion of outpatient visits and hospitalizations. Infants and young children almost uniformly experience multiple episodes of both types of illness, regardless of where they live. The identified risk factors for enteric infections and ARIs (e.g., poverty, crowding, lack of parental education, malnutrition, low birth weight, and lack of breastfeeding) overlap substantially, and most are difficult to change in the absence of major social change. Further, both enteric infections and ARIs are caused by a multitude of distinct microbial agents, for most of which no vaccine currently exists or is likely to be available in the near future. As a result, the overall approach to minimizing morbidity and mortality from both enteric infections and ARIs has been virtually identical— acceptance of the fact that such infections and illnesses will occur, combined with attempts to ensure that prompt and appropriate care is sought and given.

Enteric Infections

Overview

Enteric infections encompass those viral, bacterial, and parasitic infections of the gastrointestinal tract that are, with the exception of typhoid fever, generally manifested as diarrhea, either alone or in combination with fever, vomiting, and abdominal pain. Although most episodes of diarrheal disease are mild and self-limited, the loss of fluids and salts accompanying severe diarrhea can be life threatening. Also, not all episodes of diarrheal disease are self-limited: Studies suggest that anywhere from 3% to 23% of diarrheal illnesses in infants and young children persist for longer than 2 weeks (Black, 1993). Both self-limited and persistent diarrhea can have a substantial negative impact on the growth of a child, through malabsorption of nutrients and reduced intake due to vomiting, loss of appetite, and undesirable changes in feeding practices in response to diarrheal illness. Thus repeated episodes of diarrhea and persistent diarrhea often lead to malnutrition, which can in turn increase the likelihood of diarrhea persisting and producing a fatal outcome (El Samani, Willett, & Ware, 1988). It has been estimated that diarrheal disease has a more profound impact on the growth of children worldwide than any other infectious disease.

Cholera, while in a sense just one of many causes of watery diarrhea, is in many ways a disease unto itself. It can produce the most dramatic fluid losses of any enteric infection and, in the absence of appropriate replacement of fluid and salts, can cause death within 24 to 48 hours of its onset. Cholera epidemics and pandemics can produce enormous numbers of cases and large numbers of deaths, resulting in profound social disruption. As a result, cholera has been accorded a special status by public health officials and agencies.

Many episodes of diarrheal disease in children in low- and middle-income countries are accompanied by bloody stools or frank dysentery (abdominal cramps; painful, strained defecation; and frequent stools containing blood and mucus), which is usually the result of an invasive infection that produces local tissue damage and inflammation in the intestinal mucosa. Although the fluid loss that accompanies such episodes is generally not profound, life-threatening local intestinal and systemic complications can result. Damage to the intestinal mucosa can also lead to substantial losses of protein, resulting in growth retardation. The clinical management of such episodes poses a number of distinctive challenges (see "Current Approaches to Prevention and Control" later in this section).

On average, children younger than the age of 5 in low- and middle-income countries experience two to three episodes of diarrhea each year (Kosek, Bern, & Guerrant, 2003). The burden of disease attributable to diarrheal diseases worldwide is enormous, despite the impressive accomplishments of diarrheal disease control programs. The Global Burden of Disease project estimated that children younger than 5 years collectively experience more than 2.5 billion episodes of diarrhea annually and that diarrheal disease causes approximately 1.5 million deaths each year. Thus, like ARIs, diarrheal disease accounts for roughly 20% to 25% of all deaths among those persons younger than 5 years of age (Black, Morris, & Bryce, 2003).

Typhoid fever, which results from an enteric infection and, therefore, shares many individual- and community-level risk factors with diarrheal disease, is not accompanied by diarrhea. Although it can be life threatening, this disease has its most profound public health impact through its debilitating effects on school-aged children, causing substantial morbidity and absenteeism from school and work (Medina & Yrarrazaval, 1983).

Etiologic Agents

As noted earlier, diarrheal disease can be caused by a wide variety of viral, bacterial, and parasitic infections. In cases of endemic diarrheal disease, one or more etiologic agents can be identified in 70% to 80% of patients when state-of-the-art laboratory testing is performed. However, many of these agents can also be found in the stools of children who do not have diarrhea, and multiple infectious agents may be present in the same child with diarrhea. Thus the presence of a given causative agent in a stool sample may not mean that it is the cause of that episode of diarrhea.

These complications notwithstanding, the most important etiologic agents in young children in low- and middle-income countries are rotavirus, enterotoxigenic *Escherichia coli* (ETEC), *Shigella* species, *Campylobacter jejuni,* and *Cryptosporidium parvum.* Rotavirus is the single leading cause of nonbloody diarrhea in infants and accounts for an estimated 40% of hospital admissions for diarrhea among children younger than 5 years of age (Parashar, Hummelman, Bresee, Miller, & Glass, 2003), whereas *Shigella* species appear to be the leading cause of bloody diarrhea. Amebiasis (infection with *Entamoeba histolytica*), although frequently diagnosed, appears to be an extremely infrequent cause of bloody diarrhea in young children in low- and middle-income countries. *Vibrio cholerae* is the cause of a substantial proportion of cases of nonbloody diarrhea in endemic areas such as Bangladesh and India (Cholera Working Group, 1993; Nair et al., 1994); it is also the cause of large numbers of cases when epidemics of cholera occur in other regions, such as Africa and Latin America (Glass, Libel, & Brandling-Bennett, 1992; Goodgame & Greenough, 1975). Typhoid fever is caused by *Salmonella typhi.*

Descriptive Epidemiologic Features and Risk Factors

Children experience the highest risk of diarrheal illness between 6 and 11 months of age; the risk declines steadily thereafter (Figure 5-2) (Bern, Martines,

de Zoysa, & Glass, 1992). This age pattern is largely explained by the established risk factors for diarrheal disease and the likely sources of exposure to the causative agents.

The risk of diarrheal disease in young infants is determined in part by the feeding and hand-washing practices of the mother or other childcare providers. Breastfeeding and lack of exposure to contaminated food, water, and other environmental sources are protective factors. As infants grow and become mobile, however, they begin to encounter numerous potential sources of infection with the agents of diarrheal disease, including contaminated water and weaning foods, as well as human and animal waste that has not been disposed of properly. Some evidence also indicates that uncontrolled fly populations can contribute to the risk of diarrheal illnesses—particularly those illnesses caused by etiologic agents requiring a small infectious dose (e.g., shigellosis). Overall, it is estimated that almost 90% of deaths due to diarrheal disease are attributable to unsafe water, inadequate sanitation, and poor hygiene (Black et al., 2003).

As noted earlier, diarrheal disease and malnutrition are intricately intertwined in infants and young children. Although it is not clear that malnutrition is associated with an increased incidence of diarrheal disease, strong evidence indicates that malnutrition increases the likelihood that a child with diarrhea will die or develop persistent diarrhea, and diarrhea in turn has a negative impact on nutritional status and growth. Furthermore, strong evidence supports the contention that deficiencies of vitamin A and zinc are associated with increased morbidity and mortality from diarrheal disease.

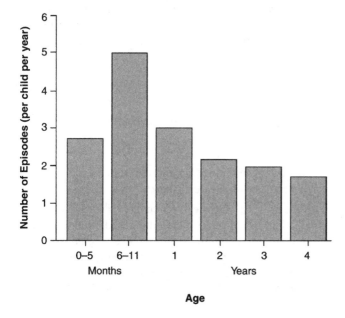

Figure 5-2 Estimated Median Diarrheal Morbidity for Under-Five-Year-Olds, Based on the Results from 18 Studies in Developing Countries. *Source:* C. Bern, J. Martines, I. de Zoysa, and R.I. Glass, "The Magnitude of the Global Problem of Diarrhoeal Disease: A ten year update." 1992, Bulletin of the World Health Organization, 70(6), p. 707. Copyright 1992 by the World Health Organization. Reprinted with Permission.

Unlike diarrheal disease, typhoid fever has long been thought to be a problem primarily in school-aged children. However, infections with *S. typhi* clearly occur in infants and preschool-aged children, and such infections in this younger age group may be substantially underreported (Sinha et al., 1999). More than 20 million new cases of typhoid fever are believed to occur worldwide each year, with the highest rates seen in South and Southeast Asia (Crump, Luby, & Mintz, 2004). *S. typhi* infection is primarily acquired from contaminated food and water.

Current Approaches to Prevention and Control

Unlike the case with ARIs (discussed later in this chapter), a number of approaches to the primary prevention of diarrheal illness have been studied and found to be successful at lowering the rate of diarrheal illness in the community. These measures include providing communities with a protected source of clean drinking water, making home treatment and safe storage of drinking water inexpensive and technologically feasible, improving sanitation through the provision of latrines, promoting hand washing and other personal hygiene habits, reducing the fly population in the community, promoting breastfeeding and proper weaning practices, providing vitamin A supplementation, and various combinations of these interventions (Huttly, Morris, & Pisani, 1997).

Although these approaches have been shown to be effective in well-funded research studies, the feasibility of fostering and sustaining such improvements across large areas and populations is directly linked to the availability of the financial resources and the political will to do so. Many children still lack access to these interventions (Black et al., 2003). In addition, such interventions can generally succeed only when the community is invested in making them work and when they are designed and introduced within a culturally acceptable framework (see Chapter 2).

In parallel with the testing of such primary prevention approaches to reduce the risk of diarrheal disease, since the early 1980s enormous efforts have been directed toward ensuring that infants and children who develop diarrhea suffer a minimum of morbidity and mortality. These efforts have focused on prevention and early treatment of dehydration through proper case management in the home, maintenance of adequate nutritional intake to minimize the impact on growth, and appropriate treatment of infants and children who are brought to health facilities. Mothers and other caretakers of children are educated to use fluids available in the home to prevent dehydration, to use oral rehydration solutions (ORS) or cereal-based

alternative solutions to prevent and treat dehydration, and to continue to breastfeed babies when they have diarrhea. ORS packets are now manufactured in many countries and widely distributed.

At the same time, mothers and healthcare providers have been discouraged from using the wide range of largely ineffective, often expensive, and sometimes dangerous antimicrobial and antidiarrheal agents that are available. Care providers should reserve these antimicrobial agents for the treatment of cholera and of dysentery suspected to be caused by shigellosis and limit the use of intravenous fluids to those who are severely dehydrated. Although promoting and sustaining such changes in diverse countries and in the face of sometimes powerful cultural barriers requires a major effort, studies from Egypt and elsewhere suggest that morbidity and mortality from diarrheal disease have been reduced substantially by such efforts (El-Rafie et al., 1990).

Perhaps in part because of the emphasis given to primary prevention and proper case management for diarrheal disease, the role of vaccines in reducing morbidity and mortality from diarrhea has been quite limited until recently. Vaccines against cholera and typhoid that represent substantial improvements over older vaccines are now available (Sur, Lopez, et al., 2009; Sur, Ochial, et al., 2009), as are newly licensed vaccines against rotavirus that have been shown to be efficacious in Africa, Latin America, and elsewhere (Madhi et al., 2010; Richardson et al., 2010). Although a few countries in which typhoid fever is a major public health problem in school-aged children have begun to administer typhoid vaccines to members of this age group, a longstanding debate has focused on the proper role for vaccines against typhoid, cholera, and other enteric infections and the circumstances under which they should be given routinely in low- and middle-income countries (Keusch & Cash, 1997). The availability of these new vaccines is leading to renewed discussion of how best to use typhoid and cholera vaccines (Levine, 2009; Sridhar, 2009), and rotavirus vaccines are already becoming or soon will become part of the EPI in many countries (Santosham, 2010).

Obstacles to Prevention and Control and Directions for Future Research

The greatest obstacle to reducing further the toll taken by diarrheal disease in low- and middle-income countries is the difficulty and expense of ensuring that everyone has regular access to clean, safe drinking water and adequate sanitation. Although WHO at one point envisioned reaching this goal by 1990, it is now clear that the obstacles to doing so are immense and extraordinarily complex. Substantial investments are needed to improve antiquated and increasingly inadequate water treatment and sewage treatment facilities in the rapidly expanding urban centers of many low- and middle-income countries. The problems associated with ensuring a safe drinking water supply and adequate sanitation in rural areas, although different, are equally challenging to overcome.

Acute Respiratory Infections
Overview

Acute respiratory infections comprise infections of various parts of the respiratory tract, ranging from mild viral and bacterial infections of the upper respiratory tract (e.g., the common cold, viral and group A streptococcal pharyngitis, and middle ear infections) to life-threatening infections of the lower respiratory tract (e.g., bronchiolitis and pneumonia caused by a variety of bacterial and viral agents). Although upper respiratory tract infections globally cause substantial minor morbidity and economic loss through lost time at work, they rarely result in severe morbidity or in mortality. Interestingly, studies suggest that the incidence of upper respiratory tract infections, although varying with age and season, is remarkably similar in free-living populations throughout the world. Because they do not pose a major public health problem and because no effective interventions against them exist, upper respiratory tract infections will not be discussed further in this chapter, except for group A streptococcal pharyngitis, which can lead to rheumatic fever and is discussed later in this section.

Lower respiratory tract infections, in contrast, are the cause of enormous morbidity and of mortality, particularly among infants and young children living in low- and middle-income settings, even when those settings are within generally industrialized countries. In low- and middle-income countries, particularly those with good childhood immunization and oral rehydration therapy programs, lower respiratory tract infections in general, and pneumonias in particular, are typically one of the leading causes of death among infants and children younger than 5 years (Graham, 1990). An estimated 2 million children younger than 5 years die annually from pneumonia and other lower respiratory tract infections, most of them in low-income countries (Rudan, Boschi-Pinto, Biloglav, Mulholland, & Campbell, 2008). This number excludes deaths due to respiratory tract infections that are preventable with vaccines historically included in the EPI (e.g., measles

and pertussis), discussed earlier. However, the accuracy of such estimates is questionable for several reasons: establishing a diagnosis of lower respiratory tract infection or pneumonia is difficult, particularly in settings where chest radiography is not available; many children die outside of hospitals; and other illnesses, such as malaria, make verbal autopsies (i.e., postmortem interviews of next-of-kin to determine the most likely cause of death), an unreliable means of establishing a definitive diagnosis.

Although pneumonia and other lower respiratory tract infections also cause substantial morbidity and mortality in older children and adults, this section focuses on these infections in infants and young children. Pneumonia in adults is discussed briefly later, as is influenza, an important cause of lower respiratory tract infections in children and adults.

Etiologic Agent, Clinical Features, and Vaccine Characteristics

Lower respiratory tract infections can be caused by a variety of viral and bacterial agents, either singly or in combination. Numerous studies conducted in various countries around the world show similar results concerning the etiologic agents responsible for these infections in infants and young children. Excluding respiratory tract infections caused by agents included among the EPI vaccines, the most important viral causes of lower respiratory tract infections are influenza, parainfluenza, respiratory syncytial virus, and adenovirus (Avila et al., 1990). The most important bacterial causes of pneumonia, as determined by lung aspirate studies (in which a needle is passed through the chest wall into affected lung parenchyma, thereby avoiding contamination of samples by flora in the upper airway), are *Streptococcus pneumoniae*, *Haemophilus influenzae*, and *Staphylococcus aureus* (Shann, 1986). Many infants and young children have evidence of dual infections (e.g., a virus and a bacterium), however. Moreover, in as many as one-third of the cases, no etiologic agent can be found using state-of-the-art laboratory techniques.

Descriptive Epidemiologic Features and Risk Factors

Infants and young children living in low- and middle-income environments consistently have been found to experience high incidence rates of pneumonia (Selwyn, 1990). For example, in the Highlands of Papua New Guinea, cumulative incidence rates in the range of 250 to 300 cases per 1,000 infants per year have been observed, compared with a rate in the range of 10 cases per 1,000 infants per year among upper-middle-income children in the United States. At the same time, elevated incidence rates mirroring those in Papua New Guinea have been observed among Native American children living in poverty in the United States. Verbal autopsy studies suggest that 25% to 50% of deaths in children younger than age 5 in low- and middle-income countries are due to pneumonia and other forms of lower respiratory tract infection (Sutrisna, Reingold, Kresno, Harrison, & Utomo, 1993).

The single most important predictor of a child's risk of developing pneumonia or other lower respiratory tract infection is age. The cumulative incidence of lower respiratory tract infections is highest among young infants and drops rapidly with increasing age, reaching markedly lower levels among children by the time they reach 2 or 3 years of age (Selwyn, 1990). Another important predictor of an increased risk of morbidity and mortality from lower respiratory tract infections is low birth weight. Other risk factors for either morbidity or mortality include exposure to indoor air pollution (from cooking, heating, and cigarette smoke), not breastfeeding, and malnutrition, including vitamin A deficiency. These factors are closely intertwined with poverty, inadequate access to health care, and with one another, so their independent effects can be difficult to disentangle (Berman, 1991). HIV infection is almost certainly another important risk factor, although its role in lower respiratory tract infections in infants and young children has not been well studied.

Rheumatic fever following group A streptococcal pharyngitis occurs in a setting of poverty and household crowding. School-aged children are primarily affected acutely, but the damage done to heart valves with this disease is usually permanent, producing life-threatening disability. Population-based data concerning the incidence of acute rheumatic fever and the prevalence of rheumatic heart disease in low- and middle-income countries are infrequently available.

Current Approaches to Prevention and Control

In the 1980s, WHO, together with various partners, began a multifaceted research program intended to develop an approach to reducing the substantial morbidity and mortality due to lower respiratory tract infections in infants and young children (WHO, 1981). This research program and the ARI control program that was subsequently developed were premised on the following observations:

- Upper respiratory tract infections, although frequently occurring, are almost always benign and require only supportive care at home.
- At the time of the program's inception, many lower respiratory tract infections in infants and

young children were not preventable with existing vaccines.

- The major known risk factors for morbidity and mortality from lower respiratory tract infections (e.g., age, low birth weight, malnutrition, and indoor air pollution) are impossible or difficult to change.
- Most morbidity and mortality from lower respiratory tract infections occur in locales where access to medical care is limited and where there are few, if any, diagnostic facilities (i.e., the ability to perform chest x-rays, microbiologic cultures, and other tests).

Given these circumstances, it was decided that an ARI control program based on a triage performed by minimally trained village health workers according to readily observable clinical signs might be feasible, inexpensive, and effective at reducing at least mortality. As a result, a large body of multidisciplinary research relating to the various aspects of such a control program was commissioned and completed. Particularly important was research relating to which readily observable clinical manifestations (e.g., cough, fever, respiratory rate, and chest indrawing), singly or in combination, best distinguished infants or young children with various levels of severity of respiratory tract infection (initially classified as mild, moderate, and severe, but later as no pneumonia, pneumonia, and severe pneumonia).

Based on this research, intervention programs were developed. These efforts were intended to train village health workers or their equivalents in how to assess and classify into one of these categories an infant or young child with signs of a respiratory tract infection. Based on their assessment, the village health workers were to recommend supportive care at home in cases of mild ARI (no pneumonia), provide an oral antimicrobial drug (either ampicillin or cotrimoxazole) and education about home care and follow-up in cases of moderate ARI (pneumonia), or refer the child immediately to the nearest hospital for assessment and inpatient care in cases of severe ARI (severe pneumonia). Well-designed intervention trials were carried out in a variety of countries to assess the efficacy of this approach in reducing mortality due to lower respiratory tract infections. As a meta-analysis of these trials showed, they were almost all successful, reducing mortality due to lower respiratory tract infections and all-cause mortality in infants and in children aged 1 to 4 years (Sazawal & Black, 1992). One caveat should be noted: Almost all of these trials assessed an intervention that included regular household visits by the village health workers in search of infants and children with signs of a respiratory tract infection.

Based on these favorable results, WHO promoted and supported the implementation of ARI control programs largely based on the model of having village health workers (or their equivalent) assess infants and young children with suspected ARI, classify them by severity of illness, and treat or refer them. The impact of such programs on mortality, as distinct from the impact seen in the intervention trials, has not been adequately assessed. These ARI control programs do not include a proactive, outreach component that ensures early case detection (i.e., regular household visits), as was present in the intervention trials, but instead rely solely on maternal recognition of illness and appropriate, timely care seeking; thus they are not likely to have as large an impact as reported in the earlier trials. On the other hand, programs that include some form of regular household visits are likely to be difficult to sustain over the long term.

For a variety of reasons, the emphasis given to ARI control programs (and vertical disease-specific programs in general) by WHO and others has diminished in recent years, and attention has shifted to ensuring that any sick infant or child, regardless of his or her other signs and symptoms, receives appropriate evaluation and care. This approach, referred to as the Integrated Management of Childhood Illness (IMCI), is described in Exhibit 5-3 (Gove, 1997; Lambrechts, Bryce, & Orinda, 1999; Perkins, Broome, Rosenstein, Schuchat, & Reingold, 1997; Weber, Mulholland, Jaffar, Troedsson, Gove, & Greenwood,

1997). Table 5-3 summarizes the interventions included in the IMCI program (Gove, 1997). While a recent study failed to find an effect of the IMCI program on child mortality (Arifeen et al., 2009), improvements in health worker skills and family and community practices (e.g., exclusive breastfeeding and care seeking for illness) were noted.

Prevention of rheumatic fever depends on the recognition of streptococcal pharyngitis and treatment with an appropriate antimicrobial agent (e.g., penicillin or erythromycin). In populations with high rates of acute rheumatic fever, school-based and other programs to detect and treat streptococcal pharyngitis have been suggested as means to combat this disease (Bach et al., 1996).

Obstacles to Prevention and Control and Directions for Future Research

Primary prevention of lower respiratory tract infections, while in part requiring improvements in living conditions and socioeconomic status, is increasingly possible due to the growing availability of affordable vaccines against the major etiologic agents. The safe, highly effective conjugate vaccine against *H. influenzae* type b that led to the virtual disappearance of invasive infections caused by this organism in the United States and other high- and middle-income countries, is now recommended by WHO for inclusion in the EPI of all countries. In turn, funding from the GAVI Alliance is making it possible for the world's poorest countries to introduce this vaccine. It is uncertain what

---

Exhibit 5-3	Integrated Management of Childhood Illness

Throughout the 1970s and 1980s, concerted efforts were made to develop case management strategies for each of the infectious diseases that collectively accounted for the majority of morbidity and mortality among infants and young children in low- and middle-income countries—measles, malaria, diarrheal disease, and acute respiratory infections. Although each of these disease-specific case management strategies has been shown to be effective at reducing severe morbidity and mortality when properly implemented, implementing multiple distinct disease-specific programs that all target the same healthcare providers can lead to overlap, inefficiency, and competition for the attention of an overworked healthcare worker. As a result, various programs within WHO and UNICEF have collaborated in the development of the Integrated Management of Childhood Illness (IMCI), which attempts to pull together into a single, more efficient program the approaches of the various disease-specific control programs (Gove, 1997).

The IMCI program includes both preventive strategies and case management approaches for the illnesses that collectively account for the majority of severe morbidity, mortality, and healthcare provider visits among infants and young children (see Table 5-3). The results of early field assessments of the IMCI algorithm in selected countries suggest that it can be an effective tool, although some modifications may be needed to maximize its usefulness (Lambrechts et al., 1999; Perkins et al., 1997; Weber et al., 1997). A recent evaluation of IMCI programs has shown that they do improve the knowledge of and the quality of the care given by healthcare providers, although an effect on mortality has yet to be demonstrated (Arifeen et al., 2009).

Table 5-3	Child Health Interventions Included in Integrated Management of Childhood Illness	
Case Management Interventions	**Preventive Interventions**
Pneumonia	Immunization during sick child visits (to reduce missed opportunities)
Diarrhea	Nutrition counseling
Dehydration	Breastfeeding support (including the assessment and corrections of
Persistent diarrhea	breastfeeding technique)
Dysentery	
Meningitis, sepsis	
Malaria	
Measles	
Malnutrition	
Anemia	
Ear infection	

Source: Gove, S. (1997). Integrated management of childhood illness by outpatient health workers: Technical basis and overview. *Bulletin of World Health Organization*, 75(suppl 1), 7–24. Copyright 1997 by the World Health Organization. Reprinted with permission.

proportion of morbidity and mortality related to lower respiratory tract infections in such countries will be prevented by this vaccine, because serotype b accounts for only a fraction of all *H. influenzae* infections. Nevertheless, results from a study in Gambia suggest that conjugate *H. influenzae* b vaccine can prevent approximately 20% of radiologically confirmed pneumonias (Mulholland et al., 1997).

Similarly, conjugate pneumococcal vaccines including the most important serotypes of *S. pneumoniae* have been tested and have shown excellent efficacy and safety. A conjugate pneumococcal vaccine including the seven serotypes that collectively accounted for approximately 80% of invasive infections in infants in the United States was approved for use in that country in 2000 and subsequently in other wealthy countries; its widespread use had a profound impact on the rate of invasive pneumococcal infections among infants in the high-income world. Conjugate pneumococcal vaccines with an expanded number of serotypes are now becoming available, and funding from the GAVI Alliance is also making them affordable for the world's poorest countries, many of which have plans in place to introduce conjugate pneumococcal vaccine over the next few years (Frist & Sezibera, 2009). When (or, indeed, if) vaccines against the various viruses (other than influenza) that cause lower respiratory tract infections in infants and small children will become available is uncertain.

Several barriers exist to reducing morbidity and mortality due to lower respiratory tract infections through means other than vaccination and the improvement of living conditions. The first set of barriers relates to ensuring that the parents or guardians of a sick child will seek and have access to appropriate care in a timely fashion. A detailed discussion of care-seeking practices and obstacles to obtaining medical care is beyond the scope of this chapter, but suffice it to say that the obstacles are multifaceted and difficult to overcome. Many challenges also arise in ensuring that those ill infants and children who are brought to medical care facilities receive timely and appropriate care, including adequate assessment, treatment, and follow-up. Finally, concerns have focused on the likelihood that increased use of currently effective and inexpensive antimicrobial agents—particularly use of inappropriate or inadequate regimens—may lead to the development of resistant strains of bacteria (particularly *S. pneumoniae*), which may then not respond to these inexpensive, oral treatment regimens.

Bacterial Meningitis

Overview

Meningitis is a nonspecific term that encompasses inflammation of the meninges (the membranous lining that covers the brain and spinal cord), which can be caused by a wide variety of infectious and noninfectious agents. Such inflammation, regardless of its cause, tends to produce a similar clinical picture—headache, stiff neck, fever, and variable other features. There is substantial overlap between the manifestations of meningitis, which is sometimes referred to as spinal meningitis or cerebrospinal meningitis, and those of many other infectious diseases. Although meningitis can be caused by a wide variety of viruses and other infectious agents (e.g., mycobacteria and parasites), the disease caused by certain bacteria poses a substantial public health threat. Therefore, this section is confined to a discussion of bacterial meningitis, excluding tuberculous meningitis, which is discussed briefly later in the section on tuberculosis.

From a public health perspective, it is important to subdivide bacterial meningitis into its endemic and epidemic forms. Endemic bacterial meningitis, while differing in a number of subtle ways with regard to its descriptive epidemiologic features and the distribution of etiologic agents in low- and middle-income countries versus high-income countries, poses a similar set of challenges in these two different settings. Epidemic bacterial meningitis, for reasons that remain unexplained, has virtually ceased to be a public health problem in industrialized countries since World War II, although small clusters of cases or hyperendemic disease can still be a vexing problem. However, in a number of low- and middle-income countries, particularly those in the "meningitis belt" of sub-Saharan Africa, periodic epidemics of bacterial meningitis continue to occur on a scale never documented in high-income countries. These epidemics can be of such a magnitude and geographic scope as to be properly called public health disasters.

In high-income countries, suspected bacterial meningitis is considered a medical emergency, requiring appropriate clinical specimens for diagnostic testing to be obtained and parenteral antimicrobial therapy in a hospital to be initiated immediately. Even under these ideal conditions, case fatality ratios for bacterial meningitis range from 3% to 25%, with the ratio depending primarily on the specific etiologic agent and the age of the patient. Further, many patients who survive the acute episode will be left with one or more serious sequelae, including deafness, blindness, mental retardation, and seizure disorders. Although the clinical outcomes of hospitalized cases of bacterial meningitis do not, in general, differ between low- and middle-income and high-income countries, the resources available for treating such patients are obviously much more limited in low- and middle-income countries. Furthermore, epidemics involving tens of thousands of such cases obviously cannot be dealt with easily by countries with extremely constrained health budgets and facilities.

Endemic Meningitis

Etiologic Agents

Studies of the etiology of endemic bacterial meningitis in low- and middle-income countries have been hampered by the need for a reasonably well-equipped and staffed microbiology laboratory to conduct such studies. Even so, a number of hospital-based studies have been conducted in areas where or in time periods when epidemic meningitis has not been present. These studies are in general agreement that the leading causes of endemic bacterial meningitis in these settings are *S. pneumoniae, H. influenzae,* and *Neisseria meningitidis*; before the introduction of conjugate *H. influenzae* b and pneumococcal vaccines, these same pathogens were responsible for most cases of bacterial meningitis in high-income countries. Recent reviews have documented the important role of *H. influenzae* b and *S. pneumoniae* in bacterial meningitis (and other syndromes) in low- and middle-income countries (O'Brien et al., 2009; Watt et al., 2009). Other organisms that account for a reasonable proportion of cases in high-income countries, such as group B *Streptococcus* and *Listeria monocytogenes,* appear to be infrequent causes of meningitis in low- and middle-income countries, although this apparent difference may be artifactual. At the same time, meningitis due to *Salmonella* species appears to be more common in low- and middle-income countries than in high-income ones.

Descriptive Epidemiologic Features and Risk Factors

The overall cumulative incidence of endemic bacterial meningitis in low- and middle-income countries appears to be four or five times that in high-income countries, although the data are limited. Somewhere between 1 in 60 and 1 in 300 children die of bacterial meningitis before the age of 5 in nonepidemic areas (Greenwood, 1987). Endemic bacterial meningitis is primarily a problem in infants and young children, although age-specific incidence rates vary with the etiologic agent. Notably, meningitis caused by *H. influenzae* occurs almost exclusively during the first 12 to 24 months of life. Although the highest rates of meningitis due to *S. pneumoniae* and endemic meningitis due to *N. meningitidis* occur in the first 12 to 24 months of life, cases also occur in older children and adults. Endemic bacterial meningitis probably occurs at approximately equal rates among males and females.

Because the three leading causes of endemic bacterial meningitis are all spread via respiratory droplets, poverty and the resulting crowding increase the risk for this disease. Failure to breastfeed has been shown to be a risk factor in high-income countries and probably increases the risk in low- and middle-income countries as well. Host factors also play an important role in determining the risk of endemic bacterial meningitis, most notably sickle cell disease and HIV infection. Sickle cell disease is associated with a markedly increased risk of infection with *S. pneumoniae*. Meningitis due to *S. pneumoniae*, like that caused by *Salmonella*, also occurs at a substantially increased rate among HIV-infected children and adults. In addition, malnutrition and anemia have been suspected to be risk factors for bacterial meningitis.

Current Approaches to Prevention and Control

Until recently, little or nothing was done to prevent endemic bacterial meningitis in low- and middle-income countries. However, bacterial meningitis due to *H. influenzae* b and many serotypes of S. pneumoniae is now preventable with vaccines produced by conjugating the bacterial polysaccharide to one of several protein molecules. The widespread use of these vaccines has led to the virtual eradication of meningitis due to *H. influenzae* b and sharp reductions in the incidence of meningitis due to *S. pneumoniae* in high-income countries. Funding from the GAVI Alliance is now making these vaccines more widely available in poor countries (see Exhibit 5-2). Although a portion of the incidence of endemic meningitis attributable to *N. meningitidis* could be prevented with existing purified polysaccharide and conjugate vaccines against serogroups C, Y, and W-135 and more recently developed vaccines against serogroup B, these vaccines are not in widespread use outside selected low- and middle-income countries (e.g., Brazil and Cuba are routinely using a vaccine against serogroup B *N. meningitidis*).

Chemoprophylaxis—that is, the giving of a short course of an antimicrobial agent to individuals in close contact with someone with bacterial meningitis due to *N. meningitidis* or *H. influenzae* type b—has been used with some success in high-income countries, but has not been widely advocated in low- and middle-income countries because of the small percentage of endemic cases that occur in close contacts of a known case, the cost and availability of the antimicrobial agents, the limited duration of the protection achieved, concerns about promoting the development of antimicrobial resistance, and logistical problems related to implementation.

Obstacles to Prevention and Control and Directions for Future Research

The primary obstacle to preventing endemic meningitis due to *H. influenzae* b and *S. pneumoniae* in low- and middle-income countries has been the cost of the highly effective and safe conjugate vaccines now used in high-income countries. As economic barriers to the introduction of these vaccines in low- and middle income are removed, endemic meningitis due

to these organisms may be markedly reduced or nearly eliminated. Prevention of endemic meningococcal meningitis in most low- and middle-income countries must await the widespread availability of serogroup B and C conjugate vaccines that are effective in infants, provide protection against multiple serotypes of serogroup B, and are affordable.

Epidemic Meningitis

Etiologic Agents

Epidemic bacterial meningitis is almost always caused by *N. meningitidis*. More specifically, serogroup A *N. meningitidis* causes most such epidemics, although epidemics due to serogroup C also have been well documented. The appearance in recent years of explosive outbreaks caused by serogroup W-135 has complicated efforts to control or prevent epidemics of meningococcal meningitis using vaccines (Bertherat, Yada, Djingarey, & Koumare, 2002). Serogroup B *N. meningitidis*, one of the most important causes of endemic bacterial meningitis, has led to "epidemics" in a variety of high-income and low- and middle-income countries, but these outbreaks are never of the scope and intensity of those caused by serogroup A, differing in overall attack rates by as much as two orders of magnitude.

Descriptive Epidemiologic Features and Risk Factors

Epidemic bacterial meningitis, generally caused by serogroup A *N. meningitidis*, is one of the most interesting but least understood infectious diseases in the world. Epidemics involving hundreds of thousands of cases and cumulative incidence rates of almost 2,000 cases per 100,000 total population have been observed in the "meningitis belt" of Africa (Figure 5-3) for more than 100 years (Moore, 1992). An epidemic there in the 1990s was one of the largest ever recorded and extended into parts of Africa not previously considered to be in the meningitis belt. In this region of Africa, epidemics in a given area last for 2 or 3 years and recur every 5 to 15 years. They occur only during the hot, dry season (January to April) and dissipate when the rains and cooler weather arrive, only to return the next dry season. The interepidemic period can vary from a few years to a decade or more, probably reflecting a combination of the time it takes to reaccumulate enough susceptible individuals to sustain an epidemic, the introduction of a new virulent strain of *N. meningitidis*, prior use of polysaccharide meningococcal vaccine in the population, and other poorly defined factors (Moore, 1992).

Epidemics of meningococcal meningitis have also occurred in Asia and Latin America. In western

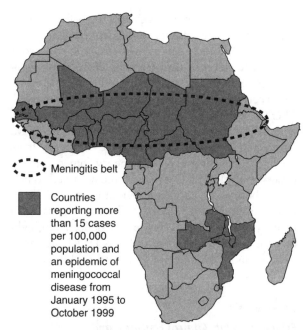

Meningitis belt

Countries reporting more than 15 cases per 100,000 population and an epidemic of meningococcal disease from January 1995 to October 1999

Figure 5-3 The Meningitis Belt of sub-Saharan Africa. *Source:* WHO Report on Global Surveillence of Epidemic-prone Infectious Diseases. WHO/CDS/CSR/ISR/2000.1 http://www.who.int/csr/resources/publications/surveillance/ WHO_CDS_CSR_ISR_2000_1/en/. Copyright 2009 by the World Health Organization. Reprinted with permission.

China and Nepal, the epidemics follow a pattern similar to that seen in Africa, except that they occur during a cold, dry season rather than a hot, dry season. In Latin America, Brazil has borne the brunt of such epidemics due to both serogroups A and C. Epidemics have also occurred in countries in the Middle East (e.g., Saudi Arabia) and the Pacific (e.g., New Zealand).

Current Approaches to Prevention and Control

Historically, efforts to reduce morbidity and mortality from epidemic meningococcal meningitis have been reactive in nature. That is, once an epidemic is detected, a vaccination campaign is implemented as rapidly as possible, and the antimicrobial agents and other materials needed to treat cases appropriately are made available in the affected area. This approach has been rightly criticized on the grounds that seemingly unavoidable delays arise when mounting such campaigns, during which time many cases (and resulting morbidity and mortality) occur. Such reactive vaccination campaigns are almost inevitably disruptive of other health programs, and the extent to which they actually reduce the size of the epidemic is often

debated. Furthermore, shortages of the purified polysaccharide vaccine used in these campaigns continue to occur (Wakabi, 2009).

One approach to improving the control of such epidemics that has been suggested is enhanced surveillance for bacterial meningitis in areas susceptible to epidemics (e.g., the meningitis belt of Africa), use of a predetermined threshold rate of cases to declare an epidemic and mount a vaccination campaign, and stockpiling of vaccines and other supplies and equipment in the immediate area (WHO, 1995). Unfortunately, projections suggest that even these steps would result in the prevention of no more than 40% to 50% of the cases that would otherwise occur, and initial attempts to establish such early detection and response capabilities have demonstrated the limitations of this approach.

Others have proposed routinely vaccinating all infants, children, and young adults in areas at risk of such epidemics with meningococcal A polysaccharide vaccine (Robbins, Towne, Gotschlich, & Schneerson, 1997). However, the need to give three or more doses of this vaccine, and at least one of these at age 3 or 4 years to possibly achieve long-term protection, has raised concerns about the costs and feasibility of such an approach (Perkins et al., 1997). Furthermore, the recent large outbreak of meningococcal meningitis caused by serogroup W-135 suggests that any meningococcal vaccine used routinely in this part of the world may need to protect against at least three serogroups—A, C, and W-135.

Obstacles to Prevention and Control and Directions for Future Research

Recognizing the limitations of an approach to controlling or preventing epidemic meningococcal meningitis epidemics based on the existing purified polysaccharide vaccines against serogroup A, a group of vaccine manufacturers and philanthropic organizations has developed a monovalent (i.e., serogroup A only) conjugate vaccine using an approach similar to that employed in making the *H. influenzae* b and *S. pneumoniae* vaccines used to successfully immunize infants. This vaccine, which is being produced in India and made available in large quantities at a very low price, has been shown in clinical trials to be immunogenic. Current plans call for its use in the countries in the meningitis belt of Africa in population-wide campaigns focused on children and young adults, followed by its introduction into the routine infant immunization schedules of these countries; the first such campaign occurred in Burkina Faso at the end of 2010. While this program, if fully funded and successfully implemented, is expected to prevent the devastating epidemics caused by serogroup A *N. meningitidis,* it is uncertain whether other *N. meningitidis* serogroups capable of causing epidemics, especially serogroups C and W-135, will become more common causes of endemic or epidemic disease in this region.

Mycobacterial Infections

Overview

Although many species of mycobacteria can infect people, only two cause sufficient human illness in low- and middle-income countries to warrant discussion here—*Mycobacterium tuberculosis,* the cause of tuberculosis (TB), and *Mycobacterium leprae,* the cause of leprosy. Although *Mycobacterium bovis* (which is closely related to *M. tuberculosis*) can cause TB in humans, it accounts for only a small percentage of cases, and these cases are generally not distinguishable from or in need of different treatment than cases caused by *M. tuberculosis.* Other than *M. leprae,* the various nontuberculous mycobacteria cause opportunistic infections that occur almost exclusively in immunocompromised individuals. Whereas these nontuberculous mycobacteria—particularly *Mycobacterium avium* complex—have caused substantial morbidity and mortality among AIDS patients in high-income countries, they appear to be uncommon in AIDS patients in low- and middle-income countries.

Tuberculosis and infection with *M. tuberculosis* are, by every indicator available, among the most important public health problems in the world. Approximately one-third of the world's population (2 billion persons) is believed to be infected with *M. tuberculosis,* and in 2008 there were 9.4 million new cases of TB and 1.8 million deaths from TB, including 500,000 deaths of people with HIV (WHO, 2009a). Because suppression of the body's immune system is the most important determinant of which individuals infected with *M. tuberculosis* will subsequently develop TB, the AIDS epidemic has had disastrous consequences for the control of TB, which was underfunded and inadequate in most low- and middle-income countries even before the arrival of HIV. In recognition of the gravity of the problems posed by it, WHO declared TB to be a global emergency in 1993.

A disease that many believe to have been leprosy was described in the Old Testament of the Bible. Leprosy occupies a unique position among human diseases, in part because of the disfigurement that it

can produce and in part because of the belief in many cultures that it represents some form of divine punishment. Although leprosy was endemic to Europe during the eleventh through thirteenth centuries, it had virtually disappeared from there by the eighteenth century, long before modern medicine arrived. There is speculation that the rise of TB and infection with *M. tuberculosis* produced cross-immunity to *M. leprae* and led to the disappearance of leprosy from Europe. Some support for this theory comes from the observation that BCG—the vaccine intended to prevent tuberculosis—appears to be at least partially effective in preventing leprosy. Whatever the cause of its near-total (but not complete) absence from high-income countries, leprosy today is largely confined to a shrinking number of low- and middle-income countries.

Tuberculosis

Etiologic Agent, Clinical Features, and Vaccine Characteristics

Compared with other bacteria, mycobacteria are slow growing and have special nutritional needs. *M. tuberculosis* can be recovered from clinical specimens, particularly those from the respiratory tract, when appropriate artificial media and techniques are used, but the process takes many weeks and requires a laboratory with a modest level of sophistication and resources. Furthermore, it can be difficult to obtain a specimen of respiratory tract secretions, particularly from a child. As a result, most cases of TB in low- and middle-income countries are diagnosed and treated based on examination of respiratory tract secretions under a microscope, radiologic findings on chest x-ray, or clinical grounds.

Descriptive Epidemiologic Features and Risk Factors

M. tuberculosis is spread via respiratory droplets produced when an individual with active pulmonary TB, particularly smear-positive TB (in which more organisms are present in the sputum), coughs or sneezes. Individuals in close contact with a person with untreated TB—particularly household contacts—are at highest risk of becoming infected. In low- and middle-income countries, the highest incidence rates of pulmonary TB occur in men and women of reproductive age, meaning that there are often infants and young children in the household in close contact with individuals with active pulmonary TB. As a result, a high proportion of individuals will be exposed to and infected with *M. tuberculosis* in childhood.

Although a small proportion of infected infants and children will develop pulmonary or extrapulmonary TB soon after becoming infected, in most instances the immune system successfully walls off, but does not kill, all the *M. tuberculosis* organisms. As these infected children grow up, various factors—particularly HIV infection and malnutrition—can reduce the ability of the immune system to keep the organisms in check, and reactivation TB can occur. Before the AIDS epidemic, it was estimated that 5% of persons infected as children developed TB soon after infection and another 5% developed TB at some point later in life. However, untreated HIV infection is such a potent inhibitor of cell-mediated immunity (the part of the immune system that holds *M. tuberculosis* infection in check) that a high proportion of untreated dually infected individuals (i.e., infected with both HIV and *M. tuberculosis*) can be expected to develop TB unless they die of something else first or receive preventive therapy.

Almost 2 million people die from TB and 8 to 10 million people experience the onset of the disease each year, with the vast majority of these deaths and illnesses occurring in low-income countries (WHO, 2009a). Although TB is a major public health problem in virtually every low-income country, the burden of disease attributable to it varies by region and country, in part because of longstanding historical differences in the incidence of TB and the prevalence of infection with *M. tuberculosis,* in part because of local differences in the adequacy of TB control programs, and in part because of differences in the extent of the HIV/AIDS epidemic. Based on admittedly incomplete passive surveillance for reported cases of TB and on tuberculin skin test surveys, it appears that sub-Saharan Africa has the highest average annual risk of infection with *M. tuberculosis* and the highest crude incidence rate of cases of TB (Figure 5-4). The largest numbers of cases of TB are seen in India and China, which account for 35% of TB cases globally (WHO, 2009a). Because of the HIV/AIDS epidemic and unrelated demographic changes (e.g., population growth and increases in the numbers of individuals surviving to their thirties and forties), it has been projected that the number of new TB cases will increase in coming years in low- and middle-income countries worldwide.

Although TB occurs in individuals in all socioeconomic strata, it is quintessentially a disease of poverty. Through its effect on crowding, poverty increases the risk of airborne transmission of *M. tuberculosis.* At the same time, through its negative effect on nutritional status, poverty increases the risk that someone infected with *M. tuberculosis* will develop TB. HIV infection is also more prevalent among poor popu-

lations, further increasing the likelihood that an infected individual will develop TB. Finally, through its effect on access to curative medical care, poverty increases the likelihood that a patient with symptomatic pulmonary TB will remain untreated and hence infectious for a longer period of time, which in turn increases the incidence of TB in low-income communities.

Current Approaches to Prevention and Control

Tuberculosis control programs exist in virtually all low- and middle-income countries, although enormous variability exists in terms of the resources at their disposal and their effectiveness. The current approach to controlling TB in low- and middle-income countries is based on a strategy of rapid detection of and provision of effective multidrug therapy to all infectious persons (i.e., patients with pulmonary TB, particularly smear-positive patients).

Since 1995, a key component of WHO recommendations has been directly observed treatment, short-course (DOTS), which involves the use of a standardized multidrug short-course regimen, with direct observation of drug ingestion for at least the first 2 months of treatment. In 2006, WHO adopted the Stop TB Strategy (Table 5-4), whose key components are as follows:

1. "Pursue high-quality DOTS expansion and enhancement
2. Address TB/HIV, multi-drug resistant (MDR)-TB, and the needs of poor and vulnerable populations
3. Contribute to a health system strengthening based on primary health care
4. Engage all care providers
5. Empower people with TB, and communities through partnership
6. Enable and promote research (WHO, 2006a)"

In the face of the limited resources available to ensure prompt diagnosis and treatment of infectious cases of TB among those who present spontaneously to health facilities, there has been an understandable reluctance in low- and middle-income countries to devote scarce resources to actively searching for other cases in the households of affected individuals or in the community. Similarly, prophylactic treatment of latent TB infection in the general population has not been considered a high priority or an effective use of limited resources. In addition, the use of a single drug, such as isoniazid, to reduce the likelihood of TB in

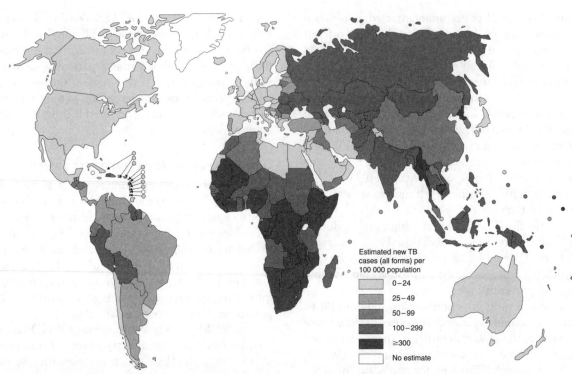

Figure 5-4A Estimated Tuberculosis Incidence Rates, 2008. *Source:* Global Tuberculosis Control: A short update to the 2009 report; http://www.who.int/tb/publications/global_report/2009/update/en/index.html; ISBN: 978-92-4-159886-6. Copyright 2009 by the World Health Organization. Reprinted with permission.

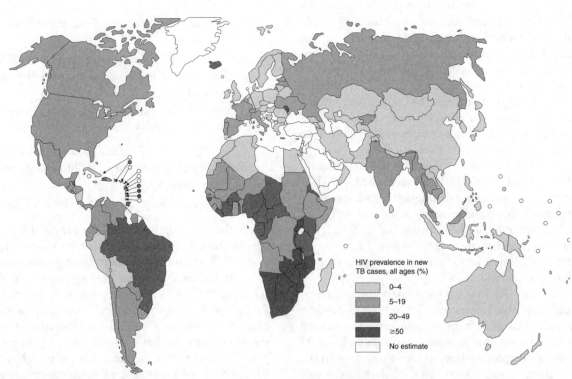

Figure 5-4B Estimated HIV Prevalence in new Tuberculosis Cases, 2008. *Source:* Global Tuberculosis Control: A short update to the 2009 report; http://www.who.int/tb/publications/global_report/2009/update/en/index.html; ISBN: 978-92-4-159886-6. Copyright 2009 by the World Health Organization. Reprinted with permission.

Table 5-4	The Stop TB Strategy at a Glance
Vision	A world free of TB.
Goal	To dramatically reduce the global burden of TB by 2015 in line with the Millennium Development Goals (MDG) and the Stop TB Partnership targets.
Objectives	• Achieve universal access to high-quality diagnosis and patient-centered treatment. • Reduce the human suffering and socioeconomic burden associated with TB. • Protect poor and vulnerable populations from TB, TB/HIV, and multidrug-resistant TB. • Support development of new tools and enable their timely and effective use.

Target	• MDG 6, Target 8: Halt and begin to reverse the incidence of TB by 2015.
	• Targets linked to the MDGs and endorsed by the Stop TB Partnership:
	  ○ By 2005: detect at least 70% of new sputum smear-positive TB cases and cure at least 85% of these cases
	  ○ By 2015: reduce TB prevalence and death rates by 50% relative to 1990
	  ○ By 2050: eliminate TB as a public health problem (fewer than 1 case per 1 million population)

Components of the Strategy and Implementation Approaches

1. Pursue High-Quality DOTS Expansion and Enhancement
Political commitment with increased and sustained financing
Case detection through quality-assured bacteriology
Standardized treatment with supervision and patient support
An effective drug supply and management system
Monitoring and evaluation system, and impact measurement

2. Address TB/HIV, MDR-TB, and Other Challenges
Implement collaborative TB/HIV activities
Prevent and control multidrug-resistant TB
Address prisoners, refugees, and other high-risk groups, and special situations

3. Contribute to Health System Strengthening
Actively participate in efforts to improve system-wide policy, human resources, financing, management,
  service delivery, and information systems
Share innovations that strengthen systems, including the Practical Approach to Lung Health (PAL)
Adapt innovations from other fields

4. Engage All Care Providers
Public–public and public–private mix (PPM) approach
International Standards for Tuberculosis Care (ISTC)

5. Empower People with TB and Communities
Advocacy, communication, and social mobilization
Community participation in TB care
Patients' Charter for Tuberculosis Care

6. Enable and Promote Research
Programme-based operational research
Research to develop new diagnostics, drugs, and vaccines

Source: The Stop TB Strategy: Building on and Enhancing DOTS to Meet the TB-related Millenium Development Goals.
http://whqlibdoc.who.int/hq/2006/WHO_HTM_STB_2006.368_eng.pdf. Copyright 2006 by the World Health Organization. Reprinted with permission.

individuals infected with *M. tuberculosis* (as practiced in a number of high-income countries) has raised the specter of inadvertent single-drug therapy of patients with unrecognized TB and resultant promotion of the development of drug-resistant strains of *M. tuberculosis*. Preventive therapy is effective in preventing TB among HIV-infected individuals in low- and middle-income countries (Whalen et al., 1997), however, WHO recommends isoniazid preventative treatment for HIV-positive persons living in areas with high TB infection prevalence (i.e., where more than 30% of the population has latent TB infection) and for those with latent TB infection or exposure to an infectious TB case.

Immunization at birth with BCG is a standard part of the EPI in every low- and middle-income country, and BCG coverage is high in almost every such country. Infant immunization with BCG appears to be quite effective at reducing the risk of disseminated TB (e.g., tuberculous meningitis) in infants and children, but the vaccine's efficacy against pulmonary TB in this age group is probably no better than 50% to 60%. Infant immunization with BCG probably has, at best, only a modest effect on the risk of developing pulmonary TB as an adult and consequently has little or no impact on the spread of M. *tuberculosis* in the community.

Obstacles to Prevention and Control and Directions for Future Research

The rapid growth of MDR-TB (i.e., TB resistant to the first-line anti-TB drugs isoniazid and rifampicin) and the emergence of extremely drug-resistant tuberculosis (XDR-TB; i.e., TB resistant to isoniazid, rifampicin, fluoroquinolones, and kanamycin, capreomycin, or amikacin) have complicated TB control efforts. Both MDR-TB and XDR-TB require lengthy treatment with second-line drugs, which are both more expensive and more toxic than the first-line drugs. Although WHO supports universal access to treatment of drug-resistant TB, scaling up of treatment availability is not always possible due to a lack of laboratory capacity to diagnose the drug-resistant form of the disease and funds for both capacity building and treatment.

As noted earlier, demographic changes and the HIV/AIDS epidemic virtually ensure that the global burden of TB will rise over the coming years. At present, the principal obstacles to reducing TB-related morbidity and mortality in low- and middle-income countries are economic and operational in nature. Increased financial and technical assistance will be needed in many countries to ensure that currently available strategies for controlling TB are fully implemented.

At the same time, further research is needed in multiple areas if control of TB is to be achieved and sustained. Development of new drugs that are effective against M. *tuberculosis,* affordable and safe, and able to clear the infection with a shorter duration of treatment is a high priority, but such drugs are unlikely to enter the market anytime soon. Similarly, development of a vaccine against M. *tuberculosis* that can prevent pulmonary TB is a high priority, but is not currently within view. In the meantime, operational research into how to enhance case detection and en-

sure dispensing of and compliance with proper treatment is needed.

Leprosy

Etiologic Agent, Clinical Features, and Vaccine Characteristics

M. *leprae* cannot be grown on artificial media. In research laboratories, it can be isolated and propagated in the foot pad of a mouse or in armadillos, but these techniques have no relevance to diagnosing leprosy. The diagnosis of leprosy is made on clinical grounds, together with histopathologic examination of tissue biopsy material. M. *leprae* grows even more slowly than M. *tuberculosis*. Its slow growth is highly relevant to the control and prevention of leprosy because of the consequent need to treat those who are infected for prolonged periods of time (months to years) and the resulting difficulty of ensuring compliance with antimicrobial therapy long after the individual feels well.

Descriptive Epidemiologic Features and Risk Factors

Although it is clear that prolonged, close contact (e.g., living in the same household) with someone with untreated leprosy—and particularly with someone having a high burden of organisms (i.e., multibacillary leprosy)—is associated with a substantially increased risk of acquiring the disease, the routes of transmission are ill defined. It is assumed that transmission occurs primarily through skin-to-skin contact or exposure to respiratory tract (e.g., nasal) secretions. Environmental or animal reservoirs of M. *leprae* are thought to have little or no role in human infections. The exceedingly long incubation period for leprosy, which is believed to be years to decades, makes any study of transmission very difficult.

Leprosy is primarily a disease of poverty. Even within a single relatively homogeneous community, it is disproportionately seen among the lowest-income members. Leprosy has often been described as being more common in rural than in urban populations and as having an association with proximity to water (e.g., lakes) or humidity, but clear differences in the prevalence of leprosy between neighboring communities are not well explained.

In the mid-1980s, the number of cases of leprosy worldwide was estimated to be between 10 and 12 million. The incidence of leprosy was 4 to 6 cases per 1,000 population, and the prevalence in affected countries often exceeded 10 individuals per 1,000 population. By 1998, control efforts had reduced the number of prevalent cases by more than 90%, to an estimated 829,000 cases worldwide (WHO, 1998a). A decade later, WHO reported that there were 249,007 newly detected cases in 2008 (WHO, 2010a). Although leprosy previously existed throughout the world, and a handful of individuals living in high-income countries such as the United States still develop leprosy each year (a few of whom have never traveled outside the United States), leprosy is now largely confined to a shrinking number of countries. In 2006, only 4 countries—Brazil, Democratic Republic of the Congo, Mozambique, and Nepal—had a prevalence of more than 1 case per 10,000 persons (WHO, 2007a).

Current Approaches to Prevention and Control

Early attempts to control leprosy were based on case finding and prolonged (i.e., multiyear) or lifetime treatment with dapsone, which had the advantages of being inexpensive and having few side effects. However, this approach failed to control leprosy, at least in part because *M. leprae* developed resistance to dapsone and because it was difficult to ensure ongoing patient compliance with treatment over many years.

In the early 1980s, multidrug treatment with two or three effective antimicrobial agents (depending on the stage of leprosy) was introduced and has produced a greater than 90% reduction in leprosy cases. WHO had set a goal of eliminating leprosy as a public health problem (i.e., achieving a prevalence of 1 case or fewer per 10,000) by the year 2000; that goal was reached in 107 of the 122 countries that had endemic leprosy in 1985. However, further progress in achieving the stated goal has been hampered by reduced funding for treatment and control efforts. In addition, use of disease prevalence as an indicator of program success is now recognized as problematic due to the lengthy incubation period of leprosy. Currently, progress is monitored using the annual number of new cases diagnosed.

Obstacles to Prevention and Control and Directions for Future Research

Because of its extremely long incubation period and the fact that infected individuals may transmit *M. leprae* for substantial periods of time prior to becoming symptomatic and receiving treatment, it is likely that incident cases of leprosy will continue to occur in substantial numbers for years to come, even if the current leprosy control strategies substantially reduce transmission (Meima, Smith, van Oortmarassen, Richardus, & Habbema, 2004).

The role, if any, for a vaccine in the immunotherapy or the prevention of leprosy remains uncertain. Numerous studies—both experimental and observational in nature—have suggested that the BCG vaccine, which is given primarily to prevent various forms of disseminated TB in children, offers some protection against leprosy. A meta-analysis performed in 2006 showed an overall protective effect of 61% in observational studies and an overall protective effect of 26% in experimental studies, providing further evidence that BCG is modestly effective against leprosy, and that two doses of BCG are more effective against leprosy than a single dose (Setia, Steinmaus, Ho, & Rutherford, 2006). Whether other candidate mycobacterial vaccines will offer even greater protection than BCG remains uncertain, as does their role, if any, in leprosy control.

Sexually Transmitted Infections and AIDS

Overview

Sexually transmitted infections have historically been one of the most neglected areas of medicine and public health in low- and middle-income countries. Until the advent of the HIV/AIDS epidemic in the 1980s, remarkably little attention was paid to STIs in such countries, despite the fact that they collectively cause enormous morbidity, loss of productivity, and infertility, and result in substantial healthcare expenditures. The fact that human immunodeficiency virus (HIV)—the cause of AIDS and all its attendant morbidity and mortality—is transmitted sexually, together with the fact that the sexual transmission of HIV is facilitated by the presence of other STIs, has focused attention on and brought an infusion of resources into this long-neglected area.

The myriad challenges confronting the treatment and control of STIs in low- and middle-income countries are multifaceted and complex. Among the most daunting are the difficulty of changing human sexual behavior; the frequency with which STIs are asymptomatic, particularly among women; the lack of simple, inexpensive diagnostic tests for such infections; and the lack of readily accessible, inexpensive, easy-to-administer, single-dose treatment regimens for most STIs.

Etiologic Agents

A variety of viruses and bacteria can be transmitted sexually (Table 5-5), including some (e.g., HBV) that are not traditionally grouped with other STIs. In this chapter, HBV is discussed with the other viruses that cause hepatitis. Many infectious agents that are transmitted sexually can also be transmitted via contaminated blood or injection equipment, and vertically from a mother to her newborn infant.

Table 5-5	Sexually Transmitted Infections of Importance in Low- and Middle-Income Countries			
Agent	**Disease**	**Vertical Transmission To Newborn Babies**	**Transmission via Blood Products**
Bacteria			
Treponema pallidum	Syphilis	Yes	Yes
Neisseria gonorrhoea	Gonorrhea, pelvic inflammatory disease	Yes	Yes
Chlamydia trachomatis	Cervicitis, urethritis, lymphogranuloma venereum, pelvic inflammatory disease	Yes	No
Haemophilus ducreyii	Chancroid	No	No
Viruses			
Human immunodeficiency virus (HIV)	AIDS	Yes	Yes
Herpes simplex	Genital herpes	Yes	No
Human papilloma (HPV)	Genital warts, cervical dysplasia and cervical carcinoma	?	No
Hepatitis B virus[a]	Acute and chronic hepatitis, cirrhosis, and hepatocellular carcinoma	Yes	Yes
Other			
Trichomonas vaginalis	Vaginitis	No	No

[a]Discussed in the section on viral hepatitis.

Of the infectious agents transmitted sexually, some initially cause ulcerative lesions, primarily on or near the genitalia (e.g., *Herpes simplex*, *Treponema pallidum*, and *Haemophilus ducreyii*), others initially cause urethral or vaginal discharge (e.g., *Neisseria gonorrhoea*, *Chlamydia trachomatis,* and *Trichomonas vaginalis*), and others cause only systemic manifestations (e.g., HIV). HPV, selected subtypes of which cause genital warts, plays an important role in the pathogenesis of cervical dysplasia and carcinoma, as well as in carcinoma of the penis, but most HPV infections are initially silent. Asymptomatic or minimally symptomatic infection with many of the sexually transmitted agents is common, greatly exacerbating the problem of interrupting transmission and reducing the prevalence and incidence of infection.

Many of the agents transmitted sexually produce not only acute symptoms referable to the lower genital tract, but also other, often more serious manifestations. For example, untreated infections with *N. gonorrhoea* and *C. trachomatis* can ascend the genital tract and produce pelvic inflammatory disease, tubal infertility, and ectopic pregnancy. Untreated primary syphilis in young adults can lead to life-threatening cardiac and neurologic complications due to tertiary syphilis years later. In addition, congenital syphilis—the result of infection of a baby at the time of birth—produces profound systemic manifestations. As noted earlier, infection with HPV of selected subtypes is strongly associated with subsequent cervical dysplasia and cervical cancer. Finally, HIV causes profound damage to the host immune system and a virtually 100% case fatality ratio in the absence of treatment with antiretroviral drug regimens.

Descriptive Epidemiologic Features and Risk Factors

Data concerning the incidence of STIs in low- and middle-income countries are considered highly unreliable due to substantial underdiagnosis and underreporting. According to one estimate, 340 million new adult cases of curable STIs (e.g., gonorrhea, chlamydia, syphilis, and trichomoniasis) occurred worldwide in 1999, the vast majority of which were in low- and middle-income countries (Figure 5-5).

The number of noncurable STIs, including genital herpes, HPV, and HIV, is difficult to estimate. The passive surveillance for AIDS in place in most low- and middle-income countries is also not very sensitive or specific, making it necessary to estimate the preva-

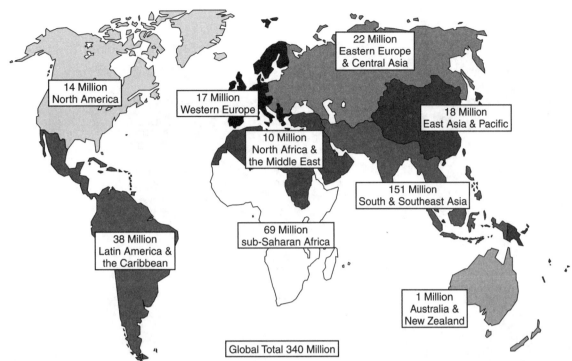

Figure 5-5 Estimated New Cases of Curable STIs Among Adults, 1999. *Source*: Global Prevalence and Incidence of Selected Curable STIs Among Adults. http://www.who.int/hiv/pub/sti/en/who_hiv_aids_2001.02.pdf Copyright 2001 by the World Health Organization. Reprinted with permission.

lence and incidence of AIDS cases. The most recent estimate is that there were 31.4 to 35.3 million persons in the world living with HIV/AIDS in 2009, including 2.6 million people who became infected in that year. While almost two-thirds of all people living with HIV in 2009 resided in sub-Saharan Africa, the incidence of new infections is rising most rapidly in selected Asian countries (e.g., China, India, Vietnam, and Indonesia) and in eastern Europe (e.g., Estonia, Latvia, Ukraine, and the Russian Federation) (Figure 5-6; UNAIDS, 2009). More than 25 million people had died of AIDS since the beginning of the epidemic through the end of 2009 (the last year for which estimates are available), and 14 million children had been orphaned (UNAIDS, 2009). The vast majority of deaths have been in low-income countries, particularly sub-Saharan Africa.

The prevalence of various STIs, particularly HIV, has been investigated in many low- and middle-income countries. The groups typically examined are those that can be studied easily and inexpensively, such as commercial sex workers, patients being treated for STIs or tuberculosis, injection drug users, pregnant women or women giving birth, and blood donors. Prevalences of HIV infection as high as 70% to 85% have been seen among commercial sex workers, and prevalences in the range of 25% to 45% have

been documented among pregnant women delivering at large urban hospitals in the worst-affected urban areas of sub-Saharan Africa (UNAIDS, 2008). Because an estimated 15% to 30% of untreated HIV-infected pregnant women will pass the virus to their newborn babies at or soon after delivery, large numbers of HIV-infected infants are also found wherever many women of reproductive age are infected. The result of widespread HIV infection among men and women of reproductive age and among infants in the most severely affected countries, in the absence of antiretroviral treatment (ART), has been a reversal of prior gains in life expectancy and prior reductions in infant and child mortality rates, an enormous increase in the number of orphaned children, and projected future declines in population size.

Given that the infectious agents under discussion are transmitted through sexual contact, it is not surprising that the highest incidence and prevalence rates of these infections are seen among men and women who are most sexually active, typically those 15 to 49 years of age. In addition, the most important risk factors for STIs—number of sexual partners, concurrency of sexual partnerships, type of sexual partners, and whether barrier protection (e.g., a male condom) is used—are directly or indirectly related to the likelihood of exposure to one of the infectious agents.

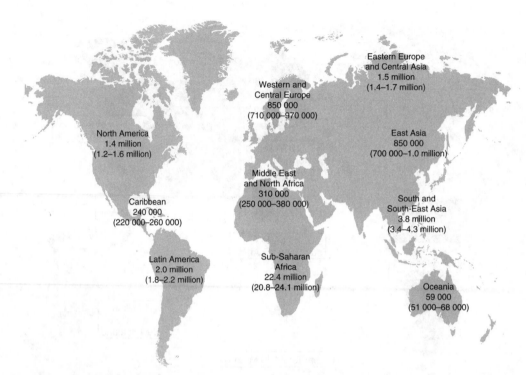

Figure 5-6 Adults and Children Estimated to Be Living with HIV/AIDS, 2008. *Source*: 09 AIDS Epidemic Update. http://data.unaids.org/pub/Report/2009/JC1700_Epi_Update_2009_en.pdf; UNAIDS/09.36E/JC1700E. Copyright 2009 by UNAIDS and WHO. Reprinted with permission.

Thus individuals with large numbers of sexual partners (e.g., commercial sex workers) who do not use barrier protection and those who have unprotected sex with such individuals, as well as those with multiple concurrent sexual partners, are at highest risk. In societies in which it is considered acceptable for men to frequent commercial sex workers or have multiple concurrent sexual partners while women are expected to have a single partner, many monogamous women acquire STIs from their husbands. Other risk factors for STIs, including HIV, have also been demonstrated, such as lack of male circumcision.

It is important to note the complex interplay between HIV infection and other STIs. There is strong evidence that infection with both ulcerative and nonulcerative STIs increases the likelihood of HIV being transmitted sexually between partners, either through the presence of disrupted mucosa or the presence in the genital tract of increased numbers of inflammatory cells and lymphocytes that can bind HIV.

Current Approaches to Prevention and Control

The current approach to the prevention and control of STIs, including HIV, focuses on improving the availability of and access to high-quality diagnostic and treatment services (especially in the case of HIV/AIDS), changing sexual practices through education and health promotion, increasing the availability and use of barrier methods that reduce transmission (e.g., male and female condoms), shortening the time between the onset of symptoms and the seeking of appropriate care, reducing the stigma attached to STIs, and improving surveillance. Recent studies demonstrating that circumcision of men reduces their risk of acquiring HIV infection (Auvert, Taljaard, Lagarde, Sobngwi-Tambekou, Sitta, & Puren, 2005; Bailey et al., 2007; Gray et al., 2007) have led to consideration of how best to promote male circumcision as a component of HIV prevention strategies. Not surprisingly, given the enormous cultural diversity that exists around the world, the approaches to delivery of risk-reduction messages (e.g., school-based programs, billboards, and radio), the groups that are targeted (e.g., the entire population; individuals of reproductive age; school-aged children; high-risk groups such as commercial sex workers, migrant workers, truck drivers), and the messages that are delivered (e.g., abstinence before marriage, monogamy, condom use) have varied greatly.

Because the laboratory facilities and trained staff needed to identify a specific etiologic agent in a given patient with a suspected STI are often lacking in many low- and middle-income countries, WHO has developed and promoted a syndromic approach to the management of STIs (WHO, 1991). This approach relies on classifying patients with a suspected STI into various groups depending on their symptoms and findings on physical examination (e.g., women with a vaginal discharge, men with urethral discharge and dysuria, and patients with genital ulcer) and then treating them with a regimen designed to cover the treatable etiologic agents that are likely to be responsible (e.g., *N. gonorrhoea* and *C. trachomatis* when a cervical or urethral discharge is present). Exhibit 5-4 provides an example of this approach.

The finding that an intensive (and expensive) regimen of AZT (zidovudine) given to HIV-infected pregnant women in the United States substantially reduced vertical transmission of HIV to their newborn babies

---

| Exhibit 5-4 | **Syndromic Management of Genital Ulcer** |

A study in Lesotho illustrates the promise and drawbacks of the syndromic approach (Htun et al., 1998). In an attempt to validate STI flowcharts for the management of genital ulcer, researchers found that syndromic protocols would have provided adequate treatment for at least 90% of their patient population, while the traditional, clinically directed protocol would have provided adequate treatment for only 62% of those same patients. At the same time, syndromic protocols would have led to the overtreatment of primary syphilis in approximately 60% of patients, while the clinically directed protocols would not have resulted in any such overtreatment.

Several similar studies have shown that syndromic case management of STIs using flowcharts often leads to both improved treatment in many patients and overtreatment in some patients. In general, to determine the appropriateness of implementing the syndromic approach in a given region, the costs of overtreatment (including the cost of the drugs themselves), the risk of promoting drug resistance, and the stigma of an STI diagnosis (which can lead to domestic violence against women) must be weighed against the benefits of improved treatment, including reductions in STI and HIV transmission, decreases in sequelae from untreated infections, and increased patient satisfaction. In view of the high prevalence of STIs in many low- and middle-income countries, this tradeoff is often considered acceptable.

---

led to trials of simpler and cheaper AZT regimens in Thailand and the Ivory Coast. These trials showed that even these simpler regimens, which are given entirely by mouth and for a shorter period of time, are partially effective in reducing vertical transmission of HIV. As a consequence, this regimen was made available in many low- and middle-income countries (Shaffer et al., 1999; Wiktor et al., 1999). Similar trials using an even simpler dosing regimen and a less expensive drug, nevirapine, also initially showed promising results (Jackson et al., 2003), but concerns about the promotion of antiretroviral drug resistance and reduced effectiveness of subsequent antiretroviral drug treatment in women treated with such regimens have arisen, suggesting that multidrug regimens may be needed to prevent mother-to-child transmission (Chi et al., 2007; Johnson et al., 2005). Safe, effective, and inexpensive approaches to preventing vertical transmission during the postpartum interval also are urgently needed, given the evidence that a substantial fraction of vertical transmission of HIV occurs via breastfeeding (Breastfeeding and HIV Transmission Study Group, 2004; Taha et al., 2007). Thus extended postpartum ART may be required to allow HIV-positive mothers to breastfeed safely and infants of such mothers to obtain the benefits of breastfeeding.

For many years, the prohibitive cost of antiretroviral drugs meant that the implementation of wide-scale AIDS treatment programs in low-income countries such as those of sub-Saharan Africa was unthinkable. As a result, fewer than 10% of people in low-income countries who needed ART had access to it in 2003. However, the introduction of generic competition in the global antiretroviral market precipitated spectacular decreases in the costs of these drugs, making it conceivable to include ART in the effort to control HIV-associated morbidity and early mortality for all affected groups. Efforts to expand access to this treatment that began several years ago, including the WHO's 3 by 5 initiative (a plan to treat 3 million people with ART by 2005); the establishment of the Global Fund to Fight HIV/AIDS, Tuberculosis, and Malaria; and the U.S. President's Emergency Plan for AIDS Relief (PEPFAR), which initially sought to treat 2 million people in selected low-income countries, are now bearing fruit. In 2009, an estimated 4.4 to 5 million HIV-infected persons were receiving ART through the Global Fund and PEPFAR, and this number is expected to rise substantially by 2013. Studies have demonstrated substantial declines in mortality among HIV-infected adults in low-income countries resulting from such treatment (Jahn et al., 2008; Mermin et al., 2008), but such efforts still require substantial expansion to meet the needs of all HIV-infected persons who could benefit from such treatment.

Obstacles to Prevention and Control and Directions for Future Research

Enormous obstacles to changing the sexual behaviors of people exist, although progress has clearly been made in reducing the frequency of high-risk sexual behaviors and the incidence of HIV infection in Thailand (Exhibit 5-5) (Celentano et al., 1996; Nelson et al., 1996; Rojanapithayakorn & Hanenberg, 1996) and Uganda (Kilian et al., 1999) in response to the AIDS epidemic. In many societies it remains socially acceptable—even desirable—for men to visit commercial sex workers and have multiple concurrent sex partners. Many men do not want to use condoms, and a woman may risk physical abuse, rejection, or loss of financial support if she tries to insist that a condom be used by her husband, boyfriend, or customer. Women who learn they are infected with HIV also risk abandonment or abuse if they share this information. Thus changing sexual behaviors requires the education of men as well as women, and reducing the incidence of STIs, including HIV, requires raising the status and improving the power of women in society. Similarly, economic and other practices that contribute to or promote risky sexual behaviors (e.g., forcing men to live apart from their wives so that they can earn a living wage) need to be rethought.

Vaccines against STIs, and particularly against HIV, are desperately needed but have proved difficult to develop. Recently licensed vaccines against HPV have been shown to be effective in preventing infection and cervical dysplasia caused by HPV types 16 and 18, and it is expected that cervical cancer caused by these types will also be prevented by use of the same vaccines (Munoz et al., 2009; Paavonen et al., 2009). However, it will be decades before declines in cervical cancer attributable to these vaccines will become apparent. In addition, only an estimated 70% of cervical cancer cases worldwide are attributable to the HPV types covered by the current vaccine.

The development of vaccines against HIV has been beset by many problems, and there is disagreement

---

Exhibit 5-5	**A Successful Public Health Program: The Declining Spread of HIV Among Thai Military Conscripts**

In the late 1980s, heterosexual commercial sex was found to contribute significantly to the rapid spread of HIV in Thailand. Thai authorities responded swiftly to this observation and implemented public health programs that substantially increased the number of commercial sex acts protected by condoms, which in turn led to significant reductions in the rate of HIV infection among young men in Thailand. This case study tells the story of this public health success.

The first national serosurvey for HIV conducted in Thailand found that HIV was exceedingly prevalent among commercial sex workers. In June 1989, 44% of sex workers in the northern province of Chiang Mai were positive for HIV, a figure that would climb to 67% by June 1993 (Celentano et al., 1996). Commercial sex in Thailand is relatively common; for example, in the period from 1991 to 1993, more than 70% of Thai military conscripts were found to have engaged in at least one commercial sex act during their period of service. Because military conscripts are selected by a national lottery, these findings are applicable to the general population of young men in Thailand; thus commercial sex was believed to be a common source of HIV infection.

To address this situation, Thai authorities implemented an HIV/AIDS prevention and control program that included the 100% Condom Campaign to promote condom use in commercial sex establishments. Under this campaign, free condoms were distributed to all sex establishments and the use of condoms was actively enforced by Thai authorities. The campaign was accompanied by mass advertising to promote condom use during commercial sex.

In the years following the initiation of the condom campaign, the use of condoms in sex establishments increased dramatically. National behavioral surveillance data revealed that the percentage of commercial sex acts in which condoms were used rose from approximately 14% in the years prior to 1989 to more than 90% by 1993 (Rojanapithayakorn & Hanenberg, 1996). Although the prevalence of HIV among sex workers has remained high, the prevalence among newly inducted military conscripts declined from more than 10% in 1991 and 1993 to approximately 7% in 1995 (Nelson et al., 1996). Further, this decline occurred in the absence of a visible AIDS epidemic (Rojanapithayakorn & Hanenberg, 1996). Experts attribute these heartening findings at least in part to the swift implementation of the Thai HIV/AIDS prevention and control program, and especially to the success of the 100% Condom Campaign.

about which type of vaccine (i.e., inactivated whole virus, subunit, genetically engineered, live, attenuated, and so on) is likely to be safe and effective. Trials of a subunit HIV vaccine begun in the United States and Thailand in 1998–1999 showed that this vaccine was not effective in preventing acquisition of HIV infection (Cohen, 2003). A more recent trial of an HIV vaccine in Thailand showed at best a modest level of protection (Rerks-Ngarm et al., 2009). Even under ideal circumstances, it is unlikely that an HIV vaccine can be available for widespread use for at least 5 to 10 years.

In the absence of vaccines against HIV and other STIs, other approaches to reducing morbidity and mortality beyond primary prevention of infection through behavior change are needed. For example, while women in high-income countries generally have access to regular screening for cervical dysplasia, which has been shown to be a highly effective tool for the secondary prevention of invasive cervical cancer, such programs are not available to most women in low- and middle-income countries because of the cost and the need for moderately sophisticated laboratory support. Studies suggest that screening for cervical dysplasia using much simpler and less expensive technology may be possible in low- and middle-income countries (University of Zimbabwe/JHPIEGO Cervical Cancer Project, 1999). Cervical cancer screening will continue to play an important role in cervical cancer prevention for years to come.

As noted earlier, universal access to antiretroviral therapy to treat HIV infection in low-income countries has become a top priority for international public health policy makers. Unfortunately, the scientific and medical community is still grappling with the many medical, technical, and logistical difficulties associated with scaling up treatment programs in areas where the public health and clinical infrastructure and resources are painfully scarce. Some of the major challenges will be to develop procedures for treating patients in the absence of laboratory-based monitoring for treatment failure and adverse events, to monitor and control emergent drug resistance, and to develop creative ways to reach populations living in rural areas.

Viral Hepatitis

Overview

Hepatitis, which means inflammation of the liver, can be caused by many different viruses (as well as bac-

teria, protozoa, chemical agents, and some noninfectious diseases). However, at least five viruses specifically infect the liver—hepatitis viruses A, B, C, D, and E. Each belongs to a different family and has unique epidemiologic features, necessitating diverse approaches to control and prevention of hepatitis.

Viral hepatitis is a major global public health problem. All five primary hepatitis viruses can cause acute disease. HBV, HCV, and hepatitis D virus (HDV) can also produce chronic infection. In many low- and middle-income countries, such persistent infections are the primary cause of serious liver disease, including chronic hepatitis, cirrhosis, and hepatocellular carcinoma; the last is a common cancer that is almost always fatal. On a worldwide basis, there are an estimated 360 million chronic carriers of HBV (WHO, 2009b) and 170 million chronic carriers of HCV (WHO, 1997a).

Hepatitis A virus (HAV) and hepatitis E virus (HEV) cause acute self-limited disease; they do not cause chronic infection. Transmitted by the fecal–oral route, these viruses are endemic in many low- and middle-income countries with suboptimal environmental sanitation. HAV infections are typically asymptomatic when they occur in infants. In older children and adults, they generally produce a self-limited illness that leads to few deaths. HEV infection results in more substantial morbidity and mortality, particularly when it occurs in pregnant women.

Etiologic Agents

The five primary hepatitis viruses (A, B, C, D, and E) account for almost all cases of viral hepatitis. Although other viruses (e.g., Epstein-Barr virus and cytomegalovirus) occasionally cause hepatitis, infections with these viruses do not principally involve the liver. GB virus C (formerly called hepatitis G virus) does not appear to cause liver disease (Bowden, 2001). The following discussion is limited to the five primary hepatitis viruses.

Descriptive Epidemiologic Features and Risk Factors

The prevalence of chronic HBV infection is moderate to high throughout low- and middle-income countries. For example, in many Asian countries HBV infection is endemic, with many individuals becoming infected during childhood and the prevalence of chronic HBV infection exceeding 8% (WHO, 2008a). The prevalence of chronic infection is also high in the Middle East, the Indian subcontinent, the Amazon Basin, and sub-Saharan Africa. In these areas, most people who acquire HBV do so at the time of birth (through vertical transmission from an infected mother) or in infancy or childhood. Most such infections produce no acute symptoms. Unfortunately, the likelihood of chronic infection and risk of progression to chronic liver disease increases significantly as the age of acquisition decreases.

The most common routes of HBV transmission in low- and middle-income settings are perinatally (from mother to child) and horizontally (from one child to another). Transmission through the use of unsterilized needles for medical injections is also thought to be significant. Less frequent modes of transmission of HBV include sexual intercourse and needle sharing among injection drug users; notably, these are the two principal modes of transmission in high-income countries. Additionally, practices such as tattooing, scarification, circumcision, body piercing, and acupuncture with unsterile instruments can spread HBV.

HDV is a defective virus, such that HDV infection can be acquired only in the presence of HBV infection. The distribution of HDV varies markedly by region but generally corresponds to the distribution of HBV, although some interesting exceptions to this pattern exist. For example, HDV infections are relatively rare in East and Southeast Asia, even though the prevalence of HBV in these regions is high (Margolis, Alter, & Hadler, 1997). The primary mode of transmission of HDV is through percutaneous exposure to blood, such as may occur through unsterile medical injections and the transfusion of unscreened blood. Perinatal and sexual transmission of HDV occur, but these routes are less efficient for spreading HBV.

HCV infection is widespread throughout the world. Although HCV is not as infectious as HBV, HCV infection is much more likely to become chronic; in fact, as many as 80% of HCV-infected persons become chronically infected (WHO, 1997b). Worldwide, the prevalence of HCV is estimated at 2% to 3%; however, in some low- and middle-income countries, the prevalence is estimated to exceed 10% (Lavanchy, 2009). The principal modes of transmission of HCV in low- and middle-income countries are believed to be the reuse of needles and syringes for medical injections and the transfusion of unscreened blood. Needle sharing among injection drug users—the main source of transmission in wealthy countries—is becoming an increasingly important route of transmission in low- and middle-income countries (Lavanchy, 2009). Some evidence suggests that HCV also can be spread perinatally and sexually, but such transmission is uncommon.

HAV infection is endemic in most low- and middle-income countries. The primary mode of transmission of this virus is via the fecal–oral route, through either person-to-person contact or the ingestion of contaminated food or water. In areas with poor environmental sanitation, HAV infection is virtually universal during the first few years of life. Infection in infancy and early childhood tends to be asymptomatic or mild and produces lifelong immunity. As sanitation improves, individuals are more likely to escape exposure to HAV in childhood. If they are infected as teenagers or adults, the clinical manifestations tend to be more severe, albeit self-limited. Fatalities from this type of hepatitis are uncommon.

HEV is also endemic in many low- and middle-income countries, where it causes substantial morbidity and mortality. HEV infection can be particularly deadly among pregnant women, with case fatality ratios approaching 30% among women infected during their last trimester (Jaiswal, Jain, Naik, Soni, & Chitnis, 2001; Khuroo, Teli, Skidmore, Sofi, & Khuroo, 1981). In endemic areas, HEV can produce cyclic outbreaks as well as sporadic cases of hepatitis. This virus is acquired through the fecal–oral route, principally through ingestion of contaminated water. Person-to-person transmission of HEV can occur but is infrequent.

Current Approaches to Prevention and Control

A safe and effective vaccine for HBV has been available since 1982. In the early 1990s, the global advisory group of EPI and WHO recommended integrating the vaccine into the national immunization programs of all countries by 1997. As of December 2006, 164 countries (85%) had achieved this goal (WHO, 2008a). In 2004, WHO released a recommendation for an infant immunization schedule calling for all infants to receive a first dose of the vaccine as soon as possible following birth, with the goal being that all children receive the vaccine within 24 hours of birth. This first dose is followed by two or three doses to complete the HBV vaccine series. As of 2008, 177 countries had introduced the infant immunization schedule with varying levels of coverage (Figure 5-7). Vaccination of older children and adults is given lower priority, with recommendations based on the epidemiologic features of HBV in the country as well as vaccination levels in children.

Chronic HBV infection can be treated with interferon or antiviral drugs such as entecavir or tenofovir. With the advent of more effective drugs with limited side effects, as well as evidence that treatment can prevent liver failure and hepatocellular carcinoma, there is now a call for treatment to be provided to individuals in low-income countries (Thursz, Cooke, & Hall, 2010).

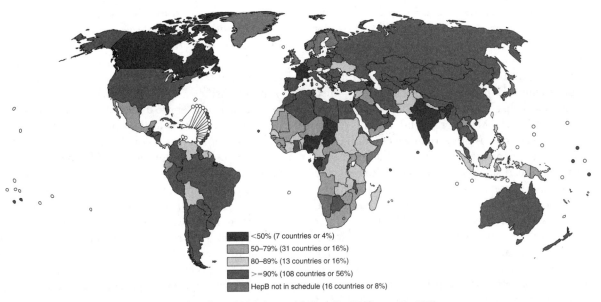

Figure 5-7 Countries Having Introduced HepB Vaccine and Infant HepB3 Coverage, 2008.
Source: World Health Organization. http://www.who.int/immunization_monitoring/diseases/hepatitis/en/.
Copyright 2009 by the World Health Organization. Reprinted with Permission.

Vaccination against HBV infection is also effective in preventing HDV coinfection. (As noted earlier, HDV infection requires the presence of HBV.) However, additional strategies are needed to prevent HDV superinfections among chronic carriers of HBV. Because there is no vaccine against HDV per se, the prevention of such superinfections depends on reducing percutaneous exposures to blood in medical and nonmedical settings among those persons who are chronically infected with HBV.

There is no vaccine against HCV at this time. Treatment of chronic HCV infection with a combination of pegylated alpha interferon and ribavirin—the currently preferred therapy in high-income countries—is effective in clearing the virus in approximately 40% of patients (Brok, Gluud, & Gluud, 2010), but such treatment is prohibitively expensive. Interrupting the transmission of HCV is currently the only feasible intervention for this form of hepatitis. WHO (1997b) recommends the following measures to prevent HCV infections:

- Screening blood and blood products worldwide
- Effectively using universal precautions and barrier techniques
- Destroying disposable needles and adequately sterilizing reusable injection materials
- Promoting public education about the risks of using unsterilized instruments to pierce the skin

The epidemiologic features of HAV infection vary by region and degree of sanitation, necessitating diverse approaches to control measures aimed at this virus. An effective vaccine against HAV is available and may prove useful in controlling the periodic outbreaks among older children and adults that occur in areas of low endemicity. This vaccine is licensed for use only in children aged 1 or older, however. In most low- and middle-income countries, HAV infection is highly endemic and routinely acquired during infancy and early childhood, when it produces little morbidity or mortality. Consequently, the prevention of HAV infection in low- and middle-income countries has not been a priority.

There is no vaccine against HEV, although a candidate vaccine performed well in a Phase II clinical trial (Shrestha et al., 2007). Improved environmental sanitation—especially the provision of clean drinking water—remains the best strategy for preventing HEV infections.

Obstacles to Prevention and Control and Directions for Future Research

Preventing HBV and HCV infections remains a major global public health goal. Universal coverage with the HBV vaccine can dramatically reduce the incidence of HBV infection and serious liver disease and represents the best hope for reducing the acute and delayed morbidity and mortality caused by this virus.

Unfortunately, the cost of supplying and distributing this relatively inexpensive vaccine in settings that have many competing needs remains a significant barrier to achieving universal immunization. Giving the first dose of the vaccine within 24 hours of birth is also a difficult goal to achieve in many low- and middle-income settings. Depending on their cost, combined vaccines may help alleviate this difficulty in the future.

Many obstacles to preventing HBV and HCV infection through means other than vaccination exist. The difficulty of ensuring safe medical injections and safe blood transfusions is a major barrier to reducing the blood-borne transmission of HBV and HCV; contaminated injections cause as many as 21 million HBV infections and 2 million HCV infections per year, according to model-based estimates (Hauri, Armstrong, & Hutin, 2004). The prevention of HEV in the absence of a vaccine is no more tractable, because the problems of securing and sustaining a clean water supply are not easily overcome in low- and middle-income countries.

Malaria and Other Arthropod-Borne Diseases

Overview

Blood-sucking arthropods—including mosquitoes, flies, bugs, fleas, mites, and ticks—are efficient vectors for a host of pathogenic protozoa, bacteria, viruses, and worms that cause tremendous suffering and death around the world. Transmitted by mosquitoes, malaria is undoubtedly the most important parasitic disease in tropical regions of low- and middle-income countries. Malaria causes an estimated 1 to 2 million deaths each year, primarily among African children (Breman, 2009; WHO, 2008b). Mosquitoes also transmit dengue fever (an estimated 50 million infections per year; WHO, 2009c), yellow fever, filariasis, and Japanese encephalitis, while various other arthropods spread trypanosomiasis, leishmaniasis, onchocerciasis (river blindness), and plague, to name but a few diseases. The public health importance of arthropod-borne diseases can scarcely be overstated—they contribute substantially to morbidity and mortality in affected countries and significantly retard social, economic, and developmental progress in those regions.

Etiologic Agents and Clinical Features

As noted earlier, arthropod-borne diseases are caused by a wide variety of pathogens. This section limits its discussion to malaria, dengue fever, yellow fever, American trypanosomiasis, and African trypanosomiasis, although many of the prevention and control issues discussed in the context of these diseases are applicable to other arthropod-borne diseases. Onchocerciasis is discussed in the section on infectious causes of blindness.

Malaria is a febrile disease caused by five species of the parasitic *Plasmodium* protozoa: *P. malariae*, *P. falciparum*, *P. vivax*, *P. ovale*, and the recently identified *P. knowlesi*. Dengue is caused by the four dengue viruses. They produce a spectrum of disease ranging from undifferentiated fever; to classic dengue fever, which is self-limiting and rarely fatal; to dengue hemorrhagic fever, which is characterized by plasma leakage and hemorrhage that can progress to shock and death. Yellow fever is caused by a virus of the same name; it is characterized by fever and, in severe cases, hemorrhage, jaundice, and liver and kidney involvement.

American trypanosomiasis (Chagas disease) is caused by the protozoan parasite *Trypanosoma cruzi*. Acute infections are usually mild, but approximately one-third of infected individuals develop more severe chronic manifestations after several years of asymptomatic infection, including gastrointestinal tract damage, neurologic involvement, and cardiac damage leading to heart failure.

African trypanosomiasis (also known as sleeping sickness) is caused by two subspecies of the protozoan parasite *Trypanosoma brucei*—namely, *T.b. rhodesiense* and *T.b. gambiense*. Individuals infected with *T.b.* rhodesiense develop symptoms within weeks to months, whereas those infected with *T.b.* gambiense develop symptoms over a period of months to years. In both cases, the disease follows a course of central nervous system derangement, coma, and certain death if left untreated.

Descriptive Epidemiologic Features and Risk Factors

Although malaria is found in 109 countries around the world, more than 80% of cases occur in tropical Africa (WHO, 2008b). The parasite is transmitted between humans (who serve as the reservoir) by the female *Anopheles* mosquito. In endemic areas, where transmission is constant, individuals who survive gradually develop immunity to severe disease. As a consequence, young children (who have not yet developed immunity) and pregnant women (who have depressed immune function) experience the highest rates of malaria morbidity and mortality. Susceptible individuals who enter endemic areas (e.g., migrant laborers, displaced persons, and travelers) are also at risk. Of the five species of malaria parasite, *P. falci-parum* causes the most severe disease, *with P. vivax, P. malariae,* and *P. ovale* causing milder forms of disease. Recent evidence suggests that infection with *P. knowlesi* may be more widely distributed than previously thought, as well as more severe, with approximately 1 out of 10 patients developing life-threatening disease (Cox-Singh et al., 2008; Daneshvar et al., 2009).

Approximately 2.5 billion people live in areas where they are at risk for dengue virus infection (Figure 5-8), resulting in an estimated 50 million infections each year and 500,000 cases of dengue hemorrhagic fever, the more severe form of the disease (WHO, 2009c). Major epidemics of dengue hemorrhagic fever have largely been limited to South and Southeast Asia and Latin America, whereas epidemics of dengue fever are more widespread.

Four dengue virus serotypes exist, all of which produce the same spectrum of clinical disease. Infection with one serotype produces lifelong immunity to that serotype, but confers only transient cross-protection against the others. Preexisting antibodies, resulting from either a prior infection with another dengue serotype or primary infection of infants with maternal dengue antibodies, are a risk factor for develop-

ing severe disease. In addition, viral virulence factors are thought to influence the clinical outcome of infection. Dengue viruses have an urban or periurban transmission cycle (human–mosquito–human) in which the mosquitoes *Aedes aegypti* and *Aedes albopictus* are the principal vectors. Frequently, multiple dengue virus serotypes cocirculate in endemic urban cycles that periodically erupt in widespread epidemics (Gubler, 1998). A rural transmission cycle is also possible, but is less important from the public health perspective.

Yellow fever virus is endemic in 32 countries in sub-Saharan Africa and 13 countries in South America (WHO, 2009d). WHO (2009d) estimates that 200,000 yellow fever cases occur annually, resulting in 30,000 deaths. Yellow fever has an urban transmission cycle in which mosquitoes (typically *A. aegypti*) transmit yellow fever virus between humans. Major epidemics of yellow fever occur when the virus is acquired by the urban vector and introduced to susceptible populations. Yellow fever also follows sylvatic and rural transmission cycles.

American trypanosomiasis occurs only in the Americas and is an important public health problem in Latin America, where it is estimated that 8 million persons are infected with *T. cruzi* (WHO, 2009e).

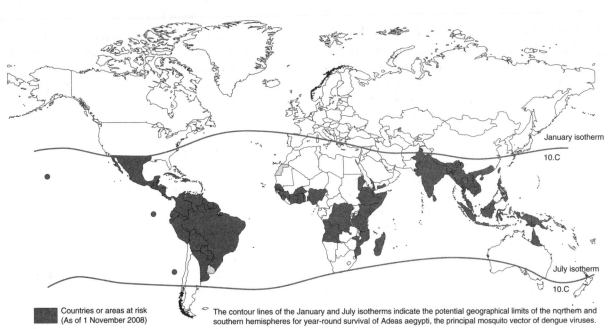

Figure 5-8 Countries/Areas at Risk of Dengue Transmission, 2008. *Source*: Dengue: Guidelines for Diagnosis, Treatment, Prevention, and Control. http://whqlibdoc.who.int/publications/2009/9789241547871_eng.pdf; ISBN: 978-92-4-154787-1. Copyright 2009 by the World Health Organization. Reprinted with Permission.

Historically, *T. cruzi* has been (and continues to be) endemic in rural areas, where a variety of wild and domestic animals serve as reservoirs for the parasite. This parasite is transmitted to humans by triatomine bugs, which infest houses built with materials that shelter the bugs (e.g., thatched roofs or cracked mud walls). In recent decades, rural migration has introduced the disease to urban areas, where *T. cruzi* then spreads via transfusions of infected blood. Congenital infection also occurs. Despite these alternative transmission routes, the triatomine vector remains the most important source of infection.

African trypanosomiasis is found exclusively in sub-Saharan Africa, where the disease occurs in rural, endemic foci in 36 countries. An estimated 50,000 to 70,000 new cases occur annually, all of which are fatal if left untreated (WHO, 2006b). Although African trypanosomiasis was nearly eliminated by the early 1960s, its incidence soared in the following decades, and devastating epidemics occurred in the wake of civil disturbance, war, and population movements. Recently, a dramatic reduction in incidence has been achieved through improved surveillance and treatment. The parasite that causes African trypanosomiasis, *T. brucei,* is transmitted to humans by the bite of the tsetse fly. Cattle and wild animals are the major reservoirs for *T.b.* rhodesiense, which is found in eastern and southern Africa, whereas humans are the major reservoir for *T.b.* gambiense, which is found in western and central Africa.

Current Approaches to Prevention and Control

The historical context of the current malaria control strategy is helpful in understanding how approaches to prevention and control evolve over time (Trigg & Kondrachine, 1998). In the 1950s, malaria prevention programs focused on parasite eradication through the use of antimalarial drugs (e.g., chloroquine) to eliminate human infection and reduce the parasite reservoir, and residual insecticides (e.g., dichloro-diphenyltrichloroethane [DDT]) to interrupt malarial transmission via its mosquito vector. By the late 1960s, the incidence of malaria had been greatly reduced in areas that implemented these programs, including Latin America and tropical Asia. These improvements proved unsustainable, however—in part because of the rigidity of the eradication program, which was vertically structured and failed to consider regional differences in malaria epidemiology and public health infrastructure. Malaria resurged in the following decades (along with other mosquito-borne diseases, including dengue fever and yellow

fever) as vector-control programs were not sustained. Global malaria eradication was declared a failure and abandoned.

In the early 1990s, the international community identified malaria as a leading public health priority (again) and began to formulate new strategies for its control. In 1998, the Roll Back Malaria (RBM) Partnership was established to coordinate an international effort to reduce the global burden of malaria—the first such campaign in more than three decades. By 2009, thousands of organizations throughout the world were participating in RBM. The discovery of artemisinin and the development of artemisinin-based combination treatments (ACTs), which can be mass-produced relatively inexpensively and are highly effective against malaria that has developed resistance to chloroquine and sulfadoxine-pyrimethamine, resulted in WHO recommending these agents as the first-line treatment for *P. falciparum* infection. A resultant increase in the deployment of ACTs (Figure 5-9) has led to enhanced control of malaria.

In 2008, the RBM released the Global Malaria Action Plan (GMAP), with the goals of halving the global burden of malaria compared to year 2000 levels by 2010, reducing malaria mortality to nearly zero, and reducing global incidence by 75% from 2000 levels by the year 2015. The GMAP uses the following key tools to control malaria:

1. "Long-lasting insecticidal nets: sleeping under insecticide-treated nets to prevent infectious mosquito bites

2. Indoor residual spraying: indoor application of long-lasting chemical insecticides to kill malarious mosquitoes

3. Intermittent preventive treatment during pregnancy: in which pregnant women, who are at increased risk for malaria infection, illness and death, receive regular preventative treatment during their pregnancies

4. Other vector (mosquito) controls: including larvaciding and environmental management

5. Diagnosis: prompt parasitological diagnosis by microscopy or rapid diagnostic tests (RDTs)

6. Treatment: prompt provision of antimalarial drugs (ACTS for *P. falciparum* and chloroquine and primaquine for *P. vivax*)" (Rollback Malaria Partnership, 2008)

Currently, there is no licensed malaria vaccine, although several are currently under development. The most promising to date is RTS,S, an adjuvanted re-

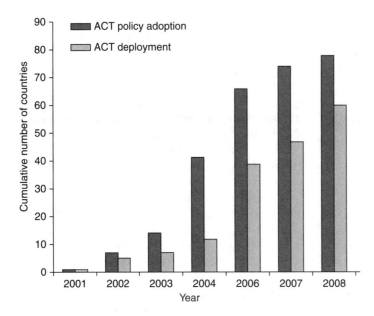

Figure 5-9 Adoption of Policy and Deployment of Artemisinin-based Therapy (ACT) by Year, Global Data, 2001–2008. *Source*: World Malaria Report 2009;http://www.who.int/malaria/world_malaria_report_2009/en/index.html; ISBN: 978-92-4-156390-1. Copyright 2009 by the World Health Organization. Reprinted with Permission.

combinant vaccine that has shown efficacy of 30% to 56% against clinical disease in Phase I/II clinical trials and 26% efficacy against all malaria episodes over a 45-month period (Alonso et al. 2004, Sacarlal et al., 2009). As yet, no data have been published indicating whether the vaccine is effective at blocking transmission of malaria (by reducing the gametocyte load)—a characteristic of the ideal malaria vaccine.

There is no specific treatment for dengue fever or dengue hemorrhagic fever beyond attentive clinical management. Moreover, there are no vaccines currently available against dengue viruses, although a number of vaccines are under development and several have shown promise in Phase I or Phase II clinical trials. Because of concerns that vaccine-induced antibody against fewer than all four serotypes could promote the development of dengue hemorrhagic fever, only a vaccine that protects against all four serotypes can be safely developed, tested, and administered to populations at risk. Thus the control and prevention of dengue fever currently depends on mosquito control, disease surveillance, and epidemic preparedness. A key component of *Aedes* control is source reduction through elimination of mosquito breeding sites.

Immunization is the most important prevention measure against yellow fever. The yellow fever vaccine, designated 17D, is safe, effective, and affordable; it requires only a single dose to provide multiple-year protection. To prevent and control yellow fever in endemic areas, WHO (1998c) recommends routine in-

fant immunization against yellow fever (within the EPI), mass immunization campaigns (e.g., preventive catch-up campaigns), vigilant case and vector surveillance, reactive immunization to contain outbreaks, and careful management of the vaccine supply. Since 2004, WHO has maintained a stockpile of 6 million doses of yellow fever vaccine for emergency response.

For American trypanosomiasis, it is currently recommended that all acute infections be treated as well as chronic infections in children. A mounting body of evidence suggests that treatment of all chronic infections may reduce the severity of illness; however, drugs used in the treatment of acute manifestations (benznidazole and nifurtimox) are toxic, so treatment of chronic infections in adults depends on each individual's health status. Prevention and control of American trypanosomiasis currently focus on interrupting vectorial transmission in addition to preventing transmission via the transfusion of infected blood. Vector-control efforts center on eradicating strictly domestic triatomine bugs and controlling domestic infestations of other (sylvatic) triatomine bugs, predominantly through indoor residual insecticide spraying in areas at high risk for American trypanosomiasis. The prevention of transfusion-related transmission is accomplished by screening all blood donors for *T. cruzi* antibodies and rejecting blood that tests positive. The results of these efforts are encouraging, with the global burden of American trypanosomiasis dropping by an estimated 50% or more between 1990 and 2006.

In 2007, WHO launched the WHO Global Network for Chagas Elimination with the goal of eliminating American trypanosomiasis by 2010. However, that goal was not met. In addition to the previously mentioned control measures, this network is working to increase surveillance and access to diagnosis and treatment, as well as to develop new treatments and improved diagnostic tests.

The current strategy for the control and prevention of African trypanosomiasis caused by *T.b.* gambiense involves active case finding and early treatment, which reduces the human reservoir by curing the infection. Passive surveillance for *T.b.* gambiense infection is problematic because infected individuals are often infectious for months to years before they develop symptoms that lead to (passive) detection. In contrast, passive surveillance and epidemic preparedness are often adequate to control the transmission of *T.b.* rhodesiense, which quickly leads to symptoms of infection. The drugs used to treat African trypanosomiasis have significant drawbacks, including high levels of toxicity. The first-stage drugs, pentamidine and suramin, and second-stage drugs, melarsoprol and eflornithine, are provided by WHO to countries in which this disease is endemic.

Obstacles to Prevention and Control and Directions for Future Research

Insecticide resistance presents a major challenge to prevention strategies based on vector control. Vectors for malaria, dengue, and yellow fever have all developed resistance to multiple insecticides, including both the classic insecticides (e.g., DDT) and their replacements (e.g., organophosphates). Alternative insecticides have been developed but are often more costly and toxic than the first-line agents. The dynamic ecology of vector-borne pathogens is an additional barrier to effective vector control. For example, changing land-use patterns, shifting weather patterns, urbanization, and population movements may result in new foci for disease transmission. Finally, national and international travel and commerce represent continuing opportunities for reinfestation, necessitating continuous surveillance even in areas that have achieved good vector control.

Drug resistance poses a serious problem for control strategies that rely on chemotherapy to treat disease and subsequently decrease transmission through the reduction of parasite load in humans. Nowhere is this problem more evident than in the history of the management of malaria. Drugs that once provided inexpensive and effective means of antimalarial prophylaxis and therapy became severely compromised by resistance in many parts of the world, resulting in substantially increased morbidity and mortality. The discovery and implementation of ACTs in combination with other interventions has resulted in a renewed ability to control malaria; however, sporadic reports of ACT-resistant malaria continue to crop up, and careful monitoring to detect drug resistance is essential for continued success.

Other barriers to the prevention and control of arthropod-borne diseases include the intermittent disruption of public health services as a consequence of civil disturbance or war and the ever-present problem of limited resources. Other problems include the difficulty of sustaining support for successful control measures (e.g., indoor insecticide spraying to control the vectorial spread of American trypanosomiasis) once the disease has been brought under control and, therefore, is no longer a public health priority.

Future prospects for the improved prevention of arthropod-borne disease rest primarily on vaccine development. Current research is focused on developing candidate tetravalent dengue fever vaccines and antimalarial vaccines.

Helminthiasis

Overview

Approximately 2 billion people are believed to be chronically infected with parasitic helminths (WHO, 2005a). The vast majority of these individuals live in low- and middle-income countries, where environmental sanitation is poor. Each parasite produces different manifestations according to the site, intensity, and length of infection. The host response also influences the clinical course of infection. In general, children experience the heaviest worm burden, and persistent infection throughout childhood is common in low- and middle-income settings. Heavy, prolonged infection adversely affects growth, development, and educational achievement, and significantly increases childhood morbidity. In adults, helminthiases can produce acute and chronic morbidity, leading to impaired productivity, chronic disability, and reduced quality of life.

In terms of global prevalence, morbidity, and mortality, the most important helminthic infections are schistosomiasis (207 million infections), ascariasis (1.2 billion infections), trichuriasis (795 million infections), hookworm (740 million infections), onchocerciasis, and lymphatic filariasis (WHO, 2006c). Although many of these infections are minimally symptomatic, the number of clinically significant cases is substantial. This section focuses on schistosomiasis and the most common intestinal helminthiases—that is, ascariasis, trichuriasis, and hookworm. Dracunculiasis, a disease of considerable historical importance, is also considered.

Etiologic Agents and Clinical Features

Human schistosomiasis (also known as bilharziasis) is caused by a group of blood trematodes (flukes) known as schistosomes. The three main species that infect humans are *Schistosoma mansoni, Schistosoma japonicum,* and *Schistosoma haematobium.* Two other species, *Schistosoma mekongi* and *Schistosoma intercalatum,* also parasitize humans, but such infections are uncommon and will not be discussed further. Acute schistosomiasis (Katayama fever) is characterized by fever and chills, abdominal pain, diarrhea, and enlargement of the spleen or other organs. Infection with *S. japonicum* is most commonly associated with acute disease, although any type of schistosomiasis can cause these symptoms. Chronic disease is initiated by the deposition of schistosome eggs in the body, which induces inflammation and scarring. Chronic infection with *S. mansoni* or *S. japonicum* can lead to hepatosplenic and intestinal involvement, although most infected individuals remain asymptomatic. Chronic infection with *S. haematobium* is associated with urinary tract disease, and a much higher proportion (50% to 70%) of infected individuals are symptomatic (WHO, 1993). *S. haematobium* infection is also associated with an increased risk of bladder cancer.

The most common intestinal helminthiases of humans are caused by *Ascaris lumbricoides, Trichuris trichiura* (whipworm), and two species of hookworm, *Ancylostoma duodenale* and *Necator americanus.* These parasites produce a diverse range of clinical manifestations, although persons with light infections generally remain asymptomatic. When worm burdens are high, *A. lumbricoides* infection is associated with malnutrition and stunted growth. *A. lumbricoides* is also the largest of the intestinal helminths, measuring 15 to 35 centimeters in length; thus single worms can cause obstruction and inflammation of the appendix, bile duct, or pancreatic duct, and a bolus of worms can cause intestinal obstruction leading to death. Trichuriasis is associated with abdominal pain, diarrhea, and general malaise when moderate worm loads are present, whereas nutritional deficiencies, anemia, and stunted growth can result from heavier worm loads. Hookworms attach to the intestinal mucosa, where they ingest 0.03 to 0.26 milliliter of blood per worm per day (Warren et al.,

1993). The major clinical manifestations of hookworm infection are iron-deficiency anemia and hypoalbuminemia resulting from chronic blood loss.

Dracunculiasis is caused by *Dracunculus medinensis* (Guinea worm), a long (60 to 90 centimeters), thin nematode. Symptoms of the disease are caused by the migration of the worm to the subcutaneous tissues and its eruption through the skin. Symptoms can include the formation of a blister or bleb at the site where the worm will emerge (usually the ankle or foot), hives, nausea, vomiting, diarrhea, and asthma. The blister ulcerates as the worm emerges, and local pain typically persists until the worm is expelled or extracted, which can take several weeks. Secondary infection of the worm track is common. Severe disability generally lasting 1 to 3 months occurs in most persons who become infected, with 0.5% of infected individuals experiencing permanent disability (Hunter, 1996). Even short-term disability can have a substantial economic impact if the worm emerges during the months when important agricultural work is performed (Hopkins, 1984).

Descriptive Epidemiologic Features and Risk Factors

Schistosomiasis is the single most important helminthic disease and the second most important parasitic disease (after malaria) worldwide. An estimated 207 million persons in 74 countries and territories harbor this infection, resulting in an estimated 4.5 million disability adjusted life-years (DALYs) lost each year (WHO, 2002a, 2010b). *S. mansoni,* the most widespread of the schistosomes, is found in parts of Africa, the Middle East, the Caribbean, and South America; *S. haematobium* is restricted to Africa and the Middle East; and *S. japonicum* is currently found only in the Western Pacific countries. Overall, the vast majority of schistosome infections (97%) occur in sub-Saharan Africa (Steinmann, Keiser, Bos, Tanner, & Utzinger, 2006).

The life cycle of the schistosome is quite complex, and a complete description is beyond the scope of this chapter. Nevertheless, a brief treatment is necessary to understand how infection plays out in human hosts. Adult worms live, mate, and deposit their eggs in the blood vessels lining the human intestines (*S. mansoni* and *S. japonicum*) or bladder (*S. haematobium*). These eggs migrate into the intestine or bladder and are passed out in the excreta. When deposited in fresh water, the eggs develop into immature parasites (miracidia) that infect fresh-water snails. The immature parasites then develop into infective larvae (cercariae). When released into the surrounding water, the larvae swim about. Those coming in contact with humans during this time penetrate through the skin and eventually reach the vascular system, completing the cycle. Thus the maintenance of schistosomes in a given area requires the presence of the intermediate host, the contamination of water with egg-laden excreta, and the exposure of humans to contaminated water.

Because schistosomes do not multiply in the human host, the intensity of infection is largely determined by the rate at which new worms are acquired. Studies have shown that the infection rate for schistosomes typically peaks during childhood and then declines with advancing age (Butterworth, Dunne, Fulford, Ouma, & Sturrock, 1996; Hagan, 1996). This finding is thought to reflect age-dependent changes in both water exposure and immunity to infection.

The public health impact of intestinal helminthiases on low- and middle-income countries is substantial. As noted earlier, *A. lumbricoides*, *T. trichiura*, and hookworm each infect 740 million to 1.2 billion individuals globally (WHO, 2006c). Although the morbidity and mortality associated with intestinal helminthiases are relatively low, the burden of illness is considerable due to the extremely high prevalence of these infections (Bundy, 1990).

A. lumbricoides, *T. trichiura*, and hookworm share a relatively simple life cycle. The parasites mature and mate in the human intestine and produce eggs that are passed out in the feces. When deposited on moist soil, these eggs develop into the infective form of the parasite. (Because this part of the life cycle is spent in soil, these worms are collectively referred to as geohelminths.) Humans acquire the parasite when contaminated soil is ingested or, in the case of hookworm, when the infective larvae in the soil penetrate exposed skin. Thus the maintenance of these helminths requires the deposition of feces in soil and the exposure of humans to that soil. For *A. lumbricoides* and *T. trichiura*, the peak intensity of infection typically occurs among young children, whereas for hookworm the peak occurs among adults (Bundy, Hall, Medley, & Savioli, 1992).

Dracunculiasis is contracted by drinking contaminated water. Parasitic larvae then migrate to the abdominal cavity, where they mature into adult worms over the course of a year. After copulation, the gravid female worm migrates through the body to the subcutaneous tissue and then secretes irritants that ulcerate the skin and expose the worm. When the affected body site is immersed in water, the worm expels clouds of larvae. The larvae are consumed by copepods (minute fresh-water crustaceans, also known as water fleas), which are in turn ingested by humans

who drink contaminated water. Dracunculiasis occurs in individuals of all ages, but is less common in very young children, possibly because breastfeeding reduces their level of water consumption (Hunter, 1996).

The global campaign to eradicate dracunculiasis was launched in the 1980s as a part of the United Nations International Drinking Water Supply and Sanitation Decade (1981–1990). Since then, the incidence of this disease has declined from 4 million reported cases in 1981 (Hopkins, Ruiz-Tiben, & Ruebush, 1997) to 3,190 confirmed cases in 2009. Endemic disease is now confined to just four African countries, and it is likely to be the next disease that is eradicated.

Current Approaches to Prevention and Control

The major strategies for the control of helminthic infections are preventative chemotherapy, environmental sanitation and health education, and control or eradication of the intermediate host. No antihelminthic vaccines are currently available.

For the control of schistosomiasis and geohelminths, WHO emphasizes controlling morbidity by reducing the intensity of infection (the number of worms per person) rather than reducing the prevalence of infection (the number of persons with worms). The former is achieved in the short term through regular deworming, despite reinfection, whereas the latter requires improved environmental sanitation, intermediate-host control (in the case of schistosomiasis, for example), or both, and is viewed as a long-term goal. WHO recommends preventative treatment for schistosomiasis, soil-transmitted helminthiasis, lymphatic filariasis, and onchocerciarsis (see Table 5-6 for current recommendations for treatment of geohelminth infections and schistosomiasis). This approach is possible because safe, effective, and inexpensive oral treatments are available for these common helminthiases. Mass drug administration, where the entire community is treated, has become a commonly used intervention, and the efficiency of this approach was improved when research showed that three of the drugs (praziquantel, ivermectin, and albendazole) could be safely administered at the same time, allowing for the treatment and control of urinary schistosomiasis, onchoceriasis, lymphatic filariasis, and several soil-transmitted helminthiases (Eigege et al., 2008; Mohammed et al., 2008).

Ultimately, most helminthiases are diseases of poor sanitation. Providing for the sanitary disposal of excreta prevents the contamination of soil and water,

Table 5-6	World Health Organization–Recommended Treatment Strategies for Geohelminth Infections and Schistosomiasis		
Community Category	**Prevalence Among School-Aged Children**[a]	**Action to Be Taken**	
Geohelminth Infections[b]			
High risk	≥50%	Treat all school-aged children (enrolled and not enrolled) twice each year	Also treat the following groups: • Preschool-aged children • Women of childbearing age, including pregnant women in the second and third trimesters and lactating women • Adults at high risk in certain occupations (e.g., tea-pickers and miners)
Low risk	≥20% and <50%	Treat all school-aged children (enrolled and not enrolled) once a year	Also treat the following groups: • Preschool-aged children • Women of childbearing age, including pregnant women in the second and third trimesters and lactating women • Adults at high risk in certain occupations (e.g., tea-pickers and miners)
Schistosomiasis			
High risk	≥50% by parasitological methods (intestinal and urinary schistosomiasis) **or** ≥30% by questionnaire for visible hematuria (urinary schistosomiasis)	Treat all school-aged children (enrolled and not enrolled) once per year	Also treat adults considered to be at risk (from special groups) or once a year to entire communities living in endemic areas
Moderate risk	≥10% but <50% by parasitological methods (intestinal and urinary schistosomiasis) **or** <30% by questionnaire for visible hematuria (urinary schistosomiasis)	Treat all school-aged children (enrolled and not enrolled) once every 2 years	Also treat adults considered to be at risk (from special groups) only
Low risk	>10% by parasitological methods (intestinal and urinary schistosomiasis)	Treat all school-aged children (enrolled and not enrolled) twice during their primary schooling age	Praziquantel should be available in dispensaries and clinics for treatment of suspected cases

a. For geohelminth infections, prevalence is of any geohelminth infection.

b. When prevalence of any geohelminth infection is less than 20%, large-scale preventive chemotherapy interventions are not recommended. Affected individuals should be dealt with on a case-by-case basis.

Source: Preventitive Chemotherapy in Human Helminthiasis; http://whqlibdoc.who.int/publications/2006/9241547103_eng.pdf; ISBN: 978-92-4-154710-9. Copyright 2006 by the World Health Organization. Reprinted with Permission.

thereby breaking the chain of transmission. However, environmental improvements must be made at the community level to be effective (Warren et al., 1993). Improvements in environmental sanitation are complemented by health education to promote healthy behaviors. For example, WHO has determined that schistosomiasis could be largely prevented by eliminating indiscriminate urination and defecation, and increasing compliance with medical interventions (WHO, 1993).

Control of the intermediate host species for certain helminths, such as snail control for schistosomiasis, can also play an important role in preventing transmission. The primary strategies for snail control include application of molluscicidal agents and environmental management. Biological control strategies, such as the introduction of competitor snails, have not proved successful and are not currently recommended (WHO, 1993). Control of the interme-diate host plays a crucial role in preventing the transmission of dracunculiasis. Much of the success of the dracunculiasis eradication campaign has been achieved by teaching people to pour drinking water through a finely woven cloth or to use a small straw-like device to filter out the tiny fleas that carry the *Dracunculus* parasite. Chemical eradicants have also played a role.

Obstacles to Prevention and Control and Directions for Future Research

Major obstacles to the effective implementation of chemotherapy-based interventions are related to the logistical and financial difficulties of treating the large number of individuals in need. In addition, chemotherapy does not address the conditions that led to the primary infection; thus reinfection is likely to occur, necessitating repeated treatments and further cost. Although widespread resistance to the antihelminthic agents in human infection has not yet emerged, resistance to benzimidazoles is often seen in veterinary practice, and some evidence suggests that limited resistance to praziquantel is possible (WHO, 2002a). As a consequence, chemotherapeutic interventions should include provisions for detecting and, if necessary, managing drug resistance.

Adequate environmental sanitation is generally viewed as the only long-term solution to the control of intestinal helminthiases and schistosomiasis. However, providing safe drinking water and adequate disposal facilities in low- and middle-income areas has proved to be an extremely difficult, costly, and lengthy process. Current control efforts emphasize targeted chemotherapeutic interventions to relieve the immediate burden of disease while maintaining universal sanitation as a long-term goal.

Zoonoses

Overview

Zoonoses are defined as diseases and infections that are naturally transmitted between vertebrate animals and humans. Zoonotic agents include a wide variety of bacteria, viruses, protozoa, and helminths, while their nonhuman hosts include wild animals and birds, food and draft animals, and household pets.

More than 200 different zoonoses are currently recognized (Hart, Trees, & Duerden, 1997). Zoonotic infections have a worldwide distribution and collectively produce significant morbidity and mortality. For example, indigenous rabies, which has a global distribution, causes more than 50,000 deaths per year (WHO, 2008c). *Yersinia pestis,* the bacterium that causes plague, remains enzoonotic in many parts of Africa, Asia, and South America, and in the southwestern United States. Although only 2,118 cases of human plague were reported to WHO (2004) in 2003, the control of human plague remains a public health priority because of its epidemic potential and relatively high case fatality ratio. In low- and middle-income settings, important zoonoses include rabies, plague, anthrax, leptospirosis, leishmaniasis, African trypanosomiasis, and a number of hemorrhagic fever viruses. Food-borne zoonoses, such as salmonellosis, campylobacteriosis, and certain *E. coli* infections, also contribute to the global burden of disease, while occupational zoonoses such as brucellosis, echinococcosis, and Q fever have regional significance. Finally, zoonotic infections are a rich source of emerging diseases, such as severe acute respiratory syndrome (SARS), avian influenza in humans, Nipah virus encephalitis, variant Creutzfeldt-Jakob disease, and Ebola hemorrhagic fever.

Although zoonoses have a worldwide distribution, low- and middle-income countries bear a greater burden of these diseases than high-income countries. This divergence reflects, in part, differences in opportunities for exposure to zoonotic pathogens. Residents of low- and middle-income countries typically experience more frequent and intimate contact with animals, and they often live in situations of suboptimal environmental sanitation (which promotes exposure to infective material such as contaminated animal excreta). In addition, many control measures that are readily available in high-income countries (e.g., mass veterinary vaccination of domesticated animals) may not be available or affordable in low- and middle-income countries.

Zoonotic pathogens are transmitted to humans by five major routes:

1. Inhalation: transmission that occurs when infective materials are aerosolized and inhaled
2. Ingestion: transmission that occurs when humans consume contaminated meat, milk,

or blood from infected animals or when food-stuffs (e.g., fruits and vegetables), drinking water, or hands are contaminated with infective materials, which are then ingested

3. Nontraumatic contact: transmission that typically occurs when pathogens enter through the skin (or mucosal surfaces or conjunctivae) as a result of direct or indirect contact with animal hides, hair, excreta, blood, or carcasses

4. Traumatic contact: transmission via animal bites or scratches

5. Arthropod: transmission by biting arthropods that feed on animals and humans

For some zoonoses, humans are incidental, dead-end hosts. Human-to-human transmission of rabies or anthrax, for example, is extremely rare. For other zoonoses, humans may serve as a reservoir for infection, transmitting pathogens to other humans or even back to animals.

Zoonoses produce a wide variety of diseases with distinct clinical and epidemiologic characteristics. In addition, they are associated with many different animals occupying a number of ecologic niches, both urban and rural. Approaches to the control and prevention of zoonoses necessarily reflect these differences. The general principles underlying these strategies often include good animal husbandry (including vaccination when appropriate), environmental sanitation, vector control, and the control or elimination of animal reservoirs (e.g., rats or other wild animals).

Rather than attempting to survey the entire range of zoonoses, this section is limited to a detailed discussion of rabies and leptospirosis, which are important zoonoses in many low- and middle-income countries.

Etiologic Agents and Clinical Features

Rabies is caused by the rabies virus, which is a Lyssavirus belonging to the Rhabdoviridae family. Typically transmitted by the bite of a rabid animal, human rabies is an acute, encephalitic disease that is almost always fatal. Following inoculation, there is an asymptomatic incubation period typically lasting 1 to 3 months, although periods as short as a few days and as long as several years have been reported (Fishbein, 1991). Postexposure prophylaxis must be initiated during this period to have an effect.

The prodromal period for rabies begins with the early signs of disease, which include nonspecific symptoms (e.g., fever and malaise) and abnormal sensations near the site of inoculation. This stage is followed by a 2- to 10-day period of acute neurologic dysfunction

that manifests as furious rabies in approximately 80% of cases and paralytic (dumb) rabies in the remainder (Fishbein, 1991). Furious rabies is characterized by periods of extreme agitation and hyperactivity interspersed with periods of normalcy. Hydrophobia, aerophobia, combativeness, and hallucination may also occur. Features of paralytic rabies include paresthesia, weakness, and paralysis. The almost inevitable final stage of rabies (both furious and paralytic) is coma followed by death.

Leptospirosis is an acute febrile disease caused by pathogenic bacteria of the genus Leptospira. The clinical course of the disease is variable: The majority of infections result in subclinical or mild disease, but 5% to 10% of those persons infected will develop more severe manifestations, including kidney failure and pulmonary hemorrhage (Levett, 2001). Ocular involvement may also occur.

Leptospira are classified serologically into 200 serovars arranged in 24 serogroups; alternatively, the organism may be classified genotypically into genomospecies (Vinetz, 2001). The serologic classification scheme is more frequently used in epidemiologic studies. Certain serovars were once thought to be associated with more severe disease, but evidence supporting this hypothesis is lacking (Levett, 2001; Vinetz, 2001).

Descriptive Epidemiologic Features and Risk Factors

Rabies is a disease of animals; humans are incidentally infected and only rarely transmit the virus. Animal reservoirs include dogs, cats, and wild animals (notably foxes, skunks, wolves, coyotes, raccoons, mongooses, and bats). Most human rabies cases are acquired from dogs, which are the major source of human infection in low- and middle-income countries. Recently, bats have emerged as a major source of rabies for humans. In fact, in South America in 2003, bats overtook dogs in transmitting fatal rabies to humans. In high-income countries, where immunization of domestic animals is common, wild animals constitute the principal reservoirs of infection and human rabies is extremely rare.

Rabies virus is present in the saliva of infected animals and is typically transmitted to humans by the bite of a rabid animal. It may also be transmitted when intact mucous membranes are exposed to infective saliva. Not every exposure results in infection. Nevertheless, if infection occurs, it is almost always fatal in the absence of postexposure prophylaxis.

Leptospirosis has a worldwide distribution, but its incidence is difficult to assess. In general, the incidence and prevalence of infection are low in high-income countries and higher in low- and middle-income countries (e.g., in some low- and middle-income countries, prevalences of antibodies to leptospirosis in the range of 18% to 48% have been reported, suggesting that exposure to the causative organism is common in such settings) (Ellis, 1998). As with rabies, human infection with Leptospira is incidental, and humans do not contribute to the transmission of the bacteria. The main animal reservoirs for Leptospira serovars that cause human disease are rats, dogs, pigs, and cattle.

Transmission of leptospires to humans typically occurs in one of two ways: (1) through contact with water that has been contaminated with the urine of infected animals or (2) through direct contact with infective animal urine. The bacteria infect humans by entering through broken skin, water-softened intact skin, mucosal surfaces, or conjunctivae. Human leptospirosis is an occupational disease among those whose professions involve contact with host animals (e.g., dairy farmers) or water (e.g., rice farmers). Home and recreational exposures are also becoming increasingly important, particularly in low- and middle-income settings. In addition, periodic flooding due to heavy rains can produce large epidemics of leptospirosis.

Current Approaches to Prevention and Control

The control of human rabies is achieved by the prevention of human exposure to the virus and the prevention of disease through postexposure prophylaxis when exposure does occur. Historically, rabies vaccines were not deemed suitable (i.e., sufficiently inexpensive, safe, and effective) for mass preexposure immunization of humans. However, WHO has encouraged research into the feasibility of incorporating rabies vaccination into the EPI for communities where rabies is a problem (WHO, 2007b).

The prevention of human exposure to rabies in low- and middle-income countries primarily depends on the control of dog rabies, which can be achieved through the widespread use of the canine rabies vaccine. The mass vaccination of pet dogs and the elimination of stray or feral dogs has been successful in many countries. For example, in the United States, the incidence of human rabies cases was reduced from 0.03 cases per 100,000 population per year in 1945 to less than 0.001 cases per 100,000 population per year in the 1980s through the successful widespread control of dog rabies (Fishbein, 1991).

The prevention of human disease once exposure to rabies virus has occurred depends on good local wound care (e.g., flushing with soap and water) and postexposure prophylaxis, which entails passive immunization with immunoglobulin and active immunization with rabies vaccine. Although the complete postexposure regimen almost always prevents disease, this regimen must be delivered during the incubation period: Neither immunization nor other treatments alter the course of disease once symptoms develop. There are no diagnostic tests that can detect rabies infection in humans prior to the onset of symptoms; thus all individuals with suspected or possible infections must receive prophylactic treatment.

The prevention of human leptospirosis focuses on interrupting the transmission of leptospires to humans. Preventive measures include the vaccination of certain host animals (e.g., cattle) or the elimination of others (e.g., rats). Human vaccination has met with limited success and is not widely applied. Environmental control strategies aimed at reducing hazards such as stagnant bodies of water or the periodic flooding of residential areas, as well as educational campaigns aimed at decreasing unnecessary water exposures, may enhance prevention efforts. Occupational improvements that curtail contact with host animals or contaminated water are also desirable. Antibiotic therapy and supportive care remain the treatment of choice, although evidence supporting the effectiveness of antibiotic therapy is incomplete.

Obstacles to Prevention and Control and Directions for Future Research

The major obstacle to the improved control of rabies is the difficulty of achieving adequate vaccine coverage among canine populations in low- and middle-income countries. WHO (2002b) estimates that 80% or greater coverage is necessary for effective control. Ensuring the delivery of vaccine to stray and feral dogs (or eliminating these dogs altogether) is especially problematic. With sustained effort, WHO considers the global elimination of urban (canine) rabies to be an attainable goal.

The future control of leptospirosis is less promising. Animal vaccination may not be economically feasible for many farmers, and vaccines are not available or appropriate for every host species. The elimination of wildlife hosts (e.g., rats) is usually not feasible. Improvements in working and living conditions to reduce contact with animals and their excreta are desirable (for many reasons), yet difficult to achieve in low- and middle-income settings. Until these difficulties are overcome, the control of leptospirosis must rely on health education to reduce risky behavior, veterinary education to promote good animal husbandry, and medical education to ensure the prompt diagnosis and treatment of leptospirosis.

Viral Hemorrhagic Fevers

Overview

The viruses that cause hemorrhagic fever (HF) belong to four different families (Table 5-7), and the illnesses they produce have distinct epidemiologic features. Despite their differences, these viruses produce a common clinical picture that is characterized by fever and hemorrhage, as their name suggests. Hemorrhagic manifestations can include petechiae, ecchymoses, bleeding gums, nosebleeds, vaginal bleeding, and bleeding from other mucosal surfaces, producing bloody urine, stool, and vomit. Complications can include cardiovascular and neurologic disturbances, shock, and death.

The spectrum of disease typically associated with each type of virus varies substantially. For example, Lassa virus infections result in inapparent or mild symptoms in many people, yet cause severe life-threatening disease in others. Ebola virus and Marburg virus, by comparison, appear to cause severe disease in virtu-

ally all those infected. The severity of the clinical illness that results from infection also varies according to differences in host response, viral virulence factors, and dose.

Infection with the HF viruses is, in general, relatively rare (Lassa virus is a notable exception). Although outbreaks are dramatic and lead to major responses on the part of public health and other officials, such infections do not have the same public health impact in terms of morbidity and mortality as the infectious diseases that more commonly afflict inhabitants of most low- and middle-income countries (WHO, 1985). However, because most HF viruses are extremely virulent and capable of causing epidemics, developing strategies to control these viruses is a public health priority. In addition, some of the viruses, such as the South American HF viruses, pose regional public health hazards within their areas of endemicity.

All HF viruses are thought to be zoonotic. These viruses have been proven or are suspected to be transmitted from animals to humans by an arthropod vector (e.g., ticks or mosquitoes) or by direct or indirect

Table 5-7	Distribution and Modes of Transmission of Viral Hemorrhagic Fevers		
Family, Genus, and Virus	**Disease**	**Principal Means of Transmission**	**Principal Locations**
Flaviviridae			
Flavivirus			
Dengue	Dengue HF	Mosquito	Asia, Latin America
Yellow fever	Yellow fever	Mosquito	sub-Saharan Africa, South America
Kyasanur Forest disease	Kyasanur Forest	Tick	India
Omsk HF	Omsk HF	Tick, muskrat	Russia
Arenaviridae			
Arenavirus			
Lassa	Lassa fever	Rodent, person-to-person	West Africa
Junin	Argentine HF	Rodent	Argentina
Machupo	Bolivian HF	Rodent	Bolivia
Guanarito	Venezuelan HF	Rodent	Venezuela
Sabio	Brazilian HF	Unknown	Brazil
Lujo		Unknown	South Africa
Bunyaviridae			
Phlebovirus			
Rift Valley fever	Rift Valley fever	Mosquito	Africa
Nairovirus			
Crimean-Congo HF	Crimean-Congo HF	Tick, person-to-person	Africa, Asia, Eastern Europe, Middle East
Hantavirus			
Hantaan, Seoul, and others	HF with renal syndrome	Rodent	Asia, Europe
Filoviridae			
Filovirus			
Marburg	Marburg HF	Person-to-person	Africa
Ebola	Ebola HF	Person-to-person	Africa

Note: HF = hemorrhagic fever.

contact with the animal reservoir (e.g., rodents or bats) of the virus (see Table 5-7). In endemic areas, the temporal distribution of many viral HFs follows seasonal changes in the activity and density of the vector or animal reservoir or seasonal changes in human activity. The age and sex distributions of infection and disease caused by some HF viruses reflect differences in exposure to the vector or reservoir, whereas other viruses affect persons of all ages and both sexes.

Several of the HFs have only recently been recognized and had their agents characterized. For example, the South American HFs, Ebola HF, and Marburg HF appear to have emerged in just the past 50 years, presumably as a result of increased human activity or settlement in areas where these viruses were already circulating among their zoonotic hosts. In some instances, such as with Argentine HF, the geographic range of the virus has expanded beyond its initial focus (Vainrub & Salas, 1994). The development of control and prevention strategies for newly emerging infections can pose special difficulties because investigators have not yet conducted the research needed to formulate treatment modalities, vaccines, vector-control strategies, and other preventive measures.

Etiologic Agents and Clinical Features

Although at least 15 different HF viruses exist (see Table 5-7), the public health significance of each virus differs substantially. The most prominent (in terms of incidence of disease) are Lassa virus, yellow fever virus, and dengue viruses. The latter two are discussed in the section on arthropod-borne diseases. Ebola virus and Marburg virus are notable for their epidemic potential and extraordinarily high case fatality ratios, whereas the South American HFs caused by the Junin, Machupo, and Guanarito viruses have regional public health importance. Detailed discussion of the remaining HF viruses is beyond the scope of this chapter.

Descriptive Epidemiologic Features and Risk Factors

Ebola HF emerged in 1976 when concurrent epidemics occurred in Democratic Republic of Congo (formerly Zaire) and Sudan. These outbreaks were caused by distinct subtypes of the virus and were characterized by high case fatality ratios (88% in Democratic Republic of Congo and 53% in Sudan). In total, 602 persons were infected and 431 died in the two outbreaks. Sudan experienced a second, smaller outbreak in 1979, and Gabon experienced three small outbreaks (each involving 60 or fewer cases) in the 1990s. A large outbreak occurred in Kikwit, Democratic Republic of

Congo, in 1995, resulting in 315 cases and 244 deaths, yielding a case fatality ratio of 77%. The largest outbreak to date was in Uganda in 2000–2001, involving 425 cases and 224 deaths (case fatality ratio of 53%). Smaller outbreaks recurred in Gabon, Democratic Republic of Congo, and Sudan between 2000 and 2004, resulting in a total of 317 cases and 260 deaths (case fatality ratio of 82%). A large outbreak occurred in Democratic Republic of Congo in 2007, with 264 cases and 187 deaths (case fatality ratio of 71%). A new strain of Ebola virus caused an outbreak in Uganda in 2007–2008, producing 149 cases and 37 deaths (case fatality ratio of 25%).

The first recognized outbreak of Marburg HF occurred in Marburg, Germany, in 1967 among laboratory workers (and their contacts), who acquired the infection from monkeys imported from Uganda. Since then, small numbers of cases have been reported in South Africa (1975), Kenya (1980 and 1987), and Uganda (2007 and 2008); in addition, more than 200 cases were identified in Democratic Republic of Congo in the period from 1998 to 2000 (Bausch et al., 2003). In 2004–2005, the largest outbreak to date occurred in Angola, involving 252 cases and 227 deaths (case fatality ratio of 90%) (Towner et al., 2006). The case fatality ratio of Marburg HF ranges from 21% to 90%.

Epidemics of Ebola HF have been sustained by person-to-person transmission through direct physical contact with infected patients or corpses (or with their bodily fluids or tissues) and the use of unsterile needles for medical injections. Person-to-person transmission is not very efficient, with secondary attack rates of only 16% being noted among household contacts of infected individuals (Dowell, Mukunu, Ksiazek, Khan, Rollin, & Peters, 1999). Marburg virus is also transmitted by person-to-person contact. Fortunately, airborne transmission does not appear to be common for either virus. Recent evidence suggests that several species of bats may be a reservoir for Ebola (Leroy et al., 2005; Pourrut, Délicat, Rollin, Ksiazek, Gonzalez, & Leroy 2007), but it is unclear whether direct bat-to-human transmission occurs or whether other hosts, such as nonhuman primates, play an intermediate role. Some evidence suggests that bats may also play a role in the transmission of Marburg virus (Towner et al., 2007).

Lassa virus is widely distributed across West Africa, where it causes substantial morbidity and mortality. Although its precise incidence is unknown, it has been estimated as many as 300,000 to 500,000 new infections occur each year, with an overall case fatality ratio of 1% to 2% (McCormick, Webb, Krebs, Johnson, & Smith, 1987; WHO, 2005b). Maternal death, fetal death, and permanent deafness are common complications of this disease (Cummins et al., 1990; Monson, Cole, Frame, Serwint, Alexander, & Jahrling, 1987; Richmond & Baglole, 2003).

Lassa virus is maintained in a rodent reservoir that is commonly found in the home. Virus is shed in rodent urine and droppings, and rodent-to-human transmission is believed to occur by aerosolization or ingestion of rodent excreta or by inoculation through broken skin. Rodent-to-human transmission may also occur when infected rodents are consumed as food (Ter Meulen et al., 1996). Person-to-person transmission occurs in community and hospital settings, and makes a substantial contribution to epidemics of Lassa fever. This mode of transmission requires direct contact with infected persons. Person-to-person airborne transmission occurs rarely, if ever. Sexual transmission can occur, but the importance of this mode of transmission is unknown.

Argentine HF, which is caused by Junin virus, was first described in 1955 in agricultural workers in the Argentine pampas. Several hundred cases of Argentine HF occur each year in large, primarily agricultural regions of the pampas. The region of endemicity is expanding, and is now nearly 10 times larger than its initial compass (Vainrub & Salas, 1994).

Bolivian HF, which is caused by Machupo virus, was subsequently described in northeastern Bolivia, which is the only known endemic area. Outbreaks of Bolivian HF occurred in the 1960s and early 1970s, including large epidemics that affected hundreds of individuals. Although no cases were reported from 1976 to 1992, possibly due to effective host control, a small outbreak in 1994, outbreaks in 2007 and 2009, and recent sporadic cases have marked its reemergence (Aguilar, 2009; "Re-emergence of Bolivian Hemorrhagic Fever," 1994).

Venezuelan HF, which is caused by Guanarito virus, was first recognized in 1989. During the period from September 1989 to January 1997, 165 cases were reported within the small region of central Venezuela where Guanarito virus is endemic (De Manzione et al., 1998).

For infections caused by the Argentine, Bolivian, and Venezuelan HF viruses, the case fatality ratio is in the range of 15% to 33% (De Manzione et al., 1998; Doyle, Bryan, & Peters, 1998). Each of these viruses is associated with a rodent reservoir that maintains the virus in the wild. As with Lassa fever, rodent-to-human transmission occurs by the aerosolization or ingestion of virus-laden rodent excreta or by inoculation through broken skin. The rodent that carries Junin virus typically dwells in agricultural fields, whereas the rodent that carries Machupo virus readily enters the home. Rodent-control strategies must take such differences into account. Person-to-person transmission of Junin, Machupo, and Guanarito viruses is considered rare, and nosocomial outbreaks are uncommon.

Current Approaches to Prevention and Control

Field trials have demonstrated that a live, attenuated Junin virus vaccine is safe and provides effective protection against Argentine HF (Maiztegui et al., 1998); it may also provide cross-protection against Bolivian HF. Vaccines are not available for Lassa fever, Ebola HF, or Marburg HF, although several candidate Lassa fever vaccines are under development.

In the absence of vaccines, reducing the morbidity and mortality caused by HF viruses depends on preventing primary transmission by limiting exposures to virus reservoirs and vectors and controlling secondary transmission (e.g., person-to-person transmission in the hospital, household, or community setting) through patient isolation and barrier nursing. In addition, the use of antiviral drugs or convalescent serum is effective in some instances.

Strategies to limit exposure to the virus are determined by the unique characteristics of the associated animal reservoir or vector and the distinct ways in which each of the viruses is transmitted. For example, the rodent that carries Machupo virus is frequently found in and around the home, and aggressive rodent eradication measures through trapping and poisoning appear to have been quite successful in controlling Bolivian HF (Kilgore et al., 1995). Conversely, the rodent reservoir of Junin virus lives in crop fields, where trapping and poisoning are difficult, necessitating the development of alternative rodent abatement strategies. Eradication (or even control) of the rodent reservoir of Lassa virus in West Africa is not considered feasible due to the density and wide distribution of the rodent that carries the virus. Thus preventing the primary transmission of Lassa virus has relied on educating at-risk communities about ways to reduce opportunities for exposure, such as never leaving food items uncovered and never consuming rodents as food.

Historically, nosocomial and person-to-person transmission of Lassa fever, Ebola HF, and Marburg HF have contributed significantly to devastating outbreaks of these diseases. (The South American HF viruses are rarely transmitted by these routes.) Field experience indicates that epidemic control is readily achieved through simple barrier nursing techniques (e.g., wearing gloves, gowns, and masks; sterilizing equipment; and isolating patients), and epidemiologic studies support this conclusion. For example, serologic studies in Sierra Leone found that hospital personnel who used barrier techniques when caring for patients with Lassa patients had no greater risk of infection than the local population (Helmick, Webb, Scribner, Krebs, & McCormick, 1986).

At present, few specific treatments are available for the viral HFs. Ribavirin (an antiviral drug) is effective in the treatment of Lassa fever (McCormick et al., 1986). Laboratory data suggest that ribavirin may also be effective in treating South American HFs, although clinical data supporting this usage are incomplete (Doyle et al., 1998). Ribavirin is unlikely to be beneficial in treating Ebola HF or Marburg HF. Convalescent serum is useful in the treatment of Argentine HF (WHO, 1985), but donors are not plentiful. Most people in low- and middle-income countries are not able to afford these therapies.

Obstacles to Prevention and Control and Directions for Future Research

The major obstacle to containing outbreaks of viral HFs (especially Ebola HF, Marburg HF, and Lassa fever) is inadequate disease surveillance, which results in delayed response and increased opportunity for epidemic spread. In many low- and middle-income countries, disease surveillance is impeded by the difficulty of making an early diagnosis in areas where illnesses with similar initial manifestations (e.g., malaria, influenza, typhoid fever, leptospirosis, meningococcemia, and hepatitis) are prevalent. The lack of ready access to diagnostic laboratories exacerbates this difficulty. In addition, because epidemics are unpredictable in time and place, surveillance efforts are difficult to maintain. Other obstacles to the control and prevention of viral HFs include the costliness of sustaining readiness for infection control measures (e.g., maintaining supplies for barrier nursing), lack of information about the vectors and reservoirs of the Ebola and Marburg viruses, the difficulties of developing and maintaining vector- and rodent-control programs, and the limited availability of ribavirin (especially for the treatment of Lassa fever).

Infectious Causes of Blindness

Overview

Severely decreased visual acuity or complete blindness is profoundly disabling in any setting, but perhaps even more so in low- and middle-income countries. Among the known causes of blindness, two infectious agents play important etiologic roles in selected regions of the world: *C. trachomatis*, the cause of trachoma, and *Onchocerca volvulus*, the cause of onchocerciasis, also known as river blindness.

Trachoma
Etiologic Agents

C. trachomatis is a small bacterium that lives within selected types of human cells and is difficult to grow in the laboratory. Although *C. trachomatis* is also the cause of STIs, as discussed previously, different immunotypes of the bacterium cause trachoma and genital tract infections. Those that cause trachoma are spread via a person-to-person route, most probably through eye and possibly nasal secretions on the hands. *C. trachomatis* is also spread mechanically by flies and probably by fomites such as washrags and handkerchiefs. Repeated episodes of infection in young (preschool) children lead to scarring of the eyelids, which in turn causes in-turned eyelashes that abrade the corneal surface, leading to subsequent corneal opacification and reduced visual acuity or blindness in adults.

Descriptive Epidemiologic Features and Risk Factors

Trachoma is an important cause of preventable blindness in the world. It is estimated that 40 million people are infected with *C. trachomatis*, of whom approximately 8.2 million have trachomatous trichiasis, the blinding stage of the disease (Mariotti, Pascolini, & Rose-Nussbaumer, 2009). Trachoma is a disease of poverty that was described by the ancient Egyptians and previously was found throughout the world. It disappeared from Europe and virtually all of the United States long before antimicrobial agents became available in the 1930s and 1940s; improved standards of living and personal hygiene are credited with its disappearance.

Trachoma is not a reportable condition, and what is known of its descriptive epidemiologic features comes from numerous surveys. This disease persists in hot, low- and middle-income countries, particularly in North Africa, the Middle East, sub-Saharan Africa, and drier regions of India and Southeast Asia. In hyperendemic areas, infection of the eye is virtually universal in children by their fifth birthday, but active disease is seen largely in older children. Repeated reinfection in children leads to the permanent damage to the eyes that results in subsequent blindness or visual impairment in adulthood. Although infection in childhood appears to be equally common in boys and girls, the blinding complications appear to be more common in women, perhaps because of repeated exposure to infected children.

Risk factors for trachoma in children largely relate to facial cleanliness, the presence of flies, and cultural practices that lead to an increased likelihood of person-to-person transmission of the etiologic agent, such as sharing washcloths and ways in which eye makeup is applied.

Current Approaches to Prevention and Control

Intervention studies have demonstrated that mass treatment with a variety of topical or oral antimicrobial agents and health educational programs that lead to improved facial cleanliness can substantially reduce the prevalence of trachoma in a community, as can fly control (Emerson et al., 2004; House et al., 2009). Reductions in disease incidence in low- and middle-income countries in the absence of a specific control program have also been documented as access to water, access to health care, and hygiene have improved.

The current approach to reducing trachoma-associated blindness in endemic areas is summarized by the acronym SAFE, which stands for (1) surgery to correct eyelid deformity, (2) antibiotics to treat acute eye infection and reduce sources of infection in the community, (3) facial cleanliness, and (4) environmental change that enhances availability of water and reduces the prevalence of flies. Studies have demonstrated that the SAFE approach can be highly effective (Ngondi et al., 2006). In 1997, WHO launched a new trachoma control program—called Global Elimination of Trachoma by 2020 (GET 2020)—based on this approach.

Obstacles to Prevention and Directions for Future Research

Trachoma is likely to remain a persistent problem in endemic areas until rising socioeconomic conditions result in better access to water, improved personal hygiene and sanitation, reductions in the numbers of flies, and improved access to healthcare services. Although community-wide treatment with antimicrobial agents can lead to reduced trachoma in such areas, these reductions have proven difficult to sustain unless such treatment is made a routine part of regularly available health services and is accompanied by improvements in hygiene. Although a vaccine against trachoma has been discussed for many years, it remains unclear whether an effective vaccine can or will ever be developed.

Onchocerciasis
Etiologic Agents

O. volvulus is a filarial parasite that is spread through the bite of one of several species of *Simulium* black flies. During the bite of an infected female fly, larvae enter the body. There, they ultimately develop into adult worms that form nodules, usually over bony prominences. Adult worms can survive inside these nodules for as long as 15 years. The female adult worm produces microfilariae that migrate to the skin and the eye and are ingested by female flies when they bite an infected person, thereby completing the cycle.

In the skin, an inflammatory response to dead and dying microfilariae can lead to incapacitating itching and various types of degenerative, often unsightly, skin changes. In the eye, heavy and prolonged infection of the cornea with the microfilariae leads to opacification and reduced visual acuity or total blindness. The microfilariae can be detected by taking small snips of skin, immersing them in saline, and examining the saline microscopically.

Descriptive Epidemiologic Features and Risk Factors

Onchocerciasis is found only in a band of sub-Saharan African countries, parts of Central America, the northern part of South America, and the Arabian peninsula. Nearly 18 million persons worldwide are believed to be currently infected with the parasite, and more than 750,000 individuals are either blind or have severe visual impairment as a result of their infection; the vast majority of these individuals live in Africa, especially Nigeria, Cameroon, Uganda, Congo, and Ethiopia (WHO, 2001). Within these affected regions, onchocerciasis occurs in clusters, largely determined by distance from the black fly breeding sites. The intensity of infection (and hence the risk of visual impairment) increases with age, as the burden of adult female worms producing microfilariae increases. This burden tends to be greater in men than in women, perhaps reflecting work-related exposures to the flies.

Current Approaches to Prevention and Control

Approaches to the control of onchocerciasis and prevention of the blindness it causes have included vector control, mass treatment of infected individuals, and nodulectomy (removal of nodules to reduce the source and number of microfilariae that migrate to the eyes). Early attempts to control onchocerciasis targeted the *Simulium* flies that serve as vectors, the immature stages of which require running water (e.g., rivers and streams) for their development. Initially, DDT was the pesticide added to rivers that served as the breeding grounds for the vector. Beginning in the 1970s, other agents that target the larval stages of the fly (e.g., temephos) were used with great success, particularly in West Africa. These programs permitted resettlement of fertile areas that had been abandoned because of onchocerciasis, but the flies' development of resistance to temephos required switching to other larvacidal agents in some areas.

The control of onchocerciasis was revolutionized in the late 1980s with the introduction of ivermectin, a single dose of which eliminates microfilariae for a number of months. Because ivermectin does not kill the adult worms, repeated treatment (e.g., every 6 to 12 months) of infected individuals over many years is needed to provide continued suppression of the number of microfilariae and to prevent visual damage. Treatment every 3 months may be even more effective at reducing both the number of female worms in nodules and the severity of symptoms (Gardon, Boussinesq, Kamgno, Gardon-Wendel, Demanga-Ngangue, & Duke, 2002). In a noteworthy humanitarian gesture, the manufacturer of ivermectin has made a commitment to provide the drug free "for as long as necessary to as many as necessary." Given the now widespread availability of ivermectin, countries affected by onchocerciasis have developed control programs that identify endemic areas (typically by conducting nodule surveys) and then make the drug available in those areas (Pacqué, Muñoz, Greene, & Taylor, 1991). To date, nearly 100 million people have received ivermectin treatment. Various approaches to making the drug available have been used (e.g., passive health center–based programs and active community-based programs), and each has advantages and disadvantages.

Obstacles to Prevention and Directions for Future Research

Although it may be possible in some endemic areas to eradicate onchocerciasis through vector control or mass ivermectin treatment programs, in the most heavily affected parts of Africa complete eradication is not likely in the foreseeable future. The effectiveness of a new drug, moxidectin, is now being tested in hopes that this agent may be able to eliminate onchocerciasis with shorter-duration treatment (Lawrence, 2009).

Emergence of New Infectious Disease Threats

The availability of a growing number of antimicrobial agents and vaccines beginning in the 1950s and continuing through the 1970s simultaneously led to the burgeoning infectious disease prevention and control activities described earlier in this chapter and to a widely shared assumption that infectious disease threats to human (and animal) health would diminish over time. A sobering note was injected into this otherwise optimistic conversation with the unexpected emergence of new infectious diseases and the reemergence of previously controlled diseases that became apparent in the 1980s and 1990s. Their appearance made it clear that efforts to control existing infectious diseases needed to be accompanied by an improved global capacity for early detection and rapid response to newly emergent or reemergent infectious diseases. Concern about the possible intentional release of infectious agents in a deliberate effort to frighten, harm, or kill gave added impetus to efforts in this area.

The concept of emerging and reemerging infections, which began receiving prominent attention after the U.S. Institute of Medicine released a report entitled *Emerging Infections: Microbial Threats to Health in the United States* in 1992, encompasses several distinct phenomena that can produce unexpected and sometimes urgent infectious disease threats. Included under the rubric of emerging and reemerging infectious disease threats are diseases caused by microbial agents not previously known to cause illness in humans (e.g., SARS, Nipah virus encephalitis, and H5N1 [avian] influenza in humans), the appearance in a new location of an infectious agent (e.g., the spread of West Nile virus to the United States), the appearance of a new epidemiologic pattern of disease caused by an infectious agent (e.g., epidemic meningococcal meningitis caused by serogroup W-135 *N. meningitidis*), the appearance or spread of new variants of an infectious agent (e.g., multidrug- and extensively drug-resistant *M. tuberculosis*), and the resurgence of an infectious disease previously under good control (e.g., diphtheria in parts of the former Soviet Union).

The 1992 report by the Institute of Medicine, together with a follow-up report in 2003 (Smolinski, Hamburg, & Lederberg, 2003), outlined a number of factors that could promote the emergence or reemergence of infectious disease threats. In addition to microbial adaptation and change in response to selection pressures, numerous human and environmental factors may contribute to the emergence or reemergence of infectious diseases—for example, increased human susceptibility to infection; human demographic conditions and behaviors; international travel and commerce; economic development and land use; technologic change; climate and ecologic factors; breakdown of public health measures; war and famine; poverty and social inequality; lack of political will;

and intent to harm. Individually and collectively, these factors may increase the likelihood that humans will come in contact with various infectious agents, produce a greater susceptibility to infection, enhance and accelerate the spread of infectious agents, and reduce the capacity of communities to detect and respond effectively to infectious disease threats. Although the result can be dramatic outbreaks that command widespread public attention and political response (e.g., SARS), other equally serious infectious disease threats (e.g., multidrug- and extensively drug-resistant tuberculosis) often go largely unnoticed by the general public and decision makers because they do not produce explosive epidemics.

A dramatic example of an emerging infectious disease threat in recent years was the appearance of SARS. This life-threatening form of pneumonia appears to have originated in southern China in late 2002 (CDC, 2003). Before the significance of these cases of pneumonia became apparent, the illness had spread to multiple other parts of Asia and eventually to Europe, North America, and elsewhere. By the middle of 2003, more than 8,400 probable cases of SARS and more than 800 SARS-related deaths had been reported from 30 countries, with China, Hong Kong, and Taiwan bearing the brunt of the epidemic. SARS is caused by a previously unknown member of the Coronaviridiae family that almost certainly originated in one or more animal reservoirs and initially spread to humans through direct exposure to infected animals in southern China. The virus then proved to be transmissible from person to person, particularly in healthcare settings. Spread of the SARS-associated coronavirus was also documented on commercial airplanes, and the ease of modern travel from one part of the world to another clearly facilitated the rapid dissemination of the virus across the globe.

In addition to the morbidity and mortality it caused, the SARS epidemic had an enormous economic impact. It has been estimated that the total cost of this epidemic to Asian economies alone was approximately $60 billion. In the absence of a vaccine, preventing further spread of the SARS epidemic required stringent isolation of patients, quarantine of exposed individuals, restrictions on travel, and various other measures that were highly disruptive of commerce, travel, and other aspects of life.

More recent experience with influenza demonstrates many of the challenges related to detecting and responding rapidly to an emergent infectious disease threat. The appearance in Hong Kong in 1997 of human cases of influenza caused by the highly pathogenic avian influenza virus A (H5N1) heralded widespread epizootics (i.e., epidemics in animals) in domestic poultry and widespread infection (often asymptomatic) in many species of wild birds that ultimately reached much of Asia and parts of Africa, Europe, and the Middle East. By 2008, several hundred human infections with H5N1 had been documented in Asia (Vietnam, Thailand, Cambodia, Indonesia, and China), as had a smaller number of infections in Egypt and Turkey (Writing Committee of the Second World Health Organization Consultation on Clinical Aspects of Human Infection with Avian Influenza A [H5N1] Virus, 2008).

The H5N1 influenza virus is highly pathogenic in people. More than 50% of the people with documented illnesses died from their disease, prompting well-justified concern about a human epidemic or pandemic caused by this virus and resulting in efforts to make and stockpile a safe and effective H5N1 vaccine. To date, however, there have been very few instances of person-to-person transmission of H5N1 virus (virtually all human cases are the result of animal-to-human transmission), and it remains uncertain whether this virus is capable of both retaining its high pathogenicity and becoming readily transmissible from person to person.

While public health officials and vaccine manufacturers were preparing for a possible H5N1 influenza pandemic, a novel H1N1 influenza A virus of swine origin arose. Although this H1N1 virus was first detected in ill individuals in southern California and in Mexico in early 2009 (Novel Swine-Origin Influenza A [H1N1] Virus Investigation Team, 2009), its origins remain unknown. By the time the virus was first detected, it undoubtedly had undergone many generations of transmission among humans and had already become widely disseminated, making attempts to contain it futile. Within a short period of time after its discovery, the novel H1N1 influenza A virus was circulating and causing disease throughout North America, Europe, and Asia in the northern hemisphere and causing large epidemics in numerous countries in South America, Southern Africa, and Australia and New Zealand in the southern hemisphere. Although a vaccine containing this virus was developed and produced with exceptional speed, neither the vaccine nor other approaches (e.g., antiviral drugs, isolation and quarantine, and social distancing measures) could prevent a pandemic from unfolding.

Fortunately, this influenza A virus has proved to be no more virulent than the influenza A and B viruses that cause annual epidemics, although it has still produced widespread morbidity and mortality. A more virulent influenza A virus would have produced

Exhibit 5-6	Global Outbreak Alert and Response Network

Throughout the 1970s, 1980s, and 1990s, outbreaks of novel or high-impact infectious diseases (e.g., Ebola, cholera, and meningococcal meningitis) in poor- and middle-income countries often led to ad hoc responses by multiple national, international, academic, research, and private-sector organizations. Unfortunately, many of these efforts were uncoordinated and sometimes duplicative or even competing in nature. Although countries often looked to the World Health Organization for leadership and technical assistance in such instances, WHO historically had very limited trained personnel and resources to devote to such efforts, as well as political and legal constraints that could limit its access.

In recognition of these problems, in 2000 WHO created the Global Outbreak Alert and Response Network (GOARN), which has its headquarters in Geneva, Switzerland. GOARN, which is intended to be an early warning system, receives a steady stream of daily reports concerning possible outbreaks from a global network of informants. It also uses a newly developed software system to monitor news sources on the Internet. GOARN staff receive 10 to 20 leads each day, which they evaluate and, when appropriate, follow up. The network has proven useful as SARS, avian influenza, swine influenza, and other outbreaks have appeared since 2000. Recent revisions to the International Health Regulations that give WHO improved access when important outbreaks occur should improve the functioning of this system.

substantially more morbidity and mortality, and would have been equally difficult to contain.

As these examples demonstrate, there is an ongoing threat of new infectious agents entering and causing disease in human populations, particularly from animal sources. Even as progress is made in eradicating or controlling historically important infectious diseases, the need persists for vigilance, preparedness, and a high level of international cooperation to detect and respond to new infectious disease threats that might emerge. WHO and others are working to improve global capacity in this area (see Exhibit 5-6).

Conclusion

The current status of infectious diseases in low- and middle-income countries reflects both the dramatic progress that has been made in controlling some diseases and the disappointing results to date in controlling others. The eradication of smallpox, the expected imminent eradication of polio, and impressive gains made against measles and neonatal tetanus all demonstrate what can be accomplished even in the lowest-income countries with an effective vaccine when concerted efforts are made to ensure that the vaccine reaches those in need. Similar progress in reducing morbidity from dracunculiasis and onchocerciasis demonstrates that, under the right conditions and with available resources, infectious diseases can be controlled through a combination of vector control and avoidance and treatment. At the same time, the reductions in the morbidity and mortality from diarrheal diseases and acute respiratory infections that have been achieved are clear evidence that a combi-

nation of improved knowledge and access to reasonably inexpensive treatment modalities can also be highly effective.

Far less encouraging has been the progress made against malaria, dengue, TB, and AIDS, all of which continue to exact a substantial toll on populations across the globe. For diseases such as TB, much can be accomplished simply by improving diagnosis and treatment of cases using tried-and-true methods that have been available for many years. For diseases such as AIDS, behavior change and improved access to treatment of other STIs can reduce the risk of acquiring HIV infection, and expanded use of antiretroviral drugs can dramatically improve the lives of HIV-infected individuals and reduce vertical transmission of the virus. Nevertheless, development and widespread use of an effective vaccine is the only realistic long-term solution to the HIV/AIDS pandemic. For vector-borne diseases such as dengue and malaria, either new approaches to vector control or effective vaccines are urgently needed.

The progress made to date in controlling the morbidity and mortality from infectious diseases in low- and middle-income countries demonstrates that much can be accomplished even in the absence of marked improvements in socioeconomic conditions. Ultimately, however, widespread improvements in education and socioeconomic conditions will be needed if such progress is to be maintained.

Acknowledgments

The authors acknowledge Christina Phares for her assistance in the preparation of this chapter.

• • • Discussion Questions

1. What are the major types of approaches that have been used to prevent morbidity and mortality from infectious diseases in low- and middle-income countries?

2. What are the major obstacles that have had and remain to be overcome in implementing various approaches to preventing morbidity and mortality from infectious diseases in low- and middle-income countries?

3. In the current year, which infectious diseases account for the most mortality in low-income countries? The most morbidity?

4. If you were working in the Ministry of Health of a low-income country and needed to set priorities concerning resource allocation, how could you go about determining the relative importance of various infectious diseases as causes of mortality in your country? The causes of morbidity/disability?

• • • References

Aaby, P., Samb, B., Simondon, F., Knudsen, K., Seck, A. M., Bennett, J., et al. (1994). Sex-specific differences in mortality after high-titre measles immunization in rural Senegal. *Bulletin of the World Health Organization, 72,* 761–770.

Aguilar, P. V., Camargo, W., Vargas, J., Guevara, C., Roca, Y., Felices, V., et al. (2009). Reemergence of Bolivian hemorrhagic fever, 2007–2008. *Emerging Infectious Diseases, 15,* 1526–1528.

Alonso, P.L., Sacarlal, J., Aponte, J.J., Leach, A., Macete, E., Milman, J., et al. (2004). Efficacy of the RTS,S/AS02A vaccine against Plasmodium falciparum infection and disease in young African children: randomised controlled trial. *Lancet, 364,* 1411–1420.

Arifeen, S. E., Hoque, D. M. E., Akter, T., Rahman, M., Hoque, M. E., Begum, K., et al. (2009). Effect of the integrated management of childhood illness strategy on childhood mortality and nutrition in a rural area in Bangladesh: A cluster randomized trial. *Lancet, 374,* 393–403.

Auvert, B., Taljaard, D., Lagarde, E., Sobngwi-Tambekou, J., Sitta, M., & Puren, A. (2005). Randomized, controlled intervention trial of male circumcision for reduction of HIV infection risk: The ANRS 1265 trial. *PLoS Med, 2,* 1112–1122.

Avila, M., Salomón, H., Carballal, G., Ebekian, B., Woyskovsky, N., Cerqueiro, M. C., et al. (1990). Role of viral pathogens in acute respiratory tract infections. *Reviews of Infectious Diseases, 12,* S974–S981.

Bach, J. F., Chalons, S., Forier, E., Elana, G., Jouanelle, J., Kayemba, S., et al. (1996). 10-year educational programme aimed at rheumatic fever in two French Caribbean islands. *Lancet, 347,* 644–648.

Bailey, R. C., Moses, S., Parker, C. B., Agot, K. & Ndinya-Achola, J.O. (2007). Male circumcision for HIV prevention in young men in Kisumu, Kenya: A randomized controlled trial. *Lancet, 369,* 643–656.

Banatvala, J. E., & Brown, D. W. G. (2004). Rubella. *Lancet, 363,* 1127–1137.

Bausch, D. G., Borchert, M., Grein, T., Roth, C., Swanepoel, R., Libande, M. L., et al. (2003). Risk factors for Marburg hemorrhagic fever, Democratic Republic of the Congo. *Emerging Infectious Diseases, 9*(12), 1531–1537.

Berman, S. (1991). Epidemiology of acute respiratory infections in children of developing countries. *Reviews of Infectious Diseases, 13,* S454–S462.

Bern, C., Martines, J., de Zoysa, I., & Glass, R. I. (1992). The magnitude of the global problem of diarrhoeal disease: A ten-year update. *Bulletin of the World Health Organization, 70,* 705–714.

Bertherat, E., Yada, A., Djingarey, M. H., & Koumare, B. (2002). First major epidemic caused by *Neisseria meningitidis* serogroup W-135 in Africa. *Tropical Medicine, 62,* 301–304.

Black, R. E. (1993). Persistent diarrhea in children of developing countries. *Pediatric Infectious Disease Journal, 12,* 751–761.

Black, R. E., Morris, S. S., & Bryce, J. (2003). Where and why are 10 million children dying every year? *Lancet, 361,* 2226–2234.

Bowden, S. (2001). New hepatitis viruses: Contenders and pretenders. *Journal of Gastroenterology and Hepatology, 16*(2), 124–131.

Breastfeeding and HIV Transmission Study Group. (2004). Late postnatal transmission of HIV-1 in breast-fed children: An individual patient data meta-analysis. *Journal of Infectious Diseases, 189,* 2154–2166.

Breman, J. G. (2009). Eradicating malaria. *Science Progress, 92,* 1–38.

Brok, J., Gluud, L. L., & Gluud, C. (2010). Ribavirin plus interferon versus interferon for chronic hepatitis C. *Cochrane Database Systematic Review, 1,* CD005445.

Bundy, D. A. (1990). New initiatives in the control of helminths. *Transactions of the Royal Society of Tropical Medicine and Hygiene, 84,* 467–468.

Bundy, D. A., Hall, A., Medley, G. F., & Savioli, L. (1992). Evaluating measures to control intestinal parasitic infections. *World Health Statistics Quarterly, 45,* 168–179.

Butterworth, A. E., Dunne, D. W., Fulford, A. J., Ouma, J. H., & Sturrock, R. F. (1996). Immunity and morbidity in *Schistosoma mansoni* infection: Quantitative aspects. *American Journal of Tropical Medicine and Hygiene, 55,* 109–115.

Celentano, D. D., Nelson, K. E., Suprasert, S., Eiumtrakul, S., Tulvatana, S., Kuntolbutra, S., et al. (1996). Risk factors for HIV-1 seroconversion among young men in northern Thailand. *Journal of the American Medical Association, 275,* 122–127.

Centers for Disease Control and Prevention (CDC). (1996). Progress toward elimination of neonatal tetanus: Egypt, 1988–1994. *Morbidity and Mortality Weekly Report, 45,* 89–92.

Centers for Disease Control and Prevention (CDC). (2002). Progress toward global eradication of poliomyelitis. *Morbidity and Mortality Weekly Report, 52,* 366–369.

Centers for Disease Control and Prevention (CDC). (2003). Outbreak of severe acute respiratory syndrome—worldwide, 2003. *Morbidity and Mortality Weekly Report, 52,* 226–228.

Centers for Disease Control and Prevention (CDC). (2004). Measles mortality reduction—West Africa, 1996–2002. *Morbidity and Mortality Weekly Report, 53,* 28–30.

Centers for Disease Control and Prevention (CDC) (2009a). Global measles mortality, 2000–2008. *Morbidity and Mortality Weekly Report, 58,* 1321–1326.

Centers for Disease Control and Prevention (CDC). (2009b). Progress toward measles control—African region, 2001–2008. *Morbidity and Mortality Weekly Report, 58,* 1036–1041.

Centers for Disease Control and Prevention (CDC). (2009c). Wild poliovirus type 1 and type 3 importations—15 countries, Africa, 2008–2009. *Morbidity and Mortality Weekly Report, 58,* 357–362.

Chi, B. H., Sinkala, M., Mbewe, F., Cantrell, R. A., Kruse, G., Chintu, N., et al. (2007). Single-dose tenofovir and emtricitabine for reduction of viral resistance to non-nucleoside reverse transcriptase inhibitor drugs in women given intrapartum nevirapine for perinatal HIV prevention: An open-label randomized trial. *Lancet, 370,* 1698–1705.

Cholera Working Group, International Centre for Diarrhoeal Diseases Research, Bangladesh. (1993). Large epidemic of cholera-like disease in Bangladesh caused by *Vibrio cholerae* O139 synonym Bengal. *Lancet, 342,* 387–390.

Cohen, J. (2003). AIDS vaccine still alive as booster after second failure in Thailand. *Science, 302,* 1309–1310.

Cox-Singh, J., Davis, T. M., Lee, K. S., Shamsul, S. S., Matusop, A., Ratnam, S., et al. (2008). *Plasmodium knowlesi* malaria in humans is widely distributed and potentially life threatening. *Clinical Infectious Diseases, 46,* 165–71.

Crump, J. A., Luby, S. P., & Mintz, E. D. (2004). The global burden of typhoid fever. *Bulletin of the World Health Organization, 82,* 346–353.

Cummins, D., McCormick, J. B., Bennett, D., Samba, J. A., Farrar, B., Machin, S. J., et al. (1990). Acute sensorineural deafness in Lassa fever. *Journal of the American Medical Association, 264,* 2093–2096.

Cutts, F. T., & Vynnycky, E. (1999). Modelling the incidence of congenital rubella syndrome in developing countries. *International Journal of Epidemiology, 28,* 1176–1184.

Daneshvar, C., Davis, T. M., Cox-Singh, J., Rafa'ee, M. Z., Zakaria, S. K., Divis, P. C., et al. (2009). Clinical and laboratory features of human *Plasmodium knowlesi* infection. *Clinical Infectious Diseases, 49,* 852–860.

De Manzione, N., Salas, R. A., Paredes, H., Godoy, O., Rojas, L., Araoz, F., et al. (1998). Venezuelan hemorrhagic fever: Clinical and epidemiological studies of 165 cases. *Clinical Infectious Diseases, 26,* 308–313.

de Quadros, C. A., Izurieta, H., Venczel, L., & Carrasco, P. (2004). Measles eradication in the Americas: Progress to date. *Journal of Infectious Diseases, 189,* S227–S235.

Dowdle, W. R., & Hopkins, D. R. (1998). *The eradication of infectious diseases: Report of the Dahlem Workshop on the Eradication of Infectious Diseases, Berlin, March 16–22, 1997.* Chichester, UK: John Wiley & Sons.

Dowell, S. F., Mukunu, R., Ksiazek, T. G., Khan, A. S., Rollin, P. E., & Peters, C. J. (1999). Transmission of Ebola hemorrhagic fever: A study of risk factors in family members, Kikwit, Democratic Republic of the Congo, 1995. Commission de Lutte contre les Epidémies à Kikwit. *Journal of Infectious Diseases, 179,* S87–S91.

Doyle, T. J., Bryan, R. T., & Peters, C. J. (1998). Viral hemorrhagic fevers and hantavirus infections in the Americas. *Infectious Disease Clinics of North America, 12,* 95–110.

Eigege, A., Pede, E., Miri, E., Umaru, J., Ogbu Pearce, P., Jinadu, M. Y., et al. (2008). Triple drug administration (TDA), with praziquantel, ivermectin and albendazole, for the prevention of three neglected tropical diseases in Nigeria. *Annals of Tropical Medicine and Parasitology, 102,* 177–179.

Ellis, W. A. (1998). Leptospirosis. In S. R. Palmer, E. J. L. Soulsby, & D. I. H. Simpson (Eds.), *Zoonoses: Biology, clinical practice, and public health control* (pp. 115–126). New York: Oxford University Press.

El-Rafie, M., Hassouna, W. A., Hirschhorn, N., Loza, S., Miller, P., Nagaty, A., et al. (1990). Effect of diarrhoeal disease control on infant and childhood mortality in Egypt: Report from the National Control of Diarrheal Diseases Project. *Lancet, 335,* 334–338.

El Samani, E. F., Willett, W. C., & Ware, J. H. (1988). Association of malnutrition and diarrhea in children aged under five years: A prospective follow-up study in a rural Sudanese community. *American Journal of Epidemiology, 128,* 93–105.

Emerson, P. M., Lindsay, S. W., Alexander, N., Bah, M., Dibba, S.-M., Faal, H. B., et al. (2004). Role of flies and pro-vision of latrines in trachoma control: Cluster-randomized controlled trial. *Lancet, 363,* 1093–1098.

Fine, P. E. M., Oblapenko, G., & Sutter, R. W. (2004). Polio control after certification: Major is-sues outstanding. *Bulletin of the World Health Organization, 82,* 47–52.

Fishbein, D. B. (1991). Rabies in humans. In G. M. Baer (Ed.), *The natural history of rabies* (2nd ed., pp. 519–549). Boca Raton, FL: CRC Press.

Frist, B., & Sezibera, R. (2009). Time for renewed global action against childhood pneumonia. *Lancet, 374,* 1485–1486.

Gardon, J., Boussinesq, M., Kamgno, J., Gardon-Wendel, N., Demanga-Ngangue, B., & Duke, O. L. (2002). Effects of standard and high doses of ivermectin on adult worms on *Onchocerca volvulus*: A randomized controlled trial. *Lancet, 360,* 203–210.

Glass, R. I., Libel, M., & Brandling-Bennett, A. D. (1992). Epidemic cholera in the Americas. *Science, 256,* 1524–1525.

Goodgame, R. W., & Greenough, W. B. (1975). Cholera in Africa: A message for the West. *Annals of Internal Medicine, 82,* 101–106.

Gove, S. (1997). Integrated management of childhood illness by outpatient health workers: Technical basis and overview. The WHO Working Group on Guidelines for Integrated Management of the Sick Child. *Bulletin of the World Health Organization, 75,* 7–24.

Graham, N. M. (1990). The epidemiology of acute respiratory infections in children and adults: A global perspective. *Epidemiologic Reviews, 12,* 149–178.

Gray, R. H., Kigozi, G., Serwadda, D., Makumbi, F., Watya, S., Nalugoda, F., et al. (2007). Male circumcision for HIV prevention in men in Rakai, Uganda: A randomized trial. *Lancet, 369,* 657–666.

Greenwood, B. M. (1987). The epidemiology of acute bacterial meningitis in tropical Africa. In J. D. Williams & J. Burnie (Eds.), *Bacterial meningitis* (pp. 61–91). London: Academic Press.

Gubler, D. J. (1998). Dengue and dengue hemorrhagic fever. *Clinical Microbiology Reviews, 11,* 480–496.

Hagan, P. (1996). Immunity and morbidity in infection due to *Schistosoma haematobium. American*

Journal of Tropical Medicine and Hygiene, 55, 116–120.

Hart, C. A., Trees, A. J., & Duerden, B. I. (1997). Zoonoses. *Journal of Medical Microbiology, 46,* 4–6.

Hauri, A. M., Armstrong, G. L., & Hutin, Y. J. (2004). The global burden of disease attributable to contaminated injections given in health care settings. *International Journal of STD and AIDS, 15*(1), 7–16.

Helmick, C. G., Webb, P. A., Scribner, C. L., Krebs, J. W., & McCormick, J. B. (1986). No evidence for increased risk of Lassa fever infection in hospital staff. *Lancet, 2,* 1202–1205.

Hopkins, D. R. (1984). Eradication of dracunculiasis. In P. G. Bourne (Ed.), *Water and sanitation: Economic and sociological perspectives* (pp. 93–114). Orlando, FL: Academic Press.

Hopkins, D. R., Ruiz-Tiben, E., & Ruebush, T. K. (1997). Dracunculiasis eradication: Almost a reality. *American Journal of Tropical Medicine and Hygiene, 57,* 252–259.

House, J., Ayele, F., Porco, T. C., Zhou, Z., Hong, K.C., Gebre, T., et al. (2009). Assessment of herd protection against trachoma due to repeated mass antibiotic distributions: A cluster-randomised trial. *Lancet, 373,* 1111–1118.

Htun, Y., Morse, S. A., Dangor, Y., Fehler, G., Radebe, F., Trees, D. L., et al. (1998). Comparison of clinically directed, disease specific, and syndromic protocols for the management of genital ulcer disease in Lesotho. *Sexually Transmitted Infections, 74,* S23–S28.

Hull, H. F., Ward, N. A., Hull, B. P., Milstien, J. B., & de Quadros, C. (1994). Paralytic poliomyelitis: Seasoned strategies, disappearing disease. *Lancet, 343,* 1331–1337.

Hunter, J. M. (1996). An introduction to Guinea worm on the eve of its departure: Dracunculiasis transmission, health effects, ecology and control. *Social Science and Medicine, 43,* 1399–1425.

Hussey, G. D., & Klein, M. (1990). A randomized, controlled trial of vitamin A in children with severe measles. *New England Journal of Medicine, 323,* 160–164.

Huttly, S. R., Morris, S. S., & Pisani, V. (1997). Prevention of diarrhoea in young children in developing countries. *Bulletin of the World Health Organization, 75,* 163–174.

Institute of Medicine. (1992). *Emerging infections: Microbial threats to health in the United States.* Washington, DC: National Academy Press.

Jackson, J. B., Musoke, P., Fleming, T., Guay, L. A., Bagenda, D., Allen, M., et al. (2003). Intrapartum and neonatal single-dose nevirapine compared with zidovudine for prevention of mother-to-child transmission of HIV-1 in Kampala, Uganda: 18-month follow-up of the HIVNET 012 randomised trial. *Lancet, 362*(9387), 859–868.

Jahn, A., Floyd, S., Crampin, A. C., Mwaungulu F., Mvula, H., Munthali, F., et al. (2008). Population-level effect of HIV on adult mortality and early evidence of reversal after introduction of antiretroviral therapy in Malawi. *Lancet, 371,* 1603–1611.

Jaiswal, S. P., Jain, A. K., Naik, G., Soni, N., & Chitnis, D. S. (2001). Viral hepatitis during pregnancy. *International Journal of Gynaecology and Obstetrics, 72*(2), 103–108.

Johnson, J. A., Li, J-F., Morris, L., Martinson, N., Gray, G., McIntyre, J., et al. (2005). Emergence of drug-resistant HIV-1 after intrapartum administration of single-dose nevirapine is substantially underestimated. *Journal of Infectious Diseases, 192,* 16–23.

Keusch, G. T., & Cash, R. A. (1997). A vaccine against rotavirus: When is too much too much? [Editorial]. *New England Journal of Medicine, 337,* 1228–1229.

Khuroo, M. S., Teli, M. R., Skidmore, S., Sofi, M. A., & Khuroo, M. I. (1981). Incidence and severity of viral hepatitis in pregnancy. *American Journal of Medicine, 70,* 252–255.

Kilgore, P. E., Peters, C. J., Mills, J. N., Rollin, P. E., Armstrong, L., Khan, A. S., et al. (1995). Prospects for the control of Bolivian hemorrhagic fever [Editorial]. *Emerging Infectious Diseases, 1,* 97–100.

Kilian, A. H., Gregson, S., Ndyanabangi, B., Walusaga, K., Kipp, W., Sahlmuller, G., et al.

(1999). Reductions in risk behaviour provide the most consistent explanation for declining HIV-1 prevalence in Uganda. *AIDS, 13,* 391–398.

Kosek, M., Bern, C., & Guerrant, R. L. (2003). The global burden of diarrhoeal disease, as estimated from studies published between 1992 and 2000. *Bulletin of the World Health Organization, 81,* 197–204.

LaForce, F. M., Lichnevski, M. S., Keja, J., & Henderson, R. H. (1980). Clinical survey techniques to estimate prevalence and annual incidence of poliomyelitis in developing countries. *Bulletin of the World Health Organization, 58,* 609–620.

Lambrechts, T., Bryce, J., & Orinda V. (1999). Integrated management of childhood illness: A summary of first experiences. *Bulletin of the World Health Organization, 77,* 582–594.

Lavanchy, D. (2009). The global burden of Hepatitis C. *Liver International, 29,* 74–81.

Lawrence, D. (2009). WHO launches test of new drug for river blindness (Newsdesk). *Lancet, 9,* 533.

Leroy, E. M., Kumulungui, B., Pourrut, X., Rouquet, P., Hassanin, A., Yaba, P., et al. (2005). Fruit bats as reservoirs of Ebola virus. *Nature, 438,* 575–576.

Levett, P. N. (2001). Leptospirosis. *Clinical Microbiology Reviews, 14*(2), 296–326.

Levine, M. M. (2009). Typhoid vaccines ready for implementation. *New England Journal of Medicine, 361,* 403–404.

Madhi, S. A., Cunliffe, N. A., Steele, D., Witte, D., Kirsten, M., Louw, C., et al. (2010). Effect of human rotavirus vaccine on severe diarrhea in African infants. *New England Journal of Medicine, 362,* 289–298.

Maiztegui, J. I., McKee, K. T. Jr., Barrera Oro, J. G., Harrison, L. H., Gibbs, P. H., Feuillade, M. R., et al. (1998). Protective efficacy of a live attenuated vaccine against Argentine hemorrhagic fever. AHF Study Group. *Journal of Infectious Diseases, 177,* 277–283.

Margolis, H. S., Alter, M. J., & Hadler, S. C. (1997). Viral hepatitis. In A. S. Evans & R. A.

Kaslow (Eds.), *Viral infections of humans: Epidemiology and control* (4th ed., pp. 363–418). New York: Plenum Medical Books.

Mariotti, S. P., Pascolini, D., & Rose-Nussbaumer, J. (2009). Trachoma: Global magnitude of a preventable cause of blindness. *British Journal of Ophthalmology, 93,* 563–568. doi: 10.1136/bio .2008.148494. pmid: 19098034.

Markowitz, L. E., Nzilambi, N., Driskell, W. J., Sension, M. G., Rovira, E. Z., Nieburg, P., et al. (1989). Vitamin A levels and mortality among hospitalized measles patients, Kinshasa, Zaire. *Journal of Tropical Pediatrics, 35,* 109–112.

McCormick, J. B., King, I. J., Webb, P. A., Scribner, C. L., Craven, R. B., Johnson, K. M., et al. (1986). Lassa fever: Effective therapy with ribavirin. *New England Journal of Medicine, 314,* 20–26.

McCormick, J. B., Webb, P. A., Krebs, J. W., Johnson, K. M., & Smith, E. S. (1987). A prospective study of the epidemiology and ecology of Lassa fever. *Journal of Infectious Diseases, 155,* 437–444.

Medina, E., & Yrarrazaval, M. (1983). Typhoid fever in Chile: Epidemiological considerations. *Revista Medica de Chile, 111,* 609–615.

Meima, A., Smith, W. C. S., van Oortmarassen, G. J., Richardus, J. H., & Habbema, J. D. F. (2004). The future incidence of leprosy: A scenario analysis. *Bulletin of the World Health Organization, 82,* 373–380.

Mermin, J., Were, W., Ekwaru, J. P., Moore, D., Downing, R., Behumbiize, P., et al. (2008). Mortality in HIV-infected Ugandan adults receiving antiretroviral treatment and survival of their HIV-uninfected children: A prospective cohort study. *Lancet, 371*(9614), 752–759.

Modlin, J. F. (2010). The bumpy road to polio eradication. *New England Journal of Medicine, 362*(25), 2346–2349.

Mohammed, K. A., Haji, H. J., Gabrielli, A. F., Mubila, L., Biswas, G., Chitsulo, L., et al. (2008). Triple co-administration of ivermectin, albendazole and praziquantel in Zanzibar: A safety study. *PLoS Neglected Tropical Diseases, 2,* e171.

Monson, M. H., Cole, A. K., Frame, J. D., Serwint, J. R., Alexander, S., & Jahrling, P. B. (1987). Pediatric Lassa fever: A review of 33 Liberian cases. *American Journal of Tropical Medicine and Hygiene, 36,* 408–415.

Moore, P. S. (1992). Meningococcal meningitis in sub-Saharan Africa: A model for the epidemic process. *Clinical Infectious Diseases, 14,* 515–525.

Mulholland, K., Hilton, S., Adegbola, R., Usen, S., Oparaugo, A., Omosigho, C., et al. (1997). Randomised trial of *Haemophilus influenzae* type b tetanus protein conjugate for prevention of pneumonia and meningitis in Gambian infants. *Lancet, 349,* 1191–1197.

Munoz, N., Manalastas, R. Jr., Pitisuttithum, P., Tresukosol, D., Monsonega, J., Ault, K., et al. (2009). Safety, immunogenicity, and efficacy of quadrivalent human papillomavirus (types 6, 11, 16, 18) recombinant vaccine in women aged 24–45 years: A randomized, double-blind trial. *Lancet, 373,* 1949–1957.

Nair, G. B., Ramamurthy, T., Bhattacharya, S. K., Mukhopadhyay, A. K., Garg, S., Bhattacharya, M. K., et al. (1994). Spread of *Vibrio cholerae* O139 Bengal in India. *Journal of Infectious Diseases, 169,* 1029–1034.

Nelson, K. E., Celentano, D. D., Eiumtrakol, S., Hoover, D. R., Beyrer, C., Suprasert, S., et al. (1996). Changes in sexual behavior and a decline in HIV infection among young men in Thailand. *New England Journal of Medicine, 335,* 297–303.

Ngondi, J., Onsarigo, A., Matthews, F., Reacher, M., Brayne, C., Baba, S., et al. (2006). Effect of 3 years of SAFE (surgery, antibiotics, facial cleanliness, and environmental change) strategy for trachoma control in southern Sudan: A cross-sectional study. *Lancet, 368,* 589–595.

Novel Swine-Origin Influenza A (H1N1) Virus Investigation Team. (2009). Emergence of a novel swine-origin influenza A (H1N1) virus in humans. *New England Journal of Medicine, 360,* 2605–2615.

O'Brien, K. L., Wolfson,, L., Watt, J. P., Henkle, E., Deloria-Knoll, M., McCall, N., et al. (2009). Burden of disease caused by *Streptococcus pneu-moniae* in children younger than 5 years: Global estimates. *Lancet, 374,* 893–902.

Otten, M. W. Jr., Deming, M. S., Jaiteh, K. O., Flagg, E. W., Forgie, I., Sanyang, Y., et al. (1992). Epidemic poliomyelitis in the Gambia following the control of poliomyelitis as an endemic disease. I. Descriptive findings. *American Journal of Epidemiology, 135,* 381–392.

Paavonen, J., Naud, P., Salmeron, J., Wheeler, C. M., Chow, S-N., Apter, D., et al. (2009). Efficacy of human papillomavirus (HPV)-16/18 AS04–adjuvanted vaccine against cervical infection and precancer caused by onocogenic HPV types (PA-TRICIA): Final analysis of a double-blind, randomized study in young women. *Lancet, 374,* 301–314.

Pacqué, M., Muñoz, B., Greene, B. M., & Taylor, H. R. (1991). Community-based treatment of on-chocerciasis with ivermectin: Safety, efficacy, and acceptability of yearly treatment. *Journal of Infectious Diseases, 163,* 381–385.

Pan America Health Organization. (1994, October). Measles elimination by the year 2000. *EPI Newsletter, 16,* 1–2.

Parashar, U. D., Hummelman, E. G., Bresee, J. S., Miller, M. A., & Glass, R. I. (2003). Global illness and deaths caused by rotavirus disease in children. *Emerging Infectious Diseases, 9,* 565–572.

Patriarca, P. A., Wright, P. F., & John, T. J. (1991). Factors affecting the immunogenicity of oral poliovirus vaccine in developing countries: Review. *Reviews of Infectious Diseases, 13,* 926–939.

Perkins, B. A., Broome, C. V., Rosenstein, N. E., Schuchat, A., & Reingold, A. L. (1997). Meningococcal vaccine in sub-Saharan Africa. [Letter]. *Lancet, 350,* 1708.

Pourrut, X., Délicat, A., Rollin, P. E., Ksiazek, T. G., Gonzalez, J. P., & Leroy, E. M. (2007). Spatial and temporal patterns of Zaire ebolavirus antibody prevalence in the possible reservoir bat species. *Journal of Infectious Diseases, 196,* S176–S183.

Re-emergence of Bolivian hemorrhagic fever. (1994). *Epidemiological Bulletin, 15,* 4–5.

Rerks-Ngarm, S., Pitisuttithum, P., Nitayaphan, S., Kaewkungwal, J., Chiu, J., Paris, R., et al. (2009). Vaccination with ALVAC and AIDSVAX to prevent HIV-1 infection in Thailand. *New England Journal of Medicine, 361,* 2209–2220.

Richardson, V., Hernandez-Pichardo, J., Quintanar-Solares, M., Esparza-Aguilar, M., Johnson, B., Gomez-Altamirano, et al. (2010). Effect of rotavirus vaccination on death from childhood diarrhea in Mexico. *New England Journal of Medicine, 362,* 299–305.

Richmond, J. K., & Baglole, D. J. (2003). Lassa fever: Epidemiology, clinical features, and social consequences. *British Medical Journal, 327,* 1271–1275.

Robbins, J. B., Towne, D. W., Gotschlich, E. C., & Schneerson, R. (1997). Love's labours lost: Failure to implement mass vaccination against group A meningococcal meningitis in sub-Saharan Africa. *Lancet, 350,* 880–882.

Rojanapithayakorn, W., & Hanenberg, R. (1996). The 100% Condom program in Thailand. *AIDS, 10,* 1–7.

Rollback Malaria Partnership. (2008). Key facts, figures and strategies: The Global Malaria Action Plan. Retrieved from http://www.rollbackmalaria .org/gmap/GMAP_Advocacy-ENG-web.pdf

Rudan, I., Boschi-Pinto, C., Biloglav, Z., Mulholland, K., & Campbell, H. (2008). Epidemiology and etiology of childhood pneumonia. *Bulletin of the World Health Organization, 86,* 408–416.

Sacarlal, J., Aide, P., Aponte, J. J., Renom, M., Leach, A., Mandomando, I., et al. (2009). Long-term safety and efficacy of the RTS,S/AS02A malaria vaccine in Mozambican children. *Journal of Infectious Diseases, 200,* 329–336.

Santosham, M. (2010). Rotavirus vaccine: A powerful tool to combat deaths from diarrhea. *Lancet, 362,* 358–360.

Sazawal, S., & Black, R. E. (1992). Meta-analysis of intervention trials on case-management of pneumonia in community settings. *Lancet, 340,* 528–533.

Schofield, F. (1986). Selective primary health care: Strategies for control of disease in the developing

world. XXII. Tetanus: A preventable problem. *Reviews of Infectious Diseases, 8,* 144–156.

Selwyn, B. J. (1990). The epidemiology of acute respiratory tract infection in young children: Comparison of findings from several developing countries. Coordinated Data Group of BOSTID Researchers. *Reviews of Infectious Diseases, 12,* S870–S888.

Senior, K. (2009). Childhood vaccination and progress towards MDG4. *Lancet, 9,* 730.

Setia, M. S., Steinmaus, C., Ho, C. S., & Rutherford, G. W. (2006). The role of BCG in prevention of leprosy: A meta-analysis. *Lancet Infectious Diseases, 6,* 162–170.

Shaffer, N., Chuachoowong, R., Mock, P. A., Bhadrakom, C., Siriwasin, W., Young, N. L., et al. (1999). Short-course zidovudine for perinatal HIV-1 transmission in Bangkok, Thailand: A randomised controlled trial. *Lancet, 353,* 773–780.

Shann, F. (1986). Etiology of severe pneumonia in children in developing countries. *Pediatric Infectious Disease, 5,* 247–252.

Shrestha, M. P., Scott, R. M., Joshi, D. M., Mammen, M. P. Jr., Thapa, G. B., Thapa, N., et al. (2007). Safety and efficacy of a recombinant hepatitis E vaccine. *New England Journal of Medicine, 356,* 895–903.

Sinha, A., Sazawal, S., Kumar, R., Sood, S., Reddaiah, V. P., Singh, B., et al. (1999). Typhoid fever in children aged less than 5 years. *Lancet, 354,* 734–737.

Smolinski, M. S., Hamburg, M. A., & Lederberg, J. (Eds.). (2003). *Microbial threats to health: Emergence, detection, and response.* Institute of Medicine. Washington, DC: National Academies Press.

Sridhar, S. (2009). An affordable cholera vaccine: An important step forward. *Lancet.* doi: 10.1016/ S0140-6736(09)61418-5.

Stanfield, J. P., & Galazka, A. (1984). Neonatal tetanus in the world today. *Bulletin of the World Health Organization, 62,* 647–669.

Steinmann, P., Keiser, J., Bos, R., Tanner, M., & Utzinger, J. (2006). Schistosomiasis and water resources development: Systematic review, meta-analysis, and estimates of people at risk. *Lancet Infectious Diseases, 6,* 411–425.

Sur, D., Lopez, A. L., Kanungo, S., Paisley, A., Manna, B., Ali, M., et al. (2009). Efficacy and safety of a modified killed whole cell oral cholera vaccine in India: An interim analysis of a cluster-randomised, double-blind, placebo-controlled trial. *Lancet, 374,* 1694–1702.

Sur, D., Ochial, R. L., Bhattacharya, S. K., Ganguly, N., Ali, M., Manna, B., et al. (2009). A cluster-randomized effectiveness trial of Vi typhoid vaccine in India. *New England Journal of Medicine, 361,* 335–344.

Sutrisna, B., Reingold, A., Kresno, S., Harrison, G., & Utomo, B. (1993). Care-seeking for fatal illnesses in young children in Indramayu, West Java, Indonesia. *Lancet, 342,* 787–789.

Sutter, R. W., Cáceres, V. M., & Mas Lago, P. (2004). The role of routine polio immunization in the post-certification era. *Bulletin of the World Health Organization, 82,* 31–39.

Sutter, R. W., Patriarca, P. A., Brogan, S., Malankar, P. G., Pallansch, M. A., Kew, O. M., et al. (1991). Outbreak of paralytic poliomyelitis in Oman: Evidence for widespread transmission among fully vaccinated children. *Lancet, 338,* 715–720.

Taha, T. E., Hoover, D. R., Kumwenda, N. I., Fiscus, S. A., Kafulafula, G., Nkhoma, C., et al. (2007). Late postnatal transmission of HIV-1 and associated factors. *Journal of Infectious Diseases, 196,* 10–14.

Ter Meulen, J., Lukashevich, I., Sidibe, K., Inapogui, A., Marx, M., Dorlemann, A., et al. (1996). Hunting of peridomestic rodents and consumption of their meat as possible risk factors for rodent-to-human transmission of Lassa virus in the Republic of Guinea. *American Journal of Tropical Medicine and Hygiene, 55,* 661–666.

Thursz, M., Cooke, G. S., & Hall, A. J. (2010). Hepatitis B treatment in resource poor settings: Time for action. *Tropical Medicine and International Health, 15,* 2–4.

Towner, J. S., Khristova, M. L., Sealy, T. K., Vincent, M. J., Erickson, B. R., Bawiec, D. A., et al. (2006). Marburgvirus genomics and association with a large hemorrhagic fever outbreak in Angola. *Journal of Virology, 80,* 6497–6516.

Towner, J. S., Pourrut, X., Albariño, C. G., Nkogue, C. N., Bird, B. H., Grard, G., et al. (2007). Marburg virus infection detected in a common African bat. *PLoS One, 2,* e764.

Trigg, P. I., & Kondrachine, A. V. (1998). Commentary: Malaria control in the 1990s. *Bulletin of the World Health Organization, 76,* 11–16.

UNAIDS. (2008). *Report on the global HIV/AIDS epidemic 2008.* Geneva, Switzerland: UNAIDS/WHO.

UNAIDS. (2009). *AIDS Epidemic Update.* Geneva, Switzerland: UNAIDS/WHO.

University of Zimbabwe/JHPIEGO Cervical Cancer Project. (1999). Visual inspection with acetic acid for cervical cancer screening: Test qualities in a primary-care setting. *Lancet, 353,* 869–873.

Vainrub, B., & Salas, R. (1994). Latin American hemorrhagic fever. *Infectious Disease Clinics of North America, 8,* 47–59.

Vinetz, J. M. (2001). Leptospirosis. *Current Opinion in Infectious Diseases, 14*(5), 527–538.

Wakabi, W. (2009). West African meningitis outbreak strains vaccine supplies. *Lancet, 373,* 1836.

Walsh, J. A. (1983). Selective primary health care: Strategies for control of disease in the developing world. IV. Measles. *Reviews of Infectious Diseases, 5,* 330–340.

Warren, K. S., Bundy, D. A., Anderson, R. M., Davis, A. R., Henderson, D. A., Jamison, D. T., et al. (1993). Helminth infection. In D. T. Jamison, W. H. Mosley, A. R. Measham, & J. L. Bobadilla (Eds.), *Disease control priorities in developing countries* (pp. 131–160). New York: Oxford University Press.

Watt, J. P., Wolfson, L. J., O'Brien, K. L., Henkle, E., Deloria-Knoll, M., McCall, N., et al. (2009). Burden of disease caused by *Haemophilus influenzae* type b in children younger than 5 years: Global estimates. *Lancet, 374,* 903–911.

Weber, M. W., Mulholland, E. K., Jaffar, S., Troedsson, H., Gove, S., & Greenwood, B. M. (1997). Evaluation of an algorithm for the integrated management of childhood illness in an area with seasonal malaria in the Gambia. *Bulletin of the World Health Organization, 75,* 25–32.

Whalen, C. C., Johnson, J. L., Okwera, A., Hom, D. L., Huebner, R., Mugyenyi, P., et al. (1997). A trial of three regimens to prevent tuberculosis in Ugandan adults infected with the human immunodeficiency virus. Uganda–Case Western Reserve University Research Collaboration. *New England Journal of Medicine, 337,* 801–808.

Wiktor, S. Z., Ekpini, E., Karon, J. M., Nkengasong, J., Maurice, C., Severin, S. T., et al. (1999). Short-course oral zidovudine for prevention of mother-to-child transmission of HIV-1 in Abidjan, Côte d'Ivoire: A randomised trial. *Lancet, 353,* 781–785.

World Health Organization (WHO). (1981). Clinical management of acute respiratory infections in children: A WHO memorandum. *Bulletin of the World Health Organization, 59,* 707–716.

World Health Organization (WHO). (1985). *Viral haemorrhagic fevers: Report of a WHO Expert Committee* (WHO Technical Report No. 721). Geneva, Switzerland: Author.

World Health Organization (WHO). (1991). *Management of patients with sexually transmitted diseases: Report of a WHO Study Group* (WHO Technical Report No. 810). Geneva, Switzerland: Author.

World Health Organization (WHO). (1993). *Control of schistosomiasis: The second report of the WHO Expert Committee* (WHO Technical Report No. 830). Geneva, Switzerland: Author.

World Health Organization (WHO). (1994). Expanded programme on immunization, Global Advisory Group. Part II. Achieving the major disease control goals. *Weekly Epidemiological Record, 69,* 29–31, 34–35.

World Health Organization (WHO). (1995). *Control of epidemic meningococcal disease: WHO practical guidelines.* Lyon, France: WHO and Foundation Marcel Mérieux.

World Health Organization (WHO). (1997a). Hepatitis C: Global prevalence. *Weekly Epidemiological Record, 72,* 341–344.

World Health Organization (WHO). (1997b). Hepatitis C. *Weekly Epidemiological Record, 72,* 65–69.

World Health Organization (WHO). (1998a). *Action programme for the elimination of leprosy: Status report 1998* (Document WHO/LEP/98.2). Geneva, Switzerland: Author.

World Health Organization (WHO). (1998b). *EPI information system: Global summary, September 1998* (Document WHO/EPI/GEN/98.10). Geneva, Switzerland: Author.

World Health Organization. (WHO) (1998c). *Yellow fever technical consensus meeting* (Document WHO/EPI/GEN/98.08). Geneva, Switzerland: Author.

World Health Organization (WHO). (2001). Onchocerciasis (river blindness): Report from the Tenth InterAmerican Conference on Onchocerciasis, Guayaquil, Ecuador. *Weekly Epidemiological Record, 76,* 205–212.

World Health Organization (WHO). (2002a). *Prevention and control of schistosomiasis and soil-transmitted helminthiasis* (WHO Technical Report No. 912). Geneva, Switzerland: Author.

World Health Organization (WHO). (2002b). Rabies vaccines. *Weekly Epidemiological Record, 77*(14), 109–120.

World Health Organization (WHO). (2004). Human plague in 2002 and 2003. *Weekly Epidemiological Record, 79*(33), 301–306.

World Health Organization (WHO). (2005a). *Deworming for health and development.* Geneva, Switzerland: Author.

World Health Organization (WHO). (2005b). Lassa fever: Fact Sheet No. 179. Retrieved from http://www.who.int/mediacentre/factsheets/fs179/en/index.html

World Health Organization (WHO). (2006a). *The Stop TB strategy: Building on and enhancing DOTS to meet the TB-related Millennium Development Goals.* Geneva, Switzerland: Author.

World Health Organization (WHO). (2006b). Human African trypanosomiasis (sleeping sickness): Epidemiological update. *Weekly Epidemiological Record, 81,* 71–80.

World Health Organization (WHO). (2006c). *Preventive chemotherapy in human helminthiasis: Coordinated use of anthelminthic drugs in control interventions: A manual for health professionals and programme managers.* Geneva, Switzerland: Author.

World Health Organization (WHO). (2007a). Global leprosy situation. *Weekly Epidemiological Record, 82,* 225–232.

World Health Organization (WHO). (2007b). Rabies vaccines: WHO position paper. *Weekly Epidemiological Record, 82,* 425–435.

World Health Organization (WHO). (2008a). Hepatitis B: Fact Sheet No. 204. Retrieved from http://www.who.int/mediacentre/factsheets/fs204/en/index.html

World Health Organization (WHO). (2008b). *World malaria report 2008* (Document WHO/HTM/GMP/2008.1). Geneva, Switzerland: Author.

World Health Organization (WHO). (2008c). Rabies: Fact Sheet No. 99. Retrieved from http://www.who.int/mediacentre/factsheets/fs099/en/index.html

World Health Organization (WHO). (2009a). Global tuberculosis control: A short update to the 2009 report. Retrieved from http://www.who.int/tb/publications/global_report/en/

World Health Organization (WHO). (2009b). Hepatitis B vaccines: WHO position paper. *Weekly Epidemiological Record, 84*(40), 405–419.

World Health Organization (WHO). (2009c). Dengue and dengue hemorrhagic fever: Fact Sheet No. 117. Retrieved from http://www.who.int/mediacentre/factsheets/fs117/en/

World Health Organization (WHO). (2009d). Yellow fever: Fact Sheet No. 100. Retrieved from http://www.who.int/mediacentre/factsheets/fs100/en/index.html

World Health Organization (WHO). (2009e). Chagas disease: Control and elimination. Retrieved from http://apps.who.int/gb/ebwha/pdf_files/A62/A62_17-en.pdf

World Health Organization (WHO). (2010a). Leprosy: Fact Sheet No. 101. Retrieved from http://www.who.int/mediacentre/factsheets/fs101/en/index.html

World Health Organization (WHO). (2010b). Schistosomiasis: Fact Sheet No. 115. Retrieved from http://www.who.int/mediacentre/factsheets/fs115/en/index.html

Writing Committee of the Second World Health Organization Consultation on Clinical Aspects of Human Infection with Avian Influenza A (H5N1) Virus. (2008). Update on avian influenza A (H5N1) virus infection in humans. *New England Journal of Medicine, 358,* 261–272.

Nutrition

KEITH P. WEST, JR., CHRISTINE P. STEWART, BENJAMIN CABALLERO, AND ROBERT E. BLACK

Nutritional concerns in low-income countries are diverse, ranging from deprivation, hunger, and consequent deficiencies that impair health, quality of life, and survival, to a rising tide of obesity and ensuing risks of chronic disease in some regions. All can coexist within the same population. Undernutrition, reflected by high prevalences of wasting, stunting, and micronutrient deficiencies, is the predominant form of malnutrition throughout southern Asia and most of sub-Saharan Africa, while overweight status and obesity, often in the presence of stunting and micronutrient malnutrition, is now a public health problem in regions of Latin America, northern Africa, the Middle East, and Central and East Asia

Undernutrition has long been considered a consequence and cause of poor human health, development, and achievement throughout life (Administrative Committee on Coordination/SubCommittee on Nutrition [ACC/SCN], 2000; World Bank, 1993; World Health Organization [WHO], 2002). For this reason, its prevention has been identified as fundamental to achieving the first Millennium Development Goal (MDG) to halve the burden of hunger between 1990 and 2015 (United Nations, 2000). Efforts directed toward this MDG will also help in reaching the fourth and fifth MDGs—reducing child and maternal mortality, respectively—given the well-known, often causal, associations between survival and adequate nutrition (Black et al., 2008; Pelletier, 1994; Sommer & West, 1996).

While severe wasting malnutrition, as evidenced by classical clinical signs such as very thin or edematous extremities and hair signs, can profoundly affect risks of morbidity and mortality, this form of undernutrition is becoming less common beyond areas of conflict and famine. More prevalent are "hidden" forms of undernourishment with respect to energy, protein, and micronutrients that can stunt child growth and development, impair resistance to infection, and decrease chances of survival. The groups at highest risk of undernutrition are impoverished and food-insecure populations who lack resources to adequately feed and care for themselves. Within a population, groups at highest risk of undernutrition are those who, at critical stages in life, are exposed to its causes and most vulnerable to its consequences: the fetus, infants, and preschool-aged children; women of reproductive age, especially during pregnancy; and older persons. Indeed, the elderly population, which is the most rapidly growing demographic group in the world, remains outside the view and reach of most nutrition policy initiatives. The nutritional relationship across these life stages is becoming increasingly apparent as evidence accrues linking poor nutrition in utero and during infancy to risks of chronic disease; this understanding is amplifying interest in the role of early life nutrition in endowing lifelong health.

In contrast to undernutrition, overnutrition affects societies caught in a "nutrition transition"—a process marked by a shift in diet away from traditional staple diets, often accompanied by seasonally available vegetables, fruits, and animal foods, and toward more processed, refined foods and sweetened beverages of higher energy (calorie) density, which incorporate added fat and sugar, but include decreased dietary fiber. These dietary changes are often coupled with lifestyle changes that lead to reductions in physical activity and energy expenditure, as well as patterns featuring more frequent meals (ACC/SCN, 2000; Popkin, 2009). The nutrition transition is occurring in parallel with the rapid economic, demographic, and health transitions now under way in many low- and middle-income societies. While the rise from dietary deficit to one of relative adequacy in society has likely contributed to improved health and longevity across the globe (Popkin, 1999), continued and excessive shifts toward overconsumption and inactivity, along with other exposures of industrialization, appear to be increasing many populations' risks of degenerative, cardiovascular, and neoplastic (i.e., noncommunicable) diseases. These diseases are rapidly becoming leading causes of adult morbidity and mortality throughout low- to middle-income countries (James et al., 2004; Mathers, Boerma, & Ma Fat, 2009; Victora et al., 2008).

The diversity and breadth of nutritional status in practically all countries, and the urgency to act to correct malnutrition, have been brought to the global stage at a series of reinforcing international conferences seeking to improve food, agricultural, and nutritional conditions in the world via declarations of intent or goals, strategic plans of action, follow-up planning sessions, and protocols for monitoring compliance. Initial momentum was provided by the World Food Conference in Rome in 1974, whose attendees issued a global call to abolish hunger and malnutrition (United Nations, 1982). This action stimulated the National Academy of Sciences in the United States to conduct the World Food and Nutrition Study in 1975, which reached the following conclusion: "In developing countries, effective nutrition interventions are likely to have more of an effect on human health than comparable investments in medical care" (National Research Council, 1977). These and other early convenings motivated efforts to focus global attention, commitment, and action to improve nutritional conditions through venues such as the World Summit for Children in 1990, International Conference on Nutrition in 1992, World Food Congress in 1996, and Millennium Development Summit in 2000. From the last emerged eight MDGs, three of which, calling to reduce hunger, and child and maternal mortality (MDGs 1, 4, and 5, respectively), can be argued to depend heavily on improving nutritional conditions in the world (Exhibit 6-1).

The various conferences addressing worldwide nutrition have drawn on an expanding base of research evidence on the impact and cost-effectiveness of interventions that, in 2008, were summarized in a

---

Exhibit 6-1	The Art of Nutrition Policy Making and Advocacy within the United Nations

Over the past 25 years, United Nations agencies have pressed the world to pay attention the health and nutrition of children and women, motivated by recognized opportunities to improve health, survival, and quality of life, especially in disadvantaged societies. During the International Year of the Child in 1978, UNICEF rallied global attention around the neglect and nutritional plight of children, especially those in poor societies. A decade later, at the World Summit for Children, sponsored by UNICEF in New York in September 1989, 179 heads of state gathered to craft, sign, and commit to the principles and action plan of the Declaration on the Rights of the Child (UNICEF, 1990), which specified health and nutritional goals for the year 2000 that included a reduction in child mortality.

At the first-ever International Conference on Nutrition (ICN) held in Rome in 1992, and during the three years of national and regional preparations that preceded it, the Food and Agricultural Organization of the United Nations (FAO) and WHO seized the global momentum to secure ministerial commitments and signatures from 159 countries to a World Declaration and Plan of Action to develop goals for improving the nutritional health in their citizenry, especially vulnerable groups. Governments pledged, before the year 2000, (1) to eliminate famine and famine-related deaths, (2) to eliminate starvation and nutritional-deficiency diseases in communities affected by natural and human-made disasters, (3) to eliminate iodine and vitamin A deficiencies, and (4) to develop and implement national nutrition plans based on situational analyses within each country, using the ICN Plan of Action as a guide (FAO, 1992).

The World Food Summit, hosted by FAO in Rome in 1996, seized on the momentum from the ICN and extended the timeline (to 2015) for governments to reduce the number of undernourished people in the world by half, using 1990–1992 as the "baseline period" (FAO, 1996), and giving a sense of progress achieved toward a repackaged and longer-term goal. In September 2000, this goal was further leveraged as the first of eight Millennium Development Goals (MDGs)—to "halve the proportion of people who suffer from hunger by the year 2015"—that were adopted by world leaders at the United Nations Millennium Summit in September 2000 (United Nations, 2000). The World Bank and International Monetary Fund's Millennium Project—a network of policy makers, experts, and task forces—now meets annually to manage and oversee strategies for achieving the MDGs (United Nations, 2004).

Notwithstanding difficulties in definition and measurement, this advocacy process has led many countries to adopt and implement elements of national nutrition policies that did not exist two decades ago.

major series of reports on undernutrition in *The Lancet* (http://www.thelancet.com/series/maternal-and-child-undernutrition). These reports offered a common basis and language for scientific, policy, and program communications about nutrition intervention and research priorities.

This chapter addresses nutritional problems of low-income countries that are motivating concern, research, and policy and program responses. These issues include the extent and causes of undernutrition, involving protein-energy malnutrition and micronutrient deficiencies at vulnerable stages of life (especially in infancy, early childhood, and adolescence; in women during pregnancy and lactation; and at older ages). They also include the food insecurity that surrounds malnutrition in most societies; interactions of nutrition and infection that have public health consequences; roles of breastfeeding and complementary feeding in assuring healthy children; and rapidly evolving facets of the nutrition transition, including evidence of its origins in early life and its adult manifestations of obesity and noncommunicable diseases. Throughout the chapter, attention is drawn to approaches to prevent malnutrition, where possible, taking into consideration the epidemiologic and resource context in which they occur.

Food Security

Food security exists when all people have reliable access to a sufficient amount of nutritious, safe, and culturally appropriate food (FAO, 1992). *Food insecurity* refers to a state of chronic, deprived economic or physical access to food, either in quantity or quality, such that dietary intake fails to meet nutritional needs or otherwise support the health of all individuals in a household or community. This concept may be extended to entire populations and regions. Indeed, this level of focus came to the forefront following a global financial crisis that swept through the world in 2008, in which combined effects of droughts, restrictive trade, surging oil prices, crop diversion for biofuel production, increasing food demand, and speculation appeared to converge and leave poor and undernourished populations of the world less food secure than they were earlier in the decade (Institute of Medicine [IOM], 2010).

Food security reflects a quality of life with dietary, health, socioeconomic, and behavioral dimensions that are evaluated many ways, each of which provides different views of risk and adequacy. An accepted approach to assessment is through the evaluation of food balance sheets maintained by the FAO, which offer composite estimates of status and trends in national and regional food sufficiency (FAO-STAT, 2004). Estimates of kilocalories of energy and grams of protein per capita provide population growth-adjusted proxies for total food availability, while the latter also addresses a facet of nutritional quality of the food supply.

Table 6-1 indicates that, over a 10-year period from 1992 and 2002, world food production and availability increased by approximately 5% on a per capita basis, with regional estimates ranging from no apparent change in caloric availability in Central America to an 8% gain in North America. Protein availability increased by a similar percentage (6%) globally, with the largest relative gains seen in South America (12% increase) and low-income countries in general (10% increase). Unfortunately, regional disparities in calorie and protein availability that were evident in the early 1990s were virtually the same a decade later. For example, the per capita energy supply for sub-Saharan African remained just below 80% of the world average over the 1992–2002 period, at 2,346 kilocalories (kcal) or approximately 12% more than a full daily ration defined under disaster feeding conditions (WHO, 2000, p. 63), while the corresponding supply for the European Union remained constant at 127% of the global average. Only in industrialized North America was there a substantial increase in food energy, from 129% to 134% of the world average, reflecting a per capita food energy supply that is 70% greater than that found in sub-Saharan Africa. Thus, while overall availability of food increased relative to population growth and improved in quality in most regions of the world, gross inter-regional inequities remained unaltered.

Global food balance estimates of dietary quality similar to those in Table 6-1 are not yet available from the FAO for the period following the recent global economic crisis (IOM, 2010), although the 11% rise in the number of hungry people from 2008 (915 million) to 2009 (1.02 billion) (FAO, 2009) suggests that poorest regions of the world have became less food secure in the latter half of the decade. While informative, food balance data remain crude indicators because the FAO regional divisions, as defined for these estimates, mask extensive within-region variation in food security as well as socioeconomic and other micro-level disparities in access.

Food insecurity can vary according to degree of urban–rural residence, the severity of usual socioeconomic pressures (e.g., prevailing food prices and adequacy of local food production), adequacy of

Table 6-1	Energy and Protein Supply on a per Capita per Day Basis, by Region of the World, Based on Food Balance Sheets of the Food and Agricultural Organization					
	Energy Supply (kcal)			Protein Supply (g)		
Region	**1992**	**2002**	**% +/−**	**1992**	**2002**	**% +/−**
World	2,708 (100%)	2,804 (100%)	+4[1]	71 (100%)	75 (100%)	+6
Africa	2,346 (87%)[2]	2,425 (86%)	+3	58 (82%)	61 (81%)	+5
Sub-Saharan Africa	2,126 (78%)	2,207 (79%)	+4	51 (72%)	54 (72%)	+6
Asia	2,581 (95%)	2,696 (96%)	+4	65 (92%)	70 (93%)	+8
South America	2,703 (100%)	2,851 (102%)	+5	69 (97%)	77 (103%)	+12
North and Central America	3,260 (120%)	3,449 (123%)	+6	96 (135%)	101 (135%)	+5
North America, Developed	3,492 (129%)	3,756 (134%)	+8	108 (152%)	113 (150%)	+5
Central America	2,935 (108%)	2,941 (105%)	0	77 (108%)	83 (111%)	+8
European Union	3,445 (127%)	3,522 (127%)	+2	104 (146%)	108 (144%)	+4
High-Income Countries	3,221 (119%)	3,414 (122%)	+6	98 (138%)	100 (133%)	+2
Low- and Middle-Income Countries	2,550 (94%)	2,666 (95%)	+5	63 (89%)	69 (92%)	+10

1. Percent change in from 1992 to 2002.
2. Percentage of the world figures for 1992 and 2002, respectively.
Source: FAOSTAT data for 2004.

transport infrastructure (Bouis & Hunt, 1999), vulnerability to economic shocks such as those that occurred in 2007–2008 (Bloem, Semba, & Kraemer, 2010; de Pee et al., 2010; IOM, 2010; Webb, 2010), and degrees of disruption due to civil instability and conflict (Toole & Waldman, 1993; Yip & Sharp, 1993). Although inequities in feeding patterns within a household can themselves lead to nutritional vulnerabilities (e.g., for female children in some cultures), variation in undernutrition can usually be more readily traced to chronic food insecurity at household, community, or larger aggregates of society. It is also apparent that financial crises that lead to sustained rises in food prices, losses of jobs, and lower real income initially create short-term adjustments and asset losses, which may then be followed by extended

nutritional consequences (Alderman, 2010). These complex patterns of causation highlight the utility of conceptualizing food insecurity and malnutrition in present and intergenerational contexts.

Conceptual Models

Two conceptual models in common use help to visualize the continuum from food insecurity to undernutrition, the causal factors involved, and the consequences of such failure to provide full nutrition. One model, which is adapted from a model developed by UNICEF (Figure 6-1), unites diverse basic (or root), underlying, and immediate causes of food insecurity and disease into a hierarchical causal path to undernutrition and its effects on health and disease (UNICEF, 1997). Implied in this model is the real-

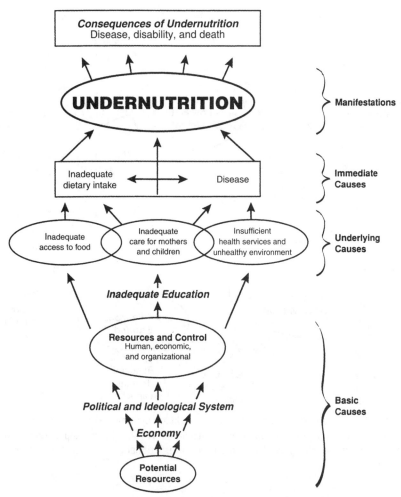

Figure 6-1 UNICEF Conceptual Model of the Causation of Undernutrition, Modified
To Include Consequences (UNICEF, 1997)
Source: UNICEF, *The State of the World's Children 1998* (New York: Oxford University
Press, 1997), p. 24. Reprinted with permission.

ization that there is no single cause of undernourishment, but rather a set of contributing factors that vary in intensity, duration, specificity, and proximity to the undernourished individual. Another approach is to view the interacting forces as "component causes" that can unite to form a "completed" cause of undernutrition (Rothman & Greenland, 1998). Which forces operate and how they interact determine the type and severity of malnutrition, as well as the health or functional consequences, and offer insight into prevention.

For example, wasting malnutrition (defined later in this chapter) can result from a diet chronically lacking energy as well as density of protein and other nutrients, intensified by frequent or prolonged bouts of diarrhea. Improving either of these determinants could,

therefore, prevent or lessen the severity and health consequences of undernutrition. Unfortunately, both conditions arise from impoverished, food-insecure, and unhygienic conditions in the home, or poor access to treatment for illnesses, stemming from lack of family resources. This lack can be a result of poor education and unemployment, or it may reflect inadequate community facilities (nonavailability of health care, poorly stocked food markets). Improvement in these underlying causes could potentially lower exposure to diarrheal pathogens or improve quality of diet. Such underlying causes occur, in part, because of individuals' membership in social, cultural, or economic classes that have little influence on governance and flow of resources within the society. Typically, immediate and underlying causes operate through

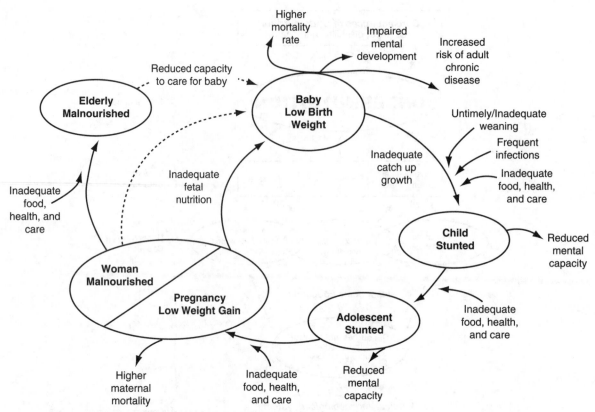

Figure 6-2 A Conceptual Model of the Intergenerational Cycle of Undernutrition. Adapted from the ACC/SCN, 2000
Source: Administrative Committee on Coordination/Subcommittee on Nutrition, Fourth Report on the World Nutrition
Situation: Nutrition Throughout the Life Cycle (Washington, DC: International Food Policy Research Institute, 2000).
Reprinted with permission.

women, who as mothers serve as caretakers, allocators of food, and managers of resources in the household. This relationship suggests that improving the status, education, and economic and political empowerment of women—addressing gender-related causes at nearly every level—could interrupt causal pathways of malnutrition (Haddad, 1999).

The second model illustrates a set of causes that affect individuals across the various stages of life, from generation to generation, within impoverished and food-insecure families and communities (Figure 6-2). In this model, infants who may be growth restricted and developmentally delayed at birth, due to maternal undernutrition, face a sequence of nutritional, health, and developmental insults, mediated by socioeconomic constraints, which stunt their growth throughout early life. These exposures may continue through adolescence and the reproductive years; if they occur among women, then, they can affect their offspring. Deprivation can also persist into vulnerable older years of life (ACC/SCN, 2000). This model identifies times in the life cycle when malnutrition occurs, as well as potentially responsive causes and intermediate outcomes that could be altered by effective and timely intervention.

Population Spectrum of Nutritional Status

Although individuals are typically exposed to poor diet, disease, and neglect over time to become malnourished, viewing the spectrum of nutritional status at a point in time (cross-sectionally) provides the basis for quantifying the types and extent of malnutrition in the population. In this respect, the term "malnutrition" does not differentiate undernutrition from overnutrition: The former refers to deficiency states of energy, protein, or micronutrients, whereas the latter typically refers to states of excess energy stores as body fat. Thus, in a single population, three distributions can be envisioned: those who are (1) normal, (2) undernourished or deficient, and (3) overnourished or obese (Figure 6-3). The overarching bell-shaped curve in Figure 6-3 represents the status of all individ-

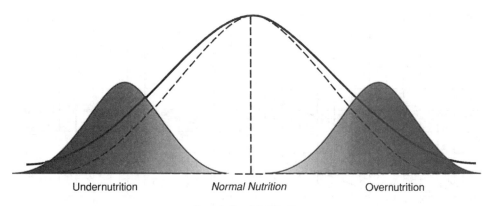

Figure 6-3 Spectrum of Nutritional Status in a Hypothetical Population
Source: Merson, M.H., Black, R.E., & Mills, A.J. (Eds). "International Public Health," 2001: Jones and Bartlett Publishers, Sudbury, MA. www.jbpub.com. Reprinted with permission.

Undernutrition   *Normal Nutrition*   Overnutrition

Population Distribution

uals in the population with respect to a continuous measure of nutritional status. The dashed curve indicates the normally nourished subgroup, including those with normal low or high nutritional values, while the smaller curves depict undernourished and overnourished individuals. The intensity of the shading reflects the severity of malnutrition within each group. The sizes of these three population groups can vary by region, socioeconomic status, age, gender, and other factors.

Because of their overlapping distributions, neither malnourished group in Figure 6-3 can be perfectly identified because it is difficult to know where individuals lie with respect to their "true" status. On the population level, making this determination necessitates reliance on indicators with cutoffs applied to define and estimate the prevalence of malnutrition and, when combined with population data, the numbers affected by each condition. A cutoff line can be drawn through either tail of the overall distribution to estimate proportions. While truly malnourished and normal individuals will often be correctly identified, a proportion of each group will also be misclassified; that is, some normal persons will be classified as malnourished (false positives), and vice versa (false negatives). This example illustrates the challenges of nutritional assessment when the aim is to estimate prevalence, screen individuals for treatment or prevention, monitor shifts in proportions malnourished over time, or evaluate community program impact on malnutrition, given that "true" distributions are rarely known.

While accuracy in measurement and careful analyses can minimize misclassification, no nutritional indicator is free of such errors. Prior to applying cutoffs to classify the "malnourished," a referent population is needed for comparison. As an example,

populations of children across a variety of ethnicities, genetic backgrounds, and geographic regions exhibit similar growth potential if raised in a supportive environment (WHO Multicentre Growth Reference Study, 2006a). Thus, low weight or height in relation to a reference distribution of relatively well-nourished children is likely to reflect undernutrition. Choice of a referent population should be guided by sample representativeness, adequacy of general health and nutritional well-being, and international availability to facilitate comparison of findings across populations.

One early, international child growth standard arose through the National Center for Health Statistics (NCHS), which combined data from the Fels Longitudinal Study in the state of Ohio with the national Health Examination Surveys in the United States to create an age- and sex-specific reference that allowed distributional comparisons based on standard deviation (*z*-score) distances from a median (Hamill, Drizd, Johnson, Reed, & Roche, 1977). Among the drawbacks of this standard was its reliance on growth patterns of American children, most of whom had been formula fed in infancy; this practice is now known to favor child growth patterns that differ from those found in adequately breastfed populations (Nommsen-Rivers & Dewey, 2009).

In response to this shortcoming, between 1997 and 2003 WHO launched a multinational child growth assessment study to develop a referent depicting presumed healthy growth of children, suitable for global population comparisons. The WHO Multicentre Growth Reference Study collected data on approximately 8,500 children representing the regions of North America (the United States), Latin America (Brazil), Africa (Ghana), Asia (India), Europe (Norway), and the Middle East (Oman) (WHO

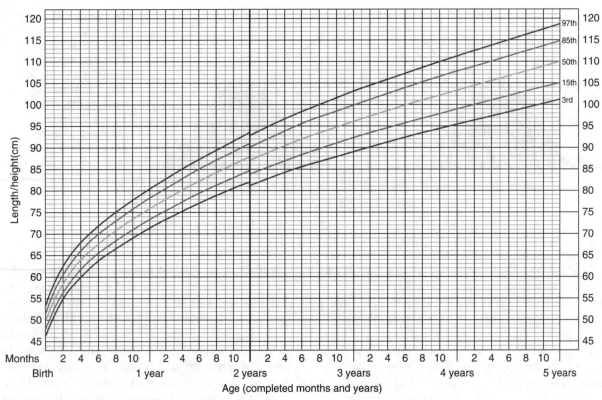

Figure 6-4 WHO Growth Chart for Length/Height for Age Percentiles for Boys 0–5 Years of Age
Source: World Health Organization. The WHO Child Growth Standards, Chart Catalogue, Boys Percentile, page 5.

Multicentre Growth Reference Study Group, 2006b). Among the resulting standard's advantages are that it reflects patterns of growth among children exposed to healthy environments, such as having been reared in nonsmoking households, provided with appropriate breastfeeding and complementary feeding practices, and rendered standard pediatric care, such as immunizations and care during illness. As such, this standard is considered prescriptive, revealing how child populations should grow, and it firmly establishes the breastfed infant as the model for normative growth and development. In addition, referent distributions for childhood body mass index (BMI) are included to enable monitoring of early life patterns of obesity by this conventional overweight indicator.

Using the WHO growth standard, age–sex cutoffs can be set on the basis of percentiles or z-scores below or above the median to classify individuals as malnourished. Weight for age, height or length for age, weight for length or height, and BMI for age percentiles and z-scores can be calculated and compared for local and cross-population purposes. A z-score less than zero serves as an indicator value below the reference median; the converse is true for a z-score greater than

zero. WHO has also developed growth charts using percentiles and z-scores to monitor child growth (www.who.int/childgrowth/en/). The child length or height percentile chart for boys is shown in Figure 6-4. The slight disjuncture in the curve at the age of 2 years is due to recumbent length having been measured prior to this age and standing height thereafter.

Anthropometry is also used to characterize an adult population's risk of being underweight, overweight, or stunted, based on BMI [weight (in kilograms) / height^2 (in meters)] cutoffs that can be used to indicate either overnutrition or undernutrition in adults, with both states being associated with increased health risks and elevated mortality (Bray & Gray, 1988). Unlike child anthropometric cutoffs, the BMI classification scheme is independent of age and gender. As shown in Table 6-2, a BMI between 18.5 and 25 kg/m^2 is considered normal. A BMI less than 18.5 kg/m^2 reflects underweight and one less than 16 kg/m^2 indicates severe thinness. BMI values of 25 or greater and 30 and greater are used to identify overweight and obese subjects, respectively (NHBLI, 1998; WHO, 1995b), although these cutoffs can vary by purpose and country.

Table 6-2	Common Anthropometric Indicators with Cross-sectional Cutoffs for Classifying Children and Adults by Severity of Undernutrition of Overweight/Obesity		
Indicator	**Cutoff Values**	**Interpretation**	**References**
Adults			
Body mass index	<16	Severe thinness	(NHBLI, 1998; WHO 1995b)
	<18.5	Underweight	
	18.5 to 24.9	Normal Range	
	25.0 to 29.9	Pre-obese/overweight	
	≥30.0	Obese	
Children			
Weight for age z-score	<−3.0	Severe underweight	(WHO, 1995a)
	−3.0 to −2.0	Moderate underweight	
	−2.0 to −1.0	Mild underweight	
Height for age z-score	<−3.0	Severe stunting	(WHO, 1995a)
	−3.0 to −2.0	Moderate stunting	
	−2.0 to −1.0	Mild stunting	
Weight for height z-score	<−3.0	Severe wasting	(WHO, 1995a)
	−3.0 to −2.0	Moderate wasting	
	−2.0 to −1.0	Mild wasting	
Mid-upper arm circumference	<11.5	Severe wasting	(West et al., 1991)
	11.5 to 12.5	Moderate wasting	
	12.5 to 13.5	Mild wasting	

Notes: The moderate to severe cutoff of less than −2 for z-scores is conventionally used to define the prevalence of underweight, stunting, and wasting. The WHO growth standard can be used for analyzing the status of local child populations using the resources available at http://www.who.int/childgrowth/en.

One caveat applies: While BMI is a useful indicator of obesity, the percentage of body weight as fat and the patterns of trunk and limb fat distributions can vary markedly at a given BMI across populations. For example, evidence shows that Asian populations have a higher percentage of body fat than Caucasian populations at the same BMI (WHO Expert Consultation, 2004). Notwithstanding this confounding factor, the WHO has recommended that the same BMI cutoffs be used for all populations to facilitate international comparisons. A similar challenge has arisen for waist circumference as a measure of central obesity, and a risk factor for cardiovascular disease and type 2 diabetes (NHBLI, 1998), but for which there is presently no consensus on cutoffs to be used across populations.

More sophisticated measures exist to measure body composition (e.g., percent body fat), such as underwater weighing, dual x-ray absorptiometry, isotope dilution techniques, and air displacement plethysmography (Lee & Gallagher, 2008). Nevertheless, due to their relatively high cost and technical requirements, these methods are presently rarely used in population assessment. By comparison, bioelectrical impedance analysis (BIA), which measures a low-voltage electrical current passing through tissues of varying impedance, offers a portable and relatively inexpensive method for partitioning fat from fat-free mass that, once validated by more sophisticated methods, can be readily applied to assess body composition in populations (Prins et al., 2008). Currently, BIA application is limited by a lack of population-specific validation equations.

Undernutrition

The term "undernutrition" usually indicates combined deficiencies in energy, protein, and essential fatty acids that typically present as anthropometric deficits and, likely, altered body composition. If severe, the individual may have clinical signs of protein-energy malnutrition (e.g., pedal edema or hair changes). Undernutrition may coexist with low-micronutrient nutriture, reflected by low plasma micronutrient concentrations or specific manifestations, such as night blindness (if vitamin A deficient), impaired host defenses, and infectious comorbidity that may be exacerbated by deficiencies and contribute to a worse state of malnutrition. This last interaction has been postulated to lead to a "vicious cycle," representing a synergy between infection and malnutrition as

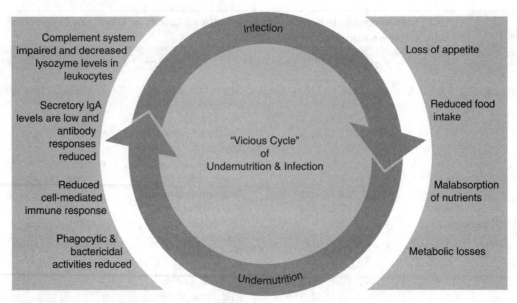

Figure 6-5 The Cycle of Undernutrition and Infection.

conceptualized by Scrimshaw, Taylor, and Gordon (1968), and depicted in Figure 6-5. In this model, frequent or extended infections depress appetite, food intake, and absorption of nutrients and increased metabolism; these factors slow growth and lead to undernutrition, which in turn impairs innate and adaptive immunity, worsening the severity and toll of an infection. These bidirectional effects are addressed later in this chapter.

Growth faltering is often detected by a lower than median referent weight gain, but principally refers to deceleration in linear (statural) growth over time, detectable by a child's widening deficit in height for age in relation to the median line of a WHO

growth chart (see Figure 6-4). The consequence of growth deceleration in the first two years of life, relative to the WHO median, is depicted in Figure 6-6 as age-specific mean height for age *z*-scores for children 1 to 59 months of age who were surveyed across the Latin American, African, and Southeast Asian regions. These data also reflect a global order of increasing severity of stunting. Irrespective of region, two key observations are the steadfast decline in attained length through the second year of life, occurring at a rate of approximately –0.10 *z*-score per month, and the lack of statural catch-up thereafter (Victora, de Onis, Hallal, Blossner, & Shrimpton, 2010). This pattern emphasizes the importance of

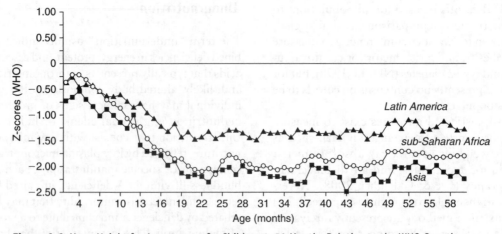

Figure 6-6 Mean Height for Age *z*-scores for Children 1–59 Months Relative to the WHO Growth Standard. Geographic groupings are based on the WHO regions for Latin America and the Caribbean, South Asia, and sub-Saharan Africa. Adapted from Victora et al., 2010.

promoting adequate fetal and postnatal linear growth in children through 2 years of age as critical to resolving lifelong, intergenerational stunting in the developing world.

Protein-Energy Malnutrition

Protein-energy malnutrition (PEM), either acute or chronic, is considered the dominant cause of undernutrition. Universally, assessment of mild-to-moderate PEM relies on comparative anthropometry—that is, standardized procedures for measuring weight, length or height, mid-upper arm circumference (MUAC), and skinfolds at mostly the tricipital and subscapular sites (Cameron, 1978; Gibson, 1990; Lohman, Roche, & Martorell, 1988).

Although low weight alone does not differentiate thinness (wasting) from stunting, a low weight for age (less than −2 z-scores) remains the dominant nutritional contributor to disease burden (Ezzati et al., 2002). Child length (for children younger than 2 years) or height (for children older than 2 years), compared to the referent gender-value for age, reveals the adequacy of linear growth (Hamill et al., 1979; WHO, 1995b). Inadequate linear growth leading to stunting (i.e., having a height for age less than −2 z-scores below the median) reflects a growth consequence of chronic PEM (Waterlow et al., 1977). Because linear growth deceleration is a gradual process, stunting is often associated with other indicators of poverty, food insecurity, and neglect (Martorell, Mendoza, & Castillo, 1988; Zere & McIntyre, 2003). Wasting, revealed by a child's weight being less than 2 z-scores below the referent weight for the same length or height, identifies acute PEM (Waterlow et al., 1977), although in undernourished populations wasting can also persist in children for long periods of time. A MUAC detects a thin arm (e.g., less than 12.5 cm in children 1 to 5 years of age) and is an alternative indicator of wasting (Jelliffe, 1966; WHO, 1995b). Traditional cutoff values and interpretation of these indicators are shown in Table 6-2.

Although milder stages of PEM are often clinically inapparent (Figure 6-7, left child), severe PEM refers to two clinically distinct presentations, marasmus and kwashiorkor, and a mixed form, marasmic kwashiorkor. *Marasmus,* which typically occurs in infancy, is marked by severe wasting, grossly clinically evident accompanied by a weight for height usually less than −3 z-scores. In a preschool child, it is diagnosed based on a MUAC less than 11.5 cm, from loss of muscle and adipose; a resultant "baggy" appearance to the skin; moderate to severe stunting from a near cessation of linear growth; soft, sparse

hair; absence of edema; alertness; and hunger (Reddy, 1991) (Figure 6-7, right child). *Kwashiorkor* is a term from the Ghanian language, Ga, for a condition that was initially observed to have developed when an older child was displaced from the breast (Williams, 1933). As implied by the term, children 2 to 3 years of age are at highest risk of this condition. Evidence of kwashiorkor includes edema (an essential feature), milder wasting, reddish hair changes, enlarged liver, frequent dermatosis (flaky paint rash), and a state of misery and disinterest in food (Reddy, 1991). Children with either marasmus or kwashiorkor are at high risk for corneal xerophthalmia due to severe vitamin A deficiency (Sommer & West, 1996). While both conditions are considered to result from severe deficiencies in energy and protein, their distinct clinical and biochemical profiles (Torun & Chew, 1999) suggest that

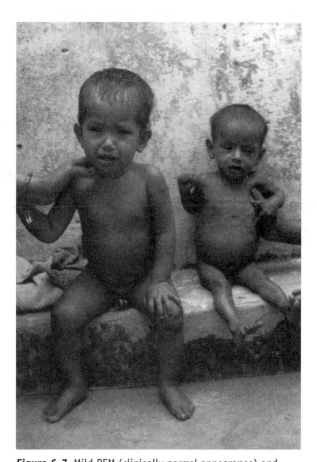

Figure 6-7 Mild PEM (clinically normal appearance) and marasmus (evident by extreme wasting of limbs and torso) in 1-year-old Bangladeshi children; child on left is a boy, child on right is a girl. Photo: KP West, Jr.
Source: West, K.P. Jr., Caballero, B. & Black, R.E. (2001). Nutrition. In: Merson, M.H., Black, R.E., Mills, A.J. (eds) "International Public Health." Gaithersburg, MD: Aspen Publishers, Inc. Chapter 5, p. 229 Figure 5-7.

this description is an oversimplification, with differences in other nutrient deficiencies and oxidative stress offering potential explanations for their occurrence (Golden, 2002).

The case fatality rate for severe wasting malnutrition is high (Brown et al., 1981). Nevertheless, outside of famine and other complex emergency conditions (Young, Borrel, Holland, & Salama, 2004), its prevalence tends to be low.

Extent of Undernutrition

The general magnitude of preschool child undernutrition can be gauged, nationally and by region, by indicators of prevalence of underweight, wasted, stunted, and overweight status (Table 6-3). Low- and middle-income countries are home to an estimated 178 million stunted children, representing 32% of all children younger than 5 years of age living in these settings (Black et al., 2008). Although the highest prevalence of stunting occurs in Eastern and Central Africa, where 50% and 42% of children are stunted,

respectively, the largest number of children who are stunted—74 million children—live in South Asia. Ten percent of children (55 million) have a weight for height z-score that is less than –2.

The highest prevalence of wasting and the largest number of children in this category are found in South-Central Asia, where 16% of children younger than 5 years are wasted. Severe wasting (weight for height z-score of less than –3) is rare, with only 3.5% of children in this category globally. Significant geographic clustering is observed, however. Of the 19.3 million children suffering from wasting malnutrition, 10.3 million live in South-Central Asia.

In 2005, 20% of children were estimated to be underweight (weight for age z-score of less than –2), with the highest prevalence in South-Central Asia and Africa. The geographic distribution of child underweight is illustrated in Figure 6-8, which shows the area of the country as being proportional to the number of underweight children living within it. Roughly half of all underweight children live in South-Central Asia.

Table 6-3	Regional Prevalence and Numbers of Underweight, Stunted, and Wasted Preschool-Aged Children					
	Underweight		**Stunted**		**Severely Wasted**	
UN Region[2]	Percentage	Number (millions)	Percentage	Number (millions)	Percentage	Number (millions)
Africa	21.9	31.1	40.1	56.9	3.9	5.6
Eastern	28.0	13.7	50.0	24.4	3.6	1.8
Middle	22.5	4.5	41.5	8.4	5.0	1.0
Northern	6.8	1.5	24.5	5.4	3.3	0.7
Southern	11.4	0.7	30.2	1.8	2.7	0.2
Western	23.9	10.7	37.7	16.8	4.3	1.9
Asia	22.0	78.6	31.3	111.6	3.7	13.3
Eastern	5.1	4.8	14.5	13.7	0.7	0.7
South-Central	33.1	60.1	40.7	73.8	5.7	10.3
South-Eastern	20.7	11.4	34.3	18.9	3.6	2.0
Western	8.9	2.2	20.6	5.2	1.6	0.4
Latin America and the Caribbean	4.8	2.7	16.1	9.2	0.6	0.3
Caribbean	5.1	0.2	8.2	0.3	1.0	0.03
Central America	6.2	1.0	23.1	3.7	0.6	0.1
South America	4.1	1.5	23.1	3.7	0.6	0.2
Low- and Middle-Income Countries	20.2	112.4	32.0	117.7	3.5	19.3

Note: Prevalence is the percentage below –2 standard deviations below the WHO growth standard value of weight for age (underweight), height for age (stunted), and weight for height (wasted) of children younger than 5 years.

Source: Black et al., 2008.

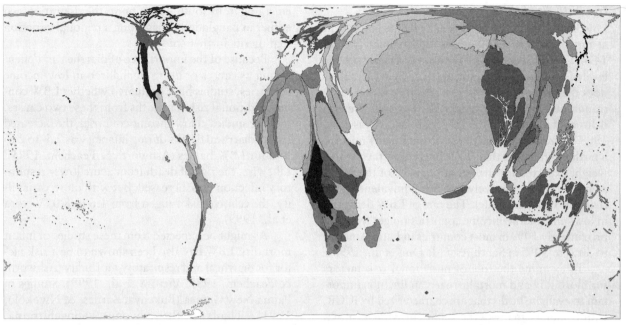

Figure 6-8 The Global Burden of Undernutrition: each country is sized in proportion to the number of underweight children who live within it
Source: Worldmapper. Underweight Children, Map No. 182. Sheffield, UK: SASI Group. University of Sheffield.

Despite the continued burden of undernutrition, the prevalence of low weight for age among preschool-aged Asian children is projected to decline by the year 2015 to half of the levels observed in 1990 (de Onis, Blossner, Borghi, Morris, & Frongillo, 2004), signaling the potential for this massive region to achieve its Millennium Development target of reducing the prevalence of preschool-child undernutrition by 50%. While all subregions appear poised to contribute to an anticipated global reduction, the greatest progress toward this goal is expected to occur in Eastern Asia, where the prevalence is projected to fall 84%, from 19% in 1990 to a virtually normal level of 3% in 2015 (de Onis, Blossner, et al., 2004). In an ironic twist, the rapidity and extent of shift upward in the region's child weight distribution has now raised concerns about obesity becoming a public health problem over the next two decades in this region of the world (Du, Lu, Zhai, & Popkin, 2002).

In contrast to Asia, nutritional conditions have deteriorated over the past decade across most of sub-Saharan Africa, including eastern, middle and western Africa, plus the Sudan (de Onis, Frongillo, & Blossner, 2000; de Onis, Wijnhoven, & Onyango, 2004). While early childhood wasting rates generally remain lower in Africa than in South Asia, the HIV/AIDS epidemic in Africa is expected to continue taking its nutritional toll on infected children, their families, new generations of orphans, and communities that have become economically decimated by the disease (Anabwani & Navario, 2005). These effects, along with the toll of conflict (Salama et al., 2004), other governance and infrastructural problems, and extended economic and food security stresses following the global financial crisis of 2008 (Brinkman et al., 2010), suggest that child nutritional status in many areas of Africa will either change little or continue to deteriorate through 2015, especially in eastern and sub-Saharan areas of Africa (de Onis, Blossner, et al., 2004).

Undernutrition as a Risk Factor for Infection and Related Mortality

Undernutrition is a risk factor for infectious morbidity and associated case fatality among children in low-income countries. Among neonates, given that gestational age and age-adjusted size at birth are often correlated with nutritional status during early childhood, it is appropriate to consider these factors as part of a continuum of risk between nutrition and infection. Nevertheless, studies have generally examined separately the risk of mortality related to status at birth in the neonatal or infant period and the risk related to nutritional status throughout childhood, at least up to age 5 years.

Low Birth Weight

Low birth weight (LBW) is usually defined as weight at birth less than 2,500 grams (approximately 5 lb, 14 oz). The incidence of LBW varies inversely with the level of economic development (ACC/SCN, 1992), as does the proportion of these births that is due to intrauterine growth restriction (IUGR) versus preterm delivery of less than 37 weeks' gestation (de Onis et al., 1998). Intrauterine growth restriction usually refers to a birth weight more than 2 z-scores below the median weight expected for the gestational age of the infant at birth (or, alternatively but not equivalently, less than the 10th percentile). The rate of LBW deliveries in low- and middle-income countries ranges from approximately 10% in most countries in Latin America to 30% to 50% in South Asia (de Onis et al., 1998).

To examine the role of nutritional risk factors for morbidity and mortality early in life, it is important to evaluate births that are characterized by IUGR. Unfortunately, many of the studies provide information only on LBW births rather than distinguishing these births by the cause of the low weight.

LBW babies have the largest increase in risk during the neonatal period, and they continue to have additional risk in the postneonatal period of infancy. In high-income countries, birth weights of 3,500 to 4,500 grams (7 lb, 11 oz to 9 lb, 14 oz) are associated with the lowest risk of neonatal mortality. The relative risk of neonatal mortality increases with birth weights less than 2,500 grams and increases even more for very LBW babies of less than 1,500 grams (3 lb, 3 oz) (Ashworth, 1998). In low-income countries, the data are more limited due to the difficulty of obtaining accurate birth weight measurements for deliveries, which occur predominantly in the home. In these settings, the neonatal mortality rates typically range as high as 50 deaths per 1,000 live births, and increase with decreasing birth weight.

In two studies that were able to cross-classify births by nutritional status for gestational age (to determine whether the newborn was growth restricted) and gestational age, the results varied. In Brazil, babies with IUGR had a fivefold increase in the risk of neonatal death (Barros, Victora, Vaughan, Teixeira, & Ashworth, 1987), while in Bangladesh the risk was only slightly increased (El-Arifeen, 1997). During the postneonatal period, LBW infants continued to have higher mortality than babies born with a higher weight. Again, the data are limited, but in Brazil babies born with IUGR had a fourfold increase in postneonatal mortality, and such births in Bangladesh were associated with a 50% increase in postneonatal deaths (Barros et al., 1987; El-Arifeen, 1997). Data

emerging from South Asia support the risk ratios seen earlier in Bangladesh, suggesting a regional variation that merits further study.

Because of the importance of diarrhea and pneumonia as causes of death in children in low-income countries, studies have evaluated whether LBW confers additional risk for deaths from these two causes. In three studies in low-income countries, the increased risk of diarrheal deaths during infancy was 2.5- to 2.8-fold for LBW babies (Ashworth & Feachem, 1985). Likewise, the risk of death from acute lower respiratory infection was increased, but with more variability; the relative risk ranged from 1.6 to 8.0 (Victora et al., 1999).

As might be expected from these studies of infant mortality, LBW has also been shown to be a risk factor for diarrheal and respiratory morbidity (Ashworth & Feachem, 1985; Victora et al., 1999). Studies in Papua New Guinea (Bukenya, Barnes, & Nwokolo, 1991), Thailand (Ittiravivongs, Songchitratna, Ratthapalo, & Pattara-Arechachai, 1991), and Brazil (Victora, Barros, Kirkwood, & Vaughan, 1990) found a relative risk associated with LBW, adjusted for other possible determinants of illness, ranging from 1.6 to 3.9 for acute diarrhea. Studies in China (Chen, Yu, & Li, 1988), Argentina (Cerquerio, Murtagh, Halac, Avila, & Weissenbacher, 1990), and Brazil (Victora et al., 1990; Victora, Smith, Barros, Vaughan, & Fuchs, 1989) found a relative risk ranging from 1.4 to 2.2 for acute lower respiratory infection or pneumonia hospitalization.

The consequences of low birth weight may extend into later childhood and adulthood as well. Illustrating this point, researchers in Gambia found that the risk of all-cause mortality in a cohort of individuals more than 14.5 years of age, followed from birth, was fourfold greater among individuals born during the preharvest "hungry" season than in the postharvest season. Death beyond 25 years of age was 10 times more likely among individuals who were born during the hungry season (Moore et al., 1999). Most known causes of death were reportedly infectious. The etiological importance of maternal undernutrition in hungry-season LBW incidence has been confirmed by low maternal weight gain and birth weight (Prentice, Whitehead, Watkinson, Lamb, & Cole, 1983), and the responsiveness of birth weight and neonatal survival to maternal supplementation with food (providing approximately 1,000 kcal per day) in this season (Ceesay et al., 1997). Both seasonal birth cohorts were comparable in nutritional status in their second year of life, suggesting a latent effect of gestational insult on subsequent health and survival.

Antenatal nutrition intervention trials are beginning to generate data supporting a causal role for nutritional exposures early in life altering risks of subsequent mortality (Christian et al., 2009). It has been hypothesized that intrauterine or early postnatal undernutrition may leave an "imprint" on an individual—for example, through defects of thymic and other lymphoid tissues at critical developmental periods—that could impair host resistance to infection (Moore et al., 1999; Prentice, 1998) or otherwise predispose individuals to disease (Barker, Osmond, Winter, Margetts, & Simmonds, 1989) later in life.

Childhood Undernutrition

This section focuses on the risk of infectious disease and related mortality in early childhood as a function of nutritional well-being reflected by anthropometric status. Severe malnutrition clearly carries a risk of death, but it is the potentially causal interaction of undernutrition with common infectious diseases in low-income countries that is of far greater importance. This relationship may reflect the aforementioned synergy between undernutrition and infectious diseases in which the combined conditions result in much greater mortality than either would alone (Scrimshaw, Taylor, & Gordon, 1967) (see Figure 6-5). Compromised host defenses and more severe infectious diseases in undernourished children may lead to higher case fatality rates, although an increased incidence of infectious diseases may play some role as well.

A review of the observational population studies in a large number of countries clearly reveals a monotonic increase in the risk of mortality at each progressively worse level of weight for age below the international median (Figure 6-9, Panel A) (Caulfield, de Onis, Blossner, & Black, 2004; Pelletier, Frongillo, & Habicht, 1993). Similar increases in mortality risk have been observed with decrements in MUAC, either adjusted (Sommer & Loewenstein, 1975) or unadjusted (Briend, Wojtyniak, & Rowland, 1987; Briend & Zimicki, 1986; West et al., 1991) for height, across all preschool ages, including early infancy once arm size is adjusted for age (De Vaquera, Townsend, Arroyo, & Lechtig, 1983; West et al., 1991). Stunting early in life (prior to age 3 years), adjusted for wasting, carries a disproportionate risk of mortality (Katz, West, Tarwotjo, & Sommer, 1989; Smedman, Sterky, Mellander, & Wall, 1987).

It is important to note that even mild undernutrition puts a child at increased risk of mortality. Because the greatest number of undernourished children have mild to moderate rather than severe malnutrition, most of the excess risk of death is attributable to the less severe forms of undernutrition. Also important is the observation that with worsening levels of weight for age, the mortality rate increases logarithmically (Figure 6-9, Panel B). Across studies, children have been estimated to experience an approximately 7% compound increase in risk of dying for every 1% decrease in weight for age below the referent median (Pelletier et al., 1993), suggesting the absence of an often posited "threshold" phenomenon (Pelletier, 1994). This effect is consistent with the postulated synergistic interaction between nutrition and infection, however, as nearly all of the deaths as recorded in the original studies were noted to be associated with infectious diseases. An estimated 21.4% of all childhood deaths—most of which are typically attributed to infectious diseases—can be attributed to stunting, severe wasting, or intrauterine growth restriction (Black et al., 2008).

Reductions in mortality may be achieved by improving nutritional status or reducing the severity of infectious diseases; however, improvements in both areas at the same time would be expected to have a synergetic benefit. In addition, improving nutritional well-being to reduce these excess deaths will require broad-based approaches to correct underlying inequities in impoverished communities that improve food security and dietary quality because poor screening specificity (which correctly excludes large numbers of children unlikely to die) in a mildly to moderately malnourished population could overwhelm targeted nutrition programs.

Diarrheal diseases and pneumonia are the two most important causes of death in children younger than five years of age in low-income countries. These two conditions have a higher case fatality rate in undernourished children compared to those who are well nourished. For example, malnourished children who were discharged from a hospital after treatment for diarrheal illness in Bangladesh had a 14-fold greater risk of dying compared with better-nourished controls (Roy, Chowdhury, & Rahaman, 1983). In a community-based study in rural India, severely wasted children had a 24-fold higher diarrheal case fatality rate compared with better-nourished children (Bhandari, Bhan, & Sazawal, 1992). In Mexico, undernourished children had an 8-fold greater risk of death with severe diarrhea (Tome, Reyes, Rodriguez, Guiscafre, & Gutierrez, 1996). Studies in the Philippines (Tupasi et al., 1990), Papua New Guinea (Shann, Barker, & Poore, 1989), Bangladesh (Rahman et al., 1990), and Argentina (Weissenbacher et al., 1990) of acute lower respiratory infection and pneumonia found a 2- to 3-fold increase in the case fatality rate in undernourished versus better-nourished children.

(A)

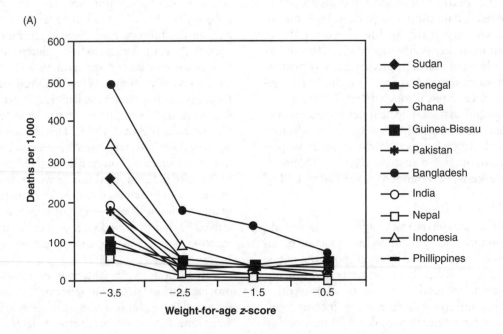

(B)

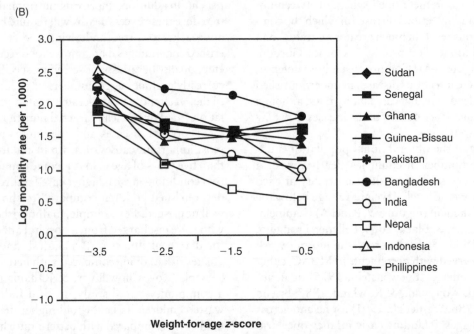

Figure 6-9 Association between Weight for Age (z-score) and Risk of All-Cause Mortality among Children 6 to 59 Months of Age at Baseline, Followed for Periods of 6 to 24 Months, in Longitudinal Population Studies in 10 Countries: Sudan, Senegal, Ghana, Guinea-Bissau, Pakistan, Bangladesh, India, Nepal, Indonesia and the Philippines. Panel (A): Deaths per 1000 per year; Panel (B): Logarithm of deaths per 1000 children per year. Sources: Pelletier, Frongillo and Habicht, 1993; Fishman et al., 2004.
Source: Fishman, S.M., Caulfield, L.E., de Onis, M., Blossner, M., Hyder, A.A., Mullany, L., & Black, R.E. (2004). Childhood and maternal undernutrition. In: Ezzati, M., Lopez, A.D., Rodgers, A., Murray, C.J.L. (Eds). Comparative Quantification of Health Risks: Global and Regional Burden of Disease Attributable to Selected Major Risk Factors (pp. 39–162). Geneva: World Health Organization.

Table 6-4	Relative Risk of Mortality Associated with Low Weight for Age			
	Weight for Age			
Cause of Death	< −3 z (95% Confidence Interval)	−2 to −3 z (95% Confidence Interval)	−1 to -2 z (95% Confidence Interval)	≥−1 z
Diarrhea	9.5 (5.5, 16.5)	3.4 (2.7, 4.4)	2.1 (1.6, 2.7)	1.0
Pneumonia	6.4 (3.9, 10.4)	1.3 (0.9, 2.0)	1.2 (0.7, 1.9)	1.0
Malaria	1.6 (1.0, 2.7)	1.2 (0.5, 3.5)	0.8 (0.2, 3.2)	1.0
Measles	6.4 (4.6, 9.1)	2.3 (1.7, 3.2)	1.3 (1.1, 1.5)	1.0
All causes	9.7 (5.2, 17.9)	2.5 (1.8, 3.6)	1.8 (1.2, 2.7)	1.0

Note: Table is based on data from Ghana, Guinea Bissau, the Philippines, India, Nepal, Bangladesh, and Pakistan.
Source: Black et al., 2008.

Prospective studies to evaluate the role of undernutrition, as assessed by anthropometry, in predisposing children to cause-specific mortality have found a progressively increased risk with worsening nutritional status (Table 6-4), particularly related to diarrheal disease, pneumonia, measles and malaria (Black et al., 2008).

Nutritional status has been assessed widely as a risk factor for the severity and incidence of diarrheal diseases. It has been estimated that underweight status has an increased relative risk of diarrhea mortality of 3.4 (95% confidence interval [CI]: 2.7–4.4) for children moderately underweight (WAZ, weight-for-age z-score, between –2 and –3) or 9.5 (95% CI: 5.5–16.5) for children severely underweight (WAZ less than –3) (Black et al., 2008). As might be expected with the reported higher case fatality rate in undernourished children, nutritional status has an association with disease severity. One measure of this relationship is the duration of the illness. In studies in several countries, the duration of diarrhea in mild to moderately malnourished children was shown to be up to 3-fold longer than for better-nourished children (Black, Brown, & Becker, 1984b). Undernutrition is also an important risk factor for the occurrence of persistent diarrhea (Baqui et al., 1993). This relationship has also been demonstrated for specific types of diarrhea, such as episodes due to *Shigella* species and enterotoxigenic *Escherichia coli*, in which the illness duration in Bangladeshi children was 2.5-fold longer

in undernourished children (Black, Brown, & Becker, 1984b). Poorer nutritional status has also been documented to be associated with increased rate of stool output in children, leading to an increased risk of dehydration (Black et al., 1984b). These mechanisms likely explain the increased risk for hospitalization and length of hospital stay due to diarrhea in undernourished children (Man et al., 1998; Victora et al., 1990).

The effect of undernutrition on diarrheal incidence has been more variable in different settings. Some studies have not found any increased risk of overall incidence in undernourished children, whereas others have found a 30% to 70% increased risk of incident diarrhea in such children (Black, Brown, & Becker, 1984a; Checkley et al., 2002; El Samani, Willett, & Ware, 1986; Guerrant, Schorling, McAuliffe, & de Souza, 1992). Some enteropathogens causing diarrhea, such as *Cryptosporidium parvum*, may be particularly selected as a cause of infection in undernourished children (Checkley et al., 1998).

The role of undernutrition as a risk factor for severity or incidence of acute lower respiratory infections or pneumonia has also been the subject of extensive study. Children who are severely underweight have a 6.4-fold elevated risk of mortality (95% CI: 3.9–10.4) due to pneumonia (Black et al., 2008). Evidence also supports an association between undernutrition and severity of respiratory infection, with such relationships being found in both hospital-based and community-based studies. Undernutrition has been found to increase the likelihood that a child will have bacteremia, pleural effusion, and other complications (Johnson, Aderele, & Gbadero, 1992). Studies in the Philippines, Costa Rica (James, 1972), and Brazil (Fonseca et al., 1996; Victora et al., 1989) found a modestly increased incidence of acute lower respiratory infections in undernourished children. In contrast, studies in Papua New Guinea (Smith, Lehman, Coakley, Spooner, & Alpers, 1991), Uruguay (Selwyn, 1990), and Guatemala (Cruz et al., 1990) did not find any such relationship. A meta-analysis found that underweight status (less than –2 z-scores weight for age) has an increased relative risk of pneumonia of 1.86 (95% CI: 1.06–3.28) (Fishman et al., 2004). One study in Gambia found that the development of pneumococcal infection was associated with a history of poor weight gain prior to the illness compared with other children in the community (O'Dempsey et al., 1996).

It has long been observed that measles is associated with undernutrition in children in low-income countries. This association and the apparent higher case fatality rate for measles in malnourished children led many to conclude that a synergistic relationship between these two entities exists. There is a significant relationship between weight for age and measles mortality, with that risk doubling for children who are moderately wasted and being 6.4-fold higher for children with severe wasting (Black et al., 2008). The observation in several African settings that vitamin A supplementation during acute measles can substantially reduce the severity and case fatality of measles (Barclay, Foster, & Sommer, 1987; Coutsoudis, Kiepiela, Coovadia, & Broughton, 1992; Hussey & Klein, 1990) also highlights the importance of nutritional risk factors in affecting survival from this disease.

The role of undernutrition in predisposing children to malaria is controversial. Early observations from the nineteenth century reported that malaria was more frequent in those persons with inadequate diets or with undernutrition (Garnham, 1954). Later, studies in the latter part of the twentieth century appeared to show that malnutrition could be actually protective against malaria. This contention was based on observational studies (Hendrickse, Hasan, Olumide, & Akinkunmi, 1971) or on interventions such as the refeeding of famine victims (Murray, Murray, Murray, & Murray, 1975) in which an exacerbation of malaria appeared to occur. Animal studies seemed to support the suppressive effects of a poor diet on malaria, leading to the belief that undernourished children are less susceptible to the infection and consequences of malaria.

More recent studies, however, indicate strongly that the relationship between nutritional status and malaria is complex and that undernutrition serves as a risk factor for increased malaria mortality and morbidity. For example, severe underweight has been found to be associated with a 60% increased risk of malaria mortality (Black et al., 2008). Additional studies indicate that specific micronutrients, such as vitamin A, zinc, iron, and others, affect the risk of infection and severity of illness with malaria as well (Caulfield, Richard, & Black, 2004). While it is now believed that undernutrition is a risk factor for malaria, it is also a consistent observation that refeeding a malaria-infected, starved host can reactivate the low-grade infection and lead to more severe disease. One implication of this finding is that antimalarial measures should be included during nutritional rehabilitation of famine victims who are likely to have malaria infection.

Contributions of Infection to Undernutrition

Infections in childhood have long been recognized to influence physical growth and rates of malnutrition among children in low- and middle-income countries. After initial observation of the relationship, more recent work has assessed the size of this effect and moderating influences. This research has been done largely through prospective community-based studies, which use intensive surveillance to assess episodes of illness and growth performance. These studies have examined the most frequent childhood infectious diseases, especially diarrhea and respiratory diseases. Some have assessed the effects of measles, malaria, and other infections, such as those of the skin. It is clear from the studies to date that infectious morbidity—particularly diarrheal disease—has an important effect on weight gain. A similar effect on linear growth has generally been observed in these studies.

The negative effect of diarrhea on weight and often height gain of children during and after an episode of acute diarrhea has been documented in diverse low-income country settings. Nevertheless, the magnitude of the effect on growth faltering has varied widely in these studies (Black, Brown, & Becker, 1983). Some studies, such as those conducted in Guatemala (Martorell, Yarbrough, Lechtig, Habicht, & Klein, 1975), Mexico (Condon-Paoloni, Joaquin, Johnston, deLicardi, & Scholl, 1977), and Bangladesh (Black et al., 1984a) have reported that 10% to 24% of the growth faltering could be explained statistically by the prevalence of diarrhea. By comparison, studies in other countries such as Uganda (Cole & Parkin, 1977), Gambia (Rowland, Cole, & Whitehead, 1977), and Sudan (Zumrawi, Dimond, & Waterlow, 1987) have reported that diarrhea could explain as much as 40% to 80% of observed faltering. In nearly all instances, these percentages of growth faltering explained by diarrhea were higher than those explained by other infectious diseases, again demonstrating the quantitative importance of the diarrhea-growth faltering relationship. In a pooled analysis of data from nine community-based studies, Checkley et al. (2008) determined the effects of diarrhea prior to 24 months of age on stunting at 24 months. The probability of stunting increased by 2.5% per episode of diarrhea; 25% of all stunting at 24 months of age was attributable to having at least five episodes of diarrhea in the first two years of life.

Infectious diseases generally result in poorer weight gain or weight loss, which may be due to either loss of appetite (Brown, Black, Robertson, & Becker, 1985) or increased metabolism. With diarrhea, there may also be intentional withholding of food, as well as malabsorption of ingested food in the damaged intestine (Behrens, Lunn, Northrop, Hanlon, & Neale, 1987; Lunn, Northrop-Clewes, & Downes, 1991). Variation in these factors may explain some of the differences in the magnitude of effect in various low-income country settings, but it also is necessary to consider factors such as the etiology of diarrhea, the age pattern of infection, the feeding pattern and dietary intake, treatment practices, and the length of the convalescent period.

To date, relatively few studies have examined the differential effect of diarrhea due to specific etiologic agents on growth. In Bangladesh, enterotoxigenic *Escherichia coli* and *Shigella* species were found to have the strongest effects on growth, while rotavirus and other enteropathogens, in part due to their lower prevalence, did not have a significant effect (Black et al., 1984a). The seasonal pattern of particular enteropathogens causing diarrhea may explain part of the seasonality in growth seen in some low-income country settings. In regard to clinical syndromes, dysentery (bloody diarrhea) and persistent diarrhea (defined by WHO as an episode lasting more than 14 days) have particularly important adverse effects on the growth of children (Black, 1993). As one might expect, the magnitude of the weight deficit is inversely related to the duration of the diarrheal episode. Persistent diarrheal episodes usually occur in children who also have a higher burden of diarrhea, so that both the persistent episodes and the high prevalence of diarrhea adversely affect growth.

Both asymptomatic and symptomatic infections can have an adverse effect on growth. Infection with *C. parvum,* with or without illness, in Peruvian children was associated with a reduction in weight gain,

after controlling for other variables (Checkley et al., 1998). Even though the effect size was smaller with asymptomatic infections than with symptomatic ones, because of their higher prevalence asymptomatic infections had a greater overall impact on growth than symptomatic infections. After experiencing an illness, children have the potential to grow more rapidly than they were growing previously; this phenomenon is known as "catch-up growth." Children with a *C. parvum* infection in the first 6 months of life did not have catch-up growth, showing that this disease had a long-lasting adverse effect on linear growth, whereas children with infections at an older age did show some catch-up growth.

There may be a substantial effect on the growth of children due to asymptomatic infection in the small intestine in a disorder referred to as tropical enteropathy. This disorder is characterized by crypt hyperplasia, villous atrophy, inflammation, increased intestinal permeability, and malabsorption (Humphrey, 2009). The continuous ingestion of large quantities of fecal bacteria in settings with poor sanitation and hygiene may be critical in the pathogenesis of tropical enteropathy. An accelerated immune response triggered by the increased small bowel permeability may divert nutrients to acute-phase proteins and other immune factors instead of supporting growth (Campbell, Elia, & Lunn, 2003). Reduced nutrient absorption, along with poor-quality diet, may also contribute to growth faltering in this disorder.

The feeding practices of a child at the time of illness can modify the effect of diarrhea on growth. Infants who are exclusively or predominantly breastfeeding tend to experience fewer adverse effects of diarrhea (Launer, Habicht, & Kardjati, 1990). This relationship may arise because breastfeeding ameliorates the severity of the illness or because breastfeeding generally seems to be continued without reduction in most circumstances during illness (Brown et al., 1985; Hoyle, Yunus, & Hen, 1980), whereas other foods may be reduced due to medical or cultural practices or anorexia because of the illness. Children in the first 6 months of life who are exclusively or predominantly breastfed may have less severe consequences of diarrhea or other infectious diseases (Khin-Maung-U et al., 1985; Launer et al., 1990; Rowland, Rowland, & Cole, 1988). Conversely, if very young children get diarrhea, they may experience long-term height deficits—effects that may be greater than if they developed diarrhea at an older age (Checkley, Epstein, Gilman, Cabrera, & Black, 2003).

There is also a modifying effect of diet on the relationship between diarrhea and growth (Brown et al., 1988). Diarrhea has a lesser effect among children whose usual dietary intake is greater or of better quality and among children who receive food supplements, compared to children with poorer diets or those not receiving food supplements in the same setting (Lutter et al., 1989).

Appropriate treatment of diarrheal illnesses may reduce the adverse effects of diarrhea on growth. The replacement of fluid and electrolytes with oral rehydration therapy may restore appetite and improve bowel function. Also, continued feeding during the illness has been demonstrated in clinical trials to result in improved weight gain in comparison to partial withholding of food during the acute phase (Brown et al., 1988). While antibiotics are not necessary for most cases of acute diarrhea, appropriate antibiotic treatment of dysentery would be expected to shorten the illness and, therefore, minimize the period of adverse effects on growth. The administration of zinc orally in treatment of diarrhea has been shown to reduce the severity and duration of diarrheal episodes, which would be expected to reduce the corresponding negative effects of diarrhea on growth (Sazawal, Black, Bhan, Bhandari, Sinha, & Jalla, 1995). Zinc supplementation for 10 to 14 days in therapy of diarrhea is recommended by WHO and UNICEF and is being widely implemented (Fischer Walker, Fontaine, Young, & Black, 2009).

Catch-up growth after a diarrheal episode seems possible without specific supplementary feeding programs, due to the child's increased consumption of available food. Even so, some diarrheal disease control programs recommend additional feeding in the convalescent period after illness. Unfortunately, the opportunity for catch-up growth may be limited by the duration of the healthy period between illnesses. Studies in Bangladesh (Black et al., 1983) and Zimbabwe (Moy, Marshall, Choto, McNeish, & Booth, 1994) have shown that, following a bout of diarrhea, children take 2 weeks to recover to their pre-illness weight and approximately 4 weeks to reach the weight that would have been expected if these children had continued their rate of growth prior to the illness. If another illness occurs during this month-long convalescent period, it may result in insufficient time for catch-up growth to occur and could add further nutritional insult. The net effect in the long term is a reduction in both ponderal and linear growth.

Acute respiratory infections—predominantly upper respiratory infections—have a high prevalence worldwide. Children in low-income countries, while having a similar prevalence of upper respiratory infections as children in higher-income countries, have a substantially higher rate of acute lower respiratory infections or pneumonia (Graham, 1990). Most of

the studies of the effect of acute respiratory infections on growth have included both upper and lower respiratory infections and have generally not found an effect of the illnesses on growth. In a Gambian study, children younger than 2 years of age with acute lower respiratory infections diagnosed by a pediatrician lost 14.7 grams of weight per day of illness, slightly but not significantly greater than the weight reduction observed with diarrheal diseases (Rowland et al., 1988). However, the prevalence of diarrhea was much higher than the prevalence of acute lower respiratory infections, so that diarrheal diseases explained half and respiratory infections only one-fourth of the observed weight deficit. Other studies in the Philippines (Adair et al., 1993), Papua New Guinea (Smith et al., 1991), Guatemala (Cruz et al., 1990), and Brazil (Victora et al., 1990) have also shown that acute lower respiratory infections adversely affect growth.

Acute respiratory illnesses are associated with a 10% to 20% reduction in food intake, possibly due to a reduction in the child's appetite (Brown et al., 1985; Mata, Cromal, Urrutia, & Garcia, 1977). As with other illnesses, catabolism may also play a role in this effect. Further studies are required to assess the magnitude of the adverse effects of acute lower respiratory infections on growth and to document whether modifying factors, like those found with diarrheal diseases, exist.

A few studies have attempted to document whether malaria has an adverse effect on growth in children in low-income countries. In Gambia, malaria prevalence was shown to adversely affect weight gain but not linear growth (Rowland et al., 1977). Subsequent studies in Uganda (Cole & Parkin, 1977) and Gambia (Rowland et al., 1988) were not able to demonstrate any effect of malaria on the growth of children. A recent trial of intermittent preventive antimalaria treatment of preschool-age children in Senegal found a benefit in weight gain but no effect on height increments (Ntab et al., 2007).

Although it has been believed for many years that measles causes a reduction in growth, this relationship has been difficult to document on a population basis. This difficulty arises in part because of the low incidence of measles found in prospective studies, which in some cases was due to the administration of measles vaccine in the study cohort. Older studies suggest that children with measles lose weight or have reduced growth velocity (Reddy, 1991). Nevertheless, measles has been best recognized as an illness that precipitates severe clinical forms of malnutrition. In children with previous undernutrition, measles can precipitate kwashiorkor or marasmus (DeMaeyer & Adiels-Tegman, 1985) as well as xerophthalmia (Sommer, 1982). Measles can also predispose patients to subsequent diarrhea and pneumonia, both of which will have additional adverse effects on nutritional status.

Intestinal helminthic infections, especially with *Acaris lumbricoides*, in children in low- and middle-income countries have been associated with poor growth (Rousham & Mascie-Taylor, 1994). In such populations, periodic deworming of children using a mass treatment approach has been demonstrated to improve growth (Adams, Stephenson, Latham, & Kinoti, 1994; Stoltzfus et al., 1998; Willett, Kilama, & Kihamia, 1979). Because children are reinfected rapidly after treatment, such approaches should be routine and combined with environmental sanitation and hygiene education.

Diet and Undernutrition

Diet in childhood should be adequate to meet all normal energy and nutrient requirements to support tissue growth, maintenance and function, and physical activity. Health and developmental consequences can occur when diet continually fails to meet these nutritional demands. Family and mealtime conditions under which food is eaten often reflect broader issues of child care and nurturing in the home that can influence child development. Most childhood undernutrition results directly from a diet that is chronically inadequate in quantity, conventionally taken to mean low in energy and protein and quality, reflecting poor biological value of protein (e.g., low amino acid score), low or imbalanced micronutrient density, or poor bioavailability due to high "antinutrient" content (e.g., phytate, fiber, oxalates). Poor quality may also refer to nonhygienic aspects of food preparation or storage, which could lead to food contamination and increased disease risk. Often the diet of the undernourished encompasses most of these features. Nutrient supplements are generally not viewed as part of the diet. Fortified food, although still rare in the diets of most low-income people, is increasingly being viewed as contributing to dietary quality. Dietary needs and the major ways these needs are met in infancy and early childhood are the focus of this section.

The Breastfeeding to Complementary Feeding Continuum

The infant-to-child feeding continuum should be viewed as a process, involving first breastfeeding and then transitional feeding, that results in adequate nourishment of children to support normal growth, health, and development from birth through early childhood. The process of establishing exclusive breastfeeding, followed by phasing in complementary feeding and the eventual transition to family foods, is illustrated in Figure 6-10 and provided as a series of steps and principles in Exhibit 6-2.

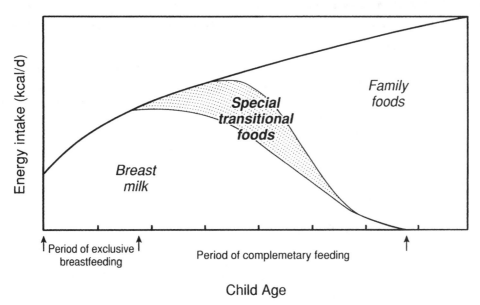

Figure 6-10 Illustration of the Sequential Phases of Early Childhood Feeding
Source: K. H. Brown, K. Dewey, and L. Allen, *Complementary Feeding of the Young Children in Developing Countries: A Review of Current Scientific Knowledge,* WHO/NUT/98 (Geneva, Switzerland: World Health Organization, 1998). Reprinted with permission.

Exhibit 6-2	Promoting Successful Breast and Complementary Feeding

Ten Steps to Successful Breastfeeding

Every facility providing maternity services and care for newborn infants should:

1. Have a written policy that is routinely communicated to all healthcare staff.
2. Train all healthcare staff in skills necessary to implement this policy.
3. Inform all pregnant women about the benefits and management of breastfeeding.
4. Help mothers initiate breastfeeding within a half-hour of birth.
5. Show mothers how to breastfeed, and how to maintain lactation even if they should be separated from their infants.
6. Give newborn infants no food or drink other than human milk, unless medically indicated.
7. Practice rooming-in (i.e., allowing mothers and infants to remain together 24 hours a day).
8. Encourage breastfeeding on demand.
9. Give no artificial teats or pacifiers to breastfeeding infants.
10. Foster the establishment of breastfeeding support groups and refer mothers to them on discharge from the hospital or clinic.

WHO Guiding Principles for Breastfeeding and Complementary Feeding

1. Practice exclusive breastfeeding from birth to 6 months of age, and introduce complementary foods at 6 months of age while continuing to breastfeed.
2. Continue frequent, on-demand breastfeeding until the child reaches 2 years of age or beyond.
3. Practice responsive feeding, applying the principles of psychosocial care.
4. Practice good hygiene and proper food handling.
5. Start at 6 months of age with small amounts of food and increase the quantity as the child gets older, while maintaining frequent breastfeeding.
6. Gradually increase food consistency and variety as the infant becomes older, adapting to the infant's requirements and abilities.
7. Increase the number of times that the child is fed complementary foods as he or she becomes older.
8. Feed a variety of nutrient-rich foods to ensure that all nutrient needs are met.
9. Use fortified complementary foods or vitamin–mineral supplements for the infant as needed.
10. Increase fluid intake during illness, including more frequent breastfeeding, and encourage the child to eat soft, varied, appetizing, favorite foods. After illness, give food more often than usual and encourage the child to eat more.

Source: E. G. Piwoz, S. L. Huffman, and V. J. Quinn, "Promotion and Advocacy for Improved Complementary Feeding: Can We Apply the Lessons Learned from Breastfeeding?" 2003, Food and Nutrition Bulletin, 24, pp. 29–44. Reprinted with permission.

This concept is advanced by clear definitions of indicators of feeding states (WHO, 2008a). Thus exclusive and predominant breastfeeding are differentiated owing to the risk of pathogen exposure and infection that accompanies the latter (Labbok & Krasovec, 1990). Partially breastfed infants can be classified by their patterns of consumption of non-human milk, solid foods, and frequency of breastfeeding or based on the percentage of total daily energy consumed from breast milk (Piwoz, Creed de Kanashiro, Lopez de Romana, Black, & Brown, 1996).

Complementary feeding begins with the introduction of foods and liquids other than human milk into an infant's diet at an age when human milk alone is no longer sufficient to meet nutritional requirements, which begins with the onset of partial breastfeeding (PAHO, 2003). Complementary foods are meant to adequately nourish infants as they transition to the family diet, while minimizing the displacement of human milk. It has been suggested that the term "weaning food" be avoided, as it may convey the wrong goal of displacing human milk with another—even if nutritious—food (Brown, Dewey, & Allen, 1998).

The complementary feeding period passes when an infant is fully weaned from the breast, although infrequent ("token") breastfeeding may persist prior to complete cessation, with likely little nutritional or growth benefit (Labbok & Krasovec, 1990; Piwoz et al., 1996). By that age, often 3 to 4 years, a child has passed through the period of highest risk for growth faltering, serious infectious illness, and mortality. Dietary progression to a full household diet is likely to follow patterns established during complementary feeding.

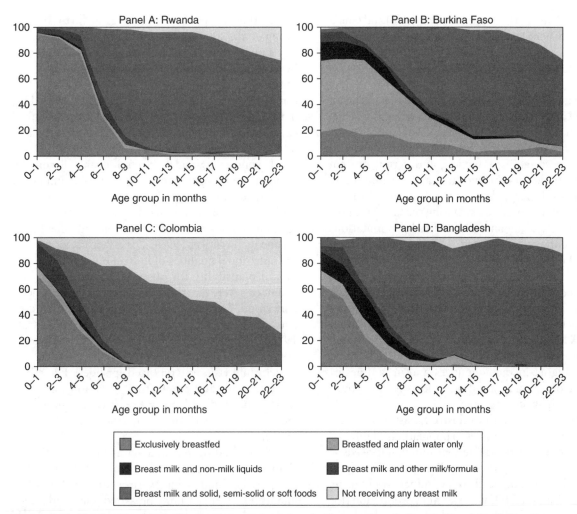

Figure 6-11 Distribution of breastfeeding and complementary feeding practices in Rwanda (Panel A), Burkina Faso (Panel B), Colombia (Panel C), and Bangladesh (Panel D). Data from Demographic and Health Surveys 2003–2007. *Source*: WHO (2010). Indicators for assessing infant and young child feeding practices: Part 3 Country profiles. Geneva, Switzerland: World Health Organization. Figures for infant and young child feeding practices by age (%): page 17, Bangladesh; page 19, Burkina Faso; page 21, Colombia; and page 36, Rwanda.

Striking differences in infant and young child feeding practices are noted both across and within regions. Different and typical patterns of breastfeeding initiation, introduction of complementary foods, and graduation to a household diet with cessation of breastfeeding, as observed in four countries, are illustrated in Figure 6-11 (WHO, 2010). The data from Rwanda (Panel A) reveals a pattern in which more than 90% of infants exclusively breastfeed shortly after birth, with a high proportion continuing to exclusively receive human milk through age 6 months. Beyond that age, most infants begin to receive solid, semi-solid, or soft foods with human milk. In contrast, in Burkina Faso (Panel B), fewer than 20% of infants are exclusively breastfed at birth. In this culture, most young infants receive either plain water or

other non-milk liquids in addition to regular breastfeeding during the first 6 months of life, beyond which solid, semi-solid, or soft foods are introduced while breastfeeding continues. Although patterns suggest a small proportion of infants continue to be exclusively or predominately breastfed well into their second year of life, such a practice fails to meet the nutritional needs of growing infants of this age. South and Southeast Asian mothers tend to partially breastfeed their infants for a longer duration, indicated by a prevalence of any breastfeeding of 50% to 80% during the third year of life (Panel D) (Brown, Black, & Becker, 1982; Grummer-Strawn, 1996; Huffman, Chowdhury, Chakraborty, & Simpson, 1980; Khatry et al., 1995), whereas a more rapid transition to the family diet is evident in Latin

America (Panel C) (Grummer-Strawn, 1996) and China (Taren & Chen, 1993).

Breastfeeding

WHO and UNICEF (2003) recommend that exclusive breastfeeding be practiced for the first 6 months of life, based on the consensus view that, on average, breastfeeding can provide adequate energy, nutrients, and fluid; protect against infection; and permit normal growth for infants through this age. Feeding early nutrient- and energy-dense, bacteriostatic colostrum is important in this process. During the first 6 months of life, average human milk intakes for populations of infants have been noted to range between 700 and 800 mL per day in both low-income and higher-income countries (Brown, Dewey, & Allen, 1998; Dewey & Brown, 2003); this amount is adequate to meet the average child's nutritional needs. This point has now been firmly established with the publication of the WHO growth standards, which demonstrated that the growth of exclusively breastfed infants reared in both higher-income countries and in families of high socioeconomic standing in low-income countries was highly comparable.

While the 6-month exclusive breastfeeding recommendation safely applies to populations of infants, it is important to recognize that individual needs—whether due to malnutrition, disease, or other factors—will inevitably lead to individual adjustments (Black & Victora, 2002). Lower milk production (for example, 400 to 600 mL per day), as has been observed in some malnourished settings (Jelliffe & Jelliffe, 1978), may indicate a need to introduce complementary foods closer to 4 months than 6 months of age. The degree to which frequent exposure to infection, as often occurs among young infants in poor societies, changes energy and nutrient requirements and the consequent ability of exclusive breastfeeding to meet increased nutritional needs remain unknown (Brown, Dewey, & Allen, 1998; Butte, 1996). In some studies, infection has been noted to have relatively little effect on human milk intake during early infancy (Brown et al., 1985; Brown, Stallings, Creed de Kanashiro, Lopez de Romana, & Black, 1990). Interaction with infection, however, could partly explain the frequent occurrence of growth failure among non-exclusively breastfed infants during the first 3 to 6 months of life in poorly nourished groups (Rivera & Ruel, 1997).

Micronutrient adequacy may also become limiting prior to 6 months of age in areas where maternal deficiencies are common during pregnancy. Infants of iron-deficient mothers may be at risk of iron defi-

ciency themselves if iron reserves at birth are low (Yang et al., 2007), given that human milk is generally a poor source of iron. Vitamin D deficiency may be a concern for young infants with limited exposure to sunlight and whose mothers are deficient in this vitamin (Kovacs, 2008). In populations where these maternal micronutrient deficiencies are thought to exist, giving supplemental iron or vitamin D in early infancy might be warranted.

Beyond energy and nutrients, human milk contains a repertoire of antimicrobial and anti-inflammatory factors, hormones, digestive enzymes, transport molecules, and growth modulators that appear to confer substantial protection from infection and other harmful agents (Prentice, 1996). These factors, along with the nutritional qualities of human milk, provide biological plausibility for observed reductions in persistent or severe diarrheal morbidity (Victora, Fuchs, Kirkwood, Lombardi, & Barros, 1992), including episodes of cholera and shigellosis (Clemens et al., 1986; Clemens et al., 1990), among breastfed versus non-breastfed infants and young children. Lower risk of sick child visits and reported episodes of diarrhea, ear infection, and respiratory infection have also been associated with early breastfeeding in higher-income countries (Raisler, Alexander, & O'Campo, 1999).

Breastfeeding markedly improves an infant's chances of surviving the first months of life. When compared to infants who were exclusively breastfed, infants who were partially breastfed (any food or water in addition to human milk) had a 2.4- to 2.8-fold increased risk of mortality due to diarrheal disease or lower respiratory tract infection in the first 5 months of life (Lauer, Betran, Barros, & de Onis, 2006). These data are also supported by findings of a multipronged breastfeeding education trial in India that led to approximately 17-fold higher odds of sustained exclusive breastfeeding to 6 months of age and, among intervened communities, a 30% lower prevalence of diarrhea at 3 months of age (Bhandari et al., 2003).

The timing of initiation of breastfeeding is also critical for neonatal survival in poor communities. In Nepal and Ghana, initiating breastfeeding more than 24 hours after birth was associated with a 2.4- to 3-fold increased risk of neonatal mortality compared to breastfeeding within 24 hours. The lowest risk of mortality was observed among infants breastfed within the first hour of birth (Edmond et al., 2006; Mullany et al., 2008). Continued breastfeeding through 6 to 23 months of life has also been associated with protection. Infants who are not breastfed during that period have been observed to incur a 3.7-fold increased risk of mortality over those who continued breastfeeding (Black et al., 2008). Breastfeeding into the third year of life has been shown to disproportionately benefit the survival of severely malnourished children (Briend & Bari, 1989; Briend, Wojtyniak, & Rowland, 1988) and, more broadly, children of low socioeconomic means (e.g., those living in homes with high maternal illiteracy and poor sanitation). Extended, partial breastfeeding has also been consistently associated with protection from severe vitamin A deficiency, as evidence by increased protection against risk of xerophthalmia (Mahalanabis, 1991; Sommer & West, 1996; West et al., 1986).

Research has shown that breastfed infants grow differently than their formula-fed peers, as demonstrated by less weight gain and, in some studies, a shorter stature by 1 year of age (Brakohiapa et al., 1988; Castillo, Atalah, Riumallo, & Castro, 1996; Caulfield, Bentley, & Ahmed, 1996; Grummer-Strawn, 1996; Victora, Vaughan, Martines, & Barcelos, 1984). This finding has persisted despite repeated attempts to adjust studies for multiple potential confounding factors. Researchers have not yet developed plausible explanations for how breastfeeding could depress physical growth, while simultaneously improving survival and reducing risks of micronutrient deficiencies, given the lack of evidence indicating that breastfeeding specifically increases the risk of infection or reduces appetite and, therefore, nutrient delivery to the infant. Instead, this association is more likely to be explained by factors related to (1) cross-sectional study designs that cannot reveal the temporal dimension of the breastfeeding–nutritional status relationship; (2) residual confounding factors, despite adjustment for multiple factors as measured that may influence both the mother's decision to breastfeed and the nutritional health of children; and (3) reverse causality, which could lead mothers to continue breastfeeding their children because they are malnourished (Caulfield et al., 1996).

More plausible findings emerged from a prospective study in Kenya that assessed the growth of 264 partially breastfed children, 14 to 20 months of age, by their breastfeeding and weaning habits observed over a 6-month period. Children who continued to breastfeed for the entire follow-up period gained more height (+0.6 cm) and weight (+230 g) than children who were breastfed for a medium duration (50% to 99% of the children seen in the 6-month follow-up) and 3.4 cm and 370 g more in height and weight, respectively, than children who breastfed for the shortest duration (fewer than 50% of the children seen in the follow-up period) (Onyango, Esrey, & Kramer, 1999). These findings agree with two other longitudinal studies of breastfeeding and growth (Adair et al., 1993; Marquis, Habicht, Lanata, Black, & Rasmussen, 1997).

Another possible explanation for the weight gain differences between breastfed and formula-fed infants is that the weight gain among formula-fed infants represents excessive growth. This view is supported by studies revealing an association between formula feeding and obesity in later life (Gillman et al., 2006; Grummer-Strawn & Mei, 2004; Owen, Martin, Whincup, Smith, & Cook, 2005; Toschke et al., 2007).

Infant feeding in the context of HIV infection presents a complex problem that is framed by the influence of infant feeding practices on child survival coupled with a higher risk of vertical transmission of HIV from mother to child through human milk. Previously, greater emphasis was placed on preventing HIV transmission by recommendations to replace breastfeeding when safe alternative feeding options are available (UNAIDS, UNICEF, & WHO, 1998). To implement this recommendation, it is critical that replacement feeding options are affordable, feasible, acceptable, sustainable, and safe (referred to with the acronym AFASS), to which one might add nutritious human milk substitutes. Unfortunately, this approach is neither feasible nor safe in many low-income settings because of unsafe water supplies, poor hygiene, and inadequate availability of suitable, low-cost replacement foods. While replacement feeding prevents transmission of HIV through human milk and is likely the best option in higher-income countries, in poor settings it can place infants at increased risk of death from other exposures and causes.

A series of studies have demonstrated that early exclusive breastfeeding is protective against postnatal transmission compared to mixed feeding (Coovadia et al., 2007; Iliff et al., 2005). In addition, two randomized trials suggested that disease-free survival was comparable between infants randomized to formula feeding or breastfeeding from birth (Thior, Lockman, & Shapiro, 2006) and between infants randomized to continued breastfeeding or abrupt weaning at 4 months of age (Kuhn et al., 2008). Continued breastfeeding beyond 6 months has also been associated with reduced risk of gastroenteropathy and mortality (Kafulafula et al., 2010; Onyango-Makumbi et al., 2010).

Where available, antiretroviral drugs have been shown to reduce the risk of mother-to-child transmission of HIV (Volmink, Siegfried, van der Merwe, & Brocklehurst, 2007). Recognizing this fact, WHO released a new set of infant feeding guidelines in 2009 (Exhibit 6-3) (WHO, 2009b) in tandem with new guidelines on the use of antiretroviral drugs for the prevention of vertical HIV transmission (WHO, 2009c).

Exhibit 6-3	WHO Key Recommendations for HIV and Infant Feeding

1. Mothers should be provided with lifelong therapy or antiretroviral (ARV) prophylaxis interventions to reduce HIV transmission through breastfeeding.
2. Mothers should exclusively breastfeed their infants for the first 6 months of life, introducing appropriate complementary foods thereafter, and continue breastfeeding for the first 12 months of life. Breastfeeding should stop only when a nutritionally adequate and safe diet without human milk can be provided.
3. Mothers who decide to stop breastfeeding at any time should stop gradually within 1 month. Mothers or infants who have been receiving ARV prophylaxis should continue ARV prophylaxis for 1 week after breastfeeding is fully stopped. Stopping breastfeeding abruptly is not advisable.
4. When mothers decide to stop breastfeeding at any time, infants should be provided with safe and adequate replacement feeds to enable normal growth and development.
5. Mothers should give commercial infant formula milk as a replacement food to their infants only when conditions for formula feeding are affordable, feasible, acceptable, sustainable, and safe.
6. Mothers may consider expressing and heat-treating human milk as an interim feeding strategy.
7. If the infants and young children are known to be HIV infected, mothers are strongly encouraged to exclusively breastfeed for the first 6 months of life and continue breastfeeding as per the recommendations for the general population—that is, up to 2 years or longer.

Source: WHO, 2009b.

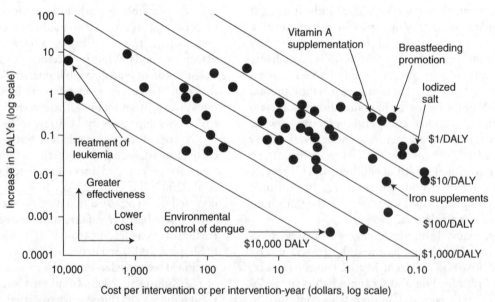

Figure 6-12 Comparison of the Cost-Effectiveness of Several Nutrition Interventions (Labeled as Vitamin A Supplementation, Breastfeeding Promotion, and Iodized Salt) in Relation to Other Public Health and Treatment Programs in Terms of Disability-Adjusted Life Years (DALYs) Gained (Horton et al., 1996), a Summary Measure of "Life Years Lost Due to Premature Mortality and Years Lived with Disability Adjusted for Severity" (Murray & Lopez, 1997). Note: Calculated DALYs gained due to vitamin A did not consider impact on child mortality (World Bank, 1993), leading to an underestimate of effectiveness.

Source: T. G. Sanghvi and J. Murray, *Improving Health Through Nutrition: The Nutrition Minimum Package* (Arlington, VA: Basic Support for Institutionalizing Child Survival [BASICS] Project, for the U.S. Agency for International Development, 1997), p. 6. Reprinted with permission.

Breastfeeding promotion and support programs have been shown to increase rates of exclusive breastfeeding. For example, a randomized program evaluation in India, implemented by Anganwadi workers, traditional birth attendants, and other local providers, reported 17-fold increased odds of exclusive breastfeeding to 6 months of age and a 30% lower prevalence of diarrhea at 3 months of age in communities that received the intervention (Bhandari et al., 2003).

The most widely adopted program to date has been the global "Baby Friendly Hospital Initiative" developed and promoted by WHO and UNICEF (Sanghvi & Murray, 1997). A hospital can be certified as "Baby Friendly" when it does not accept free or low-cost human milk substitutes, feeding bottles, or teats and has implemented the 10 steps to support successful breastfeeding (see Exhibit 6-2). It has been estimated that breastfeeding promotion, if scaled up to virtually complete coverage in the highest-priority countries, could reduce infant deaths by 12%, and deaths from 1 to 3 years of age by 9%, thus averting nearly 22 million disability-adjusted life-years (DALYs—a quantitative index of burden of disease) (Bhutta et al., 2008). Promotion and adoption of "Baby Friendly" breastfeeding practices may be one of the most cost-effective interventions for preventing DALYs in low-income countries (Horton et al., 1996; Murray & Lopez, 1997; Sanghvi & Murray, 1997; World Bank, 1993) (Figure 6-12).

Complementary Feeding

While agreement exists about the value of exclusive breastfeeding through 6 months of age and basic sequences of early childhood feeding, opinions vary about specific foods infants can tolerate, their order of introduction, frequency and mode of feeding, preparation, nutrient composition, and the degrees to which variation in these facets of child feeding affect health, growth, body composition, and development of children (Dewey & Brown, 2003). Most evidence relates to effects of diverse feeding interventions on growth and development.

The total energy requirements for healthy, breastfed infants are roughly 615 kcal/day for 6- to 8-month-olds and go up to 894 kcal/day at 12 to 23 months of age (Dewey & Brown, 2003). The added energy requirements from complementary foods for infants with "average" human milk intakes are 200 kcal/day at 6 to 8 months of age, rising to 550 kcal/day at 12 to 23 months of age (PAHO, 2003). While breastfeeding by itself is not sufficient to provide this energy for children beyond 6 months of age, much of this energy need can be met through

human milk. It is difficult to provide highly prescriptive guidelines for complementary feeding, given differences in locally available foods, individual differences in human milk intake, and other factors. Nevertheless, a series of guiding principles exists to guide practitioners and caregivers about complementary feeding practices (Exhibit 6-2). These principles highlight the importance of safe preparation and storage of foods, quantities and varieties of foods likely to meet a growing child's energy and nutrient needs, responsive infant feeding, continued feeding during and after illness, and provision of micronutrient supplements in populations at risk of deficiency.

Impact on Growth

Growth is expected to improve to an optimal level when undernourished children are adequately fed, although only modest evidence supports such an impact. Approaches employed to increase quantity, quality, or variety of complementary foods have included educational interventions, either alone or coupled with supplemental food, the delivery of fortified or unfortified foods, and dietary modifications to increase energy density of complementary foods. In general, in populations with sufficient means to procure food, education alone can have a positive impact on child growth; in contrast, in food-insecure settings, education should be combined with food supplements to have a positive impact (Bhutta et al., 2008).

In studies where complementary feeding was the only intervention, effect sizes on growth have been both modest and inconsistent (Dewey & Adu-Afarwuah, 2008). For example, a well-known study by the Instituto Nutricional de Central America y Panama (INCAP), conducted from 1969 to 1977, showed that infants fed a high-protein, multinutrient supplement (*atole*) daily for 3 years had increased linear growth by 2.5 cm relative to children given a low-calorie supplement (*fresca*). Most of this improvement occurred in late infancy, and the effect persisted into adolescence (Ruel, Rivera, Habicht, & Martorell, 1995). In Ghana, the efficacy of "Weanimix," a cereal-legume transitional food (containing maize, soybean, and groundnut) developed by UNICEF, was tested without and fortified with added vitamins and minerals, and against two other mixes using fish powder and koko, a fermented maize porridge. Six-month-old infants randomized to consume one of four mixtures daily had comparable growth and morbidity over the 6-month period of intervention, although fortification improved iron and vitamin A status, based on changes in plasma ferritin and retinol concentrations (Lartey, Manu, Brown, Peerson, & Dewey, 1999).

In a well-described trial in Colombia, mothers were randomized in the third trimester of pregnancy to receive a family food package each week, including a skim milk and vegetable protein mixture for their infants starting at 3 months of age (providing 670 kcal and 23 g of protein daily). Supplemented infants exhibited 0.6 cm and 162 g increases in length and weight, respectively, over controls by 6 months of age (Lutter et al., 1990; Mora, Herrera, Suescun, de Navarro, & Wagner, 1981). Breastfeeding patterns were not reported in this study, so the effect may have been partly influenced by improved maternal intake during pregnancy and lactation. Continued supplementation with the protein-calorie gruel further increased weight (+110 g) and length (+0.45 cm) while the children were between 9 and 12 months of age, with smaller increments observed through 36 months of age (Lutter et al., 1990).

In Jamaica, children 9 to 24 months of age given a weekly take-home milk formula (providing approximately 100 kcal/day above usual home intakes) showed improved weight, length, and head circumferential growth over controls during an initial 6-month period, but not thereafter (Walker, Powell, Grantham-McGregor, Himes, & Chang, 1991).

In recent years, lipid-based ready-to-use therapeutic food products (RUTF) have been found to be effective in treating severely wasted (acutely malnourished) infants and young children. These interventions can be delivered in community settings. However, because they have been designed to meet most of an individual child's daily energy and nutrient needs, the quantity required is large: 200 to 300 g per child per day (Chaparro & Dewey, 2010).

More recently, attention has focused on developing lipid-based nutrient supplements (LNS) to prevent early childhood undernutrition using a lower-dose product designed to enrich, but not replace, locally available complementary foods. In Ghana, for example, a 20-g daily dose (108 kcal/day) of a product ("Nutributter") that contained the full complement of micronutrients plus added essential fatty acids and milk (casein) protein was found to promote greater weight and length gains compared to micronutrient supplementation alone (Adu-Afarwuah et al., 2007). In Malawi, children who received a similar type of LNS gained more weight between 6 and 12 months of age compared to children who received a fortified porridge product (Lin et al., 2008), while the prevalence of severe stunting (less than −3 z-scores in height for age, or HAZ) was

reduced from 12.5% to 0% in children supplemented with LNS from 6 to 18 months of age (Phuka et al., 2008). In a 3-month intervention in children 6 to 60 months of age in Niger led to a reduction in wasting (less than −2 z-scores in weight for height, or WHZ) over an 8-month surveillance period (Isanaka et al., 2009).

The effectiveness of complementary feeding programs to improve child growth or reduce protein-energy malnutrition may be difficult to discern. To date, six large programs providing food supplements with education have been evaluated in Senegal, Bangladesh, Ecuador, Peru, Mexico, and Vietnam (Dewey & Adu-Afarwuah, 2008). Overall, the effect size across programs was a 0.21 standard deviation (SD) increase in weight (95% CI: 0.18–0.66) and 0.09 SD increase in length (95% CI: 0.0–0.14). The relatively small effect sizes have been attributed to technical and logistical difficulties in implementation (Dewey & Adu-Afarwuah, 2008) or other child care and feeding practices influenced by maternal socioeconomic status, education, and nutritional status (Hossain, Duffield, & Taylor, 2005); seasonality; and, possibly, chronic exposure to unsanitary conditions and pathogen exposure that can lead to inefficient nutrient utilization (Humphrey, 2009).

Development Effects

Delivery of additional nutritious, complementary feeding early in life may improve child development. In the INCAP study, *atole* recipients later in childhood were found to register higher scores on aptitude and cognitive tests than in children given *fresco* (Pollitt, Gorman, Engle, Rivera, & Martorell, 1995). When participants were followed up in adulthood, it was found that those who had received *atole* as children had improved scores on reading comprehension and cognitive ability tests and that women completed an average of 1.2 more years of education compared to those who had received *fresca* (Maluccio et al., 2009). Among men, the effect of the intervention was found to be associated with a 46% increase in wages in adulthood (Hoddinott, Maluccio, Behrman, Flores, & Martorell, 2008).

In the study in Ghana, the children who received LNS from 6 to 12 months of age had improved motor development, as measured by a greater proportion of infants who could walk independently at 12 months of age, compared to children in the control group (Adu-Afarwuah et al., 2007). Four years after completion of the Jamaican growth trial, children who had been supplemented with a milk formula (100 kcal/day) between 9 to 24 months of age showed a modest gain in perceptual–motor scores over those who had not received such supplementation. Irrespective of supplement exposure, however, children who had been stunted and had a smaller head circumference at the outset of the trial had lower intelligence scores (Grantham-McGregor, Walker, Chang, & Powell, 1997), possibly indicating early cognitive loss extending to the intrauterine period of growth restriction (Villar, Smeriglio, Martorell, Brown, & Klein, 1984).

There are also potential effects of iodine, iron, and zinc supplementation on early childhood cognition and development (Walker et al., 2007), suggesting that a usual dietary intake of foods rich in such micronutrients could provide benefit. This possibility represents an important area for additional research.

Micronutrient Deficiencies

Essential micronutrients comprise vitamins and minerals derived only from diet that are required by the body in minute amounts to support virtually all facets of molecular and cellular functions—cellular signaling, functioning and structures; cellular processes involved in proliferation, differentiation, respiration, growth, function, maturation, and death; and tissue growth, development, structure, function maintenance, repair, and loss. Micronutrient deficiencies, frequently accompanied by degrees of PEM, impair normal physiologic processes, leading to different health consequences depending on their timing, severity, multiplicity, and interactions, as well as the individual's stage of life. Historically, the severity of micronutrient deficiencies has been equated to the stages of clinical signs (for example, mild eye signs of xerophthalmia = mild vitamin A deficiency), with little attention given to systemic, subacute deficiencies, similar to the historic neglect of the extent and consequences of mild undernutrition (Pelletier et al., 1993). However, increasingly sensitive biochemical and functional indicators, greater cognizance that clinical signs reflect moderate to severe nutrient depletion ("tip of the iceberg"), and revelations about the morbidity and mortality risks associated with subacute stages of deficiency have motivated increased efforts to assess and prevent the full spectrum of micronutrient deficiencies.

Estimates of the extent of deficiencies vary widely. Based on modest data, estimates range from 20% of the world's population (more than 1 billion persons) being deficient in one or more essential micronutri-

ents (Trowbridge et al., 1993) to more than 2 billion being iron deficient alone (UNICEF, 1997). Despite this imprecision, dietary deficits or imbalances in essential micronutrients are very likely to constitute a substantial human burden, termed "hidden hunger" (Ramalingaswami, 1995), with their greatest public health consequences likely to affect mostly low-income societies (Howson, Kennedy, & Horwitz, 1998). Deficiencies in vitamin A, iron, iodine, and zinc have continued to dominate public health concerns over the past few decades, and are addressed in this section, as are advances in recent years made toward addressing multiple, concurrent micronutrient deficiencies and reducing their potential health consequences. Other deficiencies such as those of vitamin D, vitamins B_6 and B_{12}, folate, and selenium are drawing increased research attention, and will likely be viewed with greater public health evidence-based attention in the near future.

Vitamin A Deficiency

Vitamin A deficiency is the leading cause of preventable pediatric blindness and a major determinant of childhood morbidity and mortality in low-income countries (Rice, West, & Black, 2004; Sommer & West, 1996). Based on national survey data compiled by WHO from each region, an estimated 190 million preschool-aged children and 19.1 million pregnant women are living with vitamin A deficiency in lower-income countries, as defined by a plasma retinol concentration less than 0.70 µmol/L (20 µg/dL) (WHO, 2009a). Approximately one-third of the global pediatric burden of this deficiency is in India. Roughly 5.2 million of the preschool-aged children and 9.8 million of the pregnant women with vitamin A deficiency have night blindness, an ocular manifestation of xerophthalmia (WHO, 2009a). The latest WHO global map of vitamin A deficiency, based on hyporetinolemia (serum retinol < 0.70 µmol/L), shows that vitamin A deficiency remains a major public health problem across southern Asia and sub-Saharan Africa and, at a less severe level, in the Western Pacific, Central and South American, and Caribbean regions (Figure 6-13). While the annual number of new cases of potentially blinding corneal xerophthalmia is suspected to be lower than the half-million estimated by Sommer and colleagues in the early 1980s (Sommer, Tarwotjo, Hussaini, Susanto, & Soegiharto, 1981), there are no recent, reliable population cohort data that can be used as a basis to change this estimate.

More sparse are prevalence data for older children and adolescents. For example, based on a limited number of reports, approximately 23% of children 5

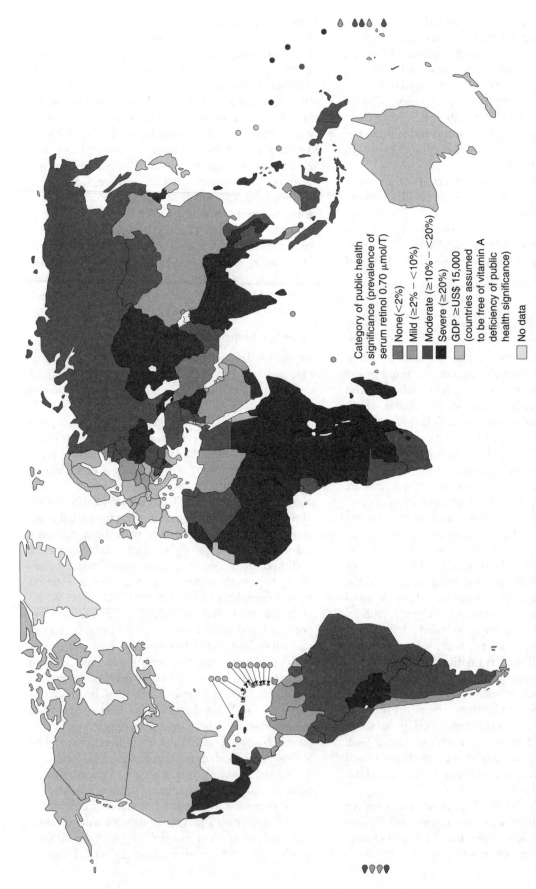

Figure 6-13A Countries categorized by the public health significance of the prevalence of vitamin A deficiency (Panel A), anemia (Panel B), iodine (Panel C), and zinc (Panel D) in children. Categories of vitamin A deficiency is based on the prevalence of low serum retinol in preschool children (≤0.70 μmol/L); *Source:* WHO, 2009. Anemia prevalence is based on low hemoglobin (<110 g/L) in preschool children; *Source:* WHO, 2008. Iodine deficiency is based on median urinary iodine concentration in school aged children; *Source:* de Benoist et al, 2008. The risk of zinc deficiency is based on the joint distribution of stunting and the adequacy of absorbable zinc in the food supply; *Source:* Black et al, 2008. *Source:* WHO (2009a). Global prevalence of vitamin A deficiency in populations at risk 1995–2005. WHO Global Database on Vitamin A Deficiency. Geneva, Switzerland: World Health Organization, page 13, Figure 2b (Biochemical vitamin A deficiency (retinol). B) countries and areas with survey data and regression-based estimates).

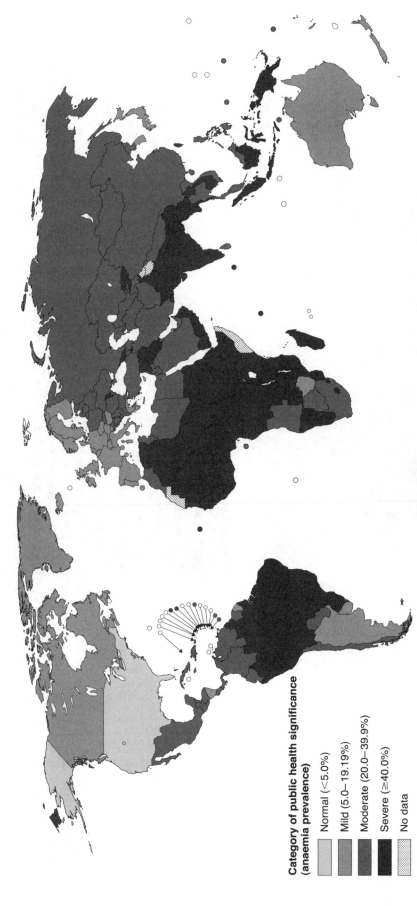

Figure 6-13B Countries categorized by the public health significance of the prevalence of vitamin A deficiency (Panel A), anemia (Panel B), iodine (Panel C), and zinc (Panel D) in children. Categories of vitamin A deficiency is based on the prevalence of low serum retinol in preschool children (≤0.70 µmol/L); *Source:* WHO, 2009. Anemia prevalence is based on low hemoglobin (<110 g/L) in preschool children; *Source:* WHO, 2008. Iodine deficiency is based on median urinary iodine concentration in school aged children; *Source:* de Benoist et al, 2008. The risk of zinc deficiency is based on the joint distribution of stunting and the adequacy of absorbable zinc in the food supply; *Source:* Black et al, 2008. *Source:* WHO (2008b). Worldwide prevalence of anaemia 1993–2005, WHO Global Database on Anaemia. Geneva, Switzerland: World Health Organization, pg 9, figure 3-1a (Anaemia as a public health problem by country: preschool-age children).

Category of public health significance (anaemia prevalence)

- Normal (<5.0%)
- Mild (5.0—19.19%)
- Moderate (20.0—39.9%)
- Severe (≥40.0%)
- No data

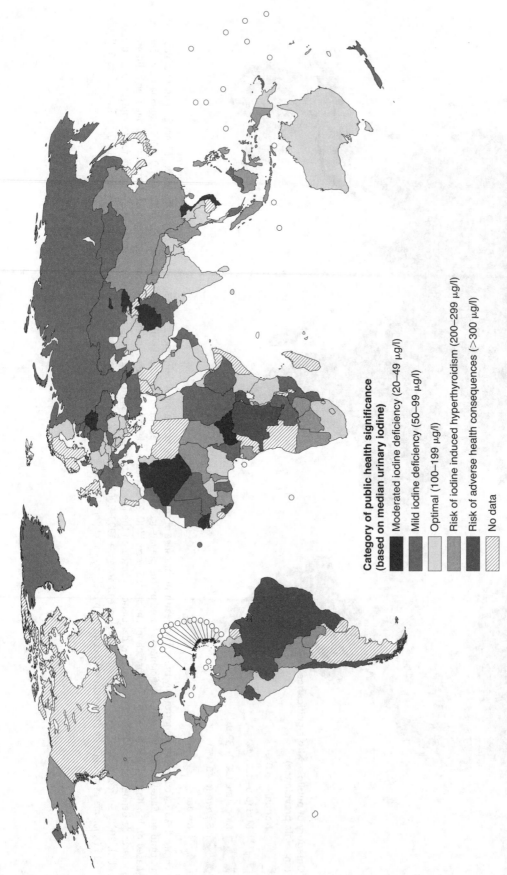

Figure 6-13C Countries categorized by the public health significance of the prevalence of vitamin A deficiency (Panel A), anemia (Panel B), iodine (Panel C), and zinc (Panel D) in children. Categories of vitamin A deficiency is based on the prevalence of low serum retinol in preschool children (≤0.70 µmol/L); *Source:* WHO, 2009. Anemia prevalence is based on low hemoglobin (<110 g/L) in preschool children; *Source:* WHO, 2008. Iodine deficiency is based on median urinary iodine concentration in school aged children; *Source:* de Benoist et al, 2008. The risk of zinc deficiency is based on the joint distribution of stunting and the adequacy of absorbable zinc in the food supply; *Source:* Black et al, 2008. *Source:* de Benoist, B., McLean, E., Andersson, M., & Rogers, L. (2008). Iodine deficiency in 2007: Global progress since 2003. Food and Nutrition Bulletin, 29, 195–202.

**Category of public health significance
(based on median urinary iodine)**

Moderated iodine deficiency (20–49 µg/l)

Mild iodine deficiency (50–99 µg/l)

Optimal (100–199 µg/l)

Risk of iodine induced hyperthyroidism (200–299 µg/l)

Risk of adverse health consequences (>300 µg/l)

No data

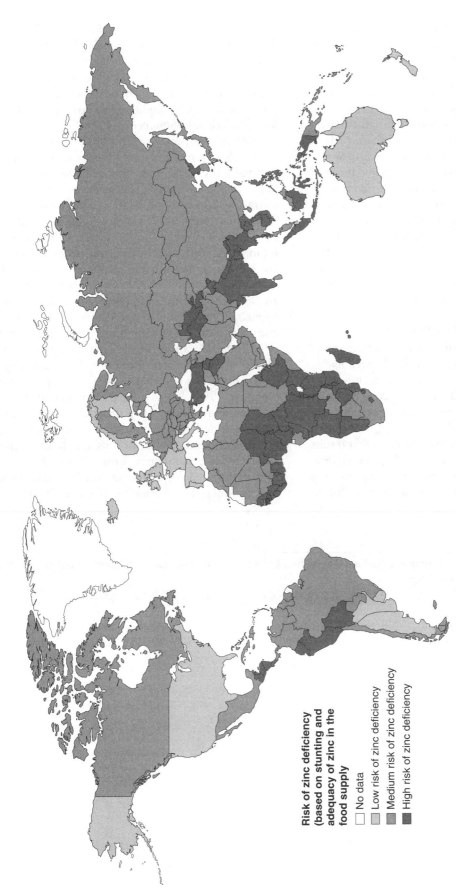

Figure 6-13D Countries categorized by the public health significance of the prevalence of vitamin A deficiency (Panel A), anemia (Panel B), iodine (Panel C), and zinc (Panel D) in children. Categories of vitamin A deficiency is based on the prevalence of low serum retinol in preschool children (≤0.70 µmol/L); *Source:* WHO, 2009. Anemia prevalence is based on low hemoglobin (<110 g/L) in preschool children; *Source:* WHO, 2008. Iodine deficiency is based on median urinary iodine concentration in school aged children; *Source:* de Benoist et al, 2008. The risk of zinc deficiency is based on the joint distribution of stunting and the adequacy of absorbable zinc in the food supply; *Source:* Black et al, 2008. *Source:* Black et al, 2008. "Maternal and child undernutrition: global and regional exposures and health consequences." *The Lancet* 371–9608.

Risk of zinc deficiency (based on stunting and adequacy of zinc in the food supply)

☐ No data

Low risk of zinc deficiency

Medium risk of zinc deficiency

High risk of zinc deficiency

to 15 years of age in South-East Asia (83 million children) are estimated to be vitamin A deficient, based on a plasma retinol concentration below 0.70 μmol/L, among whom 11% (2.6% of all children in the region) have mild xerophthalmia (Singh & West, 2004). Corneal xerophthalmia appears to be virtually absent at this age. Limited reports suggest that the magnitude of adolescent deficiency in sub-Saharan Africa can be expected to be at least as prevalent as in South-East Asia. Surveys in undernourished populations of South Asia, rural Africa, and Latin America typically report 10% to 20% of women experiencing night blindness during pregnancy (Christian et al., 1998a; Kamal, Ahsan, & Salam, 1998; Katz et al., 1995; Pradhan, Aryal, Regmi, Ban, & Govindasamy, 1997; West, 2002); this condition is attributed largely to vitamin A deficiency (Christian et al., 1998b; Dixit, 1966; Mandal, Nanda, & Bose, 1969).

Function, Requirements, and Assessment

Vitamin A is an essential nutrient that participates in the visual cycle and, at the genomic level, in regulating cell proliferation and differentiation (Blomhoff & Blomhoff, 2006). Normally, rod and cone photoreceptor cells in the retina of the eye produce photosensitive pigments that respond to light, triggering neural impulses along the optic nerve to the brain that results in vision. Rhodopsin ("visual purple") is the vitamin A–dependent photosensitive pigment that accumulates in rod cells, enabling vision under conditions of low illumination (scotopic vision) (Wald, 1955). Vitamin A deficiency leads to decreased availability of retinaldehyde (retinal) and decreased production of rhodopsin, raising the minimum threshold of light required to see in the dark. This impairment of rod function leads to "night blindness," a condition that is recognized by affected individuals (Sommer & West, 1996).

Other, more pervasive functions of vitamin A draw on its role in gene regulation, most readily detectable in rapidly dividing, bipotential cells. Within the nucleus, vitamin A metabolic intermediates (retinoic acids) interact with receptor proteins, which in turn influence gene transcription by activating or inhibiting response elements of nearby target genes (Blomhoff & Blomhoff, 2006), thereby directing protein synthesis and cell differentiation and proliferation. Thus adequate vitamin A nutriture helps to maintain, for example, the function and stability of mucus-secreting, epithelial, immunologic, and osteogenic cells in the body. Deficiency of vitamin A can change the types of cells produced, causing keratinizing metaplasia of epithelial surfaces, evident by xerotic (drying) changes on ocular surfaces that lead to xerophthalmia (Sommer, 1995). These cellular changes may disrupt the "barrier function" of epithelial surfaces. Further, vitamin A deficiency can alter the expression and function of immune effector cells and diminish their ability to clear pathogens (Ross, 1996). Over time, these pathophysiologic processes can lead to impaired host resistance to infection (Stephensen, 2001).

Table 6-5	WHO Classification and Minimum Prevalence Criteria for Xerophthalmia and Vitamin A Deficiency as a Public Health Program	
Definition (Code)	**Minimum Prevalence (%)**	**Highest-Risk Groups**
Night blindness (XN)		
Children 2 to 5 years of age	1.0%	Entire age group
Women during recent pregnancy	5.0%	Women with previous episode of XN
Conjunctival xerosis (X1A)	—	
Bitot's spots (X1B)	0.5%	
Corneal xerosis (X2)		
Corneal ulceration keratomalacia (X3)	0.01%	Children 1 to 3 years of age
Xerophthalmic corneal scar (XS)	0.05%	Cumulative over more than 1 year
Serum retinol <0.70 mol L	15.0%	
Abnormal CIC/RDR/MRDR	20.0%*	

*Provisional cut-offs above which community interventions may be warranted.

Notes: CIC = conjunctival impression cytology; RDR = relative dose response; MRDR = modified RDR.

Source: A. Sommer and F. R. Davidson, "Assessment and Control of Vitamin A Deficiency: The Annecy Accords," 2002, Journal of Nutrition, 132, pp. 2845S–2850S. Reprinted with permission.

Vitamin A status is commonly assessed by clinical, biochemical, and functional indicators. Assessment and staging of xerophthalmic eye signs, following a widely accepted WHO classification system (Table 6-5; Sommer, 1995), provide standardized criteria for evaluating the extent of moderate to severe deficiency, screening individuals for treatment, and, because xerophthalmia occurs in clusters (Katz, Zeger, & Tielsch, 1988; Katz, Zeger, West, Tielsch, & Sommer, 1993), identifying communities at risk. Biochemical and functional indicators, in the absence of clinical signs, are best applied toward estimating levels of deficiency in groups of individuals.

Serum (plasma) retinol is the most commonly measured biochemical indicator of vitamin A status. Although homeostatically controlled within a broad range of nutritional adequacy, plasma retinol concentration falls progressively with liver and total body vitamin A depletion (Olson, 1992; Underwood, 1990). Plasma retinol can also decline in response to inflammation—for example, due to infection. This relationship requires that nutritional and disease contexts be considered when interpreting plasma retinol distributions in populations (Thurnham, McCabe, Northrop-Clewes, & Nestel, 2003). Serum retinol eluted from a filter paper blood spot has shown promise as a practical and inexpensive field approach to population assessment (Craft et al., 2000). Serum retinol response tests following receipt of a standard, small oral dose of vitamin A are based on retinol kinetics (relative dose response [RDR] and modified RDR) that allow relative liver adequacy of vitamin A to be estimated (Flores, Campos, Araujo, & Underwood, 1984; Loerch, Underwood, & Lewis, 1979; Tanumihardjo et al., 1990).

Other functional, preclinical measures for evaluating community vitamin A status include retinol concentration in human milk (Stoltzfus & Underwood, 1995), conjunctival impression cytology (Natadisastra et al., 1988; Stoltzfus, Miller, Hakimi, & Rasmussen,

Table 6-6	Recommended Dietary Allowances (RDA) for Selected Micronutrients				
			Zinc (mg/day)		
			With a Mixed or Refined Vegetarian Diet	With an Unrefined Cereal-Based Diet	
	Vitamin A (μg/day)[2]	Iron (mg/day)			Iodine (μg/day)
Infants					
0–6 months	400	0.27	4	5	110
7–12 months	500	11	4	5	130
Children					
1–3 years	300	7	3	3	90
4–8 years	400	10	4	5	90
Boys					
9–13 years	600	8	6	9	120
14–18 years	900	11	10	14	150
Girls					
9–13 years	600	8	6	9	120
14–18 years	700	15	9	11	150
Men					
19–70 years	900	8	13	19	150
Women					
19–70 years	700	18[3]	8	9	150
Pregnant	770	27	10	13	220
Lactating	1300	9	9	10	290

1. RDA values adapted from Institute of Medicine (2006) for all nutrients except zinc, for which modified estimates judged to be more appropriate for dietary conditions in lower-income countries have been obtained from the International Zinc Nutrition Consultative Group (IZiNCG) (Hotz & Brown, 2004).

2. Expressed as Retinol Activity Equivalents that allow for a dietary carotenoid-to-vitamin A conversion ratio of 12:1 for beta-carotene and 24:1 for other provitamin A carotenoids.

3. Value for perimenopausal women; RDA decreases to 8 mg/day for women older than 50 years of age.

1993; Wittpenn, Tseng, & Sommer, 1986) and dark adaptometry (Congdon & West, 2002). Cutoffs established by WHO, the International Vitamin A Consultative Group (IVACG), and other provisional cutoffs for evaluating community risk by various means are shown in Table 6-5 (Congdon & West, 2002; Sommer & Davidson, 2002; WHO, 1996a).

It is becoming increasingly important to characterize and compare adequacy of vitamin A intake distributions in populations so as to develop evidence-based food-oriented strategies, for which the Dietary Reference Intakes can serve as a reference. The Recommended Dietary Allowance (RDA) for vitamin A, expressed as retinol activity equivalents, is 300 to 600 μg/day for children up to 13 years of age, and 700 to 900 μg/day thereafter for both sexes, including women during pregnancy (Table 6-6). The RDA increases substantially (to 1,300 μg/day) during lactation (IOM, 2006).

Health Consequences

Consequences of vitamin A deficiency that are of public health importance in low-income countries relate to increased risks of xerophthalmia and its blinding sequelae, infectious morbidity and mortality, and, to some extent, poor growth.

Xerophthalmia. Active stages of xerophthalmia, due to vitamin A deficiency, include night blindness, conjunctival xerosis (dryness), usually with Bitot's spots, corneal xerosis, ulceration, and necrosis ("keratomalacia" or softening of the cornea). Corneal lesions may heal to form a scar (leukoma), become

phthisic (shrunken globe), or form a staphyloma (bulging eye) (Sommer, 1995). Noncorneal xerophthalmia indicates mild eye disease but moderate to severe deficiency, revealed by a low serum retinol concentration and increased risks of morbidity and mortality (Sommer & West, 1996). Corneal involvement is a medical emergency, as it is potentially blinding and associated with a case fatality rate of 5% to 25% (Sommer, 1982).

WHO has classified stages of xerophthalmia and provided prevalence estimates as minimum criteria for defining vitamin A deficiency as a public health problem (Table 6-5). The vitamin A treatment schedule for xerophthalmia is well standardized (Table 6-7) (Sommer, 1995; WHO, UNICEF, & IVACG, 1997).

Morbidity and Mortality. A dose-responsive, strong and consistent association has been shown to exist between clinical vitamin A deficiency—represented by mild xerophthalmic eye signs—and short-term risk of child mortality (Sommer, Hussaini, Tarwotjo, & Susanto, 1983; Sommer & West, 1996). The causality of this association has been borne out by eight community intervention trials, enrolling more than 165,000 children, conducted in South and Southeast Asia and Africa (Figure 6-14). These findings show reductions of 23% to 34% in preschool-child mortality following vitamin A prophylaxis by direct supplementation or routine consumption of vitamin A–fortified food (Beaton et al., 1993; Bishai et al., 2005; Fawzi, Chalmers, Herrera, & Mosteller, 1993; Glasziou & Mackerras, 1993; Tonascia, 1993).

Table 6-7	Vitamin A Treatment and Prevention Schedules			
			Prevention	
Age	**Treatment at Diagnosis*** **(Dosage)**	**Dosage**	**Frequency**	
Younger than 6 months				
Shortly after birth	50,000 IU	50,000 IU	Once[‡]	
Postneonatally	50,000 IU	50,000 IU	6, 10, and 14 weeks of age	
6–12 months	100,000 IU	100,000 IU	Every 4–6 months	
1 year or older	200,000 IU	200,000 IU	Every 46 months	
Women	200,000 IU[†]	400,000 IU	Less than 6 weeks after delivery	

*Treat all cases of xerophthalmia and measles with the same age-specific dosage on the next day and again 1 to 4 weeks later.

[†]For women of reproductive age, give 200,000 IU only for corneal xerophthalmia; for milder eye signs (night blindness or Bitot's spots), give women 5,000 to 10,000 IU per day or up to 25,000 IU per week for 4 weeks or longer.

[‡]Provisional recommendation for non-HIV areas, based on recent trials from Indonesia (Humphrey et al., 1996), India (Rahmathullah et al., 2003), and Bangladesh (Klemm et al., 2008) showing the potential for this regimen to reduce infant mortality in southern Asia. Definitive studies of newborn vitamin A supplementation are currently under way in Africa.

Source: A. Sommer and F. R. Davidson, "Assessment and Control of Vitamin A Deficiency: The Annecy Accords," 2002, Journal of Nutrition, 132, pp. 2845S–2850S. Reprinted with permission.

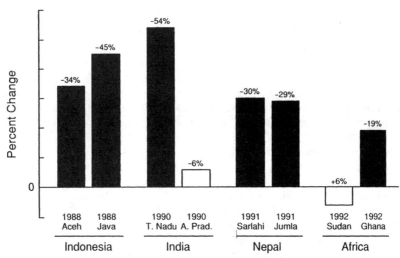

Figure 6-14 Summary of Percent Change in Mortality of Children (~>=6 mo to 72 mo) Receiving Vitamin A versus No Vitamin A (controls) in Eight Field Intervention Trials. Black bars represent statistically significant reductions, white bars nonsignificant change. Total N (across trials) >165,000 children. Meta-analyses show overall 23% to 34% reductions in mortality with vitamin A.
Source: A. Sommer and K. P. West, Jr., Vitamin Deficiency: Health, Survival, and Vision (New York: Oxford University Press, 1996), Figure 2.5, p. 30. Reprinted with permission of Oxford University Press, Inc.

Embedded in this impact on all-cause death are likely to be strong effects of vitamin A supplementation in reducing the severity and case fatality of measles, as seen in both community (Rahmathullah et al., 1990; West et al., 1991) and hospital-based clinical trials (Barclay et al., 1987; Coutsoudis et al., 1992; Ellison, 1932; Hussey & Klein, 1990), diarrhea and dysentery (Arthur et al., 1992; Banajeh, 2003), and *Plasmodium falciparum* malaria (Shankar, Genton, Semba, et al., 1999). While vitamin A programs have made substantial progress, an estimated 650,000 preschool-aged children continue to die each year from measles, malaria, diarrhea, and other infections that could be averted by preventing underlying vitamin A deficiency (Rice, West, & Black, 2004). This number is down from the estimated 1.9 million deaths occurring from these causes 20 years ago (Humphrey, West, & Sommer, 1992)—a decline plausibly attributed, in large measure, to a sustained increase in global vitamin A program activity (Exhibit 6-4).

Newborn supplementation with 50,000 IU within days following birth represents a new potential child survival approach. So far, three randomized trials in Southern Asia—one in Indonesia (Humphrey et al.,

1997) , one in Southern India (Rahmathullah et al., 2003) and one in Bangladesh (Klemm et al., 2008)—have reported reductions of 64%, 23% and 15%, respectively, in mortality by 6 months of age among infants following large-dose vitamin A receipt compared to placebo controls. The Indian site represents an area of South Asia where early infantile keratomalacia has been reported (Rahmathullah & Chanravathi, 1997). Plausible, responsive infectious diseases that may be attenuated by newborn vitamin A supplementation include pneumonia, reflected by indications of delayed pneumococcal colonization of the respiratory tract (Coles et al., 2001), and diarrheal disease (Tielsch & Rahmathullah et al., 2007).

In Harare, Zimbabwe, a large trial failed to find an infant survival benefit from either newborn or postpartum maternal vitamin A supplementation among infants of either HIV-positive or -negative mothers. Notwithstanding the high burden of HIV infection among mothers and infants, this population was otherwise adequately vitamin A nourished (Malaba et al., 2005), suggesting that the presence of vitamin A deficiency and other malnutrition and illness risk differences could explain differences in effects

| Exhibit 6-4 | The Vitamin A "Campaign" Trail |

Field research has shown that vitamin A supplementation can reduce preschool-child mortality by 25% to 35% and can virtually eliminate nutritional blindness in many low- and middle-income countries (Sommer & West, 1996). In recent years, high-potency vitamin A delivery has been redesigned as a semiannual national campaign, with widely advocated, highly organized distribution days set 6 months apart. On 2 days each year, government, communities, and local, national, and international agencies focus on distributing a $0.02 vitamin A capsule (VAC) to children. Integration of VAC distribution into the WHO Expanded Programme for Immunization or National Immunization Days (NIDs) during the late 1990s and first years of the twenty-first century (WHO, 1998) provided an ideal opportunity for delivery of this supplementation and as a means to raise community awareness and demand for this service.

Since 2002, as NIDs has undergone its planned phase-out, demand and program momentum have motivated governments and service agencies to set up new semiannual mechanisms through which to sustain VAC distribution such as "Operation Timbang," a national child-weighing day program in the Philippines (Klemm et al., 1997); "National Vitamin A Week" in Bangladesh, where VACs have been distributed since 1973 (Helen Keller International, 1998); and various forms of National Child Health or Vitamin A Days or Weeks in several countries throughout Africa, southern Asia, and Latin America. In the latter regions, VAC delivery has been combined with other services such as immunizations, deworming, oral rehydration solution distribution, and health education to create a semiannual community-based health event (Mora, Bonilla, Navas, & Largaespada, 2004).

In mountainous Nepal, a "model" national program was launched in 1993, with the support of USAID and UNICEF, that was organized around community mobilization from its outset. As of 2004, all 75 districts of the country had achieved semiannual coverage of approximately 90% among more than 2.5 million children through the efforts of approximately 25,000 local female community health volunteers. Recent program evaluations, combining coverage estimates with data from periodic Demographic Health Surveys, reflect a reduction in child mortality that is consistent with the declines observed by two previous randomized trials in the country (Shrestha et al., 2004).

Knowledge that vitamin A saves lives, coupled with a reinvigorated campaign approach to VAC delivery, has led vitamin A delivery to be considered an essential component of child survival strategies.

---

of newborn vitamin A observed to date between South Asian and sub-Saharan African populations.

Finally, maternal vitamin A deficiency may be a cause of pregnancy-related morbidity and mortality in high-mortality, vitamin A–deficient settings. A trial in the southern plains of Nepal reported maternal night blindness to be associated with increased risks of infectious and reproductive morbidity, general malnutrition (Christian et al., 1998b), and prolonged mortality risk for as long as 2 years following pregnancy (Christian et al., 2000). In this rural South Asian setting, routine, low-dose vitamin A or beta-carotene supplementation of women reduced mortality related to pregnancy by roughly 40% (West et al., 1999), with plausible pathways affected being those related to infections, obstetric hemorrhage, hypertensive illness, and anemia (Faisal & Pittrof, 2000). There was no overall effect on early infant death (Katz et al., 2000), although infant mortality was approximately 25% lower among women prone to night blindness given vitamin A (Christian et al., 2001). Follow-up of the surviving offspring 9 to 13 years later revealed improved lung function in those born to mothers given vitamin A compared to children of mothers who had received placebo (Checkley et al., 2010).

This influence of vitamin A is likely to depend on many nutritional, disease, and healthcare exposures. For example, the same weekly vitamin A or beta-carotene supplement dosages, but begun in the first trimester among better-nourished pregnant women, in a population of mothers in rural Bangladesh with markedly lower mortality risk, had no effect on maternal or infant mortality (Christian et al., 2007). Similarly, in Ghana, continuous weekly vitamin A supplementation had no effect in a population with moderately high maternal mortality (albeit a lower rate than that in Nepal), but little clinically evident vitamin A deficiency, evident by a virtual absence of night blindness (Kirkwood et al., 2010).

Poor Growth. Vitamin A is required for mammalian growth. The discovery of vitamin A early in the twentieth century was prompted by observations that young animals deprived of an ether-soluble fraction in egg yolk and milk ("fat-soluble factor A") failed to gain weight and eventually died (McCollum & Davis, 1915). Preschool-aged children, who wax and wane in vitamin A nutriture, decelerate in linear growth as they enter a mildly xerophthalmic state, only to recover height growth more slowly relative to weight as apparent vitamin A intake improves

(Tarwotjo, Katz, West, Tielsch, & Sommer, 1992). Thus different rates of recovery by aspect of growth might explain, in part, a rather consistent association between mild xerophthalmia and stunting (Khatry et al., 1995; Mele et al., 1991; Sommer & West, 1996). However, growth responses to population-based vitamin A supplementation have been mixed, with many studies finding no such effect (Fawzi et al., 1997; Kirkwood et al., 1996; Lie, Ying, En-Lin, Brun, & Geissler, 1993; Rahmathullah, Underwood, Thulasiraj, & Milton, 1991; Ramakrishnan, Latham, & Abel, 1995). Others have reported improved weight without height gain (Bahl, Bhandari, Taneja, & Bhan, 1997; West et al., 1988), height without weight gain (Humphrey et al., 1998; Muhilal, Permeisih, Idjradinata, Muherdiyantiningsih, & Karyadi, 1988), or acceleration in both aspects in high-risk subgroups (Donnen et al., 1998; Hadi et al., 2000; West et al., 1997). The presence of infection may also blunt a potential growth response (Hadi et al., 1999), which could explain observed seasonal differences in growth response to vitamin A (Hadi, Dibley, & West, 2004). On balance, it appears that aspects of growth may improve with vitamin A supplementation among children for whom, or during seasons when, vitamin A deficiency is moderate to severe and, therefore, "growth limiting" among competing nutrition and disease factors.

Prevention

Prevention of vitamin A deficiency should be guided by epidemiologic insight. For example, mild xerophthalmia has been observed to cluster by region (Cohen et al., 1987), community (Katz et al., 1988; Mele et al., 1991; Sommer, 1982), and household, where siblings of cases have been reported to be 7 to 13 times more likely to also have or develop xerophthalmia (Katz et al., 1993) and twice as likely to die (Khatry et al., 1995) than children living in homes with no history of xerophthalmia. The clustering of deficiency was observed intergenerationally in Cambodia, whereby mothers or preschool-age children were 4 to 9 times more likely to have xerophthalmia if the other had this disease (Semba, de Pee, Panagides, Poly, & Bloem, 2004). Vitamin A deficiency also often exhibits seasonality (Sinha & Bang, 1973). Knowledge of spatial, temporal, and generational patterns of clustering can help target high-risk groups and seasons for programs.

Three broad strategies exist to prevent vitamin A deficiency: direct supplementation with high-potency vitamin A, food fortification, and a wide range of dietary approaches to increase vitamin A intake. In addition, measures taken to prevent and control infection, which depletes vitamin A stores through increased use and excretion in the body (Campos, Flores, & Underwood, 1987; Mitra, Alvarez, & Stephensen, 1998), may conserve vitamin A in the body and, therefore, be viewed as an indirect way to prevent vitamin A deficiency.

High-potency vitamin A supplementation is the most common, direct strategy used to increase vitamin A intake and status. Typically, a large oral dose of vitamin A (see Table 6-7) is delivered either as a gelatinous capsule or in oily syrup to preschool-aged children on a periodic basis, providing a theoretically sufficient supply of this nutrient for a 4- to 6-month period (Bloem et al., 1995). The resulting improvement in serum retinol concentrations may vary, ranging from a few weeks to a few months, although prophylactic efficacy against xerophthalmia and child mortality can last for 6 to 12 months (Banajeh, 2003; Sommer & West, 1996).

Vitamin A can be delivered as a community-based intervention (Bloem et al., 1995), or through clinic-based treatment and prevention programs (West & Sommer, 1987). Since the early 1990s, sustained donor support has enabled the scale-up of vitamin A supplementation programs (see Exhibit 6-4). In particular, the Canadian International Development Agency (CIDA) donated approximately 4 billion vitamin A capsules to UNICEF over the course of a decade (UNICEF, 2007). Current, revised recommendations are to provide a 400,000 IU oral dose of vitamin A to women within 6 weeks after they give birth as a means to improve maternal and, via breastfeeding, infant stores of this nutrient (Table 6-7). Although effective in improving short-term vitamin A status of women and their breastfed infants, other sustained, dietary or supplementary approaches are probably also required to sustain adequate maternal and infant vitamin A status (Rice et al., 1999; Stoltzfus et al., 1993).

Fortification is assuming increasing importance as a means to improve routine intake of vitamin A. Many food "vehicles" can be technically fortified with vitamin A, in that the nutrient can be added in efficacious amounts without affecting organoleptic qualities, under ambient conditions of production and consumer use. Ideally, successful commercial food items would be produced or processed centrally in a limited number of units (to maintain quality control), have wide market penetration in high-risk areas, be consumed by target groups within a relatively narrow band of intake (to set effective and safe nutrient levels), and be produced and packaged to maintain adequate shelf life at low cost, while upholding standards set by government regulatory bodies.

To date, a few products fortified with vitamin A have been shown to be effective in improving and maintaining adequate vitamin A status in high-risk populations. Most successful has been the fortification of sugar in Guatemala and elsewhere in Central and South America, where population vitamin A status has been effectively improved over the past 2½ decades (Arroyave, Mejia, & Aguilar, 1981; Dary, 1994; Krause, Delisle, & Solomons, 1998). Monosodium glutamate fortification with vitamin A was shown to improve status and reduce child mortality in South-East Asia (Muhilal et al., 1988; Solon, Fernandez, Latham, & Popkin, 1979; Sommer & West, 1996), but organoleptic changes hindered its further use (Solon et al., 1985). Other successfully tested products include nonrefrigerated margarine (Solon et al., 1996) and centrally processed, mill-rolled wheat flour (Klemm et al., 2010), which in the Philippines has been shown to be effective in raising apparent vitamin A stores of children (Solon et al., 2000). A variety of long-standing food aid commodities such as dried skim milk powder, vegetable oil, and cereal grain flours can be fortified with vitamin A as well.

Improved intake of vitamin A through other food-based means inevitably leads to a diversified diet and increased intakes of many micronutrients (Combs, Welch, Duxbury, Uphoff, & Nesheim, 1996). Highly bioavailable, preformed vitamin A is found in liver, fish liver oil, cheese, milk, and other full-fat dairy products. Unfortunately, such foods typically account for only 10% to 15% of all food sources of vitamin A in low-income settings. Provitamin A carotenoids (for example, beta-carotene) derived from deeply colored yellow and orange fruits and vegetables, and dark green leaves, historically have been viewed as contributing more than 85% of all food-based vitamin A consumed in low- and middle-income countries (FAO, 1988). While apparently effective in preventing moderate to severe vitamin A deficiency (Sommer & West, 1996), the efficiency of bioconversion of plant-based carotenoids to retinol has been deemed to be at best half that previously calculated (i.e., from a beta-carotene:retinol conversion ratio by weight of 6:1 to 12:1) (IOM, 2006), particularly from dark green leaves (West, Eilander, & van Leishout, 2002). The new dietary conversion data suggest that poor, undernourished societies may not be able to optimize their vitamin A status while subsisting on a strictly vegetarian diet (de Pee, Bloem, Gorstein, et al., 1998; de Pee et al.,

1999; de Pee, West, Muhilal, Karyadi, & Hautvast, 1995).

Children with xerophthalmia tend to be breast-fed less frequently, weaned from the breast at an earlier age, and given foods high in vitamin A content less often than clinically normal children (Mahalanabis, 1991; Mele et al., 1991; Sommer & West, 1996; Tarwotjo, Sommer, & Soegiharto, 1982; West et al., 1986). Thus infant and child feeding approaches should encourage continued breastfeeding into the third year of life, while nutritious complementary foods such as egg, ripe mango and papaya, cooked carrot, and dark green leaves are introduced at appropriate times (de Pee, Bloem, Satoto, et al.,1998; Kuhnlein, 1992; Seshadri, 1996; Tarwotjo et al., 1982). The people with whom children eat their meals may also affect the quality of their diet. In Nepal, young children sharing a meal plate with other children and adults were more likely to eat a nutritious variety of foods at mealtime than children eating alone, particularly if the person with whom a plate was shared was an adult female (Shankar et al., 1998).

Social marketing programs have been effective in increasing household purchases and intakes of vitamin A food sources such as dark green leaves (Smitasiri, Attig, & Dhanamitta, 1992) and egg (de Pee, Bloem, Satoto, et al., 1998). Home gardening, where commonly practiced, provides an excellent means to increase the variety of provitamin A carotenoid-rich foods (Talukder, Islam, Klemm, & Bloem, 1993). Although the effects of homestead gardening on vitamin A status remain inconclusive, other food security, nutritional, and economic benefits can accrue from such programs (Marsh, 1998).

Iron Deficiency and Anemia

Iron is essential in the body for oxygen transport and cellular respiration—functions that are especially critical in red cells, brain, and muscle (Beard, 2001). Iron deficiency is considered the most common micronutrient deficiency in the world; anemia, characterized by abnormally low blood hemoglobin concentration, is its major clinical manifestation. Although anemia is not specific to iron deficiency, the two conditions are closely linked in most malnourished populations, making anemia the most frequently reported clinical index of iron deficiency in low-income countries (Yip, 1994).

An estimated 1.3 to 2 billion women, children, and men in the world are anemic (DeMaeyer & Adiels-Tegman, 1985; Stoltzfus, Mullany, & Black, 2004; WHO, 1992a). Approximately half of the global burden of anemia appears to be due solely to

Table 6-8	Prevalence of Anemia by Life Stage and Geographic Region of the World, 1993–2005					
WHO Region	**Preschool-Aged Children[1]**		**Pregnant Women**		**Nonpregnant Women**	
	Prevalence %	**Number Affected (millions)**	**Prevalence %**	**Number Affected (millions)**	**Prevalence %**	**Number Affected (millions)**
Africa	67.6	83.5	57.1	17.2	47.5	69.9
Americas	29.3	23.1	24.1	3.9	17.8	39.0
Southeast Asia	65.5	115.3	48.2	18.1	45.7	182.0
Europe	21.7	11.1	25.1	2.6	19.0	40.8
Eastern Mediterranean	46.7	0.8	44.2	7.1	32.4	39.8
Western Pacific	23.1	27.4	30.7	7.6	21.5	97.0
Global	47.4	293.1	41.8	56.4	30.2	468.4

1. Preschool-aged children (0–5 years), pregnant women (no age defined), and nonpregnant women (15–50 years).
Source: WHO, 2008b.

iron deficiency. At the same time, depletion of body iron stores with or without impaired red cell production is likely to be twice as prevalent as anemia (Cook, Finch, & Smith, 1976; Yip, 1994), leading to roughly similar global estimates of the prevalence of anemia (from all causes) and iron deficiency. The term *nutritional anemia* includes the anemia burden due to deficiency in iron plus other vitamins, particularly folate, vitamin B_{12} (Fishman, Christian, & West, 2000), and vitamin A (Sommer & West, 1996), and trace elements that participate in erythropoiesis (WHO, 1992a). Major "non-nutritional" causes of red cell mass loss or destruction and consequent anemia include hookworm (Albonico et al., 1998; Brooker et al., 1999; Hopkins et al., 1997; Stoltzfus et al., 1997; Stoltzfus et al., 1998) and malarial (Beales, 1997) infections, respectively, both of which occur in large areas of low-income countries. HIV/AIDS has also emerged as an important cause of anemia in sub-Saharan Africa (Vetter et al., 1996).

Pregnant women, infants, and young children are at highest risk of iron-deficiency anemia. Based on population surveys conducted between 1993 through 2005, roughly 1.6 billion people are estimated to be anemic, representing nearly one-fourth of the global population (Table 6-8), based on conventional hemoglobin concentration cutoffs (WHO, 2008b). On average, an even higher percentage of preschool-aged children are anemic due to iron deficiency; this condition affects 47% of such children, or an estimated 293 million worldwide. Africa and Southeast Asia share a roughly equal prevalence of anemia, and presumably iron deficiency: An estimated 65% to 68% of young children and 50% to

57% of pregnant women in those regions have anemia (see Figure 6-13). However, the largest number of people with anemia live in Southeast Asia, where 115 million children, 18 million pregnant women, and 182 million nonpregnant women are estimated to suffer from anemia. Moderate and severe maternal anemia, typically defined at hemoglobin cutoffs of less than 90 g/L or less than 100 g/L, respectively, can be expected to affect far fewer women, but its presence may differentiate, with greater clarity, populations lying along an anemia-health risk continuum (Stoltzfus, 1997). Severe anemia (hemoglobin cutoffs ranging from less than 50 g/L to less than 70 g/L) generally occurs in less than 5% of women in high-risk populations (Sharmanov, 1998; Stoltzfus, 1997).

Function, Requirements, and Assessment

In the body, iron is found in metabolically active "functional" and "storage" pools, accounting for approximately 75% and 25% of total body iron, respectively (Lynch, 1999). Approximately 80% of functional iron complexes with hemoglobin during erythropoiesis, where it plays a central role in oxygen transport to cells. Ten percent of this metabolic iron pool is incorporated into intracellular myoglobin, where oxygen is stored for use during muscle respiration and contraction. In addition, iron serves as a cofactor in more than 200 heme and nonheme enzymes involved in cellular respiration, division, neurotransmission, immunity and growth (Beard, 2001; Dallman, 1986; Ryan, 1997; Viteri, 1998). These ubiquitous functions highlight the importance of adequate iron nutriture in achieving health benchmarks as diverse as normal physical performance, pregnancy, and motor and cognitive function (Ryan, 1997; Viteri, 1998).

Metabolic and functional pathways of iron in the body provide the basis for the indicators used to assess iron status. The total body iron balance is largely regulated at the point of absorption. Approximately 12% to 25% of dietary heme iron (e.g., from red meat) is taken up by the small intestinal mucosa (Bothwell & Charlton, 1981); a much smaller fraction, typically less than 5%, of dietary nonheme iron from cereal-based diets is absorbed in this way. Absorption depends on the iron status and requirements of the host, food matrix, and the presence of dietary factors that inhibit or enhance absorption (Bothwell et al., 1982).

Newly absorbed iron as well as endogenous iron released from normal degradation of senescent red blood cells is transported to tissues by plasma transferrin. Although almost all cells require iron, approximately 80% of transferrin-bound iron is delivered to bone marrow for red cell production, a process mediated by expression of a specific transferrin receptor that reflects tissue iron need (Skikne, Flowers, & Cook, 1990). Normally, as much as 30% of the body's total iron is stored in association with ferritin, the intracellular protein from which iron can be released into circulation to maintain homeostasis, or as hemosiderin, which is a less available, longer-term intracellular storage form of tissue iron (Dallman, 1986).

During prolonged dietary deficit, iron is released from intracellular ferritin into the circulation via transferrin to support hematopoiesis, which has the effect of decreasing iron stores. As iron depletion progresses, transferrin carries and delivers a diminishing supply of iron to the marrow and other tissues. This stage of iron deficiency without anemia is reflected by increased transferrin receptor expression on cell surfaces, a low level of transferrin being satu-

rated with iron, and increased amounts of circulating erythrocyte protoporphyrin, a protein that accumulates in red blood cells lacking iron (Skikne et al., 1990). If the iron deficit continues, iron-deficiency anemia develops as hemoglobin concentration falls, red cells become smaller in size (microcytic) and more pale in color (hypochromic), and mean corpuscular volume decreases (Ryan, 1997).

Several indicators may be used to track these changes in iron status, only a few of which are commonly used and are discussed here. Assessment of hemoglobin or hematocrit concentrations, evaluating their distributions against conventional cutoffs by age, life stage, and gender (Table 6-9), is the standard approach for diagnosing and estimating the prevalence of anemia. Field assessment of hemoglobin has been advanced greatly through development and use of the HemoCue, a battery-operated portable photometer (Anglholm, Sweden) (Burger & Pierre-Louis, 2003; Yip, 1994). In populations where iron deficiency is known to be the single, major cause of anemia, comparing the distribution of hemoglobin values against a referent distribution free of iron deficiency, can reveal the total burden of anemia that should be amenable to iron intervention (Yip, 1994; Yip, Johnson, & Dallman, 1984). Estimating the prevalence of moderate to severe anemia with its greater health risk (Dallman, 1986) and responsiveness to intervention may improve the interpretation of population anemia burden relative to the use of cutoffs that define mild anemia or worse status (Stoltzfus, 1997). Assessing hemoglobin response to supplementation provides another, more accurate, but complex approach to estimating the extent of iron deficiency anemia (Yip, 1994).

Although ferritin is an intracellular iron storage protein, it also appears in the circulation, giving rise to its use as an indicator of tissue iron stores (Cook, Lipschitz, Miles, & Finch, 1974). Each 1 µg/L concentration of plasma ferritin corresponds to approx-

Table 6-9	Hemoglobin and Hematocrit Cutoff Values Used to Define Anemia	
Target Group	**Hemoglobin (g/L)**	**Hematocrit (%)**
Children 0–5 years	<110	<33
Children 5–11 years	<115	<34
Children 6–14 years	<120	<36
Nonpregnant women	<120	<36
Pregnant women	<110	<33
Men	<130	<39

Source: WHO, 2001.

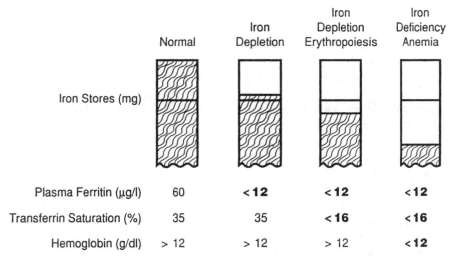

	Normal	Iron Depletion	Iron Depletion Erythropoiesis	Iron Deficiency Anemia
Plasma Ferritin (µg/l)	60	**< 12**	**< 12**	**< 12**
Transferrin Saturation (%)	35	35	**< 16**	**< 16**
Hemoglobin (g/dl)	> 12	> 12	> 12	**< 12**

Figure 6-15 Relationship between Depletion in Body Iron Stores and Change in Selected Indicators of Iron and Anemia Status. Boldvalues represent deficient status.
Source: T. H. Bothwell, & R. W. Charlton. (1981). Iron Deficiency in Women. Report from the International Nutritional Anemia Consultative Group (INACG). Washington, DC: The Nutrition Foundation.

imately 8 to 10 mg of tissue iron. Concentrations less than 12 µg/L are conventionally taken to represent a state of body iron depletion (Bothwell & Charlton, 1981), although plasma ferritin may be elevated in response to acute infection or chronic inflammation (Walter, Olivares, Pizarro, & Munoz, 1997). Measurement of soluble transferrin receptor in plasma has been shown to provide a dependable estimate of tissue iron need under conditions of chronic disease or inflammation (Ferguson, Skikne, Simpson, Baynes, & Cook, 1992), undernutrition (Kuvibidila, Warrier, Ode, & Yu, 1996), and pregnancy (Akesson, Bjellerup, Berglund, Bremme, & Vahter, 1998) but remains little used as a means of diagnosing iron deficiency in low-income countries. Another commonly used measure of iron status is percent transferrin saturation, which reflects the adequacy of iron delivery to tissues (Bothwell & Charlton, 1981). A conceptual framework developed three decades ago, illustrated with cutoffs for common serological indicators used in low-income countries, continues to provide a practical depiction of the spectrum of iron deficiency (Figure 6-15) (Bothwell & Charlton, 1981).

Simple diagnostic tools available to assess anemia in primary care settings include the clinical diagnosis of pallor (palmar, tarsal conjunctival, and nail bed), which can be used to identify severe anemia (hemoglobin less than 50 to 70 g/L or hematocrit less than 15%) with approximately 10% to 50% sensitivity and 90% to 100% specificity (Kalter et al., 1997; Luby et al., 1995; Stoltzfus et al., 1999; Zucker et al., 1997). A simple "color scale" has also been used in the field to diagnose low hemoglobin from a fresh blood spot (Lewis, Stott, & Wynn, 1998; Stott & Lewis, 1995). Inexpensive instruments for detecting anemia in primary care settings have been used as well (Robinett, Taylor, & Stephens, 1996).

The RDA for iron is based on considerations of requirements across the life stages in healthy populations, the heme to non-heme dietary iron proportions, and other factors (Table 6-6). A bioavailability of 18% is presumed for most estimates, recognizing that half to one-third of ingested iron is likely to derive from grain-based diets lacking meat, as found in most low-income countries. With this caveat in mind, an RDA has been set at 8 mg per day for men and postmenopausal women. Premenopausal intake should be 18 mg per day, with the increased amount intended to replace menstrual losses. The RDA throughout pregnancy is 27 mg per day is based on third-trimester needs, and is intended to permit iron stores to build during early gestation. The RDA for women during lactation drops to 9 mg per day to reflect the reduced requirement due to postpartum amenorrhea (IOM, 2006).

Health Consequences

The highest-risk groups in terms of both probability of becoming anemic from iron deficiency and suffering its consequences are women of reproductive age, especially during pregnancy; infants; and young children.

Pregnancy-Related Vital Outcomes. Women are at high risk of anemia due to periodic menstrual blood loss and increased requirements during pregnancy due to expanded red blood cell mass and accretion of iron in fetal tissue and the placenta. Thus gestational iron-deficiency anemia is likely to be harmful to the mother, as suggested by evidence from several observational studies over the past 40 years linking moderate anemia (hemoglobin of 40–80 g/L) to a 1.3-fold higher risk of maternal mortality (95% CI: 0.9–2.0) and severe anemia (less than 47 g/L) to a 3.5-fold higher risk (95% CI: 2–6) of maternal death compared to non-anemic gravida (Brabin, Hakimi, & Pelletier, 2001). While no experimental trials have been undertaken to demonstrate that iron supplementation reduces maternal mortality, plausible causes associated with moderate to severe anemia include puerperal cardiac failure or hemorrhage (Allen, 1997). A recent meta-analysis suggests there to be a continuous risk reduction in maternal mortality risk, reflected by a protective odds ratio of 0.75 (95% CI: 0.62–0.89), with each 10 g/L increase in blood hemoglobin concentration (Stoltzfus et al., 2004). However, data revealing the incidence and severity of maternal morbidity relative to hematologic status are lacking (Allen, 1997).

Risks of preterm delivery, low birth weight, fetal malformations, and fetal deaths have been found to follow a U-shaped curve with respect to maternal hemoglobin (hematocrit) measured early in pregnancy, with an elevated hemoglobin (e.g., more than 130 g/L) posing as much or more risk of an adverse outcome as a lower (less than 90 g/L) hemoglobin concentration (Dreyfuss, 1998; Scholl, Hediger, Fischer, & Shearer, 1992; Steer, Alam, Wadsworth, & Welch, 1995; Yip et al., 1984; Zhou et al., 1998). The causal mechanisms yielding these risks are not well understood.

Maternal iron-deficiency anemia may also place newborns at risk of low iron stores during infancy (Hokama et al., 1996; Kilbride et al., 1999; Preziosi et al., 1997). Iron supplementation during pregnancy has been found to improve newborn length, Apgar score, and survival (Christian, 1998; Preziosi et al., 1997) and lead to larger infant iron stores (plasma ferritin concentrations) at 3 months of age. In Nepal, a randomized, multiple-arm antenatal micronutrient trial found that daily supplemental iron (60 mg) and folic acid (400 µg) reduced the risk of low birth weight (less than 2,500 g) by 16% (Christian, Khatry, et al., 2003). Although there appeared to be no advantage to early infant survival through 3 months of age (Christian, West, et al., 2003), antenatal to early postnatal iron receipt was associated with a significant 31% reduction in the risk of child mortality through 7 years of age (Christian et al., 2009).

Growth. Late infancy and early childhood is a high-risk period for iron deficiency and anemia because of the high iron supplies needed to support rapid growth coupled with low dietary intake of often poorly bioavailable iron (Gibson, Ferguson, & Lehrfeld, 1998; Ryan, 1997). Although some studies have noted an association between iron-deficiency anemia and stunted growth (Chwang, Soemantri, & Pollitt, 1988), a meta-analysis of iron supplement trials failed to find an overall effect on child growth (Ramakrishnan, Aburto, McCabe, & Martorell, 2004). However, the authors did note evidence of a larger effect size—albeit not a significant one—among children who were iron deficient at baseline.

There have been some reports that iron supplementation in children may inhibit growth. Two trials in Sweden and Honduras (Dewey et al., 2002) observed linear growth deceleration and an increased occurrence of diarrhea with daily iron supplementation in non-anemic breastfed infants, whereas anemic infants may have experienced less diarrhea. In India, weight gain and linear growth appeared to be reduced in iron-replete children who were given iron (Majumdar, Paul, Talib, & Ranga, 2003), whereas in Indonesia supplemental iron mildly suppressed weight gain but had no effect on length (Idjradinata, Watkins, & Pollitt, 1994).

Taken together, these data suggest that improved child growth from increased iron intake cannot be expected, and there may be an interaction: Anemic children may benefit from such supplementation, whereas non-anemic children may be disadvantaged in their growth with iron supplement use.

Development. Evidence has been emerging in recent years regarding the developmental consequences of iron deficiency early in life, during this period of normally rapid neuronal replication, development, and maturation. Iron is essential for neurogenesis and differentiation of brain cells and regions. Deficiency likely disturbs the developing brain via at least three iron-dependant pathways: (1) disruption of oligodendrocytes, the cells responsible for producing myelin; (2) disruption of neurotransmitter synthesis and metabolism; and (3) regulation of energy metabolism in the brain (Beard, 2008). Persistent deficits in learning, psychomotor and behavioral interactions, and educational achievement have been observed more often in anemic infants and young children than in children with normal hematologic status (Aukett, Parks, Scott, & Wharton, 1986; Lozoff et al., 1998; Pollitt et al., 1995), but such abnormalities may also result from coexisting malnutrition, other health problems (Heywood, Oppenheimer, Heywood, & Jolley, 1989), and inadequate stimulation at home (Lozoff et al., 1998). Some trials have reported improved behavioral (Oski, Honig, Helu, & Howanitz, 1983), developmental (Aukett et al., 1986), and learning-achievement scores with daily iron supplementation of children (Bruner, Joffe, Duggan, Casella, & Brandt, 1996; Soemantri, Pollitt, & Kim, 1985), whereas other trials have failed to reverse early psychomotor deficits with iron (Lozoff, Wolf, & Jimenez, 1996; Walter, 1989). Recent studies have demonstrated an association between iron deficiency and reduced auditory brain stem responses (Algarin, Peirano, Garrido, Pizarro, & Lozoff, 2003), indicative of poorer nerve conduction velocity possibly due to hypomyelination. In addition, gross motor control was significantly lower in iron-deficient anemic infants than in iron-sufficient infants at 9 months of age (Shafir et al., 2008).

Prevention

Pregnant and postpartum women and infants 6 to 24 months of age represent the highest-risk groups to be targeted for prevention of iron-deficiency anemia (Stoltzfus & Dreyfuss, 1998). Women entering their reproductive years (Viteri, 1998) and preschool children represent other high-risk groups that may be

targeted by such efforts (Stoltzfus & Dreyfuss, 1998). Effective planning should establish those proportions of the anemia burden that can be attributed to iron deficiency, malaria, hookworm, or other causes (Yip, 1997), thereby enabling public health workers to develop rational and effective prevention programs. For example, anthelminthic prophylaxis may prove highly effective where hookworm and *Trichuris* are endemic (Albonico et al., 1998; Brooker et al., 1999; Christian, Khatry, & West, 2004; Hopkins et al., 1997; Stoltzfus & Dreyfuss, 1998). Malarial prophylaxis programs may also reduce risk of anemia (Beales, 1997; Huddle, Gibson, & Cullinan, 1999). Iron deficiency is the underlying cause of anemia in most populations, however, and can be directly addressed through supplementation, food fortification, or other dietary measures.

In young infants, delayed umbilical cord clamping has also been found to be an effective means of preventing anemia and iron deficiency (Hutton & Hassan, 2007). In a randomized trial in Mexico, for example, delayed cord clamping by 2 minutes resulted in a higher mean ferritin and total body iron at 6 months of age (Chaparro, Neufeld, Alavez, Cedillo, & Dewey, 2006). This greatest benefit appeared to be among infants who were born with low ferritin at delivery, those with a birth weight less than 3,000 g, and breastfed infants not receiving fortified infant formula.

Iron Supplementation. Guidelines have been developed in accordance with WHO recommendations for the use of iron and folic acid supplements to prevent and treat iron-deficiency anemia (Table 6-10) (Stoltzfus & Dreyfuss, 1998). Daily

Table 6-10	Guidelines for Supplementing Pregnant Women and Infants with Iron			
	Daily Dosage			
Prevalence of Anemia	**Iron (mg)**	**Folic Acid (μg)**	**Condition**	**Duration**
Pregnant Women				
<40%	60	400	In pregnancy	6 months*
≥40%	60	400	In pregnancy	6 months*
			Postpartum	3 months
Infants				
<40%[†]	12.5[‡]	50	Birth weight ≥ 2,500 g	6–12 months
			Birth weight < 2,500 g	2–24 months
≥40%[†]	12.5[‡]	50	Birth weight ≥ 2,500 g	6–24 months
			Birth weight < 2,500 g	2–24 months

*If 6-month duration cannot be achieved in pregnancy, continue supplement to 6 months postpartum or increase dose to 120 mg iron/day.

[†]If the prevalence in infants is not known, assume the same prevalence as observed in pregnant women in the same population.

[‡]Iron dosage based on 2 mg iron/kg body weight/day.

Source: R. J. Stoltzfus and M. L. Dreyfuss, M. L., Guidelines for the Use of Iron Supplements to Prevent and Treat Iron Deficiency Anemia (Washington, DC: ILSI Press, 1998). Reprinted with permission. Rates are based on cutoffs proposed by Stoltzfus and Dreyfuss (1998).

iron supplementation can effectively raise blood hemoglobin and plasma ferritin levels among pregnant women. Adding folic acid can guard against megaloblastic anemia, neural tube abnormalities if women are supplemented periconceptionally (MRC Vitamin Study Research Group, 1991), and other consequences of folate deficiency that may affect malnourished populations (Fishman et al., 2000).

A long-standing debate over whether prophylactic iron may be contraindicated where malaria is endemic (Menendez et al., 1997; Murray et al., 1975; Oppenheimer, 2001) has been fueled by recent findings of two randomized trials. In Zanzibar, preschool-child iron supplementation in a *falciparum* malaria-endemic area was found to be associated with a significant increase in the risk of severe illness leading to hospitalization or death and a 16% increased risk of adverse clinical events due to malaria (Sazawal et al., 2006). Stratification in a subsample suggested that these adverse effects may have been restricted to non-anemic children. In contrast, in a non-malarious area of Nepal, no adverse effects were observed from such an intervention (Tielsch et al., 2006). Given these findings, WHO has recommended that universal iron supplementation should not be implemented in malaria-endemic areas without screening individuals for iron deficiency (WHO Secretariat, 2007). As yet, however, low-cost systems remain to be implemented for routinely delivering oral iron to infants and young children in low-income countries.

Fortification. Numerous food items have been fortified with iron, including fish sauces, curry powder, sugar, salt, dairy products, and infant formulas (Stoltzfus & Dreyfuss, 1998), although few large-scale iron fortification programs exist in low- and middle-income countries (Yip, 1997). Several food-grade forms of iron are available for use, depending on the type of food vehicle, methods of preparation, storage, and other factors. For example, ferrous sulfate can be used in liquids but may discolor dry foods or make fatty foods rancid (International Nutritional Anemia Consultative Group [INACG], 1997). Iron EDTA (ethylenediaminetetraacetic acid) has been shown to permit efficient absorption of nonheme iron in the presence of dietary inhibitors of absorption (Lynch, Hurrell, Bothwell, & MacPhail, 1993).

Two primary groups are targets for fortification interventions—(1) infants and young children and (2) women—for whom different food vehicles may be considered. Powdered milk, which is frequently given to aid-recipient families, has been fortified with both iron and vitamin C and shown to improve iron status of young children in Chile (Yip, 1997). In Mexico, the government began a program to subsidize multiple-micronutrient-fortified milk for low-income children. An efficacy study conducted prior to its roll-out concluded that the intervention can reduce anemia by 37% and iron deficiency by 38% (Villalpando, Shamah, Rivera, Lara, & Monterrubio, 2006).

"Sprinkles"—single-meal sachets of lipid-encapsulated ferrous fumarate in powdered form that can be sprinkled onto porridge—offer a promising "home fortification" approach to increase iron intake in infants (Zlotkin et al., 2001). Since this approach was first proposed in 1996, nine randomized trials have been conducted in five low-income countries showing iron-fortified sprinkles to be equivalent to iron sulfate drops in curing infantile anemia (Dewey, 2007). In a trial in Haiti, children receiving take-home rations of fortified flour were randomized to receive sprinkles. After two months, the prevalence of anemia had dropped 45% in the intervention group, but only 22% in the control group (Menon et al., 2007). Several Caribbean, South American, and South Asian countries have been fortifying wheat flour with iron (Yip, 1997).

In one large, community-based wheat fortification trial in Sri Lanka, using either electrolytic or reduced iron, this intervention failed to improve hemoglobin status in either preschool- and school-aged children or nonpregnant women (Nestel et al., 2004). Conversely, in Morocco, several iron status indicators improved in school-aged children who consumed salt fortified with either iron plus iodine (Zimmerman et al., 2003) or a combination of iron, iodine, and vitamin A (Zimmerman, Wegmueller, Zeder, Chaouki, Biebinger, et al., 2004). Adverse effects have not been reported from iron fortification trials.

Dietary Approach. Typically, the iron density of diets in low-income regions ranges from 4.5 mg to 7.5 mg per 1,000 kilocalories (ACC/SCN, 1992), largely consisting of nonheme iron from grains, nuts, vegetables, and fruits, from which iron is poorly absorbed (Bothwell et al., 1982; Lynch, 1997). Phytates in foods, tannins and polyphenols in tea, calcium in dairy products and green leaves, and proteins in whole milk, cheeses, and egg whites further inhibit the absorption of nonheme iron (Hallberg, Brune, Erlandsson, Sandberg, & Rossander-Hulten, 1991; Lynch, 1997; Ryan, 1997). Concurrent intakes of ascorbic acid (e.g., from citrus) or meat, poultry, and fish (Bothwell et al., 1982; Monsen et al., 1978) can enhance nonheme absorption in a dose-response manner.

To date, dietary programs to prevent anemia in low-income countries have been few and have achieved little success (Yip, 1997). The food sources of iron with the highest bioavailability are generally of animal origin (i.e., meat, fish, and poultry), but these foods tend to be expensive, and consumed sparingly, in poor communities.

Iodine Deficiency

Iodine is an essential component of thyroid hormones that control cellular metabolism and neuromuscular tissue growth and development. Deficiency in iodine and consequent thyroid hormone production during critical periods of organogenesis can, therefore, damage the brain and nervous tissue, causing irreversible mental retardation and other developmental abnormalities. The spectrum of mild through severe health consequences causally linked to iodine deficiency at different stages of life (**Exhibit 6-5**) is collectively known as iodine-deficiency disorders (IDD) (Delange,

1994). While these effects vary in their specificity with respect to deficiency of iodine, use of this term has led to greater understanding of the multiple health and societal consequences of this nutrient deficiency. Informative treatises exist on the histories of goiter and cretinism—the two most notable clinical syndromes of iodine deficiency (Hetzel, 1989).

As an element in the Earth's crust, iodine can be either sufficient or in varying stages of depletion in areas of the world. Thus iodine adequacy of all flora and fauna, and therefore food, in a general locale depends on the adequacy of the nutrient in soil (Houston, 1999). Major mountainous regions of the world, such as the Himalayas, Andes, and Alps, are severely depleted in soil iodine, resulting from erosion due to glacier activity, rain, and deforestation (Dunn & van der Haar, 1990). In addition, plains regions of central Africa, Asia, and Europe, as well as major riverine and deltaic areas affected by frequent flooding, such as Gangetic South Asia and valleys of the Yellow, Rhine,

---

Exhibit 6-5	**Spectrum of Iodine-Deficiency Disorders**

Fetus

Abortion
Stillbirth
Congenital anomalies
Increased perinatal mortality
Increased infant mortality
Endemic cretinism
Deaf-mutism

Neonate

Neonatal goiter
Neonatal hypothyroidism
Increased susceptibility to nuclear radiation*

Child and Adolescent

Goiter
Juvenile hypothyroidism
Impaired mental function
Retarded physical development
Increased susceptibility to nuclear radiation*

Adult

Goiter with its complications
Hypothyroidism
Impaired mental function
Iodine-induced hyperthyroidism
Increased susceptibility to nuclear radiation

*Due to increased uptake of radioactive iodine by the thyroid gland.

Source: F. Delange, "The Disorders Induced by Iodine Deficiency," 1994, Thyroid, 4, pp. 107–128. Reprinted with permission.

Table 6-11	Number of Countries, Proportion of Population, and Number of Individuals with Insufficient Iodine Intake in School-Aged Children (6–12 Years) and in the General Population (All Age Groups), by WHO Region Between 1994 and 2006, and Proportion of Households Using Iodized Salt[1,2]					
		Insufficient Iodine Intake (UI < 100 μg/L)				
		School-Aged Children[4]		General Population[4]		% of Households
WHO Region[3]	Countries (number)	Proportion %	Total Number (millions)[2]	Proportion %	Total Number (millions)[2]	with Access to Iodized Salt
Africa	13	40.8	57.7	41.5	312.9	66.6
Americas	3	10.6	11.6	11.0	98.6	86.8
Southeast Asia	0	30.3	73.1	30.0	503.6	61.0
Europe	19	52.4	38.7	52.0	459.7	49.2
Eastern Mediterranean	7	48.8	43.3	47.2	259.3	47.3
Western Pacific	5	22.7	41.6	21.2	374.7	89.5
Total	47	31.5	266.0	30.6	2008.8	70.0

1. De Benoist et al., 2008.

2. WHO, UNICEF, & ICCIDD, 2007, using data from the UNICEF global database (www.childinfo.org).

3. Comprising 192 WHO member-states.

4. Based on population estimates in the year 2006.

and the Amazon, also lack iodine (Dunn & van der Haar, 1990). In some areas of Central Africa, such as Zaire, where environmental iodine and intake are marginal to low, iodine deficiency is augmented by routine consumption of goitrogenic substances, such as linamarin, a cyanide-containing compound found in the root of cassava (Delange et al., 1982). Thiocyanates, which result from detoxification of linamarin in the liver, decrease iodine uptake by the thyroid gland and suppress circulating thyroid hormone, leading to secondary iodine deficiency. Despite efforts to try to improve iodine status, iodine deficiency continues to be a problem of public health significance in 47 countries (see Figure 6-13).

As of the early 1990s, an estimated 1.6 billion persons, or nearly 30% of the world's population, were thought to be at risk of iodine deficiency (WHO, 1993), based on the documented occurrence of goiter (prevalence more than 5%) and the sizes of populations living in iodine-depleted regions of the world (Houston, 1999). Revised estimates of the extent of iodine deficiency obtained from WHO's global database for the 192 member-states of the United Nations suggest that nearly 2 billion people, including 32% of school-aged children, have an insufficient intake of iodine (de Benoist, McLean, Andersson, & Rogers, 2008) (Table 6-11). Iodine intake below the requirement is believed to occur in 73 million children in Southeast Asia and nearly 58 million children in Africa. However, the greatest proportion of children with

inadequate iodine intake live in European (52%) and the eastern Mediterranean (49%) regions. In contrast, iodine intake is more than adequate or excessive in 34 countries, emphasizing the importance of regular monitoring of national IDD prevention initiatives.

Function

Iodine, ingested as either iodide or iodate, is an essential constituent of thyroid hormones. Once in circulation, nearly all body iodide is actively trapped by follicle cells of the thyroid gland, where it is oxidized to iodine and bound to tyrosine amino acids, catalyzed by an iron-containing peroxidase, to form the thyroid hormones, T_3 (tri-iodothyronine) and T_4 (tetra-iodothyronine, or thyroxine) (Houston, 1999; Tortora & Grabowski, 1996). T_3 and T_4 are stored in the thyroid gland in association with the glycoprotein thyroglobulin.

Following stimulation from the hypothalamus, thyroid-stimulating hormone (TSH) is released from the anterior pituitary gland. It induces thyroid hormone release into circulation, where the hormone is bound to circulatory carrier proteins (Houston, 1999). As T_3 and T_4 levels rise, the hypothalamic–anterior pituitary–thyroid axis maintains homeostasis by reducing thyroid hormone release. Within target cells, thyroid hormones regulate oxygen use, basic metabolic rate, protein synthesis, and thermogenesis—a feat accomplished largely by influencing gene transcription (Stein, 1994).

During gestation, both maternal and fetally derived T_3 and T_4 contribute to the regulatory thyroxine pool that, acting in concert with other hormones (e.g., growth hormone, insulin), directs fetal tissue function, growth, and development. In particular, thyroid hormones influence the development of the brain and other neural tissue, giving rise to their, and iodine's, key role in regulating fetal and infant growth, physical and mental function, and development (Tortora & Grabowski, 1996). Paradoxically, excess buildup of iodine in the thyroid gland can suppress the release of T_3 and T_4, leading to concern about risks of toxicity associated with rapid correction of iodine deficiency in some endemic areas (Corvilain, Van Sande, Dumont, Bourdoux, & Ermans, 1998; Dunn, Semigran, & Delange, 1998; Stanbury et al., 1998), similar to the risks observed in areas of chronically high iodine intake (Konno, Makita, Yuri, Iizuka, & Kawasaki, 1994).

Health Consequences

Among the disorders caused by lack of iodine, fetal and neonatal hypothyroidism due to maternal iodine depletion is by far the most serious, with widespread consequences. This disorder permanently alters the structure and function of the brain and other nervous tissue during critical stages of development, giving rise to permanent neurological and developmental abnormalities (Hetzel, 1994; Stein, 1994). Postnatal iodine deficiency perpetuates thyroid failure that, depending on its duration and severity, can lead to continued hypothyroidism, growth retardation, sexual immaturity, and impaired cognition and motor development (Halpern, 1994).

Severe iodine deficiency can result in spontaneous abortion, stillbirth, and congenital abnormalities among surviving offspring (Pharoah, Buttfield, & Hetzel, 1971). Cretinism (**Figure 6-16**), representing the most severe clinical spectrum of the IDD, is usually manifested as severe mental and growth retardation, paraplegia, rigidity, deaf-mutism, and facial disturbances (Hetzel, 1994). The type and severity of brain and other neurological and musculoskeletal deficits appear to arise from the timing, duration, and severity of insult. For example, the central nervous system defects associated with cretinism can be linked to severe gestational iodine deficiency in the second trimester of pregnancy (DeLong et al., 1994; Halpern, 1994), a period when the cerebral cortex, basal ganglia, and cochlea undergo rapid growth and development. Normal amounts of thyroid hormone are needed for neuronal migration and myelination of the fetal brain, a process that is irreversibly damaged

with inadequate iodine (Zimmermann, 2008). Severe fetal hypothyroidism thus gives rise to the neurologic cretin. Severe growth retardation, sexual delay, and musculoskeletal deformity, with continued neurological damage, can be attributed largely to severe postnatal iodine deficiency, giving rise to the myxedemetous cretin (Boyages, 1994). For these reasons, iodine deficiency has been labeled the most common preventable cause of mental retardation (Walker et al., 2007).

Mild, biochemical, or noncretinous hypothyroidism due to iodine deficiency is a major public health concern due to its frequency in infancy and early childhood. Decreased infant survival may be a little-suspected consequence of mild neonatal hypothyroidism (Cobra et al., 1997). More fully appreciated is the observation that children living in iodine-deficient communities, who usually exhibit

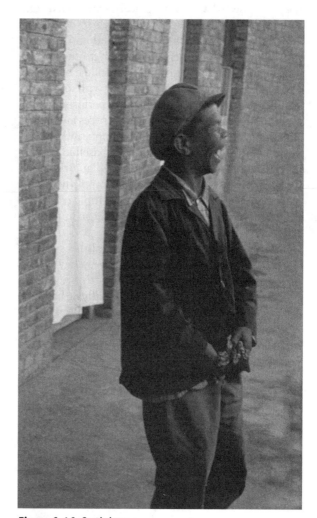

Figure 6-16 Cretinism
Source: Photograph copyright John Dunn.

one or more indications of iodine deficiency, tend to have lower intelligence quotients and perform more poorly in cognition, motor function, and school achievement tests than peers with normal status growing up under iodine-sufficient surroundings (Bleichrodt & Born, 1994; Huda, Grantham-McGregor, Rahman, & Tomkins, 1999). For example, one meta-analysis including 37 Chinese publications found that children growing up in iodine-deficient areas had IQs that averaged 12.5 points lower than children growing up in iodine-sufficient areas (Qing et al., 2005).

Historically, the strength of evidence for a unique contribution of mild iodine deficiency to impaired cognition has been tempered by lack of control in studies for community differences in nutritional, health, education, and socioeconomic factors that can also influence child stimulation and achievement. Some of these concerns for confounders are now being addressed. Two recent placebo-controlled, randomized trials among 10- to 13-year-old children have been conducted in New Zealand and Albania. In Albania, children were moderately to severely iodine deficient with a median urinary iodine of 44 µg/L and a goiter rate of 87%. Treatment with iodized oil significantly improved their cognitive performance, including measures of information processing speed, reasoning, and problem solving (Zimmermann et al., 2006). In the New Zealand study, at baseline the children were mildly deficient with a median urinary iodine concentration of 63 µg/L. After supplementation for 28 weeks, children in the intervention group had improved scores of perceptual reasoning compared to controls (Gordon et al., 2009).

Recognition and quantification of this subclinical "base of the IDD iceberg" have been key factors in motivating more vigorous efforts to prevent iodine deficiency (Hetzel, 1989). Globally, it has been estimated that IDD accounts for 2.6 million DALY lost, primarily due to cognitive and motor impairment and hearing loss associated with deficiency (Black et al., 2008).

Goiter is an enlarged thyroid gland and is the most commonly observed clinical manifestation of iodine deficiency. Chronic deficiency of iodine lowers thyroid hormone output, which in turn leads to increased TSH release from the anterior pituitary as the body attempts to stimulate increased T_3 and thyroxine production. Failure results in compensatory growth of the thyroid gland (Kavishe, 1999). Goiter size can range from barely palpable with the neck extended to grotesquely visible from a distance. An enlarged thyroid due to iodine deficiency poses a little-known health risk. Nevertheless, hyperthyroidism reflecting a state of thyrotoxicosis may serve as an indicator of cardiac risk in some elderly groups who respond abnormally to iodine prophylaxis (Corvilain et al., 1998; Dunn, Semigran, & Delange, 1998; Stanbury et al., 1998).

Assessment

Iodine status can be assessed through clinical and biochemical means. Urinary iodine concentration, goiter rate, serum TSH, and serum thyroglobulin are four methods generally recommended for assessment. They provide a complementary picture of iodine status, with urinary iodine representing a sensitive indicator of recent iodine intake, thyroglobulin responding to a change in status over a period of weeks to months, and the goiter rate usually reflective of longer-term iodine nutrition over a period of months to years (Zimmermann, 2008). Indicators with suggested cutoffs, target populations for assessment, and criteria related to severity of iodine deficiency as a public health problem have been published by WHO, UNICEF, and the International Council for the Control of Iodine Deficiency Disorders – ICCIDD (2007) (Table 6-12).

Virtually all goiter occurring in iodine-deficient areas can be attributed to iodine deficiency; thus goiter prevalence can serve as a useful population indicator of risk. The size of the thyroid gland changes inversely in response to changes in iodine intake. Nevertheless, there are practical limitations for assessing goiter in very young age groups because of the challenges in palpating the smaller thyroid gland in smaller children. Reliable thyroid examination by palpation requires well-trained observers (Peterson et al., 2000).

In 1960, WHO established a five-stage goiter classification system (Perez, Scrimshaw, & Munoz, 1960) that served as the basis for evaluating the public health significance of iodine deficiency over the subsequent three decades (WHO, 1993). The minimum clinical cutoff for estimating the total goiter rate (TGR) was a palpable glandular mass, with each lobe being at least as large as the distal phalanx of the subject's thumb. A TGR of more than 10% was set as the minimum for iodine-deficiency public health criterion (Perez et al., 1960). In 1994, WHO simplified this scheme to two clinical grades, defining goiter as a palpable mass of any size with the neck in a normal position, and it lowered the minimum TGR of public health significance to more than 5% (WHO, 1994). Although these changes were motivated by a

Table 6-12	Epidemiologic Criteria for Assessing the Severity of IDD Based on Urinary Iodine or the Total Goiter Rate in School-Aged Children and Pregnant Women				
	Urinary Iodine			**Total Goiter Rate**	
Population Group	**Median Concentration (μg/L)**	**Interpretation**		**Proportion (%)**	**Interpretation**
School-aged children	<20	Insufficient: severe iodine deficiency		≥30	Severe
	20–49	Insufficient: moderate iodine deficiency		20.0–29.9	Moderate
	50–99	Insufficient: mild iodine deficiency		5.0–19.9	Mild
	100–199	Adequate		0.0–4.9	None
	200–299	Above requirements		5.0–19.9	Mild
	≥30	Excessive			
Pregnant women	<150	Insufficient			
	150–249	Adequate			
	250–599	Above requirements			
	≥500	Excessive			

Source: WHO, UNICEF & ICCIDD, 2007.

desire to improve diagnostic reliability, the reverse may have occurred by changing the minimum cutoff to a milder, less discernible stage of thyroid enlargement (Peterson et al., 2000).

Thyroid volume is more reliably and accurately assessed by ultrasonography than by palpation, providing a clear method of choice where resources permit (Pardede et al., 1998; Tajtakova et al., 1990). In recent years, normative standards have been developed for evaluating ultrasound-derived thyroid volume distributions in adults (Delange et al., 1997) and in school-aged children for screening and population assessment (Zimmermann, Hess, et al., 2004). Thus, while the TGR remains an important population indicator of iodine deficiency risk, given the slowness and variability of goiter to respond to increased iodine intake (for example, more than 6 months' to 4 years' duration) (Elnagar et al., 1995; Hintze et al., 1988), other indicators of iodine status should be employed for surveillance and program evaluation (Zimmermann, 2004).

Urinary iodine (UI) concentration serves as the conventional, biochemical measure of current iodine intake and status of a population. Fasting morning samples of urine can be used to assess the iodine status of a community (Thomson et al., 1997; WHO, 1994), although reliable individual assessment of high day-to-day variability requires 24-hour urine collec-

tion on more than one day (Rasmussen, Ovesen, & Christiansen, 1999; Thomson et al., 1997). UI is preferably reported as micrograms per liter (μg/L; WHO, 1994), although creatinine-adjusted concentrations are occasionally used and, at least in otherwise normally nourished populations, the two measures can be equated (1 μg/L ≈ 1 μg/g) (Dunn & van der Haar, 1990). However, in populations with low protein intake, the UI/creatinine ratio is unreliable due to low creatinine excretion (WHO, UNICEF, & ICCIDD, 2007). A median UI value of more than 100 μg/L urine is considered to be reflective of a normal (average) iodine intake (that is, more than150 μg per day) and adequate status in the community (Dunn & van der Haar, 1990). Notably, median UI concentrations correlate negatively with the prevalence of goiter across communities (Bar-Andziak, Lazecki, Radwanowska, & Nauman, 1993; Caron et al., 1997; Delange et al., 1997; Kimiagar, Azizi, Navai, Yassai, & Nafarabadi, 1990; Pardede et al.,1998; Rasmussen et al., 1999) and correlate positively with iodine intake (Bar-Andziak et al., 1993; Brussard, Brants, Hulshof, Kistemaker, & Lowik, 1997; Kim, Moon, Kim, Sohn, & Oh, 1998), serving to affirm population-based assessments of risk based on this measure.

Additional iodine status indicators include serum, whole blood, or whole blood spot TSH and serum thyroglobulin concentration. TSH measurement is recommended for screening neonates for hypothyroidism, which also can indicate population iodine status (Delange, 1998; Dunn, 1996; Lixin et al., 1995). Neonatal TSH tends to be negatively correlated with maternal urinary iodine, so it reflects the status of the maternal–fetal dyad (Lixin et al., 1995). Thyroglobulin concentration reflects increased turnover of thyroid cells due to hypertrophy and hyperplasia and is reflective of iodine nutrition over a period of months or years. This measurement stands in contrast to urinary iodine concentration, which reflects more recent iodine intake. Both indicators rise with increasingly severe iodine deficiency—that is, decreasing median iodine intakes and UI excretion levels (WHO, 1994).

Prevention

Unlike other micronutrient deficiencies that might be corrected by diversifying the local diet, iodine-deficiency correction in an endemic area is largely dependent on consuming foods grown in iodine-sufficient soil or fortified with iodine (iodization). Pilot projects in China have successfully demonstrated the beneficial impact of iodinating irrigation water used for crop production on the iodine status of humans and animal herds, although this practice has not been widely implemented to date.

An average dietary iodine intake of approximately 150 µg/day is recommended for adults to maintain adequate iodine status (IOM, 2006). A usual intake of 50 µg/day is considered a minimum requirement, below which thyroid enlargement can be expected (Delange, 1994). The U.S. Institute of Medicine (2006) has set the Adequate Intake (AI) or RDA during infancy through age 3 years between 90 and 130 µg/day, premised on an adequate maternal iodine intake and breast milk iodine concentration.

Universal salt iodization (USI) remains the longest-standing, most widely adopted, and most cost-effective approach to preventing iodine deficiency and its disorders throughout the world. Begun in the United States and selected European countries in the 1920s, by the early 1990s it was estimated that fewer than 20% of households globally were consuming iodized salt. By 2000, the estimate had jumped to 70%. By 2006, USI programs were under way in at least 120 countries (UNICEF, 2008). WHO (2004) has estimated that the number of countries where IDD is a public health problem was cut in half between 1993 and 2003.

Salt iodization technology is straightforward, typically involving the dry mixing or spraying of potassium iodate or iodide with food-grade salt (Mannar & Dunn, 1995). Levels of iodization vary across and within countries, after considering salt consumption patterns, iodine gap in the diet, ambient exposures, packaging, transport, and other conditions. The recommended iodine concentration ranges from 20 to 40 parts per million (ppm) of iodine so as to provide 150 µg of iodine per person per day (WHO, UNICEF, & ICCIDD, 2007).

Several trials have demonstrated an ability of salt fortified with iodine plus iron (Zimmermann et al., 2003; Zimmermann, Wegmueller, Zeder, Chaouki, Rohner, et al., 2004) and iodine, iron, and vitamin A (Zimmermann, Wegmueller, Zeder, Chaouki, Biebinger et al., 2004) to improve the status of all three nutrients in school-aged children, opening up possibilities for salt to serve as a vehicle for preventing multiple micronutrient deficiencies. In addition to the expected efficacy of the intended dosage, the success of salt iodization rests on numerous other political, legislative, management, marketing, and salt use factors that must be synchronous to be effective (Exhibit 6-6). Failure in these other program elements has led to disappointingly small changes in iodine status in many settings, even after decades of salt iodization (Langer, Tajtakova, Podoba, Kostalova, & Gutekunst, 1994; Lindberg, Andersson, & Lamberg, 1989; Metges et al., 1996; Syrenicz et al., 1993). Even so, USI remains a viable goal in most countries in need of iodine deficiency control.

Where salt iodization is not practical, other means must be found to deliver adequate iodine to high-risk groups (Solomons, 1998). Annual or biannual supplementation with iodized oil improves iodine status (Peterson et al., 2000) and has been shown to markedly lower risk of maternal hypothyroidism, cretinism, and fetal/infant mortality (Pharoah et al., 1971). An annual dose of 200 mg of iodine has been shown to optimize iodine status while minimizing the risk of toxicity in adults (Peterson et al., 2000). Iodine can also be given as potassium iodide or potassium iodate drops or tablets in monthly 30-mg tablets or bimonthly 8-mg tablets (Zimmermann, Jooste, & Pandav, 2008).

Irrespective of the choice of iodine intervention, sound programming principles must be followed. These concepts include involving key stakeholders (ranging from government to the private sector) in planning, educating the targeted public (especially important with voluntary salt iodization), proper monitoring, and taking adequate steps to solve problems and ensure sustainability (Dunn, 1996).

Exhibit 6-6	Salt Iodization: Ensuring Quality, Maintaining Impact

Salt remains a common dietary item for people of all ages, cultures, and geographic and socioeconomic bounds. Higher-income countries have had iodized salt to prevent iodine deficiency for several decades, yet the full impact of salt iodization has yet to be achieved in most low- and middle-income countries. Iodizing salt is straightforward, but many factors may impede progress on this front.

Key steps for cost-effective salt iodization were laid out in a 1996 quality assurance workshop for producers, policy makers, scientists, and programmers (Quality Assurance Workshop for Salt Iodized Programs, 1997):

• **Producers:** Upgrade raw salt production through quality control and training; batch process salt and iodate by a mechanized, noncorrosive blender or mixer, with manual backup for power outage; or for continuous processing, use screw/auger mixer during or after adding iodate dosing pumps and spray methods for uniform iodization; package bulk salt in lined or laminated bags weighing less 50 kg, using semiautomated filling, sealing, and stitching procedures; label bulk bags with "Use No Hooks," "Iodized Salt," the producer's name and address, and bag weight; retail salt in smaller (less than 1 kg), heat-sealed bags; support government efforts to monitor and achieve iodized salt standards; monitor iodine levels with salt test kits; self-police through producer associations.

• **Governments:** Pass and review as needed enabling salt iodization legislation (setting ranges versus absolute concentrations for iodine content) that includes packaging, labeling, transport, and marketing policies; hold "stakeholder" meetings to provide updates on IDD control and discuss new technology; develop methods for small producers to meet standards; create a national database of producers to ensure training; strictly monitor and provide incentives for compliance, focusing on low-coverage areas; modernize test laboratories; accelerate consumer demand for small (less than 1 kg) retail packages; enforce policies related to national standards; monitor IDD impact.

• **Agencies:** Develop and distribute information for producers; help improve government–industry–international exchange; monitor and develop information on the potassium iodate market; help increase consumer demand for small packages of salt; assist in capacity building and quality assurance agenda.

Zinc Deficiency

Zinc is essential for many metabolic functions, growth, and survival in mammals, poultry, and some plants; thus zinc deficiency has many serious consequences (Hambidge & Krebs, 1999; Keen & Gershwin, 1990; Solomons, 1999). Even so, zinc deficiency has been one of the least "visible" micronutrient deficiencies. Evidence of some of the clinical abnormalities due to human zinc deficiency became clear in the 1960s (Prasad, 1985), but its prevalence has proved difficult to ascertain due to absence of adequate, nationally representative data on zinc status (ACC/SCN, 2000). This uncertainty, which is attributed to a lack of reliable indicators or lack of consensus with respect to their use, interpretation, and target groups to assess (Black, 1997), coupled with the limited experience with prevention programs (Gibson & Ferguson, 1998b), may have been factors that led to the near exclusion of zinc on the global micronutrient agenda until very recently ("Ending Hidden Hunger," 1992; McGuire & Galloway, 1994; Trowbridge et al., 1993).

Extensive evidence accumulated in the last decade, primarily from randomized trials of zinc supplementation in children in low-income countries, has now conclusively demonstrated the importance of zinc deficiency in these settings in regard to growth, risk of infectious disease morbidity and mortality, and other outcomes. This evidence, coupled with new estimates indicating that zinc deficiency is highly prevalent in low- and middle-income countries (Hotz & Brown, 2004), has resulted in a better appreciation of the magnitude of this problem (see Figure 6-13). It has been estimated that the global burden of disease attributable to zinc deficiency is more than 450,000 child deaths annually and nearly 4% of DALYs in children younger than 5 years of age—comparable to the burden imposed by vitamin A deficiency (Black et al., 2008; Fischer Walker, Ezzati, & Black, 2009).

With this new recognition of the magnitude of the problem has come more attention to the development of programs to prevent or rectify the deficiency.

Function, Requirements, and Assessment

Zinc, which is found in all cells, serves as a constituent of more than 200 enzymes and numerous transcription proteins (as a "zinc finger ") that regulate nucleic acid synthesis; metabolism of proteins, lipids, and carbohydrate; and cell differentiation (Cousins & Hempe, 1990; Stipanuk, 2000). These functions confer on zinc important roles in organogenesis, tissue growth, functional development, and immunity (Shankar & Prasad, 1998; Stipanuk, 2000). Such broad involvement in metabolism virtually assures zinc an important role in maintaining health.

Zinc is absorbed both by passive diffusion across a concentration gradient and by energy-dependent processes when intake is low (Stipanuk, 2000). Specific transporter proteins may facilitate its absorption (McMahon & Cousins, 1998). In mixed diets, the efficiency of this absorption can vary widely, from practically nil to 40%, with the lowest absorption associated with high grain and plant consumption and the highest with human milk and meat consumption. Absorption rates tend to be higher in individuals with zinc deficiency (Solomons, 1999). Uptake into tissues appears to be regulated in some fashion, although the mechanisms involved are poorly understood.

Approximately 85% of total body zinc resides in skeletal muscle, calcified bone, and marrow; it is mostly bound to the storage protein known as metallothionein. This leaves only a small exchangeable body pool that can respond to short-term variation in zinc intake. Less than 1% of body zinc is found in circulation (Cousins & Hempe, 1990). Although there are no large body reserves of zinc in the conventional sense, bone may serve as a passive reserve, with zinc being made available from this source during normal turnover.

Recommended Dietary Allowances for zinc in healthy individuals have been available from WHO and were updated with new values developed by the Institute of Medicine (2006) in the United States. Many critics considered the IOM values to be too low for grain-based, low-meat diets, leading to a more recent revision by the International Zinc Nutrition Consultative Group (Hotz & Brown, 2004; see Table 6-6). For children, these values range from 3 to 14 mg per day depending on age, weight, sex, and the bioavailability of dietary zinc. For adults, the rec-

ommended intakes range from 8 to 15 mg per day depending on sex and physiologic state (i.e., pregnancy or lactation). Because zinc is lost during diarrhea and may be used up more rapidly during infections, such conditions may increase the need for dietary zinc.

Zinc status may be assessed by a combination of clinical, biochemical, test-response, and dietary methods (Gibson, 1990; Gibson & Huddle, 1998). Clinical signs of moderate to severe zinc deficiency, including marked growth retardation, dermatitis and other skin changes, poor appetite, and mental lethargy, are either rare or lack sufficient specificity to be useful for population assessment. Diagnosis of more prevalent mild zinc deficiency usually rests on determining serum or plasma zinc concentration. Although unreliable for individual assessment, the distribution of serum zinc concentrations or responsiveness of the lower end of the distribution to intervention can identify groups at risk (Hotz & Brown, 2004). Serum zinc concentration varies by time of day, largely related to food ingestion, and can be lowered by infection because of cytokine-mediated shifts into the liver. Extensive recent work has resulted in suggested lower cutoffs for the assessment of serum zinc concentration depending on time of day, fasting state, age, sex, and pregnancy (Table 6-13) (Hotz & Brown, 2004).

Hair zinc concentration may be used as a static indicator to identify groups of individuals likely to be zinc deficient, with 1.68 µmol/g suggested as a cutoff (Gibson & Huddle, 1998). In comparison to serum zinc, hair zinc measurement has two advantages: (1) concentrations in hair are more stable, reflecting longer-term status, and (2) collection of hair is easier than collection of blood. The disadvantages of this approach include the limited availability of reference data and the possibility that zinc deficiency may stunt hair growth, resulting in normal hair zinc concentrations. Stable isotope dilution methods may be used to assess total body zinc stores, although the

Table 6-13	Suggested Lower Thresholds for Mean Serum Zinc Concentrations (µg/dL)* to Classify Populations at Risk of Zinc Deficiency		
		Age Group	
		10 Years or Older	
Time of Day of Blood Sample	**Younger Than 10 years**	**Nonpregnant Females**	**Males**
Morning, fasting	Unknown	70 (10.7)	74 (11.3)
Morning, other	65 (9.9)	66 (10.1)	70 (10.7)
Afternoon/evening	57 (8.7)	59 (9.0)	61 (9.3)

Note: *1 µmol/L = 6.54 µg/dL.

cost and complexity of this approach limits its use to evaluating small numbers of individuals and validating other indicators (Hambidge & Krebs, 1995; Hambidge, Krebs, & Miller, 1998).

Dietary assessment can provide valuable insight with respect to the bioavailable dietary zinc from local food resulting from concurrent estimation of zinc and phytate content, but by itself this approach cannot determine the status of an individual or population (Gibson & Ferguson, 1998a). Extensive guidelines on conducting and interpreting dietary surveys to assess the adequacy of dietary zinc intake have been published (Hotz & Brown, 2004).

Other possible measures of zinc deficiency in a population are the functional responses to zinc supplementation, such as improved growth and reduced infections, which will be considered in the following "Health Consequences" section. Because of the association of zinc deficiency with growth stunting (low height for age) as well as dietary inadequacy, the International Zinc Nutrition Consultative Group has developed a composite index consisting of the percentage of preschool-aged children who are stunted and the percentage of individuals at risk of inadequate zinc intake (from national food balance sheets) to classify countries based on their risk of zinc deficiency (see Figure 6-13D) (Hotz & Brown, 2004).

Health Consequences

As predicted by Prasad (1991), the past two decades have witnessed a vastly expanded research effort to elucidate zinc's role in health. Preschool-aged children who exhibit low serum zinc levels are more likely to develop diarrhea and experience more severe episodes of diarrhea or acute respiratory infection than children with adequate zinc status (Bahl, Bhandari, Hambidge, & Bhan, 1998). The causality of this association has been examined by quantifying the impact of zinc supplementation on the incidence, duration, and severity of acute and persistent diarrhea or dysentery (Faruque, Mahalanabis, Haque, Fuchs, & Habte, 1999; Penny et al., 1999; Rosado, Lopez, Munoz, Martinez, & Allen, 1997; Roy et al., 1999; Ruel, Rivera, Santizo, Lonnerdal, & Brown, 1997; Sazawal et al., 1995; Sazawal et al., 1996; Sazawal, Black, et al., 1997; Sazawal, Jalla, et al., 1997; Sazawal et al., 1998; Zinc Investigators' Collaborative Group, 1999), acute respiratory infections (Roy et al., 1999; Ruel et al., 1997; Sazawal et al., 1998), malaria (Shankar & Prasad, 1998), immune competence (Sazawal, Jalla, et al., 1997; Shankar & Prasad, 1998), and growth (Brown, Peerson, & Allen, 1998; Rosado et al., 1997) in young children. The number, speci-

ficity, and timeliness of these trials, coupled with an urgent need to grasp the health implications of adequate zinc nutriture for policy and program purposes, have inspired overview analyses in an attempt to better discern the health benefits of improved zinc nutriture, especially for high-risk populations.

Diarrhea. Evidence for a role of zinc in reducing the incidence, severity, and duration of diarrhea is remarkably consistent. Data from seven clinical trials evaluating the efficacy of continuous, daily zinc supplementation of preschool-aged children were pooled for analysis (Zinc Investigators' Collaborative Group, 1999). Eligible trials provided 5 to 20 mg of zinc (as sulfate, gluconate, or methionate) for periods of 12 to 54 weeks to preschoolers. The benefit of zinc supplementation was consistent across these studies, with average reductions of 18% (odds ratio = 0.82; 95% CI: 0.72–0.93) in the incidence (Figure 6-17, Panel A) and 25% (odds ratio = 0.75; 95% CI: 0.63–0.88) in the prevalence (days ill/100 person-days) (Figure 6-17, Panel B) of diarrhea. A subsequent meta-analysis of 15 trials of zinc supplementation found a reduction in diarrhea incidence (rate ratio = 0.86; 95% CI: 0.79–0.93) (Aggarwal, Sentz, & Miller, 2007). The apparent, greater impact on prevalence can be expected because prevalence includes episodic duration, which was also reduced by zinc supplementation (Faruque et al., 1999; Hambidge et al., 1998; Roy et al., 1997; Ruel et al., 1997). Zinc therapy also reduced the frequency of prolonged diarrhea (Black, 1998). Zinc supplementation has also been found to be safe in HIV-positive individuals and to reduce the incidence of diarrhea in children in South Africa (Bobat et al., 2005; Siberry, Ruff, & Black, 2002).

Zinc has also been successfully used in therapy of acute and persistent diarrhea. In a meta-analysis of 5 randomized controlled trials in acute diarrhea, the summary estimate of the effect of zinc supplements was a 16% reduction in episode duration (Zinc Investigators' Collaborative Group, 1999). Also in this systematic review of 5 trials of zinc supplements in persistent diarrhea (enrollment duration of 14 days or more), the summary estimate was a 29% reduction in duration. Many subsequent trials have confirmed the findings that zinc supplements, when used as adjunctive therapy with oral rehydration, reduce the duration and severity of the episode (Bahl et al., 2001; Baqui et al., 2002). A recent meta-analysis of 26 comparisons from 19 zinc trials found a 20% reduction in mean diarrheal duration (95% CI: 12%–28%) (Patel et al., 2010).

Results on the effect of zinc in treatment of diarrhea in infants younger than 6 months old have been

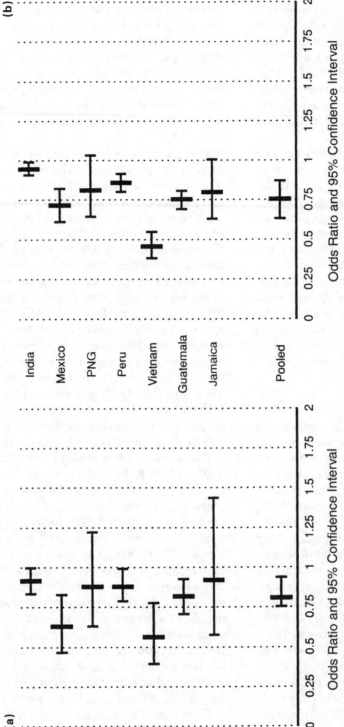

Figure 6-17 Individual and Pooled Effects (Odds Ratio and 95% Confidence Intervals) of Daily Zinc Supplementation on Incidence (Panel A) and Prevalence (Panel B) of Early Childhood Diarrhea in Seven Randomized, Double-Masked, Continuous Supplementation Trials. Sources: Zinc Investigators' Collaborative Group, 1999; Zinc Investigators' Collaborative Group, 2002.

Source: Zinc Investigators' Collaborative Group, "Prevention of Diarrhea and Pneumonia by Zinc Supplementation in Children in Developing Countries: Pooled Analysis of Randomized Controlled Trials," 1999, Journal of Pediatrics, 135, p. 693. Copyright 1999 by Mosby, Inc. Reprinted with permission.

mixed (Brooks et al., 2005; Fischer Walker, Black, & Baqui, 2008; Fischer Walker et al., 2006; Mazumder et al., 2010). Of additional interest is the finding that zinc supplements given for 2 weeks during and following diarrhea have been shown to reduce the incidence of diarrhea in the subsequent 2 to 3 months (Zinc Investigators' Collaborative Group, 1999).

Respiratory Infection. A number of studies have evaluated the effects of zinc on acute lower respiratory infection. Four zinc supplementation trials that examined this question were analyzed together (Ninh et al., 1996; Penny et al., 1999; Sazawal et al., 1998; Zinc Investigators' Collaborative Group, 1999). These studies revealed an average reduction of 41% in the incidence of pneumonia among zinc-supplemented children versus control children (odds ratio = 0.59; 95% CI: 0.41–0.83). A subsequent trial confirmed this benefit (Bhandari et al., 2002). A meta-analysis of 12 zinc trials found a reduction in the incidence of lower respiratory infections (rate ratio = 0.92; 95% CI: 0.85–0.99) (Aggarwal et al., 2007). However, further analysis of these trials demonstrated that acute lower respiratory illnesses defined by specific clinical criteria were reduced to a greater degree (incidence rate ratio = 0.65; 95% CI: 0.52–0.82) (Roth, Richard, & Black, 2010).

Zinc has also been shown to have benefits as an adjunctive therapy given along with antibiotics for pneumonia. Studies in Bangladesh and India found that children with severe pneumonia who received zinc had a shorter duration of illness and a lower rate of failure of initial antibiotic therapy (Brooks et al., 2004; Mahalanabis et al., 2004). Another study in India failed to find such a therapeutic benefit of zinc, however (Bose et al., 2006).

Malaria. Experimental zinc deficiency impairs host defenses against malarial infection (Shankar & Prasad, 1998). *Plasmodium falciparum (pf)* parasitemia has also been negatively associated with measures of zinc status or intake in Africa (Gibson & Huddle, 1998) and Southeast Asia (Gibson et al., 1991).

The public health impact of this association has been tested in four randomized, double-masked field trials. The largest study was conducted among 274 children aged 6 to 60 months in Papua New Guinea. Children who received 10 mg of zinc, 6 days per week for 10 months, experienced a 38% reduction (95% CI: 3%–60%) in *pf* malaria episodes (fever plus parasitemia of more than 9,200 organisms/µL), and a 69% reduction in episodes with heavy parasitemia (more than 100,000 organisms/µL) (Shankar, Genton & Tamja et al., 1999). Similar reductions in malarial

illness have been reported from Gambia (30%—not statistically significant) (Bates et al., 1993) and in another trial among nursery school children in Uganda, where zinc supplementation throughout the school year was associated with a 25% reduction in weekly illness event rates ($p < 0.05$), more than 80% of which were classified as malaria attacks (Kikafunda, Walker, Allan, & Tumwine, 1998). In contrast, a trial in Burkina Faso did not find an effect of zinc supplementation on the incidence of malaria, possibly because the community-based design led to early treatment and illness definitions that may not have reflected clinically important malaria (Müller et al., 2001). In addition, zinc has not been shown to be efficacious in treatment of *pf* malaria (Zinc Against Plasmodium Study Group, 2002).

Given the mounting body of evidence showing that adequate zinc nutriture can reduce the incidence and intensity of infections, it is plausible that child mortality could be reduced by preventing even "mild" zinc deficiency through supplementation or dietary enhancement, including fortification. Several trials have provided evidence suggesting that zinc supplementation may lead to a large reduction in child mortality. One trial in full-term small-for-gestational-age Indian infants, who received daily zinc supplements from 1 to 9 months of age, found a reduction by two-thirds in deaths in the group compared to infants receiving a control supplement without zinc (Sazawal et al., 2001). Large randomized controlled trials of zinc supplementation in preschool children were also conducted in Pemba, Zanzibar, and Nepal (Sazawal et al., 2007; Tielsch & Khatry et al., 2007). Although neither trial showed a benefit of zinc in children 1 to 11 months of age, both trials found a similar 18% reduction in mortality in older children (combined result relative risk = 0.82; 95% CI: 0.70–0.96).

In a large trial in Bangladesh, 50% fewer deaths were noted in preschool-aged children who received a zinc supplement along with oral rehydration therapy for diarrhea compared to children receiving oral rehydration alone (Baqui et al., 2002). Another large effectiveness trial in India found that zinc given for diarrhea treatment reduced hospitalizations for diarrhea (odds ratio = 0.69; 95% CI: 0.50–0.95) and pneumonia (odds ratio = 0.29; 95% CI: 0.15–0.54) (Bhandari et al., 2008).

Poor Growth. A recent overview has clarified the extent and type of growth response that may occur when prepubescent children are given zinc on a daily basis. Thirty-three controlled trials were included in a meta-analysis that examined the effect of giving children younger than 12 years doses of 1 to 20 mg zinc daily for periods ranging from 8 weeks to 15 months (mean of approximately 7 months) (Brown, Peerson, Rivera, & Allen, 2002). Differences in ponderal and linear growth were expressed as an "effect size" ([mean change in treatment group − mean change in control group] ÷ pooled standard deviation of the difference between groups), weighted by sample size, expressed as a standard deviation. The analysis revealed modest but statistically significant increases in weight (0.31 SD, $p < 0.001$) and height (0.35 SD, $p < 0.0001$), with larger effects seen for weight in children with lower weight for age and for height/length in more stunted children (Brown et al., 2002).

Zinc supplementation has, in some settings, also increased tricipital skinfold size (Kikafunda et al., 1998), mid-upper arm circumference (Cavan et al., 1993; Kikafunda et al., 1998), and lean body mass, supporting a role for zinc in maintaining body composition.

Reproductive Health. Zinc is required for normal maternal health, fetal growth, and development and parturition (Caulfield, Zavaleta, Shankar, & Merialdi, 1998). Although experimental zinc deficiency leads to poor pregnancy outcomes (Apgar, 1985; Bunce, Lytton, Gunesekera, Vessal, & Kim, 1994), the evidence linking human maternal zinc deficiency to intrauterine growth retardation, prematurity, low birth weight, and complications at delivery is inconsistent (Tamura, Goldenberg, Johnston, & Dubard, 2000). Several trials have reported that maternal zinc supplementation leads to modest increases (approximately 0.5 week) in length of gestation (Caulfield et al., 1998; Cherry et al., 1989; Garg, Singhla, & Arshad, 1993; Goldenberg et al., 1995; Kynast & Saling, 1986; Ross, Nel, & Naeye, 1985) and improved birth weight (Garg et al., 1993; Goldenberg et al., 1995). Other studies carried out in low-income countries have failed to find any effect on newborn size attributable to this intervention (Caulfield, Zavaleta, Figueroa, & Leon, 1999; Fawzi et al., 2005; Osendarp et al., 2000; Ross et al., 1985).

A recent meeting to review the consequences of maternal zinc deficiency concluded that the evidence is conflicting regarding its relationship with labor or delivery complications, gestational age at birth, birth weight, and fetal development (Osendarp, West, & Black, 2003). However, more subtle relationships may exist, such as improved fetal neurobehavioral development following maternal zinc supplementation (Merialdi, Caulfield, Zavaleta, Figueroa, & DiPietro, 1998).

Zinc also plays a known role in mammalian cell differentiation and turnover, ontogeny of mammalian systems, and thymic and other lymphoid tissue development and function (Cousins & Hempe, 1990). These effects could, for example, predispose individuals deprived of essential zinc in utero to permanent impairment in immunity and host resistance (Beach, Gershwin, & Hurley, 1982). Evidence from trials of zinc supplementation in pregnancy supports a beneficial effect on neonatal and infant infectious disease morbidity (Osendarp et al., 2001).

Prevention

The ubiquitous role of zinc in nature and its potential to affect many facets of health make zinc deficiency one of the most compelling of all micronutrient deficiencies to address. Yet little has been done to prevent zinc deficiency to date. Prevention strategies could employ dietary, fortification, supplementary, and agricultural approaches. Excellent sources of bioavailable zinc include red meat, liver and other organ meats, poultry, shellfish, eggs, and milk. These foods often contribute less than 10% of dietary zinc among low-income populations (Gibson & Ferguson, 1998b).

The adequacy of dietary zinc depends on both its quantity and its bioavailability, with the latter being a function of the presence of compounds in foods that inhibit absorption of zinc. These compounds include phytates, which is found abundantly in whole-grain cereals and legumes; dietary fiber; oxalates; polyphenols; and other binding compounds (Oberleas & Harland, 1981; Solomons, 1999). A dietary phytate-to-zinc molar ratio of more than 15 (Gibson, 1990), which is common in many traditional diets in low- and middle-income countries (Ferguson et al., 1993), has been associated with low zinc status (WHO, 1996b). Phytates may be reduced in some whole grains (e.g., wheat, rice, and sorghum) by milling that can remove the phytate-rich aleurone layer, or by methods that induce enzymatic (phytase) hydrolysis of phytic acid, thereby disabling its ability to complex with zinc in the gut (Lonnerdal, Sandberg, Sandstrom, & Kunz, 1989). The latter methods include soaking of cereals or legumes, and germination and fermentation of cereals and related products (Gibson, Yeudall, Drost, Mtitimuni, & Cullinan, 1998)— methods that are easily applied in rural areas. Plant breeding strategies may provide new generations of staple crops in the future that increase zinc and decrease phytic acid content, while enhancing yield (Gibson & Ferguson, 1998b; Graham, Ascher, & Hynes, 1992; Ruel & Bouis, 1998).

Fortification, either with zinc alone, but more likely along with other micronutrients, offers promise as processed staple grains and other food commodities increasingly penetrate low-income markets (Brown, Hambidge, Ranum, & Zinc Fortification Working Group, 2010). Micronutrient premixes containing zinc have been proposed for complementary and special transitional foods for children in refugee settings (Gibson & Ferguson, 1998b) based on estimated needs of infants and young (Brown, Dewey, & Allen, 1998). Direct supplementation offers the most immediate approach for improving the zinc status of mothers and children, most probably in combination with other micronutrients.

The extensive evidence that zinc supplementation started during diarrhea can reduce the severity of that episode and the incidence of subsequent episodes has led to a joint recommendation from WHO and UNICEF (2004) that zinc be used to treat all episodes of watery diarrhea and dysentery. Implementation of this recommendation has been slow but has recently been accelerating (Fischer Walker, Fontaine, et al., 2009).

Multiple Micronutrient Deficiencies

While the nutrient deficiencies covered in the preceding sections have been most extensively studied and individual interventions for them tested and scaled up, the occurrence of multiple, concurrent nutrient deficiencies beyond these four have become increasingly apparent as a public health problem. For example, in a population of Nepali pregnant women, only 14% had a single biochemical nutrient deficiency among 14 vitamins and minerals assessed; 82% had two or more deficiencies; and 18% had five or more concurrent deficiencies. Only 4% were free of deficiencies among the nutrients measured (Jiang et al., 2005). Multiple maternal deficiencies have been similarly reported from populations in India (Pathak et al., 2004). In Cambodia, 44% of stunted children aged 6 to 36 months were reported to have at least two deficiencies, and 10% were deficient in all three of the nutrients measured (zinc, iron, and vitamin A), suggesting the existence of a latent, multiply deficient population. A recent survey in Vietnam reported that 80% of children 1 to 6 years of age had two or more micronutrient deficiencies (Van Nhien et al., 2008). These studies provide a few plausible examples of multiple nutrient deficiencies likely coexisting in large proportions of generally undernourished populations where dietary quality, quantity, and diversity may be limited.

In contexts such as these, the efficacy of any single micronutrient intervention may be constrained by other concurrent deficiencies. Recognizing this

fact, interest has grown in interventions that could deliver multiple micronutrients to achieve potentially cost-effective prevention. Drawbacks of this strategy include public health workers' limited abilities to assess multiple micronutrient deficiencies, their nutrient–nutrient interactive effects on health, and their dietary determinants. These challenges have led to approaches that have assumed (a) multiple deficiencies exist where one or a few have been described in a population, (2) dietary deficits are uniformly the equivalent of an approximate recommended dietary allowance for all nutrients and individuals, and (3) multiple nutrients delivered via a single vehicle, whether a multiply fortified food or a multiple-nutrient supplement, are equivalent in efficacy to those nutrients that are distributed across several foods and beverages within typical meal patterns. Increased attention to developing concurrent, multiple micronutrient deficiency interventions and effective dietary assessment systems would, in the future, enable more informed and possibly effective public health multinutrient strategies in the future.

Prevention

Multiple nutrient deficiencies can be prevented through attempts to (1) diversify the diet to assure variety and quality and (2) fortify one or more foods with multiple nutrients, either during processing or at the point of consumption (e.g., home or school) or supplement populations with multiple-nutrient tablets. Interventions aimed at diversifying diets via small-scale agriculture and small-animal production have been implemented to a limited extent in a number of settings with promising results (Leroy & Frongillo, 2007). To date, they have proved difficult to implement and sustain at larger scales, limiting their ability to effectively improve micronutrient status at the population level (Bhutta et al., 2008). Multiple-nutrient fortification and supplementation have been variously tested in children and women of reproductive age.

Child Multiple-Micronutrient Interventions. Several supplement vehicles have been developed to deliver multiple micronutrients to infants and young children. These measures have included "foodlet" products, consisting of small dispersible tablets that can be crushed and dissolved in water or food; micronutrient powders contained in single-serving sachets that can be mixed into food; and fortified food supplements, which contain micronutrients plus protein, energy, and essential fatty acids.

The effects on child growth of a home-based micronutrient foodlet that is added to meals has been tested in a four-country trial, with the packet being given as either a daily or a weekly supplement, and compared to a placebo or iron alone (Smuts et al., 2005). Infants who received the daily micronutrient supplement gained the most weight among all intervention groups—a mean of 207 g per month compared to 186 g per month in the placebo foodlet group (a statistically significant difference). The daily supplement was also most effective in controlling anemia and iron, zinc, and riboflavin deficiencies. Provision of supplemental iron alone increased the prevalence of zinc deficiency compared to the placebo group, an outcome not observed in either of the multiple-micronutrient-recipient groups, and one of many findings in such studies that illustrate the potential for interactions that require further study.

Fortifying food products with multiple micronutrients has been shown to produce positive outcomes in children. For example, in Vietnam, school children randomized to receive a multiple-micronutrient-fortified biscuit 5 days a week for 4 months experienced 44%, 48%, and 47% reductions in their risks of anemia, zinc deficiency, and iodine deficiency, respectively, compared to children receiving a nonfortified biscuit (Nga et al., 2009). In Ghana, a fortified complementary food recipe of maize, soybean, and groundnut reduced the prevalence rates of vitamin A deficiency from approximately 34% to 10% and the rates of serum hypoferritinemia from 18% to 11% over a 6-month period (Lartey et al., 1999). In comparison, the prevalence of both vitamin A and iron deficiencies increased over the same period in a nonrandom, parallel control group who received a traditional infant porridge.

A meta-analysis examined the effect of combining multiple micronutrients with iron in improving growth, nutritional status, and mental and motor development in children (Allen, Peerson, & Olney, 2009). Overall, multiple-micronutrient supplementation was found to improve height and weight in young children. In addition, there was a 0.39 (95% CI: 0.25–0.53) standard deviation increase in mean hemoglobin concentration and a 10% to 40% reduction in the prevalence of anemia with multiple-micronutrient supplementation. The effect size was significantly larger when the micronutrients were delivered via a fortified food product. Four trials have reported effects of supplementation on child motor development, all of which suggested that multiple-micronutrient supplementation produced significant improvements in motor and mental development (Allen et al., 2009). A separate meta-analysis concluded that multiple-micronutrient supplementation had no significant effect on cognitive performance in children; in this analysis, the researchers reviewed 20 studies, the majority of which were conducted among children 5 to 16 years of age (Eilander et al., 2010). However, it is possible that the critical period for brain development, during which time micronutrients might be expected to have their largest impact, might occur earlier in life.

Maternal Multiple-Micronutrient Interventions. WHO currently recommends that women consume an iron + folic acid supplement daily during pregnancy. In addition, there has been interest in providing a multiple-micronutrient supplement that might potentially alleviate multiple deficiencies at minimal added cost to the currently recommended supplement regimen. For this reason, multiple-micronutrient supplements have been tested in a number of settings where micronutrient deficiencies are likely to coexist.

In recent years, a series of meta-analyses have reviewed the overall effects of the multiple-micronutrient supplements on maternal anemia and micronutrient status (Allen & Peerson, 2009), size at birth and length of gestation (Fall, Fisher, Osmond, Margetts, 2009), and neonatal mortality (Ronsmans et al., 2009). Across the 12 countries studied in the meta-analysis, researchers found an overall 11% reduction in the risk of low birth weight, but no effect on other measures of size at birth, such as length, head circumference, or arm circumference (Figure 6-18) (Fall et al., 2009). There appeared to be no overall difference in pregnancy duration, suggesting that the increase in birth weight was due to improved fetal growth rather than a longer duration of gestation (Fall et al., 2009). In the pooled analyses, no statistically significant effect on the risk of stillbirth, neonatal mortality, or perinatal mortality was found with multiple-micronutrient supplementation, although a worrisome suggestion of increased mortality risk in the early neonatal period was noted (Ronsmans et al., 2009). Little evidence was found to support the idea that such supplementation might provide a greater reduction in iron deficiency or anemia in the groups who received the multiple-micronutrient supplements compared to those who received iron + folic acid alone (Allen & Peerson, 2009).

To date, only one study has examined the effects of a multiple-micronutrient supplement on changes in micronutrient status in women. Pregnant women in Nepal who received the multiple-micronutrient supplement were found to have improved plasma levels of vitamin B_6, vitamin B_{12}, riboflavin, 25-hydroxyvitamin D, and zinc relative to the controls (Christian et al., 2006).

A few trials have followed children born to randomly supplemented mothers in trials beyond the

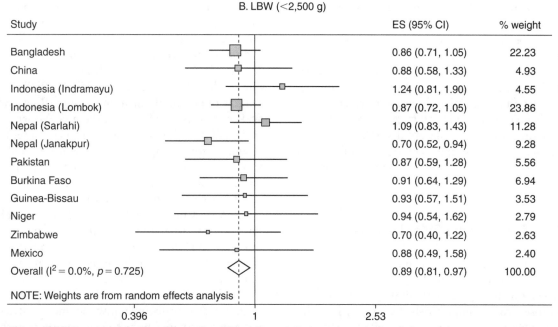

Figure 6-18 Forest plot for the effects of multiple micronutrient supplementation during pregnancy compared to controls on the risk of low birth weight. Individual (in gray boxes) and Pooled (in open diamond) Odds Ratios and 95% Confidence Intervals Are Shown.
Source: Fall, C.H., Fisher, D.J., Osmond, C., Margetts, B.M. (2009). Multiple micronutrient supplementation during pregnancy in low-income countries: a meta-analysis of effects on birth size and length of gestation. Food and Nutrition Bulletin, 30(4). S540, figure 3 B. LBW (<2,500 g) (Random-effects model forest plots for effects of MMN...)

neonatal period to look at plausible long-term health effects of supplementation. Data from a randomized trial in Nepal reported that children whose mothers had received a multiple-micronutrient supplement during pregnancy were 204 g heavier (95% CI: 27–381), and had larger head, chest, and arm circumferences relative to controls at 2.5 years of age (Vaidya et al., 2008). Children born to women in the intervention group also had a mean systolic blood pressure that was 2.5 mm Hg lower (95% CI: 0.47–4.55) than the corresponding pressure in controls. In a separate, nearby trial, Nepalese children gestationally exposed to iron + folic acid + zinc supplementation via antenatal receipt registered a modest improvement in linear growth by 6 to 8 years of age, although the effect did not appear to derive from the multiple-micronutrient supplement, which also contained iron, folic acid, and zinc (Stewart et al., 2009). Importantly, there was a reduced risk of early kidney dysfunction, represented by a urinary microalbumin:creatinine ratio of more than 3.4 mg/mmol, in children born to mothers who were supplemented antenatally with folic acid (compared to children

whose mothers did not reach such supplements), reflected by an odds ratio of 0.64 (95% CI: 0.45–0.92). This effect was comparable among children in all maternal micronutrient-recipient groups whose supplements contained folic acid. In addition, folic acid may have reduced the risk of early childhood cardiovascular disease in the children of supplement-recipient mothers (Stewart et al., 2009). In Peru, researchers found that maternal iron + folic acid + zinc supplementation was associated with greater weight, calf, and chest circumference through 12 months of age compared to supplementation with just iron + folic acid (Iannotti et al., 2008).

There is still evolving evidence about possible long-term effects on offspring morbidity and mortality associated with antenatal multiple-micronutrient use in pregnancy. In Peru (Iannotti et al., 2010) and Bangladesh (Osendarp et al., 2001), maternal supplementation with iron + folic acid + zinc reduced the risk of diarrheal illness in infants through 6 to 12 months of age. In contrast, a study in Nepal found no evidence of differences in morbidity among 6-week-old infants whose mothers had received iron + folic acid + zinc or a multiple-micronutrient supplement during pregnancy (Christian, Darmstadt, et al., 2008), suggesting either no effect or a study design that assessed infants too early in life (i.e., prior to the age of complementary food introduction, when infants begin to be especially susceptible to diarrheal illness). While the findings are inconsistent, some emerging evidence from randomized trials suggests that there are long-lasting benefits of maternal single- and combined-micronutrient supplementation on child health and survival outcomes well beyond the neonatal period.

Malnutrition Among Older Persons

A largely unrecognized group at high risk of undernutrition has been the rapidly growing segment of older persons (age greater than 60 years), particularly those living in impoverished settings where deteriorating health, strength, and capability are further stressed by the need to continue economically supporting themselves. Aging in such populations is often accompanied by decreased access to resources that are essential to maintain a minimum standard of quality of life, including adequate food, health and dental care, social and welfare services, and family support. As life expectancy continues to increase (Roubenoff, 2000; World Bank, 1993), the number of older persons will increase. By 2025, the world's older population is expected to exceed 1.2 billion, two-thirds of whom will live in low- and middle-income countries (ACC/SCN, 2000).

Undernutrition, due to coexisting primary deficiencies and secondarily to chronic disease, is believed to be common among older urban and rural people in poor societies. For example, survey data obtained from periurban slums of Mumbai, India (ACC/SCN, 2000), and rural villages of Malawi (Chilima & Ismail, 1998) indicate that 25% to 35% of free-living older persons in these areas are in a chronic state of acute undernourishment, reflected by a low body mass index (less than 18.5 kg/m^2). In a survey from rural Bangladesh, an estimated 26% of adults older than 60 years were undernourished, a factor that was significantly associated with impaired cognitive performance (Ferdous, Cederholm, Kabir, Hamadani, & Wahlin, 2010).

An undernutrition–chronic disease interaction likely exists among older persons, both originating in poverty and its determinants. Specific age-related disorders that may be exacerbated by malnutrition and disease, and likely to be of public health importance, are sarcopenia (loss of muscle mass and strength) with consequent muscle weakness, impaired mobility, and body function (Kehayias, Fiatarone, Zhuang, & Roubenoff, 1997; Roubenoff, 2000); osteoporosis with resultant bone fracture risk (Wark, 1999); and dementias of potential nutritional origin (Riggs, Spiro, Tucker, & Rush, 1996; Rosenberg & Miller, 1992; Tucker, 2000). Sarcopenia is a universal consequence of aging, with a complex etiology (Roubenoff, 2000); however, inadequate energy and protein intakes can lead to sustained negative nitrogen balance that, over time, can be an important factor in accelerated muscle loss (Kamel, 2003). Osteoporosis (loss of bone mass) may be attributable in part to chronic calcium and vitamin D insufficiency (Peacock, 1998), where a low intake is especially likely among women (Islam, Lamberg-Allardt, Karkkainen, & Ali, 2003).

Undernutrition among older persons appears to be an immense problem in low-income countries. Its magnitude provides public health workers with the impetus to estimate the extent, types, and severity of nutritional deficiencies and related disabilities and diseases in this age group; to understand causal pathways, including those that may originate early in life; and to identify resources that may better enable healthy aging.

The Nutrition Transition

The nutrition transition encompasses a series of demographic, social, and economic changes in low- and middle-income countries that have occurred over the past few decades, resulting in rapid shifts in dietary patterns and lifestyle (Cabellero & Popkin, 2002; Popkin, 1994). In turn, these changes have led to increasing prevalences of obesity, type 2 diabetes, and cardiovascular disease (Adair, 2002; Popkin, 1998) (see Chapter 7). WHO (2005) has estimated that chronic diseases account for 60% of all deaths around the world, with 80% of this mortality occurring in developing countries. Moreover, age-standardized mortality rates from chronic disease are more than 50% higher in developing countries than in developed countries (Abegunde et al., 2007).

Key elements driving the nutrition transition include improvements in communications (changing influences on eating and lifestyle), transportation (wider distribution of processed foods), income (spending more on foods and fast foods consumed outside the home), and a sedentary lifestyle. The nutrition transition can be documented in virtually every region of the world, including Latin America (Monteiro, Conde, & Popkin, 2002; Uauy, Ablbal, & Kain, 2001), northern Africa (Mokhtar et al., 2001), and China (Du et al., 2002). As discussed in this section, the resulting global profile is one in which large numbers of underweight individuals (200 million people, mostly children) co-exist with increasing numbers of overweight individuals (more than 1.6 billion people aged 15 and older).

Demographic Trends

The slowing of population growth that started several decades ago is now being manifested by a reduction in the size of the younger population and a continuing increase in the size of the older population (Zlotnik, 2002). As a consequence, an increasing proportion of the world's population is entering into those life stages where chronic diseases are more prevalent (see Chapter 1).

A second key demographic trend is urbanization. By 2025, the majority of the world's population is expected to reside in an urban area of a low- or middle-income country (Zlotnik, 2002). The urban environment affects dietary intake, physical activity, and ultimately energy balance. Some of the most energy-demanding survival activities of rural life, such as securing water and firewood, are minimal or nonexistent in the urban environment. Urban employment is predominantly sedentary—for example, office or service work. Globalization and the Internet have permitted higher-income countries to outsource many service jobs to the cheaper labor force of low- and middle-income countries (e.g., data processing, transcription, archiving). The use of mechanized transport and centralized public services also reduce energy spent on commuting to and from work. In addition, dietary energy availability and consumption tend to be higher in the urban world than in the rural environment, such that urban residents are likely to consume higher amounts of calories derived from saturated fat and refined sugars (Popkin, 1999). These conditions of increased energy intake and reduced energy output facilitate a positive energy balance and excess weight gain.

Dietary Trends

The FAO projects that per capita dietary energy production will continue to rise over the next 20 years (see Table 6-1). These estimates also anticipate a continuing increase in the contribution of fats (vegetable oils) to total caloric intake. Modest increases in meat

availability and a decline in cereal consumption are predicted as well (FAO, 2002). One interesting characteristic of this global dietary profile is that energy-dense foods, primarily due to their fat/oil content, have become widely available throughout low- and middle-income countries, usually at a relatively low price. Studies in China, for example, have shown that the rapid increase in vegetable oil consumption over the past two decades occurred equally in low- and high-income subpopulations (Ng, Zhai, & Popkin, 2008).

Consumption of caloric beverages has increased dramatically over the past decades throughout the world. In the United States, such "soft drinks" account for approximately 10% of daily calories consumed (Wang, Bleich, & Gortmaker, 2008), with similar figures being tallied in Mexico (Rivera et al., 2008). Disappearance data for sugar (i.e., the turnover of sugar stocks for a country in a given year) also show a continuing rise in consumption of caloric beverages, which have become one of the major contributors to worldwide sugar consumption (Malik, Popkin, Bray, Després, & Hu, 2010). The link between caloric beverage consumption and excess weight gain has been established in several studies (Chen et al., 2009; Schulze et al., 2004). In addition, some evidence shows that consumption of such beverages may increase an individual's risk of developing type 2 diabetes (Schulze et al., 2004).

Global production of soy, palm, and rapeseed oils rose to more than 70 million metric tons by 1996, while production of animal fat remained essentially unchanged over the same period (Popkin & Gordon-Larsen, 2004; Smil, 2002). Cultural perceptions, advertisements, and the search for convenience have also increased consumption of prepared ("fast") foods, including prepackaged foods that may have higher content of refined sugars (Drewnowski & Popkin, 1997; USDA Economic Research Service, 2001).

Notwithstanding the global epidemiologic characteristics of this transitional phenomenon, especially in lower-income sectors of lower- and middle-income countries (Blakely, Hales, Kieft, Wilson, & Woodward, 2005; Monteiro, Moura, Conde, & Popkin, 2004), obesity as a consequence of developmental and urban transition is not a "fait accompli." Consider South Korea, which has undergone a transition over the past 30 years. In this country, there has been an increase in the prevalence of adult overweight status but not obesity, attributed to retained dietary elements of high cereal grain (rice) and vegetable intakes in the population (Popkin, Horton, & Kim, 2001).

"Dual Burden" of Countries in Transition

In the early stages of the nutrition transition, obesity tends to increase first in the higher-income groups of the population. As income improves, however, the burden of obesity begins to switch toward the poor. A typical example of this trend can be seen in Brazil (Monteiro et al., 2004). This phenomenon is also illustrated by the relative risks of obesity among women by quartile of education within a series of studies across 37 developing countries (Figure 6-19). Indeed, low-income countries (e.g., those with a gross national product [GNP] per capita of less than $800 per year) generally have a low overall prevalence of obesity, because food scarcity and relatively high levels of physical activity may prevent accumulation of a surplus energy in the form of body fat. At the other end of the spectrum, upper-middle-income countries (GNP per capita of approximately $2,000 per year) show highest obesity rates in the lower-income groups.

Because many low- to middle-income countries have yet to eradicate chronic undernutrition as a public health problem, they exhibit a unique situation in which undernutrition and overnutrition often coexist within the same population group and even within the same family (Doak, Adair, Moneiro, & Popkin, 2000; Garrett & Ruel, 2003). Some estimates indicate that in some Eastern Asian and Western Pacific countries, as many as 60% of the households have at least one overweight member and one underweight member—frequently an obese mother with an underweight or stunted child (Popkin et al., 2001). This phenomenon has been termed the "dual burden" of populations in nutrition transition (Doak, Adair, Bentley, Monteiro, & Popkin, 2005).

Early Origins of Chronic Diseases and the Nutrition Transition

Observations on the impact of fetal growth and birth weight on the prevalence of diabetes and cardiovascular disease in adult life have prompted much inquiry into the effects of early nutritional factors on adult disease (Barker, 2004; Cheung, Low, Osmond, Barker, & Karlberg, 2000; Eriksson et al., 1999; Forsen et al., 2000). The "Barker hypothesis," also known as the "developmental origins of health and disease" hypothesis, proposes that undernutrition at different phases of intrauterine and postnatal growth results in an increased risk for certain noncommunicable chronic diseases in adulthood. Possible mechanisms have been explored in animal models, and point to developmental responses to stress (e.g., inadequate nutrient supply) at critical points of molecular signaling and cellular differentiation as playing a role in

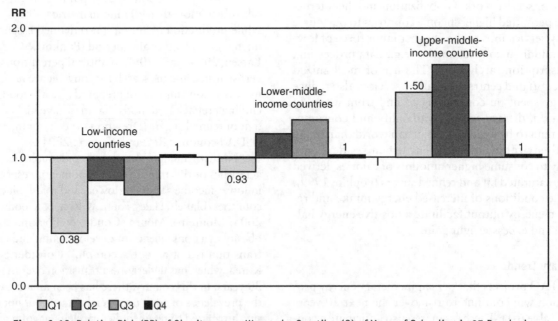

Figure 6-19 Relative Risk (RR) of Obesity among Women by Quartiles (Q) of Years of Schooling in 37 Developing (Low Income) Countries, 1992–2002.
Source: C.A. Monteiro, W.L. Conde, and B.M. Popkin, "Trends in Under- and Overnutrition in Brazil," in B. Caballero & B.M. Popkin (Eds.), The Nutrition Transition: Diet and Disease in the Developing World, Food Science and Technology International Series (London: Academic Press, 2002), pp. 224–140. Reprinted with permission.

this relationship. These responses, while needed for survival, may result in permanent changes in metabolic or regulatory systems, which later in life may prove disadvantageous (Caballero, 2006; Christian & Stewart, 2010).

For example, a restriction in energy availability to the fetus may trigger differentiation of systems in a way that would maximize energy conservation and glucose uptake. This irreversible adaptive response would become a maladaptation when this individual is exposed, as an adult, to an abundant supply of dietary energy, and would favor the development of obesity or type 2 diabetes (Eriksson et al., 1999; Forsen et al., 2000). In addition, deficiencies in micronutrients at critical stages of embryonic or fetal development may lead to alterations in the development of key hormonal regulatory pathways, the development of organ systems, or the regulation of gene expression through epigenetic pathways (Christian & Stewart, 2010).

Studies have also focused on the effects of transitions in growth velocity during childhood (i.e., slow to fast, or vice versa) on the programming of metabolic systems related to body fat accumulation and distribution, insulin sensitivity, and vascular tone (Martorell, Stein, & Schroeder, 2001; Schroeder, Martorell, & Flores, 1999; Susser & Stein, 1994). In developing countries, recent cohort studies in Brazil, Guatemala, India, South Africa, and the Philippines have illustrated that rapid weight gain in childhood is associated with elevated blood pressure in adulthood, but only to the extent that it also predicted higher BMI (Adair et al., 2009; Victora et al., 2008). Weight gain in the early childhood period did not pose any greater risk than weight gain at later ages. In Brazil, children who gained weight rapidly after the age of 20 months, but not before 20 months, had significantly lower high-density lipoprotein (HDL) cholesterol and a higher low-density lipoprotein (LDL)/HDL ratio in adolescence (Horta, Victora, Lima, & Post, 2009).

Across studies, it appears that increase in height may have no association or be protective relative to chronic disease, whereas increase in weight or BMI may be a risk factor for later adverse outcomes (Stein, Thompson, & Waters, 2005). The implications of these phenomena for low- and middle-income countries are obvious. Because of the high prevalence of impaired fetal and early postnatal growth, combined with the rapidly developing obesity epidemic in many countries, low- and middle-income countries could have large proportions of their populations at increased risk for noncommunicable diseases in adulthood.

In summary, diet-related chronic diseases are increasing at a fast pace in the developing world, particularly in middle-income countries. The major factors fueling this increase are population trends that feature an increasing number of individuals reaching older adult age; urbanization with its associated changes in diet patterns and lifestyle; changes in food availability, price, and choices leading to increases in total and fat-derived energy intake; and an increasingly sedentary lifestyle in some sectors, with consequent reduction in daily energy expenditure. These factors have already resulted in dramatic shifts in the disease burden of the urban poor, who in many middle-income countries are now bearing the dual costs of undernutrition plus obesity. WHO (2004), in collaboration with other agencies and nongovernmental organizations, has formulated a global strategy to confront the health effects of the nutrition transition. This initiative has been followed up with an implementation plan endorsed by numerous countries, an encouraging sign that obesity and related chronic diseases may be finally being recognized as major threats to the health of developing nations.

● ● ● Discussion Questions

1. The same population may be affected by multiple micronutrient deficiencies, although people at different life stages and certain socioeconomic or geographic groups may be more vulnerable to individual nutrient deficiencies. Discuss ways in which single-micronutrient deficiency prevention strategies might be combined, integrated, or coordinated to achieve cost-effective control.

2. A lower-middle-income country may be afflicted with both high rates of childhood undernutrition and a rising epidemic of obesity among its lower socioeconomic groups while undergoing a nutrition transition. Discuss the challenges that this situation poses for the country's government in developing food and nutrition policies as well as national dietary guidelines for healthy eating.

3. The Ministry of Health of a lower-income country has decided to institute a national nutrition surveillance system to monitor the country's most pressing child and maternal nutrition problems. Discuss the kinds of nutritional problems, target groups, approaches to assessment, options for routine contact in the community, and types of agencies to organize into a surveillance system to guide the ministry.

• • • References

Abegunde, D. O., Mathers, C. D., Adam, T., Ortegon, M., & Strong, K. (2007). The burden and costs of chronic diseases in low-income and middle-income countries. *Lancet, 370,* 1929–1938.

Adair, L. S. (2002). Early nutrition conditions and later risk of disease. In B. Caballero & B. M. Popkin (Eds.), *The nutrition transition: Diet and disease in the developing world* (pp. 129–145). London: Academic Press.

Adair, L. S., Martorell, R., Stein, A. D., Hallal, P. C., Sachdev, H. S., Prabhakaran, D., et al. (2009). Size at birth, weight gain in infancy and childhood, and adult blood pressure in 5 low- and middle-income-country cohorts: When does weight gain matter? *American Journal of Clinical Nutrition, 89,* 1383–1392.

Adair, L., Popkin, B. M., Van Derslice, J., Akin, J., Guilkey, D., Black, R., et al. (1993). Growth dynamics during the first two years of life: A prospective study in the Philippines. *European Journal of Clinical Nutrition, 47,* 42–51.

Adams, E. J., Stephenson, L. S., Latham, M. C., & Kinoti, S. N. (1994). Physical activity and growth of Kenyan school children with hookworm: *Trichuris trichiura* and *Ascaris lumbricoides* infections are improved after treatment with albendazole. *Journal of Nutrition, 124,* 1199–1206.

Administrative Committee on Coordination/Sub-Committee on Nutrition (ACC/SCN). (2000). *Fourth report on the world nutrition situation: Nutrition throughout the life cycle.* Washington, DC: International Food Policy Research Institute.

Adu-Afarwuah, S., Lartey, A., Brown, K. H., Zlotkin, S., Briend, A., & Dewey, K. G. (2007). Randomized comparison of 3 types of micronutrient supplements for home fortification of complementary foods in Ghana: Effects on growth and motor development. *American Journal of Clinical Nutrition, 86,* 412–420.

Aggarwal, R., Sentz, J., & Miller, M.A. (2007). Role of zinc administration in prevention of childhood diarrhea and respiratory illnesses: A meta-analysis. *Pediatrics, 119,* 1120–1130.

Akesson, A., Bjellerup, P., Berglund, M., Bremme, K., & Vahter, M. (1998). Serum transferrin receptor: A specific marker of iron deficiency in pregnancy. *American Journal of Clinical Nutrition, 68,* 1241–1246.

Albonico, M., Stoltzfus, R. J., Savioli, L., Tielsch, J. M., Chwaya, H. M., Ercole, E., & Cancrini, G. (1998). Epidemiological evidence for a differential effect of hookworm species, *Ancylostoma duodenale* or *Necator americanus,* on iron status of children. *International Journal of Epidemiology, 27,* 530–537.

Alderman, H. (2010). Safety nets can help address the risks to nutrition from increasing climate variability. *Journal of Nutrition, 140,* 148S–152S.

Algarin, C., Peirano, P., Garrido, M., Pizarro, F., & Lozoff, B. (2003). Iron deficiency anemia in infancy: Long-lasting effects on auditory and visual system functioning. *Pediatric Research, 53,* 217–223.

Allen, L. H. (1997). Pregnancy and iron deficiency: Unresolved issues. *Nutrition Reviews, 55,* 91–101.

Allen, L. H., & Peerson, J. M. (2009). Impact of multiple micronutrient versus iron–folic acid supplements on maternal anemia and micronutrient status in pregnancy. *Food and Nutrition Bulletin, 30*(4), S527–S532.

Allen, L. H., Peerson, J. M., & Olney, D.K. (2009). Provision of multiple rather than two or fewer micronutrients more effectively improves growth and other outcomes in micronutrient-deficient children and adults. *Journal of Nutrition, 139*(5), 1022–1030.

Anabwani, G., & Navario, P. (2005). Nutrition and HIV/AIDS in sub-Saharan Africa: An overview. *Nutrition, 21,* 96–99.

Apgar, J. (1985). Zinc and reproduction. *Annual Review of Nutrition, 5,* 43–68.

Arroyave, G., Mejia, L. A., & Aguilar, J. R. (1981). The effect of vitamin A fortification of sugar on the serum vitamin A levels of preschool Guatemalan children: A longitudinal evaluation. *American Journal of Clinical Nutrition, 34,* 41–49.

Arthur, P., Kirkwood, B., Ross, D., Morris, S., Gyapong, J., Tomkins, A., & Addy, H. (1992).

Impact of vitamin A supplementation on childhood morbidity in northern Ghana. *Lancet, 339,* 361–362.

Ashworth, A. (1998). Effects of intrauterine growth retardation on mortality and morbidity in infants and young children. *European Journal of Clinical Nutrition, 52,* S34–S42.

Ashworth, A., & Feachem, R. G. (1985). Interventions for the control of diarrhoeal diseases among young children: Prevention of low birthweight. *Bulletin of the World Health Organization, 63,* 165–184.

Aukett, M. A., Parks, Y. A., Scott, P. H., & Wharton, B. A. (1986). Treatment with iron increases weight gain and psychomotor development. *Archives of Diseases in Childhood, 61,* 849–857.

Bahl, R., Bhan, M. K., Bhatnagar, S., Black, R. E., Brooks, A., Cuevas, L. E., et al. (2001). Effect of zinc supplementation on clinical course of acute diarrhea. Report of a meeting, New Delhi, 7–8 May 2001. *Journal of Health Population and Nutrition, 19,* 338–346.

Bahl, R., Bhandari, N., Hambidge, K. M., & Bhan, M. K. (1998). Plasma zinc as a predictor of diarrheal and respiratory morbidity in children in an urban slum setting. *American Journal of Clinical Nutrition, 68,* 414S–417S.

Bahl, R., Bhandari, N., Taneja, S., & Bhan, M. K. (1997). The impact of vitamin A supplementation on physical growth of children is dependent on season. *European Journal of Clinical Nutrition, 51,* 26–29.

Banajeh, S. M. (2003). Is 12-monthly vitamin A supplementation of preschool children effective? An observational study of mortality rates for severe dehydrating diarrhea in Yemen. *South African Journal of Clinical Nutrition, 16,* 137–142.

Baqui, A. H., Black, R. E., El Arifee, S., Yunus, M., Chakraborty, J., Ahmed, S., & Vaughan, J. P. (2002). Effect of zinc supplementation started during diarrhea on morbidity and mortality in Bangladeshi children: Community randomized trial. *British Medical Journal, 325,* 1059–1065.

Baqui, A. H., Sack, R. B., Black, R. E., Chowdhury, H. R., Yunus, M., & Siddique, A. K. (1993). Cell-mediated immune deficiency and malnutrition are independent risk factors for persistent diarrhea in Bangladeshi children. *American Journal of Clinical Nutrition, 58,* 543–548.

Bar-Andziak, E., Lazecki, D., Radwanowska, N., & Nauman, J. (1993). Iodine intake and goiter incidence among schoolchildren living in Warsaw region (Warsaw and Ciechanow Voivodships–Warsaw Coordinating Center). *Edokrynologia Polska, 44,* 288–295.

Barclay, A. J. G., Foster, A., & Sommer, A. (1987). Vitamin A supplements and mortality related to measles: A randomised clinical trial. *British Medical Journal, 294,* 294–296.

Barker, D. J. P. (2004). The developmental origins of adult disease. *Journal of the American College of Nutrition, 23,* 588S–595S.

Barker, D. J. P., Osmond, C., Winter, P. D., Margetts, B., & Simmonds, S. J. (1989). Weight in infancy and death from ischaemic heart disease. *Lancet, 2,* 577–580.

Barros, F. C., Victora, C. G., Vaughan, J. P., Teixeira, A. M. B., & Ashworth, A. (1987). Infant mortality in southern Brazil: A population based study of causes of death. *Archives of Diseases in Childhood, 62,* 487–490.

Bates, C. J., Evans, P. H., Dardenne, M., Prentice, A., Lunn, P. G., Northrop-Clewes, C. A., et al. (1993). A trial of zinc supplementation in young rural Gambian children. *Journal of Nutrition, 69,* 243–255.

Beach, R. S., Gershwin, M. E., & Hurley, L. S. (1982). Gestational zinc deprivation in mice: Persistence of immunodeficiency for three generations. *Science, 218,* 469–471.

Beales, P. F. (1997). Anaemia in malaria control: A practical approach. *Annals of Tropical Medicine and Parasitology, 91,* 713–718.

Beard, J. L. (2001). Iron biology in immune function, muscle metabolism and neuronal functioning. *Journal of Nutrition, 131,* 568S–580S.

Beard, J. L. (2008). Why iron deficiency is important in infant development. *Journal of Nutrition, 138,* 2534–2536.

Beaton, G. H., Martorell, R., Aronson, K. J., Edmonston, B., McCabe, G., Ross, A. C., & Harvey, B. (1993). *Effectiveness of vitamin A supplementation in the control of young child morbidity and mortality in developing countries* (ACC/SCN State of the Art Series Nutrition Policy Discussion Paper No. 13). Geneva, Switzerland: Administrative Committee on Coordination/Subcommittee on Nutrition.

Behrens, R. H., Lunn, P. G., Northrop, C. A., Hanlon, P. W., & Neale, G. (1987). Factors affecting the integrity of the intestinal mucosa of Gambian children. *American Journal of Clinical Nutrition, 45,* 1433–1441.

Bhandari, N., Bahl, R., Mazumdar, S., Martines, J., Black, R. E., Bhan, M. K., & Infant Feeding Study Group. (2003). Effect of community-based promotion of exclusive breastfeeding on diarrhoeal illness and growth: A cluster randomised controlled trial. *Lancet, 361,* 1418–1423.

Bhandari, N., Bahl, R., Taneja, S., Strand, T., Molbak, K., Ulvik, R. J., et al. (2002). Effect of routine zinc supplementation on pneumonia in children aged 6 months to 3 years: Randomized controlled trial in an urban slum. *British Medical Journal, 324,* 1358–1361.

Bhandari, N., Bhan, M. K., & Sazawal, S. (1992). Mortality associated with acute watery diarrhea, dysentery, and persistent diarrhea in rural north India. *Acta Paediatrica Supplement, 381,* 3–6.

Bhandari, N., Mazumder, S., Taneja, S., Dube, B., Agarwal, R. C., Mahalanabis, D., et al. (2008). Effectiveness of zinc supplementation plus oral rehydration salts compared with oral rehydration salts alone as a treatment for acute diarrhea in a primary care setting: A cluster randomized trial. *Pediatrics, 121,* e1279–e1285.

Bhutta, Z. A., Ahmed, T., Black, R. E., Cousens, S., Dewey, K. G., Giugliani, E., et al. (2008). What works? Interventions for maternal and child survival. *Lancet, 371,* 417–440.

Bishai, D., Kumar, K. C. S., Waters, H., Koenig, M., Katz, J., Khatry, S. K., & West, K. P. Jr. (2005). The impact of vitamin A supplementation on mortality inequalities among children in Nepal. *Health Policy and Planning, 20,* 60–66.

Black, R. E. (1993). Persistent diarrhea in children of developing countries. *Pediatric Infectious Diseases Journal, 12,* 751–761.

Black, R. E. (1997). *Zinc for child health: Child Health Research Project special report.* Baltimore, MD: Johns Hopkins University.

Black, R. E. (1998). Therapeutic and preventive effects of zinc on serious childhood infectious diseases in developing countries. *American Journal of Clinical Nutrition, 68,* 476S–479S.

Black, R. E., Allen, L. H., Bhutta, Z. A., Caulfield, L. E., de Onis, M., Ezzati, M., et al. (2008). Maternal and child undernutrition: Global and regional exposures and health consequences. *Lancet, 371,* 243–260.

Black, R. E., Brown, K. H., & Becker, S. (1983). Influence of acute diarrhea on the growth parameters of children. In J. A. Bellanti (Ed.), *Acute diarrhea: Its nutritional consequences* (pp. 75–84). New York: Vevey-Raven Press.

Black, R. E., Brown, K. H., & Becker, S. (1984a). Effects of diarrhea associated with specific enteropathogens on the growth of children in rural Bangladesh. *Pediatrics, 73,* 799–805.

Black, R. E., Brown, K. H., & Becker, S. (1984b). Malnutrition is a determining factor in diarrheal duration, but not incidence, among young children in a longitudinal study in rural Bangladesh. *American Journal of Clinical Nutrition, 39,* 87–94.

Black, R. E., & Victora, C. G. (2002). Optimal duration of exclusive breast feeding in low income countries: Six months as recommended by WHO applies to populations, not necessarily to individuals. *British Medical Journal, 325,* 1252–1253.

Blakely, T., Hales, S., Kieft, C., Wilson, N., & Woodward, A. (2005). The global distribution of risk factors by poverty level. *Bulletin of the World Health Organization, 83,* 118–126.

Bleichrodt, N., & Born, M.P. (1994). A metaanalysis of research on iodine and its relationship to cognitive development. In J. B. Stanbury (Ed.), *The damaged brain of iodine deficiency* (pp. 195–200). New York: Cognizant Communication.

Bloem, M. W., Hye, A., Wijnroks, M., Ralte, A., West, K. P. Jr., & Sommer, A. (1995). The role of universal distribution of vitamin A capsules in combating vitamin A deficiency in Bangladesh. *American Journal of Epidemiology, 142,* 843–855.

Bloem, M. W., Semba, R. D., & Kraemer, K. (2010). Castel Gandolfo Workshop: An introduction to the impact of climate change, the economic crisis, and the increase in the food prices on malnutrition. *Journal of Nutrition, 140,* 132S–135S.

Blomhoff, R., & Blomhoff, H. K. (2006). Overview of retinoid metabolism and function. *Journal of Neurobiology, 66,* 606–630.

Bobat, R., Coovadia, H., Stephen, C., Naidoo, K. L., McKerrow, N., Black, R. E., & Moss, W. J. (2005). Safety and efficacy of zinc supplementation for children with HIV-1 infection in South Africa: A randomized double-blind placebo-controlled trial. *Lancet, 366,* 1862–1867.

Bose, A., Coles, C. L., Gunavathi, J. H., Moses, P., Raghupathy, P., Kirubakaran, C., et al. (2006). Efficacy of zinc in the treatment of severe pneumonia in hospitalized children < 2 y old. *American Journal of Clinical Nutrition, 83,* 1089–1096.

Bothwell, T. H., & Charlton, R. W. (1981). *Iron deficiency in women.* Report for the International Nutritional Anemia Consultative Group (INACG). Washington, DC: Nutrition Foundation.

Bothwell, T. H., Hallberg, L., Clydesdale, F. M., Van Campen, D., Cook, J. D., Wolf, W. J., & Dallman, T. R. (1982, June). *The effects of cereals and legumes on iron bioavailability.* Report for the International Nutritional Anemia Consultative Group (INACG). Washington, DC: Nutrition Foundation.

Bouis, H., & Hunt, J. (1999). Linking food and nutrition security: Past lessons and future opportunities. In J. Hunt & M. G. Quibria (Eds.), *Investing in child nutrition in Asia* (pp. 168–213). Manila: Asia Development Bank.

Boyages, S. C. (1994). The damaged brain of iodine deficiency: Evidence for a continuum of effect on the population at risk. In J. B. Stanbury (Ed.), *The damaged brain of iodine deficiency* (pp. 251–257). New York: Cognizant Communication.

Brabin, B. J., Hakimi, M., & Pelletier, D. (2001). An analysis of anemia and pregnancy-related maternal mortality. *Journal of Nutrition, 131,* 604S–615S.

Brakohiapa, L. A., Bille, A., Wuansah, E., Kishi, K., Yartey, J., Harrison, E., et al. (1988). Does prolonged breastfeeding adversely affect a child's nutritional status? *Lancet, 2,* 416.

Bray, G. A., & Gray, D. S. (1988). Obesity: Part I—Pathogenesis. *Western Journal of Medicine, 149,* 429–441.

Briend, A., & Bari, A. (1989). Breastfeeding improves survival, but not nutritional status, of 12- to 35-months-old children in rural Bangladesh. *European Journal of Clinical Nutrition, 43,* 603–608.

Briend, A., Wojtyniak, B., & Rowland, M. G. M. (1987). Arm circumference and other factors in children at high risk of death in rural Bangladesh. *Lancet, 2,* 725.

Briend, A., Wojtyniak, B., & Rowland, M. G. M. (1988). Breast feeding, nutritional state, and child survival in rural Bangladesh. *British Medical Journal, 296,* 879.

Briend, A., & Zimicki, S. (1986). Validation of arm circumference as an indicator of risk of death in one- to four-year-old children. *Nutrition Research, 6,* 249–261.

Brinkman, H-J., de Pee, S., Sanogo, I., Subran, L., & Bloem, M. W. (2010). High food prices and the global financial crisis have reduced access to nutritious food and worsened nutritional status and health. *Journal of Nutrition, 140,* 153S–161S.

Brooker, S., Peshu, N., Warn, P. A., Mosobo, M., Guyatt, H. L., Marsh, K., & Snow, R.W. (1999). The epidemiology of hookworm infection and its contribution to anaemia among pre-school children on the Kenyan Coast. *Transactions of the Royal Society for Tropical Medical Hygiene, 93,* 240–246.

Brooks, W. A., Santosham, M., Roy, S. K., Faruque, A. S. G., Wahed, M. A., Nahar, K., et al. (2005). Efficacy of zinc in young infants with acute watery diarrhea. *American Journal of Clinical Nutrition, 82,* 605–610.

Brooks, W. A., Yunus, M., Santosham, M., Wahed, M. A., Nahar, K., Yeasmin, S., & Black, R. E. (2004). Zinc for severe pneumonia in very young children: Double-blind placebo-controlled trial. *Lancet, 363,* 1683–1688.

Brown, K. H., Black, R. E., & Becker, S. (1982). Seasonal changes in nutritional status and the prevalence of malnutrition in a longitudinal study of young children in rural Bangladesh. *American Journal of Clinical Nutrition, 36,* 303–313.

Brown, K. H., Black, R. E., Robertson, A. D., & Becker, S. (1985). Effects of season and illness on the dietary intake of weanlings during longitudinal studies in rural Bangladesh. *American Journal of Clinical Nutrition, 41,* 343–355.

Brown, K.H., Dewey, K., & Allen, L. (1998). Complementary feeding of young children in developing countries: A review of current scientific knowledge. WHO/NUT/98. Geneva, Switzerland: World Health Organization.

Brown, K. H., Gastanaduy, A. S., Saavedra, J. M., Lembcke, J., Rivas, D., Robertson, A. D., et al. (1988). Effect of continued oral feeding on clinical and nutritional outcomes of acute diarrhea in children. *Journal of Pediatrics, 112,* 191–200.

Brown, K. H., Gilman, R. H., Gaffar, A., Alamgir, S. M., Strife, J. L., Kapikian, A. Z., & Sack, R. B. (1981). Infections associated with severe protein-calorie malnutrition in hospitalized infants and children. *Nutrition Research, 1,* 33–46.

Brown, K. H., Hambidge, K. M., Ranum P., & Zinc Fortification Working Group. (2010). Zinc fortification of cereal flours: Current recommendations and research needs. *Food and Nutrition Bulletin, 31,* S62–S74.

Brown, K. H., Peerson, J. M., & Allen, L. H. (1998). Effect of zinc supplementation on children's growth: A meta-analysis of intervention trials. *Bibliotheca Nutritio et Dieta, 54,* 76–83.

Brown, K. H., Peerson, J. M., Rivera, J., & Allen, L. H. (2002). Effect of supplemental zinc on the growth and serum zinc concentration of prepubertal children: A meta-analysis of randomized controlled trials. *American Journal of Clinical Nutrition, 75,* 1062–1071.

Brown, K. H., Stallings, R. Y., Creed de Kanashiro, H., Lopez de Romana, G., & Black, R. E. (1990). Effects of common illnesses on infants' energy intakes from breastmilk and other foods during longitudinal community-based studies in Huascar (Lima), Peru. *American Journal of Clinical Nutrition, 52,* 1005–1013.

Bruner, A. B., Joffe, A., Duggan, A. K., Casella, J. F., & Brandt, J. (1996). Randomised study of cognitive effects of iron supplementation in non-anaemic iron-deficient adolescent girls. *Lancet, 348,* 992–996.

Brussard, J. H., Brants, H. A. M., Hulshof, K. F. A. M., Kistemaker, C., & Lowik, M. R. H. (1997). Iodine intake and urinary excretion among adults in the Netherlands. *European Journal of Clinical Nutrition, 51,* S59–S62.

Bukenya, G. B., Barnes, T., & Nwokolo, N. (1991). Low birthweight and acute childhood diarrhoea: Evidence of their association in an urban settlement of Papua New Guinea. *Annals of Tropical Paediatrics, 11,* 357–362.

Bunce, G. E., Lytton, F., Gunesekera, B., Vessal, M., & Kim, C. (1994). Molecular basis for abnormal parturition in zinc deficiency in rats. In L. Allen, J. King, & B. Lonnerdal (Eds.), *Nutrient regulation during pregnancy, lactation, and infant growth* (pp. 209–214). New York: Plenum Press.

Burger, S., & Pierre-Louis, J. (2003). *A procedure to estimate the accuracy and reliability of HemoCue™ measurements of survey workers.* Washington, DC: International Life Sciences Institute.

Butte, N. F. (1996). Energy requirements of infants. *European Journal of Clinical Nutrition, 50,* S24–S36.

Caballero, B. (2006). Obesity as a consequence of undernutrition. *Journal of Pediatrics, 149,* S97–S99.

Caballero, B., & Popkin, B. M. (2002). *The nutrition transition: Diet and disease in the developing world.* Food Science and Technology, International Series. London: Academic Press.

Cameron, N. (1978). The methods of auxological anthropometry. In F. Falkner & J. M. Tanner

(Eds.), *Human growth: A comprehensive treatise. Vol. 3. Methodology, ecological, genetic, and nutritional effects on growth* (2nd ed., pp. 3–46). New York: Plenum Press.

Campbell, D. I., Elia, M., & Lunn, P. G. (2003). Growth faltering in rural Gambian infants is associated with impaired small intestinal barrier function, leading to endotoxemia and systemic inflammation. *Journal of Nutrition, 133*, 1332–1338.

Campos, F. A., Flores, H., & Underwood, B. A. (1987). Effect of an infection on vitamin A status of children as measured by the relative dose response (RDR). *American Journal of Clinical Nutrition, 46*, 91–94.

Caron, P., Hoff, M., Bazzi, S., Dufor, A., Faure, G., Ghandour, I., et al. (1997). Urinary iodine excretion during normal pregnancy in healthy women living in the southwest of France: Correlation with maternal thyroid parameters. *Thyroid, 7*, 749–754.

Castillo, C., Atalah, E., Riumallo, J., & Castro, R. (1996). Breast-feeding and the nutritional status of nursing children in Chile. *Bulletin of the Pan American Health Organization, 30*, 125–132.

Caulfield, L. E., Bentley, M. E., & Ahmed, S. (1996). Is prolonged breastfeeding associated with malnutrition? Evidence from nineteen demographic and health surveys. *International Journal of Epidemiology, 25*, 693–703.

Caulfield, L. E., de Onis, M., Blossner, M., & Black, R. E. (2004). Undernutrition as an underlying cause of child deaths associated with diarrhea, pneumonia, malaria, and measles. *American Journal of Clinical Nutrition, 80*, 193–198.

Caulfield, L. E., Richard, S. A., & Black, R. E. (2004). Undernutrition as an underlying cause of malaria morbidity and mortality in children less than five years old. *American Journal of Tropical Medicine, 71*(suppl 2), 55–63.

Caulfield, L. E., Zavaleta, N., Figueroa, A., & Leon, Z. (1999). Maternal zinc supplementation does not affect size at birth or pregnancy duration in Peru. *Journal of Nutrition, 129*, 1563–1568.

Caulfield, L. E., Zavaleta, N., Shankar, A., & Merialdi, M. (1998). Potential contribution of maternal zinc supplementation during pregnancy for maternal and child survival. *American Journal of Clinical Nutrition, 68*, S499–S508.

Cavan, K. R., Gibson, R. S., Grazioso, C. F., Isalgue, A. M., Ruz, M., & Solomons, N. W. (1993). Growth and body composition of periurban Guatemalan children in relation to zinc status: A longitudinal zinc intervention trial. *American Journal of Clinical Nutrition, 57*, 344–352.

Ceesay, S. M., Prentice, A. M., Cole, T. J., Ford, F., Weaver, L. T., Poskitt, E. M. E., & Whitehead, R. G. (1997). Effects on birthweight and perinatal mortality of maternal dietary supplements in rural Gambia: 5-year randomised controlled trial. *British Medical Journal, 315*, 786–790.

Cerqueiro, M. C., Murtagh, P., Halac, A., Avila, M., & Weissenbacher, M. (1990). Epidemiologic risk factors for children with acute lower respiratory tract infection in Buenos Aires, Argentina: A matched case-control study. *Reviews of Infectious Diseases, 12*, S1021–S1028.

Chapparo, C. M., & Dewey, K. G. (2010). Use of lipid-based nutrient supplements (LNS) to improve the nutrient adequacy of general food distribution rations for vulnerable sub-groups in emergency settings. *Maternal and Child Nutrition, 6*(suppl 1), 1–69.

Chaparro, C. M., Neufeld, L. M., Alavez, G. T., Cedillo, R. E., & Dewey, K. G. (2006). Effect of timing of umbilical cord clamping on iron status in Mexican infants: A randomized controlled trial. *Lancet, 367*, 1997–2004.

Checkley, W., Buckley, G., Gilman, R. H., Assis, A. M. O., Guerrant, R. L., Morris, S. S., et al. (2008). Multi-country analysis of the effects of diarrhea on childhood stunting. *International Journal of Epidemiology, 37*, 816–830.

Checkley, W., Epstein, L. D., Gilman, R. H., Black, R. E., Cabrera, L., & Sterling, C. R. (1998). Effects of *Cryptosporidium parvum* infection in Peruvian children: Growth faltering and subsequent catch-up growth. *American Journal of Epidemiology, 148*, 497–506.

Checkley, W., Epstein, L. D., Gilman, R. H., Cabrera, L., & Black, R. E. (2003). Effects of acute diarrhea on linear growth in Peruvian children. *American Journal of Epidemiology, 157,* 166–175.

Checkley, W., Gilman, R. H., Black, R. E., Lescano, A. G., Cabrera, L., Taylor, D. N., & Moulton, L. H. (2002). Effects of nutritional status on diarrhea in Peruvian children. *Journal of Pediatrics, 140,* 210–218.

Checkley, W., West, K. P. Jr., Wise, R. A., Baldwin, M. R., Wu, L., LeClerq, S. C., et al. (2010). Maternal vitamin A supplementation and lung function in offspring. *New England Journal of Medicine, 362,* 1784–1794.

Chen, Y., Yu, S., & Li, W. (1988). Artificial feeding and hospitalization in the first 18 months of life. *Pediatrics, 81,* 58–62.

Chen, L., Appel, L. J., Loria, C., Lin, P. H., Champagne, C. M., Elmer, P. J., et al. (2009). Reduction in consumption of sugar-sweetened beverages is associated with weight loss: The PREMIER trial. *American Journal of Clinical Nutrition, 89,* 1299–1306.

Cherry, F. F., Sandstead, H. H., Rojas, P., Johnson, L. K., Batson, H. K., & Wang, X. B. (1989). Adolescent pregnancy: Associations among body weight, zinc nutriture, and pregnancy outcome. *American Journal of Clinical Nutrition, 50,* 945–954.

Cheung, Y. B., Low, L., Osmond, C., Barker, D., & Karlberg, J. (2000). Fetal growth and early postnatal growth are related to blood pressure in adults. *Hypertension, 36,* 795–800.

Chilima, D. M., & Ismail, S. J. (1998). Anthropometric characteristics of older people in rural Malawi. *European Journal of Clinical Nutrition, 52,* 643–649.

Christian, P. (1998). Antenatal iron supplementation as a child survival strategy [Letter]. *American Journal of Clinical Nutrition, 68,* 403–404.

Christian, P., Darmstadt, G. L., Wu, L., Khatry, S. K., LeClerq, S. C., Katz, J., et al. (2008). The impact of maternal micronutrient supplementation on early neonatal morbidity in rural Nepal: A randomized, controlled community trial. *Archives of Diseases in Childhood: Fetal & Neonatal Edition, 93*(8), 660–664.

Christian, P., Jiang, T., Khatry, S. K., LeClerq, S. C., Shrestha, S. R., & West, K. P. Jr. (2006). Antenatal supplementation with micronutrients and biochemical indicators of status and sub-clinical infection in rural Nepal. *American Journal of Clinical Nutrition, 83,* 788–794.

Christian, P., Khatry, S. K., Katz, J., Pradhan, E. K., LeClerq, S. C., Shrestha, S. R., et al. (2003). Effects of alternative maternal micronutrient supplements on low birth weight in rural Nepal: Double blind randomised community trial. *British Medical Journal, 326,* 571–576.

Christian, P., Khatry, S. K., & West, K. P. Jr. (2004). Antenatal anthelmintic treatment, birthweight, and infant survival in rural Nepal. *Lancet, 364,* 981–983.

Christian, P., & Stewart, C. P. (2010). Maternal micronutrient deficiency, fetal development, and the risk of chronic disease. *Journal of Nutrition, 140,* 437–445.

Christian, P., Stewart, C. P., LeClerq, S. C., Wu, L., Katz, J., West, K. P. Jr., & Khatry, S. K. (2009). Antenatal and postnatal iron supplementation and childhood mortality in rural Nepal: A prospective follow-up in a randomized, controlled community trial. *American Journal of Epidemiology, 170,* 1127–1136.

Christian, P., West, K. P. Jr., Khatry, S. K., Katz, J., LeClerq, S., Pradhan, E. K., & Shrestha, S. R. (1998a). Vitamin A or ß-carotene supplementation reduces but does not eliminate maternal night blindness in Nepal. *Journal of Nutrition, 128,* 1458–1463.

Christian, P., West, K. P. Jr., Khatry, S. K., Katz, J., Shrestha, S. R., Pradhan, E. K., et al. (1998b). Night blindness of pregnancy in rural Nepal: Nutritional and health risks. International *Journal of Epidemiology, 27,* 231–237.

Christian, P., West, K. P. Jr., Khatry, S. K., Kimbrough-Pradhan, E., LeClerq, S. C., Katz, J., et al. (2000). Night blindness during pregnancy and subsequent mortality among women in Nepal: Effects of vitamin A and ß-carotene supplementation. *American Journal of Epidemiology, 152,* 542–547.

Christian, P., West, K. P. Jr., Khatry, S. K., LeClerq, S. C., Kimbrough-Pradhan, E., Katz, J., & Shrestha, S. R. (2001). Maternal night blindness increases risk of mortality in the first 6 months of life among infants in Nepal. *Journal of Nutrition, 131,* 1510–1512.

Christian, P., West, K. P. Jr., Khatry, S. K., LeClerq, S. C., Pradhan, E. K., Katz, J., et al. (2003). Effects of maternal micronutrient supplementation on fetal loss and infant mortality: A cluster-randomized trial in Nepal. *American Journal of Clinical Nutrition, 78,* 1194–1202.

Christian, P., West, K. P. Jr., Labrique, A. B., Klemm, R. D. W., Rashid, M., Shamim, A. A., et al. (2007). *Effects of vitamin A and ß-carotene supplementation on maternal and infant mortality in rural Bangladesh: JiVitA-1.* Micronutrient Forum, Istanbul, Turkey.

Chwang, L., Soemantri, A. G., & Pollitt, E. (1988). Iron supplementation and physical growth of rural Indonesian children. *American Journal of Clinical Nutrition, 47,* 496–501.

Clemens, J. D., Sack, D. A., Harris, J. R., Khan, M. R., Chakraborty, J., Chowdhury, S., et al. (1990). Breastfeeding and the risk of severe cholera in rural Bangladeshi children. *American Journal of Epidemiology, 131,* 400–411.

Clemens, J. D., Stanton, B., Stoll, B., Shadid, N. S., Banu, H., & Chowdhury, A. K. (1986). Breastfeeding as a determinant of severity in shigellosis: Evidence for protection throughout the first three years of life in Bangladeshi children. *American Journal of Epidemiology, 123,* 710–720.

Cobra, C., Muhilal, Rusmil, K., Rustama, D., Djatnika, Suwardi, S. S., et al. (1997). Infant survival is improved by oral iodine supplementation. *Journal of Nutrition, 127,* 574–578.

Cohen, N., Rahman, H., Mitra, M., Sprague, J., Islam, S., Leemhuis de Regt, E., & Jalil, M. A. (1987). Impact of massive doses of vitamin A on nutritional blindness in Bangladesh. *American Journal of Clinical Nutrition, 45,* 970–976.

Cole, T. J., & Parkin, J. M. (1977). Infection and its effect on the growth of young children: A comparison of the Gambia and Uganda. *Transactions of the Royal Society for Tropical Medicine and Hygiene, 71,* 196–198.

Coles, C. L., Rahmathullah, L., Kanungo, R., Thulasiraj, R. D., Katz, J., Santhosham, M., & Tielsch, J. M. (2001). Vitamin A supplementation at birth delays pneumococcal colonization in South Indian infants. *Journal of Nutrition, 131,* 255–261.

Combs, G. F. Jr., Welch, R. M., Duxbury, J. M., Uphoff, N. T., & Nesheim, M. C. (1996). *Food-based approaches to preventing micronutrient malnutrition: An international research agenda.* Ithaca, NY: Cornell International Institute for Food, Agriculture, and Development.

Condon-Paoloni, D., Joaquin, C., Johnston, F. E., deLicardi, E. R., & Scholl, T. O. (1977). Morbidity and growth of infants and young children in a rural Mexican village. *American Journal of Public Health, 67,* 651–656.

Congdon, N. G., & West, K. P. Jr. (2002). Physiologic indicators of vitamin A status. *Journal of Nutrition, 132,* 2889S–2894S.

Cook, J. D., Finch, C. A., & Smith, N. J. (1976). Evaluation of the iron status of a population. *Blood, 48,* 449–455.

Cook, J. D., Lipschitz, D. A., Miles, L. E. M., & Finch, C. A. (1974). Serum ferritin as a measure of iron stores in normal subjects. *American Journal of Clinical Nutrition, 27,* 681.

Coovadia, H. M., Rollins, N. C., Bland, R. M., Little, K., Coutsoudis, A., Bennish, M. L., & Newell, M. L. (2007). Mother-to-child transmission of HIV-1 infection during exclusive breastfeeding in the first 6 months of life: An intervention cohort study. *Lancet, 369,* 1107–1116.

Corvilain, B., Van Sande, J., Dumont, J. E., Bourdoux, P., & Ermans, A. M. (1998). Autonomy in endemic goiter. *Thyroid, 8,* 107–113.

Cousins, R. J., & Hempe, J. M. (1990). Zinc. In M. L. Brown (Ed.), *Present knowledge in nutrition* (6th ed., pp. 251–260). Washington, DC: ILSI Press.

Coutsoudis, A., Kiepiela, P., Coovadia, H. M., & Broughton, M. (1992). Vitamin A supplementation enhances specific IgG antibody levels and total lymphocyte numbers while improving morbidity in measles. *Pediatric Infectious Diseases Journal, 11,* 203–209.

Craft, N. E., Haitema, T., Brindle, L. K., Yamini, S., Humphrey, J. H., & West, K. P. Jr. (2000). Retinol analysis in dried blood spots by HPLC. *Journal of Nutrition, 130,* 882–885.

Cruz, J. R., Pareja, G., de Fernandez, A., Peralta, F., Caceres, P., & Cano, F. (1990). Epidemiology of acute respiratory tract infections among Guatemalan ambulatory preschool children. *Reviews of Infectious Diseases, 12,* S1029–S1034.

Dallman, P. R. (1986). Biochemical basis for the manifestation of iron deficiency. *Annual Review of Nutrition, 6,* 13–40.

Dary, O. (1994). Avances en el proceso de fortificacion de azucar con vitamina A en Centro America. *Boletin de la Oficina Sanitaria Pan Americana, 117,* 529–536.

de Benoist, B., McLean, E., Andersson, M., & Rogers, L. (2008). Iodine deficiency in 2007: Global progress since 2003. *Food and Nutrition Bulletin, 29,* 195–202.

de Onis, M., Blossner, M., Borghi, E., Morris, R., & Frongillo, E. A. (2004). Methodology for estimating regional and global trends of child malnutrition. *International Journal of Epidemiology, 33,* 1260–1270.

de Onis, M., Blossner, M., & Villar, J. (1998). Levels and patterns of intrauterine growth retardation in developing countries. *European Journal of Clinical Nutrition, 52,* S5–S15.

de Onis, M., Frongillo, E. A., & Blossner, M. (2000). Is malnutrition declining? An analysis of changes in levels of child malnutrition since 1980. *Bulletin of the World Health Organization, 78,* 1222–1233.

de Onis, M., Wijnhoven, T. M. A., & Onyango, A. W. (2004). Worldwide practices in child growth monitoring. *Journal of Pediatrics, 144,* 461–465.

de Pee, S., Bloem, M. W., Gorstein, J., Sari, M., Satoto, Yip, R., et al. (1998). Reappraisal of the role of vegetables in the vitamin A status of mothers in Central Java, Indonesia. *American Journal of Clinical Nutrition, 68,* 1068–1074.

de Pee, S., Bloem, M. W., Satoto, Yip, R., Sukaton, A., Tjiong, R., et al. (1998). Impact of a social marketing campaign promoting dark-green leafy vegetables and eggs in Central Java, Indonesia. *International Journal of Vitamin and Nutrition Research, 68,* 389–398.

de Pee, S., Bloem, M. W., Tjiong, R., Martini, E., Satoto, Gorstein, J., et al. (1999). Who has a high vitamin A intake from plant foods, but a low serum retinol concentration? Data from women in Indonesia. *European Journal of Clinical Nutrition, 53,* 288–297.

de Pee, S., Brinkman, H-J., Webb, P., Godfrey, S., Darnton-Hill, I., Alderman, H., et al. (2010). How to ensure nutrition security in the global economic crisis to protect and enhance development of young children and our common future. *Journal of Nutrition, 140,* 138S–142S.

de Pee, S., West, C. E., Muhilal, Karyadi, D., & Hautvast, J. G. A. J. (1995). Lack of improvement in vitamin A status with increased consumption of dark-green leafy vegetables. *Lancet, 346,* 75–81.

de Vaquera, M. V., Townsend, J. W., Arroyo, J. J., & Lechtig, A. (1983). The relationship between arm circumference at birth and early mortality. *Journal of Tropical Pediatrics, 29,* 167–174.

Delange, F. (1994). The disorders induced by iodine deficiency. *Thyroid, 4,* 107–128.

Delange, F. (1998). Screening for congenital hypothyroidism used as an indicator of the degree of iodine deficiency and of its control. *Thyroid, 8,* 1185–1192.

Delange, F., Benker, G., Caron, P., Eber, O., Ott, W., Peter, F., et al. (1997). Thyroid volume and urinary iodine in European school children: Standardization of values for assessment of iodine deficiency. *European Journal of Endocrinology, 136,* 180–187.

Delange, F., Thilly, C., Bourdoux, P., Hennart, P., Courtois, P., & Ermans, A. M. (1982). Influence of dietary goitrogens during pregnancy in humans on thyroid function of the newborn. In F. Delange, F. B. Iteke, & A. M. Ermans (Eds.), *Nutritional factors involved in goitrogenic action of cassava* (pp. 40–50). Ottawa: International Developmental Research Centre Publications.

DeLong, R., Tai, M., Xue-Yi, C., Xin-Min, J., Zhi-Hong, D., Rakeman, M. A., et al. (1994). The neuromotor deficit in endemic cretinism. In J. B. Stanbury (Ed.), *The damaged brain of iodine deficiency* (pp. 9–13). New York: Cognizant Communication.

DeMaeyer, E. M., & Adiels-Tegman, M. (1985). The prevalence of anemia in the world. *World Health Statistics Quarterly, 38*, 302–316.

Dewey, K. G. (2007). Increasing iron intake of children through complementary foods. *Food and Nutrition Bulletin, 28*, S595–S609.

Dewey, K. G., & Adu-Afarwuah, S. (2008). Systematic review of the efficacy and effectiveness of complementary feeding interventions in developing countries. *Maternal and Child Nutrition, 4*, 24–85.

Dewey, K. G., & Brown, K. H. (2003). Update on technical issues concerning complementary feeding of young children in developing countries and implications for intervention programs. *Food and Nutrition Bulletin, 24*, 5–28.

Dewey, K. G., Domellof, M., Cohen, R. J., Rivera, L. L., Hernell, O., & Lonnerdal, B. (2002). Iron supplementation affects growth and morbidity of breast-fed infants: Results of a randomized trial in Sweden and Honduras. *Journal of Nutrition, 132*, 3249–3255.

Dixit, D. T. (1966). Night blindness in third trimester of pregnancy. *Indian Journal of Medical Research, 54*, 791–795.

Doak, C. M., Adair, L. S., Bentley, M., Monteiro, C., & Popkin, B. M. (2005). The dual burden household and the nutrition transition paradox. *International Journal of Obesity and Related Metabolic Disorders, 29*, 129–136.

Doak, C. M., Adair, L. S., Monteiro, C., & Popkin, B. M. (2000). Overweight and underweight coexist within households in Brazil, China and Russia. *Journal of Nutrition, 130*, 2965–2971.

Donnen, P., Brasseur, D., Dramaix, M., Vertongen, F., Zihindula, M., Muhamiriza, M., & Hennart, P. (1998). Vitamin A supplementation but not deworming improves growth of malnourished preschool children in eastern Zaire. *Journal of Nutrition, 128*, 1320–1327.

Drewnowski, A., & Popkin, B. M. (1997). The nutrition transition: New trends in the global diet. *Nutrition Reviews, 55*, 31–43.

Dreyfuss, M. L. (1998). *Anemia and iron deficiency during pregnancy: Etiologies and effects on birth outcomes in Nepal.* Unpublished thesis, Johns Hopkins University, Baltimore, MD.

Du, S., Lu, B., Zhai, F., & Popkin, B. M. (2002). The nutrition transition in China: A new stage of the Chinese diet. In B. Caballero & B. M. Popkin (Eds.), *The nutrition transition: Diet and disease in the developing world* (Vol. 11, pp. 205–221). London: Academic Press.

Dunn, J. T. (1996). Seven deadly sins in confronting endemic iodine deficiency, and how to avoid them. *Journal of Clinical Endocrinological Metabolism, 81*, 1332–1335.

Dunn, J. T., Semigran, M. J., & Delange, F. (1998). The prevention and management of iodine-induced hyperthyroidism and its cardiac features. *Thyroid, 8*, 101–106.

Dunn, J. T., & van der Haar, F. (1990). *A practical guide to the correction of iodine deficiency.* Netherlands: International Council for Control of Iodine Deficiency Disorders.

Edmond, K. M., Zandoh, C., Quigley, M. A., Amenga-Etego, S., Owusu-Agyei, S., & Kirkwood, B. R. (2006). Delayed breastfeeding initiation increases risk of neonatal mortality. *Pediatrics, 117*, e380–e386.

Eilander, A., Gera, T., Sachdev, H. S., Transler, C., van der Knaap, H. C., Kok, F. J., & Osendarp, S. J. (2010). Multiple micronutrient supplementation for improving cognitive performance in children: Systematic review of randomized controlled trials. *American Journal of Clinical Nutrition, 91*(1), 115–130.

El Samani, F. Z., Willett, W. C., & Ware, J. H. (1986). Predictors of simple diarrhoea disease surveillance in a rural Ghanaian pre-school child population. *Transactions of the Royal Society for Tropical Medicine and Hygiene, 80,* 208–213.

El-Arifeen, S. (1997). *Birthweight, intrauterine growth retardation and prematurity: A prospective study of infant growth and survival in the slums of Dhaka, Bangladesh.* Unpublished doctoral dissertation, Johns Hopkins School of Public Health, Baltimore, MD.

Ellison, J. B. (1932). Intensive vitamin therapy in measles. *British Medical Journal, 2,* 708–711.

Elnagar, B., Eltom, M., Karlsson, F. A., Ermans, A. M., Gebre-Medhin, M., & Bourdoux, P. P. (1995). The effects of different doses of oral iodized oil on goiter size, urinary iodine, and thyroid-related hormones. *Journal of Clinical Endocrinological Metabolism, 80,* 891–897.

Ending hidden hunger: Proceedings of a policy conference on micronutrient malnutrition, Montreal, Quebec, Canada, 10–12 October 1991. (1992). Atlanta, GA: Task Force on Child Survival and Development.

Eriksson, J. G., Forsen, T., Tuomilehto, J., Reunanen, A., Osmond, C., & Barker, D. (1999). Size at birth, growth in childhood and future risk of type 2 diabetes. *Diabetes, 48,* A72.

Ezzati, M., Lopez, A. D., Rodgers, A., Vander Hoorn, S., Murray, C. J. L., & Comparative Risk Assessment Collaborating Group. (2002). Selected major risk factors and global and regional burden of disease. *Lancet, 360,* 1347–1360.

Faisal, H., & Pittrof, R. (2000). Vitamin A and causes of maternal mortality: Association and biological plausibility. *Public Health Nutrition, 3,* 321–327.

Fall, C. H., Fisher, D. J., Osmond, C., & Margetts, B. M. (2009). Multiple micronutrient supplementation during pregnancy in low-income countries: A meta-analysis of effects on birth size and length of gestation. *Food and Nutrition Bulletin, 30*(4), S533–S546.

FAOSTAT. (2004). FAO statistical databases. Retrieved from http://faostat.fao.org

Faruque, A. S. G., Mahalanabis, D., Haque, S. S., Fuchs, G. J., & Habte, D. (1999). Double-blind, randomized, controlled trial of zinc or vitamin A supplementation in young children with acute diarrhoea. *Acta Paediatrica, 88,* 154–160.

Fawzi, W. W., Chalmers, T. C., Herrera, G., & Mosteller, F. (1993). Vitamin A supplementation and child mortality: A meta-analysis. *Journal of the American Medical Association, 269,* 898–903.

Fawzi, W. W., Herrera, G., Willett, W. C., Nestle, P., El Amin, A., & Mohamed, K. A. (1997). The effect of vitamin A supplementation on the growth of preschool children in the Sudan. *American Journal of Public Health, 87,* 1359–1362.

Fawzi, W. W., Villamor, E., Msamanga, G. E., Antelman, G., Aboud, S., Urassa, W., & Hunter, D. (2005). Trial of zinc supplements in relation to pregnancy outcomes, hematologic indicators, and T cell counts among HIV-1–infected women in Tanzania. *American Journal of Clinical Nutrition, 81,* 161–167.

Ferdous, T., Cederholm, T., Kabir, Z. N., Hamadani, J. D., & Wahlin, A. (2010). Nutritional status and cognitive function in community-living rural Bangladeshi older adults: Data from the Poverty and Health in Ageing Project. *Journal of the American Geriatric Society, 58,* 919–924.

Ferguson, B. J., Skikne, B. S., Simpson, K. M., Baynes, R. D., & Cook, J. D. (1992). Serum transferrin receptor distinguishes the anemia of chronic disease from iron deficiency anemia. *Journal of Laboratory Clinical Medicine, 19,* 385–390.

Ferguson, E. L., Gibson, R. S., Opare-Obisaw, C., Ounpuu, S., Thompson, L. U., & Lehrfeld, J. (1993). The zinc nutriture of preschool children living in two African countries. *Journal of Nutrition, 123,* 1487–1496.

Fischer Walker, C. L., Bhutta, Z. A., Bhandari, N., Teka, T., Shahid, F., Taneja, S. et al. (2006). Zinc supplementation for the treatment of diarrhea in infants in Pakistan, India and Ethiopia. *Journal of Pediatric Gastroenterology and Nutrition, 42,* 357–363.

Fischer Walker, C. L., Black, R. E., & Baqui, A. H. (2008). Does age affect the response to zinc therapy for diarrhea in Bangladeshi infants? *Health Population and Nutrition, 26*, 105–109.

Fischer Walker, C., Ezzati, M., & Black, R. E. (2009). Global and regional child mortality and burden of disease attributable to zinc deficiency. *European Journal of Clinical Nutrition, 63*, 591–597.

Fischer Walker, C., Fontaine, O., Young, M. W., & Black, R. E. (2009). Zinc and low osmolarity oral rehydration salts for diarrhea: A renewed call to action. *Bulletin of the World Health Organization, 87*, 780–786.

Fishman, S., Caulfield, L. E., de Ois, M., Blossner, M., Hyder, A. A., Mullany, L., & Black, R. E. (2004). Childhood and maternal underweight. In M. Ezzati, A. D. Lopez, A. Rodgers, & C. J. L. Murray (Eds.), *Comparative quantification of health risks: Global and regional burden of disease attributable to selected major risk factors* (pp. 39–162). Geneva, Switzerland: World Health Organization.

Fishman, S. M., Christian, P., & West, K. P. Jr. (2000). The role of vitamins in the prevention and control of anaemia. *Public Health and Nutrition, 3*, 125–150.

Flores, H., Campos, F., Araujo, C. R. C., & Underwood, B. A. (1984). Assessment of marginal vitamin A deficiency in Brazilian children using the relative dose response procedure. *American Journal of Clinical Nutrition, 40*, 1281–1289.

Fonseca, W., Kirkwood, B. R., Victora, C. G., Fuchs, S. R., Flores, J. A., & Misago, C. (1996). Risk factors for childhood pneumonia among the urban poor in Fortaleza, Brazil: A case-control study. *Bulletin of the World Health Organization, 74*, 199–208.

Food and Agriculture Organization of the United Nations (FAO). (1988). *Requirements of vitamin A, iron, folate, and vitamin B$_{12}$: Report of a joint FAO/WHO expert committee.* Rome: Food and Agriculture Organization.

Food and Agriculture Organization of the United Nations (FAO). (1996). World Food Summit, 13–17 November 1996, Rome, Italy. Retrieved from http://www.fao.org/wfs/index_en.htm

Food and Agriculture Organization of the United Nations (FAO). (2002). *World agriculture: Towards 2015/2030.* Rome: Food and Agriculture Organization of the United Nations.

Food and Agriculture Organization of the United Nations (FAO). (2009). Retrieved July 11, 2010, from http://www.fao.org/news/story/en/item/20568/icode/

Food and Agriculture Organization of the United Nations (FAO) & World Health Organization (WHO). (1992). *World declaration and plan of action for nutrition.* Rome: International Conference on Nutrition.

Forsen, T., Eriksson, J., Tuomilehto, J., Reunanen, A., Osmond, C., & Barker, D. (2000). The fetal and childhood growth of persons who develop type 2 diabetes. *Annals of Internal Medicine, 133*, 176–182.

Garg, H. K., Singhla, K. C., & Arshad, Z. (1993). A study of the effect of oral zinc supplementation during pregnancy on pregnancy outcome. *Indian Journal of Physiology and Pharmacology, 37*, 276–284.

Garnham, P. C. C. (1954). Malaria in the African child. *East African Medical Journal, 31*, 155–159.

Garrett, J. L., & Ruel, M. T. (2003). *Stunted child-overweight mother pairs: An emerging policy concern?* (FCSD Discussion Paper No. 148). Washington, DC: International Food Policy Research Institute.

Gibson, R. S. (1990). *Principles of nutritional assessment.* New York: Oxford University Press.

Gibson, R. S., & Ferguson, E. L. (1998a). Assessment of dietary zinc in a population. *American Journal of Clinical Nutrition, 68*, 430S–434S.

Gibson, R. S., & Ferguson, E. L. (1998b). Nutrition intervention strategies to combat zinc deficiency in developing countries. *Nutrition Research Reviews, 11*, 115–131.

Gibson, R. S., Ferguson, E. L., & Lehrfeld, J. (1998). Complementary foods for infant feeding in developing countries: Their nutrient adequacy and improvement. *European Journal of Clinical Nutrition, 52,* 764–770.

Gibson, R. S., Heywood, A., Yaman, C., Sohlstrom, A., Thompson, L. U., & Heywood, P. (1991). Growth in children from the Wosera subdistrict, Papua New Guinea, in relation to energy and protein intakes and zinc status. *American Journal of Clinical Nutrition, 53,* 782–789.

Gibson, R. S., & Huddle, J. M. (1998). Suboptimal zinc status in pregnant Malawian women: Its association with low intakes of poorly available zinc, frequent reproductive cycling, and malaria. *American Journal of Clinical Nutrition, 67,* 702–709.

Gibson, R. S., Yeudall, F., Drost, N., Mtitimuni, B., & Cullinan, T. (1998). Dietary interventions to prevent zinc deficiency. *American Journal of Clinical Nutrition, 68,* 484S–487S.

Gillman, M. W., Rifas-Shiman, S. L., Berkey, C. S., Frazier, A. L., Rockett, H.R., Camargo, C. A. Jr, et al. (2006). Breastfeeding and overweight in adolescence: Within-family analysis [corrected]. *Epidemiology, 17,* 112–114.

Glasziou, P. P., & Mackerras, D. E. M. (1993). Vitamin A supplementation in infectious diseases: A meta-analysis. *British Medical Journal, 306,* 366–370.

Golden, M. H. N. (2002). The development of concepts of malnutrition. *Journal of Nutrition, 132,* 2117S–2122S.

Goldenberg, R. L., Tamura, T., Neggers, Y., Copper, R. L., Johnston, K. E., DuBard, M. B., & Hauth, J. C. (1995). The effect of zinc supplementation on pregnancy outcome. *Journal of the American Medical Association, 274,* 463–468.

Gordon, R. C., Rose, M. C., Skeaff, S. A., Gray, A. R., Morgan, K. M. D., & Ruffman, T. (2009). Iodine supplementation improves cognitive function in mildly iodine-deficient children. *American Journal of Clinical Nutrition, 90,* 1264–1271.

Graham, N. M. H. (1990). The epidemiology of acute respiratory infections in children and adults: A global perspective. *Epidemiologic Reviews, 12,* 149–178.

Graham, R. D., Ascher, J. S., & Hynes, S. C. (1992). Selecting zinc-efficient cereal genotypes for soils of low zinc status. *Plant and Soil, 146,* 241–250.

Grantham-McGregor, S. M., Walker, S. P., Chang, S. M., & Powell, C. A. (1997). Effects of early childhood supplementation with and without stimulation on later development in stunted Jamaican children. *American Journal of Clinical Nutrition, 66,* 247–253.

Grummer-Strawn, L. M. (1996). The effect of changes in population characteristics on breastfeeding trends in fifteen developing countries. *International Journal of Epidemiology, 25,* 94–102.

Grummer-Strawn, L. M., Mei, Z. (2004). Does breastfeeding protect against pediatric overweight? Analysis of longitudinal data from the Centers for Disease Control and Prevention Pediatric Nutrition Surveillance System. *Pediatrics, 113,* e81–e86.

Guerrant, R. I., Schorling, J. B., McAuliffe, J. F., & de Souza, M. A. (1992). Diarrhea as a cause and an effect of malnutrition: Diarrhea prevents catch-up growth and malnutrition increases diarrhea frequency and duration. *American Journal of Tropical Medicine and Hygiene, 47,* 28–35.

Haddad, L. (1999). Women's status: Levels, determinants, consequences for malnutrition, interventions, and policy. In J. Hunt & M. G. Quibria (Eds.), *Investing in child nutrition in Asia* (pp. 96–131). Manila: Asian Development Bank.

Hadi, H., Dibley, M. J., & West, K. P. Jr. (2004). Complex interactions with infection and diet may explain seasonal growth responses to vitamin A in preschool aged Indonesian children. *European Journal of Clinical Nutrition, 58,* 990–999.

Hadi, H., Stoltzfus, R. J., Dibley, M. J., Moulton, L. H., West, K. P. Jr., Kjolhede, C. L., & Sadjimin, T. (2000). Vitamin A supplementation selectively improves the linear growth of Indonesian preschool children: Results from a randomized controlled trial. *American Journal of Clinical Nutrition, 71,* 507–513.

Hadi, H., Stoltzfus, R. J., Moulton, L. H., Dibley, M. J., & West, K. P. Jr. (1999). Respiratory infections reduce the growth response to vitamin A supplementation in a randomized controlled trial.

International Journal of Epidemiology, 28, 874–881.

Hallberg, L., Brune, M., Erlandsson, M., Sandberg, A. S., & Rossander-Hulten, L. (1991). Calcium: Effects of different amounts on nonheme- and heme-iron absorption in humans. *American Journal of Clinical Nutrition, 53,* 112–119.

Halpern, J. P. (1994). The neuromotor deficit in endemic cretinism and its implications for the pathogenesis of the disorder. In J. B. Stanbury (Ed.), *The damaged brain of iodine deficiency* (pp. 15–24). New York: Cognizant Communication.

Hambidge, K. M., & Krebs, N. F. (1995). Assessment of zinc status in man. *Indian Journal of Pediatrics, 62,* 169–180.

Hambidge, K. M., & Krebs, N. F. (1999). Zinc, diarrhea, and pneumonia. *Journal of Pediatrics, 135,* 661–664.

Hambidge, K. M., Krebs, N. F., & Miller, L. (1998). Evaluation of zinc metabolism with use of stable-isotope techniques: Implications for the assessment of zinc status. *American Journal of Clinical Nutrition, 68,* 410S–413S.

Hamill, P. V. V., Drizid, T. A., Johnson, C. L., Reed, R. B., Roche, A. F., & Moore, W. M. (1979). Physical growth: National Center for Health Statistics percentiles. *American Journal of Clinical Nutrition, 32,* 607–629.

Hamill, P. V., Drizd, T. A., Johnson, C. L., Reed, R. B., & Roche, A. F. (1977). NCHS growth curves for children birth–18 years, United States. *Vital Health Statistics, 11,* i–iv, 1–74.

Helen Keller International. (1998). *Current status of preschool vitamin A capsule supplementation program in rural Bangladesh.* Bangladesh: Author.

Hendrickse, R. G., Hasan, A. H., Olumide, L. O., & Akinkunmi, A. (1971). Malaria in early childhood: An investigation of five hundred seriously ill children in whom a "clinical" diagnosis of malaria was made on admission to the children's emergency room at University College Hospital, Ibadan. *Annals of Tropical Medicine and Parasitology, 65,* 1–20.

Hetzel, B. S. (1989). *The story of iodine deficiency: An international challenge in nutrition.* Oxford, UK/Delhi, India: Oxford University Press.

Hetzel, B. S. (1994). Historical development of the concepts of the brain–thyroid relationships. In J. B. Stanbury (Ed.), *The damaged brain of iodine deficiency* (pp. 1–7). New York: Cognizant Communication.

Heywood, A., Oppenheimer, S., Heywood, P., & Jolley, D. (1989). Behavioral effects of iron supplementation in infants in Madang, Papua New Guinea. *American Journal of Clinical Nutrition, 50,* 630–640.

Hintze, G., Emrich, D., Richter, K., Thal, H., Wasielewski, T., & Kobberling, J. (1988). Effect of voluntary intake of iodinated salt on prevalence of goitre in children. *Acta Endocrinologica (Copenhagen), 117,* 333–338.

Hoddinott, J., Maluccio, J. A., Behrman, J. R., Flores, R., & Martorell, R. (2008). Effect of a nutrition intervention during early childhood on economic productivity in Guatemalan adults. *Lancet, 371,* 411–416.

Hokama, T., Takenaka, S., Hirayama, K., Yara, A., Yoshida, K., Itokazu, K., et al. (1996). Iron status of newborns born to iron deficiency anaemic mothers. *Journal of Tropical Pediatrics, 42,* 75–77.

Hopkins, R. M., Gracey, M. S., Hobbs, R. P., Spargo, R. M., Yates, M., & Thompson, R. C. A. (1997). The prevalence of hookworm infection, iron deficiency, and anaemia in an Aboriginal community in north-west Australia. *Medical Journal of Australia, 166,* 241–244.

Horta, B. L., Victora, C. G., Lima, R. C., & Post, P. (2009). Weight gain in childhood and blood lipids in adolescence. *Acta Paediatrica, 98,* 1024–1028.

Horton, S., Sanghvi, T., Phillips, M., Fiedler, J., Perez-Escamilla, R., Lutter, C., et al. (1996). Breastfeeding promotion and priority setting. *Health Policy and Planning, 11,* 156–168.

Hossain, S. M. M., Duffield, A., & Taylor A. (2005). An evaluation of the impact of a US$60 million nutrition programme in Bangladesh. *Health Policy and Planning, 20,* 35–40.

Hotz, C., & Brown, K. H. (Eds.). (2004). International Zinc Nutrition Consultative Group (IZiNCG) Technical Document No. 1: Assessment of the risk of zinc deficiency in populations and options for its control [Special issue]. *Food and Nutrition Bulletin, 25*(suppl 2), S94–S203.

Houston, R. (1999). *The Nepal national vitamin A program: Elements of success.* Kathmandu, Nepal: Nepali Technical Assistance Group and John Snow, Inc., for the Ministry of Health, U.S. Agency for International Development, and UNICEF.

Howson, C. P., Kennedy, E. T., & Horwitz, A. (1998). *Prevention of micronutrient deficiencies: Tools for policymakers and public health workers.* Washington, DC: National Academy Press.

Hoyle, B., Yunus, M., & Hen, L. C. (1980). Breastfeeding and food intake among children with acute diarrheal disease. *American Journal of Clinical Nutrition, 33,* 2365–2371.

Huda, S. N., Grantham-McGregor, S. M., Rahman, K. M., & Tomkins, A. (1999). Biochemical hypothyroidism secondary to iodine deficiency is associated with poor school achievement and cognition in Bangladeshi children. *Journal of Nutrition, 129,* 980–987.

Huddle, J. M., Gibson, R. S., & Cullinan, T. R. (1999). The impact of malarial infection and diet on the anaemia status of rural pregnant Malawian women. *European Journal of Clinical Nutrition, 53,* 792–801.

Huffman, S. L., Chowdhury, A. K. M., Chakraborty, J., & Simpson, N. K. (1980). Breastfeeding patterns in rural Bangladesh. *American Journal of Clinical Nutrition, 33,* 144–154.

Humphrey, J. H. (2009). Child undernutrition, tropical enteropathy, toilets, and handwashing. *Lancet, 374,* 1032–1035.

Humphrey, J. H., Agoestina, T., Wu, L., Usman, A., Nurachim, M., Subardja, D., et al. (1996). Impact of neonatal vitamin A supplementation on infant morbidity and mortality. *Journal of Pediatrics, 128,* 489–496.

Humphrey, J. H., Agoestina, T., Juliana, A., Septiana, S., Widjaja, H., Cerreto, M. C., et al. (1998). Neonatal vitamin A supplementation: effect on development and growth at 3 y of age. *American Journal of Clinical Nutriton, 68,* 109–117.

Humphrey, J. H., West, K. P. Jr., & Sommer, A. (1992). Vitamin A deficiency and attributable mortality among under-5-year-olds. *Bulletin of the World Health Organization, 70,* 225–232.

Hussey, G. D., & Klein, M. (1990). A randomized, controlled trial of vitamin A in children with severe measles. *New England Journal of Medicine, 323,* 160–164.

Hutton, E. K., & Hassan, E. S. (2007). Late vs early clamping of the umbilical cord in full-term neonates: Systematic review and meta-analysis of controlled trials. *Journal of the American Medical Association, 297,* 1241–1252.

Iannotti, L. L., Zavaleta, N., Leon, Z., Shankar, A. H., & Caulfield, L. E. (2008). Maternal zinc supplementation and growth in Peruvian infants. *American Journal of Clinical Nutrition, 88*(1), 154–160.

Iannotti, L. L., Zavaleta, N., Leon, Z., Huasquiche, C., Shankar, A. H., Caulfield, L. E. (2010). Maternal zinc supplementation reduces diarrheal morbidity in peruvian infants. *Journal of Pediatrics, 156,* 960–964.

Idjradinata, P., Watkins, W. E., & Pollitt, E. (1994). Adverse effect of iron supplementation on weight gain of iron replete young children. *Lancet, 343,* 1252–1254.

Iliff, P. J., Piwoz, E. G., Tavengwa, N. V., Zunguza, C. D., Marinda, E. T., Nathoo, K. J., et al. (2005). Early exclusive breastfeeding reduces the risk of postnatal HIV-1 transmission and increases HIV-free survival. *AIDS, 19,* 699–708.

Institute of Medicine (IOM). (2006). *Dietary reference intakes: Essential guide to nutrient requirements.* J. J. Otten, J. P. Hellwig, & L. D. Meyers (Eds.). Washington, DC: National Academies Press.

Institute of Medicine (IOM). (2010). *Mitigating the nutritional impacts of the global food price crisis: Workshop summary.* Washington, DC: National Academies Press.

International Nutritional Anemia Consultative Group (INACG). (1997). *Iron EDTA for food fortification.* Washington, DC: Nutrition Foundation.

Isanaka, S., Nombela, N., Djibo, A., Poupard, M., Van Beckhoven, D., Gaboulaud, V., et al. (2009). Effect of preventive supplementation with ready-to-use therapeutic food on the nutritional status, mortality, and morbidity of children aged 6 to 60 months in Niger: A cluster randomized trial. *Journal of the American Medical Association, 301,* 277–285.

Islam, M. Z., Lamberg-Allardt, C., Karkkainen, M., & Ali, S. M. K. (2003). Dietary calcium intake in premenopausal Bangladeshi women: Do socio-economic or physiological factors play a role? *European Journal of Clinical Nutrition, 57,* 674–680.

Ittiravivongs, A., Songchitratna, K. S., Ratthapalo, S., & Pattara-Arechachai, J. (1991). Effect of low birthweight on severe childhood diarrhea. *Southeast Asian Journal of Tropical Medicine and Public Health, 22,* 557–562.

James, J. W. (1972). Longitudinal study of the morbidity of diarrheal and respiratory infections in malnourished children. *American Journal of Clinical Nutrition, 25,* 690–694.

James, W. P. T., Jackson-Leach, R., Mhurchu, C. N., Kalamara, E., Shayeghi, M., Rigby, N. J., et al. (2004). Overweight and obesity (high body mass index). In M. Ezzati, A. D. Lopez, A. Rodgers, & C. J. L. Murray (Eds.), *Comparative quantification of health risks: Global and regional burden of disease attributable to selected major risk factors* (pp. 497–596). Geneva, Switzerland: World Health Organization.

Jelliffe, D. B. (1966). *The assessment of the nutritional status of the community* (WHO Monograph Series No. 53). Geneva, Switzerland: World Health Organization.

Jelliffe, D. B., & Jelliffe, E. F. P. (1978). The volume and composition of human milk in poorly nourished communities: A review. *American Journal of Clinical Nutrition, 31,* 492–515.

Jiang, T., Christian, P., Khatry, S. K., Wu, L., & West, K. P. Jr. (2005). Micronutrient deficiencies in early pregnancy are common, concurrent, and vary by season among rural Nepali pregnant women. *Journal of Nutrition, 135,* 1106–1112.

Johnson, W. B., Aderele, W. I., & Gbadero, D. A. (1992). Host factors and acute lower respiratory infections in pre-school children. *Journal of Tropical Pediatrics, 38,* 132–136.

Kafulafula, G., Hoover, D. R., Taha, T. E., Thigpen, M., Li, Q., Fowler, M. G., et al. (2010). Frequency of gastroenteritis and gastroenteritis-associated mortality with early weaning in HIV-1 uninfected children born to HIV infected women in Malawi. *Journal of Acquired Immune Deficiency Syndromes, 53,* 6–13.

Kalter, H. D., Burnham, G., Kolstad, P. R., Hossain, M., Schillinger, J. A., Khan, N. Z., et al. (1997). Evaluation of clinical signs to diagnose anaemia in Uganda and Bangladesh, in areas with and without malaria. *Bulletin of the World Health Organization, 75*(suppl), 103–111.

Kamal, M. K., Ahsan, R. I., & Salam, A. K. M. A. (1998). *Achieving the goals for children in Bangladesh.* Dhaka, Bangladesh: Bangladesh Bureau of Statistics/Ministry of Planning/Government of the People's Republic of Bangladesh/UNICEF.

Kamel, H. K. (2003). Sarcopenia and aging. *Nutrition Reviews, 61,* 157–167.

Katz, J., Khatry, S. K., West, K. P. Jr., Humphrey, J. H., LeClerq, S. C., Pradhan, E. K., et al. (1995). Night blindness is prevalent during pregnancy and lactation in rural Nepal. *Journal of Nutrition, 125,* 2122–2127.

Katz, J., West, K. P. Jr., Khatry, S. K., Pradhan, E. K., LeClerq, S. C., Christian, P., et al. (2000). Maternal low-dose vitamin A or beta-carotene supplementation has no effect on fetal loss and early infant mortality: A randomized cluster trial in Nepal. *American Journal of Clinical Nutrition, 71,* 1570–1576.

Katz, J., West, K. P. Jr., Tarwotjo, I., & Sommer, A. (1989). The importance of age in evaluating anthropometric indices for predicting mortality. *American Journal of Epidemiology, 130,* 1219–1226.

Katz, J., Zeger, S. L., & Tielsch, J. M. (1988). Village and household clustering of xerophthalmia and trachoma. *International Journal of Epidemiology, 17,* 865–869.

Katz, J., Zeger, S. L., West, K. P. Jr., Tielsch, J. M., & Sommer, A. (1993). Clustering of xerophthalmia within households and villages. *International Journal of Epidemiology, 22,* 709–715.

Kavishe, F. P. (1999). Iodine: Iodine deficiency disorders. In M. J. Sadler, J. J. Strain, & B. Caballero (Eds.), *Encyclopedia of human nutrition* (pp. 1146–1153). San Diego: Academic Press.

Keen, C. L., & Gershwin, M. E. (1990). Zinc deficiency and immune function. *Annual Review of Nutrition, 10,* 415–431.

Kehayias, J. J., Fiatarone, M. F., Zhuang, H., & Roubenoff, R. (1997). Total body potassium and body fat: Relevance to aging. *American Journal of Clinical Nutrition, 66,* 904–910.

Khatry, S. K., West, K. P. Jr., Katz, J., LeClerq, S. C., Pradhan, E. K., Wu, L. S., et al. (1995). Epidemiology of xerophthalmia in Nepal: A pattern of household poverty, childhood illness, and mortality. *Archives of Ophthalmology, 113,* 425–429.

Khin-Maung-U, Nyunt-Nyunt-Wai, Myo-Khin, Mu-Mu-Khin, Tin-U, & Thane-Toe. (1985). Effect on clinical outcome of breast feeding during acute diarrhoea. *British Medical Journal, 290,* 587–589.

Kikafunda, J. K., Walker, A. F., Allan, E. F., & Tumwine, J. K. (1998). Effect of zinc supplementation on growth and body composition of Ugandan preschool children: A randomized, controlled intervention trial. *American Journal of Clinical Nutrition, 68,* 1261–1266.

Kilbride, J., Baker, T. G., Parapia, L. A., Khoury, S. A., Shuqaidef, S. W., & Jerwood, D. (1999). Anaemia during pregnancy as a risk factor for iron-deficiency anaemia in infancy: A case-control study in Jordan. *International Journal of Epidemiology, 28,* 461–468.

Kim, J. Y., Moon, S. J., Kim, K. R., Sohn, C. Y., & Oh, J. J. (1998). Dietary iodine intake and urinary iodine excretion in normal Korean adults. *Yonsei Medical Journal, 39,* 355–362.

Kimiagar, M., Azizi, F., Navai, L., Yassai, M., & Nafarabadi, T. (1990). Survey of iodine deficiency in a rural area near Tehran: Association of food in-take and endemic goitre. *European Journal of Clinical Nutrition, 44,* 17–22.

Kirkwood, B. R., Hurt, L., Amenga-Etego, S., Tawiah, C., Zandoh, C., Danso, S., et al. (2010). Effect of vitamin A supplementation in women of reproductive age on maternal survival in Ghana (ObaapaVitA): A cluster-randomised, placebo-controlled trial. *Lancet, 375,* 1640–1649.

Kirkwood, B. R., Ross, D. A., Arthur, P., Morris, S. S., Dollimore, N., Binka, F. N., et al. (1996). Effect of vitamin A supplementation on the growth of young children in northern Ghana. *American Journal of Clinical Nutrition, 63,* 773–781.

Klemm, R. D. W., Labrique, A. B., Christian, P., Rashid, M., Shamim, A. A., Katz, J., et al. (2008). Newborn vitamin A supplementation reduced infant mortality in rural Bangladesh. *Pediatrics, 122,* 242–250.

Klemm, R. D. W., Villate, E. E., Tuason-Lopez, C., Puertollano, E. P., Triunfante, J., del Rosario, A., & Dimaano, M. V. (1997). *Integrating vitamin A capsule supplementation into child weighing: A monitoring study on Philippine OPT Plus.* Manila, Philippines: Helen Keller International and Nutrition Service, Department of Health.

Klemm, R. D. W., West, K. P. Jr., Dary, O., Palmer, A. C., Johnson, Q., Randall, P., et al. (2010). Vitamin A fortification of wheat flour: Considerations and current recommendations. *Food and Nutrition Bulletin, 31,* S47–S61.

Konno, N., Makita, H., Yuri, K., Iizuka, N., & Kawasaki, K. (1994). Association between dietary iodine intake and prevalence of subclinical hypothyroidism in the coastal regions of Japan. *Journal of Clinical Endocrinology and Metabolism, 78,* 393–397.

Kovacs, C. S. (2008). Vitamin D in pregnancy and lactation: Maternal, fetal and neonatal outcomes from human and animal studies. *American Journal of Clinical Nutrition, 88,* 520S–528S.

Krause, V. M., Delisle, H., & Solomons, N. W. (1998). Fortified foods contribute one half of recommended vitamin A intake in poor urban Guatemalan toddlers. *Journal of Nutrition, 128,* 860–864.

Kuhn, L., Aldrovandi, G. M., Sinkala, M., Kankasa, C., Semrau, K., Mwiya, M., et al. (2008). Effects of early, abrupt weaning on HIV-free survival of children in Zambia. *New England Journal of Medicine, 359*, 130–141.

Kuhnlein, H. V. (1992). Food sources of vitamin A and provitamin A. *Food and Nutrition Bulletin, 14*, 3–5.

Kuvibidila, S., Warrier, R. P., Ode, D., & Yu, L. (1996). Serum transferrin receptor concentrations in women with mild malnutrition. *American Journal of Clinical Nutrition, 63*, 596–601.

Kynast, G., & Saling, E. (1986). Effect of oral zinc application during pregnancy. *Gynecology and Obstetrics Investigations, 21*, 117–123.

Labbok, M., & Krasovec, K. (1990). Toward consistency in breastfeeding definitions. *Studies in Family Planning, 21*, 226–230.

Langer, P., Tajtakova, M., Podoba, J. Jr., Kostalova, L., & Gutekunst, R. (1994). Thyroid volume and urinary iodine in school children and adolescents in Slovakia after 40 years of iodine prophylaxis. *Experimental Clinical Endocrinology, 102*, 394–398.

Lartey, A., Manu, A., Brown, K. H., Peerson, J. M., & Dewey, K. G. (1999). A randomized, community-based trial of the effects of improved, centrally processed complementary foods on growth and micronutrient status of Ghanaian infants from 6 to 12 months of age. *American Journal of Clinical Nutrition, 70*, 391–404.

Lauer J. A., Betran, A. P., Barros, A.J.D., & de Onis, M. (2006). Deaths and years of life lost due to suboptimal breast-feeding among children in the developing world: a global ecological risk assessment. *Public Health Nutrition, 9*(6), 673–685.

Launer, L. J., Habicht, J. P., & Kardjati, S. (1990). Breast feeding protects infants in Indonesia against illness and weight loss due to illness. *American Journal of Epidemiology, 131*, 322–331.

Lee, S. Y., & Gallagher, D. (2008). Assessment methods in human body composition. *Current Opinion in Clinical Nutrition and Metabolic Care, 11*, 566–572.

Leroy, J. L., & Frongillo, E. A. (2007). Can interventions to promote animal production ameliorate undernutrition? *Journal of Nutrition, 137*(10), 2311–2316.

Lewis, S. M., Stott, G. J., & Wynn, K. J. (1998). An inexpensive and reliable new haemoglobin colour scale for assessing anaemia. *Journal of Clinical Pathology, 51*, 21–24.

Lie, C., Ying, C., En-Lin, W., Brun, T., & Geissler, C. (1993). Impact of large-dose vitamin A supplementation on childhood diarrhoea, respiratory disease, and growth. *European Journal of Clinical Nutrition, 47*, 88–96.

Lin, C. A., Manary, M. J., Maketa, K., Briend, A., & Ashorn, P. (2008). An energy-dense complementary food is associated with a modest increase in weight gain when compared with a fortified porridge in Malawian children aged 6–18 months. *Journal of Nutrition, 138*, 593–598.

Lindberg, O., Andersson, L. C., & Lamberg, B.-A. (1989). The impact of 25 years of iodine prophylaxis on the adult thyroid weight in Finland. *Journal of Endocrinology Investigations, 12*, 789–793.

Lixin, S., Zhongfu, S., Jiaxiu, Z., Qilin, M., Deming, K., Lifu, Y., & Ying, T. (1995). The measurement and application of TSH-IRMA levels among different age groups in areas with iodine deficiency disorders. *Chinese Medical Science Journal, 10*, 30–33.

Loerch, J. D., Underwood, B. A., & Lewis, K.C. (1979). Response of plasma levels of vitamin A to a dose of vitamin A as an indicator of hepatic vitamin A reserves in rats. *Journal of Nutrition, 109*, 778–786.

Lohman, T. G., Roche, A. F., & Martorell, R. (1988). *Anthropometric standardization reference manual.* Champaign, IL: Human Kinetics.

Lonnerdal, B., Sandberg, A. S., Sandstrom, B., & Kunz, C. (1989). Inhibitory effects of phytic acid and other inositol phosphates on zinc and calcium absorption in suckling rats. *Journal of Nutrition, 119*, 211–214.

Lozoff, B., Klein, N. K., Nelson, E. C., McClish, D. K., Manuel, M., & Chacon, M. E. (1998).

Behavior of infants with iron-deficiency anemia. *Child Development, 69,* 24–36.

Lozoff, B., Wolf, A. W., & Jimenez, E. (1996). Iron-deficiency anemia and infant development: Effects of extended oral iron therapy. *Journal of Pediatrics, 129,* 382–399.

Luby, S. P., Kazembe, P. N., Redd, S. C., Ziba, C., Nwanyanwu, O. C., Hightower, A. W., et al. (1995). Using clinical signs to diagnose anaemia in African children. *Bulletin of the World Health Organization, 73,* 477–482.

Lunn, P. G., Northrop-Clewes, C. A., & Downes, R. M. (1991). Intestinal permeability, mucosal injury, and growth faltering in Gambian infants. *Lancet, 338,* 907–910.

Lutter, C. K., Mora, J. O., Habicht, J. P., Rasmussen, K. M., Robson, D. S., & Herrera, M. G. (1990). Age-specific responsiveness of weight and length to nutritional supplementation. *American Journal of Clinical Nutrition, 51,* 359–364.

Lutter, C. K., Mora, J. O., Habicht, J. P., Rasmussen, K. M., Robson, D. S., Sellers, S. G., et al. (1989). Nutritional supplementation: Effects on child stunting because of diarrhea. *American Journal of Clinical Nutrition, 50,* 1–8.

Lynch, S. R. (1997). Interaction of iron with other nutrients. *Nutrition Reviews, 55,* 102–110.

Lynch, S. R. (1999). Iron: Physiology, dietary sources, and requirement. In M. J. Sadler, J. J. Strain, & B. Caballero (Eds.), *Encyclopedia of Human Nutrition* (pp. 1153–1159). San Diego: Academic Press.

Lynch, S. R., Hurrell, R. F., Bothwell, T. H., & MacPhail, A. P. (1993). *Iron EDTA for food fortification.* A report of the International Nutritional Anemia Consultative Group. Washington, DC: Nutrition Foundation.

Mahalanabis, D. (1991). Breast feeding and vitamin A deficiency among children attending a diarrhoea treatment centre in Bangladesh: A case-control study. *British Medical Journal, 303,* 493–496.

Mahalanabis, D., Lahiri, M., Paul, D., Gupta, S., Gupta, A., Wahed, M. A., & Khaled, M. (2004). Randomized, double-blind, placebo-controlled clinical trial of the efficacy of treatment with zinc or vitamin A in infants and young children with severe acute lower respiratory infection. *American Journal of Nutrition, 79,* 430–436.

Majumdar, I., Paul, P., Talib, V. H., & Ranga, S. (2003). The effect of iron therapy on the growth of iron-replete and iron-deplete children. *Journal of Tropical Pediatrics, 49,* 84–88.

Malaba, L. C., Iliff, P. J., Nathoo, K. J., Marinda, E., Moulton, L. H., Zijenah, L. S., et al. (2005). Effect of postpartum maternal or neonatal vitamin A supplementation on infant mortality among infants born to HIV-negative mothers in Zimbabwe. *American Journal of Clinical Nutrition, 81,* 454–460.

Malik, V. S., Popkin, B. M., Bray, G. A., Després, J. P., & Hu, F. B. (2010). Sugar-sweetened beverages, obesity, type 2 diabetes mellitus, and cardiovascular disease risk. *Circulation, 121,* 1356–1364.

Maluccio, J. A., Hoddinott, J., Behrman, J. R., Martorell, R., Quisumbing, A. R., & Stein, A. D. (2009). The impact of improving nutrition during early childhood on education among Guatemalan adults. *Economic Journal, 119,* 734–763.

Man, W. D., Weber, M., Palmer, A., Schneider, G., Wadda, R., Jaffar, S., et al. (1998). Nutritional status of children admitted to hospital with different diseases and its relationship to outcome in the Gambia, West Africa. *Tropical Medicine and International Health, 3,* 678–686.

Mandal, G. S., Nanda, K. N., & Bose, J. (1969). Night blindness in pregnancy. *Journal of Obstetrics and Gynecology of India, 19,* 453–458.

Mannar, M. G. V., & Dunn, J. T. (1995). *Salt iodization for the elimination of iodine deficiency.* Amsterdam, Netherlands: International Council for Control of Iodine Deficiency Disorders.

Marquis, G. S., Habicht, J. P., Lanata, C. F., Black, R. E., & Rasmussen, K. M. (1997). Breast milk or animal-product foods improve growth of Peruvian toddlers consuming marginal diets. *American Journal of Clinical Nutrition, 66,* 1102–1109.

Marsh, R. (1998). Building on traditional gardening to improve household food security. *Food, Nutrition, and Agriculture, 22*, 4–14.

Martorell, R., Mendoza, F., & Castillo, R. (1988). Poverty and stature in children. In J. C. Waterlow (Ed.), *Linear growth retardation in less developed countries* (pp. 57–73). Nestle Nutrition Workshop Series, Vol. 14. New York: Vevey-Raven Press.

Martorell, R., Stein, A. D., & Schroeder, D. G. (2001). Early nutrition and later adiposity. *Journal of Nutrition, 131*, 874S–880S.

Martorell, R., Yarbrough, C., Lechtig, A., Habicht, J. P., & Klein, R. E. (1975). Diarrheal diseases and growth retardation in preschool Guatemalan children. *American Journal of Physical Anthropology, 43*, 341–346.

Mata, L. J., Cromal, R. A., Urrutia, J. J., & Garcia, B. (1977). Effect of infection of food intake and the nutritional state: Perspectives as viewed from the village. *American Journal of Clinical Nutrition, 30*, 1215–1227.

Mathers, C. D., Boerma, T., & Ma Fat, D. (2009). Global and regional causes of death. *British Medical Bulletin, 92*, 7–32.

Mazumder, S., Taneja, S., Bhandari, N., Dube, B., Agarwal, R. C., Mahalanabis, D., et al. (2010). Effectiveness of zinc supplementation plus oral rehydration salts for diarrhea in infants aged less than 6 months in Haryana state, India. *Bulletin of the World Health Organization.* Retrieved from http://www.who.int/bulletin/online_first/10-075986.pdf

McCollum, E. V., & Davis, M. (1915). The essential factors in the diet during growth. *Journal of Biological Chemistry, 23*, 231–254.

McGuire, J., & Galloway, R. (1994). *Enriching lives: Overcoming vitamin and mineral malnutrition in developing countries.* Washington, DC: World Bank.

McMahon, R. J., & Cousins, R. J. (1998). Mammalian zinc transporters. *Journal of Nutrition, 128*, 667–670.

Mele, L., West, K. P. Jr., Kusdiono, Pandji, A., Nendrawati, H., Tilden, R. L., et al. (1991). Nutritional and household risk factors for xerophthalmia in Aceh, Indonesia: A case-control study. *American Journal of Clinical Nutrition, 53*, 1460–1465.

Menendez, C., Kahigwa, E., Hirt, R., Vounatsou, P., Aponte, J. J., Font, F., et al. (1997). Randomised placebo-controlled trial of iron supplementation and malaria chemoprophylaxis for prevention of severe anaemia and malaria in Tanzanian infants. *Lancet, 350*, 844–850.

Menon, P., Ruel, M. T., Loechl, C. U., Arimond, M., Habicht, J. P., Pelto, G., & Michaud, L. (2007). Micronutrient sprinkles reduce anemia among 9–24 month old children when delivered through an integrated health and nutrition program in rural Haiti. *Journal of Nutrition, 137*, 1023–1030.

Merialdi, M., Caulfield, L. E., Zavaleta, N., Figueroa, A., & DiPietro, J. A. (1998). Adding zinc to prenatal iron and folate tablets improves fetal neurobehavioral development. *American Journal of Obstetrics and Gynecology, 180*, 483–490.

Metges, C. C., Greil, W., Gartner, R., Rafferzeder, M., Linseisen, J., Woerl, A., & Wolfram, G. (1996). Influence of knowledge on iodine content in foodstuffs and prophylactic usage of iodized salt on urinary iodine excretion and thyroid volume of adults in southern Germany. *Zeitschrift Ernahrungswiss, 35*, 6–12.

Mitra, A. K., Alvarez, J. O., & Stephensen, C. B. (1998). Increased urinary retinol loss in children with severe infections. *Lancet, 351*, 1033–1034.

Mokhtar, N., Elati, J., Chabir, R., Bour, A., Elkari, K., Schlossman, N. P., et al. (2001). Diet culture and obesity in northern Africa. *Journal of Nutrition, 131*, 887S–892S.

Monsen, E. R., Hallberg, L., Layrisse, M., Hegsted, D. M., Cook, J. D., Mertz, W., & Finch, C. A. (1978). Estimation of available dietary iron. *American Journal of Clinical Nutrition, 31*, 134–141.

Monteiro, C. A., Conde, W. L., & Popkin, B. M. (2002). Trends in under- and overnutrition in Brazil.

In B. Caballero & B. M. Popkin (Eds.), *The nutrition transition: Diet and disease in the developing world* (pp. 224–140). Food Science and Technology International Series. London: Academic Press.

Monteiro, C. A., Moura, E. C., Conde, W. L., & Popkin, B. M. (2004). Socioeconomic status and obesity in adult populations of developing countries: A review. *Bulletin of the World Health Organization, 82,* 940–946.

Moore, S. E., Cole, T. J., Collinson, A. C., Poskitt, E. M. E., McGregor, I. A., & Prentice, A. M. (1999). Prenatal or early postnatal events predict infectious deaths in young adulthood in rural Africa. *International Journal of Epidemiology, 28,* 1088–1095.

Mora, J., Bonilla, J., Navas, G. E., & Largaespada, A. (2004). *Vitamin A deficiency is virtually under control in Nicaragua.* Paper presented at the twenty-second IVACG meeting, Lima, Peru.

Mora, J. O., Herrera, M. G., Suescun, J., de Navarro, L., & Wagner, M. (1981). The effects of nutritional supplementation on physical growth of children at risk of malnutrition. *American Journal of Clinical Nutrition, 34,* 1885–1892.

Moy, R. J. D., Marshall, T. F. de C., Choto, R. G. A. B., McNeish, A. S., & Booth, I. W. (1994). Diarrhoea and growth faltering in rural Zimbabwe. *European Journal of Clinical Nutrition, 48,* 810–821.

MRC Vitamin Study Research Group. (1991). Prevention of neural tube defects: Results of the Medical Research Council vitamin study. *Lancet, 338,* 131–137.

Muhilal, Permeisih, D., Idjradinata, Y. R., Muherdiyantiningsih, & Karyadi, D. (1988). Vitamin A–fortified monosodium glutamate and health, growth, and survival of children: A controlled field trial. *American Journal of Clinical Nutrition, 48,* 1271–1276.

Mullany, L. C., Katz, J., Li, Y. M., Khatry, S. K., LeClerq, S. C., Darmstadt, G. L., & Tielsch, J. M. (2008). Breast-feeding patterns, time to initiation, and mortality risk among newborns in southern Nepal. *Journal of Nutrition, 138,* 599–603.

Müller, O., Becher, H., van Zweeden, A. B., Ye, Y., Diallo, D. A., Konate, A. T., et al. (2001). Effect of zinc supplementation on malaria and other causes of morbidity in West African children: Randomized double blind placebo controlled trial. *British Medical Journal, 322,* 1567–1571.

Murray, C. J. L., & Lopez, A. D. (1997). Global mortality, disability, and the contribution of risk factors: Global burden of disease study. *Lancet, 349,* 1436–1442.

Murray, M. J., Murray, N. J., Murray, A. B., & Murray, M. B. (1975). Refeeding-malaria and hyperferraemia. *Lancet, 1,* 653–654.

Natadisastra, G., Wittpenn, J. R., Muhilal, West, K. P. Jr., Mele, L., & Sommer, A. (1988). Impression cytology: A practical index of vitamin A status. *American Journal of Clinical Nutrition, 48,* 695–701.

National Heart, Blood and Lung Institute (NHBLI). (1998). *Clinical guidelines on the identification, evaluation, and treatment of overweight and obesity in adults.* NIH Publication No. 98-4083. Bethesda, MD: National Institutes of Health.

National Research Council. (1977). *World food and nutrition study: The potential contributions of research.* Washington, DC: National Academy of Sciences.

Nestel, P., Nalubola, R., Sivakaneshan, R., Wickramasinghe, A. R., Atukorala, S., Wickramanayake, T., & Flour Fortification Trial Team. (2004). The use of iron-fortified wheat flour to reduce anemia among the estate population in Sri Lanka. *International Journal of Vitamin and Nutrition Research, 74,* 35–51.

Ng, S. W., Zhai, F., & Popkin, B. M. (2008). Impacts of China's edible oil pricing policy on nutrition. *Social Science and Medicine, 66,* 414–426.

Nga, T. T., Winichagoon, P., Dijkhuizen, M. A., Khan, N. C., Wasantwisut, E., Furr, H., & Wieringa, F. T. (2009). Multi-micronutrient–fortified biscuits decreased prevalence of anemia and improved micronutrient status and effectiveness of deworming in rural Vietnamese school children. *Journal of Nutrition, 139*(5), 1013–1021.

Ninh, N. X., Thissen, J. P., Collette, L., Gerard, G. G., Khoi, H. H., & Ketelslegers, J. M. (1996). Zinc supplementation increases growth and circulating insulin-like growth factor I (IGF-I) in growth-retarded Vietnamese children. *American Journal of Clinical Nutrition, 63,* 514–519.

Nommsen-Rivers, L. A., & Dewey, K. G. (2009). Growth of breastfed infants. *Breastfeeding Medicine, 4,* S45–S49.

Ntab, B., Cisse, B., Boulanger, D., Sokhna, C., Targett, G., Lines, J., et al. (2007). Impact of intermittent preventive anti-malarial treatment on the growth and nutritional status of preschool children in rural Senegal (West Africa). *American Journal of Tropical Medicine and Hygiene, 77,* 411–417.

Oberleas, D., & Harland, B. F. (1981). Phytate content of foods: Effect on dietary zinc bioavailability. *Journal of the American Dietetic Association, 79,* 433–436.

O'Dempsey, T. J., McArdle, R. F., Lloyd-Evans, N., Baldeh, I., Lawrence, B. E., Secka, O., & Greenwood, B. (1996). Pneumococcal disease among children in a rural area of West Africa. *Pediatric Infectious Disease Journal, 15,* 431–437.

Olson, J. A. (1992). Measurement of vitamin A status. *Netherlands Journal of Nutrition, 53,* 163–167.

Onyango, A. W., Esrey, S. A., & Kramer, M. S. (1999). Continued breastfeeding and child growth in the second year of life: A prospective cohort study in western Kenya. *Lancet, 354,* 2041–2045.

Onyango-Makumbi, C., Bagenda, D., Mwatha. A., Omer, S. B., Musoke, P., Mmiro, F., et al. (2010). Early weaning of HIV-exposed uninfected infants and risks of serious gastroenteritis: Findings from two perinatal HIV prevention trials in Kampala, Uganda. *Journal of Acquired Immune Deficiency Syndromes, 53,* 20–27.

Oppenheimer, S. J. (2001). Iron and its relation to immunity and infectious disease. *Journal of Nutrition, 131,* 616S–635S.

Osendarp, S. J. M., van Raaij, J. M. A., Arifeen, S. E., Wahed, M. A., Baqui, A. H., & Fuchs, G. J. (2000). A randomized, placebo-controlled trial of the effect of zinc supplementation during pregnancy on pregnancy outcome in Bangladeshi urban poor. *American Journal of Clinical Nutrition, 71,* 114–119.

Osendarp, S. J. M., van Raaij, J. M. A., Darmstadt, G. L., Baqui, A. H., Hautvast, J. G. A., & Fuchs, G. J. (2001). Zinc supplementation during pregnancy and effects on growth and morbidity in low birth-weight infants: A randomized placebo controlled trial. *Lancet, 357,* 1080–1085.

Osendarp, S. J. M., West, C. E., & Black, R. E., on behalf of the Maternal Zinc Supplementation Study Group. (2003). The need for maternal zinc supplementation in developing countries: An unresolved issue. *Journal of Nutrition, 133,* 817S–827S.

Oski, F. A., Honig, A. S., Helu, B., & Howanitz, P. (1983). Effect of iron therapy on behavior performance in nonanemic, iron-deficient infants. *Pediatrics, 71,* 877–880.

Owen, C. G., Martin, R. M., Whincup, P. H., Smith, G. D., & Cook, D. G. (2005). Effect of infant feeding on the risk of obesity across the life course: A quantitative review of published evidence. *Pediatrics, 115,* 1367–1377.

Pan American Health Organization (PAHO). (2003). *Guiding principles for complementary feeding of the breastfed child.* Washington, DC: Pan American Health Organization/World Health Organization.

Pardede, L. V. H., Hardjowasito, W., Gross, R., Dillion, D. H. S., Totoprajogo, O. S., Yosoprawoto, M., et al. (1998). Urinary iodine excretion is the most appropriate outcome indicator for iodine deficiency at field conditions at district level. *Journal of Nutrition, 128,* 1122–1126.

Patel, A., Mamtani, M., Dibley, M. J., Badhoniya, N., & Kulkarni, H. (2010). Therapeutic value of zinc supplementation in acute and persistent diarrhea: A systematic review. *PLoS ONE, 5,* e10386.

Pathak, P., Kapil, U., Kapoor, S. K., Saxena, R., Kumar, A., Gupta, N., et al. (2004). Prevalence of multiple micronutrient deficiencies amongst pregnant women in a rural area of Haryana. *Indian Journal of Pediatrics, 71,* 1007–1014.

Peacock, M. (1998). Effects of calcium and vitamin D insufficiency on the skeleton. *Osteoporosis International, 8,* S45–S51.

Pelletier, D. L. (1994). The potentiating effects of malnutrition on child mortality: Epidemiologic evidence and policy implications. *Nutrition Reviews, 52,* 409–415.

Pelletier, D. L., Frongillo, E. D., & Habicht, J. P. (1993). Epidemiologic evidence for a potentiating effect of malnutrition on child mortality. *American Journal of Public Health, 83,* 1130–1133.

Penny, M. E., Peerson, J. M., Marin, M., Duran, A., Lanata, C. F., Lonnerdal, B., et al. (1999). Randomized, community-based trial of the effect of zinc supplementation, with and without other micronutrients, in the duration of persistent childhood diarrhea in Lima, Peru. *Journal of Pediatrics, 135,* 208–217.

Perez, C., Scrimshaw, S., & Munoz, A. (1960). Technique of endemic goitre surveys. In *Endemic goitre* (pp. 360–383). Geneva, Switzerland: World Health Organization.

Peterson, S., Sanga, A., Eklof, H., Bunga, B., Taube, A., Gebre-Medhin, M., & Rosling, H. (2000). Classification of thyroid size by palpation and ultrasonography in field surveys. *Lancet, 355,* 106–110.

Pharoah, P. O. D., Buttfield, I. H., & Hetzel, B. S. (1971). Neurological damage to the fetus resulting from severe iodine deficiency during pregnancy. *Lancet, 1,* 308–310.

Phuka, J. C., Maleta, K., Thakwalakwa, C., Cheung, Y. B., Briend, A., Manary, M. J., & Ashorn, P. (2008). Complementary feeding with fortified spread and incidence of severe stunting in 6- to 18-month-old rural Malawians. *Archives of Pediatric Adolescent Medicine, 162,* 619–626.

Piwoz, E. G., Huffman, S. L., and Quinn, V. J. (2003). Promotion and Advocacy for Improved Complementary Feeding: Can We Apply the Lessons Learned from Breastfeeding? *Food and Nutrition Bulletin, 24,* 29–44.

Piwoz, E. G., Creed de Kanashiro, H., Lopez de Romana, G., Black, R. E., & Brown, K. H. (1996). Feeding practices and growth among low-income Peruvian infants: A comparison of internationally recommended definitions. *International Journal of Epidemiology, 25,* 103–114.

Pollitt, E., Gorman, K. S., Engle, P. L., Rivera, J. A., & Martorell, R. (1995). Nutrition in early life and the fulfillment of intellectual potential. *Journal of Nutrition, 125,* 1111S–11118S.

Popkin, B. M. (1994). The nutrition transition in low-income countries: An emerging crisis. *Nutrition Reviews, 52,* 285–298.

Popkin, B. M. (1998). The nutrition transition and its health implications in lower-income countries. *Public Health and Nutrition, 1,* 5–21.

Popkin, B. M. (1999). Urbanization, lifestyle changes, and the nutrition transition. *World Development, 27,* 1905–1915.

Popkin, B. M. (2009). Global changes in diet and activity patterns as drivers of the nutrition transition. In S. C. Kalhan, A. M. Prentice, & C. S. Yajnik (Eds.), *Emerging societies: Coexistence of childhood malnutrition and obesity* (pp. 1–14). Nestle Nutrition Institute Workshop Series Pediatric Program. Basel, Switzerland: Nestec & Vevey/S. Karger.

Popkin, B. M., & Gordon-Larsen, P. (2004). The nutrition transition: Worldwide obesity dynamics and their determinants. *International Journal of Obesity and Related Metabolic Disorders, 28,* S2–S9.

Popkin, B. M., Horton, S. H., & Kim, S. (2001). The nutrition transition and prevention of diet-related diseases in Asia and the Pacific. *Food and Nutrition Bulletin, 22,* 3–57.

Pradhan, A., Aryal, R. H., Regmi, G., Ban, B., & Govindasamy, P. (1997). *Nepal Family Health Survey 1996.* Kathmandu, Nepal/Calverton, MD: Ministry of Health (Nepal), New ERA, & Macro International.

Prasad, A. S. (1985). Clinical manifestations of zinc deficiency. *Annual Review of Nutrition, 5,* 341–363.

Prasad, A. S. (1991). Discovery of human zinc deficiency and studies in an experimental human model. *American Journal of Clinical Nutrition, 53,* 403–412.

Prentice, A. M. (1996). Constituents of human milk. *Food and Nutrition Bulletin, 17,* 305–312.

Prentice, A. M. (1998). Early nutritional programming of human immunity. In *Annual Report, 1998* (pp. 53–64). Laussanne: Nestle Foundation for the Study of Problems of Nutrition in the World.

Prentice, A. M., Whitehead, R. G., Watkinson, M., Lamb, W. H., & Cole, T. J. (1983). Prenatal dietary supplementation of African women and birthweight. *Lancet, 1,* 489–492.

Preziosi, P., Prual, A., Galan, P., Daouda, H., Boureima, H., & Hereberg, S. (1997). Effect of iron supplementation on the iron status of pregnant women: Consequences for newborns. *American Journal of Clinical Nutrition, 66,* 1178–1182.

Prins, M., Hawkesworth, S., Wright, A., Fulford, A. J., Jarjou, L. M., Prentice, A. M., & Moore, S. E. (2008). Use of bioelectrical impedance analysis to assess body composition in rural Gambian children. *European Journal of Clinical Nutrition, 69,* 1065–1074.

Qing, M., Wang, D., Watkins, W. E., Gebski, V., Yan, Y. Q., Li, M., & Chen, Z. P. (2005). The effects of iodine on intelligence in children: A meta-analysis of studies conducted in China. *Asia Pacific Journal of Clinical Nutrition, 14,* 32–42.

Quality Assurance Workshop for Salt Iodized Programs. (1997). Program Against Micronutrient Malnutrition, Opportunities for Micronutrient Interventions, and John Snow, Inc.

Rahman, M. M., Huq, F., Sack, D. A., Butler, T., Azad, A. K., Alam, A., et al. (1990). Acute lower respiratory infections in hospitalized patients with diarrhea in Dhaka, Bangladesh. *Reviews of Infectious Diseases, 12,* S899–S906.

Rahmathullah, L., & Chandravathi, T. S. (1997). Aetiology of severe vitamin A deficiency in children. *National Medical Journal of India, 10,* 62–65.

Rahmathullah, L., Tielsch, J. M., Thulasiraj, R. D., Katz, J., Coles, C., Devi, S., et al. (2003). Impact of supplementing newborn infants with vitamin A on early infant mortality: Community based randomized trial in southern India. *British Medical Journal, 327,* 254–259.

Rahmathullah, L., Underwood, B. A., Thulasiraj, R. D., & Milton, R. C. (1991). Diarrhea, respiratory infections, and growth are not affected by a weekly low-dose vitamin A supplement: A masked, controlled field trial in children in southern India. *American Journal of Clinical Nutrition, 54,* 568–577.

Rahmathullah, L., Underwood, B. A., Thulasiraj, R. D., Milton, R. C., Ramaswamy, K., Rahmathullah, R., & Babu, G. (1990). Reducing mortality among children in southern India receiving a small weekly dose of vitamin A. *New England Journal of Medicine, 323,* 929–935.

Raisler, J., Alexander, C., & O'Campo, P. (1999). Breastfeeding and infant illness: A dose-response relationship. *American Journal of Public Health, 89,* 25–30.

Ramakrishnan, U., Aburto, N., McCabe, G., & Martorell, R. (2004). Multimicronutrient interventions but not vitamin A or iron interventions alone improve child growth: Results of 3 meta-analyses. *Journal of Nutrition, 134,* 2592–2602.

Ramakrishnan, U., Latham, M. C., & Abel, R. (1995). Vitamin A supplementation does not improve growth of preschool children: A randomized, double-blind field trial in south India. *Journal of Nutrition, 125,* 202–211.

Ramalingaswami, V. (1995). New global perspectives on overcoming malnutrition. *American Journal of Clinical Nutrition, 61,* 259–263.

Rasmussen, L. B., Ovesen, L., & Christiansen, E. (1999). Day-to-day and within-day variation in urinary iodine excretion. *European Journal of Clinical Nutrition, 53,* 401–407.

Reddy, V. (1991). Protein-energy malnutrition. In P. Stanfield, M. Brueton, M. Chan, M. Parkin, & T. Waterston (Eds.), *Diseases of children in the subtropics and tropics* (4th ed., pp. 335–357). London: Hodder & Stoughton.

Rice, A. L., Stoltzfus, R. J., de Francisco, A., Chakraborty, J., Kjolhede, C. L., & Wahed, M. A. (1999). Maternal vitamin A or ß-carotene supplementation in lactating Bangladeshi women benefits mothers and infants but does not prevent subclinical deficiency. *Journal of Nutrition, 129,* 356–365.

Rice, A. L., West, K. P. Jr., & Black, R. E. (2004). Vitamin A deficiency. In M. Ezzati, A. D. Lopez, A. Rodgers, & C. J. L. Murray (Eds.), *Comparative quantification of health risks: Global and regional burden of disease attributable to selected major risk factors* (pp. 211–256). Geneva, Switzerland: World Health Organization.

Riggs, K. M., Spiro, A. L. I., Tucker, K., & Rush, D. (1996). Relations of vitamin B_{12}, vitamin B_6, folate, and homocysteine to cognitive performance in the Normative Aging Study. *American Journal of Clinical Nutrition, 63,* 306–314.

Rivera, J. A., Munoz-Hernandez, O., Rosas-Peralta, M., Guilar-Salinas, C. A., Popkin, B. M., & Willett, W. C. (2008). Beverage consumption for a healthy life: Recommendations for the Mexican population. *Revista de Investigacion Clinica, 60,* 157–180.

Rivera, J., & Ruel, M. T. (1997). Growth retardation starts in the first three months of life among rural Guatemalan children. *European Journal of Clinical Nutrition, 1,* 92–96.

Robinett, D., Taylor, H., & Stephens, C. (1996). *Anemia detection in health services: Guidelines for program managers* (2nd ed.). Seattle: Program for Appropriate Technology in Health.

Ronsmans, C., Fisher, D. J., Osmond, C., Margetts, B. M., & Fall, C. H. (2009). Multiple micronutrient supplementation during pregnancy in low-income countries: A meta-analysis of effects on stillbirths and on early and late neonatal mortality. *Food and Nutrition Bulletin, 30*(4), S547–S555.

Rosado, J. L., Lopez, P., Munoz, E., Martinez, H., & Allen, L. H. (1997). Zinc supplementation reduced morbidity, but neither zinc nor iron supplementation affected growth or body composition of Mexican preschoolers. *American Journal of Clinical Nutrition, 65,* 13–19.

Rosenberg, I. H., & Miller, J. W. (1992). Nutritional factors in physical and cognitive functions of elderly people. *American Journal of Clinical Nutrition, 55,* 1237S–1243S.

Ross, A. C. (1996). The relationship between immunocompetence and vitamin A status. In A. Sommer & K. P. West, Jr. (Eds.), *Vitamin A deficiency: Health, survival, and vision* (pp. 251–273). New York: Oxford University Press.

Ross, S. M., Nel, E., & Naeye, R. (1985). Differing effects of low- and high-bulk maternal dietary supplements during pregnancy. *Early Human Development, 10,* 295–302.

Roth, D. E., Richard, S. A., & Black, R. E. (2010). Zinc supplementation for the prevention of acute lower respiratory infection in children in developing countries: Meta-analysis and meta-regression of randomized trials. *International Journal of Epidemiology, 39,* 795–808.

Rothman, K. J., & Greenland, S. (1998). Causation and causal inference. In K. J. Rothman & S. Greenland (Eds.), *Modern epidemiology* (2nd ed., pp. 7–28). Philadelphia: Lippincott-Raven.

Roubenoff, R. (2000). Sarcopenia and its implications for the elderly. *European Journal of Clinical Nutrition, 54,* S40–S47.

Rousham, E. K., & Mascie-Taylor, C. G. (1994). An 18-month study of the effect of periodic anthelminthic treatment on the growth and nutritional status of pre-school children in Bangladesh. *Annals of Human Biology, 21,* 315–324.

Rowland, M. G. M., Cole, T. J., & Whitehead, R. G. (1977). A quantitative study into the role of infection in determining nutritional status in Gambian village children. *British Journal of Nutrition, 37,* 441–450.

Rowland, M. G. M., Rowland, S. G. J. G., & Cole, T. J. (1988). Impact of infection on the growth of children from 0 to 2 years in an urban West African community. *American Journal of Clinical Nutrition, 47,* 134–138.

Roy, S. K., Chowdhury, A. K., & Rahaman, M. M. (1983). Excess mortality among children discharged from hospital after treatment for diarrhoea in rural Bangladesh. *British Medical Journal, 287,* 1097–1099.

Roy, S. K., Tomkins, A. M., Akramuzzaman, S. M., Behrens, R. H., Haider, R., Mahalanabis, D., & Fuchs, G. (1997). Randomised controlled trial of zinc supplementation in malnourished Bangladeshi children with acute diarrhoea. *Archives of Diseases in Childhood, 77,* 196–200.

Roy, S. K., Tomkins, A. M., Haider, R., Behrens, R. H., Akramuzzaman, S. M., Mahalanabis, D., & Fuchs, G. J. (1999). Impact of zinc supplementation on subsequent growth and morbidity in Bangladeshi children with acute diarrhoea. *European Journal of Clinical Nutrition, 53,* 529–534.

Ruel, M. T., & Bouis, H. E. (1998). Plant breeding: A long-term strategy for the control of zinc deficiency in vulnerable populations. *American Journal of Clinical Nutrition, 68,* 488S–494S.

Ruel, M. T., Rivera, J., Habicht, J. P., & Martorell, R. (1995). Differential response to early nutrition supplementation: Long-term effects on height at adolescence. *International Journal of Epidemiology, 24,* 404–412.

Ruel, M. T., Rivera, J. A., Santizo, M.-C., Lonnerdal, B., & Brown, K. H. (1997). Impact of zinc supplementation on morbidity from diarrhea and respiratory infections among rural Guatemalan children. *Pediatrics, 99,* 808–813.

Ryan, A. S. (1997). Iron-deficiency anemia in infant development: Implications for growth, cognitive development, resistance to infection, and iron supplementation. *Yearbook of Physical Anthropology, 40,* 25–62.

Salama, P., Spiegel, P., Talley, L., & Waldman, R. (2004). Lessons learned from complex emergencies over the past decade. *Lancet, 364,* 1801–1813.

Sanghvi, T., & Murray, J. (1997). *Improving child health through nutrition: The Nutrition Minimum Package.* Arlington, VA: Basic Support for Institutionalizing Child Survival (BASICS) Project, for the U.S. Agency for International Development.

Sazawal, S., Black, R. E., Bhan, M. K., Bhandari, N., Sinha, A., & Jalla, S. (1995). Zinc supplementation in young children with acute diarrhea in India. *New England Journal of Medicine, 333,* 839–844.

Sazawal, S., Black, R. E., Bhan, M. K., Jalla, S., Bhandari, N., Sinha, A., & Majumdar, S. (1996). Zinc supplementation reduces the incidence of persistent diarrhea and dysentery among low socioeconomic children in India. *Journal of Nutrition, 126,* 443–450.

Sazawal, S., Black, R. E., Bhan, M. K., Jalla, S., Sinha, A., & Bhandari, N. (1997). Efficacy of zinc supplementation in reducing the incidence and prevalence of acute diarrhea: A community-based, double-blind, controlled trial. *American Journal of Clinical Nutrition, 66,* 413–418.

Sazawal, S., Black, R. E., Jalla, S., Mazumdar, S., Sinha, A., & Bhan, M. K. (1998). Zinc supplementation reduces the incidence of acute lower respiratory infections in infants and preschool children: A double-blind controlled trial. *Pediatrics, 102,* 1–5.

Sazawal, S., Black, R. E., Menon, V. P., Dhingra, P., Caulfield, L. E., Dhingra, U., & Bagati, A. (2001). Zinc supplementation in infants born small for gestational age reduces mortality: A prospective randomized controlled trial. *Pediatrics, 108,* 1280–1286.

Sazawal, S., Black, R. E., Ramsan, M., Chwaya, H. M., Dutta, A., Dhingra, U., et al. (2007). Effect of zinc supplementation on mortality in children aged 1–48 months: A community-based randomized placebo-controlled trial. *Lancet, 369,* 927–934.

Sazawal, S., Black, R. E., Ramsan, M., Chwaya, H. M., Stoltzfus, R. J., Dutta, A., et al. (2006). Effects of routine prophylactic supplementation with iron and folic acid on admission to hospital and mortality in preschool children in a high malaria transmission setting: Community-based, randomised, placebo-controlled trial. *Lancet, 367*(9505), 133–143.

Sazawal, S., Jalla, S., Mazumder, S., Sinha, A., Black, R. E., & Bhan, M. K. (1997). Effect of zinc supplementation on cell-mediated immunity and lymphocyte subsets in preschool children. *Indian Pediatrics, 34,* 589.

Scholl, T. O., Hediger, M. L., Fischer, R. L., & Shearer, J. W. (1992). Anemia vs iron deficiency:

Increased risk of preterm delivery in a prospective study. *American Journal of Clinical Nutrition, 55,* 985–988.

Schroeder, D. G., Martorell, R., & Flores, R. (1999). Infant and child growth and fatness and fat distribution in Guatemalan adults. *American Journal of Epidemiology, 149,* 177–185.

Schulze, M. B., Manson, J. E., Ludwig, D. S., Colditz, G. A., Stampfer, M. J., Willett, W. C., et al. (2004). Sugar-sweetened beverages, weight gain, and incidence of type 2 diabetes in young and middle-aged women. *Journal of the American Medical Association, 292,* 927–934.

Scrimshaw, N. S., Taylor, C. E., & Gordon, J. E. (1968). *Interactions of nutrition and infection* (WHO Monograph Series). Geneva, Switzerland: World Health Organization.

Selwyn, B. J. (1990). The epidemiology of acute respiratory tract infection in young children: Comparison of findings from several developing countries. *Reviews of Infectious Diseases, 12,* S870–S888.

Semba, R. D., de Pee, S., Panagides, D., Poly, O., & Bloem, M. W. (2004). Risk factors for xerophthalmia among mothers and their children and for mother–child pairs with xerophthalmia in Cambodia. *Archives of Ophthalmology, 122,* 517–523.

Seshadri, S. (Ed.). (1996). *Use of carotene-rich foods to combat vitamin A deficiency in India: A multicentric study* (Scientific Report No. 12). New Delhi: Nutrition Foundation of India.

Shafir, T., Angulo-Barroso, R., Jing, Y., Angelilli, M. L., Jacobson, S. W., & Lozoff, B. (2008). Iron deficiency and infant motor development. *Early Human Development, 84,* 479–485.

Shankar, A. H., Genton, B., Semba, R. D., Baisor, M., Paino, J., Tamja, S., et al. (1999). Effect of vitamin A supplementation on morbidity due to *Plasmodium falciparum* in young children in Papua New Guinea: A randomised trial. *Lancet, 354,* 203–209.

Shankar, A. H., Genton, B., Tamja, S., Arnold, S., Wu, L., Baisor, M., et al. (1999). Zinc supplementation can reduce malaria-related morbidity in preschool children. *American Journal of Tropical Medicine and Hygiene, 57,* A434.

Shankar, A. H., & Prasad, A. S. (1998). Zinc and immune function: The biological basis of altered resistance to infection. *American Journal of Clinical Nutrition, 68,* 447S–463S.

Shankar, A. V., Gittelsohn, J., West, K. P. Jr., Stallings, R., Gnywali, T., & Faruque, F. (1998). Eating from a shared plate affects food consumption in vitamin A–deficient Nepali children. *Journal of Nutrition, 128,* 1127–1133.

Shann, F., Barker, J., & Poore, P. (1989). Clinical signs that predict death in children with severe pneumonia. *Pediatric Infectious Disease Journal, 8,* 852–855.

Sharmanov, A. (1998). Anaemia in Central Asia: Demographic and health survey experience. *Food and Nutrition Bulletin, 19,* 307–317.

Shrestha, R., Pandey, P., Whalley, A., Pandey, S., Mathema, P., Quinley, J., & Dharampal, R. (2004). *Scaling-up child health services: A decade's experience of the Nepal National Vitamin A Program (NVAP).* Paper presented at the twenty-second IVACG Meeting, Lima, Peru.

Siberry, G. K., Ruff, A. J., & Black, R. (2002). Zinc and human immunodeficiency virus infection. *Nutrition Research, 22,* 527–538.

Singh, V., & West, K. P. Jr. (2004). Vitamin A deficiency and xerophthalmia among school-aged children in southeastern Asia. *European Journal of Clinical Nutrition, 58,* 1342–1349.

Sinha, D. P., & Bang, F. B. (1973). Seasonal variation in signs of vitamin-A deficiency in rural West Bengal children. *Lancet, 2,* 228–231.

Skikne, B. S., Flowers, C. H., & Cook, J. D. (1990). Serum transferrin receptor: A quantitative measure of tissue iron deficiency. *Blood, 75,* 1870–1876.

Smedman, L., Sterky, G., Mellander, L., & Wall, S. (1987). Anthropometry and subsequent mortality in groups of children aged 6–59 months in Guinea-Bissau. *American Journal of Clinical Nutrition, 46,* 369–373.

Smil, V. (2002). Food production. In B. Caballero & B. M. Popkin (Eds.), *The nutrition transition: Diet and disease in the developing world* (pp. 25–50). London: Academic Press.

Smitasiri, S., Attig, G. A., & Dhanamitta, S. (1992). Participatory action for nutrition education: Social marketing vitamin A–rich foods in Thailand. *Ecology of Food and Nutrition, 28,* 199–210.

Smith, T. A., Lehman, D., Coakley, C., Spooner, V., & Alpers, M. P. (1991). Relationships between growth and acute lower-respiratory infections in children < 5 years in a highland population of Papua New Guinea. *American Journal of Clinical Nutrition, 53,* 963–970.

Smuts, C. M., Lombard, C. J., Benadé, A. J., Dhansay, M. A., Berger, J., Hople, T., et al. (2005). Efficacy of a foodlet-based multiple micronutrient supplement for preventing growth faltering, anemia, and micronutrient deficiency of infants: The four country IRIS trial pooled data analysis. *Journal of Nutrition, 135*(3), 631S–638S.

Soemantri, A. G., Pollitt, E., & Kim, I. (1985). Iron deficiency anemia and educational achievement. *American Journal of Clinical Nutrition, 42,* 1221–1228.

Solomons, N. W. (1998). There needs to be more than one way to skin the iodine deficiency disorders cat: Novel insights from the field in Zimbabwe. *American Journal of Clinical Nutrition, 67,* 1104–1105.

Solomons, N. W. (1999). Malnutrition: Secondary malnutrition. In M. J. Sadler, J. J. Strain, & B. Caballero (Eds.), *Encyclopedia of Human Nutrition* (pp. 1254–1259). San Diego, CA: Academic Press.

Solon, F. S., Fernandez, T. L., Latham, M. C., & Popkin, B. M. (1979). An evaluation of strategies to control vitamin A deficiency in the Philippines. *American Journal of Clinical Nutrition, 32,* 1445–1453.

Solon, F. S., Klemm, R. D. W., Sanchez, L., Darnton-Hill, I., Craft, N. E., Christian, P., & West, K. P. Jr. (2000). Efficacy of a vitamin A–fortified wheat-flour bun on the vitamin A status of Filipino school children. *American Journal of Clinical Nutrition, 72,* 738–744.

Solon, F. S., Latham, M. C., Guirriee, R., Florentino, R., Williamson, D. F., & Aguilar, J. (1985). Fortification of MSG with vitamin A: The Philippines experience. *Food Technology, 39,* 71–79.

Solon, F. S., Solon, M. S., Mehansho, H., West, K. P. Jr., Sarol, J., Perfecto, C., et al. (1996). Evaluation of the effect of vitamin A–fortified margarine on the vitamin A status of preschool Filipino children. *European Journal of Clinical Nutrition, 50,* 720–723.

Sommer, A. (1982). *Nutritional blindness: Xerophthalmia and keratomalacia.* New York: Oxford University Press.

Sommer, A. (1995). *Vitamin A deficiency and its consequences: A field guide to detection and control* (3rd ed.). Geneva, Switzerland: World Health Organization.

Sommer, A., & Davidson, F. R. (2002). Assessment and control of vitamin A deficiency: The Annecy Accords. *Journal of Nutrition, 132,* 2845S–2850S.

Sommer, A., Hussaini, G., Tarwotjo, I., & Susanto, D. (1983). Increased mortality in children with mild vitamin A deficiency. *Lancet, 2,* 585–588.

Sommer, A., & Loewenstein, M. S. (1975). Nutritional status and mortality: A prospective validation of the QUAC stick. *American Journal of Clinical Nutrition, 28,* 287–292.

Sommer, A., Tarwotjo, I., Hussaini, G., Susanto, D., & Soegiharto, T. (1981). Incidence, prevalence, and scale of blinding malnutrition. *Lancet, 1,* 1407–1408.

Sommer, A., & West, K. P. Jr. (1996). *Vitamin A deficiency: Health, survival, and vision.* New York: Oxford University Press.

Stanbury, J. B., Ermans, A. E., Bourdoux, P., Todd, C., Oken, E., Tonglet, R., et al. (1998). Iodine-induced hyperthyroidism: Occurrence and epidemiology. *Thyroid, 8,* 83–100.

Steer, P., Alam, M. A., Wadsworth, J., & Welch, A. (1995). Relation between maternal haemoglobin concentration and birthweight in different ethnic groups. *British Medical Journal, 310,* 489–491.

Stein, A. D., Thompson, A. M., & Waters, A. (2005). Childhood growth and chronic disease: Evidence from countries undergoing the nutrition transition. *Maternal and Child Nutrition, 1,* 177–184.

Stein, S. A. (1994). Molecular and neuroanatomical substrates of motor and cerebral cortex abnormalities in fetal thyroid hormone disorders. In J. B. Stanbury (Ed.), *The damaged brain of iodine deficiency* (pp. 67–102). New York: Cognizant Communication.

Stephensen, C. B. (2001). Vitamin A, infection, and immune function. *Annual Review of Nutrition, 21,* 167–192.

Stewart, C. P., Christian, P., LeClerq, S. C., West, K. P. Jr., & Khatry, S. K. (2009). Antenatal supplementation with folic acid + iron + zinc improves linear growth and reduces peripheral adiposity in school-age children in rural Nepal. *American Journal of Clinical Nutrition, 90,* 132–140.

Stipanuk, M. H. (2000). *Biochemical and physiological aspects of human nutrition.* Philadelphia: WB Saunders.

Stoltzfus, R. J. (1997). Rethinking anaemia surveillance. *Lancet, 349,* 1764–1766.

Stoltzfus, R. J., Albonico, M., Chwaya, H. M., Tielsch, J. M., Schulze, K. J., & Savioli, L. (1998). Effects of the Zanzibar school-based deworming program on iron status of children. *American Journal of Clinical Nutrition, 68,* 179–186.

Stoltzfus, R. J., Chwaya, H. M., Tielsch, J. M., Schulze, K. J., Albonico, M., & Savioli, L. (1997). Epidemiology of iron deficiency anemia in Zanzibari school children. *American Journal of Clinical Nutrition, 65,* 153–159.

Stoltzfus, R. J., & Dreyfuss, M. L. (1998). *Guidelines for the use of iron supplements to prevent and treat iron deficiency anemia.* International Nutrition Anemia Consultative Group/World Health Organization/United Nations Children's Fund. Washington, DC: ILSI Press.

Stoltzfus, R. J., Edward-Raj, A., Dreyfuss, M. L., Albonico, M., Montresor, A., Thapa, M. D., et al. (1999). Clinical pallor is useful to detect severe anemia in populations where anemia is prevalent and severe. *Journal of Nutrition, 129,* 1675–1681.

Stoltzfus, R. J., Hakimi, M., Miller, K. W., Rasmussen, K. M., Dawiesah, S., Habicht, J. P., & Dibley, M. J. (1993). High-dose vitamin A supplementation of breast feeding Indonesian mothers: Effects on the vitamin A status of mother and infant. *Journal of Nutrition, 123,* 666–675.

Stoltzfus, R.J., Miller, K.W., Hakimi, M., & Rasmussen, K.M. (1993). Conjunctival impression cytology as an indicator of vitamin A status in lactating Indonesian women. *American Journal of Clinical Nutrition, 58,* 167–173.

Stoltzfus, R. J., Mullany, L., & Black, R. E. (2004). Iron deficiency anaemia. In M. Ezzati, A. D. Lopez, A. Rodgers, & C. J. L. Murray (Eds.), *Comparative quantification of health risks: Global and regional burden of disease attributable to selected major risk factors* (Vol. 1, 163–209). Geneva, Switzerland: World Health Organization.

Stoltzfus, R. J., & Underwood, B. A. (1995). Breast-milk vitamin A as an indicator of the vitamin A status of women and infants. *Bulletin of the World Health Organization, 73,* 703–711.

Stott, G. J., & Lewis, S. M. (1995). A simple and reliable method for estimating haemoglobin. *Bulletin of the World Health Organization, 73,* 369–373.

Susser, M., & Stein, Z. (1994). Timing in prenatal nutrition: A reprise of the Dutch Famine Study. *Nutrition Reviews, 52,* 84–94.

Syrenicz, A., Napierala, K., Celibala, R., Majewska, U., Krzyzanowska, B., Gulinska, M., et al. (1993). Iodized salt consumption, urinary iodine concentration, and prevalence of goiter in children from four districts of northwestern Poland (Szczecin

Coordinating Center). *Endokrynologia Polska, 44,* 343–350.

Tajtakova, M., Hancinova, D., Langer, P., Tajtak, J., Foldes, O., Malinovsky, E., & Varga, J. (1990). Thyroid volume by ultrasound in boys and girls 6–16 years of age under marginal iodine deficiency as related to the age of puberty. *Klinisce Wochenschrift, 68,* 503–506.

Talukder, A., Islam, N., Klemm, R., & Bloem, M. (1993). *Home gardening in South Asia: The complete handbook.* Dhaka, Bangladesh: Helen Keller International.

Tamura, T., Goldenberg, R. L., Johnston, K. E., & Dubard, M. (2000). Maternal plasma zinc concentrations and pregnancy outcome. *American Journal of Clinical Nutrition, 71,* 109–113.

Tanumihardjo, S. A., Muhilal, Yuniar, Y., Permaeshi, D., Sulaiman, Z., Karyadi, D., & Olson, J. A. (1990). Vitamin A status in preschool-age Indonesian children as assessed by the modified relative-dose-response assay. *American Journal of Clinical Nutrition, 52,* 1068–1072.

Taren, D., & Chen, J. (1993). A positive association between extended breast-feeding and nutritional status in rural Hubei Province, People's Republic of China. *American Journal of Clinical Nutrition, 58,* 862–867.

Tarwotjo, I., Katz, J., West, K. P. Jr., Tielsch, J. M., & Sommer, A. (1992). Xerophthalmia and growth in preschool Indonesian children. *American Journal of Clinical Nutrition, 55,* 1142–1146.

Tarwotjo, I., Sommer, A., & Soegiharto, T. (1982). Dietary practices and xerophthalmia among Indonesian children. *American Journal of Clinical Nutrition, 35,* 574–581.

Thior, I., Lockman, S., & Shapiro, R. L. (2006). Breastfeeding plus infant zidovudine prophylaxis for 6 months vs formula feeding plus infant zidovudine for 1 month to reduce mother-to-child HIV transmission in Botswana: A randomized controlled trial: The Mashi Study. *Journal of the American Medical Association, 296,* 794–805.

Thomson, C. D., Colls, A. J., Conaglen, J. V., Macormack, M., Stiles, M., & Mann, J. (1997). Iodine status of New Zealand residents as assessed by urinary iodide excretion and thyroid hormones. *British Journal of Nutrition, 78,* 891–912.

Thurnham, D. I., McCabe, G. P., Northrop-Clewes, C. A., & Nestel, P. (2003). Effects of subclinical infection on plasma retinol concentrations and assessment of prevalence of vitamin A deficiency: Meta-analysis. *Lancet, 362,* 2052–2058.

Tielsch, J. M., Khatry, S. K., Stoltzfus, R. J., Katz, J., LeClerq, S. C., Adhikari, R., et al. (2007). Effect of daily zinc supplementation on child mortality in southern Nepal: A community-based, cluster randomized, placebo-controlled trial. *Lancet, 370,* 1230–1239.

Tielsch, J. M., Khatry, S. K., Stoltzfus, R. J., Katz, J., LeClerq, S. C., Adhikari, R., et al. (2006). Effect of routine prophylactic supplementation with iron and folic acid on preschool child mortality in southern Nepal: Community-based, cluster randomized, placebo-controlled trial. *Lancet, 367,* 144–152.

Tielsch, J. M., Rahmathullah, L., Thulasiraj, R. D., Katz, J., Coles, C., Sheeladevi, S., et al. (2007). Newborn vitamin A dosing reduces the case fatality but not incidence of common childhood morbidities in South India. *Journal of Nutrition, 137,* 2470–2474.

Tome, P., Reyes, H., Rodriguez, L., Guiscafre, H., & Gutierrez, G. (1996). Death caused by acute diarrhea in children: A study of prognostic factors. *Salud Publica de Mexico, 38,* 227–235.

Tonascia, J. A. (1993). Meta-analysis of published community trials: Impact of vitamin A on mortality. In Helen Keller International (Ed.), *Bellagio meeting on vitamin A deficiency and childhood mortality: Proceedings of Public Health Significance of Vitamin A Deficiency and Its Control* (pp. 49–51). New York: Helen Keller International.

Toole, M. J., & Waldman, R. J. (1993). Refugees and displaced persons: War, hunger, and public health. *Journal of the American Medical Association, 270,* 600–605.

Tortora, G. J., & Grabowski, S. R. (1996). The endocrine system. In G. J. Tortora & S. R. Grabowski

(Eds.), *Principles of anatomy and physiology* (8th ed., pp. 501–550). New York: HarperCollins.

Torun, B., & Chew, F. (1999). Protein-energy malnutrition. In M. E. Shils, J. A. Olson, M. Shike, & A. C. Ross (Eds.), *Modern nutrition in health and disease* (pp. 963–988). Baltimore, MD: Williams & Wilkins.

Toschke, A. M., Martin, R. M., von Kries, R., Wells, J., Smith, G. D., & Ness, A. R. (2007). Infant feeding method and obesity: Body mass index and dual-energy X-ray absorptiometry measurements at 9–10 y of age from the Avon Longitudinal Study of Parents and Children (ALSPAC). *American Journal of Clinical Nutrition, 85,* 1578–1585.

Trowbridge, F. L., Harris, S. S., Cook, J., Dunn, J. T., Florentino, R. F., Kodyat, B. A., et al. (1993). Coordinated strategies for controlling micronutrient malnutrition: A technical workshop. *Journal of Nutrition, 123,* 775–787.

Tucker, K. (2000). B vitamins, homocysteine, heart disease, and cognitive function. *SCN News, 19,* 30–33.

Tupasi, T. E., Mangubat, N. V., Sunico, M. E., Magdangal, D. M., Navarro, E. E., Leonor, Z. A., et al. (1990). Malnutrition and acute respiratory tract infections in Filipino children. *Review of Infectious Diseases, 12,* S1047–S1054.

Uauy, R., Albala, C., & Kain, J. (2001). Obesity trends in Latin America: Transiting from under- to overweight. *Journal of Nutrition, 131,* 893S–899S.

UNAIDS, UNICEF, & World Health Organiztion (WHO). (1998). *HIV and infant feeding: Guideline for decision-makers.* Geneva, Switzerland: WHO & UNAIDS.

Underwood, B. A. (1990). Methods for assessment of vitamin A status. *Journal of Nutrition, 120,* 1459–1463.

UNICEF. (1990). *The world summit for children.* New York: Author.

UNICEF. (1997). *The state of the world's children 1998.* New York: Oxford University Press.

UNICEF. (2007). *Vitamin A supplementation: A decade of progress.* UNICEF Working Paper. New York: Author.

UNICEF. (2008). *Sustainable elimination of iodine deficiency.* New York: Author.

United Nations. (1982, December 21). *Food problems* (A/RES/37/247). New York: Author.

United Nations. (2000, September 8). *United Nations Millennium Declaration* (A/RES/55/2). New York: Author.

United Nations. (2004, August 27). *Implementation of the United Nations Millennium Declaration* (A/59/282). New York: Author.

USDA Economic Research Service. (2001). *Changing structure of global food consumption and trade.* Washington, DC: United States Department of Agriculture/ARS.

Vaidya, A., Saville, N., Shrestha, B. P., de L Costello, A. M., Manandhar, D. S., & Osrin, D. (2008). Effects of antenatal multiple micronutrient supplementation on children's weight and size at 2 years of age in Nepal: Follow-up of a double-blind randomised controlled trial. *Lancet, 371,* 492–499.

Van Nhien, N., Khan, N. C., Ninh, N. X., Van Huan, P., Hople, T., Lam, N. T., et al. (2008). Micronutrient deficiencies and anemia among preschool children in rural Vietnam. *Asia Pacific Journal of Clinical Nutrition, 17*(1), 48–55.

Vetter, K. M., Djomand, G., Zadi, F., Diaby, L., Brattegaard, K., Timite, M., et al. (1996). Clinical spectrum of human immunodeficiency virus disease in children in a West Africa city: Project RETRO-CI. *Pediatric Infectious Disease Journal, 15,* 438–442.

Victora, C. G., Adair, L., Fall, C., Hallal, P. C., Martorell, R., Richter, L., et al. (2008). Maternal and child undernutrition: Consequences for adult health and human capital. *Lancet, 371,* 340–357.

Victora, C. G., Barros, F. C., Kirkwood, B. R., & Vaughan, J. P. (1990). Pneumonia, diarrhea, and growth in the first 4 years of life: A longitudinal study of 5914 urban Brazilian children. *American Journal of Clinical Nutrition, 52,* 391–396.

Victora, C. G., de Onis, M., Hallal, P. C., Blossner, M., & Shrimpton, R. (2010). Worldwide timing of growth faltering: revisiting implications for interventions. *Pediatrics, 125,* e473–e480.

Victora, C. G., Fuchs, S. C., Kirkwood, B. R., Lombardi, C., & Barros, F. C. (1992). Breastfeeding, nutritional status, and other prognostic factors for dehydration among young children with diarrhoea in Brazil. *Bulletin of the World Health Organization, 70,* 467–475.

Victora, C. G., Kirkwood, B. R., Ashworth, A., Black, R. E., Rogers, S., Sazawal, S., et al. (1999). Potential interventions for the prevention of childhood pneumonia in developing countries: Improving nutrition. *American Journal of Clinical Nutrition, 70,* 309–320.

Victora, C. G., Smith, P. G., Barros, F. C., Vaughan, J. P., & Fuchs, S. C. (1989). Risk factors for deaths due to respiratory infections among Brazilian infants. *International Journal of Epidemiology, 18,* 918–925.

Victora, C. G., Vaughan, J. P., Martines, J. C., & Barcelos, L. B. (1984). Is prolonged breast-feeding associated with malnutrition? *American Journal of Clinical Nutrition, 39,* 307–314.

Villalpando, S., Shamah, T., Rivera, J. A., Lara, Y., & Monterrubio, E. (2006). Fortifying milk with ferrous gluconate and zinc oxide in a public nutrition program reduced the prevalence of anemia in toddlers. *Journal of Nutrition, 136,* 2633–2637.

Villar, J., Smeriglio, V., Martorell, R., Brown, C. H., & Klein, R. E. (1984). Heterogeneous growth and mental development of intrauterine growth-retarded infants during the first 3 years of life. *Pediatrics, 74,* 783–791.

Viteri, F. E. (1998). A new concept in the control of iron deficiency: Community-based preventive supplementation of at-risk groups by the weekly intake of iron supplements. *Biomedical and Environmental Sciences, 11,* 46–60.

Volmink, J., Siegfried, N., van der Merwe, L., & Brocklehurst, P. (2007). Antiretrovirals for reduc-

ing the risk of mother to child transmission of HIV infection. *Cochrane Database Systematic Reviews,* CD003510.

Wald, G. (1955). The photoreceptor process in vision. *American Journal of Ophthalmology, 40,* 18–41.

Walker, S. P., Powell, C. A., Grantham-McGregor, S. M., Himes, J. H., & Chang, S. M. (1991). Nutritional supplementation, psychosocial stimulation, and growth of stunted children: The Jamaican study. *American Journal of Clinical Nutrition, 54,* 642–648.

Walker, S. P., Wachs, T. D., Gardner, J. M., Lozoff, B., Wasserman, G. A., Pollitt, E., et al. (2007). Child development: Risk factors for adverse outcomes in developing countries. *Lancet, 369,* 145–157.

Walter, T. (1989). Infancy: Mental and motor development. *American Journal of Clinical Nutrition, 50,* 655–666.

Walter, T., Olivares, M., Pizarro, F., & Munoz, C. (1997). Iron, anemia, and infection. *Nutrition Reviews, 55,* 111–124.

Wang, Y. C., Bleich, S. N., & Gortmaker, S. L. (2008). Increasing caloric contribution from sugar-sweetened beverages and 100% fruit juices among US children and adolescents, 1988–2004. *Pediatrics, 121,* e1604–e1614.

Wark, J. D. (1999). Osteoporosis: A global perspective. *Bulletin of the World Health Organization, 77,* 424–426.

Waterlow, J. C., Buzina, R., Keller, W., Lane, J. M., Nichaman, M. Z., & Tanner, J. (1977). The presentation and use of height and weight data for comparing the nutritional status of groups of children under the age of 10 years. *Bulletin of the World Health Organization, 55,* 489–498.

Webb, P. (2010). Medium- to long-run implications of high food prices for global nutrition. *Journal of Nutrition, 140,* 143S–147S.

Weissenbacher, M., Carballal, G., Avila, M., Salomon, H., Harisiadi, J., Catalano, M., et al. (1990). Hospital-based studies on acute respiratory tract infection in young children. *Review of Infectious Diseases, 12,* S889–S898.

West, C. E., Eilander, A., & van Lieshout, M. (2002). Consequences of revised estimates of carotenoid bioefficacy for dietary control of vitamin A deficiency in developing countries. *Journal of Nutrition, 132,* 2920S–2926S.

West, K. P. Jr. (2002). Extent of vitamin A deficiency among preschool children and women of reproductive age. *Journal of Nutrition, 132,* 2857S–2866S.

West, K. P. Jr., Chirambo, M., Katz, J., Sommer, A., & Malawi Survey Group. (1986). Breast-feeding, weaning patterns, and the risk of xerophthalmia in southern Malawi. *American Journal of Clinical Nutrition, 44,* 690–697.

West, K. P. Jr., Djunaedi, E., Pandji, A., Kusdiono, Tarwotjo, I., Sommer, A., & Aceh Study Group. (1988). Vitamin A supplementation and growth: A randomized community trial. *American Journal of Clinical Nutrition, 48,* 1257–1264.

West, K. P. Jr., Katz, J., Khatry, S. K., LeClerq, S. C., Pradhan, E. K., Shrestha, S. R., et al. (1999). Double blind, cluster randomised trial of low-dose supplementation with vitamin A or ß-carotene on mortality related to pregnancy in Nepal. *British Medical Journal, 318,* 570–575.

West, K. P., Jr., LeClerq, S. C., Shrestha, S. R., Wu, L. S.-F., Pradhan, E. K., Khatry, S. K., et al. (1997). Effects of vitamin A on growth of vitamin A–deficient children: Field studies in Nepal. *Journal of Nutrition, 127,* 1957–1965.

West, K. P. Jr., Pokhrel, R. P., Katz, J., LeClerq, S. C., Khatry, S. K., Shrestha, S. R., et al. (1991). Efficacy of vitamin A in reducing preschool child mortality in Nepal. *Lancet, 338,* 67–71.

West, K. P. Jr., & Sommer, A. (1987). *Delivery of oral doses of vitamin A to prevent vitamin A deficiency and nutritional blindness* (Nutrition Policy Discussion Paper No. 2). Rome: United Nations Administrative Committee on Coordination, Sub-Committee on Nutrition.

Willett, W. C., Kilama, W. L., & Kihamia, C. M. (1979). Ascaris and growth rates: A randomized trial of treatment. *American Journal of Public Health, 69,* 987–991.

Williams, C. D. (1933). A nutritional disease of childhood associated with a maize diet. *Archives of Diseases in Childhood, 8,* 423–433.

Wittpenn, J. R., Tseng, S. C. G., & Sommer, A. (1986). Detection of early xerophthalmia by impression cytology. *Archives of Ophthalmology, 104,* 237–239.

World Bank. (1993). *World development report 1993: Investing in health.* New York: Oxford University Press.

World Health Organization (WHO). (1992). *Maternal health and safe motherhood programme. The prevalence of anaemia in women: A tabulation of available information* (2nd ed.) (WHO/MCH/MSM/92.2). Geneva, Switzerland: Author.

World Health Organization. (1993). Global prevalence of iodine deficiency disorders. MDIS Working Paper No. 1. Geneva, Switzerland: Micronutrient Deficiency Information System/World Health Organization.

World Health Organization (WHO). (1994). Indicators for assessing iodine deficiency disorders and their control through salt iodization (WHO/NUT/94.6). Geneva, Switzerland: Author.

World Health Organization (WHO). (1995a). *The global prevalence of vitamin A deficiency* (MDIS Working Paper No. 2; WHO/NUT/95.3). Geneva, Switzerland: Author.

World Health Organization (WHO). (1995b). *Physical status: The use and interpretation of anthropometry: Report of a WHO expert committee.* WHO Technical Report Series 854. Geneva, Switzerland: Author.

World Health Organization (WHO). (1996a). *Indicators for assessing vitamin A deficiency and their application in monitoring and evaluating intervention programs* (WHO/NUT/96.10). Geneva, Switzerland: Author.

World Health Organization (WHO). (1996b). *Trace elements in human health and nutrition.* Geneva, Switzerland: Author.

World Health Organization (WHO). (1998). *Integration of vitamin A supplementation with immunization: Policy and programme implications. Report of a meeting 12–13 January, 1998, New York.* Geneva, Switzerland: WHO, Global Program for Vaccines and Immunization, Expanded Program on Immunization.

World Health Organization (WHO). (2000). *The management of nutrition in major emergencies.* Geneva, Switzerland: Author.

World Health Organization (WHO). (2001). *Iron deficiency anaemia: assessment, prevention and control.* (WHO/NHD/01.3). Geneva, Switzerland: Author.

World Health Organization (WHO). (2002). *The world health report 2002: Reducing risks, promoting healthy life.* Geneva, Switzerland: Author.

World Health Organization (WHO). (2004). Global strategy on diet, physical activity and health. Retrieved 2010 from http://www.who.int/dietphysicalactivity/strategy/eb11344/en/index.html

World Health Organization (WHO). (2005). *Preventing chronic diseases: A vital investment: WHO global report.* Geneva, Switzerland: Author.

World Health Organization (WHO). (2008a). *Indicators for assessing infant and young child feeding practices: Part 1. Definitions.* Geneva, Switzerland: Author.

World Health Organization (WHO). (2008b). *Worldwide prevalence of anaemia 1993–2005.* Geneva, Switzerland: Author.

World Health Organization (WHO). (2009a). *Global prevalence of vitamin A deficiency in populations at risk 1995–2005.* Geneva, Switzerland: Author.

World Health Organization (WHO). (2009b). *HIV and infant feeding: Revised principles and recommendations.* Geneva, Switzerland: Author.

World Health Organization (WHO). (2009c). *Use of antiretroviral drugs for treating pregnant women and preventing HIV infection in infants.* Geneva, Switzerland: Author.

World Health Organization (WHO). (2010). *Indicators for assessing infant and young child feeding practices: Part 3. Country profiles.* Geneva, Switzerland: Author.

World Health Organization (WHO) & UNICEF. (2003). *Global strategy for infant and young child feeding.* Geneva, Switzerland: WHO.

World Health Organization (WHO) & UNICEF. (2004). *Clinical management of acute diarrhea.* Geneva, Switzerland: United Nations Children's Fund and WHO.

World Health Organization (WHO), UNICEF, & ICCIDD. (2007). *Assessment of iodine deficiency disorders and monitoring their elimination: A guide for program managers* (3rd ed.). Geneva, Switzerland: WHO.

World Health Organization (WHO), UNICEF, & IVACG. (1997). *Vitamin A supplements: A guide to their use in the treatment and prevention of vitamin A deficiency and xerophthalmia* (2nd ed.). Geneva, Switzerland: WHO.

World Health Organization (WHO) Expert Consultation. (2004). Appropriate body-mass index for Asian populations and its implications for policy and intervention strategies. *Lancet, 363,* 157–163.

World Health Organization (WHO) Multicentre Growth Reference Study Group. (2006a). Assessment of differences in linear growth among populations in the WHO Multicentre Growth Reference Study. *Acta Paediatrica, 450* (suppl), 56–65.

World Health Organization (WHO) Multicentre Growth Reference Study Group. (2006b). *WHO child growth standards for length/height-for-age, weight-for-age, weight-for-length, weight-for-height and body mass index-for-age: Methods and development.* Geneva, Switzerland: WHO.

World Health Organization (WHO) Secretariat. (2007). Conclusions and recommendations of the WHO consultation on prevention and control of iron deficiency in infants and young children in malaria-endemic areas. *Food and Nutrition Bulletin, 28*(4 suppl), S621–S631.

Yang, Z., Lonnerdal, B., Adu-Afarwuah, S., Brown, K. H., Chaparro, C. M., Cohen, R. J., et al. (2007). Prevalence and predictors of iron deficiency in fully breastfed infants at 6 mo of age: Comparison of data from 6 studies. *American Journal of Clinical Nutrition, 89*, 1433–1440.

Yip, R. (1994). Iron deficiency: Contemporary scientific issues and international programmatic approaches. *Journal of Nutrition, 124*, 1479S–1490S.

Yip, R. (1997). The challenge of improving iron nutrition: Limitations and potentials of major intervention approaches. *European Journal of Clinical Nutrition, 51*, S16–S24.

Yip, R., Johnson, C., & Dallman, P. R. (1984). Age-related changes in laboratory values used in the diagnosis of anemia and iron deficiency. *American Journal of Clinical Nutrition, 39*, 427–436.

Yip, R., & Sharp, T. W. (1993). Acute malnutrition and high childhood mortality related to diarrhea: Lessons from the 1991 Kurdish refugee crisis. *Journal of the American Association, 270*, 587–590.

Young, H., Borrel, A., Holland, D., & Salama, P. (2004). Public nutrition in complex emergencies. *Lancet, 364*, 1899–1909.

Zhou, L.-M., Yang, W.-W., Hua, J.-Z., Deng, C.-Q., Tao, X., & Stoltzfus, R. J. (1998). Relation of hemoglobin measured at different times in pregnancy to preterm birth and low birthweight in Shanghai, China. *American Journal of Epidemiology, 148*, 998–1006.

Zimmermann, M. B. (2004). Assessing iodine status and monitoring progress of iodized salt programs. *Journal of Nutrition, 134*, 1673–1677.

Zimmermann, M. B., Connolly, K., Bozo, M., Bridson, J., Rohner, F., & Grimci, L. (2006). Iodine supplementation improves cognition in iodine-deficient schoolchildren in Albania: A randomized, controlled double-blind study. *American Journal of Clinical Nutrition, 83*, 108–114.

Zimmermann, M. B., Hess, S. Y., Molinari, L., de Benoist, B., Delange, F., Braverman, L. E., et al. (2004). New reference values for thyroid volume by ultrasound in iodine-sufficient schoolchildren: A World Health Organization/Nutrition for Health and Development Iodine Deficiency Study Group report. *American Journal of Clinical Nutrition, 79*, 231–237.

Zimmermann, M. B., Jooste, P. L., & Pandav, C. S. (2008). Iodine deficiency disorders. *Lancet, 372*, 1251–1262.

Zimmermann, M. B., Wegmueller, R., Zeder, C., Chaouki, N., Biebinger, R., Hurrell, R. F., & Windhab, E. (2004). Triple fortification of salt with microcapsules of iodine, iron, and vitamin A. *American Journal of Clinical Nutrition, 80*, 1283–1290.

Zimmermann, M. B., Wegmueller, R., Zeder, C., Chaouki, N., Rohner, F., Saissi, M., et al. (2004). Dual fortification of salt with iodine and micronized ferric pyrophosphate: A randomized, double-blind, controlled trial. *American Journal of Clinical Nutrition, 80*, 952–959.

Zimmermann, M. B., Zeder, C., Chaouki, N., Saad, A., Torresani, T., & Hurrell, R. F. (2003). Dual fortification of salt with iodine and microencapsulated iron: A randomized, double-blind, controlled trial in Moroccan school children. *American Journal of Clinical Nutrition, 77*, 425–432.

Zinc Against Plasmodium Study Group. (2002). Effect of zinc on the treatment of *Plasmodium falciparum* malaria in children: A randomized controlled trial. *American Journal of Clinical Nutrition, 76*, 805–812.

Zinc Investigators' Collaborative Group. (1999). Prevention of diarrhea and pneumonia by zinc supplementation in children in developing countries: Pooled analysis of randomized controlled trials. *Journal of Pediatrics, 135*, 689–697.

Zinc Investigators' Collaborative Group. (2002). Therapeutic effects of oral zinc in acute and persistent diarrhea in children in developing countries: Pooled analysis of randomized controlled trials. *American Journal of Clinical Nutrition, 72*, 1516–1522.

Zlotkin, S. H., Arthur, P., Antwi, K. Y., & Yeung, G. (2001). Treatment of anemia with microencapsulated ferrous fumarate p lus ascorbic acid supplied as "sprinkles" to complementary (weaning) foods. *American Journal of Clinical Nutrition, 74,* 791–795.

Zlotnik, H. (2002). Demographic trends. In B. Caballero & B. M. Popkin (Eds.), *The nutrition transition: Diet and disease in the developing world* (pp. 71–108). London: Academic Press.

Zucker, J. R., Perkins, B. A., Jafari, H., Otieno, J., Obonyo, C., & Campbell, C. C. (1997). Clinical

signs for the recognition of children with moderate or severe anaemia in western Kenya. *Bulletin of the World Health Organization, 78*(suppl), 97–102.

Zumrawi, F. Y., Dimond, H., & Waterlow, J. C. (1987). Effects of infection on growth in Sudanese children. *Human Nutrition: Clinical Nutrition, 41,* 453–461.

7

Chronic Diseases and Risks

A DEREK YACH, GEORGE A. MENSAH, CORINNA HAWKES,
JOANNE E. EPPING-JORDAN, AND KRISELA STEYN

Chronic diseases include a heterogeneous group of conditions that usually emerge in middle age after a long exposure to adverse social, environmental, behavioral, and lifestyle factors. To a large extent, chronic diseases have common underlying characteristics: a few common risk factors that act independently and synergistically, a long latency between cumulative exposure to risk and disease outcomes, a high degree of preventability, a low cure rate necessitating decades of treatment and care coordination, considerable comorbidity, and strong linkages to poverty and socioeconomic development. They are predominantly caused by noninfectious diseases.

This chapter focuses on the leading chronic disease killers: cardiovascular diseases (mainly ischemic heart disease and stroke), common cancers, chronic respiratory diseases (mainly chronic obstructive pulmonary disease and asthma), and diabetes. Other chronic diseases are covered in Chapter 9. Emphasis is given to unhealthy consumption and activity patterns—tobacco use, unhealthy diets, and physical inactivity—and the resulting intermediate risks, such as high blood pressure, obesity, and abnormal glucose and lipid metabolism. The epidemiology, demography, current and future trends, and economic implications of these chronic diseases and their risks are briefly summarized. The policy responses and impediments to progress in addressing chronic diseases are described as well.

Epidemiologic Trends: Disease Mortality and Burden

Worldwide, approximately 58 million deaths occurred in 2005, of which chronic diseases in adults accounted for 60% (see the World Health Organization's website: http://www.who.int/topics/chronic_disease/en/; World Health Organization [WHO], 2005). Cardiovascular diseases (CVD)—principally coronary heart disease (CHD) and stroke—caused 17.5 million deaths; cancer, 7.6 million deaths; chronic respiratory disease, 4.1 million deaths; and diabetes, 1.1 million deaths (see Figure 7-1). In high-income countries, 8 out of the 10 leading causes of death are chronic diseases, which account for 93% of total deaths in these countries (Table 7-1) (WHO, 2008). Similarly, 7 out of the 10 leading causes of death in middle-income countries are chronic diseases, which account for 91% of total deaths; in low-income countries, ischemic heart disease, stroke, and chronic obstructive lung disease rank second, fifth, and sixth, respectively, among the 10 leading killers (WHO, 2008).

The majority of chronic disease deaths, nearly 80%, occur in low- and middle-income countries (Figure 7-2) (WHO, 2008, 2009a) and, relative to higher-income nations, are more likely to occur among younger people (Leeder, Raymond, Greenberg, Liu, & Esson, 2004). In addition, the age-specific death rates are higher in low- and low-middle-income countries relative to upper-middle- and high-income countries (Leeder et al., 2004; WHO, 2008). Not surprisingly, as shown in Figure 7-3 and Table 7-2, the high prevalence of risk factors in low- and middle-income countries contribute to chronic disease–related deaths and disability-adjusted life-years in low- and middle-income countries (WHO, 2009a).

---

[1] Statements made and opinions expressed in this chapter are those of the authors and should not be construed as necessarily representing an official position of PepsiCo, Inc.

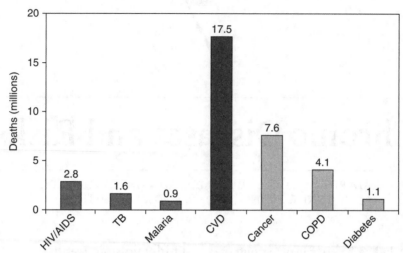

Figure 7-1 Projected global deaths by cause, 2005. *Source:* Modified from WHO, 2005. Preventing chronic diseases: a vital investment: WHO global report. http://www.who.int/chp/chronic_disease_report/full_report.pdf

Table 7-1	The Ten Leading Causes of Deaths in the World, and in Low-, Middle-, and High-Income Countries, 2004					
Disease or injury	Deaths (millions)	Percent of total deaths	Disease or injury	Deaths (millions)	Percent of total deaths
World			*Low-income countries[a]*		
1. Ischemic heart disease	7.2	12.2	1. Lower respiratory infections	2.9	11.2
2. Cerebrovascular disease	5.7	9.7	2. Ischaemic heart disease	2.5	9.4
3. Lower respiratory infections	4.2	7.1	3. Diarrhoeal diseases	1.8	6.9
4. COPD	3.0	5.1	4. HIV/AIDS	1.5	5.7
5. Diarrhoeal diseases	2.2	3.7	5. Cerebrovascular disease	1.5	5.6
6. HIV/AIDS	2.0	3.5	6. COPD	0.9	3.6
7. Tuberculosis	1.5	2.5	7. Tuberculosis	0.9	3.5
8. Trachea, bronchus, lung cancers	1.3	2.3	8. Neonatal infections[b]	0.9	3.4
9. Road traffic accidents	1.3	2.2	9. Malaria	0.9	3.3
10. Prematurity and low birth weight	1.2	2.0	10. Prematurity and low birth weight	0.8	3.2
Middle-income countries			*High-income countries*		
1. Cerebrovascular disease	3.5	14.2	1. Ischaemic heart disease	1.3	16.3
2. Ischaemic heart disease	3.4	13.9	2. Cerebrovascular disease	0.8	9.3
3. COPD	1.8	7.4	3. Trachea, bronchus, lung cancers	0.5	5.9
4. Lower respiratory infections	0.9	3.8	4. Lower respiratory infections	0.3	3.8
5. Trachea, bronchus, lung cancers	0.7	2.9	5. COPD	0.3	3.5
6. Road traffic accidents	0.7	2.8	6. Alzheimer and other dementias	0.3	3.4
7. Hypertensive heart disease	0.6	2.5	7. Colon and rectum cancers	0.3	3.3
8. Stomach cancer	0.5	2.2	8. Diabetes mellitus	0.2	2.8
9. Tuberculosis	0.5	2.2	9. Breast cancer	0.2	2.0
10. Diabetes mellitus	0.5	2.1	10. Stomach cancer	0.1	1.8

[a]Countries grouped by gross national income per capita – low income ($825 or less), high income ($10,066 or more).

[b]This category also includes other non-infectious causes arising in the perinatal period, which are responsible for about 20% of deaths shown in this category.

Source: Reproduced with permission from the World Health Organization, 2008. The global burden of disease: 2004 update. Geneva: World Health Organization. Available at: http://www.who.int/entity/healthinfo/global_burden_disease/GBD_report_2004update_full.pdf

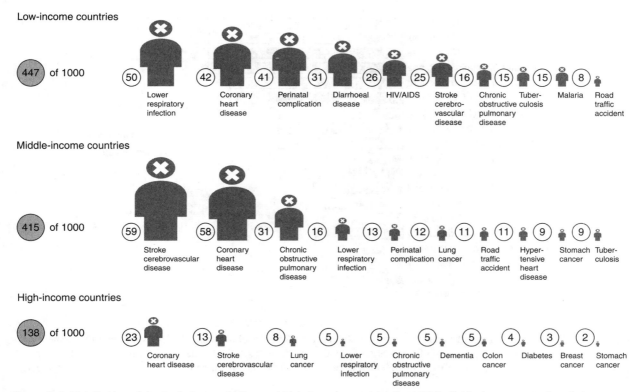

Figure 7-2 Distribution of deaths in low-, middle-, and high-income countries for 1000 individuals representative of the women, men and children from all over the globe who died in 2004. *Source:* Reproduced from WHO, 2008. http://www.who.int/mediacentre/factsheets/fs310_2008.pdf

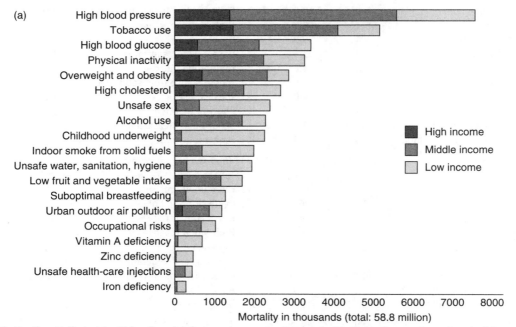

Figure 7-3A Deaths attributed to 19 leading risk factors, by country income level, 2004. *Source:* Reproduced with permission from: World Health Organization, 2009. Global health risks: mortality and burden of disease attributable to selected major risks. http://www.who.int/healthinfo/global_burden_disease/GlobalHealthRisks_report_full.pdf

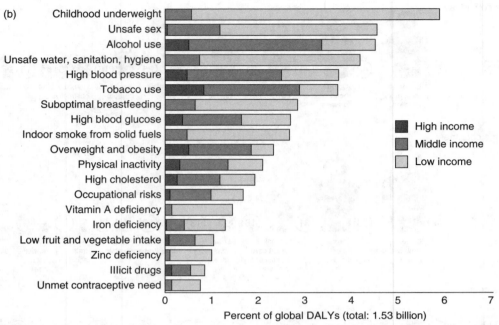

Figure 7-3B Percentage of disability-adjusted life years (DALYs) attributed to 19 leading risk factors, by country income level, 2004. *Source:* Reproduced with permission from: World Health Organization, 2009. Global health risks: mortality and burden of disease attributable to selected major risks. http://www.who.int/healthinfo/global_burden_disease/GlobalHealthRisks_report_full.pdf

Table 7-2			Ranking of Selected Risk Factors: 10 Leading Risk Factor Causes of Death by Income Group, 2004		
Risk factor	**Deaths (millions)**	**Percentage of total**	**Risk factor**	**Deaths (millions)**	**Percentage of total**
World			*Low-income countries[a]*		
1. High blood pressure	7.5	12.8	1. Childhood underweight	2.0	7.8
2. Tobacco use	5.1	8.7	2. High blood pressure	2.0	7.5
3. High blood glucose	3.4	5.8	3. Unsafe sex	1.7	6.6
4. Physical inactivity	3.2	5.5	4. Unsafe water, sanitation, hygiene	1.6	6.1
5. Overweight and obesity	2.8	4.8	5. High blood glucose	1.3	4.9
6. High cholesterol	2.6	4.5	6. Indoor smoke from solid fuels	1.3	4.8
7. Unsafe sex	2.4	4.0	7. Tobacco use	1.0	3.9
8. Alcohol use	2.3	3.8	8. Physical inactivity	1.0	3.8
9. Childhood underweight	2.2	3.8	9. Suboptimal breastfeeding	1.0	3.7
10. Indoor smoke from solid fuels	2.0	3.3	10. High cholesterol	0.9	3.4
Middle-income countries[a]			*High-income countries[a]*		
1. High blood pressure	4.2	17.2	1. Tobacco use	1.5	17.9
2. Tobacco use	2.6	10.8	2. High blood pressure	1.4	16.8
3. Overweight and obesity	1.6	6.7	3. Overweight and obesity	0.7	8.4
4. Physical inactivity	1.6	6.6	4. Physical inactivity	0.6	7.7
5. Alcohol use	1.6	6.4	5. High blood glucose	0.6	7.0
6. High blood glucose	1.5	6.3	6. High cholesterol	0.5	5.8
7. High cholesterol	1.3	5.2	7. Low fruit and vegetable intake	0.2	2.5
8. Low fruit and vegetable intake	0.9	3.9	8. Urban outdoor air pollution	0.2	2.5
9. Indoor smoke from solid fuels	0.7	2.8	9. Alcohol use	0.1	1.6
10. Urban outdoor air pollution	0.7	2.8	10. Occupational risks	0.1	1.1

[a]Countries grouped by gross national income per capita – low income (US$ 825 or less), high income (US$ 10 066 or more).

Source: Reproduced with permission from: World Health Organization, 2009. Global health risks: mortality and burden of disease attributable to selected major risks. http://www.who.int/healthinfo/global_burden_disease/GlobalHealthRisks_report_full.pdf

Overall, the burden of disease and loss of economic output associated with chronic diseases is substantial (Abegunde, Mathers, Adam, Ortegon, & Strong, 2007). In one study of 23 countries that accounted for approximately 80% of the total burden of chronic disease mortality in the low- and middle-income world, researchers demonstrated that chronic diseases were responsible for 50% of the total disease burden in 2005 (Abegunde et al., 2007). For 15 of the selected countries for which death registration data were available, the estimated age-standardized death rates for chronic diseases in 2005 were 54% higher

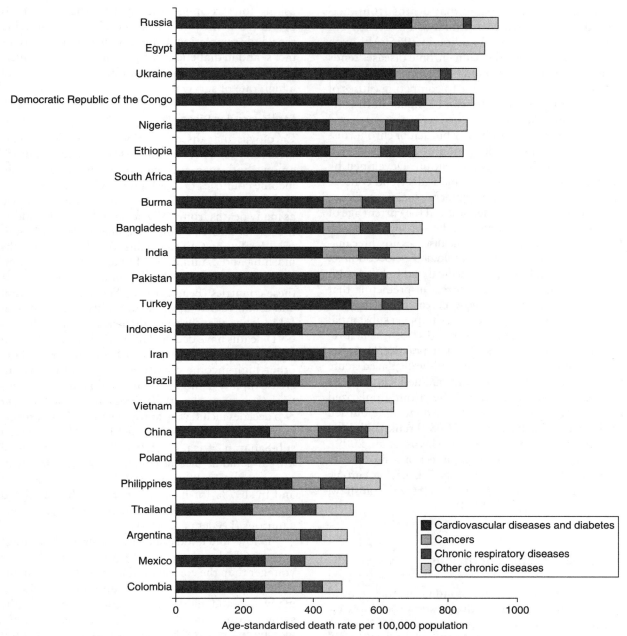

Figure 7-4 Projected age-standardized death rates for 2005 from chronic diseases (per 100,000), for all ages and both sexes in 23 selected countries. *Source:* Reprinted from *The Lancet*, 370, Dele O Abegunde, Colin D Mathers, Taghreed Adam, Monica Ortegon, Kathleen Strong, "The burden and costs of chronic diseases in low-income and middle income countries" 1929–38, 2007 with permission from Elsevier.

for men and 86% higher for women than those for men and women in high-income countries (Figure 7-4) (Abegunde et al., 2007).

The shift toward a higher burden of chronic diseases in low- and middle-income nations is well illustrated by China. By the late 1990s, 83% of rural deaths in that country were already caused by chronic diseases (Bumgarner, 2003). Age-specific death rates increased rapidly between 1986 and 1999 for CVD and cancers. It is predicted that deaths from diet-related chronic diseases in China will increase from 5 million in 1995 to 15.3 million in 2025. Although the percentage of deaths from chronic diseases tends to be lower in low- and middle-income countries than in high-income countries due to competing causes of death, absolute death rates can be higher in the former (Unwin et al., 2001).

The trend toward a higher burden of chronic diseases in low- and middle-income countries has been termed the epidemiologic transition. Developed by Omran (1971), the theory behind this trend conceptualizes three ages of disease epidemiologies: pestilence and famine, receding epidemics, and the current age of degenerative and human-made chronic diseases. Driving the transition to chronic diseases are three major sets of determinants: ecobiologic; socioeconomic, political, and cultural; and medical and public health interventions. Omran was correct in predicting that chronic diseases would impose a greater burden in the coming decades. In Africa, for example, a substantial increase in the amount of chronic disease was first reported in the 1970s (Reis, 1978). In practice, however, chronic diseases have not smoothly displaced acute infectious diseases in low- and middle-income countries. Rather, these countries suffer from a polarized and protracted double, triple, or quadruple burden of disease (Bradshaw et al., 2003; Frenk, Bobdilla, Sepulveda, & Cervantes, 1989; Mayosi et al., 2009). For example, in South Africa, infectious diseases account for 28% of years of life lost (YLLs), while chronic diseases account for 25% of YLLs (Steyn, Bradshaw, Norman, & Laubscher, 2003).

Common Chronic Conditions

The most common chronic conditions, their typical clinical features, and the diagnostic procedures required to identify them are presented in Table 7-3. The prevalence of these conditions varies significantly around the world, but is mainly determined by the extent to which populations have progressed along the timeline of the epidemiologic, nutrition, and other health transitions. All of the conditions listed in Table 7-3 occur more frequently in middle-aged and older people and, with the exception of cancers, occur more frequently in urban than rural settings. Some chronic disease risk factors, such as high blood pressure and high blood lipid and blood sugar levels, can be present without any signs or symptoms; therefore, their diagnoses depend either on regular screening by motivated healthcare providers or on the population asking for screening—usually after they have been prompted by health education initiatives targeting the whole population. Patients with strokes, heart attacks, and in diabetic coma present as medical emergencies requiring immediate hospitalization to ensure a high rate of survival.

Cardiovascular Diseases

Cardiovascular diseases, principally ischemic heart disease and stroke, remain the leading cause of death among both men and women in low- and middle-income countries (as for high-income countries); see Figure 7-5 and Table 7-1. In absolute numbers, twice as many deaths from CVD occur in low- and middle-income countries as high-income developed countries. Each year, CVD accounts for 2.8 million deaths in China and 2.5 million in India, dwarfing the combined totals of all deaths from infectious diseases in these countries (Beaglehole & Yach, 2003). In rural and urban Tanzania, stroke mortality rates are threefold higher than in the United Kingdom. Whereas CVD deaths have declined by 50% since the 1960s in the United States, the United Kingdom, and many other high-income countries, they continue to increase rapidly in most low- and middle-income countries (Leeder et al., 2004). Predictions for the next two decades include a near tripling of CHD and stroke mortality in Latin America, the Middle East, and even sub-Saharan Africa. Projected CHD mortality for all low- and middle-income countries is anticipated to increase between 1990 and 2020 by 120% for women and by 137% for men, compared with age-related increases of between 30% and 60% in high-income countries (Leeder et al., 2004).

In low- and middle-income countries, the average ages at which people die of CVD are significantly younger than the corresponding ages in high-income countries. CVD rates for 30- and 40-year-olds in many low- and middle-income countries are now the same as those for 40- and 50-year-olds in high-income countries (WHO, 2003d). In India and South Africa, CVD death rates in working-age women are higher today than they were in U.S. women in the 1950s (Leeder et al., 2004). In Pakistan, the overall

Table 7-3	Clinical Features of Common Chronic Conditions and Their Risk Factors	
Conditions	**Typical Clinical Features**	**Diagnostic Requirements**
Hypertension	No obvious symptoms	Measure blood pressure following standardized procedures (e.g., WHO guidelines)
High blood lipid	No obvious symptoms	Measure total cholesterol, high-density lipoprotein cholesterol, and triglyceride levels in fasting blood samples
Obesity	Obviously overweight, often associated with tiredness, daytime somnolence, excessive snoring, and possibly arthritis	Measure height (meters) and weight (kilograms); calculate body mass index (BMI)=weight/height^2; measure waist circumference
Diabetes	Malaise, excessive thirst, excessive urination, hunger, blurred vision, and tendency to develop infections	Measure fasting or random blood glucose, possibly glucose tolerance test
Asthma	Wheezing, difficulty with breathing, and coughing (bronchospasm) relieved by asthma medication	Peak flow measurements and other lung function tests, chest x-ray, and relief of symptoms with bronchodilators
Chronic bronchitis	Productive cough for 3 months per year in two consecutive years, shortness of breath, and frequent chest infections	Lung function tests, chest x-ray
Myocardial infarction (heart attack)	Sudden onset of severe crushing chest pain that could radiate down left arm, to the neck or jaw, with associated sweating, faintness, shortness of breath, and nausea	Emergency, hospitalization, clinical examination, electrocardiograph, blood tests for cardiac enzyme
Cerebrovascular disease (stroke)	Sudden weakness; loss of motor or sensory function, usually unilateral; inability to speak; vision disturbances; or unconsciousness	Emergency, hospitalization, neurologic and full clinical examination, consider CAT scan, identify underlying causes
Angina	Central chest pain precipitated by exertion and relieved by resting	Electrocardiograph, pain relieved by angina medication
Transient ischemic attack	Same presentation as stroke—weakness, loss of motor or sensory function, inability to speak, or vision disturbance—but resolving within 24 hours	Neurological and full clinical examination, identify underlying causes
Cancers in general	Unexplained loss of weight, malaise, and tiredness	Full clinical examination, special investigations
Breast cancer	A painless lump in the breast or discharge from the nipple or breast deformity	Regular self-examination and by a doctor to identity a lump early, mammogram, biopsy of lump for pathology diagnosis
Cervical cancer	Unexplained vaginal discharge or bleeding, pain on intercourse	Clinical examination, Pap smear, cytological diagnosis
Lung cancer	Unexplained shortness of breath, chronic cough could be blood stained, and could have enlarged lymph nodes in neck	Clinical examination, sputum examination, chest x-ray, bronchoscopy, lung biopsy
Prostate cancer	Difficulty or pain with urination, frequent urination with dribbling	Clinical rectal examination, prostate-specific antigen (PSA) blood test, biopsy, prostatectomy, pathology diagnosis
Colon cancer	Ongoing abdominal pain or discomfort, change in bowel habits	Clinical examination, test for blood in the stool, barium enema, colonoscopy; surgery and pathology
Stomach cancer	Dyspepsia, ongoing upper abdominal pain or discomfort, nausea and vomiting	Clinical examination, barium meal, gastroscopy, surgery, and pathology

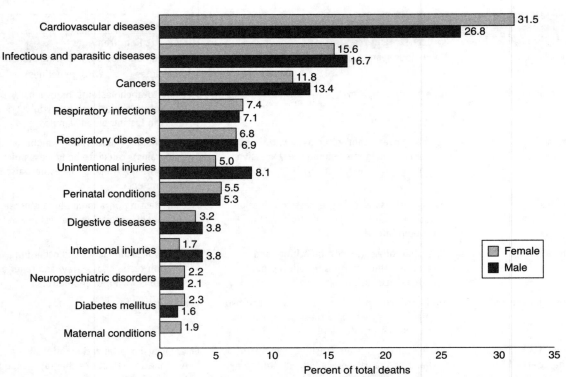

Figure 7-5 Distribution of deaths by leading cause groups, males and females, world, 2004. *Source:* Reproduced with permission from the World Health Organization, 2008. The global burden of disease: 2004 update. Geneva: World Health Organization. Available at: http://www.who.int/entity/healthinfo/global_burden_disease/GBD_report_2004update_full.pdf

prevalence of coronary artery disease is 26.9% in men and 30.0% in women; this rate translates to one in four middle-aged adults with prevalent coronary artery disease. The risk is uniformly higher in the young and in women (Nishtar, 2003). In rural Vietnam, CVD accounted for approximately 20% of all deaths in 2000, with more than 40% of these deaths occurring among people younger than 70 years (Minh, Byass, & Wall, 2003).

Diabetes

The global prevalence of diabetes among all age groups was estimated at 171 million (2.8% of the global population) in 2000, which is projected to increase to 366 million (6.5%) in 2030; 298 million of those affected will live in low- and middle-income countries (Wild, Roglic, Green, Sicree, & King, 2004). The projected increase in the prevalence of diabetes over this period in low- and middle-income countries will be 147%, compared with 54% for established market economies (Table 7-4) (Wild et al., 2004). By 2030, most people with diabetes in low- and middle-income countries will be between 45 and 64 years old. In high-income countries, by contrast, most people with diabetes will be older than 65 years. These projections consider demographic changes and some

Table 7-4	Projected Increase in Diabetes in Developing Countries		
Region	**Estimated Number of People with Diabetes, 2000**	**Estimated Number of People with Diabetes, 2030**	**Percentage Change**
India	31,705	79,441	151
China	20,757	42,321	104
Other Asia and Islands	22,238	58,109	148
Sub-Saharan Africa	7,146	18,645	161
Latin America and the Caribbean	13,307	32,959	148
Middle Eastern Crescent	20,051	52,794	163

Source: S. Wild, G. Roglic, A. Green, R. Sicree, and H. King, "Global Prevalence of Diabetes: Estimates for 2000 and Projections for 2003," 2004, *Diabetes Care,* 27, pp. 1047–1053. Reprinted with permission.

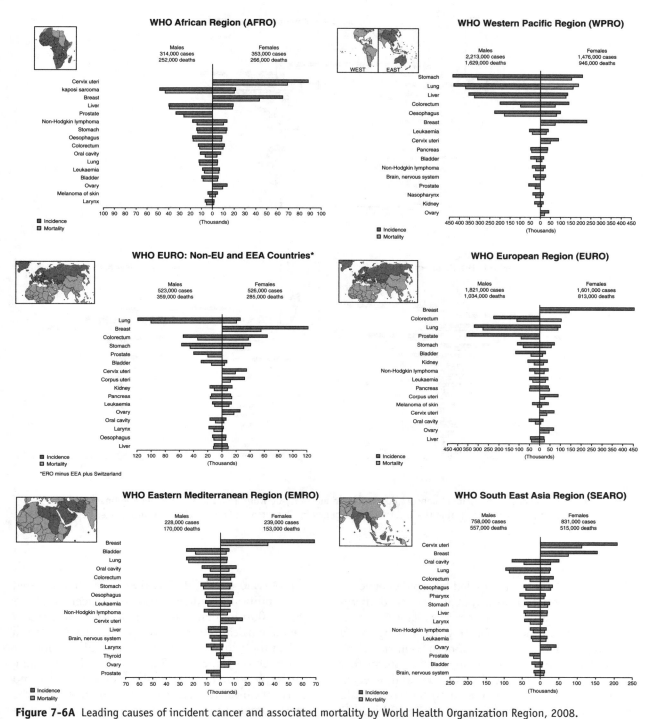

Figure 7-6A Leading causes of incident cancer and associated mortality by World Health Organization Region, 2008.
Source: Reproduced with permission from the International Agency for Research on Cancer (2008). World Cancer Report. Lyons, France: IARC Press.

aspects of urbanization, but not current increases in childhood and adult obesity in most urban settings, which will increase the prevalence of type 2 diabetes even more (Wild et al., 2004).

One example of rapid change and diabetes prevalence comes from the Pacific region. Diabetes was virtually nonexistent in populations indigenous to the Pacific who maintained a traditional lifestyle.

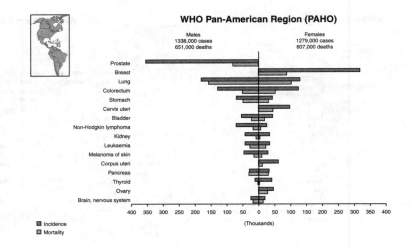

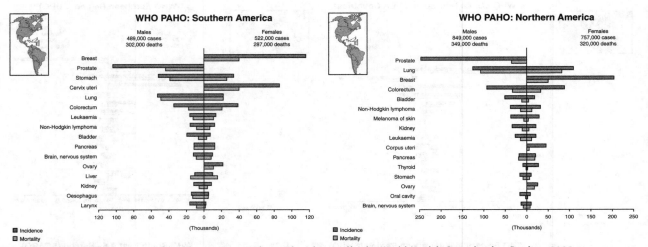

Figure 7-6B Leading causes of incident cancer and associated mortality by World Health Organization Region, 2008.
Source: Reproduced with permission from the International Agency for Research on Cancer (2008). World Cancer Report. Lyons, France: IARC Press.

However, in recent years, fueled by rapid changes in diet and a reduction in physical activity, diabetes prevalence in this region has soared (Foliaki & Pearce, 2003). A similar picture is emerging in many island states and even in some of the poorest countries of the world. For example, epidemiologic data indicate that diabetes prevalence in adults (35 years and older) in urban areas of Tanzania is at least 10% (Aspray et al., 2000). In China, a survey carried out in 2000–2001 showed that 5.2% of men aged 35 to 74 years (12.7 million) and 5.8% of women of the same age group (13.3 million) have diabetes (diagnosed and undiagnosed)—far higher rates than previously reported (Gu et al., 2003).

Cancer

Figure 7-6 shows the distribution of incident cases and mortality from cancer in men and women by WHO regions. Worldwide, there were an estimated 12.4 million incident cases of cancer in 2008 (6,672,000 in men and 5,779,000 in women) and 7.6 million deaths from cancer (4.3 million in men and 3.3 million in women) (International Agency for Research on Cancer [IARC], 2008). Globally, lung cancer was the most common incident cancer and cause of cancer-related deaths in men. In women, the most common incident cancer and cause of cancer-related death was breast cancer (IARC, 2008).

The International Agency for Research on Cancer (http://www.iarc.fr/) estimates that cancer incidence increased 19% between 1990 and 2000 (Stewart & Kleihaus, 2003). The major causes of cancer are (1) tobacco use in both high-income and low- and middle-income countries, (2) chronic infections in low- and middle-income countries, and (3) a complex array of diet and physical activity factors. The prevalence of different types of cancers varies between high-income and low- and middle-income countries.

Lung cancer, which is the most frequently occurring cancer worldwide and a type of cancer that is primarily due to tobacco use, accounts for 1.2 million deaths each year— 2.3% of all cancer deaths. Cancers caused by tobacco are increasing in most low- and middle-income countries and among women in almost all countries. In a few high-income countries, tobacco-related cancer incidence has started to decline as men smoke less. In contrast, cancers caused by chronic infections and food contaminants and preparation methods have been in decline in low- and middle-income countries for decades. There has been little change in the incidence of the two most common cancers in women—breast and cervix—over the last few decades. Survival rates remain very low for lung, liver, and stomach cancers, although they have increased for many other cancers in recent years, due mainly to early detection and increasingly effective treatments (Stewart & Kleihaus, 2003).

It is estimated that the overall number of cancer cases will rise by 50% in the next 20 years, leading to a total of 15.3 million new patients with cancer per year—60% of whom will be living in low- and middle-income countries (Ullrich et al., 2004).

Chronic Respiratory Diseases

Chronic respiratory diseases include two major groups of diseases: chronic obstructive pulmonary disease (COPD) and asthma. COPD accounts for 4.8% of all deaths worldwide (2.7 million deaths annually); 50% of those deaths occur in China and countries in the western Pacific, and a further 24% occur in India (WHO, 2003d). Major risk factors for COPD include tobacco use, a range of occupational exposures, indoor air pollution from biomass fuel, and childhood exposure to respiratory infections (Ait-Khaled, Enarson, & Bousquet, 2001). These risk factors are substantially more common among people living in low- and middle-income countries, and in poor communities in high-income countries.

Comorbid Conditions

Comorbidity refers to simultaneous occurrence in a person of two or more disorders. A notable form of comorbidity is between diabetes and CVD. Heart attacks, for example, are significantly more common in people with diabetes, as are deaths following a first heart attack (International Diabetes Federation, 2003). In addition, important comorbidities exist between some mental disorders and other chronic diseases: Persons with chronic conditions have a greater probability of developing mental disorders such as

depression (WHO, 2003c). The proportion of patients with depression who also have other common chronic diseases, such as CVD, diabetes, and cancer, ranges from 22% to 33% (WHO, 2003c).

There are also interactive effects between certain infectious and noninfectious diseases. Several infectious agents cause cancer: Hepatitis B virus causes liver cancer; human papillomavirus (HPV) causes cervical cancer; *Helicobacter pylori* causes stomach cancer; human immunodeficiency virus (HIV) causes several cancers, including Kaposi's sarcoma and non-Hodgkin's lymphoma; and *Schistosoma haematobium* causes bladder cancer (Stewart & Kleihaus, 2003). All of these cancers are common in low- and middle-income countries, especially in the poorest countries where resources for treatment are extremely inadequate. Vaccines to prevent these infections and effective drugs to treat them could greatly reduce the cancer burden in these countries.

Finally, there are interactions between risk factors and death rates from other diseases. Tobacco increases the death rate from tuberculosis (TB)—a classic disease of poverty—in those persons already infected. In India, smokers are 4.5 times more likely to die of TB than nonsmokers (Gajalakshmi, Peto, Kanaka, & Jha, 2003). An estimated 80% of TB-infected patients smoke. As a result, tobacco is probably the major cause of death in treated TB patients (Yach & Raviglione, 2004).

Risk Factors

Major Risk Factors

Over the last 50 years, epidemiologic studies have provided evidence of which risk factors promote the development of chronic diseases. This chapter focuses mainly on three major risk factors—tobacco, diet, and physical activity—which collectively explain the incidence of most chronic diseases.

Many risk factors are common to several chronic diseases, and most are modifiable. The strength of the evidence and the quality of studies have been highest for tobacco. Since the first Surgeon General's report on smoking in 1964 (U.S. Department of Health, Education, and Welfare, 1964) the criteria for deciding whether tobacco causes a disease have been refined, the evidence of the impact of tobacco on specific causes has strengthened, and the number of diseases and conditions listed as being causally related to tobacco has lengthened. The recent 50-year follow-up of doctors has quantified the long-term impact of tobacco in a unique way; in particular, it showed that smoking continues to pose substantial risks well into the eighth decade of life and, conversely, that quitting confers life-extending benefits at advanced ages (Doll, Peto, Boreham, & Sunderland, 2004). In the Surgeon General's report of 2004 (U.S. Department of Health and Human Services [DHHS], 2004), several diseases were added to previous lists of smoking-caused conditions.

In contrast, there have not been as many major reviews of the impact of specific dietary factors and physical activity on specific outcomes. One of the most recent international reviews on the topic is sum-

marized in Table 7-5. The causal criteria differ from those used for tobacco, and there have been substantially fewer cohort studies of long duration in the areas of diet and nutrition compared with tobacco. Taken together, the results of causal studies of tobacco, diet, and physical activity indicate that several major diseases are closely and negatively associated with just these three risk factors.

In the most recent analysis of global mortality and burden of disease attributable to selected major risk factors, six chronic disease risk factors—tobacco, high blood pressure, high blood glucose, indoor air

Table 7-5	A Selective Summary of the Evidence for Obesity, Type 2 Diabetes, Cardiovascular Disease, Cancer, Dental Disease, and Osteoporosis					
	Obesity	Type 2 Diabetes	CVD	Cancer	Dental Disease	Osteoporosis
Energy and Fats						
High intake of energy-dense foods	C+					
Saturated fats		P+	C+			
Trans-fatty acids			C+			
Dietary cholesterol			P+			
Fish and fish oils			P−			
Carbohydrate						
High intake of dietary fiber	C−	P−	P−			
Free sugars					C+	
Vitamins						
Vitamin D					C−	C−
Minerals						
High intake of sodium			C+			
Fluoridation of local water supply					C−	
Fruits and Vegetables	C−	P−	C−	P−		
Beverages, non-alcoholic						
Sugar-sweetened soft drinks	P+				P+	
Beverages, alcoholic						
High alcohol intake			C+	C+		C+
Low to moderate alcohol intake			C−			
Weight and physical activity						
Overweight and obesity		C+	C+	C+		
Voluntary weight loss		C−				
Regular physical activity	C−	C−	C−	C−		C−
Physical inactivity	C+	C+				
Other factors						
Exclusive breastfeeding	P+					
Environmental factors						
Heavy marketing of energy-dense foods and fast-food outlets	P+					

C+: Convincing increasing risk; C−: Convincing decreasing risk; P+: probable increasing risk; P−: probable decreasing risk.

Source: World Health Organization, *Diet, Nutrition, and the Prevention of Chronic Diseases*, Technical Report No. 916 (Geneva, Switzerland: World Health Organization, 2003). Reprinted with permission.

pollution, physical inactivity, and high cholesterol—are among the 10 leading risk factors contributing to the burden of mortality in low-income countries (Table 7-2) (WHO, 2009c). In contrast, in both middle- and high-income countries, all 10 leading risk factors contributing to overall mortality are chronic disease risk factors (WHO, 2009c).

It is clear from the global analyses that tobacco and high blood pressure are major universal threats to health. Diet-related risks dominate in all parts of the world, albeit with varying contributions coming from under-consumption and over-consumption in different parts of the world. A lack of fruit and vegetables is evident in most countries and has implications not just for chronic noncommunicable disease, but also for infectious diseases.

Risk Factor Trends

Trends in risk factors for chronic diseases in developing countries are not encouraging. The number of cigarettes smoked has more than doubled since 1960 (Mackay, Eriksen, & Shafey, 2006). There have been positive dietary trends over the past decades that are reducing the levels of undernutrition, but the supply of fat increased by 28% between 1977 and 1997–1999, while the Food and Agriculture Organization (FAO) of the United Nations predicts further increases in total per capita consumption of vegetable oils, sugar,

and meat and declines in cereal consumption (WHO, 2003b). Importantly, children are increasingly exposed to risk factors, portending a massive increase in chronic disease occurrence in future decades. Alcohol abuse is becoming more widespread among youth. Age of uptake of smoking is showing a trend toward the early teenage years, and young people exhibit high usage of other tobacco products.

A survey of 1 million 13- to 15-year-olds demonstrated that tobacco use occurs in one in five children in almost all of the more than 100 countries surveyed (Global Youth Tobacco Survey Collaborating Group, 2003) (Table 7-6). Moreover, almost as many girls as boys smoke, and in some areas more girls smoke than boys. This trend can be linked with advertising and marketing practices, which target both girls and women by associating smoking with independence, glamour, and romance. In the most recent assessment of the 100 countries surveyed, 61 reported no change over time in prevalence of cigarette smoking (Warren, Lea, Lee, Jones, Asma, & McKenna, 2009). Similarly, in 50 of the 97 sites with data on use of other tobacco products there was no change. However, 34 countries reported an increase in other tobacco use, which the authors attributed to use of waterpipes, an emerging trend in tobacco use (Warren et al., 2009). Again, the recent evidence showed an increasing trend of tobacco use among adolescent girls (Warren et al., 2009).

Table 7-6	Percentage of Students Aged 13 to 15 Who Currently Smoke Cigarettes		
	Boys	**Girls**	**Boys/Girls Ratio**
Overall (Median)	**15.0**	**6.6**	**1.9:1.0**
Africa	10.4	4.6	2.2:1.0
Burkina Faso	28.6	9.6	3.0:1.0
South Africa	21.0	10.6	2.0:1.0
The Americas	**16.6**	**12.2**	**1.2:1.0**
Columbia	31.0	33.4	0.9:1.0
United States	17.7	17.8	1.0:1.0
Eastern Mediterranean	**22.8**	**5.3**	**4.3:1.0**
Jordan	22.0	9.9	2.2:1.0
Europe	33.9	29.0	1.2:1.0
Bulgaria	26.0	39.4	0.7:1.0
Czech Republic	34.0	35.1	1.0:1.0
Southeast Asia	**13.5**	**3.2**	**4.2:1.0**
Indonesia	38.9	4.7	8.3:1.0
Myanmar	19.0	3.2	5.9:1.0
Western Pacific	**11.0**	**6.4**	**1.7:1.0**
Palau	20.0	23.3	0.9:1.0

Source: Global Youth Tobacco Survey Collaborating Group, "Differences in Worldwide Tobacco Use by Gender: Findings from the Global Youth Tobacco Survey," 2003, *Journal of School Health, 73,* pp. 207–215. Reprinted with permission.

Table 7-7	Prevalence of Overweight and Obesity Among School-Aged Children in Global Regions		
	Percentage of All Children		
	Obesity	**Overweight**	**Obesity and Overweight**
Worldwide	2.7	7.6	10.3
Americas	8.2	23.6	31.8
Europe	4.6	15	19.6
Near/Middle East	6.2	9.7	15.9
Asia-Pacific	1	4.1	5.1
Sub-Saharan Africa	0.2	1.1	1.3

Source: T. Lobstein, L. Baur, and R. Uauy, "Obesity of Children and Young People: A Crisis in Public Health," 2004, *Obesity Reviews, 5*(Suppl. 1), pp. 4–85. Reprinted with permission.

Obesity and overweight are becoming more prevalent among young people (Table 7-7). Ten percent of the world's school-aged children are now estimated to be carrying excess body fat (Lobstein, Bauer, & Uauy, 2004). Of these overweight children, one-fourth are obese. Although the prevalence of overweight is dramatically higher in high-income regions, it is rising significantly in most parts of the world. The International Obesity Taskforce (http://www.iotf.org/) attributes rising levels of overweight and obesity to a range of factors, including greater availability and marketing of energy-dense foods and decreased opportunities for physical activity.

Kelly et al. (2008) recently estimated the overall prevalence and absolute burden of overweight and obesity in the world and in various regions in 2005 and provided projections of the global burden in 2030. An estimated 23.2% of the world's adult population in 2005 was overweight (24.0% of men and 22.4% of women) and 9.8% was obese (7.7% of men and 11.9% of women). Overall, the total numbers of overweight and obese adults in 2005 were 937 million (range of 922 million to 951 million) and 396 million (range of 388 million to 405 million), respectively. These authors' projections suggest that by 2030, the respective number of overweight and obese adults will be 1.35 billion and 573 million individuals without adjusting for secular trends. In fact, if recent secular trends continue unchanged, the absolute numbers will total 2.16 billion overweight individuals and 1.12 billion obese individuals (Kelly et al., 2008).

The examples of China and South Africa illustrate the accumulation of risk factors in both adults and children. In 2003, there were 320 million smokers in China older than the age of 15, compared with 250 million smokers in 1986. If current smoking patterns remain unchanged, it is predicted that 100 million men who are now younger than age 30 will die of smoking-related diseases (Zhang & Baiqiang, 2003). Dietary intake in China has also changed significantly over the past decades: The percentage of energy obtained from fat for 20- to 25-year-old adults rose from 19.3% in 1989 to 27.3% in 1997 (Du, Lu, Zhai, & Popkin, 2002). In the same time period, the overall prevalence of obesity among children aged 2 to 6 years increased from 4.2% to 6.4% (1.5% to 12.6% in cities) (Luo & Hu, 2002). In Beijing, 18.2% of local primary and middle school students suffer from obesity, a rate far higher than the 10.6% recorded in 1991 (Chinese Center for Disease Control and Prevention, 2004).

In South Africa, the results of the 1999 National Food Consumption Survey of 1- to 8-year-olds showed that 19.3% of children were stunted (i.e., had a height for age less than or equal to 2 standard deviations of the National Center for Health Statistics' 50th percentile) and that the prevalence of overweight and obesity (body mass index [BMI] greater than or equal to 25) was 17.2%, with levels of overweight being significantly higher in children from urban areas and those living in homes with refrigerators, stoves, and television sets (Steyn, Labadarios, Nel, & Lombard, 2005). In adults, a strong gender difference is evident with respect to underweight and overweight. Data from the nationally representative South African Demographic and Health Survey of 1998 showed that 12.9% of men and 4.8% of women aged 15 to 65 were underweight (BMI less than 18.5). In contrast, 25.4% of men and 68.5% of women were overweight or obese (Bourne, Lambert, & Steyn, 2002). Not surprisingly, reports have cited increased prevalence of type 2 diabetes and high levels of hypertension in South Africa.

Although emphasis in this chapter has been placed on tobacco use, unhealthy diets, physical inactivity, and obesity, a number of intermediate risk factors deserve mention because of the important

Exhibit 7-1	**Hypercholesterolemia and Hypertension in Africa**

After many decades of scientific debate and data published from large community-based trials in the 1970s and 1980s, high total blood cholesterol levels were proven to be an independent major risk factor for atherosclerosis-related chronic diseases such as coronary heart disease and cerebrovascular disease (strokes). Total blood cholesterol levels vary considerably between populations with different dietary patterns. Most people of Africa still following traditional diets have far lower blood cholesterol levels than those found in people of Europe or the United States, or in people of India who migrated and adopted typical Western lifestyles. These differences among people with different lifestyles are present from a young age. In Johannesburg and Soweto, Steyn and associates (2000) found that the mean total cholesterol level in African and colored 5-year-old children was 3.9 mmol/L, compared with 4.1 mmol/L for Indian and 4.4 mmol/L for white children. These group differences in total cholesterol profiles tend to continue into adolescence and adulthood. Several African studies have shown that total cholesterol levels usually differ between urban and rural settings, reflecting the effects of urbanization on increasing total cholesterol levels (Knuiman, Hermus, & Hautvast,1980; Seftel et al.,1993; Swai et al.,1993).

It is estimated that between 10 million and 20 million people in sub-Saharan Africa alone have hypertension and, further, that adequate hypertension treatment could prevent approximately 250,000 deaths in this region (Cappuccio, Plange-Rhule, Phillips, & Eastwood, 2000). Unfortunately, hypertension is universally under-diagnosed or inadequately treated, or both, with the result that extensive end-organ damage and premature death is often seen. Furthermore, hypertension is frequently coexistent with other noncommunicable disease risk factors, such as diabetes.

Early surveys in sub-Saharan African countries showed that the lowest prevalence of hypertension occurred in the poorest countries; as affluence increased, however, the prevalence increased. Researchers also found that hypertension was more common in urban than rural settings in the region (Nissinen, Bothig, Granroth, & Lopez, 1988). The elegant Kenyan Luo migration study of Poulter and colleagues (1990) was the first to show that migration of people living in traditional rural villages on the northern shores of Lake Victoria to the urban settings of Nairobi was associated with an increase in blood pressure. The urban migrants had higher body weights, pulse rates, and urinary sodium–potassium ratios than those who remained in the rural areas. This suggests a marked change in the diet of the new arrivals in Nairobi, including a higher salt and calorie intake, along with a reduced potassium intake due to consumption of fewer fruits and vegetables.

A high intake of sodium is common in sub-Saharan Africa, as salt is widely used to preserve food or to make food tastier. For example, Cappuccio and associates (2000) described the diet in Ghana as consisting mostly of unprocessed food and highly salted fish and meat. Substantial amounts of salt are added to food while cooking, and monosodium glutamate–based flavoring cubes or salts are often used to give food taste. In addition to a high salt intake, people in sub-Saharan Africa frequently eat few fruits and vegetables, resulting in low potassium intakes.

pathophysiological roles they play in the causation of chronic diseases, especially cardiovascular diseases and cancer. The major intermediate risk factors include high blood pressure; high blood levels of total and low-density lipoprotein (LDL) cholesterol; low levels of high-density lipoprotein (HDL) cholesterol; insulin resistance, impaired glucose tolerance and abnormal glucose metabolism; and abnormal plasma concentrations of fibrinogen, factor VII coagulant activity, and plasminogen activator inhibitor-1 (PAI-1) (Daae, Kierulf, Landaas, & Urdal, 1993; Grant, 2007; Hsueh & Law, 1998; Mertens & Van Gaal, 2002). Many of these intermediate risk factors typically cluster in persons with diabetes, cardiovascular disease, and chronic diseases (Daae et al., 1993; Grant, 2007; Hsueh & Law, 1998).

Additionally, several biomarkers of inflammation and oxidative stress—often referred to as "emerging risk factors"—have been associated with the pathogenesis of cardiovascular diseases, diabetes, and cancer (Khatami, 2007; Schenk et al., 2010; Solenski, 2007; Theuma & Fonseca, 2003). Often, however, it remains uncertain whether the observed associations with chronic diseases are truly causal and independent from possible confounding factors and to what extent these markers (separately and in combination) provide incremental predictive value (Danesh et al., 2007). Exhibit 7-1 describes major trends and implications related to some of these risk factors in the poorest region of the world, Africa.

Accumulation of Risks over the Lifecourse

The current burden of chronic diseases reflects cumulative risks over people's lifetimes. Figure 7-7 indicates that the future global burden of chronic disease will be determined by current population exposures to the major chronic disease risk factors. Most importantly, it shows that the accumulation of chronic disease risk begins in fetal life, and then marches forward inexorably starting early in infancy

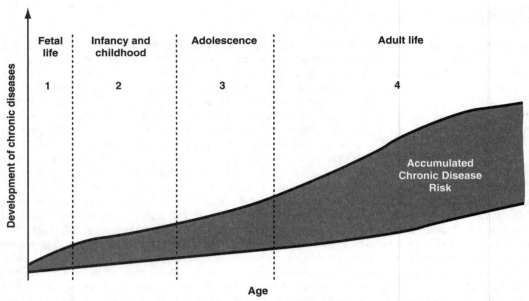

Figure 7-7 A Life Course Approach to Chronic Disease Prevention. *Source:* I. Aboderin, A. Kalache, Y. Ben-Shlomo, J. W. Lynch, C. D. Yajnik, D. Kuh, and D. Yach, Life Course Perspectives in Coronary Heart Disease, Stroke and Diabetes: Key Issues and Implications for Policy and Research (Geneva, Switzerland: World Health Organization, 2001). Reprinted with permission.

and childhood. Thus the emerging evidence supports starting health promotion efforts during pregnancy and early childhood and continuing prevention efforts throughout the lifecourse (Institute of Medicine, 2010).

The major risks for cancer, CVD, and diabetes accumulate beginning early in fetal life. Early-life risk factors—such as suboptimal diet, early termination of breastfeeding, exposure to tobacco and alcohol, exposure to indoor air pollution from biomass fuels, and repeated respiratory infections—are important for the development of chronic diseases in adulthood. Recent research derived from birth cohort studies has documented how and when these lifecourse influences happen (Aboderin et al., 2001; Batty & Leon, 2002). The risk of developing CVD or diabetes, for example, is influenced by biological and social factors at all stages of the life course, from fetal life to adulthood. Some lifecourse influences are disease specific, whereas others are cohort specific. Known risk factors remain the most firmly established link to many major chronic diseases. For example, 80% to 90% of patients who develop clinically significant CHD and more than 95% of patients who have experienced a fatal CHD event have at least one of the major cardiac risk factors—smoking, diabetes, hypertension, or hypercholesterolemia (Canto & Iskandrian, 2003). The link between infant nutrition and chronic dis-

ease has been the subject of much research and debate. Studies indicate that early postnatal nutrition permanently affects the major components of the metabolic syndrome that determine the individual's propensity to CVD (Singhal & Lucas, 2004) and that influences in fetal life and early childhood are related to systolic blood pressure (Levitt et al., 1999).

COPD and lung function in adults are also the result of cumulative exposures that start early in life. South African studies have shown that what were assumed to be racial or genetic differences in lung size are probably due to early childhood respiratory infections occurring in crowded homes where biomass fuel is used, combined with tobacco use and adverse occupational exposures (Goldin, Louw, & Joubert, 1996). More recent analyses of the determinants of chronic bronchitis based on a population survey of 5,671 men and 8,155 women in South Africa estimated the following population-attributable fractions in men: 25% for tobacco use, 14% for occupational exposure, and 10% for past TB. In women, these fractions were 14% for use of smoky domestic fuel, 10% for past TB, and 11% for tobacco use (Ehrlich et al., 2004). This study demonstrates how multiple assaults on the lung—including infectious agents, fuel use, exposure at work, and tobacco use—are important in chronic lung disease. All of these factors have been shown to be related to poverty as well.

Economic Impacts and Health Inequalities

Economic Costs of Selected Chronic Diseases and Risks

Chronic diseases have a significant impact on national economies by disabling and killing the working-age population (Leeder et al., 2004). This results in high direct costs (e.g., health care and treatment) and indirect costs (e.g., number of productive years lost, social security costs, and pension costs). Owing to the relatively high rates of chronic disease among people with potential to contribute to economic productivity, the economic impact of chronic diseases resulting from lost productivity is likely to be particularly significant in low- and middle-income countries.

Evidence is already emerging that the growing burden of chronic disease in low- and middle-income countries is having a significant impact on healthcare costs and lost productivity. For example, Popkin and associates (2001) estimated that diet-related chronic diseases (cancer, coronary heart disease, stroke, hypertension, and diabetes) accounted for 22.6% of healthcare costs (primarily state costs) in China in 1995, while the estimated cost of lost productivity owing to these diseases was 0.5% of gross domestic product (GDP). In India, diet-related chronic diseases accounted for 13.9% of healthcare costs (primarily individual expenditures) and 0.7% of GDP in lost productivity in 1995. These estimates of lost productivity are inevitably underestimates because they are based on mortality and do not consider the lost productivity resulting from morbidity. Estimates have also been made for specific diseases and risk factors.

Cardiovascular Disease

As the recent report from the Institute of Medicine (2010) makes clear, the economics of CVD in low- and middle-income countries has not been heavily studied and methods and data are not uniform; as a result, little evidence has been gathered to show estimates that are often not comparable. Nevertheless, the totality of the existing evidence is convincing: Over time, CVD has significant economic consequences (Institute of Medicine, 2010).

In the United States, CVD accounts for approximately 61% of all healthcare spending (DHHS, 2001). For example, in 2004, the top three most expensive conditions billed to Medicare were all cardiovascular diseases—coronary atherosclerosis, congestive heart failure, and acute myocardial infarction (Russo & Andrews, 2006). Together with costs associated with heart rhythm disorders and acute stroke, cardiovascular conditions accounted for five of the top 10 most expensive conditions billed to Medicare (Russo & Andrews, 2006). Similarly, six of the 20 most expensive conditions treated in the United States in 2004 were cardiovascular conditions (Russo & Andrews, 2006). In the United Kingdom, the total cost of coronary heart disease in 1999 was $11.45 billion, comprising $2.81 million costs to the U.K. healthcare system, $3.92 million in informal care, and $4.72 million in friction period-adjusted productivity loss (friction period is the period of employee absence before replacement by another worker) (24.1% due to mortality and 75.9% to morbidity) (Liu, Maniadakis, Gray, & Rayner, 2002).

The potential economic costs of CVD are potentially even higher in emerging economies owing to the burden of CVD mortality and morbidity among the workforce that occurs at a relatively young age. Leeder and associates (2004) have provided compelling information on the macroeconomic costs of CVD in Brazil, China, India, Russia, and South Africa:

- Potentially productive years of life lost (PPYLL, meaning years lost by people in the age range 35 to 64 years): In the five countries, 33.7 million PPYLL are expected by 2030, an increase from 20.5 million in 2000. Compared with 2000, the number of PPYLL attributable to cardiovascular disease will increase in 2030 by 64% in Brazil, 57% in China, and 95% in India. These growth rates compare with the 20% increase expected in the United States and the 30% increased expected in Portugal over the same period.

- Payroll losses: In India, payroll losses in a single year (2000) from CVD were estimated at $198 million (not including healthcare costs).

- Social security costs arising from disability: Based on the conservative assumption that disability from CVD lasts on average three years, in India the wage losses due to disability that disrupts gainful employment is calculated at $30 million over the three-year period. In South Africa, it is estimated that the disabled workforce cost $64 million in public disability payments in 2000, predicted to rise to $550 million in 2040.

- Direct healthcare costs: In South Africa, direct health systems costs from CVD amounted to $230 million to $300 million in 1991 ($310 million to $470 million at more current values); data from a region of Brazil indicate that patients admitted for circulatory disease account for 10.5% of hospital days but 20% of costs. In China, hospital costs attributable to cardiovascular conditions totaled more than $9.6 billion in 1998 (20% of all costs).

Diabetes

There have been numerous estimates of the healthcare costs of diabetes. The direct healthcare costs of diabetes, including the treatment of complications, range from 2.5% to 15% of national annual healthcare budgets, depending on diabetes prevalence and the level of treatment available (WHO, 2003c). For example:

- In Latin America and the Caribbean, the direct healthcare costs of diabetes were estimated at $10.7 billion in 2000 (Barceló, Aedo, Rajpathak, & Robles, 2003). Indirect costs were more than five times higher than the direct costs, estimated at $54.9 billion. Thus the total costs of diabetes for the region were $65.2 billion (Barceló et al., 2003).

- In the United States, the direct costs of diabetes for people of all age groups were estimated at $91.8 billion in 2002 (American Diabetes Association [ADA], 2003), an increase from $44 billion in 1997 (ADA, 1998).

- Studies in India estimate that, for a low-income Indian family with an adult with diabetes, as much as 25% of family income can be devoted to diabetes care (Shobana et al., 2000).

- In WHO's Western Pacific region, an analysis of healthcare expenditure showed that 16% of hospital expenditures were devoted to people with diabetes (WHO, 2002a). In the Republic of the Marshall Islands, this figure was 25%. Twenty percent of offshore expenditures on health by Fiji—instances where facilities for care were not available in Fiji, so patients had to travel elsewhere—was attributable to diabetes-related complications.

Many estimates have been made on the costs of diabetes in Sweden. Most recently, direct and indirect costs per person were estimated at approximately $8,500 per year, taking into account comorbidity (Norlund, Apelqvist, Bitzen, Nyberg, & Scherstén, 2001). Twenty-eight percent of the costs were for health care, 41% for lost productivity, and 31% for the municipality and for relatives.

Although there are few data on diabetes-related costs in African or Middle Eastern countries, studies from the early 1990s again suggest such costs are high. In Tunisia, an estimate from the early 1990s

placed the total annual costs of medication and outpatient care for people with diabetes at 2.6 times that for people without diabetes—$179 versus $68 (Chale, Swai, Mujinja, & McLarty, 1992).

The International Diabetes Federation (2003) has estimated the annual direct healthcare costs of diabetes worldwide and expressed them in international dollars. (International dollars are a common currency unit that takes account of the relative purchasing power of various currencies.) For people in the 20 to 79 age bracket, costs are at least 153 million international dollars, and may be as much as 286 billion international dollars or more. If the prevalence of diabetes continues to climb, total direct healthcare expenditures for this disease are expected to be between 213 billion and 396 billion international dollars in 2025. This means that the proportion of the world healthcare budget devoted to diabetes care in 2025 will be between 7% and 13%, with high-prevalence countries spending as much as 40% of their budget on caring for diabetic patients. Estimates of the indirect costs of this disease are just as high—or even higher—as the direct costs.

The cost of treating CVD is the largest identifiable proportion (26.4%) of the overall diabetes healthcare expenditure. This dominance reflects two factors: Patients with CVD are more likely to be hospitalized and consume more medicines, and CVD is highly prevalent in people with diabetes (Simpson, Corabian, Jacobs, & Johnson, 2003).

Asthma

Asthma is associated with significant healthcare expenditures that include both direct medical costs and indirect economic costs from absenteeism and the loss of future potential earnings secondary to both morbidity and mortality (Bahadori et al., 2009). In a recent systematic review of the economic burden of asthma, Bahadori and colleagues (2009) showed that hospitalization and medications were the most important cost drivers of direct costs, while work and school loss accounted for the greatest percentage of indirect costs. Most importantly, the evidence collected by these researchers suggested that these costs are increasing.

The medical costs for asthma are considerable. For example, they constitute 1.3% of Singapore's total healthcare cost ($33.93 million per year), and 1.4% of direct healthcare costs ($2.86 million) in Estonia, where medication expenses are 53% of the total (Chew, Goh, & Lee, 1999; Kiivet, Kaur, Lang, Aaviksoo, & Nirk, 2001). In Spain, Martinez-Moragon and colleagues (2009) estimated that the average annual direct and indirect cost of asthma in adults were $2,354 per patient, with an average per capita cost to the National Health Service of $2,091.

Risk Factors

Tobacco has many negative economic impacts. The most authoritative review of the economic impact of tobacco by the World Bank provided estimates from low- and middle-income and high-income countries of the annual healthcare costs associated with use of this product (Table 7-8). The substantial economic impact of tobacco in low- and middle-income countries led major development agencies, including the European Commission, to conclude that tobacco was truly a poverty-related issue requiring urgent attention. More recently this position was restated by the United Nations' Economic and Social Council (2004).

National healthcare spending attributable to obesity has been estimated to range from 2% and 6% for high-income countries (Finkelstein, Fiebelkorn, & Wang, 2003, 2004; Kuchler & Ballenger, 2002; Thompson & Wolf, 2001). These estimates deal only with direct healthcare spending rather than decreased productivity and other indirect measures. The data referred to earlier in relation to the costs of diet-related chronic diseases in China and India include the impact of obesity (Popkin et al., 2001).

Macroeconomic Impacts

Indirect productivity losses incurred because of chronic diseases have the potential to affect the global macro economy. A growing body of evidence shows that premature death and disability from chronic diseases affect national emerging economies by dampening the engine of productivity and reducing economic growth (Leeder et al., 2004). This hypothesis can also be extended to the global level, because workers in emerging markets are generating growth not only in their home economies, but also in high-income nations. In fact, some economists argue the potential returns for high-income-country investors from emerging markets could be higher than the returns from Organization for Economic Cooperation and Development (OECD) countries over the long term, especially in the light of low expected returns in mature markets (Clark & Hebb, 2002; Heller, 2003; Kimmis, Gottchalk, Armendariz, & Griffith-Jones, 2002). If chronic diseases do diminish productivity as predicted, then investor returns in low- and middle-income countries will likewise be affected, with corresponding impacts on growth in OECD countries.

Both transnational corporations (TNCs) and pension funds face risks from this source. Where TNCs are direct employers with health insurance liabilities, the lesson of the HIV/AIDS pandemic is

Table 7-8	Total Economic Cost Attribute to Tobacco Use, 2005 or Latest Available Data
Country	**Total Costs***
Australia	$14.19 billion
Bangladesh	$424 billion
Canada	$12.89 billion
China	$4.29 billion
Denmark	$828 billion
Finland	$240 billion
France	$16.44 billion
Germany	$24.38 billion
Hong Kong SAR	$33.80 billion
India	$63.16 billion
Netherlands	$2.93 billion
New Zealand	$17.03 million
Norway	$1.62 billion
Puerto Rico	$97 billion
Republic of Korea	$3.33 billion
South Africa	$103 billion
Switzerland	$9.58 billion
United Kingdom	$2.30 billion
United States	$184.54 billion
Venezuela	$284 billion

Note: Total economic cost is defined as direct healthcare costs plus indirect economic burden, including productivity loss, absenteeism, and other socioeconomic costs.

Source: J. Mackay, M. Eriksen, O. Shafey. The Tobacco Atlas, Second Edition (Atlanta, GA: American Cancer Society, 2006).

that chronic conditions can place heavy financial burdens on a company, especially when treatment is expensive. U.S.-based TNCs already face huge health-care costs at home. Indeed, a recent study put the health and productivity expenses incurred by six large employers in the United States at $3,524 per eligible employee in 1999 (Goetzel, Hawkins, Ozminkowski, & Wang, 2003). Although "short-termism" is still endemic in pension fund investments, recent trends show a growing interest in more long-term value investing, and some companies with direct investments overseas are themselves debating the need to incorporate longer-term upfront investments into their business practice in low- and middle-income countries to sustain profitability over the long term (Clark & Hebb, 2002).

Impact on Health Inequalities

As aptly stated by Gunnar Myrdal (1952), the Nobel Prize winner for economics in the 1950s, people are sick because they are poor, and they become poorer because they are sick. This downward spiral occurs with chronic diseases. Increased cumulative exposure to risk factors over the lifecourse, combined with social and economic inequalities, leads to the levels of inequalities seen in later adult life (see Figure 7-7).

Chronic diseases impose a significant burden on low-income populations. In high-income countries, the relationships among poverty and cardiovascular disease, cancer, diabetes, and their associated risk factors are well described. It is also firmly established that chronic diseases explain health inequalities by social class, ethnicity, and gender (Aboderin et al., 2001; Batty & Leon, 2002; Brands & Yach, 2001; Kogevinas, Pearce, Susser, & Boffetta, 1997; Mackenbach et al., 2000; Marmot, Adelstein, Robinson, & Rose, 1978; Wong, Shapiro, Boscardin, & Ettne, 2002).

Chronic diseases are not common among the very poorest people in low- and middle-income countries, but neither do they affect only the affluent. As risks accumulate over the lifecourse and over generations, this trend will become more evident. In high-income countries, exposure to risk factors (e.g., tobacco, alcohol, poor diet, little physical activity) is directly associated with poverty, social class, and level of education. These risks, when aggregated, result in the higher rates of chronic diseases found among poorer populations. The same relationship applies in Europe's poorest countries. In low- and middle-income countries, the poorest populations already exhibit the highest risks for tobacco and alcohol use (Jha & Chaloupka, 2000), but the relationship with inter-mediate risk factors and diseases is complex and varies between countries.

- India: Currently, rates of hypertension, cholesterol, diabetes, and cardiovascular disease increase directly with socioeconomic status (Singh et al., 1999; Vikram, Pandey, Misra, Sharma, Devi, & Khanna, 2003). Yet, high rates of hypertension and LDL cholesterol are now being measured in urban slums (Misra, Pandey, Devi, Sharma, Vikram, & Khanna, 2001), and tobacco consumption is higher among the most poorly educated. Death rates from TB—a disease associated with poverty—are four times higher among people who smoke relative to nonsmokers (Gajalakshmi et al., 2003). Poorer people also suffer from relatively higher rates of complications from diabetes, owing to their propensity to be exposed to multiple risk factors (Ramachandran, Snehalatha, Vijay, & King, 2002).

- Brazil: In urban Brazil, an inverse relationship between socioeconomic status and smoking and alcohol consumption in men and women was measured in the 1980s (Duncan, Schmidt, Achutti, Polanczyk, Benia, & Maia, 1993). Also identified were inverse links between socioeconomic status and hypertension in men, and between sedentary lifestyle and obesity in women.

- Jamaica: Obesity increases with income level strongly in men and weakly in women (owing to high levels of obesity among the poorest women) (Mendez, Cooper, Luke, Wilks, Bennett, & Forrester, 2004). The relationship between income, diabetes, and hypertension, however, is nonlinear. In women, plotting diabetes and hypertension prevalence against income forms a U-shaped curve, with the highest rates of diabetes being found in the poorest women. Obesity and diabetes are strongly related, especially among poor women. The lack of a strong income gradient in hypertension or diabetes—despite a strong relationship between income and obesity—might be partly attributable to greater adverse effects of obesity among the poor.

- China: In China, there is a U-shaped relationship between socioeconomic status and hypertension in women. This result in part reflects the fact that poorer women tend to have lower body mass indices and to smoke less but engage in less physical activity; the reverse is true for the wealthiest group (Bell, Adair, & Popkin, 2004).

Owing to the long and often variable lag times between exposure to risk factors and disease onset, exposure to chronic disease risks in low- and middle-income countries has yet to fully develop into a direct relationship among poverty, intermediate risk factors, and chronic disease. Over time, accumulation of risk among poorer groups will increase as availability and marketing of products associated with a Western lifestyle (e.g., higher-fat, higher-calorie foods) increases with economic development. There are concerns that over the long term, this trend will lead to a pronounced association between chronic diseases and poverty.

Data on obesity illustrate that the risk factor gradient will increasingly tilt toward poorer groups as economies develop. Until the late 1980s, socioeconomic status and obesity tended to be inversely related in high-income populations and directly related in low- and middle-income populations (Sobal & Stunkard, 1989). In other words, in low- and middle-income economies, obesity was associated with more affluent groups. More recently, however, work from Brazil has shown that over time female obesity shifts toward lower-income groups in economically more developed regions and urban areas. Although low socioeconomic status still confers protection from obesity in low-income nations, when national GNP reaches a value of approximately $2,500 per capita, obesity rates become directly associated with low socioeconomic status (Monteiro, Conde, Lu, & Popkin, 2004; Peña & Bacallao, 2000).

A recent study comparing the relationship between social class and consumption patterns in the United States and China illustrates this point (Kim, Symons, & Popkin, 2004). Using a composite lifestyle index (LI) that included data on diet, smoking, alcohol, and physical activity, the authors showed that an inverse relationship exists between socioeconomic status and the LI in the United States, but a direct relationship exists between the two in China. China is on the ascending limb of economic growth, whereas the U.S. population is considered to on the descending limb. This phenomenon suggests that policy makers in low- and middle-income countries should not wait for a social class gradient to appear in the occurrence of chronic disease (or risk factors) before implementing strong disease-preventive and health-promoting policies.

An increasingly important and emerging challenge is the issue of health inequalities among the elderly. As the global population ages, with the population aged 60 years and older being forecast to more than triple in the next 45 years, the burden of health inequalities in the elderly is expected to increase substantially (WHO, 2008). In low- and middle-income countries where the proportion of older people is growing even faster than in high-income countries, the lack of contributory pension schemes and deteriorating traditional social security arrangements act together to worsen the burden of health inequalities (Commission on Social Determinants of Health, 2008). Although health inequalities in the elderly tend to be smaller in magnitude than those observed among younger populations, they remain an important public health challenge, whose underlying determinants are not completely understood (von dem Knesebeck, 2010). Older women, especially widows, are affected significantly because they tend to be poorer, have higher rates of impoverishment and destitution, and are more susceptible to chronic diseases (Women and Gender Equity Knowledge Network [WGEKN], 2007).

Determinants of Major Chronic Diseases

Demographic Change

This section addresses aging and urbanization, two powerful demographic factors affecting chronic disease.

Aging

The aging of populations, due mainly to a decline in fertility rates and a higher proportion of children living into adulthood, is an important underlying determinant of chronic disease epidemics (Beaglehole & Yach, 2003). Although demographic change has been well described in respect to high-income countries, the pace and impact of aging in low- and middle-income countries is only just beginning to be appreciated. Recent United Nations projections suggest that the population share of those older than 60 years of age will rise from the range of 5% to 6% to that 14% to 15% over two decades in Algeria, Egypt, Iran, South Africa, and Tunisia. High-income countries are already under pressure to address the pensions and social insurance demands of aging populations; low- and middle-income countries will soon have to do so, albeit from a starting base of substantially fewer resources (Heller, 2003).

Aging need not be a risk factor per se for increased morbidity caused by chronic diseases. Fries first postulated in 1980 that if health promotion and disease prevention programs were successful, it would be possible to have continued increases in longevity without a concomitant increase in morbidity and disability. In his model of "compression of morbidity," Fries (1980) theorized that the means are available to modify and improve the quality of aging. This model proposes that sufficient postponement can mean the avoidance of chronic symptoms until the natural life span has run its course—in which case chronic disease is effectively prevented. As the rates of premature death decline, the survival curve becomes increasingly rectangular in this model. Evidence is emerging that such has been the case in the United States for the last decade (Fries, 2003). During this time, mortality rates dropped by 1% per year and disability rates by 2% per year, suggesting that compression of morbidity with longevity is possible. Increases in life expectancy past the age of 65 years have been, and are expected to remain, modest.

The decline in disability in people older than the age of 65 has been much more dramatic and continues at a relatively rapid rate. The avoidance of health risks, such as smoking, lack of exercise, and obesity, has been shown to be a major factor in the postponement of disability, leading to the conclusion that health enhancement interventions for the elderly and the implementation of disability postponement measures within healthcare systems as part of broad health policy initiatives are the best means to facilitate the further compression of morbidity (Fries, 2003). The expected cumulative health expenditures in healthier elderly persons, despite their greater longevity, were similar to those for less healthy persons (Lubitz, Cai, Kamarow, & Lentzner, 2003). These relatively recent findings suggest that risk factor prevention and health promotion will save both lives and money.

Urbanization

At the beginning of the twentieth century, just 16 cities in the world had population of more than 1 million people; today, approximately 400 meet this criterion, three-fourths of which are in low- and middle-income countries (Cohen, 2004). Further dramatic expansion of giant metropolises in the low- and middle-income world is predicted (Heller, 2003), and long-term projections show that, on a global scale, urban populations will soon exceed rural populations.

Urbanization can stimulate chronic disease prevention efforts by improving access to a wider variety of foods, to health systems for early diagnosis and

effective treatment, and to knowledge and information about healthy living. At the same time, urban areas are magnets for the flow of goods, investment, technology, and marketing, which subsequently attract flows of people from rural areas. Urbanization thus does not cause chronic diseases per se, but rather creates conditions in which a mass of people are exposed to different products, technologies, marketing, and working and social environments. For example, urban populations develop high levels of branded cigarette consumption following exposure to advertising (Yach, Mathews, & Buch, 1990). Diets in urban areas tend to be higher in fat, animal products, and processed foods (Popkin, 1999). Urbanization also distances people from the point of food production, which has implications for dietary intake (WHO, 2003b). When people move to urban areas, they adopt less physically demanding types of employment, such as manufacturing and services (Popkin & Doak, 1998), and unplanned urban sprawl may not be conducive to pedestrian activity.

Evidence from South Africa in the 1960s suggests urbanization is associated with the development of diabetes (Seftel & Schultz, 1961), while more recent data point to an association with an earlier incidence of stroke (Vorster, 2002). In Thailand, city dwellers have higher blood pressure, BMIs, and cholesterol levels (InterASIA Collaborative Group, 2003).

Economic Factors

Economic Development

The world economy is now more integrated than ever before, with increased trade, investment, and communications flowing between countries. Changes on this front could be even more dramatic over the next 50 years, as Brazil, China, India, and Russia become much larger economic forces (Wilson & Purushothaman, 2003).

With economic growth comes the potential for better health: Average life expectancy has increased in the past 30 years as average incomes have risen. At the same time, growth brings with it economic, cultural, and social shifts. Among these shifts are the spread of risk factors for chronic diseases. This spread is not inevitable, but is probable if unchecked, and will lead to a deterioration of chronic disease profiles.

This process can be conceptualized by a chronic disease consumption curve, based on both empirical data and well-founded assumptions (Figure 7-8). Empirical data show increasing levels of tobacco use and obesity with economic development (Popkin & Doak, 1998; Yach, 1990); lag times between uptake of risk factors and onset of disease; and declines in

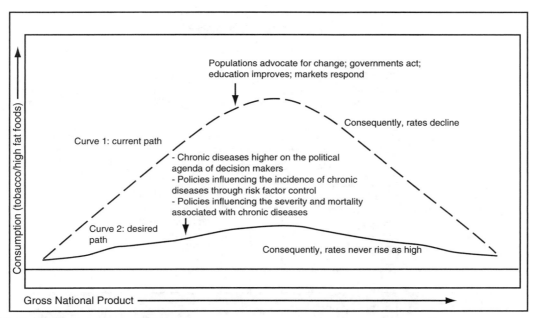

Figure 7-8 Chronic Disease Consumption Curve.

mortality and morbidity from chronic disease in the OECD countries (Leeder et al., 2004). Data on tobacco use and obesity apply more widely to other risks associated with consumption behavior, while declining mortality from chronic diseases is associated with very high levels of social and economic development. Thus, in the absence of policy actions, consumption of tobacco, alcohol, and foods high in fat, salt, and sugar grows with GNP, to be followed by associated increases in chronic diseases decades later (curve 1 in Figure 7-8). This pattern contrasts with that for infectious diseases, which in general decline with economic growth (McKeown, 1988). Chronic disease risk rates do not begin to fall until high levels of wealth and literacy are reached, whereupon governments are more likely to respond to public health concerns and use a broad range of policy instruments to influence consumption trends.

Globalization

Globalization is part of the process of global economic development. Important processes in globalization—trade, foreign investment, marketing, and the spread of technologies—have implications for the spread and alleviation of chronic diseases. These flows drive, and are driven by, the process of globalization and the development of global production systems. Flows of tobacco are always negative; flows concerning food, alcohol, and goods and services related

to physical activity can be both positive and negative. Together, these systemic drivers have tremendous implications on overall consumption and physical activity patterns, which in turn affect chronic disease incidence, prevalence, morbidity, and mortality (Institute of Medicine, 2010). As shown in Figure 7-9, these systemic drivers, defined as "broad processes that ultimately have an effect on classically defined individual risk factors," are influenced by country-specific social, political, and economic factors (Institute of Medicine, 2010). These factors may also present opportunities for modification of traditional risk factors in the comprehensive prevention and control of chronic diseases. A detailed discussion of the relationship between globalization and chronic diseases appears in Chapter 15.

Policy Responses to the Growing Burden of Chronic Diseases

There are many impediments to addressing chronic diseases, not least of which are the myths perpetuated regarding the burden of chronic diseases and the most appropriate way to control them (Table 7-9). These myths create a policy-making environment in which it is all too easy to justify neglect.

Key stakeholders have met the growing burden of chronic diseases with a patchwork of responses.

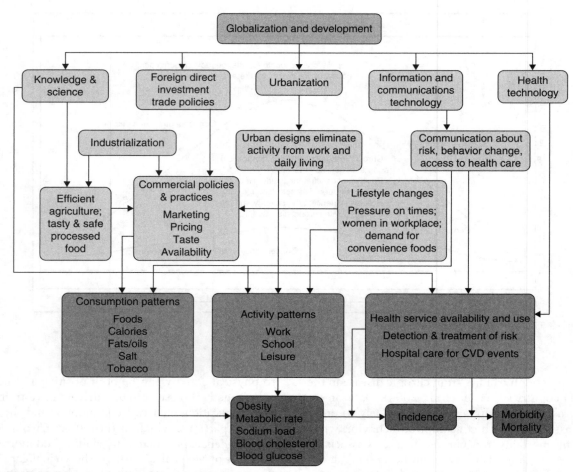

Figure 7-9 Globalization and Development. *Source:* Valentin Fuster and Bridget B. Kelly, Editors; Committee on Preventing the Global Epidemic of Cardiovascular Disease: Meeting the Challenges in Developing Countries; Institute of Medicine *Promoting Cardiovascular Health in the Developing World: A Critical Challenge to Achieve Global Health* Figure 3.2, page 130.

Overall, there is a lack of policy coherence between different stakeholders, which is merely exacerbated by the absence of adequate global governance of chronic diseases (Yach, Hawkes, Gould, & Hofman, 2004). Table 7-10 summarizes the range of policy responses to chronic diseases.

Governments

At a national level, many ministries of health do recognize chronic disease prevention and control as a significant health priority, but this has not translated into comprehensive policy development or fiscal and human resources (Alwan, Maclean, & Mandil, 2001). In a review of government policies and actions in 185 countries (Alwan et al., 2001), the following conclusions emerged:

- The capacity of health systems to prevent and treat chronic diseases is generally low.

- Few countries have developed comprehensive national plans to address chronic diseases.

- Needed legislative and fiscal policies to support health promotion and prevention are not in place.

- Most governments do not provide a budget line item for chronic disease control.

- Few countries have essential medicines for chronic disease management readily available in their primary care settings.

World Health Organization

The World Health Organization has responsibility for addressing the global burden of chronic diseases. Many WHO functions and goals are directly related to chronic disease control, including "strengthen health services," "control endemic and other diseases," and "propose conventions, agreements and

Table 7-9	**Eight Myths of Chronic Disease Burden and Control**

Myth 1: We can wait until infectious diseases are controlled.
Reality: As development progresses, chronic diseases do not smoothly displace acute diseases. Many countries have a double burden of disease; thus we must deal with both and develop the health system accordingly. Further, some infectious diseases are chronic in nature (e.g., HIV/AIDS).

Myth 2: Economic growth will improve all health conditions.
Reality: Economic development can improve health in low- and middle-income countries. Yet, economic growth can also exacerbate chronic diseases.

Myth 3: Chronic diseases are diseases of affluence.
Reality: Chronic diseases are not solely diseases of affluence in high-income and most low- and middle-income countries. Low socioeconomic status leads to cumulative exposure to risk factors, greater comorbidity, and decreased access to quality health care.

Myth 4: Chronic diseases are diseases of the elderly.
Reality: Chronic diseases in low- and middle-income countries are no longer just diseases of the elderly. Chronic diseases in these countries affect a much higher proportion of people during their prime working years, compared to high-income countries.

Myth 5: Chronic diseases result from freely adopted risks.
Reality: Chronic diseases cannot be blamed solely on the failure of individual responsibility, because the cultural and environmental context in any society or community inevitably affects personal choices. Thus governments, industry, and others play a role in their incidence.

Myth 6: Benefits of chronic disease control accrue only to individuals.
Reality: Chronic disease control fosters positive social development and benefits societies economically, thereby benefiting the public as a whole. Like acute disease control, chronic disease control is an appropriate public investment.

Myth 7: Acute, infectious disease models are applicable to chronic diseases.
Reality: Interventions for acute diseases are relatively simple, whereas chronic diseases require a planned, proactive approach to health care, and the active participation of patients, families, and communities.

Myth 8: Treating individuals in the health sector is the only appropriate chronic disease strategy.
Reality: The medical community has focused on using traditional approaches to screen "high-risk" individuals—that is, those with a high probability of contracting chronic diseases. Yet, prevention requires a multisectoral commitment in addition to more comprehensive health service interventions for clinical prevention.

regulations" (Article 2). WHO member states first requested action on chronic diseases at the Ninth World Health Assembly in 1956, when a resolution from India requesting that the Director General establish an expert committee on CVD and hypertension (WHO, 1956). Since then, member states from both high-income and low- and middle-income countries have demanded action, including the global strategy on the prevention and control of noncommunicable diseases in 2000; the landmark resolution on the Framework Convention on Tobacco Control (FCTC) in 2003; and a resolution and strategy on diet, physical activity, and health in 2004.

Donor Agencies

Health has not traditionally been a priority area for many donors, and chronic diseases in low- and middle-income countries have received substantially less attention than other health issues. Although official development assistance for health has increased significantly in the last decade, these resources have been almost entirely devoted to the HIV/AIDS pandemic in sub-Saharan Africa. Bilateral aid agencies rarely prioritize chronic disease or related risk factors. A recent analysis of current trends in global funding showed that chronic diseases are the least funded area in global health, receiving less than 3% of all development assistance for health from 2001 through 2007 (Nugent & Feigl, 2010). This finding is consistent with several earlier analyses showing that donor assistance for health is heavily skewed toward infectious diseases, especially HIV/AIDS (Sridhar & Batniji, 2008; Stuckler et al., 2008; Yach, Hawkes, Gould & Hofman, 2004).

The Institute of Medicine (2010) has pointed out that the trend is now at least in the right direction for cardiovascular diseases. Global donor funding for cardiovascular diseases and other chronic diseases

Table 7-10	Summary of Key Players' Policy Responses to the Global Burden of Chronic Disease	
Key Players	**Policy Responses**	
	Positive	**Neutral or Negative**
Heads of state	• G8: Recognition that "health is the key to prosperity" and "poor health drives poverty" • G77: Recent support for the FCTC	• G8: Mobilization of resources for Global Fund in 2001 but no commitment to chronic diseases • G77: No concerted effort on chronic diseases; critical of the draft global strategy on diet, physical activity, and health
Health ministries	• High recognition of problem of chronic diseases	• Inadequate capacity and budget for chronic disease prevention and control in most countries
World Health Organization	• 46 chronic disease resolutions since 1956 • Noncommunicable disease cluster established in 1998 and capacity later developed in regions	• Commitment not followed by funding or high-level advocacy
International donors	• Modest support for tobacco control • Increased health support by donors mostly directed toward HIV/AIDS pandemic	• Minimal support for chronic diseases
World Bank and regional development banks	• World Bank recognizes impact of risk factors on poor and is developing a "Policy Note" on chronic diseases • Policies on chronic diseases and risks emerging in some regional development banks	• Not yet reflected by coherent policy response, investment, or inclusion in poverty reduction strategies • Regional development banks' health-sector strategies concentrate on communicable diseases and funding is minimal or nonexistent
United Nations initiatives related to health and development	• World Summit of Sustainable Development Plan of Implementation includes chronic diseases • WHO Commission on Macroeconomics and Health now giving greater consideration to chronic disease threat • International Labor Organization's SOLVE program addresses chronic disease risks in the workplace	• Millennium Development Goals exclude chronic diseases • UN Population Fund (UNFPA) does not include chronic diseases or risk factors in strategy on population and development (Intertional Conference on Population and Development) • UNICEF's goal-setting program does not make reference to risk factors for chronic diseases among children • ILO report to the World Commission on the Social Dimension of Globalization and MNE Declaration does not refer to chronic diseases
International nongovernmental organizations (NGOs)	• High potential for national capacity building and wide geographic reach • GLOBALink and Framework Convention Alliance supporting Framework Convention Tobacco Control (FCTC) was effective	• Integrated support by NGOs for chronic diseases has been is insufficiently mobilized
Agricultural and trade sectors	• Links made between tobacco production and health • Increasing research into relationships among agriculture, trade, and chronic diseases	• Linkages among agriculture, trade, and chronic disease are insufficiently recognized • Research is receiving insufficient support
Business and investment community	• Some companies developing new business models for chronic disease prevention • Investment community warning of risks associated with chronic diseases	• Companies' efforts are largely restricted to corporate social responsibility initiatives, which rarely refer to chronic diseases • Powerful commercial interests have attempted to thwart chronic disease prevention initiatives
Academic health centers, research institutions, and journals	• Active research and development programs between low- and middle-income countries, high-income and research groups • International committees recognize chronic disease research is necessary • Recent editions suggest major journal editors are giving more attention to chronic disease in low- and middle-income countries	• U.S. academic health centers and international schools of public health have not adequately incorporated chronic diseases in teaching or research • Funding for research is not proportionally allocated • Only a tiny proportion of low- and middle-country researchers publish papers on chronic diseases

Table 7-11	Official Development Assistance (ODA) Funding for Health and Disease Areas per 2008 DALY		
	2008 DALYs, LMICs (million)***	Health Development Assistance 2007	Funding per DALY
Infectious diseases	518	US$ 6,516 mill*	US$ 12.5
Noncommunicable chronic diseases	646	US$ 503 mill**	78 cents
All conditions	1,338	US$ 2,791 mill*	US$ 16.4

*Source for 'Infectious Disease' and 'All conditions' funding: Ravishankar, N., P. Gubbins, R. J. Cooley, K. Leach-Kemon, C. M. Michaud, D. T. Jamison, and C. J. Murray. 2009. Financing of global health: Tracking development assistance for health from 1990 to 2007. *Lancet* 373(9681):2113–2124.;
**Source for 'NCD' Funding: CGD Funding Analysis;
*** Source for 2008 DALYs: WHO, 2008. 2008. *The global burden of disease : 2004 update*. Geneva:World Health Organization.

Source: Institute of Medicine (2010). Preventing the Global Epidemic of Cardiovascular Disease: Meeting the Challenges in Developing Countries. Washington, DC: National Academies Press. Reproduced with permission.

increased from $236 million in 2004 to more than $618 million in 2008 in real terms. Of this amount, approximately $10 million (in 2007) is directly identifiable as CVD funding. As shown in Table 7-11, in 2007, $0.78/DALY (disability-adjusted life years) of external health funding was spent on noncommunicable diseases in low- and middle-income countries, compared to $12.5/DALY on infectious diseases (HIV/AIDS, TB, and malaria combined) (Institute of Medicine, 2010). Overall development assistance for health was $16.4/DALY for all conditions combined (Nugent & Feigl, 2010).

United Nations Agencies

United Nations (UN) health and development reports play a major role in setting priorities for global health. Persistent problems that hinder development, such as infant and maternal mortality, malnutrition, and HIV/AIDS, have appropriately received priority in the poorest countries. Despite their impact in low- and middle-income countries, chronic diseases are not recognized as a health and development issue. Millennium Development Goal (MDG) 6 is "Combat HIV/AIDS, malaria, and other diseases" (United Nations Development Program [UNDP], 2001). Although "other diseases" theoretically includes chronic diseases, in practice these conditions tend to be ignored when resources are allocated to health and when countries report on how they are addressing MDG goals (UNDP, 2001). The UN Population Fund (UNFPA, 1995) does not mention chronic illnesses in its strategy on population and development. Likewise the recent goal-setting program of the UN Children's Fund (UNICEF), A World Fit for Children, excludes risk factors for chronic conditions for children from the 25 action points proposed to "promote healthy lives," despite strong global evidence

that tobacco use and obesity are ubiquitous risks among children in low- and middle-income countries (UN General Assembly, 2002). The Plan of Action of the World Summit on Sustainable Development (WSSD, 2002) does, however, state that it will "develop or strengthen, where applicable, preventive, promotive and curative programs to address noncommunicable diseases and conditions . . . and associated risk factors, including alcohol, tobacco, unhealthy diets and lack of physical activity."

The World Bank has been active in health for decades and is aware of the need to address chronic diseases. It was instrumental in defining the economic basis for action against tobacco (World Bank, 1999). However, of the $4.25 billion allocated to loans for health between 1997 and 2002, only 2.5% was explicitly devoted to chronic disease control programs.

Nongovernmental Organizations

Nongovernmental organizations (NGOs) have a wide geographic spread and the ability to build capacity. At a national level, NGOs are reported to play a variety of roles in chronic disease control, but their precise roles and effectiveness in various countries are not well known (Alwan et al., 2001). There is only limited advocacy at the global level for a chronic disease prevention and control agenda. The most effective advocates for prevention have focused on specific diseases or risks. Internationally, NGOs proved critical in the development of the WHO FCTC. Nevertheless, there has been no concerted effort to promote and develop a comprehensive prevention and management approach to chronic diseases by NGOs. NGOs concerned with diet and nutrition in high-income countries have not built capacity in low- and middle-income countries, for example. International consumer group input is inadequate. Initiatives such as "sustainable development" and "corporate social responsibility" have not been applied to chronic diseases.

Private Sector

Sustained engagement by the private sector in prevention of chronic diseases has been insufficient to date, although new business models are emerging as investors warn of risks (Table 7-12) and enlightened companies recognize that profitability and public health can coexist. In recent years, tobacco companies such as Philip Morris and BAT have developed corporate social responsibility (CSR) initiatives aimed at persuading the public that their products are less dangerous. Their efforts are not supported by public health authorities. CSR criteria have to date focused on environmental factors, labor standards, and human rights, rather than on health considerations. If health were to be considered a key factor when deciding on whether a CSR program was really responsible, tobacco companies would be immediately excluded.

Certain TNCs and associated lobbyists have actively tried to thwart action by national governments and WHO in addressing risk factors. The tobacco industry has asserted that WHO should not focus on the "lifestyle issues" of affluent Western countries. It has also attempted to redirect WHO policies on tobacco, alleging that WHO is misspending its budget "at the expense of more urgent public health needs, particularly in developing countries, such as prevention of malaria and other communicable diseases" (WHO, 2000). Lobbyists for tobacco, sugar, and some other food interests have worked hard to keep attention away from the need to address consumption patterns that drive chronic diseases (Brownell & Hagen, 2004).

Self-regulatory guidelines on marketing adopted by alcohol companies have proved useful in some ways, but tend to fall short of their claims (Babor et al., 2003). Several food and beverage companies have issued guidelines on marketing to children and reducing the number of beverage calories available to children during the school day (Alliance for a Healthier Generation, 2006; Hawkes, 2004a). As a result of these guidelines, the industry committed to changing the beverage mix in schools across the United States by removing full-calorie soft drinks and providing for lower-calorie, nutritious beverage options in age-appropriate portions by the beginning of the 2009–2010 school year (American Beverage Association, 2010). As shown in Figure 7-10, the volume of full-calorie carbonated soft drink shipments—which are not permitted in any U.S. schools under this new policy—fell the most sharply, by 95%. (American Beverage Association, 2010). Water, which is permitted under the guidelines, is the only item among the beverages that has not experienced a significant reduction in shipment volume since the guidelines were put in place. These results highlight how alliances and partnerships with the food industry can achieve good results in altering risk factors for chronic diseases.

There are currently few private–public partnerships addressing chronic disease prevention. One new such initiative is the Oxford Health Alliance (www.oxha.org), which brings together academics, non-governmental organizations, international health groups, and the private sector. Novo Nordisk has played an initiating role with Oxford and Yale Universities in this endeavor. New community-based research projects to determine how best to prevent chronic diseases in 20 low- and middle-income and high-income countries are being supported through the Alliance, which regularly convenes major players involved in chronic disease prevention in an effort to find practical means of increasing advocacy and funding. The focus of this partnership is on reducing tobacco use, improving diets, and increasing levels of

---

Table 7-12	Equity and Market Research into the Future of the Tobacco and Food Industry

- Moody's Investors Service (2003): "FDA regulation is a real possibility and would transform the industry. Easing the introduction of reduced-risk products would be an advantage to Philip Morris."
- Swiss Reinsurance Company (2004): "The increasing prevalence of obesity has financial implications for consumers of life insurance products and society as a whole . . . As consumers' body mass index goes up, so too will their premiums."
- JP Morgan (2003): The food industry should "review its marketing practices and transform itself."
- UBS Warburg (2002): "There are risks associated with obesity that have not yet been factored into share prices."
- Datamonitor (2002): "[Food] manufacturers have a great opportunity for product leadership and category reinvention."
- JP Morgan (2004): "R&D [research and development] is making safer cigarettes a reality."

Source: Razaire et al., 2003; Swiss Reinsurance Company, 2004; Langlois et al., 2003, p. 1; Streets et al., 2002 p. 1; Datamonitor, 2002; JP Morgan, 2004.

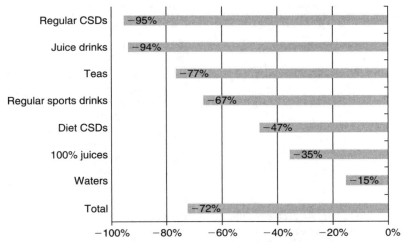

Figure 7-10 Percent Change in Total Volume of Beverage Shipments All Schools, 2004 to 2009–2010. *Source:* Reproduced with permission from the American Beverage Association. Alliance School Beverage Guidelines Final Progress Report, 2010; www.ameribev.org.

physical activity so as to make an impact on cardiovascular disease, certain cancers, diabetes, and chronic respiratory diseases.

The Institute of Medicine (2010) recently emphasized that many intervention approaches designed to address chronic diseases are more likely to succeed if public education and government policies and regulations are complemented by the voluntary collaboration of the private sector. The full language of the two recommendations addressing the private sector appears in Table 7-13. In addition to the Institute of Medicine, several national and international health organizations have made recommendations to the private sector for reducing the risk of chronic diseases. The specific recommendations from the WHO are shown in Table 7-14. The food industry has taken these recommendations seriously, and examples of the spectrum of their responses are also shown in Table 7-14.

As a concrete example of the role the food industry could play in supporting individuals and populations reduce the risk for chronic diseases, PepsiCo unveiled a new set of 11 goals and commitments that form the core of its human sustainability effort. The goals are built around three pillars that embrace product reformulation, changes in marketing and information campaigns, and ways to improve the affordability and accessibility of products in underserved communities. PepsiCo put into place global nutrition criteria based on established national and international recommendations contained in reports from WHO, FAO, and the Institute of Medicine, as well as the U.S. Dietary Guidelines for Americans

(Mirmiran, Noori, Zavareh, & Azizi, 2009; Stampfer, Hu, Manson, Rimm, & Willett, 2000; Xu et al., 2006).

Several other companies in the food and beverage industry have made similar commitments to undertake strategies to reduce the risk of chronic diseases. For example, in May 2008, 10 companies—Ferrero, General Mills, Grupo Bimbo, Kellogg's, Kraft Foods, Mars, Nestlé, PepsiCo, The Coca-Cola Company, and Unilever—established the International Food and Beverage Alliance (IFBA) to explicitly answer WHO's call to action by committing to the following goals: (1) food reformulation; (2) consumer information; (3) responsible marketing; (4) promotion of healthy lifestyles; and (5) public–private partnerships (IFBA, 2009). These 10 multinational companies account for approximately 80% of the global advertising spending by the food and beverage industry and collectively have revenues in excess of $350 billion annually (Yach, Khan, Bradley, Hargrove, Kehoe, & Mensah, 2010). They are also present collectively in more than 200 countries and thus have to reach to impact millions of lives in this endeavor.

Academic and Research Community

The academic response to chronic disease prevention and control in low- and middle-income countries has been mixed. Few courses on chronic disease epidemiology and control in such countries exist anywhere in the world, and few research institutes support research into chronic disease risks and prevention programs in these areas. Notably, there is a paucity of research conducted on chronic diseases by

Table 7-13	Institute of Medicine Recommendations on Collaboration with the Private Sector
Recommendation 8: Collaborate to improve diets	WHO, the World Heart Federation, the International Food and Beverage Association, and the World Economic Forum, in conjunction with select leading international NGOs and select governments from developed and developing countries, should coordinate an international effort to develop collaborative strategies to reduce dietary intake of salt, sugar, saturated fats, and trans-fats in both adults and children. This process should include stakeholders from the public health community and multinational food corporations as well as the food services industry and retailers. This effort should include strategies that take into account local food production and sales.
Recommendation 9: Collaborate to improve access to CVD diagnostics, medicines, and technologies	National and sub-national governments should lead, negotiate, and implement a plan to reduce the costs of and ensure equitable access to affordable diagnostics, essential medicines, and other preventive and treatment technologies for CVD. This process should involve stakeholders from multilateral and bilateral development agencies; CVD-related professional societies; public and private payers; pharmaceutical, biotechnology, medical device, and information technology companies; and experts on health care systems and financing. Deliberate attention should be given to public–private partnerships and to ensuring appropriate, rational use of these technologies.

Table 7-14	World Health Organizations Global Strategy on Diet, Physical Activity, and Health	
Specific Recommendation to the Food Industry	**Food Industry Response**	
■ Promote healthy diets and physical activity in accordance with national guidelines and international standards and the overall aims of the global strategy	■ Under way through the commitments made by International Food and Beverage Alliance (IFBA) to address the areas of food reformulation, consumer information, responsible marketing, promotion of health lifestyles, and public–private partnerships. ■ IFBA has also established food and beverage industry groups in more than 15 countries/regions, including the 27 countries of the European Union and the 6 countries of the Cooperation Council for the Arab States of the Gulf, to allow industry to react according to the different needs and concerns of different member states rapidly and individually as well as expand company participation at the local and regional level, to optimize the local impact, and to ensure that industry efforts take into consideration regional and national differences. ■ More groups are being established in many more countries.	
■ Limit the levels of saturated fats, trans-fatty acids, free sugars, and salt in existing products	■ Since the global strategy was launched in 2004, the food and beverage industry has taken significant steps toward creating measurable improvements, including major reductions in the marketing of products high in fat, sugar, and salt to children younger than12 years of age. ■ IFBA companies have reformulated or introduced more than 28,000 nutritionally enhanced products globally. These ef-	

continued

Table 7-14	*continued*

	forts include specifically reducing or eliminating trans-fat in approximately 18,000 products. Calories were reduced and saturated fats, sugar, carbohydrates, and sodium were also eliminated or reduced in a significant number of products. At the same time, many products were fortified with vitamins, minerals, whole grains, and/or fiber.
■ Continue to develop and provide affordable, healthy, and nutritious choices to consumers	■ IFBA members are also developing product formulations that compensate for chronic micronutrient shortages sometimes found in the low- and middle-income world, where chronic shortages of iron, vitamin A, and iodine in particular can have far-reaching health consequences. ■ IFBA members have increased investments in R&D aimed at achieving this goal. Each company employs scientists, nutritionists, and engineers to develop innovative foods and beverages. The IFBA has also established processes for internal and external expert and scientific review of its nutrition standards, which are then used to drive product innovation.
■ Provide consumers with adequate and understandable product and nutrition information	■ Ongoing efforts continue but require closer government oversight and interaction to have a major impact. ■ IFBA companies have increased their use of consumer information tools, including websites, help lines, in-store leaflets, and brochures.
■ Practice responsible marketing that supports the global strategy, particularly with regard to the promotion and marketing of foods high in saturated fats, trans-fatty acids, free sugars, or salt, especially to children	■ Considerable progress has been made through the IFBA pledge, which is being implemented globally and is subject to external audit. ■ IFBA companies engaged Accenture to provide a global "snapshot" of companies' compliance with their marketing commitments. Accenture tested compliance in 12 markets around the world and reported a 98.17% compliance rate for TV advertising, 100% compliance for print advertising, and only one instance of noncompliance on the Internet.
■ Issue simple, clear, and consistent food labels and evidence-based health claims that will help consumers to make informed and healthy choices with respect to the nutritional value of foods	■ Requires clarity from WHO on the optimal way forward. Many individual company efforts are under way. ■ Many IFBA companies have improved the labeling on their packaging to provide easily understandable nutritional information, including guideline daily amounts (GDAs) or Daily Values, ingredient listings, and key nutrients. IFBA companies have also made significant progress in implementing full nutritional labeling on a voluntary basis in countries where full nutritional labeling is not compulsory. ■ For example, 88% of companies surveyed in Kenya, South Africa, and Uganda are already exceeding the legal labeling requirements and 75% plan on adding more nutritional labeling in the next 24 months.
■ Provide information on food composition to national authorities	■ Under way in countries whose governments have clearly stated norms.

Source: Adapted from WHA 57.17; article 61

researchers in low- and middle-income countries. This can be explained by the levels of investment in health research for chronic disease prevention and control. At the global level, approximately $10 billion was spent on CVD disease research and a further $1.6 billion on diabetes research in 2000–2001. Of that the total amount, roughly 75% was spent in the United States, Japan, United Kingdom, France, and Italy. Further, more than 95% of this spending goes toward new drug development; very little is devoted to community-based prevention research. There are few significant funding sources for chronic disease research in low- and middle-income countries. One such funder, the Fogarty International Center of the National Institutes of Health (NIH; www.fic.nih.gov), supports tobacco control research in low- and middle-income countries.

Against this backdrop, it is not surprising that authors from the United States and United Kingdom dominated research output in all chronic disease and risk categories, accounting for 80% of research on tobacco and cancer, 75% on diabetes and cardiovascular disease, and 60% on obesity. India and China produced less than 3.5% of research publications in all categories, despite being home to 40% of the world's population and a large share of the chronic disease burden. Articles about tobacco with authors from Africa, China, Europe, India, and the United Kingdom declined as a percentage of total papers, but increased by more than 20% relative to the output by authors from the United States.

Preventing and Managing Chronic Diseases: What Needs to Be Done

To make real progress in chronic disease control, the following elements are required: solid evidence of what should be done; acknowledgment by key players of their roles and responsibilities; and recognition of the actions that are required at local, national, and international levels.

Several approaches as to what should be done have been proposed, usually summarized as involving either the promotion of healthy lifestyles for the whole population or the early diagnosis and cost-effective management of risk factors and disease. In reality, it is useful to split this distinction further because it has implications for who should take responsibility for actions. Thus three sets of actions are necessary:

1. Health promotion aimed at shifting the entire distribution of risks in populations through intersectoral actions

2. Prevention programs aimed at reducing the prevalence of specific major risks, especially tobacco use and unhealthy diets

3. Health service programs to identify and reduce risk for patients with risk behaviors and/or preclinical signs of chronic diseases, and programs to prevent the onset of complications in those with disease

These three interrelated actions are described in the following subsections.

Systems That Promote Health

Over the years, the phrase "health systems" has been used to refer to all forms of treatments for diseases, some aspects of rehabilitation, and a few aspects of primary prevention or health promotion. Health departments of countries manage healthcare systems and receive "health" budgets to do so. This narrow perspective leads to public confusion and a lack of clarity about who is really responsible for broader aspects of health promotion.

For chronic diseases such as HIV/AIDS, TB, cancer, diabetes, and cardiovascular disease, there is a long lag between exposure to risks for disease and the occurrence of clinical disease. Acting on risks will reduce incidence, and effective treatment will prevent serious complications and death. Approximately half of the decline in CVD mortality in the United States over the last two decades is ascribed to better treatment, and half to better prevention of risks. For a few cancers, treatment has led to dramatic increases in survival. Such has not been the case, however, with two major tobacco-related cancers: lung and larynx.

Advocacy groups for patients' rights to treatment have successfully changed drug pricing policies and improved access to diagnosis and treatment for a range of diseases, such as HIV/AIDS, breast cancer, and epilepsy. In contrast, the voices calling for prevention and health promotion are relatively mute. The political pressure for greater investments in prevention and health promotion has until recently been lacking. Stronger systems are needed to promote health and prevent risk, and better healthcare systems are needed to address failures of prevention and conditions for which causes (and successful interventions) remain unknown (McGinnis, Williams-Russo, & Knickman, 2002).

How Is a System for Health Promotion Broader Than a Healthcare System?

The goals of a system concerned with health promotion would be broader and focused more on determinants and underlying causes of ill health and on ways of promoting health, compared with healthcare systems. Healthcare systems usually focus on providing treatment within a system that emphasizes quality of care, cost-effectiveness, and equity in access to lifelong care. Within government, many sectors play a role in promoting health or causing disease. A system for health promotion would recognize this complexity and ensure that all policies were evaluated in relation to their impact on health and not just from a narrow sectoral perspective. Healthcare systems are funded mainly from health department budgets, some form of social insurance, and private out-of-pocket expenditures. In contrast, a system for health promotion could tap into funding within many sectoral departments—from agriculture and sports to education and welfare. Healthcare system debates at a national level tend to focus on whether programs should be vertical or horizontal, and ways to achieve cost-containment and equity goals. Debates within government on systems for health promotion would address complex and profound issues involving tradeoffs between development priorities and between allocations that would benefit current as opposed to future generations. Policy impact evaluations would be required to ensure that decisions are made in a transparent manner.

The principle of policy impact assessments is well accepted in relation to the environment or in relation to long-term impacts on budgets, but has generally been neglected from a health perspective. The result has been profoundly negative for health promotion. For example:

- Urban design decisions rarely consider the impact on physical activity—and, consequently, on obesity, diabetes, and CVD incidence.

- Agricultural policies are not developed from a health perspective but primarily for short-term commercial and political reasons. Thus subsidies may be provided for products harmful to health, such as tobacco; to protect high-income countries' farmers at the cost of low- and middle-income countries' economies; and with few incentives for farmers to grow more fruits and vegetables.

- Trade policies often place protection of patents ahead of public health concerns—particularly those of the poorest countries and communities.

- Decisions related to foreign direct investment (FDI) are usually neutral with regard to the effects of new investments on health outcomes. It is often assumed that FDI will bring new jobs and economic growth and, therefore, is always good for societies. Contrary evidence suggests that certain types of FDI promote rapid acquisition of unhealthy consumption patterns for products such as tobacco; foods with high fat, sugar, and salt content; and alcohol (Table 7-15).

Systems for health promotion would be governed at the national level by the cabinet as a whole and not just by the ministry or department of health. In a few countries, ministries of health are often mandated to take the lead on all issues related to health. This situation usually occurs when there is a strong and dynamic minister.

Table 7-15	Foreign Direct Investment: Foreign Assets and Employment of Tobacco, Alcohol, Food, and Retail Companies in the World's Largest 100 Transnational Corporations, 2001			
Sector	Corporation	Home Economy	Foreign Assets (Rank) US$ billion	Foreign Employment
Food and Beverage	Hutinson Whampoa Limited	Hong Kong	40.9 (17)	53,478
	Nestle SA	Switzerland	33.1 (21)	223,000
	Unilever	UK/Netherlands	30.5 (25)	204,000
	Diageo	UK	19.7 (47)	60,000
	Procter & Gamble	USA	17.3 (58)	43,381
	Coca-Cola Company	USA	17.1 (59)	26,000
	McDonalds	USA	12.8 (79)	251,000
	Danone Group SA	France	11.4 (86)	88,000
Retail	Carrefour SA	France	29.3 (29)	235,894
(food and drink)	Wal-Mart Stores	USA	26.3 (24)	303,000
	Royal Ahold NV	Netherlands	19.9 (44)	183,851
Alcohol	Diageo	UK	19.7 (47)	60,000
Tobacco	Phillip Morris	USA	19.3 (49)	39,000
	BAT	UK	10.4 (92)	59,000

Note: Eleven automobile and 10 pharmaceutical companies are also among the top 100 transnational corporations.

Source: United Nations Conference on Trade and Development, *World Investment Report 2003* (Geneva and New York: UNCTAD, 2003). Reprinted with permission.

The report by Derek Wanless (2004) entitled *Securing Good Health for the Whole Population* provides detailed guidance to sectoral ministries on how they could contribute to improving health overall, and especially how they could reduce inequalities in health. What makes Wanless's work so important is that it was commissioned and coordinated by the U.K. Treasury, albeit by drawing heavily on public health expertise. This report must rank as one of the most important contributions to public health anywhere, and it certainly has implications for how one can take a step-by-step approach to building true systems for health promotion. Unlike so many of the other reports cited by Wanless and produced over the last few decades, this one is likely to be backed by government finance and, where required, legislation and taxation; it is already strongly supported by a newly activated public health community.

Which Types of Conflicts Occur?

Progress in much of infectious disease control is achievable with additional funding for surveillance, effective treatment, and new drugs and vaccines where existing ones are ineffective or are not available; it also requires general improvements in housing and related infrastructure (water, sanitation, and energy). All of these investments are now regarded as noncontentious. Even the tough issues of improving access to drugs in poor countries are being addressed nationally and internationally within the context of the World Trade Organization's Doha trade round. Those conflicts that do remain are subsiding, and the move is now to seek funds for effective action.

In contrast, progress in promoting health often involves WHO and public health agencies urging individuals to stop smoking; eat less fat, sugar, and salt; engage in more physical activity; and eat more fruits, vegetables, nuts, and grains. They do so knowing that individual responsibility without supportive government and multisectoral action rarely leads to sustained change. Further, unless "healthy choices are made," in the words of the Ottawa Charter, "the easy choices"—such as unhealthy consumption patterns—will persist, especially among the poor, where they often become entrenched as the easiest and most affordable choices.

Table 7-16 summarizes a number of policy issues that require resolution at a level of government outside of the health department. The table lists some traditional opponents to healthy public policies, along with possible supporters of change. As noted earlier, tobacco use and diet/physical activity shortcomings are major contributors to the burden of disease in both high-income and low- and middle-income countries.

Because of their disproportionate impact, special emphasis is given to the nature of conflicts and tradeoffs that have occurred in these areas. Notably, the call to stop smoking has unified a variety of opposition groups—the tobacco industry itself, the hospitality and entertainment industries, farmers, advertising companies, and often the media. All are told a simple message: If people smoke less, they will all lose jobs. It has taken decades of policy work by economists, public health advocates, and practitioners to correct myths propagated by the tobacco industry surrogates. Examples of such myths include the following:

- Restaurants and pubs will go bankrupt if smoke-free policies are introduced. The opposite is the truth.

- Finance departments will lose revenue from smuggling and reduced tax receipts if excise taxes increase. Actually, although smuggling may have a small impact on revenue, the solution is not to condone crime, but rather to strengthen customs and excise controls.

Table 7-16	Supporters and Opponents of Selected Policy Issues		
Major Risk Factor	**Policy Issue**	**Supporters**	**Opponents**
Tobacco	Excise tax	Finance, World Bank	Tobacco industry
	Advertising bans	N/A	Advertisers, media, libertarians
	Smoke-free areas	Restaurants	Hospitality and restaurant sector
	Agricultural subsidies	Enlightened countries	Farmers, rural voters
	Advertising to children	N/A	Advertisers, multinational food companies, media
Diet, nutrition	Commodity changes, sugar	Fruit, vegetable farmers	Sugar farmers, producers, lobbyists
	promotion to children	Sports, gyms	Sports, toys, fast food industries

N/A = not applicable.

- Tobacco farmers in countries such as Zimbabwe and Malawi will be unemployed in a few years as tobacco consumption declines. Unfortunately, from a public health perspective, consumption does not fall at a rate faster than 5% per year, and usually rates of 2% have been regarded as impressive if maintained for years. At those rates, and in the face of continued population growth, the demand for leaf tobacco will remain high for many decades. The immediate threat to African tobacco farmers comes more from the introduction of mechanization locally and subsidies in high-income countries than from less smoking.

Like the tobacco issue, the public health statement "Consume sugar sparingly," which seems like common sense to most people, evokes strong responses from a wide range of special interests. During the development of the WHO Global Strategy on Diet, Physical Activity and Health, the full range of possible arguments against this simple message about sugar emerged (A. Waxman, 2004; H. Waxman, 2004). Soda manufacturers have led the global efforts to deny that sugar causes obesity or dental caries, or that specific levels of sugars are desirable. Sugarcane farmers in low- and middle-income countries are concerned that if new WHO/FAO guidelines on sugar consumption were applied globally, they would lose their jobs. The economic stakes are much more substantive for sugar as opposed to tobacco; the size of the lobbying community is far greater and the evidence base on the economics of sugar use is not as well described as it is for tobacco.

For several years, proponents of antismoking campaigns made efforts to be prepared for critique of any efforts to control tobacco use. These included engaging with the Food and Agriculture Organization, the World Bank, the IMF, UNICEF, and other UN partners and jointly agreeing that the key policy goal in relation to tobacco was demand reduction. Supply-related issues would need to be addressed but should not block action on making public health gains. In the process, new research by the World Bank showed that tobacco control was sound economic and health policy, and the FAO showed that farmers' short-term fears were exaggerated. Within the UN family, policy coherence was achieved. This harmony was later reflected in increased policy coherence within governments. Similar work is yet to emerge with respect to many food policy issues. They are inherently more complex, involve a wider array of players, and will need to address the reality that there may be some losers over the long term, but that these are likely to be more than offset by winners, particularly in the fruit, vegetable, and nuts sectors. As with tobacco, and opposite to what lobbyists maintain, there will only be very modest impacts on the demand for sugar over the next few decades even if the WHO recommendations are fully implemented (LMC International, 2004).

Specific Prevention Programs to Address Tobacco, Diet, and Physical Activity

Tobacco

Since the first major reports of tobacco-related harm surfaced in the early 1960s, there has been an evolution in the development of policies to tackle tobacco. This evolution has unfolded in different ways in different geographic regions. By the early 1970s, the content of a comprehensive package of interventions to address tobacco had been accepted as the way forward and had been incorporated into national law in several Nordic countries, as well as in Singapore, Australia, and New Zealand. A very similar package was adopted three decades later as the basis for global action—the WHO FCTC (http://www.who.int/tobacco/framework/en). None of the early-adopter countries was home to multinational tobacco companies, however, and all had a strong history of open and critically transparent parliamentary processes that gave emphasis to health.

In the United States, tobacco company efforts ensured that few attempts by the federal government succeeded and that tobacco control was based on a strong educational component. Innovation was left to the states and, increasingly, to local cities and towns. In California, for example, the freedom that came with statehood stimulated local initiatives that were well funded and politically supported. Sensing the threat posed by the increasing evidence that interventions were effective in reducing smoking, the tobacco industry hired large numbers of consultants, including economists, journalists, advertisers, physicians, and philosophers, to dispute this evidence. This led to the strange situation whereby tobacco control experts could discover what really made a difference simply by studying where opposition was strongest. Thus taxes, advertisement bans, smoke-free policies, and litigation, which the industry argued would "not work," should be emphasized. In contrast, industry-favored policies such as education at schools, voluntary agreements on advertising, and accommodation between smokers and nonsmokers are largely ineffective. In many cases, the tobacco industry actively commissioned research that was either methodologically flawed or simply fraudulent to give weight to its arguments. The same approaches, although in some cases at lower levels of intensity, were adopted by major tobacco companies based in Japan, Germany, and the United Kingdom.

Paradoxically, some of the earliest countries to act against tobacco introduced effective policies even though the evidence from research was not yet available. Randomized control studies of advertising bans or tax increases were not possible. Rather, professional judgment and common sense played a key role in their programs. Decades later, low- and middle-income countries introducing these same measures are being challenged by tobacco companies that dispute their now well-established effectiveness.

The accumulation of experience from many countries means that it is now much clearer what works and what does not in terms of tobacco control. It confirms the wisdom of the early adopters: Be comprehensive; keep the debate alive, interesting, and provocative in the media; incrementally tighten laws as public support and demand for action increases; move to make smoking an unacceptable and antisocial behavior; and globalize action to counter the global reach and strategies of tobacco companies—particularly their marketing and investment practices. International consensus of what constitutes the key elements of a comprehensive approach to tobacco control is now enshrined in the text of the FCTC, which by August 2004 had been adopted by 192 countries, signed by 170, and ratified by 29.

Diet/Physical Activity

With the enormous contemporary focus on obesity, it is easy to ignore the profound changes that have occurred with respect to many other aspects of healthy diets. Salt levels in processed foods have declined in many countries, often stimulated by government regulations; consumption of saturated fat has been reduced in many high-income countries as a result of education, better product choices provided by companies, and media coverage (although this achievement took three decades); and the need for all people to eat more fruits and vegetables is now accepted widely even though consumption remains far below suggested levels. The combined effects of these dietary changes have led to a striking reduction in the incidence of CVD in high-income countries, with the impact especially apparent in the former communist countries of eastern Europe, now members of the European Union, where change proceeded rapidly after the breakup of the Soviet bloc after 1990.

Unfortunately, at the same time as the progress just described has occurred, some aspects of diet have worsened. More sugar is consumed by children in many countries, and physical activity levels have collapsed. In low- and middle-income countries, a more rapid nutrition transition is under way than ever occurred in high-income countries, with "bads" increasingly displacing "goods."

Governments worldwide are now struggling to develop effective approaches to obesity. The recently adopted WHO Global Strategy on Diet, Physical Activity, and Health proposes a range of key elements of a comprehensive approach (WHO, 2004). However, this issue is only just now reaching the policy agenda; compared with the moves to address tobacco use, the level of active intervention and support by many governments has been low.

Table 7-17 considers which key elements of the FCTC have implications for diet and physical activity. A few points are worth noting:

- Increasing prices through excise tax works well for tobacco control but remains technically doubtful as a means of influencing food choices. Currently, taxes on soft drinks are used to raise revenue for health promotion. Measures to make fruits and vegetables more affordable may be a better alternative.

- Several recent studies suggest that fear works in tobacco control communications directed toward adults and children. In contrast, this approach seems to have limited use in influencing food choices or in promoting physical activity.

- Few of the interventions related to tobacco use and diet/physical activity have been explicitly designed or evaluated in terms of their impact on reducing risks among the poorest communities and their impact on minorities. Evidence suggests that most tobacco control measures have mainly benefited the most educated and the wealthiest subpopulations in countries. This issue requires serious research and policy attention because chronic diseases already contribute to inequalities in survival by social class and area.

- The success of tobacco taxation as a very effective policy tool for reducing CVD risk in a broad range of countries has led some authors to propose taxing other products such as food and beverages as a strategy for reducing the risks of chronic diseases (Brownell & Frieden, 2009). However, the evidence is insufficient with respect to effectiveness or health impact of this approach (Institute of Medicine, 2010).

- There is preliminary evidence suggesting that a "thin subsidy" to lower the price of healthy

Table 7-17	Potential Relevance of FCTC Provisions to Diet and Physical Activity	
Measure	**FCTC Tobacco Provision**	**Application to Diet and Physical Activity**
Pricing and taxes	Increase price by raising excise taxes and through prohibitions or restrictions on sales/imports of tax and duty-free tobacco products	Use price measures to make fruits and vegetables more affordable; conduct research to consider whether taxing certain foods will promote healthier eating
Exposure to environmental tobacco smoke	Measures aimed at protecting the public from exposure to environmental tobacco smoke	Not applicable
Packaging and labeling requirements	Provisions address the size of health warnings and labeling, especially with respect to misleading language (Article 11)	Health warnings and disclosure of nutritional information: adherence to Codex nutrition labeling guidelines and science-based criteria for health claims
Product content	Guidelines for testing, measuring and regulating the contents and emissions of tobacco products (Article 9)	Regulation of harmful ingredients; labeling that discloses significant ingredients; food safety regulations
Education campaigns	Promotion of public awareness of health risks of tobacco use/exposure to tobacco smoke, and of the benefits of cessation of tobacco use and of tobacco-free lifestyles	Educational campaigns in schools, workplaces, primary healthcare settings, and other sites reaching the general public; information and skill building to encourage optimal nutrition and physical activity
Restrictions on advertising, sponsorship, and promotion	Restrictions—preferably a complete ban—on advertising, sponsorship, and promotion of tobacco products	Restrictions on advertising, sponsorship, and promotion of some food products to children; discouragement of sedentary behavior and unhealthy lifestyles
Clinical interventions	Cessation programs; diagnosis and treatment of tobacco dependence	Clinical interventions based on collaborative goal setting, skill building, self-monitoring, personalized feedback, planned follow-up, and links to community resources

Source: D. Yach, C. Hawkes, J. E. Epping-Jordan, and S. Galbraith, "The World Health Organization's Framework Convention on Tobacco Control: Implications for the Global Epidemics of Food-Related Deaths and Disease," 2003, *Journal of Public Health Policy, 24 (2–3)*, pp. 274–290.

foods in the United States would be a cost-effective intervention for CHD and stroke (Cash, Sunding, & Zilberman, 2005; Institute of Medicine, 2010).

Have Risk Factor–Specific Policies Made a Difference?

The impact of policies on tobacco use, and on the health consequences that follow, has been well documented. In many high-income countries, male smoking rates reached 50% to 60% by the early 1960s, but are now approximately 20% to 30%; in some places, such as California, they have fallen as low as 11%. Cardiovascular disease, lung cancer, and other tobacco-related diseases have declined in these countries. In some cases, the declines have been rapid and substantial. There is growing evidence that the intense public and media debates over several decades

have themselves played a powerful role in changing behaviors.

Much less progress has been made in reducing smoking rates among women. In some high-income countries, women's smoking rates are still increasing—and along with them, CVD and, after a further lag period, lung cancer rates. Among adults, the greatest declines in tobacco use have occurred among members of higher social classes, with very modest progress evident among manual workers, marginalized groups, and people with the lowest levels of education. In addition, smoking prevalence among children in many high-income countries remains high. In many countries, girls are more likely to smoke than boys, portending future reversals of the traditional female advantage in life expectancy.

Several low- and middle-income countries and countries in transition have also made real progress, but in only a few, such as Poland, has this achievement so far translated into fewer deaths from tobacco-related causes. A World Bank review of strategies and successes in tobacco control in Brazil, South Africa, Thailand, Poland, Bangladesh, and Canada showed that a range of policies and regulations had contributed to reduced smoking prevalence (de Beyer & Brigden, 2003).

For many low- and middle-income countries, the fundamental challenge is different from that in high-income countries: how to stop an increase in smoking against a backdrop of historically relatively low rates (especially among women and children). In high-income countries, the goal has primarily been to reduce already high rates among men, while in countries in transition it is also important to prevent the rise in female smoking. The different policy approaches called for when the goal is to stop an increase compared to when it is to reduce already high rates have not been carefully distinguished. Taxes, advertising bans, and early introduction of smoke-free policies may well be most effective and cost-effective in settings where education levels are low; where health services, including cessation programs, are underdeveloped; and where the unchecked impact of the tobacco industry is greatest.

Overall, however, "considerable progress" has been made against the global tobacco epidemic, as demonstrated in the most recent WHO country-level analysis (WHO, 2009b). Nearly 400 million people are now newly covered by tobacco control measures because of the actions taken by 17 countries to fight the tobacco epidemic (WHO, 2009b). The most common of these measures introduced is the establishment of smoke-free environments. Figure 7-11 shows the state of selected tobacco control policies and compliance in the world as of 2008. Seven countries, most of which are middle-income nations, newly adopted comprehensive smoke-free laws in 2008. Of real importance is the fact that several of these countries progressed from having either no national smoke-free law or only minimal protection in some types of public places or workplaces to full protection in all types of places. Nevertheless, as the WHO report details, only 9% of countries mandate smoke-free bars and restaurants, and 65 countries report no implementation of any smoke-free policies on a national level.

Achievements in relation to diet have been less clear-cut. Although increased consumption of micronutrients, especially from fresh fruits and vegetables, and reductions in consumption of saturated fat

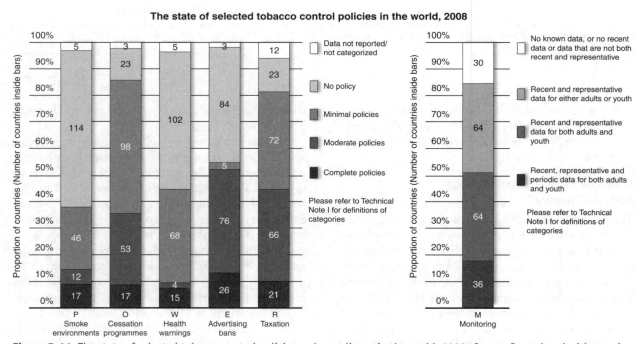

Figure 7-11 The state of selected tobacco control policies and compliance in the world, 2008. *Source:* Reproduced with permission from the World Health Organization (2009). WHO report on the global tobacco epidemic, 2009: implementing smoke-free environments. Geneva: World Health Organization.

have led to declines in stroke and CVD, the growth of obesity has fueled an epidemic of type 2 diabetes. As time passes, this trend can be expected to reverse the earlier gains, with the decline this time being driven not by consumption of saturated fat, but rather by excessive calories, carbohydrates, hypertension, and diabetes itself.

The Limitations of Studies on Cost-Effectiveness for Chronic Disease Prevention

Many interventions for chronic disease prevention and health promotion have been tried and tested, notably by the Cochrane collaboration process. As summarized in Table 7-18, Cochrane reviews of several interventions are now available (Riemsma et al., 2002), and a global task force has identified additional priority areas for future research (Doyle et al., 2005). As identified in the lessons learned from the tobacco experience (Exhibit 7-2), success in health promotion and chronic disease prevention depends on having a comprehensive set of interventions that taken collectively make it possible for healthy choices to be easy choices. Several studies carried out in school, workplace, or healthcare settings have demonstrated short-term effects in relatively small groups of people, but those effects are rarely replicated across large populations. Further, the types of interventions with the greatest probability of influencing the behavior of populations—namely, those involving regulatory actions, changes in fiscal policy, or intersectoral actions—do not lend themselves to randomized control studies of the type usually reported in Cochrane reviews.

More complex approaches are needed to evaluate such interventions. One recent initiative by WHO researchers provides an example of what could be done more broadly. A comprehensive review that applies to all countries, at all levels of development, used methods that could be applied to the full range of chronic diseases and risks (Murray et al., 2003). The study used the output of systematic reviews as a basis for developing evidence on effectiveness and costs of interventions to lower population-wide measures of systolic blood pressure and cholesterol. The results showed that nonpersonal health interventions, including government action to stimulate a reduction in the salt content of processed foods, are cost-effective ways to limit CVD. Combination treatment is also cost-effective for people whose risk of a CVD event over the next 10 years is greater than 35%. Taken together, personal and nonpersonal health interventions (excluding those related to tobacco) could lower the global incidence of CVD events by as much as 50% (Murray et al., 2003).

Management of Chronic Diseases by Healthcare Systems

Healthcare Quality and Access

Universally, healthcare systems are not organized to provide effective and efficient prevention and care for chronic diseases. Countries often struggle with the complexity of insufficient resources combined with inadequate access to necessary drugs and technologies. The chemotherapeutic agents that are most effective against the 10 leading cancers are not available in many low- and middle-income countries,

Exhibit 7-2	**Twelve Lessons from the Experience of Tobacco That May Be Applicable to Policy Development Relating to Diet and Nutrition**

1. Address the issue of individual responsibility versus collective/environmental action early and often. This issue pervades debates on the role of government versus the role of the individual. Both sides of the issue need to be addressed, with emphasis being given to the Ottawa Charter statement that "healthy choices need to be the easy choices."
2. Evidence of harm is necessary but not sufficient to motivate policy change. There is a need for some essential epidemiologic gaps to be closed in relation to diet and outcomes in low- and middle-income countries, but there is already sufficient knowledge to act now, rather than using the call for more research as an excuse for delaying action.
3. Decisions to act need not wait for evidence of the effectiveness of interventions. For example, the initial tobacco control interventions were not evidence based but rather represented sound judgment at the time. We know now what has worked for tobacco and can adapt some elements immediately. For others, we should introduce interventions in such a way that their effectiveness can be critically evaluated and appropriate adjustments can be made over time.

(continued)

Exhibit 7-2	*continued*

4. The real and perceived needs and concerns of low- and middle-income countries need to be addressed even if they involve going beyond the initial scope of the risk being addressed. For tobacco control, this meant addressing all forms of tobacco use, not just cigarettes, and considering the concerns of tobacco farmers and providing convincing evidence that their livelihoods did not face an immediate threat. For the diet/nutrition area, approaches will be more complex and require that close interaction be sought between those working to address hunger, micronutrient deficiencies, and undernutrition in general and those working to develop policies for overweight and chronic disease prevention. The goal should be to promote the optimal diet for all. It also requires that the complex agricultural issues related to subsidies and decisions about what gets cultivated receive greater attention.

5. The more comprehensive the package of measures considered, the greater the impact. Most approaches currently discussed in relation to diet and physical activity tend to emphasize very narrow approaches—more exercise at schools or more education at work, for example. Few take a broad perspective. Within a comprehensive package, those working in tobacco and diet/physical activity need to understand where governments have constraints and help authorities to address them. For example, some countries have a constitutional impediment to a complete ban on tobacco advertisement.

6. Broad-based vertical and horizontal coalitions, that are effectively networked, are key. Vertical coalitions include all those parties involved in public health—from the local health department to the regional and national authority to WHO. What has become increasingly clear is that a wide array of players outside the traditional boundaries of health need to be engaged and to lead on certain aspects of the problem. Health-oriented entities still need to provide overall direction and leadership, however. This feat has been achieved for the FCTC process within the UN, among NGOs, and to a limited extent across departments inside many governments. It remains to be done for diet and physical activity.

7. Media-savvy individual and institutional leadership matters. Say no more!

8. Change in support for tobacco control took decades of dedicated effort by all. The global breakthrough came when the then Director General of WHO, Dr. Gro Harlem Brundtland, proved willing to tackle an unpopular topic by speaking out often to heads of state, major donors, and those in the industry about tobacco use being a real global concern. Progress had been happening well before this point, however, in developing the basis for having content that would work in the FCTC, and in having a network of advocates and NGOs ready to rally in support.

9. Modest, well-spent funds can have a massive impact, but without clear goals any gains achieved in this way may not be sustainable. For both tobacco and diet, there are no agreed targets or internationally accepted indicators of progress. Moreover, some countries have set targets for tobacco control but then did not provide resources for their attainment.

10. Complacency that past actions will serve well as strategies in the future may retard future progress. Despite all the progress in tobacco control, the bottom line remains that global consumption continues to increase, albeit slowly; few countries have achieved sustained declines of more than 2% prevalence per year for a decade (Canada has come close, and South Africa has reported a 65% decline per year for eight years). Such slow rates of decline must mean that we need to reconsider our policies and interventions and consider what is needed to reach an 8% to 10% decline per year and then to maintain levels well below 10% in all subgroups. Perhaps stronger emphasis on smoke-free policies combined more tightly with access to cessation programs and increased prices could achieve such levels of decline. New approaches, including the use of plain packaging, need to be considered as well. For diet issues, and especially obesity, investment in large-scale community-based research is needed to yield the first signs of progress.

11. Rules of engagement with the tobacco and food industries need to be different and continually under review. Until now, the public health community has not officially met with the tobacco industry—exceptions being the Centers for Disease Control and Prevention (CDC) and WHO as part of their on-the-record interactions in relation to product regulation. As time passes, there will be a need to meet with tobacco industry scientists to review their progress on potentially reduced-risk products and to consider which criteria should be used to judge their claims of reduced harm. A new set of rules for engagement is required to extract possible areas of progress. At this stage, interaction in relation to youth smoking, marketing, taxes, and smoke-free public places does seem warranted. With respect to the food industry, the issues are more complex, and at this stage an agreed set of rules for engagement should be developed that could include guidance on how to find common solutions to issues related to marketing to children, product content and safety, joint action to promote physical activity and healthy eating, and support for priority research.

12. Risk factor envy is harmful. As the media shift their attention and focus on obesity, funders are shifting their emphasis, too. There is a real danger that one major health problem will be displaced by another. An urgent need exists to build synergies between those active in tobacco and others addressing diet and physical activity, as well as diseases associated with these risk factors. A grand coalition of the willing could do more good for public health by pushing for sustained policy and financial change together than by competing against one another.

Table 7-18	Cochrane Reviews of Effective Interventions in Chronic Disease Risk Factors		
Risk Factor Area	Examples of Published Cochrane Reviews	Cochrane Reviews in Progress (Published Protocol or Registered Title)	Examples of Interventions Needing Review
Tobacco	• Community interventions for preventing smoking in young people • Impact of tobacco advertising and promotion on increasing adolescent smoking behaviors • Workplace interventions for smoking cessation	• Stage-based interventions for smoking cessation • Mass-media interventions for smoking cessation in adults (registered title only)	• Interventions targeted by gender to decrease tobacco initiation • Interventions utilizing marketing strategies to promote healthy behaviors in young people, focusing on tobacco
Obesity	• Advice on low-fat diets for obesity • Interventions for preventing childhood obesity	• Exercise for obesity	
Diet	• Reduced or modified dietary fat for preventing cardiovascular disease	• Interventions for promoting the initiation of breastfeeding	• Interventions utilizing marketing strategies to promote healthy behaviors in young people, focusing on food[*] • Interventions for healthier food choices[*] (e.g., sales promotion strategies of supermarkets to increase healthier food purchase and/or pricing policies to increase healthy food choices)
Physical activity	• Exercise for preventing and treating osteoporosis in postmenopausal women • Exercise to improve self-esteem in children and young people	• Interventions for promoting physical activity • Interventions implemented through sporting organizations for increasing participation in sport (registered title only) • School-based physical activity programs for promoting physical activity and fitness in children and adolescents aged 6–18 (registered title only)	• Physical exercise to improve mental health outcomes for adults[*] • Interventions to minimize the impact of urban sprawl on physical activity[*] • Interventions to increase the supply of sidewalks and walking trails for the public • Healthy cities project to reduce cardiovascular risk factors[*] (could apply to all risk factors)

[a] Identified as priority topics for review by the Cochrane Collaboration process.

Source: R.P. Riemsma, J. Pattenden, C. Bridel, A.J. Sowden, L. Mather, I.S. Watt, and A. Walker, "A systematic review of the Effectiveness of Interventions Based on a Stages-of-Change Approach to Promote Individual Behavior Change," 2002, *Health Technology Assessment, 6(24)*, pp. 1–231.

where they are often subject to high import duties (IARC, 2003). Likewise, inhaled beclomethasone is often not available or affordable in low- and middle-income countries, placing patients with COPD and asthma at considerable risk for premature death (Ait-Khaled et al., 2001).

Opportunities for secondary prevention are being missed. The WHO PREMISE study of secondary prevention of CHD and cerebrovascular disease showed that knowledge and treatment of these diseases are underutilized in the care of patients in low- and middle-income countries. Most patients were aware of the preventive effects of lifestyle factors, such as quitting smoking, eating a healthier diet, and performing physical activity, but did not necessarily follow these recommendations. Many patients were not receiving preventive medication such as aspirin. Measurement of cardiovascular risk factors, such as blood sugar and blood cholesterol levels and blood pressure, was not sufficiently regular. Inadequate resources and facilities of healthcare systems in low- and middle-income countries are largely responsible for the insufficiencies of secondary prevention (WHO PREMISE, in press).

Quality gaps extend beyond medication availability, however. In the Caribbean, for example, a medical record review of more than 1,600 patients attending healthcare clinics for diabetes indicated that over a 12-month period, fewer than one-third had received dietary advice and only 5% had received exercise advice (Gulliford, Alert, Mahabir, Ariyanayagam-Baksh, Fraser, & Picou, 1996). Similar findings have been reported in South Africa (Beattie, Kalk, Price, Rispel, Broomberg, & Cabral, 1998) and India (Raheja et al., 2001). This phenomenon is not limited to low- and middle-income countries. In one study of the quality of health care delivered to adults in the United States, McGlynn et al. (2003) showed that participants received only 54.9% of recommended care; moreover, these researchers found little difference among the proportion of recommended preventive care provided (54.9%), the proportion of recommended acute care provided (53.5%), and the proportion of recommended care provided for chronic conditions (56.1%). In essence, adults in the United States received the appropriate recommended quality health care from their caregivers only half the time.

Underlying Drivers of the Problem

Most healthcare systems have not kept pace with the decline in acute health problems and the increase in chronic disease and are still trying to manage chronic problems using acute care mentality, methods, and systems. Because current healthcare systems developed in response to acute problems and the urgent needs of patients, they are designed to address pressing concerns. As such, healthcare interactions are characterized by one-to-one visits with healthcare workers whose purpose is to diagnose and treat a patient's pressing complaint. Testing, diagnosing, relieving symptoms, and expecting cure are characteristic of this kind of health care, and these functions fit the needs of patients experiencing acute and episodic health problems.

The application of this typical visit format to chronic conditions brings obvious problems, however. One problem is the discrete nature of the interactions, which belies the importance of promoting planned and proactive care. Clearly, chronic conditions are not a series of disconnected complaints, yet people with chronic disease are frequently treated as if this were the case. This approach is wasteful and inefficient given that complications and the eventual outcomes of poorly managed chronic conditions follow a known and predictable course. Chronic diseases require health care that is proactive and organized around the concepts of planned care and prevention.

A second major problem is that healthcare workers frequently fail to recognize the importance of empowering patients to become active participants in their ongoing care. There is substantial evidence—in the form of more than 400 published articles—that interventions designed to promote patients' roles in the prevention and management of chronic diseases are associated with improved outcomes. What patients do for themselves on a daily basis— engage in regular physical activity, eat properly, avoid tobacco use, sleep regularly, adhere to treatment plans—influences their health far more than biomedical interventions alone. There is also ample scientific evidence demonstrating that successful healthcare interventions do exist for changing patients' health behavior and for increasing their adherence to treatments. Unfortunately, these interventions, which could prevent many chronic diseases and improve their management once they occur, are all too often missing from current systems of care.

Characteristics of Effective Systems of Care for Chronic Diseases

Health care for patients with chronic conditions requires a fundamental change in perspective from the familiar acute care model. The magnitude of the challenge is eased somewhat by the fact that chronic conditions share many common features. Whereas biomedical management changes depending on the unique features of the specific disease, the general components of care organization and delivery for patients with chronic conditions are essentially the same. These components include a well-defined care plan, patient self-management, scheduled follow-up appointments, monitoring of outcome and adherence, and stepwise treatment protocols. Collectively, these approaches represent a significant shift in healthcare practices. The differences between typical current and desired future approaches are described in the following subsections.

Patient-Centered Care

Patient-centered care recognizes the patient as a person; fully informs patients about the risks and benefits of treatment options; tailors decision making in response to individual patients' values, needs, and expressed preferences; shares power and responsibility among patients and providers; and develops patients' abilities to participate in their care. Across its multiple meanings, research shows that patient-centered care is crucial for obtaining good outcomes for chronic conditions.

Several experiences within low- and middle-income countries have demonstrated the utility of patient-centered care across diverse cultures and resource contexts. WHO's Integrated Management of Adult Illness (IMAI) general principles of chronic care, for example, focus on equipping first-level healthcare workers to provide patient-centered health care. Specifically, the guidelines and related training materials prepare such workers to solicit patients' concerns and preferences, work in collaboration with patients to decide specific goals and treatment plans, and support patients in their daily efforts regarding prevention, medication adherence, and self-management.

Early results indicate that this approach is understandable and usable by first-level health workers. To date, physicians, nurses, and lay providers have been trained in this approach in Burkina Faso, Burundi, Ethiopia, Sudan, and Uganda. In Shanghai, China, a community-based chronic disease self-management program has been shown to improve health status and reduce hospitalizations among patients with hypertension, heart disease, chronic lung disease, arthritis, stroke, and diabetes. Participants learn to take responsibility for the day-to-day management of their disease and the physical and emotional problems caused by their disease. The program is led by lay people with chronic conditions, who follow a detailed leader's manual throughout the program (Fu et al., 2003).

Emphasis on Primary Health Care

In low- and middle-income countries, patients with chronic conditions present and need to be managed mainly at the primary healthcare level. This represents a departure from the approach used in healthcare systems that are driven by tertiary care, specialty settings. Oman has successfully made the shift to a decentralized primary healthcare system, with health programs and activities in this country now being coordinated with the regional health services via referrals and linkages (WHO, 2002c). Similarly, the health policy of the Islamic Republic of Iran is based on primary health care, with particular emphasis on the expansion of health networks and programs in rural areas.

Population-Based Care

Health care for chronic conditions is most effective when policies, plans, and practices prioritize the health of a defined population rather than the single unit of a patient seeking care. A population focus implies that healthcare systems assess and monitor the health of communities, emphasize prevention and promote healthy behavior, assure universal access to appropriate and cost-effective services, and contribute to the evidence base for effective treatments and systems of care.

Cuba's family doctor program is a notable application of population-based care. Each family doctor is responsible for the general health of the entire population in a small, defined area. Physicians are expected to provide preventive, maternal, and curative services to children and adults, and to monitor all patients with chronic conditions. They live in the communities that they serve, often residing in the same apartment block as their patients. In addition to medical consultations, Cuba's family doctors play an active role in promoting health among the communities they serve. They provide informal advice and counseling to community members, and they run regular prevention and self-management groups concerning a range of issues. They are also expected to set a positive example for their patients in the conduct of their day-to-day lives (Warman, 2001).

Proactive Care

Proactive care anticipates patients' needs rather than relying on a patient-initiated, often acute care–focused interaction. In rural South Africa, a proactive noncommunicable disease management program for hypertension, diabetes, asthma, and epilepsy was established within primary health care. This program emphasized planned care: Clinic-held treatment cards and registries were introduced, and diagnostic and management protocols were followed, which included regular, planned follow-up with a clinic nurse. Using this proactive care approach, nurses were able to achieve good disease control among most of the patient population—68% of patients with hypertension,

82% of those with diabetes, and 84% of those with asthma (Coleman, Gill, & Wilkinson, 1998).

A Model of Care: Innovative Care for Chronic Conditions

A model based on these approaches has been developed by WHO. The Innovative Care for Chronic Conditions (ICCC) framework provides a road map for decision makers who want to improve their health system's capacity to manage chronic conditions (WHO, 2002b) (Figure 7-12). This framework is composed of fundamental components within the levels of patient interactions, organization of health care, community, and policy. These components are described as building blocks that can be used to help decision makers progressively create or redesign a healthcare system to expand its capacity to manage long-term health problems. Although the framework does not prescribe specific changes that must be tailored to unique needs and resources, it highlights the need for comprehensive system design or change in the requirements for effective care.

Barr et al. (2003) have also proposed an expanded chronic care model (Figure 7-13) that em-phasizes the inclusion of elements of the population health promotion field so that broad-based prevention efforts, recognition of the social determinants of health, and enhanced community participation can all be part of the work of health system teams as they address the prevention and control of chronic diseases. Table 7-19 compares the components of the expanded chronic care model with those of the chronic care model developed by Wagner and colleagues (1996).

Comprehensive Care Applied to Clinical Prevention

The preponderance of the evidence suggests that effective healthcare strategies for reducing risk do exist, but tend to be weakly implemented (Coffield et al., 2001). Many professional competencies for delivering effective clinical prevention are outside the scope and culture of clinical medicine, so healthcare professionals frequently have little or no training in the skills required to improve care (Glasgow, Orleans, & Wagner, 2001).

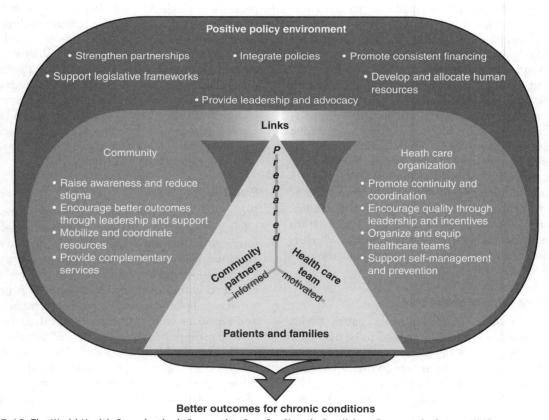

Figure 7-12 The World Health Organization's Innovative Care for Chronic Conditions Framework. *Source:* WHO.

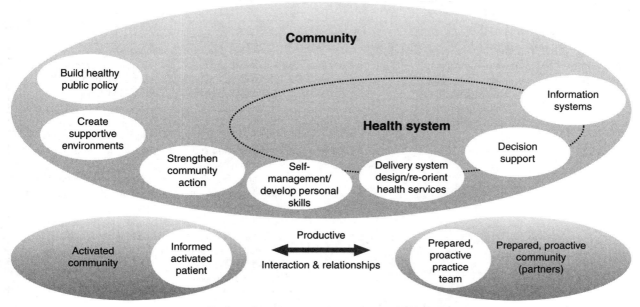

Figure 7-13 The expanded Chronic Care Model. *Source:* Reproduced with permission from Barr, V. J., Robinson, S., Marin-Link, B., Underhill, L., Dotts, A., Ravensdale, D. et al. Hosp.Q. 2003; 7: 73–82.

Table 7-19	Comparison of the Chronic Care Model with the Expanded Chronic Care Model		
Components of the Chronic Care Model		**Components of the Expanded Chronic Care Model**	**Examples**
Health System-Organization of Healthcare	Program planning that includes measurable goals for better care of chronic illness		
Self-Management Support	Emphasis on the importance of the central role that patients have in managing their own care	Self-Management/ Develop Personal Skills — Enhancing skills and capacities for personal health and wellness	• Smoking prevention and cessation programs • Seniors' walking programs
Decision Support	Integration of evidence-based guidelines into daily clinical practice	Decision Support — Integration of strategies for facilitating the community's abilities to stay healthy	• Development of health promotion and prevention "best practice" guidelines
Delivery System Design	Focus on teamwork and an expanded scope of practice to support chronic care	Delivery System Design/Re-orient Health Services — Expansion of mandate to support individuals and communities in a more holistic way	• Advocacy on behalf of (and with) vulnerable populations

Clinical Information Systems	Developing information systems based on patient populations to provide relevant client data	Information System — Creation of broadly-based information systems to include community data beyond the health-care system	• Emphasis in quality improvement on health and quality of life outcomes, not just clinical outcomes
			• Use of broad community needs assessments that take into account:
			  • poverty rates
			  • availability of public transportation
			  • violent crime rate

(continued)

Table 7-19		continued		
Components of the Chronic Care Model		**Components of the Expanded Chronic Care Model**		**Examples**

Community Resources and Policies	Developing partnerships with community organizations that support and meet patients' needs	Build Healthy Public Policy	Development and implementation of policies designed to improve population health	• Advocating for/developing:
				  • smoking bylaws
				  • walking trails
				  • reductions in the price of whole wheat flour
				• Maintaining older people in their homes for as long as possible
				• Work towards the development of well-lit streets and bicycle paths
				• Supporting the community in addressing the need for safe affordable housing

		Create Supportive Environments	Generating living and employing conditions that are safe, stimulating, satisfying and enjoyable	
		Strengthen Community Action	Working with community groups to set priorities and achieve goals that enhance the health of the community	

Source: Reproduced with permission from Barr, V. J., Robinson, S., Marin-Link, B., Underhill, L., Dotts, A., Ravensdale, D. et al. Hosp.Q. 2003; 7: 73–82.

Many opportunities for better integration of the treatment of chronic diseases and the prevention of risk factor behaviors remain largely untapped. For example, stronger support for smoking cessation among TB patients would save lives in the long term, and smoking cessation among patients with CHD is the single most effective intervention for reducing mortality in these patients who smoke. As demonstrated by the 36% reduction in the relative risk of mortality among CHD patients who quit tobacco use, smoking is at least as important as other secondary prevention measures such as use of statins (a 29% reduction), aspirin (15%), beta blockers (23%), or angiotensin-converting enzyme (ACE) inhibitors (23%) (Critchley & Capewell, 2003). Smoking cessation is also a priority for people with mental disorders. In one of the major studies on comorbidity between tobacco use and depression, researchers found that people with mental disorders are almost twice as likely to smoke as individuals without such disorders. Further, they found that people with a mental disorder had consumed 44.3% of all cigarettes smoked by a nationally representative sample in the previous days (Lasser, Boyd, Woolhandler, Himmelstein, McCormick, & Bor, 2000).

Another challenge is that effective clinical prevention services must extend beyond the mere provision of information to patients. The era of exhortation by healthcare professionals to "eat better" or "drop some weight" is long past: Modern, evidence-based interventions emphasize shared decision making and collaborative goal setting among providers and patients (Serdula, Khan, & Dietz, 2003). The clearer and more personalized the goal, the better (Estabrooks, Glasgow, & Dzewaltowski, 2003). Skill building to overcome barriers, self-monitoring, personalized feedback, and systematic links to community resources such as peer support groups are other important elements for success (Steptoe, Perkins-Porras, McKay, Rink, Hilton, & Cappuccio, 2003). Many healthcare settings deliver these kinds of interventions in group formats, which enhances the efficiency of healthcare professionals and provides the added element of social support (Noel & Pugh, 2002).

Comprehensive Care Applied to Adherence

The ICCC framework recognizes the importance of treatment adherence as a primary determinant of the effectiveness of treatment. Good adherence confers both health and economic benefits. Adherence has been associated with improved blood pressure control

(Luscher, Vetter, Sigenthaler, & Vetter, 1985) and lessened complications of hypertension (Morisky, Levine, Green, Shapiro, Russell, & Smith, 1983; Psaty, Koepsell, Wagner, Lo Gerfo, & Inui, 1990). Despite the clear importance of treatment adherence, a number of rigorous reviews have found that in high-income countries, adherence among patients with chronic diseases averages only 50%; it is even lower in low- and middle-income countries. In Gambia, China, and the United States, for example, only 27%, 43%, and 51%, respectively, of patients adhere to their medication regimen for high blood pressure. Similar patterns have been reported for other conditions, such as depression (range of 40% to 70%), asthma (43% for acute treatments and 28% for maintenance), and HIV/AIDS (range of 37% to 83%) (WHO, 2003a).

Adherence is a complex behavioral process that is influenced by five interacting dimensions: social and economic factors, healthcare system factors, condition-related factors, therapy-related factors, and patient-related factors. Because each dimension plays an important role in determining adherence rates (WHO, 2003a), all of them should be considered when designing interventions to improve outcomes. The most effective interventions have been shown to be multilevel, targeting more than one factor with more than one intervention (Dickinson, Wilkie, & Harris, 1999).

Contemporary perspectives have pointed out the importance of conceptualizing adherence as the active, voluntary involvement of the patient in the management of his or her disease, including a mutually agreed-upon course of treatment and sharing of responsibility between the patient and healthcare providers (Flood & Chiang, 2001). According to this perspective, adherence is an active, responsible, and flexible process of self-management, in which the person strives to achieve good health by working in close collaboration with healthcare staff instead of simply following rigidly prescribed rules.

Summary of Effective Health Care

Reviews of interventions to improve health care for chronic conditions have demonstrated the importance of using multifaceted approaches as opposed to "magic bullet" or "single lever" interventions (Grimshaw et al., 2001; Renders, Valk, Griffin, Wagner, Eijk, & Assendelft, 2002; Wagner et al., 2001). Models of integrated, coordinated care, such

as the ICCC framework, capture this complexity in an organized way.

Several key concepts have emerged from research within this area. First, it is necessary to work across multiple levels in a coordinated fashion to effect meaningful change in health care for chronic diseases. Second, organized systems of care—not just individual healthcare workers—are essential in producing positive outcomes for chronic disease. Third, it is crucial to work across the disease continuum in a comprehensive way. Comprehensive care for chronic conditions must span the full range of phases from clinical prevention, to treatment, to rehabilitation, to palliation.

The Role of National Governments

Primary prevention and health promotion requires a careful balance between individual, family, and community responsibility; government regulations and policies; and multisectoral actions by government, industry, and civil society (Yach, 2005).

A key role for government is to embrace strategies that reduce exposure to risk factors and attempt to influence individual behavior (Leeder et al., 2004). The range of scales at which government can operate to influence the degree of risk exposure has been conceptualized by WHO as a stepwise approach to chronic disease control (Table 7-20). Examples of these levels include population-based cross-sectoral interventions, fiscal policies, and regulations on the information provided to consumers. Some examples of how effective such approaches can be when governments provide leadership over a sustained period of time are described in the following subsections.

Comprehensive Community-Based Programs of Prevention and Health Promotion

Finland provides one such example of success that is applicable to both high-income and low- and middle-income countries. Health promotion efforts in Finland began in 1972 in the province of North Karelia, where rates of heart disease were double those found in the rest of the country, at a time when Finland was not the wealthy country it is now. Taking a population-wide approach, the North Karelia project encouraged change across sectors: diversification of agriculture away from meat and dairy; encouragement of individual lifestyle shifts to better diets, more exercise, and less smoking; and training of medical professionals to increase monitoring of blood pressure. The program was expanded to the rest of Finland in 1977. Although the introduction of cholesterol-lowering drugs may

Table 7-20	Stepwise Policy and Program Targets for National Prevention and Control of Chronic Diseases		
	Population Approaches		
Resource Level	**National Level**	**Community Level**	**Individual High-Risk Approaches**
Step 1: Core	WHO Framework Convention on Tobacco Control (FCTC) is ratified in every country. Tobacco control legislation consistent with the elements of the FCTC is enacted and enforced. A national nutrition and physical activity policy consistent with the global strategy is developed and endorsed at the cabinet level, including laws. Health impact assessment of public policy is carried out; priority areas include transport, urban planning, taxation, trade, and agriculture	Local infrastructure plans include the provisions and maintenance of accessible and safe sites for physical activity (such as parks and pedestrian-only areas). Health-promoting community projects include participatory actions to cope with the environmental factors that increase individuals' risk of chronic diseases—inactivity, unhealthy diet, and tobacco and alcohol use. Active health promotion programs focusing on chronic diseases are implemented in different settings: villages, schools, and workplaces, and explicitly aim to reach poor communities.	Context-specific guidelines for chronic disease prevention and control have been adopted and are used at all healthcare levels. A sustainable, accessible, and affordable supply of appropriate medication is assured for priority chronic diseases. A system exists for the consistent, high-quality application of clinical guidelines and for the clinical audit of services offered. A proactive follow-up system for patients with diabetes and hypertension is in operation.
Step 2: Expanded	Tobacco legislation provides for incremental increases in taxes on tobacco, and a proportion of the revenue is earmarked for health promotion. Food standards legislation is enacted and enforced; it includes nutrition labeling. Sustained, well-designed, national programs (counter-advertising) are in place to promote nonsmoking lifestyles, consumption of fruits and vegetables, and physical activity. Country standards are established that regulate marketing of unhealthy food to children.	Sustained, well-designed programs are in place to promote tobacco-free lifestyles (e.g., smoke-free public places, smoke-free sports). Healthy diets (e.g. low-cost, low-fat foods, fresh fruit and vegetables). Physical activity (e.g., "movement") in different domains (occupational and leisure).	Systems are in place for selective and targeted prevention aimed at high-risk populations, based on absolute levels of risk. Publicly financed "quit-line" for smokers; weight control line.
Step 3: Optimal	Policies shown to work for chronic disease prevention and control are implemented. There is policy coherence between agricultural systems and chronic diseases. Country standards are established that regulate marketing of unhealthy food to children.	Recreational and fitness centers are available for community use.	Opportunistic screening, case-finding, and management programs are implemented. Self-management groups are fostered for tobacco cessation and overweight reduction. Appropriate diagnostic and therapeutic interventions are implemented.

Source: Adapter from: World Health Organization, *World Health Report, 2003* (Geneva, Switzerland: World Health Organization, *2003*).

also have played a role, in the past 30 years deaths from heart disease and deaths from lung cancer in North Karelia have each fallen by approximately 70%. Male life expectancy has increased, as has per capita vegetable consumption. Under the auspices of WHO, pilot projects based on North Karelia have been developed in regions of China and in Chile, Iran, and Oman.

Governments have been successful in introducing some elements of the comprehensive approach as well. Raising the tobacco excise tax can reduce consumption effectively, increase government revenue, and reduce the burden of disease (de Beyer & Brigden, 2003; Guindon, Tobin, & Yach, 2002). A precedent has been set by Thailand, which has identified health promotion as a priority area to reduce the incidence of chronic disease (WHO Thailand, 2010). The Thai government set up the Thai Health Promotion Foundation (ThaiHealth) in April 2001, sustained by a dedicated 2% surcharge tax on alcohol and tobacco products. Although inevitably prone to shifts in the tax regime, this arrangement provides a relatively sustainable source of funding.

The power of advocacy supported by government and executed by NGOs has been demonstrated by the work of Heartfile in Pakistan (Nishtar, 2003), an organization created to focus on CVD prevention and health promotion. Heartfile's tactics for targeting cardiovascular disease have been wide ranging. Community intervention programs have been composed of print and electronic media campaigns and other public health promotion campaigns carried out in various aspects of the community, such as restaurants. Other activities have been directed at the reorientation of health services, research, and advocacy to highlight CVD in the government agenda. Heartfile has been successful in establishing strong and effective links at regional, national, and international levels, paving the way for private-sector–based initiatives, collaboration with health service providers, and more effective dissemination of information in the future. In more countries—and globally—this kind of strong and broad alliance of major health professional organizations, consumer groups, enlightened businesses and industries, and academic institutions is needed to better prioritize prevention strategies against chronic disease in developing countries.

Specific regulations can be implemented to control the information environment regarding risk factors, thereby diminishing chronic disease over the long term. Reducing the marketing of tobacco products is known to reduce consumption, for example (World Bank, 1999). By providing information to consumers, warnings and labels can also affect consumption. Warnings on cigarette packages have been shown to be effective, while for food, evidence from middle- and high-income countries indicates that consumers use nutrition labels to make food choices (Hawkes, 2004b).

Reorientation of Health Services to Address Chronic Disease

Many lives continue to be lost prematurely because of inadequate treatment and long-term management of chronic diseases, even though simple and inexpensive approaches to address these diseases exist. Even in wealthy countries, the full potential of these interventions is not being realized. The situation in both poorer countries and poor communities within rich countries is even less satisfactory. In most countries, for example, effective means of preventing, treating, and providing palliative care for cancer exist, but are not broadly implemented. There are many opportunities for coordinated risk reduction, care, and long-term management of chronic disease. For example, smoking cessation is a priority for all patients who smoke; dietary and physical activity information and skill building should be provided to most patients in virtually all healthcare settings. Unfortunately, few efforts have been made to explicitly target poor communities with such interventions.

Considerable progress has been made in improving access to, and reducing the prices of, antiretroviral agents for HIV/AIDS, drugs to treat TB, and several vaccines. Similar progress has yet to be made for essential drugs that are required to improve survival for treatable cancers, diabetes, and CVD. A patient with heart disease in a poor nation has the same right to effective drug treatment as a patient with malaria, tuberculosis, or HIV/AIDS. Nongovernmental organizations have yet to advocate as effectively for better access to chronic disease treatment as they have for selected infectious diseases, despite the huge savings in lives and suffering that would result from broader access to such health care.

Continued strengthening of certain aspects of infectious disease control, particularly those related to chronic infectious diseases such as TB and HIV/AIDS, will in turn benefit the control of CVD, diabetes, and cancer. The same transformation of healthcare systems is required to address prevention and long-term disease management for both infectious and noninfectious chronic diseases. In sub-Saharan African countries, an opportunity exists to ensure that the new platforms for health service delivery that are being built to expand access to treatment for HIV/AIDS also address noninfectious chronic diseases. The marginal increased investments required to provide this more comprehensive infrastructure would in all likelihood yield substantial gains for public health among poor communities whose members already suffer from CVD, diabetes, and cancer.

Promotion of Broader Societal Changes

Many aspects of chronic disease prevention require legislative, financial, and engineering approaches to redress unmet needs. These aspects, which are often not under the control of health departments, can complement educational programs. Unfortunately, educational programs have a limited impact, especially among poor and illiterate populations. Implementation of the following measures can bring about a disproportionately large positive impact for poor populations: infrastructural changes that promote public transport and physical activity, laws that ban tobacco advertising and smoking in public places, tax policies that raise excise taxes on tobacco, and agricultural policies that provide schools and poor communities with easy, government-funded access to fruits, vegetables, and other food staples.

Global Action to Achieve Sustained National Benefits

In an era of globalization, national governments need to act together to address several global threats to health and to maximize the potential benefits that accrue through globalization. Some of these actions that relate specifically to chronic diseases are described here. Further details are contained in Chapter 15.

Redirection of Investment

The tremendous financial inflows into chronic disease risk factors in low- and middle-income nations have the potential to be reoriented to investments that assist in the prevention of chronic diseases, rather than increase their prevalence. Flows of certain goods, technology, marketing, and FDI into weakly regulated markets are undermining healthy public policy. These investments could be shifted away from financing that promotes behaviors associated with development of chronic diseases and toward products, marketing, and services that are better aligned with public health goals. This is essentially a process of making markets work for chronic disease prevention. For example, businesses could make core business investments that are positive for health, encouraged by conditionalities placed on investment in risk-creating products. It is in both governments' and companies' self-interest to channel their financial resources ways that reduce chronic diseases. Equity research

has already shown, for example, that it is in the tobacco and food industries' interest to invest in healthier products and more responsible marketing (see Table 7-12).

Implementing Global Norms and Standards

Global norms and standards have an important role to play in the prevention of chronic diseases. Many low- and middle-income countries lack the basic human resources necessary to develop and implement laws and regulations, as well as the tax policies that are so important to many aspects of chronic disease control. For them, international support is often the spur to national action, and global norms provide the umbrella of legitimacy that they need to develop and implement national laws. There is also an increasing need to establish global norms in a wide range of spheres that affect transnational influences on chronic diseases—from marketing and trade to human resource flows. Such norms can balance the otherwise unrestrained influences of powerful actors and can assist countries that have limited national public health and regulatory ability. To do so, public health capacities in trade and political science must be strengthened so as to (1) effectively participate in the World Trade Organization, where health issues are increasingly considered, and (2) develop stronger norms that could be used as the basis for resolving trade disputes concerning products associated with adverse health impacts.

The FCTC is one example of a global norm that can protect low- and middle-income countries from industry pressures as they introduce effective tobacco control. This framework represents the first time WHO has used its treaty-making right to advance public health goals. The FCTC was adopted by all the countries in the world (all 192 WHO member states) in May 2003. The pioneering convention aims to protect health and save the lives of billions in present and future generations through tobacco advertising bans, larger health warning labels on tobacco products, measures to protect against secondhand smoke, tobacco tax and price increases, and efforts to eliminate illicit trade (see Table 7-17). Other norms that are important for noncommunicable disease control include the International Code of Marketing of Breast-milk Substitutes and the Codex Alimentarius Commission (with its likely increased focus on food labeling and health claims).

Treaties are probably not the solution to the complex issues related to nutrition transition or physical inactivity. At the global level, combinations of multiple-stakeholder and intergovernmental codes are better options to pursue in this case, especially in relation to restricting the marketing of alcohol and foods to young children. Such approaches are already being used in many ways in many low- and middle-income countries to improve labor conditions, improve environmental quality, and protect human rights. These approaches are cheaper and quicker to implement than traditional legislative approaches, but require strong independent oversight to ensure they have the desired impact.

Globalization of Civil Society

NGOs have a set of potentially critical abilities: to unite both high-income and low- and middle-income country interests in the face of common threats over a wide geographic range, to build national capacity, to channel individual concerns into productive societal change, and to place on the ground "connectors" who can implement policy and technical advice provided by national and international authorities. Another characteristic of NGOs is that their advocacy activities calling for government action can somewhat offset the argument that a government is a "nanny state" if it institutes regulations designed to facilitate pro-health choices (Leeder et al., 2004). A global network of the various categories of NGOs, all of which are committed to chronic disease prevention and control, could lobby governments and WHO and would be a useful force to support global and national advocacy, enhance national capacity, and have a wide geographic reach.

Several elements of such a network already exist. The International Union Against Cancer (UICC) hosts Globalink, an Internet-based network of more than 4,000 tobacco advocates and policy makers who together have moved the FCTC process ahead, and influenced many national and local initiatives in tobacco control by combining forces across the world. ProCOR, an email- and Internet-based service for chronic disease researchers and policy makers in low- and middle-income countries, provides practical and essential educational material to people involved in policy and program development (Lown, 2004).

The UN High Level Meeting on Non-Communicable Diseases, to be held in September 2011, will be an unprecedented opportunity to bring NCDs to the international arena and stress the need for global action. NCD advocates hope that the meeting will have a lasting impact, similar to the UN General Assembly Special Session on HIV/AIDS in 2001.

• • • Discussion Questions

1. What are the leading risk factors that contribute to death and disability in low- and middle-income countries, and how do they differ from those found in high-income countries?

2. Given current trends in risk factors, what are likely to be the major causes of death and disability in low- and middle-income countries in the 2020s and beyond?

3. Which policies and actions taken over the next decade at national and international levels could influence these trends, and which factors might facilitate their implementation?

4. Outline major gaps in knowledge and research that hamper progress in chronic disease control in low- and middle-income countries.

5. Describe how globalization could be positively harnessed for chronic disease prevention. In doing so, consider how public–private partnerships involving major multinational corporations could play a more effective role in health promotion and chronic disease prevention.

• • • References

Abegunde, D. O., Mathers, C. D., Adam, T., Ortegon, M., & Strong, K. (2007). The burden and costs of chronic diseases in low-income and middle-income countries. *Lancet, 370*(9603), 1929–1938.

Aboderin, I., Kalache, A., Ben-Shlomo, Y., Lynch, J. W., Yajnik, C. D., Kuh, D., & Yach, D. (2001). *Life course perspectives on coronary heart disease, stroke and diabetes: Key issues and implications for policy and research.* Geneva, Switzerland: World Health Organization.

Ait-Khaled, N., Enarson, D., & Bousquet, J. (2001). Chronic respiratory diseases in developing countries: The burden and strategies for prevention and management. *Bulletin of the World Health Organization, 79*(10), 971–979.

Alliance for a Healthier Generation. (2006). Alliance for a Healthier Generation school beverage guidelines. Retrieved from http://www.pepsiproductfacts.com/pdfs/School_Beverage_Guidelines.pdf

Alwan, A., Maclean, D., & Mandil, A. (2001). *Assessment of national capacity for noncommunicable disease prevention and control.* Geneva, Switzerland: World Health Organization.

American Beverage Association. (2010). Alliance school beverage guidelines final progress report, 2010. Retrieved from www.ameribev.org

American Diabetes Association (ADA). (1998). Economic consequences of diabetes mellitus in the U.S. in 1997. *Diabetes Care, 21,* 296–309.

American Diabetes Association (ADA). (2003). Economic consequences of diabetes mellitus in the U.S. in 2002. *Diabetes Care, 26,* 917–932.

Aspray, T. J., Mugusi, F., Rashid, S., Whiting, D., Edwards, R., Alberti, K. G., & Unwin, N. C. (2000). Essential Non-Communicable Disease Health Intervention Project. Rural and urban differences in diabetes prevalence in Tanzania: The role of obesity, physical inactivity and urban living. *Transactions of the Royal Society of Tropical Medicine and Hygiene, 94*(6), 637–644.

Babor, T., Caetano, R., Casswell, S., Edwards, G., Giesbrecht, N., Graham, K., et al. (2003). *Alcohol: No ordinary commodity.* Oxford, UK: Oxford University Press.

Bahadori, K., Doyle-Waters, M. M., Marra, C., Lynd, L., Alasaly, K., Swiston, J., et al. (2009). Economic burden of asthma: A systematic review. *BMC Pulmonary Medicine, 9,* 24.

Barceló, A., Aedo, C., Rajpathak, S., & Robles, S. (2003). The cost of diabetes in Latin America and the Caribbean. *Bulletin of the World Health Organization, 81*(1), 19–27.

Barr, V. J., Robinson, S., Marin-Link, B., Underhill, L., Dotts, A., Ravensdale, D., et al. (2003). The expanded Chronic Care Model: An integration of concepts and strategies from population health promotion and the Chronic Care Model. *Hospital Quarterly, 7,* 73–82.

Batty, G. D., & Leon, D. A. (2002). Socio-economic position and coronary heart disease risk factors in children and young people. *European Journal of Public Health, 12,* 263–272.

Beaglehole, R., & Yach, D. (2003). Globalisation and the prevention and control of non-communicable disease: The neglected chronic diseases of adults. *Lancet, 362,* 903–908.

Beattie, A., Kalk, W. J., Price, M., Rispel, L., Broomberg, J., & Cabral, J. (1998). The management of diabetes at primary level in South Africa: The results of a facility-based assessment. *Journal of the Royal Society of Health, 118*(6), 338–345.

Bell, A. C., Adair, A. S., & Popkin, B. M. (2004). Understanding the role of mediating risk factors and proxy effects in the association between socio-economic status and untreated hypertension. *Social Science and Medicine, 59,* 275–283.

Bourne, L. T., Lambert, E. V., & Steyn, K. (2002). Where does the black population of South Africa stand on nutrition transition? *Public Health Nutrition, 5*(1A), 157–162.

Bradshaw, D., Groenewald, P., Laubscher, R., Nannan, N., Nojilana, B., Norman, R., et al. (2003). Initial burden of disease estimates for South Africa, 2000. *South African Medical Journal, 93*(9), 682–688.

Brands, A., & Yach, D. (2001). *Noncommunicable diseases and gender.* Geneva, Switzerland: World Health Organization.

Brownell, K. D., & Frieden, T. R. (2009). Ounces of prevention–the public policy case for taxes on sugared beverages. *New England Journal of Medicine, 360*(18), 1805–1808.

Brownell, K. D., & Hagen, K. B. (2004). *Food fight: The inside story of the food industry. America's obesity crisis, and what we can do about it.* Chicago: Contemporary Books.

Bumgarner, R. (2003). *China: Non-communicable disease issues and options revisited.* Geneva, Switzerland: World Health Organization.

Canto, J. G., & Iskandrian, A. E. (2003). Major risk factors for cardiovascular disease. Debunking the "only 50%" myth. *Journal of the American Medical Association, 290,* 947–949.

Cappuccio, F. P., Plange-Rhule, J., Phillips, R. O., & Eastwood, J. B. (2000). Prevention of hypertension and stroke in Africa. *Lancet, 356,* 677–678.

Cash, S., Sunding, D., & Zilberman, D. (2005). Fat taxes and thin subsidies: Prices, diet, and health outcomes. *Acta Agriculturae Scandinavica, Section C—Economy, 2,* 167–174.

Chale, S. S., Swai, A. B., Mujinja, P. G., & McLarty, D. G. (1992). Must diabetes be a fatal disease in Africa? Study of costs of treatment. *British Medical Journal, 304,* 1215–1218.

Chew, F. T., Goh, D. Y., & Lee, B. W. (1999). The economic cost of asthma in Singapore. *Australian and New Zealand Journal of Medicine, 29*(2), 228–233.

Chinese Center for Disease Control and Prevention, cited in Xinhua News Agency. (2004, January 24). Unhealthy lifestyles cause disease among one third of Beijing residents.

Clark, G. L., & Hebb, T. (2002). *Understanding pension fund corporate engagement in a global arena.* Paper prepared for the seminar Understanding Pension Fund Corporate Engagement in a Global Arena, November 24–26, 2002, Oxford University, Oxford, UK.

Coffield, A. B., Maciosek, M. V., McGinnis, J. M., Harris, J. R., Caldwell, M. B., Teutsch, S. M., et al. (2001). Priorities among recommended clinical preventive services. *American Journal of Preventive Medicine, 21*(1), 1–9.

Cohen, B. (2004). Urban growth in developing countries: A review of current trends and a caution regarding existing forecasts. *World Development, 32*(1), 23–51.

Coleman, R., Gill, G., & Wilkinson, D. (1998). Noncommunicable disease management in resource-poor settings: A primary care model from rural South Africa. *Bulletin of the World Health Organization, 76*(6), 633–640.

Commission on Social Determinants of Health. (2008). *Closing the gap in a generation: Health equity through action on the social determinants of health.* Geneva, Switzerland: World Health Organization.

Critchley, J., & Capewell, S. (2003). Mortality risk reduction associated with smoking cessation in patients with coronary heart diseases: A systematic review. *Journal of the American Medical Association, 290,* 86–97.

Daae, L. N., Kierulf, P., Landaas, S., & Urdal, P. (1993). Cardiovascular risk factors: Interactive effects of lipids, coagulation and fibrinolysis. *Scandinavian Journal of Clinical and Laboratory Investigation, 215*(suppl), 19–27.

Danesh, J., Erqou, S., Walker, M., Thompson, S. G., Tipping, R., Ford, C., et al. (2007). The Emerging Risk Factors Collaboration: Analysis of individual data on lipid, inflammatory and other markers in over 1.1 million participants in 104 prospective studies of cardiovascular diseases. *European Journal of Epidemiology, 22,* 839–869.

Datamonitor. (2002). *Childhood obesity 2002: How obesity is shaping the U.S. food and beverage markets.* New York: Author.

de Beyer, J., & Brigden, L. W. (2003). *Tobacco control policy: Strategies, successes and setbacks.* Washington, DC: World Bank/Research for International Tobacco Control.

Dickinson, D., Wilkie, P., & Harris, M. (1999). Taking medicines: Concordance is not compliance. *British Medical Journal, 319*(7212), 787.

Doll, R., Peto, R., Boreham, J., & Sunderland, I. (2004). Mortality in relation to smoking: 50 years' observations of male British doctors. *British Medical Journal, 328,* 1519–1528.

Doyle, J., Waters, E., Yach, D., McQueen, D., De Francisco, A., Stewart, T., et al. (2005). Global priority setting for Cochrane systematic reviews of health promotion and public health research. *Journal of Epidemiology and Community Health, 59,* 193–197.

Du, S., Lu, B., Zhai, F., & Popkin, B. M. (2002). A new stage of the nutrition transition in China. *Public Health Nutrition, 5*(1A), 169–174.

Duncan, B. D., Schmidt, M. I., Achutti, A. C., Polanczyk, C. A., Benia, L. R., & Maia, A. A. (1993). Socioeconomic distribution of noncommunicable disease risk factors in urban Brazil: The case of Pôrto Alegre. *Bulletin of the Pan American Health Organization, 27*(4), 337–349.

Economic and Social Council. (2004). *Ad hoc interagency task force on tobacco control: Report of the Secretary-General* (E/2004/55). New York: United Nations.

Ehrlich, R. I., White, N., Norman, R., Laubscher, R., Steyn, K., Lombard, C., & Bradshaw, D. (2004). Predictors of chronic bronchitis in South African adults. *International Journal of Tuberculosis and Lung Disease, 8*(3), 369–376.

Estabrooks, P. A., Glasgow, R. E., & Dzewaltowski, D. A. (2003). Physical activity promotion through primary care. *Journal of the American Medical Association, 289*(22), 2913.

Finkelstein, E. A., Fiebelkorn, I. C., & Wang, G. (2003). National medical spending attributable to overweight and obesity: How much, and who's paying? *Health Affairs,* W3-219–W3-226.

Finkelstein, E. A., Fiebelkorn, I. C., & Wang, G. (2004). State-level estimates of annual medical expenditures attributable to obesity. *Obesity Research, 12*(1), 18–24.

Flood, R. G., & Chiang, V. W. (2001). Rate and prediction of infection in children with diabetic ketoacidosis. *American Journal of Emergency Medicine 19,* 270–273.

Foliaki, S., & Pearce, N. (2003). Prevention and control of diabetes in Pacific people. *British Medical Journal, 327,* 437–439.

Frenk, J., Bobdilla, J. L., Sepulveda, J., & Cervantes, L. M. (1989). Health transition in middle income countries: New challenges for health care. *Health Policy and Planning, 4*(1), 29–39.

Fries, J. F. (1980). Ageing, natural death, and the compression of morbidity. *New England Journal of Medicine, 303,* 130–135.

Fries, J. F. (2003). Measuring and monitoring success in compressing morbidity. *Annals of Internal Medicine, 139,* 455–459.

Fu, D., Fu, H., McGowan, P., Shen, Y., Zhu, L., Yang, H., et al. (2003). Implementation and quantitative evaluation of chronic disease self-management programme in Shanghai, China: Randomized controlled trial. *Bulletin of the World Health Organization, 81*(3), 174–182.

Gajalakshmi, V., Peto, R., Kanaka, T. S., & Jha, P. (2003). Smoking and mortality from tuberculosis and other diseases in India. *Lancet, 362,* 507–515.

Glasgow, R. E., Orleans, C. T., & Wagner, E. H. (2001). Does the chronic care model serve also as a template for improving prevention? *Milbank Quarterly, 79*(4), 579–612.

Global Youth Tobacco Survey Collaborating Group. (2003). Differences in worldwide tobacco use by gender: Findings from the Global Youth Tobacco Survey. *Journal of School Health, 73,* 207–215.

Goetzel, R. Z., Hawkins, K., Ozminkowski, R. J., & Wang, S. (2003). The health and productivity cost burden of the "top 10" physical and mental health conditions affecting six large US employers in 1999. *Journal of Occupational and Environmental Medicine, 45,* 5–14.

Goldin, J. G., Louw, S. J., & Joubert, G. (1996). Spirometry of healthy adult South African men.

Part I. Interrelationship between socio-environmental factors and "race" as determinant of spirometry. *South African Medical Journal, 86*(7), 820–826.

Grant, P. J. (2007). Diabetes mellitus as a pro-thrombotic condition. *Journal of Internal Medicine, 262,* 157–172.

Grimshaw, J. M., Shirran, L., Thomas, R., Mowatt, G., Fraser, C., Bero, L., et al. (2001). Changing provider behavior: An overview of systematic reviews of interventions. *Medical Care, 39,* 112–145.

Gu, D., Reynolds, K., Duan, X., Xin, X., Chen, J., Wu, X. et al. (2003). Prevalence of diabetes and impaired fasting glucose in the Chinese adult population: Interna-tional Collaborative Study of Cardiovascular Disease in Asia (InterASIA). *Diabetologia, 46*(9), 1190–1198.

Guindon, G. E., Tobin, S., & Yach, D. (2002). Trends and affordability of cigarette prices: Ample room for tax increases and related health gains. *Tobacco Control, 11,* 35–43.

Gulliford, M. C., Alert, C. V., Mahabir, D., Ariyanayagam-Baksh, S. M., Fraser, H. S., & Picou, D. I. (1996). Diabetes care in middle-income countries: A Caribbean case study. *Diabetic Medicine, 13*(6), 574–581.

Hawkes, C. (2004a). *Marketing food to children: The global regulatory environment.* Geneva, Switzerland: World Health Organization.

Hawkes, C. (2004b). *Nutrition labels and health claims: The global regulatory environment.* Geneva, Switzerland: World Health Organization.

Heller, P. S. (2003). *Who will pay? Coping with aging societies, climate change, and other long-term fiscal challenges.* Washington, DC: International Monetary Fund.

Hsueh, W. A., & Law, R. E. (1998). Cardiovascular risk continuum: Implications of insulin resistance and diabetes. *American Journal of Medicine, 105,* 4S–14S.

Institute of Medicine. (2010). *Preventing the global epidemic of cardiovascular disease: Meeting the challenges in developing countries.* Washington, DC: National Academies Press.

InterASIA Collaborative Group. (2003). Cardiovascular risk factors levels in urban and rural Thailand: The International Collaborative Study of Cardiovascular Diseases in Asia (InterASIA). *European Journal of Cardiovascular Prevention and Rehabilitation, 10*(4), 249–257.

International Agency for Research on Cancer (IARC). (2003). *World cancer report.* Lyon, France: IARC Press.

International Agency for Research on Cancer (IARC). (2008). *World cancer report.* Lyons, France: IARC Press.

International Diabetes Federation. (2003). *Diabetes atlas* (2nd ed.). Brussels: International Diabetes Federation.

International Food and Beverage Alliance (IFBA). (2009). *Progress report on the food and beverage alliance's five commitments to action under the 2004 global strategy on diet, physical activity, and health.* Retrieved from: https://www.ifballiance.org/sites/default/files/IFBA's%20Progress%20Report%20to%20DG%20Dr%20Chan%20(November%202009).pdf

Jha, P., & Chaloupka, F. J. (Eds.). (2000). *Tobacco control in developing countries.* New York: Oxford University Press.

JP Morgan. (2004, July 26). *The path to a safer cigarette: Global equity research.* New York: Author.

Kelly, T., Yang, W., Chen, C. S., Reynolds, K., & He, J. (2008). Global burden of obesity in 2005 and projections to 2030. *International Journal of Obesity (London), 32,* 1431–1437.

Khatami, M. (2007). Standardizing cancer biomarkers criteria: data elements as a foundation for a database. Inflammatory mediator/M-CSF as model marker. *Cell Biochemistry and Biophysics, 47*(2), 187–198.

Kiivet, R. A., Kaur, I., Lang, A., Aaviksoo, A., & Nirk, L. (2001). Costs of asthma treatment in Estonia. *European Journal of Public Health, 11*(1), 89–92.

Kim, S., Symons, M., & Popkin, B. M. (2004). Contrasting socioeconomic profiles related to healthier lifestyles in China and the United States. *American Journal of Epidemiology, 159*(2), 184–191.

Kimmis, J., Gottchalk, R., Armendariz, E., & Griffith-Jones, S. (2002). *Making the case for UK pension fund investment in developing country assets.* Unpublished manuscript, Institute for Development Studies, University of Sussex, Brighton, England.

Knuiman, J. T., Hermus, R. J. J., & Hautvast, J. G. A. J. (1980). Serum total and high-density lipoprotein (HDL) cholesterol concentrations in rural and urban boys from 16 countries. *Atherosclerosis, 36,* 529–537.

Kogevinas, M., Pearce, N., Susser, M., & Boffetta, P. (Eds.). (1997). *Social inequalities and cancer* (IARC Scientific Publications No. 138). Lyon, France: IARC.

Kuchler, F., & Ballenger, N. (2002). Societal costs of obesity: How can we assess when federal interventions will pay? *Food Review, 25*(3), 33–37.

Langlois, A., Adam, V., & Powell, A. (2003). *Food manufacturing. Obesity: The big issue.* London: JP Morgan European Equity Research.

Lasser, K., Boyd, J. W., Woolhandler, S., Himmelstein, D. U., McCormick, D., & Bor, D. H. (2000). Smoking and mental health: A population-based prevalence study. *Journal of the American Medical Association, 284,* 2606–2610.

Leeder, S., Raymond, S., Greenberg, H., Liu, H., & Esson, K. (2004). *A race against time: The challenge of cardiovascular disease in developing countries.* New York: Trustees of Columbia University.

Levitt, N. S., Steyn, K., de Wet, T., Morrell, C., Edwards, R., Ellison, G. T. H., & Cameron, N. (1999). An inverse relationship between blood pressure and birth weight among 5 year old children from Soweto, South Africa. *Journal of Epidemiology and Community Health, 53,* 264–268.

Liu, J. L. Y., Maniadakis, N., Gray, A., & Rayner, M. (2002). The economic burden of coronary heart disease in the UK. *Heart, 88,* 597–603.

LMC International. (2004, May). *Implications of the WHO/FAO expert consultative report on the sugar market.* Unpublished manuscript, LMC International, London.

Lobstein, T., Baur, L., & Uauy, R. (2004). Obesity in children and young people: A crisis in public health. *Obesity Reviews, 5*(suppl 1), 4–85.

Lown, B. (2004, June 16). *A cardiologist's perspective on the crisis and challenges of biotechnology.* Plenary address to the fifth International Heart Health Conference, Milan, Italy.

Lubitz, J., Cai, L., Kamarow, E., & Lentzner, H. (2003). Health, life expectancy, and health care spending among the elderly. *New England Journal of Medicine, 349*(11), 1048–1055.

Luo, J., & Hu, F. B. (2002). Time trends of obesity in pre-school children in China from 1989 to 1997. *International Journal of Obesity, 26*(4), 553–558.

Luscher, T. F., Vetter, H., Sigenthaler, W., & Vetter, W. (1985). Compliance in hypertension: Facts and concepts. *Journal of Hypertension, 3,* 3–9.

Mackay, J., Eriksen, M., & Shafey, O. (2006). *The tobacco atlas.* Atlanta, GA: American Cancer Society.

Mackenbach, J. P., Cavelaars, A. E. J. M., Kunst, A. E., et al. (2000). Socio-economic inequalities in cardiovascular disease mortality: An international study. *European Heart Journal, 21,* 1141–1151.

Marmot, M. G., Adelstein, A. M., Robinson, N., & Rose, G. A. (1978). Changing social-class distribution of heart disease. *British Medical Journal, 2*(6145), 1109–1112.

Martinez-Moragon, E., Serra-Batlles, J., De, D. A., Palop, M., Casan, P., Rubio-Terres, C., et al. (2009). Economic cost of treating the patient with asthma in Spain: The AsmaCost study. *Archives of Bronconeumology, 45,* 481–486.

Mayosi, B. M., Flisher, A. J., Lalloo, U. G., Sitas, F., Tollman, S. M., & Bradshaw, D. (2009). The burden of non-communicable diseases in South Africa. *Lancet, 374,* 934–947.

McGinnis, J. M., Williams-Russo, P., & Knickman, J. R. (2002). The case for more active policy attention to health promotion. *Health Affairs, 21*(2), 78–93.

McGlynn, E. A., Asch, S. M., Adams, J., Keesey, J., Hicks, J., DeCristofaro, A., et al. (2003). The quality of health care delivered to adults in the United States. *New England Journal of Medicine, 348,* 2635–2645.

McKeown, T. (1988). *The origins of human disease.* Oxford, UK: Basil Blackwell.

Mendez, M. A, Cooper, R. S., Luke, A., Wilks, R., Bennett, F., & Forrester, T. (2004). Higher income is more strongly associated with obesity than with obesity-related metabolic disorders in Jamaican adults. *International Journal of Obesity, 28*(4), 543–550.

Mertens, I., & Van Gaal, L. F. (2002). Obesity, haemostasis and the fibrinolytic system. *Obesity Review, 3,* 85–101.

Minh, H. V., Byass, P., & Wall, S. (2003). Mortality from cardiovascular diseases in Bavi District, Vietnam. *Scandinavian Journal of Public Health, S62,* 26–31.

Mirmiran, P., Noori, N., Zavareh, M. B., & Azizi, F. (2009). Fruit and vegetable consumption and risk factors for cardiovascular disease. *Metabolism, 58*(4), 460–468.

Misra, A., Pandey, R. M., Devi, J. R., Sharma, R., Vikram, N. K., & Khanna, N. (2001). High prevalence of diabetes, obesity and dyslipidaemia in urban slum populations in northern India. *International Journal of Obesity, 25,* 1–8.

Monteiro, C. A., Conde, W. L., Lu, B., & Popkin, B. M. (2004, June 22). Obesity and health inequities in the developing world [Advance online version]. *International Journal of Obesity, 1–6.*

Morisky, D. E., Levine, D. M., Green, L. W., Shapiro, S., Russell, R. P., & Smith, C. R. (1983). Five year blood pressure control and mortality following health education for hypertensive patients. *American Journal of Public Health, 73,* 153–162.

Murray, J. L., Lauer, J. A., Hutaberry, R. C. W., Niessen, L., Tamijuma, N., Rodgen, A., et al.

(2003). Effectiveness and costs of interventions to lower systolic blood pressure and cholesterol: A global and regional analysis on reduction of cardiovascular disease rate. *Lancet, 361,* 717–725.

Myrdal, G. (1952). *Economic aspects of health.* Address to the World Health Assembly, World Health Organization, Geneva, Switzerland.

Nishtar, S. (2003). Cardiovascular disease prevention in low resource settings: Lessons from the Heartfile experience in Pakistan. *Ethnicity & Disease, 13,* S138–S148.

Nissinen, A., Bothig, S., Granroth, H., & Lopez, A. D. (1988). Hypertension in developing countries. *World Health Statistics Quarterly, 41,* 141–154.

Noel, P. H., & Pugh, J. A. (2002). Management of overweight and obese adults. *British Medical Journal, 325*(7367), 757–761.

Norlund, A., Apelqvist, J., Bitzen, P. O., Nyberg, P., & Schersten, B. (2001). Cost of illness of adult diabetes mellitus underestimated if comorbidity is not considered. *Journal of Internal Medicine, 250,* 57–65.

Nugent, R. A. & Feigl, A. B. (2010). A closer look at non-communicable disease funding: Why so little? Working Paper 282, Center for Global Development.

Omran, A. R. (1971). The epidemiologic transition: A theory of the epidemiology of population change. *Milbank Memorial Fund Quarterly, 49,* 509–538.

Peña, M., & Bacallao, J. (2000). Obesity among the poor: An emerging problem in Latin America and the Caribbean. In M. Peña & J. Bacallao (Eds.), *Obesity and poverty: A new public health challenge* (Scientific Publication No. 576, pp. 3–10). Washington, DC: Pan American Health Organization.

Popkin, B. M. (1999). Urbanization, lifestyle changes and the nutrition transition. *World Development, 27*(11), 1905–1916.

Popkin, B. M., & Doak, C. M. (1998). The obesity epidemic is a worldwide phenomenon. *Nutrition Reviews, 56*(4), 106–114.

Popkin, B. M., Horton, S., Kim, S., Mahal, A., & Shuigao, J. (2001). Trends in diet, nutritional status and diet-related noncommunicable diseases in China and India: The economic costs of nutrition transition. *Nutrition Reviews, 59,* 379–390.

Poulter, N., Khaw, K. T., Hopwood, B. E., Mugambi, M., Peart, W. S., Rose, G., & Sever, P. S. (1990). The Kenyan Luo migration study: Observations on the initiation of a rise in blood pressure. *British Medical Journal, 300,* 967–972.

Psaty, B. M., Koepsell, T. D., Wagner, E. H., Lo Gerfo, J. P., & Inui, T. S. (1990). The relative risk of incident coronary heart diseases associated with recently stopping the use of β-blockers. *Journal of the American Medical Association, 73,* 1653–1657.

Raheja, B. S., Kapur, A., Bhoraskar, A., Sathe, S. R., Jorgensen, L. N., Moorthi, S. R., et al. (2001). DiabCare Asia—India Study: Diabetes care in India—current status. *Journal of the Association of Physicians of India, 49,* 717–722.

Ramachandran, A., Snehalatha, C., Vijay, V., & King, H. (2002). Impact of poverty on the prevalence of diabetes and its complications in urban southern India. *Diabetic Medicine, 19,* 130–135.

Razaire, C. (2003). *Industry outlook: Tobacco.* New York: Moody's Investor Service.

Reis, C. S. (1978). Demographic and epidemiological transition in Africa. *Tropical Doctor, 8,* 229–233.

Renders, C. M., Valk, G. D., Griffin, S. M., Wagner, E. H., Eijk, J. T., & Assendelft, W. J. (2002). Interventions to improve the management of diabetes in primary care, outpatient and community settings: A systematic review. *Diabetes Care, 24,* 1821–1833.

Riemsma, R. P., Pattenden, J., Bridle, C., Sowden, A. J., Mather, L., Watt, I. S., & Walker, A. (2002). A systematic review of the effectiveness of interventions based on a stages-of-change approach to promote individual behaviour change. *Health Technology Assessment, 6*(24), 1–231.

Russo, C. A., & Andrews, R. M. (2006, September). *The national hospital bill: The most expensive conditions, by payer, 2004* (HCUP Statistical Brief #13). Rockville, MD: Agency for Healthcare Research and Quality. Retrieved from http://www.hcup-us .ahrq.gov/reports/statbriefs/sb13.pdf

Schenk, J. M., Kristal, A. R., Neuhouser, M. L., Tangen, C. M., White, E., Lin, D. W., et al. (2010). Biomarkers of systemic inflammation and risk of incident, symptomatic benign prostatic hyperplasia: Results from the prostate cancer prevention trial. *American Journal of Epidemiology, 171,* 571–582.

Seftel, H., Asvat, M. S., Joffe, B. I., Raal, F. J., Panz, V. R., Vermaak, W. J. H., et al. (1993). Selected risk factors for coronary heart disease in male scholars from the major South African population groups. *South African Medical Journal, 83,* 891–897.

Seftel, H. C., & Schultz, E. (1961). Diabetes mellitus in the urbanised Johannesburg African. *South African Medical Journal, 35,* 66–70.

Serdula, M. K., Khan, L. K., & Dietz, W. H. (2003). Weight loss counseling revisited. *Journal of the American Medical Association, 289*(14), 1747–1750.

Shobana, R., Rama Rao, P., Lavanya, A., Williams, R., Vijay, V., & Ramachandran, A. (2000). Expenditure on health care incurred by diabetic subjects in a developing country: A study from southern India. *Diabetes Research and Clinical Practice, 48,* 37–42.

Simpson, S., Corabian, P., Jacobs, P., & Johnson, J. A. (2003). The cost of major comorbidity in people with diabetes mellitus. *Canadian Medical Association Journal, 168,* 1661–1667.

Singh, R. B., Beegom, R., Mehta, A. S., Niaz, M. A., et al. (1999). Social class, coronary risk factors and undernutrition, a double burden of diseases, in women during transition, in five Indian cities. *International Journal of Cardiology, 69*(2), 139–147.

Singhal, A., & Lucas, A. (2004). Early origins of cardiovascular disease: Is there a unifying hypothesis? *Lancet, 363,* 1642–1645.

Sobal, J., & Stunkard, A. J. (1989). Socioeconomic status and obesity: A review of the literature. *Psychological Bulletin, 105*(2), 260–275.

Solenski, N. J. (2007). Emerging risk factors for cerebrovascular disease. *Current Drug Targets, 8,* 802–816.

Sridhar, D. & Batniji, R. (2008). Misfinancing global health: A case for transparency in disbursements and decision making. *Lancet, 372*(9644), 1185–1191.

Stampfer, M. J., Hu, F.B., Manson, J. E., Rimm, E. B., & Willett, W. C. (2000). Primary prevention of coronary heart disease in women through diet and lifestyle. *New England Journal of Medicine, 343*(1), 16–22.

Steptoe, A., Perkins-Porras, L., McKay, C., Rink, E., Hilton, S., & Cappuccio, F. P. (2003). Behavioural counselling to increase consumption of fruit and vegetables in low income adults: Randomised trial. *British Medical Journal, 326*(7394), 855.

Stewart, B. W., & Kleihaus, P. (Eds.). (2003). *World cancer report.* Lyon, France: IARC Press.

Steyn, K., Bradshaw, D., Norman, R., & Laubscher, R. (2003). *Determinants and treatment of hypertension in South Africa/determinants of hypertension and its treatment in South Africa during 1998: The first Demographic and Health Survey* [Draft]. Tygerburg, South Africa: South Africa Medical Research Council.

Steyn, K., de Wet, T., Richter, L., Cameron, N., Levitt, N. S., & Morrell, C. (2000). Cardiovascular disease risk factors in five-year-old urban South African children: The Birth to Ten study. *South African Medical Journal, 90*(7), 719–726.

Steyn, N. P., Labadarios, D., Nel, J., & Lombard, C. (2005). Secondary data analysis of the National Food Consumption Survey in South Africa: Prevalence of stunting and overweight. *Nutrition, 21*(1), 4–13.

Streets, J., Levy, C., Erskine, A., & Hudson, J. (2002). *Absolute risk of obesity.* London: UBS Warburg Global Equity Research.

Stuckler, D., King, L., Robinson, H. & McKee, M. (2008). WHO's budgetary allocations and burden of disease: a comparative analysis. *Lancet, 372*(9649), 1563–1569.

Swai, A. B., McLarty, D. G., Kitange, H. M., Kilima, P. M., Tatalla, S., Keen, N., et al. (1993). Low prevalence of risk factors for coronary heart disease in rural Tanzania. *International Journal of Epidemiology, 22*(4), 651–659.

Swiss Reinsurance Company. (2004). *Too big to ignore: The impact of obesity on mortality trends.* Zurich: Author.

Theuma, P. & Fonseca, V. A. (2003). Inflammation and emerging risk factors in diabetes mellitus and atherosclerosis. *Current Diabetes Reports, 3,* 248–254.

Thompson, D., & Wolf, A. M. (2001). The medical-care cost burden of obesity. *Obesity Reviews, 2,* 189–197.

Ullrich, A., Sepulveda, C., Waxman, A., Costa e Silva, V. L., Beaglehole, R., Bettcher, D., & Vestal, G. (2004). Cancer prevention in the political arena: The WHO perspective. *Annals of Oncology, 15*(suppl 4), 249–256.

United Nations Development Program (UNDP). (2001). *Implementing the Millennium Declaration.* New York: Author. Retrieved from http://www .undp.org/mdg/goal6.pdf

United Nations General Assembly. (2002, October 11). *A world fit for children* (S-27/2). New York: United Nations.

United Nations Population Fund (UNFPA). (1995). *State of the world's population 1996. Changing places: Population, development, and the urban future. Annual report.* New York: Author. Retrieved from http://www.unfpa.org/swp/1996/index.htm

Unwin, N. C., Setel, P., Rashid, S., Mugusi, F., Mbanya, J. C., Kitange, H., et al. (2001). Non-communicable diseases in sub-Saharan Africa: Where do they feature in the health research agenda? *Bulletin of the World Health Organization, 79*(10), 947–953.

U.S. Department of Health and Human Services (DHHS). (2001). *The Surgeon General's call to action to prevent and decrease overweight and obesity.* Rockville, MD: Author.

U.S. Department of Health and Human Services (DHHS). (2004). *The health consequences of smoking: A report of the Surgeon General.* Atlanta, GA: Centers for Disease Control and Prevention.

U.S. Department of Health, Education and Welfare. (1964). *Smoking and health: Report of the Advisory Committee to the Surgeon General of the Public*

Health Service (PHS Publication No. 1103). Washington, DC: Author.

Vikram, V. M., Pandey, R. M., Misra, A., Sharma, R., Devi, J. R., & Khanna, N. (2003). Non-obese (body mass index, 25 kg/m^2) Asian Indians with normal waist circumference have high cardiovascular risk. *Nutrition, 19*(6), 503–509.

von dem Knesebeck O. (2010, May 18). Health inequalities in ageing societies. *International Journal of Public Health.55*(6), 523–524.

Vorster, H. H. (2002). The emergence of cardiovascular disease during urbanisation of Africans. *Public Health Nutrition, 5*(1A), 239–243.

Wagner, E. H., Austin, B. T., & Von Korff, M. (1996). Improving outcomes in chronic illness. *Managed Care Quality, 4,* 12–25.

Wagner, E. H., Glasgow, R. E., Davis, C., Bonomie, A. E., Provost, L., McCulloch, D., et al. (2001). Quality improvement in chronic illness care: A collaborative approach. *Joint Commission Journal on Quality Improvement, 27,* 63–80.

Wanless, D. (2004). *Securing good health for the whole population: Final report.* London: Her Majesty's Treasury. Retrieved from http://www.hm-treasury.gov.uk/consult_wanless04_final.htm

Warman, A. (2001). Living the revolution: Cuban health workers. *Journal of Clinical Nursing, 10*(3), 311–319.

Warren, C. W., Lea, V., Lee, J., Jones, N. R., Asma, S., & McKenna, M. (2009). Change in tobacco use among 13–15 year olds between 1999 and 2008: Findings from the Global Youth Tobacco Survey. *Global Health Promotion, 16,* 38–90.

Waxman, A. (2004). The WHO Global Strategy on Diet, Physical Activity and Health: The controversy on sugar. *Development, 47*(2), 75–83.

Waxman, H. A. (2004). Politics of international health in the Bush administration. *Development, 47*(2), 24–30.

WHO PREMISE (Phase I) Study Group. (In press). Gaps in secondary prevention of myocardial infarction and stroke: World Health Organization study

on Prevention of Recurrences of Myocardial Infarction and Stroke (WHO PREMISE) in low and middle income countries. *Bulletin of the World Health Organization.*

Wild, S., Roglic, G., Green, A., Sicree, R., & King, H. (2004). Global prevalence of diabetes: Estimates for 2000 and projections for 2030. *Diabetes Care, 27,* 1047–1053.

Wilson, D., & Purushothaman, R. (2003). *Dreaming with BRICS: The path to 2050.* New York: Goldman Sachs.

Women and Gender Equity Knowledge Network (WGEKN). (2007). *Unequal, unfair, ineffective and inefficient gender inequity in health: Why it exists and how we can change it. Final report of the Women and Gender Equity Knowledge Network of the Commission on Social Determinants of Health.* Geneva, Switzerland: World Health Organization.

Wong, M. D., Shapiro, M. F., Boscardin, W. J., & Ettner, S. L. (2002). Contribution of major diseases to disparities in mortality. *New England Journal of Medicine, 347*(20), 1585–1592.

World Bank. (1999). *Curbing the epidemic: Governments and the economics of tobacco control.* Washington, DC: Author.

World Health Organization (WHO). (1956). *Cardiovascular diseases and hypertension* (WHA9.31 21). Geneva, Switzerland: Author.

World Health Organization (WHO). (2000). *Tobacco company strategies to undermine tobacco control activities at the World Health Organization: Report of the Committee of Experts on Tobacco Industry Documents.* Geneva, Switzerland: Author.

World Health Organization (WHO). (2002a). *The cost of diabetes* (WHO Fact Sheet 236). Geneva, Switzerland: Author.

World Health Organization (WHO). (2002b). *Innovative care for chronic conditions: Building blocks for action.* Geneva, Switzerland: Author.

World Health Organization (WHO). (2002c). *WHO report on the consultative meeting on primary health care policy review in the Eastern*

Mediterranean Region, Muscat, Oman, 28–30 January 2002. Cairo, Egypt: Author.

World Health Organization (WHO). (2003a). *Adherence to long-term therapies: Evidence for action.* Geneva, Switzerland: Author.

World Health Organization (WHO). (2003b). *Diet, nutrition and the prevention of chronic diseases* (Technical Report No. 916). Geneva, Switzerland: Author.

World Health Organization (WHO). (2003c). *Investing in mental health.* Geneva, Switzerland: Author.

World Health Organization (WHO). (2003d). *World health report, 2003.* Geneva, Switzerland: Author.

World Health Organization (WHO). (2004). *Global strategy on diet, physical activity and health.* Geneva, Switzerland: Author.

World Health Organization (WHO). (2005). *Preventing chronic diseases: A vital investment.* Geneva, Switzerland: Author.

World Health Organization (WHO). (2008). The global burden of disease: 2004 update. Retrieved from http://www.who.int/healthinfo/global_burden_disease/GBD_report_2004update_full.pdf

World Health Organization (WHO). (2009a). *Global health risks: Mortality and burden of disease attributable to selected major risks.* Geneva, Switzerland: Author.

World Health Organization (WHO). (2009b). *WHO report on the global tobacco epidemic, 2009: Implementing smoke-free environments.* Geneva, Switzerland: Author.

World Health Organization (2009). Global health risks: mortality and burden of disease attributable to selected major risks. http://www.who.int/healthinfo/global_burden_disease/GlobalHealth Risks_report_full.pdf

World Health Organization (WHO) Thailand. (2010). Health promotion. Retrieved from http://www.whothailand.org/en/Section3/Section116.htm

World Summit on Sustainable Development (WSSD). (2002). Plan of implementation. Retrieved from http://www.johannesburgsummit.org/html/documents/summit_docs/2309_planfinal.htm

Xu, J., Eilat-Adar, S., Loria, C., Goldbourt, U., Howard, B. V., Fabsitz, R. R. et al. (2006). Dietary fat intake and risk of coronary heart disease: the Strong Heart Study. *American Journal of Clinical Nutrition, 84*(4), 894–902.

Yach, D. (1990). Tobacco-induced diseases in South Africa. *International Journal of Epidemiology, 19*(4), 1122–1123.

Yach, D. (2005). Chronic diseases: Cardiovascular disease, cancer, and diabetes. In B. S. Levy & V. W. Sidel (Eds.), *Social injustice and public health (pp.253-276).* Oxford, UK: Oxford University Press.

Yach, D., Hawkes, C., Epping-Jordan, J. E., & Galbraith, S. (2003). The World Health Organization's Framework Convention on Tobacco Control: Implications for the global epidemics of food-related deaths and disease. *Journal of Public Health Policy, 24*(2–3), 274–290.

Yach, D., Hawkes, C., Gould, C. L., & Hofman, K. J. (2004). The global burden of chronic diseases: Overcoming impediments to prevention and control. *Journal of the American Medical Association, 291*(21), 2616–2622.

Yach, D., Khan, M., Bradley, D., Hargrove, R., Kehoe, S., & Mensah, G. (2010, May). The role and challenges of the food industry in addressing chronic disease. *Global Health, 6*(10), 10.

Yach, D., Mathews, C., & Buch, E. (1990). Urbanisation and health: Methodological difficulties in undertaking epidemiological research in developing countries. *Social Science and Medicine, 31*(4), 507–514.

Yach, D., & Raviglione, M. (2004). TB and tobacco. *Evidence-Based Health Care, 8,* 28.

Zhang, H., & Baiqiang, C. (2003). The impact of tobacco on lung health in China. *Respirology, 8,* 17–21.

Unintentional Injuries and Violence

ROBYN NORTON, ADNAN A. HYDER, AND ALEXANDER BUTCHART

Introduction

Injuries are no "accident" and violence does not just happen. Recognition that a scientific approach to the prevention and control of injuries and violence can be effective has significantly raised these conditions' profile on the public health agenda. Twenty years ago, injuries and violence hardly received mention in the curricula of most schools of public health, whereas today their prevention and control is an integral part of a well-balanced training in public health in most high-income countries and in increasing numbers of low- and middle-income countries.

Injuries have traditionally been defined as physical damage to a person caused by an acute transfer of energy (mechanical, thermal, electrical, chemical, or radiation energy) or by the sudden absence of heat or oxygen. It is now recognized, however, that this definition is too narrow and should be broadened to include impacts that result in psychological harm, maldevelopment, or deprivation (Krug, Dahlberg, Mercy, Zwi, & Lozano, 2002).

Injuries can be grouped in various ways, but most commonly are categorized with reference to the presumed underlying intent—that is, into injuries of unintentional, intentional, and undetermined intent. Unintentional injuries are those where there is no evidence of predetermined intent. They include injuries sustained as a result of road traffic crashes, poisonings, falls, burns, and drowning, as well as occupational and sports injuries.

Intentional injuries result from violence, defined as "the intentional use of physical force or power, threatened or actual, against oneself, another person, or against a group or community, that either results in or has a high likelihood of resulting in injury, death,

psychological harm, maldevelopment or deprivation" (Krug et al., 2002, p. 5). In addition to intentional injuries, victims of violence are at increased risk of a wide range of psychological and behavioral problems, including depression, alcohol abuse, smoking, anxiety, and suicidal behavior, as well as reproductive health problems such as unwanted pregnancy, sexually transmitted diseases, and sexual dysfunction (Krug et al., 2002). Violence can be categorized as self-directed violence (violence a person inflicts upon himself or herself), interpersonal violence (violence inflicted by another individual or a small group of individuals), or collective violence (violence inflicted by larger groups such as states, organized political groups, religious groups, militia groups, and terrorist organizations). Self-directed violence includes completed suicides, attempted suicides, suicidal ideation and suicidal behaviors, and self-harm. Interpersonal violence includes child maltreatment, intimate-partner violence, and elder abuse—all forms that occur largely between family members; youth violence and sexual violence, which occur largely in the community between people who are unrelated and may or may not be acquainted; and collective violence, which can be subdivided into social, political, and economic violence.

It is not always clear whether an injury has occurred from violence or an unintended cause. In such cases, the injury is classified as being of undetermined intent, although for legal or social reasons, it may well be classified as an unintentional injury.

This chapter considers unintentional injuries and violence, including issues relating to a number of cause-specific injuries. The latter include those injuries that are routinely analyzed and for which statistics are published by the World Health Organization

(WHO); individually, these injuries account for the greatest injury burden in terms of mortality and disability-adjusted life-years (DALYs). They include road traffic injuries, poisonings, falls, burns and drowning, as well as self-directed violence, interpersonal violence (including child maltreatment, youth violence, intimate-partner violence, sexual violence, and elder abuse), and collective violence, including war.

The first section provides an overview of the global burden of injuries and violence. It includes discussion about data sources and the challenges of obtaining accurate data, especially in low- and middle-income countries. The next section outlines known and potential risk factors for unintentional injuries and violence. Included here is information on the extent to which knowledge about risk factors in one setting can be applied to other settings, and especially the extent to which knowledge about risk factors can be transferred from high-income settings to low- and middle-income settings.

Current evidence about effective interventions to prevent and control injuries and violence is then outlined. Again, the extent to which evidence of effectiveness from high-income countries can be extrapolated to low- and middle-income countries is considered.

The last section considers the opportunities and challenges that exist in advancing the injury and violence prevention agenda. Issues addressed include the ongoing need for advocacy for prevention, the essential role of research, the significance of a trained workforce, and the role of national and international organizations in promoting the injury and violence prevention agenda, including international societies.

The Global Burden of Injuries and Violence

Data Sources

Data on injuries and violence may be obtained from sources both within and outside the health sector. Health sector data sources include the usual data sources for other health conditions, such as health information systems, vital registration systems, and hospital discharge data, in addition to sources that are more specific to injuries and violence, such as ambulance data and trauma registries. Sources outside the health sector cover a wide spectrum, depending on the type and nature of the injuries or violence. Commonly used non-health sector data sources are police data, transport sector data, legal records, and insurance company claims. Innovative data sources for injuries have also been used, such as newspapers and consumer reports. For both unintentional injuries and violence, population-based surveys are an essential complement to service-based sources of information, especially in settings where access to services such as health care and the police is limited, and where victims may be reluctant or unable to seek help, such as in cases of child maltreatment, intimate-partner violence, and elder abuse. This diversity of data sources makes the field of injuries and violence both unique and challenging—unique, in terms of the intersectoral nature of the information, and challenging, because the biases and nature of data from each source need to be understood.

Comprehensive global data on injuries and violence are available from the WHO (http://www.who.int/violence_injury_prevention/violence/en/), especially as part of this organization's Global Burden of Disease efforts. Attempts to have consistent and internationally comparable data have been made by WHO through the Global Burden of Disease studies in 1990, 2000, and 2005 (final estimates from the latter will be produced in mid-2011). WHO data do have some limitations: Notably, the information relies on available data from around the world and in specific instances its coverage is less than desirable. For example, data on burns include only fire burns (and not scalds), and data on drowning do not include drowning due to floods. Nevertheless, its aggregation of all injuries into one unified system of information makes the WHO database most useful for public health purposes.

For specific types of injury, alternative data sources are available, and they frequently provide estimates that differ from those provided by WHO. For example, both the International Road and Traffic Accident Database (http://www.oecd.org/document/53/0,2340,en_2649_34351_2002165_1_1_1_1,00.html) and the World Bank (http://data.worldbank.org/data-catalog) provide estimates of deaths from road traffic injuries—estimates that are often somewhat lower than those provided by WHO. With respect to violence, the United Nations Organization on Drugs and Crime maintains a database that compares information on national homicide rates derived from police crime statistics with WHO vital registration data and burden of disease estimates (http://www.unodc.org/documents/data-and-analysis/IHS-rates-05012009.pdf).

The quantity and quality of data for different health outcomes from injuries and violence vary. Generally, more and better-quality data are available for deaths than for morbidity and disability. Data on the types and severity of nonfatal health outcomes are important, yet challenging to obtain, especially from low- and middle-income countries. Data on nonfatal health outcomes have primarily been derived from high-income countries, although in the past decade significant information on injuries and violence has emerged from a number of low- and middle-income countries. In general, however, the state of routine health information in low- and middle-income countries has been fragile, especially in regions such as sub-Saharan Africa and South Asia. Thus it is not surprising that these regions have little tradition of developing specific information sources for injuries and violence. Notably, population-based studies from these regions frequently suggest that the injury and violence burden is higher than reported in national official statistics, indicating that these conditions are significantly underreported in official estimates.

Estimates of Injury and Violence Mortality and Disability

In the following section, most of the data presented have been derived from WHO data and reports for the years 1998–2004 (http://www.who.int). Additionally, specific studies or sources have been quoted, to highlight recent information from low- and middle-income countries.

More than 5 million deaths occurred from all injuries worldwide in 2004, of which nearly 90% were in low- and middle-income countries. Approximately 23% of these deaths were caused by road traffic injuries, with suicide and homicide accounting for 15% and 11% of deaths, respectively (Figure 8-1). Notably, 21% of deaths were classified as "other" types of unintentional injury deaths, which include injuries such as animal bites, insect bites, and unspecified injuries. Not surprisingly, injury death rates were highest for road traffic injuries, followed by "other" unintentional injuries, suicide, and homicide (Figure 8-2). Somewhat similar patterns were observed for burden of disease rates, which include nonfatal health outcomes (using DALYs); however, falls had higher rates of nonfatal health outcomes due to the high morbidity from such injuries (Figure 8-3). Importantly, the rates were highest for all "other" unintentional injuries, which likely reflects the challenges inherent in coding the specific causes of nonfatal unintentional injuries.

Unintentional Injuries

In 2004, more than 3.9 million unintentional injury deaths occurred, which were collectively responsible for 6.6% of the global mortality burden. The vast majority (91%) of unintentional injury deaths occurred in individuals in low- and middle-income

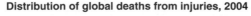

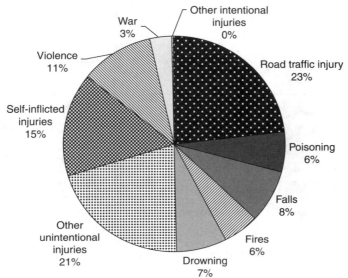

Figure 8-1 Distribution of global deaths from injury, 2004. *Source:* WHO

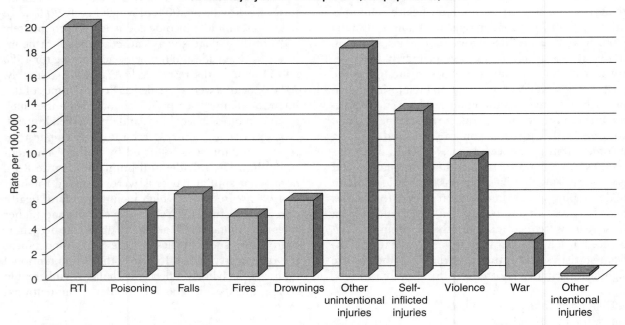

Figure 8-2 Global injury death rates per 100,000 population, 2004. *Source:* WHO

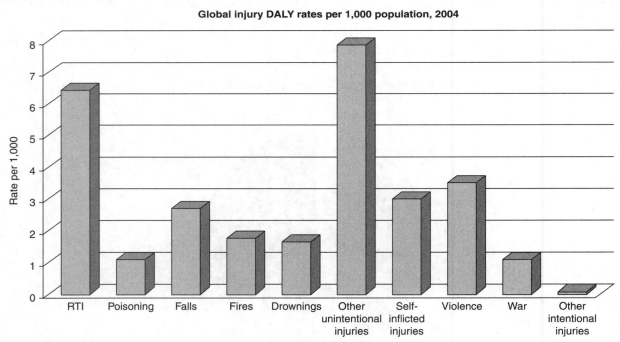

Figure 8-3 Global injury DALY rates per 1,000 population, 2004. *Source:* WHO

countries. The worldwide rate of unintentional injuries was 61 per 100,000 population; the highest rate was found in Southeast Asia (SEARO; 80 per 100,000) and the lowest rate in the Americas (AMRO; 39 per 100,000). Unintentional injuries were also responsible for more than 138 million DALYs in 2004, with 94% occurring in low- and middle-income countries and the rates being highest in those regions that include large numbers of low- and middle-income countries.

Road traffic injuries killed more than 1.2 million people in 2004, making these types of injuries the ninth leading cause of death worldwide. Road traffic injuries accounted for 2.2% of global mortality and resulted in a heavy death toll for people in all age categories. According to the Global Burden of Disease study, death and disability from road traffic injuries are projected to rise substantially in future years to become the fifth leading cause of DALYs lost worldwide by 2030 (World Health Statistics, 2008). Globally, 1.0 million of those persons killed from road traffic injuries during 2004 were from low- or middle-income countries, corresponding to 20 deaths per 100,000 population. The absolute number of fatalities and the mortality rate resulting from road traffic injuries vary considerably across countries, from 130,000 fatalities from this cause in the European region to nearly 350,000 deaths in the Western Pacific. Although all age groups are affected by fatalities resulting from road traffic injuries, young adults—particularly males—are most at risk of loss of life. Because this age group corresponds to the most economically productive segment of the population, road traffic injuries have serious implications for national economies.

Road traffic injuries are frequently defined in terms of the types of road users involved. Typically, data specify whether the users were the occupants of four-wheeled motorized vehicles or pedestrians, cyclists, or riders of motorized two-wheeled vehicles, with the latter being described as the vulnerable road users. A recent survey undertaken by WHO (2009) indicated that vulnerable road users account for 46% of all global deaths and contribute disproportionately to deaths in low- and middle-income countries.

According to WHO estimates, 346,000 *poisoning* deaths occurred in 2004. These deaths demonstrated a 2:1 male-to-female ratio. More than 90% of these deaths occurred in low- and middle-income countries.

Falls caused more than 424,000 deaths worldwide in 2004, with the majority of these fatalities occurring in low- and middle- income countries, and the male-to-female ratio being 2:1. These numbers translate to a mortality rate of 7 deaths per 100,000 population globally and a loss of 3 DALYs per 1,000 population. Clearly, falls make an important contribution to morbidity and disability on a global basis.

WHO registers data only for *burns* that result from fires; it does not tally data for scalds (water burns)—an important limitation. More than 310,000 deaths were caused by fires in 2004, resulting in more than 2 DALYs lost per 1,000 population. Unlike with other types of injuries, more females than males died from fires (male-to-female ratio of 0.6:1.00).

Drowning is the process of experiencing respiratory impairment from submersion or immersion in liquid leading to death or morbidity (WHO, 2003). In 2004, an estimated 388,000 people drowned. One-third of drownings occurred in the Western Pacific region, although the African region has the highest drowning fatality rate (Table 8-1). Overall, the male rate of drowning is more than twice that for females. The rate of drowning in the African region is more than four times, and the Western Pacific region is more than twice, that of the Americas (the region with the lowest rate). It is important to note that these data include only "accidental drowning and submersion";

Table 8-1	Drowning Deaths by Gender in Each WHO Region, 2004						
Region	**World**	**AFR**	**AMR**	**EMR**	**EUR**	**SEAR**	**WPR**
Males	262,940	46,466	18,348	21,523	27,765	63,288	85,134
Females	125,060	15,874	3,842	8,140	6,460	36,648	53,823
Total	388,000	62,340	22,190	29,663	34,225	99,936	138,957
Male-to-Female ratio	2.1:1	2.9:1	4.8:1	2.6:1	4.3:1	1.7:1	1.6:1
Percent	100	16	6	8	9	26	36
Rate*	6.0	8.5	2.5	5.7	3.9	6	8

* Rate per 100,000 people.

Note: AFR = African region of WHO, AMR = American region, EMR = Eastern Mediterranean region, EUR = European region, SEAR = Southeast Asian region, WPR = Western Pacific region.

Source: WHO

they exclude drowning due to floods (cataclysms), boating, and water transport.

Table 8-2 shows selected indices of the burden of drowning in China and India—the most populous low- and middle-income countries in the world—for 2004. Both of these countries have high drowning mortality rates, and together they contribute 49% of the world drowning deaths and 50% of the total DALYs attributed to drowning globally.

Violence

Self-directed violence caused the deaths of more than 840,000 people globally in 2004 and was associated with more than 19 million DALYs lost. These latter injuries include suicides, attempted suicide, self-destructive behaviors, and self-mutilation. Although data on self-directed injuries are challenging to obtain, case studies from several parts of the world indicate that they are being increasingly documented globally (see Exhibit 8-1).

Interpersonal violence accounted for a global total of 600,000 deaths in 2004. This form of fatal violence disproportionately affected low- and middle-income countries, where more than 90% of all interpersonal violence-related deaths were estimated to have occurred. The estimated rate of violent death in low- and middle-income countries was 10.41 per 100,000 population in 2004, compared to 2.68 per 100,000 in high-income countries.

The extent of *child maltreatment* is difficult to gauge because much, if not most, of such abuse goes unreported. Nevertheless, child maltreatment is a

Table 8-2	Drowning in China and India, 2004	
Marker	**China**	**India**
Drowning deaths	121,000	70,000
Mortality rate*	9.2	6.30%
Percentage of global unintentional drowning mortality	31	18
Rank as a leading cause of unintentional death†	4	3
Drowning DALYs	3,383,000	1,913,000
Percentage of total DALYs	32	18

*All rates per 100,000 population.

† Ranked from one to six of leading cause of disability due to unintentional injury

DALY: Disability-adjusted life-year.

Source: WHO

Exhibit 8-1	Suicides in South Asia: Case Study from Pakistan

No official data on suicides are collected in Pakistan, a conservative South Asian Islamic country with traditionally low suicide rates. As a result, national rates on suicide are neither known nor reported to WHO. Nevertheless, an accumulating body of anecdotal evidence suggests that suicide rates have been gradually increasing in Pakistan over the last few years. To date, both suicide and attempted suicide have been under-studied and under-researched subjects in this country. A general lack of trained mental health researchers in the country is partly to blame for this situation. Furthermore, a lack of interest by available researchers may be related to the generally held belief that suicide and attempted suicide are rare events in Muslim countries and, therefore, unworthy of scientific study. Other reasons behind the paucity of data may be the difficulty in gaining access to such data, as there are many legal, social, and cultural issues related to suicide and attempted suicide. Both suicide and attempted suicide are illegal acts, socially and religiously condemned, making research in this area difficult.

Police data from Sindh—one of the four provinces of Pakistan—provide a unique picture of trends of suicide over a 15-year span (1985–1999). During this period, there were 2,568 reported suicides (71% men, 39% women; ratio 1.8:1.00). The lowest number was 90 in 1987, and the highest number was 360 in 1999. Poisoning by organophosphates was the most common method of suicide, followed by hanging.

A more recent review of 23 studies found young age, male gender, marriage, and low socioeconomic status to be reported risk factors for suicides. These data, although limited in scope, provide evidence of an important public health issue of suicides in Pakistan. Firearms, hanging, and organophosphorous poisoning were the most common methods of suicide. There is urgent need for further research on suicide in Pakistan. Interventions for suicide prevention in the country can then be planned.

Selected References

Khan, M. M., & Hyder, A. A. (2006). Suicides in the developing world: Case study from Pakistan. *Suicide & Life-threatening Behavior, 36*(1), 76–81.

Khan, M. M., & Prince, M. (2003). Beyond rates: The tragedy of suicide in Pakistan. *Tropical Doctor, 33*, 67–69.

Shahid, M., & Hyder, A. A. (2008). Deliberate self-harm and suicides: A review from Pakistan. *International Journal of Injury Prevention & Safety Promotion, 15*(4), 233–241.

global problem with serious lifelong consequences for many of its victims. International studies reveal that between one-fourth and one-half of all children around the world report severe and frequent physical abuse, including being beaten, kicked, or tied up by parents, and approximately 20% of women and 5% to 10% of men report having been sexually abused as children (Runyan, Wattam, Ikeda, Hassan, & Ramiro, 2002). Additionally, many children are subject to psychological and emotional abuse and neglect, although the extent of these phenomena worldwide remains unknown. In 2004, an estimated 31,000 children younger than 15 years of age died from homicide, although this number probably underestimates the true extent of the problem. A significant proportion of deaths due to child maltreatment are missed because their maltreatment cause is not apparent to medical practitioners—that is, they appear to be a result of unintentional injuries such as falls or burning. In conflict and refugee settings, girls may be at particular risk of sexual violence, exploitation, and abuse by combatants, security forces, members of their communities, aid workers, and others.

Youth violence is defined as violence committed by or against individuals between the ages of 10 and 29 years. In 2004, an estimated 247,157 youth homicides took place globally—equivalent to 677 children and young people aged 10 to 29 years being killed every day, and a rate of 10.69 deaths per 100,000 population. Youth homicide rates vary dramatically between countries, ranging from 3.95 per 100,000 in high-income countries to 11.51 in low- and middle-income countries. The very highest rates occur in the countries of Africa and Latin America. In all countries, young males are both the main perpetrators and victims of homicide, and female rates of youth homicide are almost everywhere much lower than male rates. For every young person killed by violence, an estimated 20 to 40 more sustain injuries that require hospital treatment (Mercy, Butchart, Farrington, & Cerda, 2002).

Sexual violence also affects a significant proportion of youth, with 3% to 24% of women surveyed in the WHO multi-country study on women's health and domestic violence reporting that their first sexual experience was forced, in a majority of cases while they were adolescents (García-Moreno, Jansen, Ellsberg, Heise, & Watts, 2005). Physical fighting and bullying are also common among young people. In Africa, the Global Schools-based Student Health Survey examined exposure to physical and sexual violence among school-going youth aged 13 to 15 years in Namibia, Swaziland, Uganda, Zambia, and Zimbabwe (Brown, Riley, Butchart, & Kann, 2008).

The prevalence of exposure to physical violence during the 12 months preceding the survey was 42%, and the prevalence of lifetime exposure to sexual violence was 23%. Exposure differed across countries, with the rates of exposure to physical violence ranging from 27% to 50% and those for sexual violence ranging from 9% to 33%. After adjustment for age, exposure to physical violence was more likely among boys than girls, and exposure to sexual violence more likely among girls than boys, although differences between genders were not large (Brown et al., 2008).

A study of bullying in school-aged children in 40 countries (mainly in Europe) found that exposure to bullying varied across countries, with estimated exposure rates ranging from 8.6% to 45.2% among boys, and from 4.8% to 35.8% among girls. Adolescents in Baltic countries reported higher rates of bullying and victimization, whereas their peers in northern European countries reported the lowest prevalence. Boys reported higher rates of bullying in all countries. Rates of victimization were higher for girls in 29 of 40 countries (Craig et al., 2009).

According to WHO documents, *intimate-partner violence* is defined as "any behavior within an intimate relationship that causes physical, psychological or sexual harm to those in the relationship. Such behaviors include "acts of physical aggression—such as slapping, hitting, kicking and beating; psychological abuse—such as intimidation, constant belittlement and humiliation; forced intercourse and other forms of sexual coercion; and various controlling behaviors—such as isolating a person from their family and friends, monitoring their movements, and restricting their access to information or assistance" (Heise & García-Moreno, 2002). The true extent of intimate-partner violence is unknown. Surveys have produced a wide range of prevalence estimates, but the results are difficult to compare given cultural differences and social taboos in responding to questions.

The WHO multi-country study on women's health and domestic violence against women (García-Moreno et al., 2005) interviewed more than 24,000 women between the ages of 15 and 49 in rural and urban areas in 10 countries to provide the most comprehensive picture of the patterns of intimate-partner violence and sexual violence victimization currently available. It showed that physical abuse by a partner at some point in life up to 49 years of age was reported by 13% to 61% of interviewees across all study sites. Sexual violence by a partner at some point in life up to 49 years of age was reported by 6% to 59% of interviewees, and sexual violence by a nonpartner older than 15 years at some point in life up to 49 years of age was reported by 0.3% to 11.5% of interviewees.

Sexual violence includes rape (by either an intimate partner or a stranger), attempted rape, gang rape, and other forms of forced sexual acts in any setting (e.g., home, work). Surveys indicate that between 1% and 8% of women (females older than 16 years) report experiencing sexual violence within the past 5 years, while as many as 27% report experiencing sexual violence from an intimate partner in the past year (Jewkes, Sen, & García-Moreno, 2002).

Abuse of the elderly is a category of violence that incorporates physical, sexual, emotional, and psychological acts or neglect directed toward older people. It is an important type of violence, especially given the prediction that the global population of persons older than 65 years of age will reach more than 1 billion in the first half of the 21st century (Wolf, Daichman, & Bennett, 2002). More than 80% of these older people will reside in low- and middle-income countries, where they will represent more than 12% of the population. Abuse of the elderly occurs in both home and institutional settings and is very difficult to measure. Thus there is a persistent lack of global statistics on this issue. Surveys in high-income countries indicate a prevalence of 4% to 6% of abuse of older persons (Wolf et al., 2002).

Collective violence—including armed conflict with and between states—was estimated by WHO to cause more than 180,000 deaths worldwide in 2004. There is a 9:1 male-to-female ratio of deaths in this category. This estimate includes only deaths caused directly by war; it does not include deaths caused indirectly by war, such as those that result from disruption of the health system or those that occur after the end of war.

Estimates of the Economic and Social Costs of Injury and Violence

Loss of life and health is just one dimension in explaining why injuries and violence are an important public health problem. Other important dimensions include these conditions' social and economic toll on individuals, families, and societies. Death of loved ones, lifelong disabilities resulting in unemployment, and the staggering costs of medical care for victims are some of the other effects of injuries and violence that need to be described. In addition, factors such as lost productivity, insurance claims, replacement income activities, and family consequences are important. Unfortunately, such information is not readily available and is rarely collected in large parts of the world; as a consequence, our knowledge of the economic and social impacts of injuries and violence remains limited.

This section, while not presenting a comprehensive review of the economic and social costs of all injuries and violence, provides examples of the breadth and—importantly—the limitations of what has been documented for a few specific injuries.

Costs associated with *unintentional injuries* have been studied in some high-income countries. In one study of unintentional injuries that occurred in home settings in the United States, the total societal cost was estimated at $217 billion; falls accounted for the largest proportion (42%) of this cost (Zaloshnja, Miller, Lawrence, & Romano, 2005). In another study, focusing on childhood unintentional injuries, the total cost, which included loss of future work and quality of life, was $347 billion per year, or $17,000 per child injured (Danseco, Miller, & Spicer, 2000). A few cost-focused studies have addressed unintentional child injuries in low- and middle-income countries. For example, a recent analysis of more than 6,000 children younger than 15 years of age who were hospitalized for unintentional injuries in China showed a mean institutional cost of $166 and a mean length of stay exceeding 17 days per injury case (Jiang, Zhang, Wang, Wang, Xu, & Shang, 2010). Further, the cost associated with poisoning averaged $53 per case; for scald burns, this cost was $198 per case. A community-level analysis in Vietnam showed that the total annual cost of unintentional child injuries was more than $235,000—equivalent to the income of nearly 1,800 people in the country (Thanh, Hang, Chuc, & Lindholm, 2003). See Exhibit 8-2.

Despite the global significance of *road traffic injuries* in terms of mortality and disability, the economic and social consequences of such injuries have been documented only in the past decade, and most countries in the world report not having undertaken costing exercises (WHO, 2009). Work performed by Transport Research Laboratory (TRL), based on road crash costs from 21 high-income and low- and middle-income countries, found that the average annual cost of road crashes was approximately 1% of the gross national product (GNP) in low- and middle-income countries, 1.5% of GNP in countries in economic transition, and 2% in highly motorized countries. Based on these data, the researchers suggested that the annual burden of the economic costs of road traffic injuries globally was $518 billion in 2000, with the annual costs of road traffic injury in low- and middle-income countries being approximately $65 billion, exceeding the total annual amount received by these countries in development assistance at that time (Jacobs, Aeron-Thomas, & Astrop, 2000).

Exhibit 8-2	**Impact of Helmet Laws in Vietnam**

On December 15, 2007, a new law mandating the use of helmets among motorcycle riders and passengers took effect in Vietnam. Severe financial penalties were established to support the laws. WHO promoted helmet usage and the new law through media campaigns including print, radio, and television, in three provinces: Yen Bai, Da Nang, and Binh Duong. In addition to encouraging motorcyclists to wear helmets, the media campaign focused on the use of quality helmets.

Data on helmet usage were monitored by Hanoi School of Public Health in collaboration with WHO. In November 2007, prior to the implementation of the mandatory helmet law, the rate of correct usage of motorcycle helmets by motorcyclists was 42% among riders and 36% among passengers. A year after the law took effect, helmet usage was found to exceed 90% for both riders and passengers. However, among child passengers, helmet usage ranged from 15% to 53% (Pervin et al., 2009).

According to data collected by the National Traffic Safety Committee (NTSC), the increased usage of helmets among motorcyclists has resulted in a reduction of 1,557 deaths and 2,495 injuries in Vietnam. A study published in April 2010 reported that the increased helmet usage resulted in an 18% reduction in the risk of death and a 16% reduction in the risk of head injury among motorcyclists in the country (Passmore et al., 2010).

Selected References

Passmore, J., Tu, N. T., Luong, M. A., Chinh, N. D., & Nam, N. P. (2010). Impact of mandatory motorcycle helmet wearing legislation on head injuries in Viet Nam: Results of a preliminary analysis. *Traffic Injury Prevention, 11*(2), 202–206.

Pervin, A., Passmore, J., Sidik, M., McKinley, T., Nguyen, T. H., & Nguyen, P. N. (2009). Viet Nam's mandatory motorcycle helmet law and its impact on children. *Bulletin of the World Health Organization, 87*(5), 369–373.

More recent work has attempted to document and compare the impact of road traffic injuries on low-income households in Bangladesh and India (Aeron-Thomas, Jacobs, Sexton, Gururaj, & Rahmann, 2004). In both countries, males who provided the majority of the household income were the most common victims of road traffic fatalities; their deaths reduced household income and food consumption for the victim's family. While poor households did not report higher rates of road traffic injuries than nonpoor households, the poor were found to spend a much greater proportion of their income on funeral and/or medical costs than the nonpoor. As a consequence, road traffic injury was a contributor in tipping households into poverty.

Interpersonal violence is expensive. Estimates of the cost of violence in the United States put this figure at 3.3% of the gross domestic product (GDP). In England and Wales, the total costs from violence—including homicide, wounding, and sexual assault—amount to an estimated $40.2 billion annually. Although interpersonal violence disproportionately affects low- and middle-income countries, as a recent report shows, there is a scarcity of studies addressing the economic effects of this violence in low- and middle-income countries (Waters, Hyder, Rajkotia, Basu, Rehwinkel, & Butchart, 2004). Estimates from low- and middle-income countries indicate that the overall costs of violence are substantial (Exhibit 8-3).

Comparisons with high-income countries are complicated by the fact that economic losses related to productivity tend to be undervalued in lower-income countries because these losses are typically based on foregone wages and income. For example, a single *homicide* is calculated to cost, on average, $15,319 in South Africa, $602,000 in Australia, $829,000 in New Zealand, and more than $2 million in the United States (all monetary values have been converted to 2001 U.S. dollars to enable comparisons and to adjust for inflation and varying exchange rates).

Many of the studies detailing the costs of specific types of violence have been conducted in the United States (Waters, Hyder, Rajkotia et al., 2004). *Child abuse* results in $94 billion in annual costs to the U.S. economy, or 1% of GDP. Direct medical treatment costs per abused child have been calculated by different studies to range from $13,781 to $42,518 per child. *Intimate-partner violence* costs the U.S. economy $12.6 billion on an annual basis, or 0.1% of GDP—compared to 1.6% of GDP in Nicaragua and 2.0% of GDP in Chile. *Gun violence*—which includes suicides—has been calculated to carry a $155 billion per year cost in the United States, with lifetime medical treatment costs per victim ranging from $37,000 to $42,000.

Evidence abounds that the public sector—and thus society in general—picks up much of the tab for interpersonal violence. Several studies in the United States have shown that 56% to 80% of the costs of caring for victims of gun and stabbing injuries is either directly paid by public financing or not paid at

| Exhibit 8-3 | **Estimating the Economic Costs of Violence** |

In 2008, WHO, the U.S. Centers for Disease Control and Prevention, and the Small Arms Survey developed economic costing guidelines to assess the direct and indirect economic burden of interpersonal and self-directed violence (Butchart et al., 2008). These guidelines were subsequently tested to assess the costs of fatal and nonfatal interpersonal and self-directed violence in Brazil, Jamaica, and Thailand. In Brazil during 2004, the direct medical cost of injuries due to violence (R$519 million) amounted to 0.4% of the total health budget, while loss of productivity due to violence-related injuries (R$15.5 billion) accounted for approximately 12% of all health expenditures, or 1.2% of GDP. In Jamaica, the direct medical costs of interpersonal violence in 2006 totaled J$2.1 billion—the vast majority of which was concentrated among young males. Indirect medical costs were 10 times higher, exceeding J$27.5 billion. Direct medical costs accounted for approximately 160% of Jamaica's total health expenditure, while the combined direct and indirect impacts were equivalent to 4% of GDP. In Thailand for 2005, the direct medical cost of violence-related injuries accounted for about 4% of Thailand's total health budget, while the loss of productivity due to violence-related injuries accounted for approximately 0.4% of GDP.

References

Butchart, A., Brown., D., Khanh-Huynh, A., Corso, P., Florquin, N., & Muggah, R. (2008). *Manual for estimating the economic costs of injuries due to interpersonal and self-directed violence*. Geneva, Switzerland: World Health Organization.

all; in the latter case, the costs are absorbed by government and society in the form of uncompensated care financing and overall higher payment rates. In low- and middle-income countries, it is also probable that society absorbs much of the costs of violence, through direct public expenditures and negative effects on investment and economic growth.

Studies documenting the economic effects of interpersonal violence have used a broad range of categories to distinguish the various types of costs associated with this condition. Those estimating indirect costs—including the opportunity cost of time, lost productivity, and reduced quality of life—provide higher cost estimates than studies that limit the costs of violence to direct costs alone. Other key methodological issues include the economic values assigned to human life, lost productive time, and psychological distress. The rates at which future costs and benefits are discounted, in accounting terms, also vary across studies.

Risk Factors for Unintentional Injuries and Violence

As with most diseases, the causes of unintentional injuries and violence are considered to be multifactorial. The traditional epidemiological paradigm of host (including biological and behavioral), vector, and environmental factors, which in combination contribute to the incidence of disease, has been readily adapted

and applied in determining the causes of unintentional injury. This paradigm has been extended, however, to consider each factor in relation to the timing of the injury occurrence—that is, factors operating prior to, during, and following the injury that might be associated with both the incidence and the severity of the injury (Haddon, 1968). In determining the causes of violence, especially interpersonal violence, a somewhat different model (described as an ecological model), has more commonly been utilized, which focuses on the interplay between individual, relationship, community, and societal factors (Krug et al., 2002).

In the past two decades, the evidence base identifying risk factors for unintentional injuries and violence has expanded dramatically, as the numbers of injury researchers and research institutions have increased. The application of public health research methods, commonly used in identifying risk factors for other causes of death and disability, to the problems of unintentional injuries and violence has undoubtedly contributed to the growth in this knowledge. For example, case-control and cohort studies now likely contribute as much to the evidence base in the injury field as they do for other leading causes of death and disability, such as cancer and heart disease.

Most of this research has been undertaken in high-income countries, in large part given the preponderance of researchers and research institutions in these areas. Nevertheless, the evidence base identifying risk factors for unintentional injuries and violence in low- and middle-income countries is growing, along with the recognition that certain types of injuries and forms of violence are unique to these countries. Thus, while some risk factors may be common across a wide range of settings (e.g., alcohol misuse), other risk factors are unique to the environments in which they occur (e.g., the significance of water wells in increasing the risks of drowning in low- and middle-income countries, or the specificity of suicide by self-immolation among women in some Islamic and Asian societies).

This section summarizes known and potential risk factors for the leading cause-specific injuries. The discussion here highlights the extent to which knowledge has been obtained exclusively in high-income countries, the extent to which this knowledge might be transferred to low- and middle-income countries, and the areas where the evidence base is still minimal.

Risk Factors for Road Traffic Injuries

Not surprisingly, given the significant burden of road traffic injuries, much is known about risk factors for such injuries, as outlined in detail in *World Report on Road Traffic Injury Prevention* (Peden et al., 2004) and updated most recently in *Global Status Report on Road Safety: Time for Action* (WHO, 2009). The 2004 report describes road traffic injury risk in terms of four functions: factors affecting exposure to risk, factors influencing crash involvement, factors influencing crash injury severity, and factors influencing the severity of post-crash injuries.

Factors Influencing Exposure to Risk

Increasing motorization is, without doubt, one of the main factors contributing to the increase in road traffic injuries worldwide and especially in low- and middle-income countries. Motorization rates rise with income (Kopits & Cropper, 2003). Thus, in a growing number of low- and middle-income countries where economies are experiencing growth, there has been a corresponding increase in the numbers of motor vehicles (Bener, 2009).

Unfortunately, in some low- and middle-income countries, traffic growth has included proliferation of less safe forms of travel (i.e., motorized two-wheeled vehicles), resulting in concurrent increases in related injuries (WHO, 2009). This growth in motorized two-wheeled vehicles is not unique to low- and middle-income countries, however; high-income countries are adopting these vehicles in larger numbers as they try to find solutions to the problems of growing traffic congestion. In London, for example, due to the introduction of policies that encourage the use of such vehicles, deaths and injuries among motorized two-wheeler users are increasing (Peden et al., 2004).

Projected demographic changes in high-income countries over the next 20 to 30 years are likely to result in greater numbers of people older than the age of 65 years being exposed to traffic risks and, given their greater physical vulnerability, greater numbers sustaining injury. By comparison, in low- and middle-income countries, increasing economic growth is fueling both the aspirations of younger people to drive motor vehicles and the need to travel greater distances to work. As a consequence, in many low- and middle-income countries, this vulnerable road user group will continue to be the predominant group involved in road crashes.

Transport, land use, and road network planning have all been shown to be important in determining exposure to injury risk. While many of the technical aspects of planning, highway design, traffic engineering, and traffic management have been the hallmarks of transport systems, such planning systems are frequently absent in low- and middle-income countries, as evidenced by the fact that only one-third of countries surveyed for the global status report had a national road safety strategy (WHO, 2009). The necessity for such planning is probably even greater in low- and middle-income countries than in high-income countries, given the extremely diverse and multiple modes of traffic (both motorized and non-motorized) seen in the former countries.

Factors Influencing Crash Involvement

The overwhelming influence of speed and alcohol consumption on the risk of crash involvement has been confirmed primarily in studies undertaken in high-income countries, but also in an increasing number of studies undertaken in low- and middle-income countries. A number of other host-related factors, as outlined in this section, have also been postulated as increasing the risk of crash involvement, although evidence to support their involvement remains limited and is mostly restricted to studies undertaken in high-income countries.

There is very good evidence from high-income countries to show a strong relationship between increasing vehicle speeds and increasing risk of crash, both for motor vehicle occupants and for vulnerable road users, particularly pedestrians (Global Road Safety Partnership, 2008). This relationship is likely to hold true in low- and middle-income countries as well. Indeed, data obtained both from routinely collected police reports (Sobngwi-Tambekou, Bhatti, Kounga, Salmi, & Lagarde, 2010; Zhao et al., 2009) and from case-control studies (Donroe, Tincopa, Gilman, Brugge, & Moore, 2008) in a number of low- and middle-income countries show that speed is a leading causal factor in road traffic crashes.

The observation that alcohol is associated with an increased risk of road crashes, in studies of victims and perpetrators, has been confirmed in many studies conducted both in high-income and low- and middle-income countries (Global Road Safety Partnership, 2007; Peden et al., 2004). In particular, a survey of studies conducted in low- and middle-income countries found that alcohol was present in the blood of between 4% and 69% of injured drivers, 18% to 90% of crash-injured pedestrians and 10% to 28% of injured motorcyclists (Global Road Safety Partnership, 2007). These findings are reinforced by case-control and case cross-over studies that provide clear evidence of alcohol's association with an increase of road traffic injuries (Odero & Zwi, 1995; Woratanarat et al., 2009).

Other factors that have been shown to increase the risks of road crashes in a number of high-income countries include fatigue, use of hand-held mobile telephones, and inadequate visibility of vulnerable road users (Peden et al., 2004); these factors are equally likely to increase these risks in a number of low- and middle-income countries. Indeed, studies in China show twofold increased risks of car crash associated with driver chronic sleepiness (Liu et al., 2003). In addition, surveys of commercial and public road transport in a number of African countries have shown that drivers often work unduly long hours and go to work when exhausted (Nafukho & Khayesi, 2002), consistent with the overall evidence on the relationship between fatigue and work-related traffic crashes (Robb, Sultana, Ameratunga, & Jackson, 2008). Studies in Malaysia have clearly shown that motorcyclists who use daytime running lights have a crash risk that is 10% to 29% lower than the risk of motorcyclists who do not (Radin Umar, Mackay, & Hills, 1996).

Clearly, road-related and vehicle-related risk factors may increase the risk of crash involvement. Specific factors related to road planning that have been suggested as risk factors for crashes include through-traffic passing through residential areas, conflicts between pedestrians and vehicles near schools located on busy roads, lack of segregation of pedestrians and high-speed traffic, lack of median barriers to prevent dangerous overtaking on single-carriage roads, and lack of barriers to prevent pedestrian access onto high-speed roads. There remains a dearth of studies that have examined the risks associated with each of these factors, especially in low- and middle-income

countries. Although vehicle-related factors clearly have the potential to increase risks of injury, data from a number of African countries suggest that while these factors do contribute to crash involvement, their contribution may account for less than 5% of all such crashes (Van Schoor, van Niekerk, & Grobbelaar, 2001).

Factors Influencing Injury Severity

In-vehicle crash protection is undoubtedly a factor relating to crash injury severity. While significant improvements have been made to private vehicles in the past decade, many of these improvements have not yet made their way into vehicles in low- and middle-income countries (Odero, Garner, & Zwi, 1997). However, the issue of crash protection that reduces injury severity to vulnerable road users is probably of greater relevance, especially in low- and middle-income countries, where vulnerable road users are predominant. Few countries, whether high- or low-income countries, have established requirements to protect vulnerable road users by means of crash-worthy designs for the front of cars or buses (Mohan, 2002).

A significant risk factor for increased injury severity in motorized two-wheeled users is non-use or inappropriate use of motorcycle helmets (Liu, Ivers, Norton, Boufous, Blows, & Lo, 2008; WHO, 2009). A risk factor for increased injury severity in bicyclists is non-use of helmets (Thompson, Rivara, & Thompson, 2003). Failure to use seat belts is also a significant risk factor associated with injury severity in vehicle occupants, especially in many low- and middle-income countries that lack any requirement for seat belts to be present in vehicles or used by drivers and passengers (FIA Foundation for the Automobile and Society, 2009; WHO, 2009).

Studies in high-income countries suggest that roadside hazards, such as trees, poles, and road signs, may contribute to between 18% and 42% of road crash fatalities (Kloeden, McLean, Baldock, & Cockington, 1998). The extent to which this risk applies to low- and middle-income countries has not been determined.

Factors Influencing Severity of Post-crash Injuries

Both the availability and quality of prehospital and in-hospital care are major influences on the outcomes for patients with injuries sustained in a crash. Comparisons between high-income countries and low- and middle-income countries show clear differences in the proportions of injured individuals who die before reaching a hospital, in large part reflecting the limited access to prehospital medical services in low- and middle-income countries (Mock, Jurkovich, nii-Amon-Kotei, Arreola-Risa, & Maier, 1998). Factors that determine survival and outcome include early availability of care, the time interval between the injury and the patient's arrival at a definitive-care hospital, referral based on triage, and availability of physical and human resources.

Risk Factors for Poisonings

The global literature on unintentional poisonings includes significant information on occupational-related poisonings, especially pesticide poisonings, and a growing body of information on environmental poisoning, especially lead poisoning. The particular focus of this section, however, is on risk factors for other unintentional poisonings; occupational and environmental poisoning are covered in depth in Chapter 10 under the topic of environmental health.

The literature in this area almost exclusively considers risk factors for poisonings in young children, even though the majority of poisonings occur in adults, for whom therapeutic errors and adverse reactions to medications may well be significant issues. In high-income countries, product accessibility—in terms of both safe packaging and storage—has long been recognized as the key risk factor in unintentional poisoning (Shannon, 2000). Storage issues also appear to be risk factors for poisoning in low- and middle-income countries, including the numbers of used storage containers in the residence, the use of nonstandard containers for storage (e.g., the use of cola bottles for the storage of kerosene), and the storage of poisons at ground level (Azizi, Zulkifli, & Kasim,1993; Chatsantiprapa, Chokkanapitak, & Pinpradit, 2001; Soori, 2001).

As highlighted in the recently published *World Report on Child Injury Prevention* (Peden et al., 2008), several case-control studies conducted in low- and middle-income countries show evidence of a number of sociodemographic risk factors for unintentional poisoning, including young age of parents, residential mobility, and limited adult supervision of children (Azizi et al., 1993; Soori, 2001). Previous poisoning may also be a risk factor (Soori, 2001).

Risk Factors for Fall-Related Injuries

Fall-Related Injuries in Older People (Including Hip Fractures)

Risk factors for fall-related injuries in older people are generally considered in terms of risk factors for falling (both intrinsic and extrinsic risk factors), risk factors associated with the severity of the impact following the fall, and risk factors associated with low levels of bone mineral density, insofar as almost all fall-related injuries in older people involve broken bones. These risk factors include low bone density; poor nutritional status and low body mass index (BMI); low calcium intake; comorbid conditions, such as hypertension and diabetes; poor performance in activities of daily living (ADLs and instrumental ADLs); low levels of engagement in physical activity; poor cognitive function; poor perceived health status; poor vision; environmental factors affecting balance or gait; family history of hip fracture; and alcohol consumption (Hippisley-Cox & Coupland, 2009; Robbins et al., 2007).

While much of the research in this area has been undertaken in high-income countries, reports from low- and middle-income countries show that these studies' findings are consistent across most countries (Chew, Yong, Mas Ayu, & Tajunisah, 2010; Coutinho, Bloch, & Rodrigues, 2009). A few studies, however, have identified other factors that have not previously been identified and may be more relevant in the context of low- and middle-income countries. For example, studies in Thailand have suggested that factors associated with poor socioeconomic status may be risk factors, such as lack of electricity in the house and living in Thai-style houses or huts (Jitapunkul, Yuktananandana, & Parkpian, 2001).

Fall-Related Injuries in Younger People

The *World Report on Child Injury Prevention* (Peden et al., 2008) has systematically reviewed the available evidence on risk factors for fall-related injuries in younger people. Much of the research has sought to identify factors associated with falls from heights. In high-income countries, such falls occur from balconies and apartment windows, beds/bunks and nursery equipment (including baby walkers), and playground equipment. In contrast, in low- and middle-income countries, such falls are more likely to occur from rooftops, trees, and animals, such as in those countries where camel racing is a popular activity. Poverty appears to be a consistent underlying risk factor for falls, while the absence of protective rails/guards or similar equipment is associated with increased risk. Severity of injury appears to be associated with the height of the fall and the nature of the surface on which the child falls.

Risk Factors for Burn-Related Injuries

Burn-related injuries sustained as a result of fires account for the majority of burn-related deaths, although hot water burns are a significant cause of morbidity, especially in low- and middle-income countries.

In high-income countries, much of our knowledge about risk factors for fire-related injuries has come from cross-sectional studies and only a few case-control studies. In these studies, a number of risk factors have been consistently identified. Nonmodifiable risk factors include both young and older age, male gender, nonwhite race, low income, disability, and late night/early morning occurrence (Warda, Tenenbein, & Moffatt, 1999). Modifiable risk factors included place of residence, type of residence (such as mobile homes and homes without a smoke detector or telephone), smoking, and alcohol use (Warda et al., 1999). By comparison, few controlled studies have examined risk factors for hot water burns, and most discussion in the literature focuses on the lack of temperature controls for hot water systems or taps (Jaye, Simpson, & Langley, 2001).

Studies undertaken in low- and middle-income countries have similarly mostly focused on risk factors for burn-related injuries, with few examining risk factors for hot water–related injuries. In the majority of cases, these studies have focused on risk factors for burns in children (Peden et al., 2008). Many of the identified risk factors are related to poverty, such as low family income, lack of water supply, and overcrowding. Lack of parental supervision and history of burns in siblings are risk factors as well. By comparison, maternal education appears to be consistently protective. Not surprisingly, other protective factors relate to the knowledge about burn risks, presence of smoke detectors, and ready access to first aid services.

Risk Factors for Drowning

In high-income countries, the majority of drowning incidents are associated with recreation or leisure activities including swimming pools (Brenner, 2003), while in most low- and middle-income countries they are associated with everyday activities near bodies of water, including rivers, water wells, or buckets (Hyder, Arifeen, Begum, Fishman, Wali, & Baqui, 2003; Kobusingye, Guwatudde, & Lett, 2001).

Very few studies, in either high- or low-income countries, have examined risk factors for drowning in adults. Nevertheless, evidence does consistently show that a significant proportion of adult drowning incidents are associated with positive blood alcohol levels (Carlini-Cotrim & da Matta Chasin, 2000; Driscoll, Harrison, & Steenkamp, 2004).

Most studies in this area—although there have been few properly controlled studies—have focused on risk factors for drowning in children, as reported in *World Report on Child Injury Prevention* (Peden et al., 2008). Children living in rural areas and close to bodies of water appear to be at greatest risk, with lack of parental supervision being noted as a factor across most studies.

Risk Factors for Self-directed Violence

World Report on Violence and Health provides a comprehensive overview of known risk factors for suicidal behavior based on the findings of an extensive body of research, primarily in high-income countries, that has examined the role of psychiatric, biological, social, and environmental factors as well as factors related to an individual's life history (De Leo, Bertolote, & Lester, 2002).

Case-control studies, using psychological autopsies (information gathered after death from relatives, healthcare professionals, and medical records), have played an important role in identifying psychiatric risk factors for suicide, as have longitudinal studies. Depression is perhaps the leading psychiatric condition associated with increased risk of suicidal behaviors. Given this type of mental illness is relatively common, it is not surprising that a large proportion of all suicides are believed to be related to this condition. Other conditions associated with increased risk include schizophrenia, anxiety disorders of conduct and personality, impulsivity, and a sense of hopelessness. Alcohol and drug abuse also play significant roles, although the close relationship between the latter and depression makes it difficult to determine the independent contributions of these conditions. Without doubt, another important risk factor is previous suicidal attempt, with some studies suggesting that the risk for persons who have attempted suicide in the past could be as high as 20 to 30 times the risk seen in the general population.

Among the biological and medical markers that have been identified as risk factors, family history of suicide is one of the strongest markers, suggesting the possibility of a genetic predisposition; this contention has been supported by twin studies. Other evidence in support of a biological basis for suicide comes from studies of neurobiological processes, particularly those that have examined serotonin levels in psychiatric patients. Such investigations suggest that altered serotonin levels may, in part, be linked to greater risks of suicide. Suicide may also be the consequence of severe and painful illness, although the extent to which any such relationship is independent of psychiatric illness has not been determined as yet.

Certain negative life events may be precipitating factors for suicide for some individuals, including personal loss (whether through divorce, separation, or death), interpersonal conflict (including bullying), a broken or disturbed relationship, and legal or work-related problems. In particular, studies have shown a higher risk of suicide attempts among victims of violence between intimate partners due to unresolved conflicts, as well as in individuals with a history of physical or sexual abuse in childhood. While in many countries, marriage and children do appear to be protective factors against suicide, those who marry early may not be equally protected. Studies undertaken in Pakistan and China also suggest that married women, especially older married women, may not necessarily be protected (Khan & Reza, 1998; Yip, 1998). In contrast, individuals who are socially isolated appear to be at increased risk, including homosexual adolescents and the elderly.

Social and environmental factors that are believed to increase the risk of suicidal behavior include availability of the means of suicide; a person's place of residence, employment, or immigration status; affiliation with a religion; and economic conditions. Numerous studies, undertaken in a wide range of countries, provide clear evidence that both the ready availability of means of suicide and the lethality of those methods influence the incidence of suicide attempts and completions. Likewise, studies conducted in high-, middle-, and low-income countries show that rural residence is an important risk factor for suicide, possibly related to issues of social isolation and increased accessibility to means of suicide. While some exceptions exist, there does appear to be a consistent relationship between greater religious involvement and lower risk of suicide. Both the economic prosperity of a community and personal economic circumstances appear to be related to risk of suicide as observed in various studies.

Risk Factors for Interpersonal Violence

The quantity and nature of research on the risk factors for interpersonal violence vary across the categories of child maltreatment, intimate-partner violence, youth violence, sexual violence, and elder abuse, as does the extent to which the research has focused on risk factors associated with perpetrators versus risk factors associated with victims.

While certain risk factors are specific to these different types of interpersonal-directed violence and to perpetrators or victims, a number of common risk factors have been observed across at least three of these different categories and to some extent in both high-income and low- and middle-income countries. In terms of individual risk factors, these characteristics include being male and young, abusing alcohol and other drugs, and being a victim of

child abuse or neglect. Family risk factors include low socioeconomic status of the household, marital discord, and parental conflict involving use of violence. Community risk factors include low social capital in the community, high crime levels in the community of residence, and poor access to or inadequate medical care and situational factors. Lastly, societal risk factors include rapid social change (leading to the breakdown of traditional value and social support networks), economic inequality, poverty, weak economic safety nets, poor rule of law and high levels of corruption, a culture of violence, gender inequalities, high firearms availability, and punitive responses to perpetrators and conflict/post-conflict scenarios (Butchart, Phinney, Check, & Villaveces, 2004; Mercy, Butchart, Rosenberg, Dahlberg, & Harvey, 2008; Rosenberg, Butchart, Mercy, Narasimhan, & Waters, 2006).

The following risk factors for *child maltreatment* have been identified through research in various countries, but not all areas of the world; thus one cannot assume that they apply to all social and cultural contexts. Nevertheless, this list does provide an overview of risk factors that should be considered when attempting to understand the causes of child maltreatment in any context (WHO & International Society for Prevention of Child Abuse and Neglect, 2006). Child maltreatment risk factors include characteristics and attributes of the child, and of the parent and caregiver. Of course, while they may have risk factors, children themselves are the victims and are never to blame for the maltreatment. Age is a major risk factor among children who suffer maltreatment. Children younger than four years of age are at greatest risk of severe injury and death from maltreatment, but across all forms of child maltreatment combined, adolescents are at greatest risk. Other risk factors in children include being an unwanted infant or failing to fulfill parental expectations; having special needs, crying persistently, or having abnormal physical features; and demonstrating symptoms of mental ill health, or personality or temperament traits that are perceived as problematic.

Parental or caregiver factors that can increase the risk of child maltreatment include difficulty bonding with a newborn or not nurturing the child; having been maltreated as a child; lacking awareness of child development or having unrealistic expectations; inflicting inappropriate, excessive, or violent punishment; lacking self-control when upset or angry; misusing alcohol or drugs, including during pregnancy; involvement in criminal activity; being depressed or exhibiting feelings of low self-esteem or inadequacy;

and experiencing financial difficulties. Factors within family, friend, intimate-partner, and peer relationships that may increase the risk of child maltreatment include lack of parent–child attachment; physical, developmental, or mental health problems of a family member; family breakdown or violence; being isolated in the community or lacking a support network; breakdown of support in childrearing from the extended family; and discrimination against the family.

Characteristics of communities and societies that can increase the risk of child maltreatment include gender and social inequality; social, economic, health, and education policies that lead to poor living standards or to socioeconomic inequality or instability; lack of adequate housing or services to support families and institutions; high levels of unemployment or poverty; rapid rates of in- and out-migration to neighborhoods; the easy availability of alcohol or a local drug trade; inadequate policies and programs to prevent child maltreatment, child pornography, child prostitution, and child labor; and social and cultural norms that demand rigid gender roles, support the use of corporal punishment or severe physical punishment of children, and diminish the status of the child in parent–child relationships.

Risk factors associated with *youth violence* exist at the level of the individual, relationship, community, and society (Mercy et al., 2002). Individual-level factors include personality and behavioral traits such as hyperactivity; impulsiveness; poor behavioral control; attention problems; history of early aggressive behavior; early involvement with drugs, alcohol, and tobacco; antisocial beliefs and attitudes; low intelligence; low commitment to school and school failure; residence in a single-parent household; experiencing parental separation or divorce at a young age; and exposure to violence and conflict in the family. Additionally, studies show that drunkenness is an important immediate situational factor that can precipitate youth violence.

Factors within family, friend, intimate-partner, and peer relationships that may increase the risk of youth violence include poor monitoring and supervision of children by parents; harsh, lax, or inconsistent disciplinary practices; a low level of attachment between parents and children; low parental involvement in activities; parental substance abuse or criminality; poor family functioning and a low level of family cohesion; low family income; and witnessing violence or experiencing abuse as a child. Associating with delinquent peers has also been linked to violence in young people.

At community and societal levels, poor social cohesion within a community has been linked to higher rates of youth violence, as have rapid urbanization and unemployment leading to the social dislocation of young people and the erosion of informal social controls. Gangs and a local supply of guns and drugs represent a potent mixture that increases the likelihood of youth violence. Factors such as extreme and highly visible socioeconomic inequalities, rapid social and demographic changes in the youth population, and urbanization can also increase the risk of youth violence. The quality of a country's governance—its laws and the extent to which they are enforced, as well as policies for social protection—also has important implications for such violence.

Intimate-partner violence and *sexual violence* share a number of common risk factors, as described in the WHO and London School of Hygiene & Tropical Medicine (in press) document titled *Preventing Intimate Partner and Sexual Violence: Taking Action and Generating Evidence*. Women and men with lower levels of education are at increased risk of victimization and perpetration, respectively, of intimate-partner violence. Childhood sexual abuse is strongly associated with both the perpetration of intimate-partner violence and sexual violence by men as well as the victimization of women in the form of intimate-partner and sexual violence. A diagnosis of antisocial personality disorder is a strong risk factor for the perpetration of both intimate-partner and sexual violence. Alcohol abuse is consistently found to be associated with the perpetration of both types of violence as well. Males who have multiple sexual partners or who are suspected by their partners of infidelity are more likely to perpetrate both intimate-partner and sexual violence. In addition, attitudes that are accepting of violence are strongly associated with perpetration and victimization of such violence.

Risk factors that are specific to intimate-partner violence include a past history of violence, which for both perpetrators and victims is a strong risk factor for future intimate-partner violence. Marital discord and dissatisfaction are strongly associated with both perpetration of and victimization by this kind of violence. Likewise, ineffective court/police responses are associated with intimate-partner violence.

Risk factor research on *elder abuse* is scant. Although a variety of risk factors have been hypothesized to exist, the evidence cited to support many of these hypotheses—such as the significance of caregiver stress—is not convincing. One of the most consistent findings, however, is the important role of social isolation. Additionally, while little empirical evidence has been documented to support this contention, cultural norms relating to ageism and sexism are thought to play an important role in elder abuse.

Risk Factors for Collective Violence

As outlined in greater detail in *World Report on Violence and Health* (Krug et al., 2002), the Carnegie Commission on Preventing Deadly Conflict (1997) has identified a range of factors that either alone or in combination may precipitate the risk of political violence. In brief, these factors include political and economic factors (e.g., lack of democratic processes, unequal access to power, distribution of resources and access to resources, and control over both key natural resources and drug production or trading); societal and community factors (e.g., inequalities between groups, fueling of group fanaticism, and ready availability of weapons); and demographic factors (particularly rapid demographic change).

Interventions to Prevent Unintentional Injuries and Violence

Interventions to prevent unintentional injuries have traditionally been considered in terms of the *three E's*: education, enforcement, and engineering. Such measures are also described within the framework of the Haddon Matrix—that is, in terms of their focus on preventing the occurrence of the injury event, versus minimizing the severity of injury at the time of the injury event, versus minimizing the severity of injury following the injury event. By comparison, interventions aimed at reducing violence have addressed individual, relationship, community, and societal approaches, mirroring the ecological model outlined in the previous section.

While randomized controlled trials, whether they involve individuals or communities, represent the gold standard by which the effectiveness of preventive interventions might best be assessed, such trials remain relatively uncommon in the injury and violence field. Studies comparing the incidence of injury before and after the implementation of an intervention, sometimes with reference to a control population (i.e., a group in which the intervention has not been introduced), more commonly provide the only evidence of effectiveness. Of course, randomized controlled trials are clearly not needed for interventions whose benefits are obvious. In contrast, for other interventions, particularly those that may have modest but important benefits, rigorous evaluation methods are required.

Studies addressing the effectiveness of interventions in low- and middle-income countries, as distinct from their effectiveness in high-income countries, are also relatively uncommon. While the proven efficacy of some interventions in high-income countries does not require replication in low- and middle-income countries (e.g., the use of motorcycle helmets), strategies that may be effective in increasing the rates of helmet wearing in high-income countries may not necessarily be appropriate in low- and middle-income countries; thus specific evidence of their effectiveness is required. Tailoring of the interventions found effective in high-income countries to ensure that they are appropriate in low- and middle-income countries, with rigorous evaluation to confirm their applicability, is thus increasingly being endorsed.

Interventions to Prevent Road Traffic Injuries

"Safer systems, safer roads, safer vehicles, and safer people" is the motto employed by those working to reduce road traffic injuries (Peden et al., 2004). In the public health sector, much of the emphasis in terms of interventions has, not surprisingly, focused on the last of these elements (WHO, 2009).

Safer Systems

A focus on safer systems involves managing exposure to the risk of a road traffic injury, through appropriate transport and land use policies. In particular, it involves implementing strategies aimed at reducing motor vehicle traffic, encouraging use of safer modes of traffic, and minimizing exposure to high-risk scenarios. Reductions in motor vehicle traffic are possible through application of efficient fuel taxes, land use restrictions, and safety impact assessments of transport and land use plans; by the provision of shorter, safer routes; and through trip reduction measures, including greater emphasis on the development and use of public transport systems. Minimizing exposure to high-risk scenarios includes strategies such as restricting access to different parts of the road network, giving priority in the road network to higher-occupancy vehicles or to pedestrians and slow-moving transport, placing restrictions on speed and engine performance of motorized two-wheelers, separating different traffic modes, increasing the legal age for operating motorized two-wheelers, and introducing graduated driver licensing systems. While it seems obvious that the implementation of these strategies should lead to reductions in road traffic injuries, limited documentation of their effectiveness is available.

Safer Roads

Intervention strategies focusing on safer roads need to incorporate safety awareness in planning road networks, safety features in road design, and remedial action at high-risk crash sites. Although they may not have been examined in rigorously controlled studies, many of these strategies have been adapted and adopted over many years in both high-income and low- and middle-income countries.

Traffic calming measures are among the strategies recommended with respect to incorporating safety features into road design. Systematic reviews of the evidence confirm that traffic-calming measures do reduce road traffic injuries, although evidence from randomized controlled trials is not yet available (Bunn, Collier, Frost, Ker, Roberts, & Wentz, 2003; Retting, Ferguson, & McCartt, 2003). Although most of the evidence cited in support of these measures comes from high-income countries, a "before and after" study conducted in Ghana showed clearly that speed bumps were effective in reducing traffic injuries and especially pedestrian injuries (Afukaar, Antwi, & Ofosu-Amah, 2003).

The introduction of speed cameras (designed to capture images of drivers violating speed limits) and other speed enforcement devices has also been shown to be highly cost-effective in reducing road traffic injuries. Nevertheless, the quality of these studies remains low and relatively few have been conducted in low- and middle-income countries (ICF Consulting & Imperial College Centre for Transport Studies, 2003; Wilson, Willis, Hendrikz, & Bellamy, 2006).

Other safety features that might be incorporated into road design include provisions for slow-moving traffic and for vulnerable road users, lanes for overtaking other road users, median barriers, street lighting, advisory speed limits, and systematic removal of roadside hazards, such as trees or utility poles (Beyer & Ker, 2009; Peden et al., 2004).

Safer Vehicles

Strategies focusing on safer vehicles that have been suggested as likely to decrease the incidence of road traffic injuries include improving the visibility of vehicles, crash-protective vehicle design, and further development of *intelligent vehicles*. However, in low- and middle-income countries, strategies that simply ensure regular maintenance of older vehicles may be effective, although evidence to support this hypothesis is limited. Specifically, it has been suggested that vehicle regulation/licensing and inspection has the potential to be a cost-effective means of ensuring that safer vehicles are used in low- and middle-income countries (Peden et al., 2004).

Meta-analyses of the effects of (automatic) daytime running lights on cars have consistently shown that they decrease the frequency of road crashes, including pedestrian and cycle crashes (Elvik & Vaa,

2004). Similar positive effects of daytime running lights on motorcycles have been shown in low- and middle-income countries (Radin Umar et al., 1996; Yuan, 2000).

The installation and maintenance of seat belts in cars, including child restraint systems, is probably the most well-known and most effective crash vehicle design strategy. However, data from the surveys conducted for the Global Status Report showed that more than one-fourth of all countries that manufacture or assemble cars do not require that seat belts be fitted (Peden et al., 2009). Among other intelligent vehicle devices that might prove useful in low- and middle-income countries are speed limiters and alcohol ignition interlock devices.

Safer People

In recent decades, effective intervention strategies aimed at improving road user behavior have increasingly focused on the introduction and enforcement of relevant legislation, combined with enforcement and education, rather than advocating educational efforts alone (Poli de Figueiredo, Rasslan, Bruscagin, Cruz, & Rocha e Silva, 2001). Many of these legislative intervention strategies have addressed speeding, alcohol use and driving, motorcycle helmet use, seat belts, and child restraints (Peden et al., 2009). However, despite this focus, only 48% of countries have national and subnational laws relating to all five of these risk factors. Even when legislation has been passed, enforcement of the laws is often weak, especially in low- and middle-income countries.

A large body of research—albeit little of it conducted in low- and middle-income countries—shows that the setting and enforcement of speed limits can lead to reductions of as much as 34% in road traffic injuries (Peden et al., 2004). Similarly, numerous studies demonstrate that the setting and enforcement of legal blood alcohol limits, minimum drinking-age laws, and use of alcohol checkpoints lead to important reductions in road traffic injuries of varying magnitude (Peden et al., 2004).

Both bicycle helmets and, in particular, motorcycle helmets have been shown to have a significant impact in reducing head injuries among riders (Liu et al., 2008; Thompson et al., 2003). The introduction of mandatory seat belt laws and mandatory child restraint laws has been shown to have a major impact in reducing occupant deaths and injuries—as much as 25% decreases have been noted in some areas (FIA Foundation for the Automobile and Society, 2009). Additionally, systematic reviews have shown the greater effectiveness of enforcement strategies that allow enforcement officers to specifically stop and check seat belt use (primary enforcement) compared with strategies that allow seat belt use to be checked only when other enforcement strategies are the focus of the traffic stop (secondary prevention) (Dinh-Zarr et al., 2001; Rivara, Thompson, Beahler, & MacKenzie, 1999). Moreover, many studies have shown that enforcement needs to be selective, highly visible, and well publicized; conducted over a sufficiently long period; and repeated several times a year (Jonah, Dawson, & Smith, 1982; Jonah & Grant, 1985; Solomon, Ulmer, & Preusser, 2002).

Interventions to Prevent Poisonings

The prevention of unintentional poisonings includes consideration of both occupational and non-occupational poisonings, including household poisonings. Efforts to prevent occupational exposures include the promotion, legislation, and enforcement of nonchemical methods of pest control and the promotion of the safe use of pesticides when nonchemical methods are not feasible. Interventions such as these largely fall within the domain of specialists working in occupational and environmental health and are not considered further in this chapter.

Suggested interventions to reduce exposure to non-occupational poisonings include better storage of poisonings, in terms of both the storage position and the nature of the storage vessels (Nixon, Spinks, Turner, & McClure, 2004; Peden et al., 2008). With respect to the former, the suggested interventions include storing poisonous materials outside the home, and at levels beyond the reach of children (above head height). With respect to the nature of the storage containers, it has been suggested that efforts need to be directed toward reducing the use of *secondhand* household containers (e.g., cola bottles), including the introduction and enforcement of legislation to prohibit sales of poisons in such containers (Nhachi & Kasilo, 1994). While these interventions clearly have merit, evidence demonstrating their effectiveness is lacking.

The efficacy of child-resistant containers (CRCs) in preventing access to poisons has been demonstrated, however. According to data from a controlled "before and after" study undertaken in South Africa, the free distribution of CRCs appears to be a highly effective means of preventing poisoning in children (Krug, Ellis, Hay, Mokgabudi, & Robertson, 1994).

Other interventions that have been suggested, but not rigorously examined, include the use of warning labels on poison packaging, appropriate first aid education, and the introduction of poison control centers that are charged with monitoring the incidence of poisonings and providing appropriate preventive advice (Nixon et al., 2004; Peden et al., 2008). Likewise, home safety education and the provision of safety education have been proposed as potentially effective interventions; while the available evidence appears promising, the impact of such interventions on poisoning rates is unclear (Kendrick, Smith et al., 2008).

Interventions to Prevent Fall-Related Injuries

Fall-Related Injuries in Older People

In community-dwelling individuals, exercise interventions show the greatest promise in reducing the risk and rate of falls, including multiple-component group exercise, Tai Chi, and individually prescribed multiple-component home-based exercise (Gillespie et al., 2009). Assessment and multifactorial interventions reduce the rate of falls but not the risk of falling, as does gradual withdrawal of psychotropic medication. Overall, vitamin D supplementation does not reduce the risk of falls, although this measure may well do so in persons with lower vitamin D levels. Similarly, home safety interventions do not reduce falls overall, but are effective in preventing falls among persons with visual impairment and among others at higher risk of falling. Other effective interventions are directed toward individuals who reside in certain living environments and those with specific medical conditions (Gillespie et al., 2009).

Some evidence indicates that multifactorial interventions can reduce both number of falls and risk of falling in hospitals, and may do so in nursing care facilities as well. Vitamin D supplementation is also effective in reducing the rate of falls in nursing care facilities. By comparison, exercise in subacute hospital settings appears effective, but its effectiveness in nursing care facilities remains uncertain (Cameron et al., 2010).

Hip protectors initially appeared to be a promising intervention to reduce the impact of a fall in older people. More recently, a growing number of studies have questioned the effectiveness of these devices, given the relatively poor compliance rates that are achieved in real-life settings (Parker, Gillespie, & Gillespie, 2006).

Fall-Related Injuries in Younger People

The *World Report on Child Injury Prevention* document (Peden et al., 2008) highlights a number of areas where interventions have been shown to be effective or appear promising. These strategies include engineering measures focused on the redesign of equipment, such as nursery equipment, and environmental measures that focus on the redesign of playgrounds or buildings. Previous successes with the Children Can't Fly program in low-income areas in the United States have been replicated in low-income countries, where the use of window guards have been shown to be a promising approach to the prevention of falls from buildings. By comparison, while educational strategies for the prevention of falls in children might seem to be appealing at first glance, there is still little evidence to show the effectiveness of such approaches in reducing the rates of falls (Kendrick, Watson et al., 2008).

Interventions to Prevent Burn-Related Injuries

Limited evidence supports the effectiveness of interventions to prevent fire-related injuries, in large part reflecting the paucity of research in this area. Studies in high-income countries have focused on the effectiveness of smoke detector giveaway programs, community- and school-based educational campaigns, and community-based burns prevention measures. Unfortunately, the most rigorous of the studies—a randomized, controlled trial of a smoke detector giveaway program in inner-city London—did not demonstrate any evidence of effectiveness in terms of reduced incidence of fires and fire-related injuries (DiGuiseppi et al., 2002).

Interventions that have been proposed but not yet shown to be effective largely rely on reducing exposure to fires and flames (Peden et al., 2008). These measures include separating cooking areas from living areas (including efforts to reduce the use of indoor fires for cooking), ensuring cooking surfaces are at appropriate heights, reducing the storage of flammable substances in households, and providing for greater supervision of younger children. Some other promising interventions, involving the introduction of safer lamps and stoves, are currently being implemented in low-income countries (Peden et al., 2008).

Evidence for the effectiveness of interventions to prevent water-related burn injuries is minimal, but promising. In an increasing number of high-income countries, much effort has been directed toward measures that not only educate communities about the dangers of high tap water temperatures, but also legislate and enforce efforts to regulate the temperature of water flowing from household taps (Macarthur, 2003). In contrast, in low-income countries, scalds due to hot water are more likely to be associated with cooking and boiling of water, rather than water from taps. Consequently, interventions related to the separation of the cooking areas from living and play areas have been emphasized, as well as suggestions that cooking vessels holding water might be better designed to minimize the chances of spillage.

Finally, interventions directed at increasing awareness of burns prevention (whether fire or water related) have been proposed, especially given the success of *safe community* interventions involving a multitude of strategies (Ytterstad & Sogaard, 1995). To date, there is limited evidence to show that such interventions have been successful (Turner, Spinks, McClure, & Nixon, 2004).

Interventions to Prevent Drowning

Evidence for the effectiveness of interventions to prevent drowning, whether in high- or low-income countries, is almost nonexistent. The only data providing some evidence of effectiveness have come from case-control studies undertaken in high-income countries, suggesting that fencing of domestic swimming pools reduces the risks of drowning (Thompson & Rivara, 2000). Extrapolation of these findings to a low-income setting would suggest that measures to limit exposure to bodies of water close to dwellings might be effective in reducing drowning rates. Examples that have been proposed include covering wells with grills, fencing lakes or riverbanks that are close to residences, and building flood control embankments (Peden et al., 2008).

The effectiveness of learn-to-swim programs, while a common component of prevention programs in high-income countries and increasingly in low- and middle-income countries, has not been examined in rigorously controlled studies. Similarly, education regarding the burden and risk factors for drowning, especially the risks posed by prior consumption of alcohol, has also been postulated as a potential intervention strategy (Celis, 1991). Increased supervision of children around bodies of water and the provision of life guards at popular swimming areas have been proposed as other measures that might reduce drowning (Hyder et al., 2003).

Interventions to prevent water-related transport drowning include equipping boats with flotation devices, ensuring that boats and flotation devices are well maintained, introducing legislation and enforcing regulations relating to the maximum numbers of individuals who may be carried on specific types of boats, and providing fully trained and responsive coast guard services (WHO, 2003). However, as with the preventive measures proposed to prevent non-transport-related drowning, evidence of these interventions' effectiveness is lacking (Peden et al., 2008).

Interventions to Prevent Self-directed Violence

Although many interventions to prevent self-directed violence have been available for some time, there is very limited evidence to show their effectiveness in terms of actual reductions in suicidal behavior (Daniel & Goldston, 2009; De Leo et al., 2002). Individual approaches to prevention include both treatment approaches and behavioral approaches. Treatment approaches focus on identifying and managing (primarily with pharmacotherapy) mental disorders that have been shown to be associated with increased risk of self-directed violence. Behavioral therapy approaches seek to identify situations and issues that may place individuals at high risk and consider ways in which individuals can be better equipped to address these situations. Relationship approaches to prevention focus on enhancing social relationships so as to reduce repeated suicidal behaviors.

Community-based prevention efforts include encouraging attendance at suicide prevention centers and self-help groups and school-based interventions that involve training of school staff, community members, and healthcare providers to identify those persons at risk and refer them to treatment. By comparison, societal approaches include both restricting access to the means of suicide and managing media reports of suicides. Attempts to limit the availability of suicide means have included reducing access to sedatives, pesticides, carbon monoxide in domestic gas and in car exhausts, and handguns in the home. Safer storage, bans, and replacement of pesticides with less toxic alternatives could prevent many of the estimated 370,000 suicides caused by ingestion of these chemicals every year. Although international conventions have long attempted to manage hazardous substances, many highly toxic pesticides continue to be widely used. Research suggests, however, that bans must be accompanied by evaluations of agricultural needs and replacement with low-risk alternatives for pest control.

Interventions to Prevent Interpersonal Violence

This section is adapted from the 2009 WHO and John Moores University publication titled "Violence Prevention: The Evidence," a set of seven briefings based on rigorous reviews of the literature examining scientific evidence for the effectiveness of interventions to prevent interpersonal violence. Each briefing focuses on a broad strategy for preventing violence, and under that umbrella, reviews the evidence for the effectiveness of specific interventions.

This section summarizes the headline findings from each of the seven briefings and spotlights the specific interventions within each strategy that have the strongest evidence for preventing violence. Table 8-3 presents an overview of the results, indicating for each intervention the strength of the evidence for its effectiveness and the types of interpersonal violence it has been found to prevent.

Developing Safe, Stable, and Nurturing Relationships Between Children and Their Parents and Caregivers

Some interventions that encourage nurturing relationships between parents (or caregivers) and children in their early years have been shown to prevent child maltreatment and reduce childhood aggression (e.g., Bilukha et al., 2005; Geeraert, Van de Noortgate, Grietans, & Onghenea, 2004; Kaminski, Valle, Filene, & Boyle, 2008; MacLeod & Nelson, 2000; Nelson, Laurendeau, & Chamberland, 2001). These types of interventions also have the potential to prevent the lifelong negative consequences of child maltreatment on mental and physical health, social and occupational functioning, human capital and security, and, ultimately, social and economic development. An emerging body of evidence suggests that such measures may reduce criminal convictions and violent acts in adolescence and early adulthood, and probably help to decrease intimate-partner violence and self-directed violence in later life (Caldera, Burrell, Rodriguez, Crowne, Rohde, & Duggan, 2007; Olds et al., 1998).

High-quality trials in the United States and other developed countries have shown that both the Nurse–Family Partnership home-visiting program (Olds, Sadler, & Kitzman, 2007) and the Positive Parenting Program (Triple P; Prinz, Sanders, Shapiro, Whitaker, & Lutzker, 2009) reduce child maltreatment. In home-visiting programs, trained personnel visit parents and children in their homes and provide health advice, support, child development education, and life coaching for parents to improve child health, foster parental caregiving abilities, and prevent child maltreatment. Parenting education is usually center-based and delivered in groups; it aims to prevent child maltreatment by improving parents' childrearing skills, increasing parental knowledge of child development, and encouraging positive child management strategies. Evidence also suggests that parent and child programs—which typically incorporate parenting education along with child education, social support, and other services—may prevent child maltreatment and youth violence later in life.

As evidence for the effectiveness of these parenting and parent–child programs in high-income

Table 8-3	Overview of Violence Prevention Interventions with Some Evidence of Effectiveness, by Types of Violence Prevented					
Intervention	**Type of Violence**					
	CM	**IPV**	**SV**	**YV**	**EA**	
1. Developing safe, stable, and nurturing relationships between children and their parents and caregivers						
Parent training, including nurse home visitation	●			○		
Parent–child programs	○			○		
2. Developing life skills in children and adolescents						
Preschool enrichment programs				○		
Social development programs				●		
3. Reducing the availability and harmful use of alcohol						
Regulating sales of alcohol			○			
Raising alcohol prices			○			
Interventions for problem drinkers		●				
Improving drinking environments				○		
4. Reducing access to guns						
Restrictive firearm licensing and purchase policies				○		
Enforced bans on carrying firearms in public				○		
5. Promoting gender equality to prevent violence against women						
School-based programs to address gender norms and attitudes		●	○			
Microfinance combined with gender equity training		○				
Life-skills interventions		○				
6. Changing cultural and social norms that support violence						
Social marketing to modify social norms		○	○			
7. Victim identification, care, and support programs						
Screening and referral		○				
Advocacy support programs		●				
Psychosocial interventions			○			
Protection orders		○				

Key:
●: Well supported by evidence (multiple randomized, controlled trials with different populations)
○: Emerging evidence

Note: CM: child maltreatment; IPV: intimate-partner violence; SV: sexual violence; YV: youth violence; EA: elder Abuse.
Source: Adapted from WHO-Liverpool John Moores University, 2009.

countries continues to expand, the time is ripe to initiate their large-scale implementation and outcome evaluation in low- and middle-income countries (Mikton & Butchart, 2009).

Developing Life Skills in Children and Adolescents

Evidence shows that the life skills acquired in social development programs—which are aimed at building social, emotional, and behavioral competencies—can prevent youth violence (Botvin, Griffin, & Nichols, 2006; Hahn et al., 2007; Hawkins, Catalano, Kosterman, Abbott, & Hill, 1999; Wilson & Lipsey,

2007). In addition, preschool enrichment programs—which provide children with academic and social skills at an early age—appear promising (Nelson, Westhues, & MacLeod, 2003; Reynolds, Ou, & Topitzes, 2004; Reynolds, Temple, & Ou, 2003). Life skills help children and adolescents effectively deal with the challenges of everyday life. When such programs target children early in life, they can help prevent aggression, reduce involvement in violence, improve social skills, boost educational achievement, and improve job prospects. These effects are most pronounced in children from poor families and neighborhoods. The benefits of high-quality programs that invest early in an individual's life also have the potential to produce benefits that last well into adulthood.

To date, most of the research on life-skills programs has been conducted in high-income countries, particularly the United States. More evidence is needed on how such preschool enrichment and social development programs would affect children in low- and middle-income countries.

Reducing the Availability and Harmful Use of Alcohol

It has long been thought that violence might be prevented by reducing the availability of alcohol, through brief interventions and longer-term treatment for problem drinkers, and by improving the management of environments where alcohol is served. Evidence for the effectiveness of such interventions has rarely been obtained in randomized controlled trials; in addition, such evidence comes chiefly from high-income countries and some parts of Latin America.

Alcohol availability can be regulated by restricting the hours or days it can be sold and by reducing the number of alcohol retail outlets (Cohen, 2007; Douglas, 1998; Duailibi, Ponicki, Grube, Pinsky, Laranjeira, & Raw, 2007; Guerrero & Concha-Eastman, 2008; Nemtsov, 1998). Reduced sales hours have generally been found to be associated with reduced violence and higher outlet densities with higher levels of violence. Economic modeling strongly suggests that raising alcohol prices (e.g., through increased taxes, state-controlled monopolies, and minimum-price policies) can lower consumption and, hence, reduce violence (Grossman & Markowitz, 2001; Markowitz, 2000; Markowitz & Grossman, 1998, 2000).

Brief interventions and longer-term treatment for problem drinkers—using, for instance, cognitive behavioral therapy—have been shown in several trials to reduce several forms of violence, including child maltreatment and intimate-partner violence (Dinh-Zarr, Heitman, Roberts, & DiGuiseppi, 2004). In addition, some evidence supports the effectiveness of interventions in and around drinking establishments that target factors such as crowding, comfort levels, physical design, staff training, and access to late night transport (Bellis & Hughes, 2008; Graham & Homel, 2008).

Reducing Access to Guns

Emerging evidence suggests that limiting access to firearms can prevent homicides and injuries and reduce the costs of these forms of violence to society. More rigorous studies on this topic are needed to more fully elucidate these effects, however (Hahn, Bilukha, Crosby, Fullilove, Liberman, & Moscicki, 2003). Some evidence, for example, indicates that jurisdictions with restrictive firearms legislation and lower firearms ownership tend to have lower levels of gun violence (Conner & Zhong, 2003; Kapusta, Etzersdorfer, Krall, & Sonneck, 2007; Killias, van Kesteren, & Rindlisbacher, 2001; Miller, Hemenway, & Azrael, 2007; Rosengart, Cummings, Nathens, Heagerty, Maier, & Rivara, 2005). Restrictive firearm licensing and purchasing policies—including bans, licensing schemes, minimum ages for buyers, and background checks—have been implemented and appear to be effective in countries as diverse as Australia, Austria, Brazil, and New Zealand. Studies in Colombia and El Salvador indicate that enforced bans on carrying firearms in public may reduce homicide rates (e.g., Marinho de Souza, Macinko, Alencar, Malta, & de Morais Neto, 2007; Villaveces, Cummings, Espitia, Koepsell, McKnight, & Kellermann, 2000).

Promoting Gender Equality to Prevent Violence Against Women

Although further research in this area is needed, some evidence shows that school and community interventions can promote gender equality and prevent violence against women by challenging stereotypes and cultural norms that give men power and control over women. School-based programs can address gender norms and attitudes before they become deeply engrained in children and youth. Studies of the Safe Dates program in the United States (Foshee, Bauman, Arriaga, Helms, Koch, & Linder, 1998; Foshee, Bauman, Ennett, Suchindran, Benefield, & Linder, 2005) and the Youth Relationship Project in Canada (Wolfe et al., 2009), which also addresses dating violence, have reported positive results, for example.

Outcome evaluation studies are beginning to support community interventions that aim to prevent violence against women by promoting gender equality. Notably, some evidence suggests that programs that combine microfinance with gender equity training can reduce intimate-partner violence. Some of the strongest support for this concept has come from the IMAGE initiative in South Africa, which combines microloans and gender equity training (Kim et al., 2007; Pronyk et al., 2006). Another intervention for which evidence of effectiveness is building is the Stepping Stones program in Africa and Asia; this life-skills training program addresses gender-based violence, relationship skills, assertiveness training, and communication about HIV (Jewkes et al., 2008; Paine et al., 2002).

Changing Cultural and Social Norms That Support Violence

Rules or expectations of behavior—that is, norms—within a cultural or social group can encourage violence. Interventions that challenge cultural and social norms supportive of violence can prevent acts of violence and have been widely used, although the evidence base for their effectiveness is currently weak. Further rigorous evaluations of such interventions are required.

The effectiveness of interventions addressing dating violence and sexual abuse among teenagers and young adults by challenging social and cultural norms related to gender is supported by some evidence (e.g., Bruce, 2002; Fabiano, Perkins, Berkowitz, Linkenbach, & Stark, 2003). Other interventions also appear promising, including those targeting youth violence and education through entertainment ("edutainment") aimed at reducing intimate partner violence (e.g., Usdin, Scheepers, Goldstein, & Japhet, 2005).

Victim Identification, Care, and Support Programs

Interventions to identify victims of interpersonal violence and provide effective care and support are critical for protecting health and breaking cycles of violence from one generation to the next.[1]

Evidence of effectiveness is emerging for the following interventions: screening tools to identify victims of intimate-partner violence and refer them to appropriate services (Olive, 2007; Ramsay, Richardson, Carter, Davidson, & Feder, 2002); psychosocial interventions—such as trauma-focused cognitive behavioral therapy—to reduce mental health problems associated with violence, including post-traumatic stress disorder (Kornør et al., 2008; Roberts, Kitchiner, Kenardy, & Bisson, 2009); and protection orders, which prohibit a perpetrator from contacting the victim (Holt, Kernic, Wolf, & Rivara, 2003; McFarlane et al., 2004), to reduce repeat victimization. Several trials have shown that advocacy support programs—which offer services such as advice, counseling, safety planning, and referral to other agencies—enhance victims' safety behaviors and reduce the likelihood of their experiencing further harm (McFarlane, Groff, O'Brien, & Watson, 2005, 2006).

Interventions to Prevent Collective Violence

The prevention of collective violence involves reducing the potential for violent conflicts and providing appropriate responses to violent conflicts when they occur. Not surprisingly, scientific evidence about the effectiveness of such interventions is lacking (Zwi, Garfield, & Loretti, 2002). Nevertheless, policies that facilitate reductions in poverty, that make decision making a more accountable process, that reduce inequalities between groups, and that reduce access to biological, chemical, nuclear, and other weapons have been recommended. When planning responses to violent conflicts, recommended approaches include assessing at an early stage which populations are most vulnerable and what their needs are, coordinating the activities of the various players, and working toward global, national, and local capabilities so as to deliver effective health services during the various stages of an emergency (Zwi et al., 2002).

The Role of Health Services in Preventing Death and Disability from Unintentional Injuries and Violence

While the focus of this section has been on identifying strategies to prevent the occurrence of injuries, it is important to recognize that access to health services plays a major role in preventing death and disability from injuries and violence. Differential access to health and medical services has been identified in other fields of health as having an important bearing on long-term outcomes, and the importance of such services is now being increasingly recognized in the injury field (Razzak & Kellermann, 2002).

For example, although prehospital transport systems exist in major cities in low- and middle-income countries, the prehospital care that is delivered to trauma victims in the field is minimal or nonexistent in rural areas. This lack of quality emergency medical services care and timely transport to the hospital translates into higher mortality rates. Significant reductions in mortality have been reported as a result of improvements in trauma care (Mock, Lormand, Joshipura, Goosen, & Peden, 2004). WHO has recently suggested that even in environments where fewer resources are available, injury mortality and disability can be reduced by reorganizing systems, upgrading of the skills of health staff, and ensuring minimum physical and human resources are available (Mock, Quansah, Krishnan, Arreola-Risa, & Rivara, 2004).

---

[1]The briefing does not cover the area of prehospital and emergency medical care, as this topic is already addressed by the following sources: Mock, C., Juillard, C., Brundage, S., Goosen J., & Joshipura, M. (Eds.). (2009). *Guidelines for trauma quality improvement programmes*. Geneva, Switzerland: World Health Organization; Mock, C., Lormand, J-D., Goosen, J., Joshipura, M., & Peden, M. (2004). *Guidelines for essential trauma care*. Geneva, Switzerland: World Health Organization; Sasser, S., Varghese, M., Kellermann, A., & Lormand, J-D. (2005). *Prehospital trauma care systems*. Geneva, Switzerland: World Health Organization.

Economic Analyses of Interventions to Prevent Unintentional Injuries and Violence

Currently, there is a dearth of literature on economic evaluations of interventions for injuries, in large part reflecting the infancy of this field and the limited, but growing evidence base identifying effective preventive strategies. Unfortunately, even for interventions that are routinely used in high-income countries, proof of their cost-effectiveness is not always easy to find. The situation is even more critical in low- and middle-income countries, where evaluations of these interventions are rarely available.

Exemplifying this paucity as well as the potential importance of such data are two reviews that documented economic analyses of interventions directed at reducing road traffic injuries (Hyder, Waters, Philipps, & Rehwinkel, 2004; Waters, Hyder, & Phillips, 2004). These reviews, which relied on mostly data from high-income countries, suggest that interventions such as mandatory helmet laws, laws mandating motor vehicle inspections, installation of automatic daytime running lights, and seat belt laws are likely to provide widespread benefits with high benefit–cost ratios, even in low- and middle-income countries.

Costs of interventions for injuries were analyzed as part of the Disease Control Priorities project (www.dcp2.org; Norton, Hyder, Bishai, & Peden, 2006). Specifically, Bishai and Hyder (2006) estimated the cost-effectiveness of five interventions that could reduce injuries in lower- and middle-income countries: enforcing traffic laws more strictly, erecting speed bumps, promoting helmets for bicycles, promoting helmets for motorcycles, and storing kerosene in child-proof containers. They estimated what each intervention would cost in six world regions over a 10-year period from both governmental and societal perspectives, with costs being measured in U.S. dollars for 2001. Some data were available on the effectiveness of each intervention and were used to form models of DALYs averted by each strategy for various regions. The interventions had cost-effectiveness ratios ranging from $5 to $556 per DALY averted, depending on the region. Enhanced speeding control, for example, was found to be highly cost-effective at $93 per DALY. Similarly, at $13.98 per DALY, placing speed bumps at 25% of the most dangerous junctions turned out to be highly cost-effective, though this measure requires the identification of such intersections. Bicycle helmet legislation is not universally implemented in the high-income world, yet its cost-effectiveness ($170 per DALY) makes it an attractive option. Interestingly, motorcycle helmet legislation in East Asia was found to have a higher cost and lower benefit at $556 per DALY. At $96 per DALY, child-resistant containers are a highly cost-effective intervention that warrants serious consideration by a large part of the low- and middle-income world where paraffin (kerosene) is used, including sub-Saharan Africa, South Asia, East Asia, and parts of the Middle East.

Empirical work conducted in low- and middle-income countries remains rare; however, a recent example is a study that examined the costs and potential effectiveness of increasing traffic enforcement in Uganda, as assessed on the four major roads to the capital Kampala (Bishai, Asiimwe, Abbas, Hyder, & Bazeyo, 2008). By using monthly data on traffic citations and casualties for the years 2001 to 2005 and employing time series regression, costs were computed from the perspective of the police department. The average cost-effectiveness of better road safety enforcement in Uganda was determined to be $603 per death averted or $27 per life year saved discounted at 3% (amounting to 1.5% of Uganda's $1,800 GDP per capita).

Although relatively few economic evaluations of interventions targeting interpersonal violence have been published, the available studies suggest that behavioral, legal, and regulatory interventions cost less money than they save, in some cases by several orders of magnitude (Waters, Hyder, Rajkotia et al., 2004). A review of the costs and benefits of early intervention programs to prevent child maltreatment concluded that some home-visiting programs targeting high-risk/low-income mothers returned between $2 and $3 for each dollar spent (Aos, Lieb, Mayfield, Miller, & Pennucci, 2004). In a further review of nine early childhood programs, seven were found to be cost-effective, yielding between $2 and $17 in benefits for every dollar invested (Kilburn & Karoly, 2008). Despite this benefit, both reviews concluded that not all childhood interventions are cost-effective, with some being ineffective and very expensive. Little research has been conducted into the cost-effectiveness of preventive strategies for other types of violence; along with outcome evaluation studies, such investigations should be a research priority.

Advancing the Injury and Violence Prevention Agenda: Opportunities and Challenges

In the past decade, our knowledge about the burden of injuries and violence, as well as risk factors and effective interventions addressing these issues, has increased exponentially. In many high-income countries, the benefits of this increased knowledge have resulted in significant declines in injury and violence-related mortality and morbidity rates. In contrast, for many low- and middle-income countries, increases in rates of injury and violence are predicted over the next 20 years, as a result of both changing sociodemographic patterns and these countries' success in addressing the burden of communicable disease and maternal and child ill health. Consequently, there is an imperative to rapidly advance an injury and violence prevention agenda, while recognizing that many of the challenges faced by low- and middle-income countries will be different to those that have been faced in the previous two decades.

Advocacy for Injury and Violence Prevention

It remains critical that the global health community fully understand the health, economic, and social impacts of unintentional injuries and violence. It is equally important that the health sector recognize that clearly defined risk factors for injuries and violence exist and that effective interventions can prevent these problems and reduce the burden of death and disability they give rise to. However, despite the recent efforts by WHO and many injury and violence prevention professionals throughout the world, many governments and the wider community fail to recognize that injuries are no "accident" and that violence does not just happen—and that we can work to prevent increases in the incidence of these conditions. For this reason, targeted and evidence-based advocacy is essential at local, national, and international levels.

The key messages to be transmitted in advocacy efforts are as follows: Injuries and violence cause considerable death and disability; they are predictable events with clearly identified causes; and they can be effectively prevented. Moreover, there is a great need, especially in low- and middle- income countries, to initiate national dialogues around key injury issues and stimulate an intersectoral approach to address them. The recent WHO reports on violence and health, on road traffic injury prevention, and on child injury prevention, for example, propose such an approach to national stakeholders and stress the need for national ownership and local action (Krug et al., 2002; Peden et al., 2004; Peden et al., 2008). Some early successes can be seen at the global level. For example, at the ministerial summit on global road safety held in Moscow in 2009, national leaders pledged their support for the "decade of global road safety 2010–2020." Only months later, the United Nations General Assembly passed a resolution on global road safety in 2010. This resolution, which was cosponsored by more than 90 countries, calls on all member states to pay attention to the increasing burden of road traffic injuries and encourages governments to invest in evidence-based efforts to improve road safety.

The emergence of violence prevention as a key component of the global health agenda can in part be ascribed to the role played by the World Health Assembly and its partner organizations in highlighting violence prevention and injury prevention in general. Since the publication of *World Report on Violence and Health* in 2002, two World Health Assembly resolutions have called on countries to invest in violence prevention; by 2010, three out of six WHO regional committees (Africa, the Americas, and Europe) had adopted similar resolutions. The inclusion of violence prevention on the agenda of other multilateral agencies is also a useful indication of its emergence as a global priority. The World Bank's Disease Control Priorities, for example, included a single chapter on all types of injuries and violence in its first edition in 1993; by comparison, the second edition, which was published in 2006, had an entire chapter dedicated to interpersonal violence, another chapter addressing unintentional injuries, and a third chapter on trauma care. The United Nations General Assembly has also reviewed special reports on violence against children, violence against women, and armed violence, which have resulted in resolutions calling for greater investment in multisectoral efforts to address these forms of violence.

Research and Development Needs

To date, global investments for injury and violence research and interventions, compared with investments made in other health areas, do not match the burden of disease. For example, road traffic injuries have been identified as a highly neglected area for investments compared with the burden of disease they represent, measured in dollars per DALY (approximately $0.40 per DALY), especially when considered in relation to other major health problems (Ad Hoc Committee on Health Research Relating to Future Intervention Options, 1996). Given this fact, it is not surprising that national analyses of safety investments have demonstrated very low investment rates in low-income countries such as Pakistan and Uganda—approximately $0.07 per person in Pakistan (Bishai, Hyder, Ghaffar, Morrow, & Kobusingye, 2003). There are some notable recent exceptions, such as the investments announced in 2009 by Bloomberg Philanthropies to establish model intervention areas in 10 countries to demonstrate the impact of road traffic injury prevention and control measures. Consequently, while we already know a great deal about the burden, causes, and effective interventions for injuries and violence, significant gains in our understanding of these factors could be made if equitable resources were directed to the field.

Given that 90% of the world's population lives in low- and middle-income countries, and the burden of injuries and violence is predicted to increase in these countries, it is imperative that future research and development activities focus especially on the needs of these countries. While it would be inappropriate to outline a detailed agenda for future research and developments that is relevant to all countries, a generic framework that encompasses the types of research required can be recommended.

Epidemiological research describing the existing burden, causes, and distribution of unintentional injuries and violence is still needed in low- and middle-income countries. Assessing the loss of health and life from unintentional injuries and violence, identifying the populations affected by these conditions, and determining the specific circumstances in which they occur, represent a continuing research agenda for low- and middle-income countries. Problems of under-reporting and other biases in available data need to be addressed as well.

Of course, it is critical not only to identify the determinants of unintentional injuries and violence, but also to address them. The lack of *intervention research* in low- and middle-income countries has left a huge gap in health research globally. Scientific trials of injury and violence prevention interventions have largely not been conducted in these countries, and there is a great need to modify, adapt, and test both existing and proposed interventions in these settings. While some might argue that such research should be a priority in most low- and middle-income countries, unless the basic research on the burden and determinants of unintentional injuries and violence has been undertaken, the political and financial support for such research will not be forthcoming.

The lack of empirical information on the cost-effectiveness of injury and violence prevention interventions remains a major policy issue, especially given that interventions used in high-income countries might potentially be transferred to low- and middle-income countries without regard to their appropriateness or relevance in the latter regions. Perhaps equally important is the concern that without such research, highly cost-effective interventions will not be implemented at all. *Policy-oriented research* that identifies the barriers to implementation and translation of research findings is, therefore, an essential component in advancing the injury and violence prevention agenda.

The Significance of a Trained Workforce

Research and programs in the field of unintentional injuries and violence require trained individuals with specific skills and tools. Injury and violence prevention is a science replete with conceptual frameworks, epidemiological approaches, intervention testing methods, and analytical techniques. Well-developed training programs in high-income countries have emerged that can produce a workforce who can carry the injury and violence prevention agenda forward. At present, the general lack of such trained human resources in the low- and middle-income world means that capacity development for human resources must necessarily focus on developing capacity in these countries.

Issues of both quantity and quality arise with regard to the development of a trained workforce. Clearly, there needs to be a critical mass of trained injury and violence prevention professionals in a country if authorities there are to understand, develop, and implement interventions. At the same time, the field covers a broad range of topics, so a wide diversity of skills is needed for prevention. Epidemiology, statistics, health information systems, health policy, economics, sociology, and criminology—these are merely some of the fields that have a role in reducing the burden of disease from injuries and violence. In this context, the role of the public health sector is both to assume leadership in developing and organizing a response to injuries and violence and to facilitate the inputs provided by other fields and disciplines. For this reason, management and leadership skills are important assets for a well-trained workforce in injury and violence prevention.

Efforts to address these capacity development needs are being implemented both in high-income countries and in low- and middle-income countries. For example, WHO has created a teaching curriculum (TEACH-VIP) that may be freely used in training programs and courses and that covers all basic aspects of injury prevention and control (http://www.who.int/violence_injury_prevention/media/news/2010/13_01_2010/en/index.html). It focuses on enhancing the knowledge base of participants and their technical foundations for work in the injury field.

WHO also has a free mentoring program (MENTOR-VIP) that allows people from low- and middle-income countries to enroll in a one-year mentoring relationship with more experienced colleagues from around the world (http://www.who.int/violence_

injury_prevention/capacitybuilding/mentor_vip/en/). The mentoring program focuses on hands-on learning and the development of specific skills for practicing injury prevention and control.

Other examples of capacity building include the work by partner organizations such as the Road Traffic Injuries Research Network (www.rtirn.net), which facilitates the development of both junior and senior researchers from low- and middle-income countries who are seeking to develop their research skills in road traffic injuries research.

The Roles of National and International Organizations

The roles of national agencies (e.g., ministries of health and medical research councils), international organizations (e.g., the United Nations Development Program [UNDP], WHO, and the World Bank), and international societies (e.g., the International Society for Child and Injury Prevention [http://iscaip.net/iscaip/] and the International Society for Violence and Injury Prevention [http://www.isvip.org/]) need to be emphasized in advancing the injury and violence prevention agenda.

The roles of national organizations include the following:

- *Advocacy*: accepting ownership of the problem and promoting engagement with other national institutions
- *Implementation*: developing policy and ensuring programs are available on the ground in countries for addressing injuries and violence
- *Evaluation*: a continuous process of assessing interventions and programs, in addition to supporting nationally relevant research

The role of international organizations and societies can be summarized as follows:

- *Strategic*: first internally recognizing the toll on societies of injuries and violence, and then convincing governments externally to appreciate the same (as has been done in the case of road traffic injuries by the joint World Bank–WHO report in 2004 and for child injuries by the joint WHO–UNICEF report in 2008)
- *Facilitation*: providing technical assistance, appropriate advice, and relevant tools for national policies and action

- *Resource mobilization*: demonstrating true commitment to supporting the implementation of effective interventions in countries and promoting research in the field

The international movements currently under way for violence prevention and road traffic injuries prevention are examples of how joint global–national partnerships are needed for making change.

Conclusions

Unintentional injuries and violence represent a major global health problem, and one that will increase in magnitude unless systematic, scientifically based approaches to prevention are implemented. While the public health community has recognized the significance of the global injury epidemic only relatively recently, much new knowledge has been generated in a very short time. Much of this new knowledge has focused on the burden of injury in high-income countries, however. Thus the challenge for the future is to extend our knowledge to the growing injury and violence burden faced by low- and middle-income countries.

The international public health community has an important role to play in addressing this challenge, by facilitating the description of the problem, the development of solutions, the implementation of programs, and the analysis of effects. Moreover, the public health community can play a leadership role in galvanizing a multisectoral response to injuries and violence, advocating for investments at national and international levels, and catalyzing the sharing of experiences around the world. The large and often devastating health impacts of injuries and violence make it imperative that the international public health community not only take an interest in these issues, but also be proactive in addressing the burden of disease from injuries and violence at local, national, and international levels.

In summary, injuries are no "accident," and violence does not just happen; rather, these are highly predictable and preventable events. The international public health community has already played an important role in taking this message forward. The challenge is to continue to do so, so that the predicted epidemics of unintentional injuries and violence in low- and middle-income countries can be prevented.

• • • Discussion Questions

1. Why should public health programs in low- and middle-income countries address injuries and violence?

2. List three indicators you would expect to change as a result of a road traffic injury program in a country. Which data do you need to measure these changes? How will you obtain the data?

3. Choose a specific type of injury. Which steps can be taken to reduce the burden of this injury in low- and middle-income countries?

4. Suppose you were funding research on injuries and violence. Describe five topics or studies that would be your priority for research in low- and middle-income countries.

5. Compare and contrast how the prevention of violence and unintentional injuries differ in respect to their use of passive versus active prevention strategies.

• • • References

Ad Hoc Committee on Health Research Relating to Future Intervention Options. (1996). *Investing in health research and development.* (Document TDK/Gen/96.1). Geneva, Switzerland: World Health Organization.

Aeron-Thomas, A., Jacobs, G. D., Sexton, B., Gururaj, G., & Rahmann, F. (2004). *The involvement and impact if road crashes on the poor: Bangladesh and India case studies* (Published Project Report No. PRP 010). Crowthorne, UK: Transport Research Laboratory.

Afukaar, F. K., Antwi, P., & Ofosu-Amah, S. (2003). Pattern of road traffic injuries in Ghana: Implications for control. *Injury Control and Safety Promotion, 10*(1–2), 69–76.

Aos, S., Lieb, J., Mayfield, J., Miller, M., & Pennucci, A. (2004). *Benefits and costs of prevention and early intervention programs for youth.* Olympia, WA: Washington State Institute for Public Policy.

Azizi, B. H., Zulkifli, H. I., & Kasim, M. S. (1993). Risk factors for accidental poisoning in urban Malaysian children. *Annals of Tropical Paediatrics, 13*(2), 183–188.

Bellis, M. A., & Hughes, K. (2008). Comprehensive strategies to prevent alcohol-related violence. *IPC Review, 2,* 137–168.

Bener, A. (2009). Emerging trend in motorisation and the epidemic of road traffic crashes in an economically growing country. *International Journal of Crashworthiness, 14*(2), 183–188.

Beyer, F. R., & Ker, K. (2009). Street lighting for preventing road traffic injuries. *Cochrane Database of Systematic Reviews, 1,* CD004728.

Bilukha, O., Hahn, R. A., Crosby, A., Fullilove, M. T., Liberman, A., Moscicki, E., et al. (2005). The effectiveness of early childhood home visitation in preventing violence: A systematic review. *American Journal of Preventive Medicine, 28,* 11–39.

Bishai, D., Asiimwe, B., Abbas, S., Hyder, A. A., & Bazeyo, W. (2008). Cost-effectiveness of traffic enforcement: Case study from Uganda. *Injury Prevention, 14,* 223–227.

Bishai, D., & Hyder, A. (2006). Modeling the cost effectiveness of injury interventions in lower and middle income countries: opportunities and challenges. *Cost Effectiveness and Resource Allocation, 4*(1), 2.

Bishai, D., Hyder, A. A., Ghaffar, A., Morrow, R. H., & Kobusingye, O. (2003). Rates of public investment for road safety in developing countries: Case studies of Uganda and Pakistan. *Health Policy and Planning, 18*(2), 232–235.

Botvin, G. J., Griffin, K. W., & Nichols, T.D. (2006). Preventing youth violence and delinquency through a universal school-based prevention approach. *Prevention Science, 7,* 403–408.

Brenner, R. A. (2003). Prevention of drowning in infants, children and adolescents. *Pediatrics, 112*(2), 440–445.

Brown, D. W., Riley, L., Butchart, A., & Kann, L. (2008). Bullying among youth from eight African countries and associations with adverse health behaviours: Global school-based student health survey. *Pediatric Health, 2*(3), 289–299.

Bruce, S. (2002). *The "A Man" campaign: Marketing social norms to men to prevent sexual assault. The report on social norms* (Working paper no. 5). Little Falls, NJ: PaperClip Communications.

Bunn, F., Collier, T., Frost, C., Ker, K., Roberts, I., & Wentz, R. (2003). Traffic calming for the prevention of road traffic injuries: Systematic review and meta-analysis. *Injury Prevention, 9*(3), 200–204.

Butchart, A., Brown., D., Khanh-Huynh, A., Corso, P., Florquin, N., & Muggah, R. (2008). *Manual for estimating the economic costs of injuries due to interpersonal and self-directed violence.* Geneva, Switzerland: World Health Organization.

Butchart, A., Phinney, A., Check, P., & Villaveces, A. (2004). *Preventing violence: A guide to implementing the recommendations of the World Report on Violence and Health.* Geneva, Switzerland: Department of Injuries and Violence Prevention, World Health Organization.

Caldera, D., Burrell, L., Rodriguez, K., Crowne, S. S., Rohde, C., & Duggan, A. (2007). Impact of a statewide home visiting program on parenting and on child health and development. *Child Abuse & Neglect, 31*(8), 829–852.

Cameron, I. D., Robinovitch, S., Birge, S., Kannus, P., Khan, K., Lauritzen, J., et al. (2010). Hip protectors: recommendations for conducting clinical trials – an international consensus statement (part II). *Osteoporosis International, 21*(1), 1–10.

Carlini-Cotrim, B., & da Matta Chasin, A.A. (2000). Blood alcohol content and death from fatal injury: A study in metropolitan area of Sao Paulo, Brazil. *Journal of Psychoactive Drugs, 32*(3), 269–275.

Celis, A. (1991). Drowning in Jalisco: 1983–1989. *Saluda Publica Mexico, 33*(6), 585–589.

Chatsantiprapa, K., Chokkanapitak, J., & Pinpradit, N. (2001). Host and environment factors for exposure to poisons: A case control study of preschool children in Thailand. *Injury Prevention, 7*(3), 214–217.

Chew, F. L., Yong, C. K., Mas Ayu, S., & Tajunisah, I. (2010). The association between various visual function tests and low fragility hip fractures among the elderly: A Malaysian experience. *Age and Ageing, 39*(2), 239–245.

Cohen, A. B. (2007). *Sobering up: The impact of the 1985–1988 Russian anti-alcohol campaign on child health.* Tufts University. Retrieved from http://www.cid.harvard.edu/neudc07/docs/neudc07_s3_p01_cohen.pdf

Conner, K. R., & Zhong, Y. (2003). State firearm laws and rates of suicide in men and women. *American Journal of Preventive Medicine, 25,* 320–324.

Coutinho, E. S., Bloch, K. G., Rodrigues, L. C. (2009). Characteristics and circumstances of falls leading to severe fractures in elderly people in Rio de Janeiro, Brazil. *Cadernos de Saúde Pública, 25*(2), 455–459.

Craig, W., Harel-Fisch, Y., Fogel-Grinvald, H., Dostaler, S., Hetland, J., Simons-Morton, B., et al. (2009). A cross-national profile of bullying and victimization among adolescents in 40 countries. *International Journal of Public Health, 54*(2 suppl), 216–224.

Daniel, S. S., & Goldston, D. B. (2009). Interventions four suicidal youth: A review of the literature and developmental considerations. *Suicide & Life-threatening Behavior, 39*(3), 252–268.

Danseco, E. R., Miller, T. R., & Spicer, R. S. (2000). Incidence and costs of 1987–1994 childhood injuries: Demographic breakdowns. *Pediatrics, 105*(2), E27.

De Leo, D., Bertolote, J.M., & Lester, D. (2002). Self-directed violence. In E. Krug, L.L. Dahlberg, J.A. Mercy, A.B. Zwi & R. Lozano (Eds.), *World report on violence and health* (pp. 183–212). Geneva, Switzerland: World Health Organization.

DiGuiseppi, C., Roberts, I., Wade, A., Sculpher, M., Edwards, P., Godward, C., et al. (2002). Incidence of fires and related injuries after giving out free smoke alarms: Cluster randomized controlled trial. *British Medical Journal, 325*(7371), 995.

Dinh-Zarr, T. B., Heitman, C., Roberts, E., & DiGuiseppi, C. (2004). Interventions for preventing injuries in problem drinkers [review]. *Cochrane Database of Systematic Reviews, 3,* CD001857.

Dinh-Zarr, T. B., Sleet, D. A., Shults, R. A., Zaza, S., Elder, R. W., Nichols, J. L., et al. (2001). Reviews of evidence regarding interventions to increase the use of safety belts. *American Journal of Preventive Medicine, 21*(4 suppl), 48–65.

Donroe, J., Tincopa, M., Gilman, R. H., Brugge, D., & Moore, D. A. (2008). Pedestrian road traffic injuries in urban Peruvian children and adolescents: Case control analyses of personal and environmental risk factors. *PLoS One, 3*(9), e3166.

Douglas, M. (1998). Restriction of the hours of sale of alcohol in a small community: A beneficial impact. *Australian and New Zealand Journal of Public Health, 22,* 714–719.

Driscoll, T. R., Harrison, J. A., & Steenkamp, M. (2004). Review of the role of alcohol in drowning associated with recreational aquatic activity. *Injury Prevention, 10*(2), 107–113.

Duailibi, S., Ponicki, W., Grube, J., Pinsky, I., Laranjeira, R., & Raw, M. (2007).The effect of restricting opening hours on alcohol-related violence. *American Journal of Public Health, 97,* 2276–2280.

Elvik, R., & Vaa, T. (2004). *Handbook of road safety measures.* Amsterdam: Elsevier.

Fabiano, P. M., Perkins, H. W., Berkowitz, A., Linkenbach, J., & Stark, C. (2003). Engaging men as social justice allies in ending violence against women: Evidence for a social norms approach. *Journal of American College Health, 52*(3), 105–112.

FIA Foundation for the Automobile and Society. (2009). *Seat-belts and child restraints: A road safety manual for decision-makers and practitioners.* London: Author.

Foshee, V. A., Bauman, K. E., Arriaga, X. B., Helms, R. W., Koch, G. G., & Linder, G. F. (1998). An evaluation of Safe Dates, an adolescent dating violence prevention program. *American Journal of Public Health, 88,* 45–50.

Foshee, V. A., Bauman, K. E., Ennett, S. T., Suchindran, C., Benefield, T., & Linder, G. F. (2005). Assessing the effects of the dating violence prevention program "Safe Dates" using random coefficient regression modelling. *Prevention Science, 6,* 245–257.

García-Moreno, C., Jansen, H., Ellsberg, M., Heise, L., & Watts, C. (2005). *WHO multi-country study on women's health and domestic violence against women.* Geneva, Switzerland: World Health Organization.

Geeraert, L., Van de Noortgate, W., Grietans, H., & Onghenea, P. (2004). The effects of early prevention programs for families with young children at risk for physical child abuse and neglect: A meta-analysis. *Child Maltreatment, 9,* 277–291.

Gillespie, L. D., Robertson, M. C., Gillespie, W. J., Lamb, S. E., Gates, S., Cumming, R. G., Rowe, B. H. (2009) Interventions for preventing falls in older people living in the community. *Cochrane Database Systematic Reviews, 2,* CD007146.

Global Road Safety Partnership. (2007). *Drinking and driving: A road safety manual for decision-makers and practitioners.* Geneva, Switzerland: Author.

Global Road Safety Partnership. (2008). *Speed management: A road safety manual for decision-makers and practitioners.* Geneva, Switzerland: Author.

Graham, K., & Homel, R. (2008). Raising the bar: Preventing aggression in and around bars, pubs and clubs. Portland, OR: Willan.

Grossman, M., & Markowitz, S. (2001). Alcohol regulation and violence on college campuses. In M. Grossman & C.R. Hsieh (Eds.), *Economic analysis of substance use and abuse: The experience of developed countries and lessons for developing countries.* (pp. 257–289). Cheltenham, UK: Edward Elgar.

Guerrero, R., & Concha-Eastman, A. (2008). An epidemiological approach for the prevention of urban violence: The case of Cali, Colombia. Retrieved from http://www.longwoods.com/content/17590

Haddon, W. Jr. (1968). The changing approach to the epidemiology, prevention, and amelioration of trauma: The transition to approaches etiologically rather than descriptively based. *American Journal of Public Health and the Nation's Health, 58*(8), 1431–1438.

Hahn, R. A., Bilukha, O. O., Crosby, A., Fullilove, M. T., Liberman, A., & Moscicki, E. K. (2003). First reports evaluating the effectiveness of strategies for preventing violence: Firearms laws. *Morbidity and Mortality Weekly Report, 52*(RR14), 11–20.

Hahn, R., Fuqua-Whitley, D., Wethington, H., Lowy, J., Liberman, A., Crosby, A., et al. (2007). The effectiveness of universal school-based programs for the prevention of violent and aggressive behavior: A report on recommendations of the Task Force on Community Preventive Services. *Morbidity and Mortality Weekly Report: Recommendations and Reports, 56,* 1–12.

Hawkins, J. D., Catalano, R. F., Kosterman, R., Abbott, R., & Hill, K. G. (1999). Preventing adolescent health-risk behaviors by strengthening protection during childhood. *Archives of Pediatrics & Adolescent Medicine, 153,* 226–234.

Heise, L., & García-Moreno, C. (2002). Violence by intimate partners. In E. Krug, L. L. Dahlberg, J. A. Mercy, A. B. Zwi, & R. Lozano (Eds.), *World report on violence and health* (pp. 87–121). Geneva, Switzerland: World Health Organization.

Hippisley-Cox, J., & Coupland, C. (2009). Predicting risk of osteoporotic fracture in men and women in England and Wales: Prospective derivation and validation of QFractureScores. *British Medical Journal, 339,* b4229.

Holt, V. L., Kernic, M. A., Wolf, M. E., & Rivara, F. P. (2003). Do protection orders affect the likelihood of future partner violence and injury? *American Journal of Preventive Medicine, 24*(1), 16–21.

Hyder, A. A., Arifeen, S., Begum, N., Fishman, S., Wali, S., & Baqui, A.H. (2003). Death from drowning: Defining a new challenge for child survival in Bangladesh. *Injury Control and Safety Promotion, 10*(4), 205–210.

Hyder, A. A., Waters, H., Philipps, T., & Rehwinkel, J. (2004). *Exploring the economics of motorcycle helmet laws: Implications for low and middle-income countries.* Baltimore, MD: Johns Hopkins University.

ICF Consulting & Imperial College Centre for Transport Studies. (2003). *Cost–benefit analysis of road safety improvements: Final report.* London: ICF Consulting.

Jacobs, G., Aeron-Thomas, A., & Astrop, A. (2000). *Estimating global road fatalities* (TRL Report 445). Crowthorne, UK: Transport Research Laboratory.

Jaye, C., Simpson, J. C., & Langley, J. D. (2001). Barriers to safe hot tap water: Results from a national study of New Zealand plumbers. *Injury Prevention, 7,* 302–306.

Jewkes, R., Nduna, M., Levin, J., Jama, N., Dunkle, K., Puren, A., & Duvvury, N. (2008). Impact of stepping stones on incidence of HIV and HSV-2 and sexual behaviour in rural South Africa: Cluster randomised controlled trial. *British Medical Journal, 337,* a506. doi: 10.1136/bmj.a506

Jewkes, R., Sen, P., & Garcia-Moreno, C. (2002). Sexual violence. In E. Krug, L. L. Dahlberg, J. A. Mercy, A. B. Zwi, & R. Lozano (Eds.), *World report on violence and health* (pp. 149–181). Geneva, Switzerland: World Health Organization.

Jiang, X., Zhang, Y., Wang, Y., Wang, B., Xu, Y., & Shang, L. (2010). An analysis of 6215 hospitalized unintentional injuries among children aged 0–14 in northwest China. *Accident Analysis & Prevention, 42*(1), 320–326.

Jitapunkul, S., Yuktananandana, P., & Parkpian, V. (2001). Risk factors of hip fracture among Thai female patients. *Journal of the Medical Association of Thailand, 84*(11), 1576–81.

Jonah, B. A., Dawson, N. E., & Smith, G. A. (1982). Effects of a selective traffic enforcement program on seat belt usage. *Journal of Applied Psychology, 67*(1), 89–96

Jonah, B. A., & Grant, B. A. (1985). Long-term effectiveness of selective traffic enforcement programs for increasing seat belt usage. *Journal of Applied Psychology, 70*(2), 257–263.

Kaminski, J. W, Valle, L. A., Filene, J. H., & Boyle, C. L. (2008). A meta-analytic review of components associated with parent training program effectiveness. *Journal of Abnormal Child Psychology, 36,* 567–589.

Kapusta, N. D., Etzersdorfer, E., Krall, C., & Sonneck, G. (2007). Firearm legislation reform in the European Union: The impact on firearm availability, firearm suicide and homicide rates in Austria. *British Journal of Psychiatry, 191,* 253–257.

Kendrick, D., Smith, S., Sutton, A., Watson, M., Coupland, C., Mulvaney, C., & Mason-Jones, A. (2008). Effect of education and safety equipment on poisoning-prevention practices and poisoning: Systematic review, meta-analysis and meta-regression. *Archives of Disease in Childhood, 93*(7), 599–608.

Kendrick, D., Watson, M. C., Mulvaney, C. A., Smith, S. J., Sutton, A. J., Coupland, C. A., & Mason-Jones, A. J. (2008). Preventing childhood falls at home: Meta-analysis and meta regression. *American Journal of Preventive Medicine, 35*(4), 370–379.

Khan, M. M., & Reza, H. (1998). Gender differences in non-fatal suicidal behavior in Pakistan: Significance of sociocultural factors. *Suicide and Life-Threatening Behavior, 28,* 62–68.

Kilburn, R., & Karoly, L. A. (2008). *The economics of early childhood policy: What the dismal science has to say about investing in children* (OP-227-CFP). Santa Monica, CA: RAND Corporation. Retrieved from http://www.rand.org/pubs/occasional_papers/OP227/

Killias, M., van Kesteren, J., & Rindlisbacher, M. (2001.) Guns, violent crime, and suicide in 21 countries. *Canadian Journal of Criminology, 43,* 429–448.

Kim, J. C., Watts, C. H., Hargreaves, J. R., Ndhlovu, L. X., Phetla, G., Morison, L. A., et al. (2007.) Understanding the impact of a microfinance-based intervention on women's empowerment and the reduction of intimate partner violence in South Africa. *American Journal of Public Health*, 97(10), 1794–1802.

Kloeden, C. N., McLean, A. J., Baldock, M. R. J., & Cockington, A. J. T. (1998). *Severe and fatal car crashes due to roadside hazards: A report to the Motor Accident Commission.* Adelaide, Australia: National Health and Medical Research Council Road Accident Research Unit, University of Adelaide.

Kobusingye, O., Guwatudde, D., & Lett, R. (2001). Injury patterns in rural and urban Uganda. *Injury Prevention, 7*(1), 46–50.

Kopits, E., & Cropper, M. (2003). *Traffic fatalities and economic growth* (Policy Research Working Paper 3035). Washington, DC: World Bank.

Kornør, H., Winje, D., Ekeberg, Ø., Weisæth, L., Kirkehei, I., Johansen, K., & Steiro, A. (2008). Early trauma-focused cognitive-behavioural therapy to prevent chronic post-traumatic stress disorder and related symptoms: A systematic review and meta-analysis. *BMC Psychiatry, 8,* 81.

Krug, A., Ellis, J. B., Hay, I. T., Mokgabudi, N. F., & Robertson, J. (1994). The impact of child-resistant containers on the incidence of paraffin (kerosene) ingestion in children. *South African Medical Journal, 84*(11), 730–734.

Krug, E., Dahlberg, L. L., Mercy, J. A., Zwi, A. B., & Lozano R. (Eds.). (2002). *World report on violence and health.* Geneva, Switzerland: World Health Organization.

Liu, B. C., Ivers, R., Norton, R., Boufous, S., Blows, S., & Lo, S. K. (2008). Helmets for preventing injury in motorcycle riders. *Cochrane Database of Systematic Reviews, 1,* CD004333.

Liu, G. F., Han, S., Liang, D. H., Wang, F. Z., Shi, X. Z., Yu, J., & Wu, Z. L. (2003). Driver sleepiness and risk of car crashes in Shenyang, a Chinese northeastern city: Population-based case-control study. *Biomedical and Environmental Sciences, 16*(3), 219–226.

Macarthur, C. (2003). Evaluation of Safe Kids Week 2001: Prevention of scald and burn injuries in young children. *Injury Prevention, 9*(2), 112–116.

MacLeod, J., & Nelson, G. (2000). Programs for the promotion of family wellness and the prevention of child maltreatment: A meta-analytic review. *Child Abuse & Neglect.* 24(9), 1127-49.

Marinho de Souza Mde, F., Macinko, J., Alencar, A. P., Malta, D. C., & de Morais Neto, O. L. (2007). Reductions in firearm-related mortality and hospitalizations in Brazil after gun control. *Health Affairs, 26,* 575–584.

Markowitz, S. (2000). The price of alcohol, wife abuse, and husband abuse. *Southern Economic Journal, 67,* 279–303.

Markowitz, S., & Grossman, M. (1998.) Alcohol regulation and domestic violence towards children. *Contemporary Economic Policy, 16,* 309–320.

Markowitz, S., & Grossman, M. (2000). The effects of beer taxes on physical child abuse. *Journal of Health Economics, 19,* 271–282.

McFarlane, J. M., Groff, J. Y., O'Brien, J. A., & Watson, K. (2005). Behaviors of children following a randomized controlled treatment program for their abused mothers. *Issues in Comprehensive Pediatric Nursing, 28,* 195–211.

McFarlane, J. M., Groff, J. Y., O'Brien, J. A., & Watson, K. (2006). Secondary prevention of intimate partner violence: A randomized controlled trial. *Nursing Research, 55,* 52–61.

McFarlane, J., Malecha, A., Gist, J., Watson, K., Batten, E., Hall, I., & Smith, S. (2004). Protection orders and intimate partner violence: An 18-month study of 150 black, Hispanic, and white women. *American Journal of Public Health, 94*, 613–618.

Mercy, J. A., Butchart, A., Farrington, D., & Cerda, M. (2002). Youth violence. In E. Krug, L. L. Dahlberg, J. A. Mercy, A. B. Zwi, & R. Lozano (Eds.), *World report on violence and health* (pp. 23–56). Geneva, Switzerland: World Health Organization.

Mercy, J. A., Butchart, A., Rosenberg, M. L., Dahlberg, L., & Harvey, A. (2008). Preventing violence in developing countries: A framework for action. *International Journal of Injury Control and Safety Promotion, 15*(4), 197–208.

Mikton, C., & Butchart A. (2009). Child maltreatment prevention: A systematic review of reviews. *Bulletin of the World Health Organization, 87*(5), 353–361.

Miller, M., Hemenway, D., & Azrael, D. (2007). State-level homicide victimization rates in the US in relation to survey measures of household firearm ownership, 2001–2003. *Social Science and Medicine, 64*, 656–664.

Mock, C. J., Jurkovich, G. J., nii-Amon-Kotei, D., Arreola-Risa, C., & Maier, R. V. (1998). Trauma mortality patterns in three nations at different economic levels: Implications for global trauma system development. *Journal of Trauma, 44*(5), 804–812.

Mock, C., Lormand, J. P., Joshipura, M., Goosen, J., & Peden, M. (2004). *Guidelines for essential trauma care.* Geneva, Switzerland: World Health Organization.

Mock, C., Quansah, R., Krishnan, R., Arreola-Risa, C., & Rivara, F. (2004). Strengthening the prevention and care of injuries worldwide. *Lancet, 363*(9427), 2172–2179.

Mohan, D. (2002). Road safety in less-motorized environments: Future concerns. *International Journal of Epidemiology, 31*(3), 527–532.

Nafukho, F. M., & Khayesi, M. (2002). Livelihood, conditions of work, regulation, and road safety in the small-scale public transport sector: A case of the matatu mode of transport in Kenya. In X. Godard & I. Fatouzoun (Eds.), *Urban mobility for all: Proceedings of the Tenth International CODATU Conference, Lome, Togo, 12–15 November 2002* (pp. 241–425). Lisse, Netherlands: AA Balkema.

Nelson, G., Laurendeau, M., & Chamberland, C. (2001). A review of programs to promote family wellness and prevent the maltreatment of children. *Canadian Journal of Behavioural Science, 33*, 1–13.

Nelson, G., Westhues, A., & MacLeod, J. (2003). A meta-analysis of longitudinal research on preschool prevention programs for children. *Prevention and Treatment, 6*, 31.

Nemtsov, A. V. (1998). Alcohol-related harm and alcohol consumption in Moscow before, during and after a major anti-alcohol campaign. *Addiction, 93*, 1501–1510.

Nhachi, C. F., & Kasilo, O. M. (1994). Household chemicals poisoning admissions in Zimbabwe's main urban centres. *Human and Experimental Toxicology, 13*(2), 69–72.

Nixon, J., Spinks, A., Turner, C., & McClure, R. (2004). Community based programs to prevent poisoning in children 0–15 years. *Injury Prevention, 10*(1), 43–46.

Norton, R., Hyder, A., Bishai, D., & Peden, M. (2006). Unintentional injuries. In D. Jamison, J. Breman, A. Measham, G. Alleyne, M. Claeson, & D. Evans (Eds.), *Disease control priorities in developing countries* (pp. 737–753). New York: Oxford University Press.

Odero, W., Garner, P., & Zwi, A. B. (1997). Road traffic injuries in developing countries: A comprehensive review of epidemiological studies. *Tropical Medicine and International Health, 2*(5), 445–460.

Odero, W. O., & Zwi, A. B. (1995). Alcohol-related traffic injuries and fatalities in LMICs: A critical review of literature. In C. N. Kloeden & A. J. McLean (Eds.), *Proceedings of the 13th International Conference on Alcohol, Drugs and Traffic Safety, Adelaide, 13–18 August 1995* (pp. 713–720). Adelaide, Australia: Road Accident Research Unit.

Olds, D., Henderson, C. R. Jr., Cole, R., Eckenrode, J., Kitzman, H., Luckey, D., et al. (1998). Long-term effects of nurse home visitation on children's criminal and antisocial behavior: 15-year follow-up of a randomized controlled trial.

Journal of the American Medical Association, 280(14), 1238–1244.

Olds, D. L., Sadler, L., & Kitzman, H. (2007). Programs for parents of infants and toddlers: Recent evidence from randomized trials. *Journal of Child Psychology and Psychiatry,* 48, 355–391.

Olive, P. (2007). Care for emergency department patients who have experienced domestic violence: A review of the evidence base. *Journal of Clinical Nursing,* 16, 1736–1748.

Paine, K., Hart, G., Jawo, M., Ceesay, S., Jallow, M., Morison, L., et al. (2002). "Before we were sleeping, now we are awake": Preliminary evaluation of the Stepping Stones sexual health programme in the Gambia. *African Journal of AIDS Research,* 1, 41–52.

Parker, M. J., Gillespie, W. J., & Gillespie, L. D. (2006). Effectiveness of hip protectors for preventing hip fractures in elderly people: Systematic review. *British Medical Journal,* 332(7541), 571–574.

Peden, M., Oyebite, K., Ozanne-Smith, J., Hyder, A. A., Branche, C., Rahman, F. A. K. M., et al. (Eds.). (2008). *World report on child injury prevention.* Geneva, Switzerland: World Health Organization.

Peden, M., Scurfield, R., Sleet, D., Mohan, D., Hyder, A. A., Jarawan, E., & Matherc, C. (Eds.). (2004). *World report on road traffic injury prevention.* Geneva, Switzerland: World Health Organization.

Poli de Figueiredo, L. F., Rasslan, S., Bruscagin, V., Cruz, R., & Rocha e Silva, M. (2001). Increases in fines and driver licence withdrawal have effectively reduced immediate deaths from trauma on Brazilian roads: First-year report on the new traffic code. *Injury,* 32(2), 91–94.

Prinz, R. J., Sanders, M. R., Shapiro, C. J., Whitaker, D. J., & Lutzker, J. R. (2009). Population-based prevention of child maltreatment: The U.S. triple P system population trial. *Prevention Science.* doi: 10.1007/s11121-009-0123-3

Pronyk, P. M., Hargreaves, J. R., Kim, J. C., Morison, L. A., Phetla, G., Watts, C., et al. (2006). Effect of a structural intervention for the preven-

tion of intimate-partner violence and HIV in rural South Africa: A cluster randomised trial. *Lancet,* 368(9551), 1973–1983.

Radin Umar, R. S., Mackay, G. M., & Hills, B. L. (1996). Modelling of conspicuity-related motor cycle accidents in Seremban and Shah Alam, Malaysia. *Accident Analysis and Prevention,* 28(3), 325–332.

Ramsay, J., Richardson, J., Carter, Y. H., Davidson, L. L., & Feder, G. (2002). Should health professionals screen women for domestic violence? Systematic review. *British Medical Journal,* 325, 314.

Razzak, J. A., & Kellermann, A. L. (2002). Emergency medical care in developing countries: Is it worthwhile? *Bulletin of the World Health Organization,* 80(11), 900–905.

Retting, R. A., Ferguson, S. A., & McCartt, A. T. (2003). A review of evidence-based traffic engineering measures designed to reduce pedestrian–motor vehicle crashes. *American Journal of Public Health,* 93(9), 1456–1463.

Reynolds, A. J., Ou, S. R., & Topitzes, J. W. (2004). Paths of effects of early childhood intervention on educational attainment and delinquency: A confirmatory analysis of the Chicago child–parent centers. *Child Development,* 75, 1299–1328.

Reynolds, A. J., Temple, J. A., & Ou, S. R. (2003). School-based early intervention and child well-being in the Chicago longitudinal study. *Child Welfare,* 82, 633–656.

Rivara, F. P., Thompson, D. C., Beahler, C., & MacKenzie, E. J. (1999). Systematic reviews of strategies to prevent motor vehicle injuries. *American Journal of Preventive Medicine,* 16(1 suppl), 1–5.

Robb, G., Sultana, S., Ameratunga, S., & Jackson, R. (2008). A systematic review of epidemiological studies investigating risk factors for work-related road traffic crashes and injuries. *Injury Prevention,* 14(1), 51–58.

Robbins, J., Aragaki, A. K., Kooperberg, C., Watts, N., Wastawski-Wende, J., Jaskson, R. D., et al. (2007). Factors associated with 5-year risk of hip fracture in postmenopausal women. *Journal of the American Medical Association,* 298(20), 2389–2398.

Roberts, N. P., Kitchiner, N. J., Kenardy, J., & Bisson, J. I. (2009). Systematic review and meta-analysis of multiple-session early interventions following traumatic events. *American Journal of Psychiatry, 166,* 293–301.

Rosenberg, M., Butchart, A., Mercy, J., Narasimhan, V., & Waters, H. (2006). Interpersonal violence. In D. T. Jamison, J. G. Breman, A. R. Measham, G. Alleyne, M. Claeson, D. B. Evans, et al. (Eds.), *Disease control priorities in developing countries* (2nd ed., pp. 755–770). Washington, DC: Oxford University Press & World Bank.

Rosengart, M., Cummings, P., Nathens, A., Heagerty, P., Maier, R., & Rivara, F. (2005).An evaluation of state firearm regulations and homicide and suicide death rates. *Injury Prevention, 11,* 77–83.

Runyan, D., Wattam, C., Ikeda, R., Hassan, F., & Ramiro, L. (2002). Child abuse and neglect by parents and other caregivers. In E. Krug, L. L. Dahlberg, J. A. Mercy, A. B. Zwi, & R. Lozano (Eds.), *World report on violence and health* (pp. 59–86). Geneva, Switzerland: World Health Organization.

Shannon, M. (2000). Ingestion of toxic substances by children. *New England Journal of Medicine, 342*(3), 186–191.

Sobngwi-Tambekou, J., Bhatti, J., Kounga, G., Salmi, L. R., & Lagarde, E. (2010). Road traffic crashes on the Yaoundé-Douala road section, Cameroon. *Accident Analysis & Prevention, 42*(2), 422–426.

Solomon, M. G., Ulmer, R. G., & Preusser, D. F. (2002). *Evaluation of click it or ticket model programs* (DOT HS-809-498). Washington, DC: National Highway Traffic Safety Administration.

Soori, H. (2001). Developmental risk factors for unintentional childhood poisoning. *Saudi Medical Journal, 22*(3), 227–230.

Thanh, N. X., Hang, H. M., Chuc, N. T., & Lindholm, L. (2003). The economic burden of unintentional injuries: A community-based cost analysis in Bavi, Vietnam. *Scandinavian Journal of Public Health Supplement, 62,* 45–51.

Thompson, D. C., & Rivara, F. P. (2000). Pool fencing for preventing drowning in children. *Cochrane Database of Systematic Reviews, 2,* CD001047.

Thompson, D. C., Rivara, F. P., & Thompson, R. (2003). Helmets for preventing head and facial injuries in bicyclists. *Annals of Emergency Medicine, 41*(5), 738–740.

Turner, C., Spinks, A., McClure, R., & Nixon, J. (2004) Community-based interventions for the prevention of burns and scalds in children. *Cochrane Database Systematic Reviews, 3,* CD004335.

Usdin, S., Scheepers, E., Goldstein, S., & Japhet, G. (2005). Achieving social change on gender-based violence: A report on the impact evaluation of Soul City's fourth series. *Social Science and Medicine, 61,* 2434–2445.

Van Schoor, O., van Niekerk, J., & Grobbelaar, B. (2001). Mechanical failures as a contributing cause to motor vehicle accidents: South Africa. *Accident Analysis and Prevention, 33*(6), 713–721.

Villaveces, A., Cummings, P., Espitia, V. E., Koepsell, T. D., McKnight, B., & Kellermann, A. L. (2000). Effect of a ban on carrying firearms on homicide rates in 2 Colombian cities. *Journal of the American Medical Association, 283*(9), 1205–1209.

Warda, L., Tenenbein, M., & Moffatt, M. E. K. (1999). House fire injury prevention update. Part I: A review of risk factors for fatal and non-fatal house fire injury. *Injury Prevention, 5*(3), 145–150.

Waters, H. R., Hyder, A. A., & Phillips, T. L. (2004). Economic evaluation of interventions for reducing road traffic injuries: A review of literature with applications to low and middle-income countries. *Asia Pacific Journal of Public Health, 16*(1), 23–31.

Waters, H., Hyder, A., Rajkotia, Y., Basu, S., Rehwinkel, J. A., & Butchart, A. (2004). *The economic dimensions of interpersonal violence.* Geneva, Switzerland: World Health Organization.

Wilson, C., Willis, C., Hendrikz, J. K., & Bellamy, N. (2006). Speed enforcement detection devices for preventing road traffic injuries. *Cochrane Database of Systematic Reviews, 2,* CD004607.

Wilson, S. J., & Lipsey, M. W. (2007). School-based interventions for aggressive and disruptive behavior: Update of a meta-analysis. *American Journal of Preventive Medicine, 33,* S130–S143.

Wolf, R., Daichman, L., & Bennett, G. (2002). Abuse of the elderly. In E. Krug, L. L. Dahlberg, J. A. Mercy, A. B. Zwi, & R. Lozano (Eds.), *World report on violence and health* (pp. 125–145). Geneva, Switzerland: World Health Organization.

Wolfe, D. A., Crooks, C., Jaffe, P., Chiodo, D., Hughes, R., Ellis, W., et al. (2009). A school-based program to prevent adolescent dating violence: A cluster randomized trial. *Archives of Pediatrics & Adolescent Medicine, 163*(8), 692–699.

Woratanarat, P., Ingsathit, A., Suriyawongpaisal, P., Rattanasiri, S., Chatchaipun, P., Wattayakorn, K., & Anukarahanonta, T. (2009). Alcohol, illicit and non-illicit psychoactive drug use and road traffic injury in Thailand: A case-control study. *Accident Analysis & Prevention, 41*(3), 651–657.

World Health Organization (WHO). (2003). *Drowning fact sheet.* Geneva, Switzerland: Author.

World Health Organization (WHO). (2009). *Global status report on road safety: Time for action.* Geneva, Switzerland: Author. Retrieved from www.who.int/violence_injury_prevention/road_safety_status/2009

World Health Organization (WHO) & International Society for Prevention of Child Abuse and Neglect. (2006). *Preventing child maltreatment: A guide to taking action and generating evidence.* Geneva, Switzerland: WHO.

World Health Organization (WHO) & Liverpool John Moores University. (2009). Violence prevention: The evidence (an eight-part series of briefings). Retrieved March 31, 2010, from http://www.who.int/violence_injury_prevention/violence/4th_milestones_meeting/publications/en/index.html

World Health Organization (WHO) & London School of Hygiene & Tropical Medicine. (In press). *Preventing intimate partner and sexual violence: Taking action and generating evidence.* Geneva, Switzerland: WHO.

World Health Statistics. (2008). Retrieved from http://www.who.int/whosis/whostat/2008/en/index.html

Yip, P. S. F. (1998). Age, sex, marital status and suicide: An empirical study of East and West. *Psychological Reports, 82,* 311–322.

Ytterstad, B., & Sogaard, A. J. (1995). The Harstad injury prevention study: Prevention of burns in small children by a community-based intervention. *Burns, 21*(4), 259–266.

Yuan, W. (2000). The effectiveness of the "Ride Bright" legislation for motorcycles in Singapore. *Accident Analysis and Prevention, 32*(4), 559–563.

Zaloshnja, E., Miller, T. R., Lawrence, B. A., & Romano, E. (2005). The costs of unintentional home injuries. *American Journal of Preventive Medicine, 28*(1), 88–94.

Zhao, X. G., He, X. D., Wu, J. S., Zhao, G. F., Ma, Y. F., Zhang, M., et al. (2009). Risk factors for urban road traffic injuries in Hangzhou, China. *Archives of Orthopaedic and Trauma Surgery, 129*(4), 507–513.

Zwi, A. B., Garfield, R., & Loretti, A. (2002). Collective violence. In E. Krug, L. L. Dahlberg, J. A. Mercy, A. B. Zwi, & R. Lozano (Eds.), *World report on violence and health* (pp. 213–239). Geneva, Switzerland: World Health Organization.

Global Mental Health

VIKRAM PATEL, ALAN J. FLISHER, AND ALEX COHEN

Introduction

For the purposes of this chapter, we consider the definition of "mental health" to include all conditions that affect the nervous system that are leading causes of disease burden. Conditions with a vascular or infectious etiology, such as HIV infection of the brain or cerebrovascular diseases, are excluded here, as they are addressed in other chapters.

Based on the criteria of burden (discussed later), mental disorders include intellectual disability (or mental retardation), epilepsy, anxiety and mood disorders (AMD), psychoses (schizophrenia and bipolar disorders), substance use disorders (alcohol and drug use disorders), and dementia. Thus this list of health conditions includes disorders that clinicians may categorize as psychiatric, neurological, or substance use disorders. This chapter uses the acronym MNS disorders (meaning "mental, neurological, and substance use disorders") as proposed by the World Health Organization's Mental Health Gap Action (mhGAP) program (WHO, 2008c) to denote this group of conditions.

Collectively, between 10% and 20% of the general population suffer from one or more of the MNS disorders. These disorders have been increasingly recognized as a major contributor to the burden of global ill health and disability (Mathers & Loncar, 2006), including in low- and middle-income countries, in spite of the coexisting burden of infectious and other noncommunicable diseases. This double burden can be partly attributable to the epidemiological and demographic transitions evident in most countries, and it leads to unique challenges in securing a prominent place for mental health in global health policy. There are strong linkages between MNS disorders and other health and social concerns, including several Millennium Development Goals (MDGs)—notably, gender equity, poverty, HIV/AIDS, primary education, and maternal and child health. This evidence is the rationale for the slogan that there is "no health without mental health" (Prince et al., 2007).

Global mental health encompasses study, research, and practice endeavors that place a priority on improving mental health and achieving equity of health outcomes resulting from MNS disorders. Global mental health is concerned with promoting the quality of life of the hundreds of millions of people living with MNS disorders worldwide. Most live in low- and middle-income countries, where service provision is grossly inadequate, and treatment gaps can be as high as 90%. Stigma and discrimination linked to MNS disorders are also pervasive. Of course, these problems are by no means confined to low- and middle-income countries; however, the extent of the neglect is much more striking in these regions. In all countries, social disadvantage commonly accompanies a diagnosis of an MNS disorder. Poverty, unemployment, and impoverished social relationships increase the risk for some mental disorders, and all too often these are also preventable outcomes of these conditions arising from the failure to offer effective treatments, end discrimination, provide rehabilitation, and promote social inclusion for those affected by mental health issues.

This global health discipline has seen a substantial growth in its profile since the publication of the first Global Burden of Disease report (Murray & Lopez, 1996). Subsequent global public health documents—notably, the World Mental Health Report (Desjarlais, Eisenberg, Good, & Kleinman (1995); the Institute of Medicine's (2001) report on psychiatric, neurological and developmental disorders in developing countries; and the World Health Report of 2001 (WHO, 2001a)—have continued to emphasize the discipline. Most recently, the publication of a two ground-breaking series on global mental health—in *The Lancet* (http://www.thelancet.com/series/global-mental-health) and *PLoS Medicine* (http://www.plosmedicine.org/article/info%3Adoi%2F10.1371%2Fjournal.pmed.1000160)—have given the discipline a tremendous impetus toward expansion. These publications have collectively highlighted the global health crisis and proposed solutions to alleviate the unmet needs. Based on the twin principles of the science of cost-effective treatments and the promotion of the human rights of people affected by mental disorders, *The Lancet* series ended with a call to action, to scale up services for people living with mental disorders (Lancet Global Mental Health Group, 2007). Recent global initiatives by the WHO (mhGAP; WHO, 2008c) and the Global Alliance for Chronic Diseases (Grand Challenges in Global Mental Health), along with the launch of a new Movement for Global Mental Health (www.globalmental health.org; "Movement for Global Mental Health Gains Momentum," 2008), provide a common platform for professionals and civil society to promote this cause.

This chapter is organized in three parts. First, it presents a brief history of public mental health. Next, it discusses four pillars of evidence that are the foundations for global mental health: the concepts and classification of mental disorders; the burden and impact of mental disorders; effective prevention and treatment strategies, and the ways that these strategies can be delivered in low-resource contexts; and human rights and mental disorders. Finally, it considers the strategies for addressing global mental health issues in the immediate future.

Historical Development of Public Mental Health

The origins of public mental health can be traced back to the early Islamic world of North Africa, Spain, and the Middle East. Believing that insane people were loved by God, Islamic societies established a series of asylums—first in Baghdad in the eighth century, and later in Cairo, Damascus, and Fez (Mora, 1980). Later, between the twelfth and fifteenth centuries in the area then known as Flanders, mental hospitals were established in Ghent, Bruges, and Antwerp, as

well as the famous Colony of Gheel (Pierloot, 1975). The origins of public mental health also include a thirteenth-century priory house for the Order of Bethlehem that was transformed into Bethlem Hospital of London, which later became infamous for the brutality shown to its inmates and whose nickname—Bedlam—came to signify any asylum or person who was "mad" (Andrews, Briggs, Porter, Tucker, & Waddington, 1997).

It is probably fair to mark the beginning of modern public mental health as the late eighteenth century, when a shift in beliefs about the nature of mental illness occurred. Before this time, "madness" was associated with a loss of rationality, which meant that mentally ill individuals were considered as less than human and, in an effort to restore them to reason, were treated as brutes (Scull, 1989). "Moral treatment," which was developed simultaneously and independently in France (Pinel, 1977) and England (Digby, 1985), rejected the notion that mentally ill people lacked reason; instead, this view suggested that tolerance and confinement in a well-ordered and pleasant environment could restore a person to rationality and mental health (Grob, 1994).

In Europe and North America during the first half of the nineteenth century, this new perspective brought about a powerful movement that sought to abolish the abuses of the past and to establish public systems of mental institutions that would offer beneficent care and the prospect of recovery to mentally ill persons (Scull, 1989). However, as soon as the public asylums were opened, they were filled beyond capacity. Thus, throughout the second half of the nineteenth century, the notion of small curative institutions was forgotten under the dual pressures of increasing demands for services and a reluctance on the part of governments to allocate more funds for the care of mentally ill indigents (Grob, 1994; Scull, 1989). In addition, as conditions in the asylums grew worse, more and more physicians began to question their usefulness (Scull, MacKenzie, & Hervey, 1996). By the late nineteenth century, then, public mental health efforts were inextricably associated with the wretched, overcrowded conditions in mental asylums.

Beginning in the 1950s, and continuing through the 1960s and 1970s, efforts were made in North America and Western Europe to remove long-term patients from psychiatric facilities and to provide them with treatment and care in the community. The impetus behind this *deinstitutionalization* movement came from a convergence of several forces. First, as a result of the successes in treating soldiers traumatized by their experiences in World War II, psychiatrists became optimistic about their ability to effectively treat other mental disorders outside of hospital settings (Grob, 1994). Second, there was a growing awareness that the abusive conditions found in most state psychiatric hospitals, and the negative effects of long-term institutionalization, were at least as harmful as chronic mental disorder itself. Third, fiscal conservatives were concerned with the enormous expense of caring for patients in large institutions. Finally, the discovery in 1954 of chlorpromazine, the first effective antipsychotic medication, offered people with chronic mental disorders the prospect of living in the community rather than in hospital settings (Greenblatt, 1992). Together, these forces brought about a dramatic shift in admission and discharge practices in psychiatric hospitals. In the United States, the effects of these changes were obvious: The number of people in mental hospitals decreased from 559,000 in 1955 to 138,000 25 years later (Goldman, 1983).

Today, there is consensus that the deinstitutionalization movement in the United States has only partly achieved its aims. The odd alliance of fiscal conservatives and civil rights advocates that gave rise to the movement also meant that tens of thousands of patients were discharged from psychiatric hospitals with insufficient planning and without sufficient support services (e.g., housing and rehabilitation programs) and enough community mental health centers. Thus the setting of the neglect shifted from the asylum to the community. In fact, deinstitutionalization is a misnomer for what took place, at least in the United States; *dehospitalization* is a more accurate term. Great numbers of patients were discharged from hospitals, only to be accommodated in other institutional settings—for example, prisons, jails, single-room occupancy hotels, and adult homes for mentally disabled persons—that often replicated the worst aspects of the old asylums (Jencks, 1994; Levy, 2002).

Other countries, such as Australia, have managed the process of deinstitutionalization in a more appropriate and comprehensive manner (Whiteford, Buckingham, & Manderscheid, 2002). For example, the state of Victoria in Australia closed all of its psychiatric hospitals and, in their place, developed a wide range of community services and acute psychiatric units in general hospitals. With these efforts, opportunities for providing care in the community have expanded, and the civil rights of patients have been protected. Thus Australia has managed to avoid most of the worst experiences of deinstitutionalization in the United States.

Community-Based Mental Health Services

The community mental health movement was both an impetus for and a product of deinstitutionalization. Although the potential for treating people with mental disorders outside of hospital settings was recognized prior to the discovery of effective antipsychotic medications, the evolution of community-based services came about with the recognition that treatment and care require a range of social and rehabilitation services and involve more than just dispensing medication. Thus, while the definition of community care may have once simply meant care outside hospitals, it now encompasses professional services in community settings, social reintegration and support services (i.e., housing, employment, medical care, and welfare) (Tansella & Thornicroft, 2001).

Community-based mental health represents an ideology as much as a set of psychiatric practices (Mechanic, 2001). Indeed, the ideology has come to signify a set of principles that shape the planning and delivery of services: openness and honesty, respect, fair and equitable allocation of care and treatment, responsiveness to the changing needs of clients, and openness to learning and change (Tansella & Thornicroft, 2001). In addition, proponents of community-based care recognize that the parties involved in mental health services (e.g., government funding agencies, mental health professionals, the users of mental health services and their families, and researchers) may hold conicting values and interests, and that managing disparate views is a major challenge to providing effective services (Szmukler & Thornicroft, 2001). For example, professionals may offer efficacious medications, but patients may consider the side effects of those medications, or the need for housing and income, as more important for their well-being than the reduction of symptoms.

Colonial Psychiatry

During the nineteenth and early twentieth centuries, European colonial governments established large psychiatric institutions throughout Asia and Africa. These institutions have often been depicted as being a form of social control of indigenous populations (Good, 1992; Jackson, 1999; Schmidt, 1967; Swartz, 1999). While it may be true that the majority of colonial asylum administrators were racist and that indigenous people suffering from mental illness did not receive the best of care, it is also true that asylums in the colonies merely reflected their counterparts in Europe. After the end of European rule, the old asylums were the only mental health facilities that remained in the former colonies.

Against this background, an obvious recommendation was immediate deinstitutionalization. When such a course of action is considered, however, one must be cautious and recognize the need to replace hospital-based treatment with the development of psychiatric services in community facilities, including more inpatient services in general hospitals. At the same time, it is necessary to improve services and reform those existing psychiatric hospitals that cannot be closed and to convert them into specialist referral and training centers (Lin, Huang, Minas, & Cohen, 2009).

Culture and Classification

The classification of diseases leads, in theory, to more accurate diagnoses and more effective treatments. Valid and reliable systems of classification make it possible to determine accurate prevalence and incidence rates and, therefore, should guide decisions about the development of services. The classification of mental disorders, however, presents some unique challenges. Many authors have noted that psychiatric diagnoses do not "carve nature at the joint" and that the boundaries between different conditions may not be distinct (Blacker & Tsuang, 1992; Kendler & Gardner, 1998; Tsuang, Stone, & Faraone, 2000). Problems with classification increase when one moves from the world of academic research, clinical samples, and controlled trials to mental disorders as they occur in the community, where comorbidity is the rule, rather than the exception (Kessler et al., 1994). These problems are merely exacerbated by cultural variations in the expression of mental distress (Kleinman, 1988, 2004).

A key characteristic that differentiates the process of classification of mental disorders from the classification of other health problems is that, for most mental disorders, there are no specific and replicable pathophysiological changes that can be reliably identified in a clinical setting. Virtually all of the diagnostic categories used in psychiatry are essentially those of "illnesses" as compared to "diseases." This distinction implies that classification is based on the nature of symptoms and syndromes, rather than on their etiology (as, for example, in the case of infectious diseases) or their pathology (as, for example, in the case of vascular disease). The classification of mental disorders, therefore, is influenced by cultural factors, such as the language of emotional distress, and the ways in which these are conceptualized by a particular culture. In the absence of demonstrable disease processes, a variety of explanations are likely to arise that are heavily influenced by belief systems, notably religious beliefs. Historically, a number of classifications of mental disorders have coexisted in different cultures.

This section considers the history behind the emergence of the current, phenomenologically oriented, diagnostic system, which is largely based on descriptions of mental disorders in the United States and the United Kingdom. It also describes the role, and relevance, of alternative worldviews of understanding mental disorders.

The Evolution of Culturally Sensitive Biomedical Classifications

Historically, cross-cultural studies in psychiatric epidemiology have suffered from several problems. First, case identification techniques varied from site to site and methods were not standardized. These inconsistencies led to a movement to standardize the process of psychiatric measurement and diagnosis, albeit one driven by psychiatric classification systems originating in Euro-American societies. Standardized interviews that mimicked clinical psychiatric evaluations were developed and became the criteria for determining "caseness" in epidemiological investigations. After standardizing the interview schedules in Euro-American cultures, the interviews were subsequently used in other cultures. Most of these subsequent cross-cultural psychiatric investigations relied on implicit, largely untested assumptions:

- The universality of mental illnesses, implying that regardless of cultural variations, disorders as described in Euro-American classifications occur everywhere

- Invariance, implying that the core features of psychiatric syndromes are unchanging

- Validity, implying that although refinement is possible, the diagnostic categories of current classifications are valid clinical constructs (Beiser, Cargo, & Woodbury, 1994).

This approach, which is labeled the "etic" or universalist approach, became the most popular method for epidemiological investigations of mental illness across cultures. According to the etic approach, because mental illnesses are similar throughout the world, psychiatric taxonomies, their measuring instruments, and models of health care must also be globally applicable.

Many researchers have cautioned that there is a risk of confounding culturally distinctive behavior with psychopathology on the basis of superficial similarities of behavior patterns or phenomena in different cultures (Kleinman, 1988). It has been argued that classifications of psychiatric disorders have largely reflected American and European concepts of psychopathology based on implicit cultural concepts of normality and deviance. Critics accuse the etic approach of contributing to a worldview that "privileges biology over culture" (Eisenbruch, 1991) and ignores the cultural and social contexts of psychiatric disorders.

In contrast, the emic approach argues that the culture-bound aspects of biomedicine, such as its emphasis on medical disease entities, limit its universal applicability. More specifically, this approach suggests that culture plays such an influential role in the presentation of psychiatric disorders that it is wrong to presume a priori that Euro-American psychiatric categories are appropriate throughout the world (Littlewood, 1990). The emic approach proposes that phenomena should be evaluated within a culture and its context, aiming to understand their significance and relationship with other intra-cultural elements.

The emic approach has also drawn its share of criticism—the most fundamental complaint being that it is unable to provide data that can be compared across cultures. The emic approach has also been criticized for not suggesting plausible alternatives, such as a set of principles that would help ensure cultural sensitivity, or models upon which to fashion culturally sensitive nosologies (Beiser et al., 1994).

Both the etic and emic approaches have strengths and weaknesses, and it is widely accepted that integrating their methodological strengths is essential for the development of the "new cross-cultural psychiatry" or a culturally sensitive psychiatry (Kleinman, 1988; Littlewood, 1990). Value must be placed on both folk beliefs about mental illness and the biomedical system of psychiatry. It is important to investigate patients' "explanatory models"—that is, how patients understand their problems, including their nature, origins, consequences, and remedies, as these aspects of understanding can radically alter patient–doctor negotiations over appropriate treatment (Kleinman, 1988). Similarly, researchers should follow the example of Bolton and colleagues (2003) and examine the psychiatric symptoms of persons who are considered to be mentally ill by the local population, determining the relationship of the diagnostic system used by local populations with the psychiatric diagnostic categories. In essence, the central aim of the "new" cross-cultural psychiatry is to describe mental illness in different cultures using methods that are sensitive and valid for the local culture and result in

data that are comparable across cultures. To tackle this difficult task, psychiatric research needs to blend both ethnographic and epidemiological methods, emphasizing the unique contribution of both approaches to the understanding of mental illness across cultures.

Biomedical and Alternative Worldviews of Mental Illness

Two main biomedical systems of psychiatric classification are used today: the International Classification of Diseases (ICD; developed by the World Health Organization [WHO]) and the *Diagnostic and Statistical Manual* [DSM]; developed by the American Psychiatric Association). Diagnostic criteria of syndromes can and do change over time, as is well demonstrated by the regular revisions of international psychiatric classifications, which are considerably influenced by attitudinal, political, and historical factors.

Both major classifications of mental disorders have attempted to improve their cross-cultural and international validity in recent years. The tenth revision of the ICD (ICD-10) was developed with the explicit purpose of being an international standard. Thus efforts were made to ensure that the drafters of the ICD-10 were drawn from as many countries as was feasible, and its system of classification was field-tested by more than 700 clinicians in 39 countries from all continents, although the largest number of centers were in European or high-income countries. In these field trials, two or more clinicians rated a consecutive group of new patients presenting to the service and made an ICD-10 diagnosis according to the manual; the inter-rater reliability coefficient for each disorder was also calculated. The vast majority of ICD-10 conditions had reasonable reliability (Sartorius et al., 1993). In addition to reliability, assessment of the cultural validity of diagnostic categories has also been attempted by classifications—for example, by including guidelines for clinicians to make a "cultural formulation" of a person's mental health problem (Exhibit 9-1).

Indigenous classifications, by and large, are based on spiritual, supernatural, or humoral etiological theories (Murdock, Wilson, & Frederick, 1980) that are not tenable in the practice of biomedicine. Broadly, there is a general classification of illness into two categories: "normal" and "abnormal." Normal illnesses are perceived as being caused by physical agents (such as infections and climactic changes) and considered to be treated effectively by either biomedical or traditional treatments, whereas abnormal illnesses are perceived to be caused by spiritual or supernatural causes and, therefore, are brought principally to traditional healers.

This formulation implies the clinician provides a narrative summary of the following aspects of the disorder:

- The cultural identity of the individual (e.g., language abilities, cultural preference group, degree of involvement with other cultures in community)

- Cultural explanations of the illness (similar to the explanatory models described earlier and including prominent idioms of distress, causal models, and treatment preferences)

- Cultural factors related to the psychosocial environment and functioning (culturally relevant interpretations of social stressors, available social support and disability)

- Cultural elements of the relationship between the individual and the clinician (i.e., identify differences and similarities in cultural and social status that might influence diagnosis and treatment)

- Overall cultural assessment—a conclusion describing how these cultural considerations influence diagnosis and treatment decisions

Source: American Psychiatric Association

A further classification of "unnatural" causes is a model in which illness is brought about by supernatural forces, by other human beings, or by the behavior of an individual or his or her family. The classifications used are typically flexible and patient dependent; thus, even though phenomenology may be used by a healer to understand the nature of the illness, an etiological model is almost always provided because it gives the illness experience meaning for the patient.

There is evidence that with the influence of urbanization and other changes in society, views about illness are also changing. Thus biomedical diagnostic systems are increasingly being used in low- and middle-income countries, and multiple illness models are supported simultaneously. Indeed, it is not unusual in many low- and middle-income countries for a person with a mental illness to consult both traditional/religious and biomedical healthcare providers.

Most commonly, the explanatory models of mental illnesses equate them with psychotic or severe mental disorders. For these disorders, there is a striking similarity in the behavioral symptoms across cultures, with some behaviors such as incoherent speech, talking to oneself, disrobing, wandering, and aggression being particularly common (Patel, 1995). At the same time, there is much less emphasis on cognitive features such as delusions, which are central to the diagnosis in the biomedical model. Disorders resembling depression and anxiety, although often not perceived to be mental disorders, are still recognized by local people and traditional healers as being sources of illness, suffering, and misfortune.

Although the ICD-10 is an international system, it was not (at least initially) intended to supplant local classificatory systems. Over time, however, most countries have gradually shed any existing indigenous classification schemes. For the few that remain, there have been attempts to make them conform to the ICD as closely as possible. China is possibly the only low- and middle-income country that still has its own classification of mental disorders. The first Chinese Classification of Mental Disorders (CCMD) appeared in 1979; since then, the system has undergone several revisions. Its third and most recent version is heavily influenced by the ICD-10 and *DSM-IV* systems, but still retains certain local features. The main differences between the ICD-10 and the CCMD-3 are summarized by Lee (2001). Notable among these variations are the CCMD-3's retention of the term "neurosis" and its retention of some specific categories of neurotic disorders such as neurasthenia. Personality disorder is less often diagnosed in Chinese populations; thus two categories of personality disorder—borderline personality disorder and avoidant personality disorder—are excluded from the Chinese scheme. The CCMD also includes its own section of culture-related mental disorders such as *qigong*-induced mental disorder. *Qigong* is a trance-based form of a traditional Chinese healing system. The disorder is similar to a dissociative state, featuring identity disturbance, irritability, hallucinations, and aggressive and bizarre behaviors. These often acute, brief episodes are linked to excessive practice of *qigong* meditation by physically or psychologically ill subjects. (Exhibit 9-2).

| Exhibit 9-2 | Culture-Bound Syndromes |

ICD-10 defines culture-specific disorders as sharing two cardinal characteristics:

- They are not "easily" accommodated by the categories in established and internationally used psychiatric classifications.

- They were first described in, and subsequently closely or exclusively associated with, a particular population or cultural area.

ICD-10 includes several examples of culture-bound categories—*amok*, *dhat* syndrome, and *koro* in Asian cultures; *latah* in indigenous cultures of Scandinavia, the

---

Exhibit 9-2   *Continued*

Americas, and Asia; *susto* in Latin America; and *taijin kyofusho* in Japan. None of the culture-specific syndromes resemble severe mental disorders; all occur within the context of severe stress and are phenomenologically closest to the neurotic and dissociative disorders and neurotic disorders. Many conditions bear considerable similarity to one another and to a multitude of other conditions described in diverse cultures. *Susto* and *nervios* are folk idioms of distress, *koro* and *dhat* are related to a cultural concern regarding fertility and procreation, *latah* and *amok* are related to a cultural emphasis on learned dissociation, and *brain fag* is an example of syndromes related to acculturative stress on adolescents (the pressure of academic performance of some cultures).

The concept of "culture-bound" syndromes has been criticized because it implies that mental disorder categories predominantly based on observations made in patient populations in Euro-American cultures are "culture free." Conditions that are almost entirely seen only in such cultures—for example, anorexia nervosa or multiple personality disorders—are not classified as "culture-bound syndromes," even though they bear very similar characteristics to those conditions that given this label. It is likely that this approach of classifying mental disorders will give way to an acknowledgment that some mental disorders are more common in some cultures than others, and that the expression of all mental disorders is influenced by cultural factors.

Source: International Classification of Diseases-10

The Burden of Mental Disorders

This section will address the prevalence, impact and social determinants of mental disorders in the global context.

Prevalence of Mental Disorders

We review the evidence for six categories of mental disorders.

Anxiety and Mood Disorders

Advances in the development of valid and reliable diagnostic interviews, the initiation of multiple cross-national surveys of mental disorders, and continued research in clinical epidemiology have all improved the ability of psychiatric epidemiologists to determine prevalence rates of anxiety and mood disorders (Kessler, 2000). The best example of these advances is found in the work of the World Mental Health Survey Initiative, which has conducted surveys of the prevalence, severity, and treatment of nonpsychotic mental disorders (anxiety, depressive or mood, externalizing, and substance disorders) among nationally representative samples of persons in more than 20 countries across five of the six WHO regions. In the first publication synthesizing findings from 17 countries (Kessler et al., 2009), 12-month prevalence rates of these disorders ranged from a low of 6.0% in Nigeria to a high of 27.0% in the United States. In all but two of the countries, anxiety disorders were the most common.

The World Mental Health Survey Initiative (http://www.hcp.med.harvard.edu/wmh/) has generated a vast amount of data, and it continues to conduct surveys in more countries. Questions remain about the validity of its findings, especially regarding the large variation in cross-national prevalence rates. As acknowledged by the investigators, the instruments used in the survey were developed in studies conducted primarily in wealthy Western countries and their use in different settings may have led to measurement biases (WHO World Mental Health Survey Consortium, 2004). Nevertheless, this study represents a major advance in psychiatric epidemiology and will, for many years, inform global mental health policy development.

Psychotic Disorders

The investigation of the cross-cultural epidemiology of severe mental disorders—notably, schizophrenia—was initiated with Emil Kraepelin's visit to Java in 1904. Kraepelin (2000 [1904]) noted that he had found cases of schizophrenia and bipolar disorder among the Javanese, but that "comparison between the native and the European populations is made [difficult] by the fact that the clinical symptomatology, while broadly in agreement with that seen [in Europe], presents certain very noteworthy differences in individual instances." Since then, only one project—the WHO Determinants of Outcome of Severe Mental Disorders—has conducted epidemiological investigations into the incidence of schizophrenia in different countries (Jablensky et al., 1992). This research found that the incidence of schizophrenia ranged from 7 to 14 per 100,000 among populations at risk (ages 15 to 44 years). The extent of this variation was not statistically significant, and experts in the field concluded that the incidence of schizophrenia is similar in different populations.

More recently, however, a meta-analysis of 158 studies determined that the median value of these rates was 15.2 per 100,000, with a range of 7.7 to

43.0 per 100,000 (McGrath, Saha, Welham, El Saadi, MacCauley, & Change, 2004). From this evidence, the investigators concluded that there *are* significant differences in incidence rates of schizophrenia across populations. Furthermore, the meta-analysis determined that rates were higher among men than women, in urban areas, and in migrant groups.

Another meta-analysis of 188 studies in 46 countries reported a median point prevalence of 4.6 (range: 1.9–10.0) per 1,000 persons. The prevalence of schizophrenia was higher in migrants compared to native-born individuals (Saha, Chant, Welham, & McGrath, 2005).

Substance Abuse Disorders

The burden of substance abuse disorders varies considerably across and within countries, between subgroups in a given population, and according to the substance being abused. If dependence on tobacco (arguably the most common substance to be abused) is excluded, alcohol use disorders (AUD) are the most common substance abuse disorder in most countries. AUD refer to the entire range of health conditions associated with drinking alcohol above the recommended limit set by the WHO and include hazardous, harmful, and dependent drinking (Room, Babor, & Rehm, 2005; WHO, 1992). The large and growing burden of AUD in low- and middle-income countries has been systematically documented recently (Patel, in press; Rehm, Mathers, Patra, & Popova, 2009). Point prevalence of AUD in adults was estimated to be almost 2% globally (WHO, 2008a); the rates were almost six times higher among men than among women (WHO, 2001b). The prevalence of AUD varies widely across different regions of the world, ranging from very low levels in some Middle Eastern countries to more than 5% in North America and parts of Eastern Europe, and it is rising rapidly in some of the developing regions of the world. Economic growth has fueled the local alcohol industry (Caetano & Laranjeira, 2006) and made low- and middle-income countries the target of market expansion by an ever-growing number of transnational producers of alcoholic beverages (Bengal, 2005).

Besides tobacco and alcohol, a large number of other substances, generally grouped under the broad category of *drugs*, are also abused. These include illicit substances such as heroin, cocaine, and cannabis. The prevalence of drug abuse and dependence ranges widely between and within populations according to the type of drug, and prevalence rates are notoriously difficult to ascertain due to hidden nature of drug using populations.

Epilepsy

Epilepsy, one of the most common neurological disorders, is characterized by the occurrence of repeated seizures over an extended period of the life course. Its prevalence varies widely: 5–8 per 1,000 in Europe and North America (Forsgren, 2008); 5–75 per 1,000 in sub-Saharan Africa (Preux & Druet-Cabanac, 2005); 6–44 per 1,000 in South America (Burneo, Tellez-Zenteno, & Wiebe, 2005); and 1.5–14 per 1,000 in Asia (Mac, Tran, Quet, Odermatt, Preux, & Tan, 2007). It is assumed that the prevalence of epilepsy is relatively high in low- and middle-income countries, but, given the wide ranges of the rates, the exact ratio between low- and middle-income countries and high-income countries is difficult to determine. Epidemiological research suggests that as many as 65 million globally suffer from epilepsy and that approximately 80% of them live in low- and middle-income countries (Mbuba & Newton, 2009).

A recent population based study from Mozambique revealed a high prevalence of seizure disorders, ranging from 2% to 5% of children (Patel, Simbine, Soares, Weiss, & Wheeler, 2007). Rates of narrowly defined epilepsy range from 0.5% to 3.7% in Africa (Birbeck & Kalichi, 2004; Osuntokun et al., 1987; Rwiza et al., 1992); these rates exclude secondary seizures, such as malarial and febrile seizures, and the lower rates typically encompass only those individuals with current active epilepsy. A key finding of these studies is that the prevalence of epilepsy is greater in rural areas, where the majority of the population lives. One explanation for the higher rural prevalence is that with large numbers of people moving into cities, persons with disabilities, including epilepsy, are less likely to relocate, which results in a proportional rise in the prevalence of these disorders in rural areas (Patel, Simbine et al., 2007).

Developmental Disabilities

Developmental disabilities (DD) are limitations in function resulting from disorders of the developing nervous system (Institute of Medicine, 2001). These limitations usually become manifest during infancy or early childhood. Five major categories of DD are defined under the ICD-10: cognitive (e.g., mental retardation [MR] and specific learning disabilities [SLD]), motor (e.g., cerebral palsy), sensory (e.g., visual or hearing disabilities), language (e.g., expressive language disorder), and behavioral (e.g., pervasive developmental disorder [PDD] and attention-deficit/hyperactivity disorder [ADHD]) (Institute of Medicine, 2001; WHO, 1990). Children are frequently affected in multiple domains. The proportion of the global burden of DD is likely to be higher in low- and middle-income countries because they experience a much higher prevalence of recognized risk factors for DD, notably poor perinatal care, nutritional deficiencies, neonatal infections, and consanguineous marriages. Furthermore, as improvements in child survival occur in most low- and middle-income countries, a concomitant rise in the prevalence of DD may occur.

There are few reliable, population-based estimates of the prevalence of DD in low- and middle-income countries. However, some studies have provided prevalence estimates for severe mental handicap that suggest these rates are higher in low- and middle-income countries (Institute of Medicine, 2001). A recent population-based study of DD in India (Srinath et al., 2005) reported that 4.4% of the children had at least one of the following disabilities: MR, specific speech articulation disorder, or expressive language disorder. When ADHD was included, the prevalence of DD increased to 6.1%. The prevalence of severe mental retardation in another Indian study was reported as nearly 1.5% (in comparison to a prevalence of about 0.5% in the United States) (Narayanan, 1981).

ADHD, as defined by the American Psychiatric Association (1994), is characterized by symptoms in one or both of two core domains: inattention and hyperactivity-impulsiveness. One analysis estimated *DSM-IV* prevalence rates from studies that used either structured ratings or parent plus teacher ratings and impairment criteria (Nigg, 2006). The researchers concluded that the median prevalence rate for ADHD was 7%. The ratio of boys to girls affected by ADHD is approximately 2:1.

A growing and convincing body of evidence has emerged in the past decade that supports the conclusion that ADHD is not a cultural construct (Buitelaar et al., 2005; Faraone, Sergeant, Gillberg, & Biederman, 2003; Rohde, Szobot, Polanczyk, Schmitz, Martins, & Tramontina, 2005), although, as with all mental disorders, cultural factors do influence illness recognition and help seeking. A recent review identified 22 studies addressing ADHD prevalence rates in "non-Western" countries over the last 15 years (Flisher, Hatherill, Dhansay, & Swartz, 2007). The prevalence rates reported in these studies were, generally speaking, at least as high as those reported for Western countries.

Dementia

Dementia is a syndrome caused by disease of the brain, usually chronic and progressive, in which there is disturbance of multiple higher cortical functions, including memory, learning, orientation, language, comprehension, and judgment. Diagnosis is made on the basis of decline in cognitive function and independent living skills. Dementia mainly affects older people, with only 2% to 5% of cases starting before the age of 65 years. After this point, prevalence doubles with every five-year increment in age (Ritchie, Kildea, & Robine, 1992).

In 2005, international experts who reviewed the global evidence on prevalence of dementia estimated that 24.3 million people were affected in 2001, with 4.6 million new cases occurring annually (Ferri et al., 2005). New estimates, based on a systematic review of global prevalence, suggest that 35.5 million people were affected by dementia in 2010; these numbers were forecast to nearly double every 20 years, to 65.7 million in 2030 and 115.4 million in 2050 (Prince & Jackson, 2009).

Earlier suggestions of a lower prevalence of dementia in low- and middle-income countries than in high-income countries—strikingly so in some studies (Hendrie et al., 1995)—have not been confirmed by more recent research (Llibre Rodriguez et al., 2008; Molero, Pino-Ramirez, & Maestre, 2007). This discrepancy may have been accounted for by under-detection of mild and recent-onset cases in low- and middle-income regions. In 2010, 58% of all people with dementia worldwide lived in low- and middle-income countries; this figure is expected to rise to 71% by 2050, as proportionate increases over the next 20 years in the number of people in the higher-risk age groups will be much steeper in low- and middle-income countries compared with high-income countries. Hence, forecasts suggest a 40% increase in prevalence in Europe, 63% in North America, 77% in the southern Latin American cone, and 89% in the high-income Asia Pacific countries, compared with 117% growth in East Asia, 107% in South Asia, 134% to 146% in the rest of Latin America, and 125% in North Africa and the Middle East.

The Impact of Mental Disorders

This section considers the impact of mental disorders in three domains: disability and mortality; economic burden; and other health outcomes.

Disability and Mortality

Historically, rates of mortality dominated assessments of public health priorities. As a consequence, mental disorders, which are mainly associated with disability (rather than death), were not considered important. That all changed with the development of disability-adjusted life-years (DALYs), a measure that combines the impact of morbidity and mortality into a single statistic and makes it possible to compare the burden of disease imposed by a variety of health conditions (Murray & Lopez, 1996).

In 2004, the Global Burden of Disease study (GBD; WHO, 2008a) suggested that 13.1% of the total burden of disease was attributable to neuropsychiatric disorders. Three conditions—unipolar depressive disorders (4.3%), alcohol use disorders (1.6%), and self-inflicted injuries (1.3%; such injuries are often associated with mental illness)—were among the 20 leading causes of the global burden of disease. Among women aged 15 to 44 years, depression was the leading cause of disease burden in both high-income countries and low- and middle-income countries. Even in low-income countries that continue to experience high rates of morbidity and mortality due to infectious diseases as well as maternal, perinatal, and nutritional conditions, mental disorders accounted for 8% of the total burden of disease (WHO, 2001b).

The burden of mental disorders may be underestimated in the GBD (Prince et al., 2007), in particular due to the relatively small number of deaths attributed to mental disorders (estimated at 1.4% of years of life lost through premature mortality). However, each year nearly 1 million people commit suicide—a figure that is almost certainly a massive underestimate given the large gaps between reported suicides and the number ascertained through systematic community-based verbal autopsies of all deaths in countries such as India and China (Gajalakshmi & Peto, 2007; Phillips, Li, & Zhang, 2002). Suicide is among the three leading causes of death in young people in all regions of the world (Exhibit 9-3); accidents, many of which are fueled by substance use and abuse, are also among the three leading causes of death for this subpopulation (Patton et al., 2009). Mortality due to other reasons is also elevated in patients with psychosis, depression, and dementia. The poor quality of health care received by those with mental disorders for medical problems may explain some of this excess mortality (Prince et al., 2007).

Economic Burden

The economic burden of mental disorders is huge, not only because of the direct costs of treatment, but also because of indirect costs such as lost wages, reduced productivity, and premature mortality (Rice, Kelman, & Miller, 1992). Research from the United States indicates that, as of the mid-1990s, the eco-

nomic cost of depression totaled $53 billion (the equivalent of $75 billion in 2009) (Greenberg, Kessler, Nells, Finkelstein, & Berndt, 1996; Wang, Simon, & Kessler, 2003). Of this amount, more than 60% was the result of reduction in work productivity, while a little less than 25% represented the cost of treatment; the remaining 15% was the result of premature mortality (Greenberg et al., 1999; Greenberg, Stiglin, Finkelstein, & Berndt, 1993). The case is much the same in Europe. In 2004, the total economic burden of depression in Europe was $167.2 billion (the equivalent of about $188.5 billion in 2008) (Sobocki, Jonsson, Angst, & Rehnberg, 2006). Of this amount, treatment accounted for approximately 35%, while excess morbidity and mortality was responsible for the remainder.

Although a relatively rare condition, schizophrenia imposes a substantial economic burden. A systematic review found that treatment costs for schizophrenia account for between 1.5% and 3% of national healthcare budgets in high-income countries, with substantial additional indirect costs being associated with, for example, loss of productivity, informal care by families, and excess mortality (Knapp, Managalore, & Simon, 2004).

Alcohol use disorders also impose a great burden on society. A review of research in four high-income countries and two middle-income countries found that alcohol use disorders imposed economic costs that ranged from 1.3% to 3.3% of gross domestic product (GDP) (Rehm, Mathers, Popova, Thavorncharoensap, Teerawattananon, & Patra, 2009; WHO, 2001b). On average, indirect costs accounted for approximately 75% of the total costs.

Relatively few studies have focused on the costs of mental disorders in low- and middle-income countries (Shah & Jenkins, 2000). These investigations generally report a considerable economic impact of severe mental disorders, such as schizophrenia and depression, on household finances (Patel, Chisholm, Kirkwood, & Mabey, 2007; Westermeyer, 1984). Also, it is difficult for people with serious mental disorders to secure remunerative employment in these regions. A substantial burden of care is also attributable to mental retardation. For the individual and family, this may include attending to activities of daily living and self-care. The education system faces the challenge of providing appropriate educational services, which can range from segregated specialized residential and day schools, to special classes in regular schools, to mainstreaming or inclusive education. For the health system, there is a burden attributed to associated disabilities, such as cerebral palsy, sensory

Exhibit 9-3	Suicide

As of 2004, an estimated 800,000 people were believed to commit suicide every year, which represents 1.4% of total mortality (WHO, 2008a). The estimated annual mortality is 14.5 per 100,000, which makes suicide the tenth leading cause of death worldwide (Hawton & van Heeringen, 2009). However, these figures probably underestimate the actual number of suicides, given incomplete death registrations and sociocultural prohibitions concerning suicide.

In addition, suicide rates display wide variations according to age, gender, ethnicity, and country. In most countries, older adults have the highest rates of suicide. Nevertheless, suicide is a leading cause of death in young people in all regions of the world (Patton et al., 2009).

Men, at least in high-income countries, have suicide rates that are two to four times higher than those for women, although this is not the case in Asia, where the ratio is much smaller or even reversed. In China, women have suicide rates that are 25% higher than those of men; this is primarily due to the large numbers of young women who commit suicide in rural China (Phillips et al., 2002).

Suicide rates also vary among ethnic groups within countries. For example, African Americans in the United States and Indian women in the United Kingdom have suicide rates that are relatively low compared to the general population (Hawton & van Heeringen, 2009). Some social groups, such as unemployed persons and medical personnel, have relatively high suicide rates.

Countries undergoing rapid and traumatic social change also tend to have high rates of suicide—for example, this is true of the countries that once made up the Soviet Union. In addition, suicide rates tend to rise during times of economic distress. Notably, the economic crisis of 1997–1998 resulted in sharp increases in suicide in Japan, Hong Kong, and South Korea (Chang, Gunnell, Sterne, Lu, & Cheng, 2009).

At the same time, mental disorders have been consistently shown to be predictors of suicide. The lifetime risk for suicide among persons with depression is 4%. The rate is roughly the same for persons with schizophrenia, but is much higher for persons with bipolar disorders (10% to 15%) (Hawton & van Heeringen, 2009). Persons with alcohol use disorders and anorexia nervosa also are at high risk of suicide (Desjarlais et al., 1995; WHO, n.d., 2001b).

Given the strong evidence that sociocultural, socioeconomic, and psychiatric factors are all associated with suicide, it would seem that suicidal behavior does not constitute a syndrome or series of syndromes, nor does it occur randomly. A heuristic suicide pathway can assist in the management of suicidal people and the prevention of suicidal behavior (Flisher, 1999).

Step 1 in this pathway consists of factors that generally predispose individuals to suicidal behavior. These include demographic factors (male and female gender for completed and attempted suicide, respectively; increasing age), biological factors (family history of psychopathology, biochemical abnormalities), psychopathology (especially alcohol use and depression), social context (high community-based suicide rates, not adhering to a religion in which suicide is proscribed), and a family or personal history of suicide. In addition, certain cultures are characterized by specific patterns that may predispose their members to suicide—for example, dowry disputes in India.

Step 2 in the heuristic involves a precipitating event, which converts a predisposition toward suicidal behavior into actual behavior. Such events can include stressful life events, altered states of mind (fear, intoxication), a suicide cluster in one's social network, reports of suicide in the media, or spring season.

Step 3 in the suicide pathway refers to the opportunity that needs to be present to make a suicide attempt, such as a method of suicide and privacy. Step 4 is the actual suicidal behavior.

Strategies to prevent suicide should aim to intervene at specific points along this pathway. For example, in Step 1, one can aim to identify and provide mental health services for those deemed to be at risk—for example, people suffering from alcohol dependence or depression. In Step 2, one can increase access to crisis intervention services or provide life skills training to assist people in responding to stressful life events in an adaptive manner without resorting to suicide; implement postvention, in which one intervenes with members of a social network in which there is a suicide cluster; and work with the media to discourage glamorizing suicide. In Step 3, one can reduce opportunities by limiting access to firearms, pesticides, or fatal household gas. In Step 4, one can increase access to, and improve the quality of, emergency medical care following suicide attempts.

deficits, epilepsy, and comorbid mental disorders (Molteno & Westaway, 2001).

Impact on Other Health Outcomes

A recent review demonstrated that mental disorders interact with physical disorders in multiple ways (Prince et al., 2007). First, mental disorders are risk factors for physical health problems, which in turn increase the risk for mental disorders. There is strong evidence of comorbidity between diabetes and mood disorders (Anderson, Freeland, Clouse, & Lustman, 2001; Grigsby, Anderson, Freeland, Clouse, & Lustman, 2002), for example, and depression may increase the risk for diabetes (Eaton, Armenian, Gallo,

Pratt, & Ford, 1996). Between 10% and 20% of people with schizophrenia have type 2 diabetes (Holt, Bushe, & Citrome, 2005). Depression is a risk factor for cardiovascular diseases (CVD; Hemingway & Marmot, 1999) and stroke (Larson, Owens, Ford, & Eaton, 2001). There is also strong evidence of the increased risk for depression *after* myocardial infarction (Strik, Lousberg, Cheriex, & Honig, 2004) and stroke (Aben, Lodder, Honig, Lousberg, Boreas, & Verhey, 2006). Tuberculosis (TB) is more common among people who are heavy drinkers (Buskin, Gale, Weiss, & Nolan, 1994) and among those with serious mental illness (McQuistion, Colson, Yankowitz, & Susser, 1997). A significant proportion of HIV/AIDS cases may be attributed to injection drug use (Chander, Himelhoch, & Moore, 2006), and alcohol abuse is recognized as a risk factor for unsafe sexual behaviors. People with severe mental illness have higher rates of HIV/AIDS than the general population (Cournos, McKinnon, & Sullivan, 2005). Not surprisingly, living with HIV/AIDS is associated with a high prevalence of depression (Maj et al., 1994) and neurocognitive impairment and dementia (White, Heaton, & Monsch, 1995).

AUD are a major risk factor for other health outcomes, including road traffic injuries and cirrhosis (Desai, Nawamongkolwattana, Ranaweera, Shrestha, & Sobhan, 2003; Rehm et al., 2009; Room et al., 2005). Although dependent drinking is the most severe form of AUD, the population-level burden of alcohol-attributable health problems predominantly arises from less severe forms of AUD ("hazardous drinking") (Room et al., 2005; WHO, 2001c). Even though hazardous drinkers are predominantly men, women suffer the consequences of hazardous drinking, in the form of depression, domestic violence, and diversion of family resources from priority needs (Gil-Gonzalez, Vives-Cases, Alvarez-Dardet, & Latour-Perez, 2006; Patel, Kirkwood et al., 2006).

Second, anxiety and mood disorders and other common mental health problems (called "somatoform disorders") may present in primary health care/general medical settings with physical symptoms (Escobar, Waitzkin, Silver, Gara, & Holman, 1998; Gureje, Simon, Ustun, & Goldberg, 1997). Such symptoms, which are sometimes termed "medically unexplained" because they cannot be attributed to physical disorders, are associated with considerable disability and high levels of help seeking and associated healthcare costs (Escobar et al., 1998).

Third, the coexistence of mental and physical disorders is associated with worse outcomes of the physical disorder through a variety of mechanisms. For example, depression is associated with higher rates of reinfarction, disability, and death following myocardial infarction (Hemingway & Marmot, 1999) and stroke (Parikh, Robinson, Lipsey, Starkstein, Fedoroff, & Price, 1990). Similarly, depression is associated with worse glycemic control (Lustman et al., 2000), complications (de Groot, Anderson, Freeland, Clouse, & Lustman, 2001), and death (Katon et al., 2005) in people with diabetes. Similar findings have been reported for HIV/AIDS, where depression is associated with increased mortality (Cook et al., 2004; Ickovics et al., 2001) and more rapid disease progression (Ickovics et al., 2001). One mechanism that may potentially explain some of these associations is poor adherence to treatment regimes among people with mental disorders (Ammassari et al., 2004; Dolder, Lacro, & Jeste, 2003; Ziegelstein, Fauerbach, Stevens, Romanelli, Richter, & Bush, 2000).

The fourth mechanism is the strong association of mental disorders with a range of women's health concerns. Depression is strongly associated with dysmenorrhea, dyspareunia, and pelvic pain (Latthe, Mignini, Gray, Hills, & Khan, 2006). In some cultures in Asia, gynecological complaints, such as abnormal vaginal discharge, are associated with depression (Patel, Weiss, et al., 2006). Maternal mental illnesses are associated with a range of adverse perinatal outcomes, including low birth weight, premature birth, child undernutrition, and developmental delays (Bennedsen, Mortensen, Olesen, & Henriksen, 1999; Nilsson, Lichtenstein, Cnattingius, Murray, & Hultman, 2002; Patel, Rahman, Jacob, & Hughes, 2004).

Social Determinants of Mental Disorders

The etiology of mental disorders comprises a complex interplay between biological factors, most notably inherited predisposition, and psychosocial factors. Until the 1950s, the dominant notions about the etiology of mental disorders were environmental in nature. For example, schizophrenia was attributed to abnormal parenting, and obsessive–compulsive disorder to "anal aggression."

Beginning in the 1960s, however, a more balanced view emerged (Plomin, Owen, & McGuffin, 1994). Consensus was reached that both environmental and genetic influences contribute to the development of mental disorders. The question changed from *which* factors were relevant for a specific disorder, to *how much* each contributed to the condition (Anastasi, 1958). Ultimately, this question, too, proved to be based on an incorrect assumption— namely, that the social and genetic factors exert their influences in an additive and independent manner. There is now recognition that they exert their influences in an interactive manner. Contemporary scientists are attempting to answer the question of *how* they interact.

This section briefly reviews the evidence on four types of social determinants of mental disorders: poverty, gender, conflict, and the marginalization experienced by indigenous communities across the world.

Poverty

There is now substantial evidence demonstrating the relationship between poverty and socioeconomic inequalities with mental disorders. In the United Kingdom, for example, evidence has pointed to an association between a low standard of living and the prevalence of depression (Weich & Lewis, 1998). A recent systematic review located 115 studies in which the associations between poverty and anxiety and mood disorders in low- and middle-income countries were examined (Lund et al., 2010). Most reported positive associations between a range of poverty indicators and anxiety and mood disorders. Multivariate analyses reported that in community-based studies, 79%, 15%, and 6% reported positive, null, and negative associations, respectively. A robust association was found between anxiety and mood disorders and education, food insecurity, housing, social class, socioeconomic status, and financial stress. By comparison, the associations between anxiety and mood disorders and income, employment, and consumption were inconsistent.

Studies in developed countries have shown that mortality and morbidity rates are more affected by relative, rather than absolute, living standards. A survey in the United States, for example, showed an independent association between low income and living in income unequal states with depression in women (Kahn, Wise, Kennedy, & Kawachi, 2000). The association between poverty and poor mental health may be mediated both by individual psychological factors, such as low self-esteem and frustration, and by a breakdown in structural factors in the community, such as less social cohesion and poorer infrastructure. The lack of social support and the breakdown of kinship structures may be important stressors for the millions of migrant laborers in the urban centers of Asia, Africa, and South America, as well as the millions of dependents who are left behind in rural areas and whose primary source of income consists of the remittances relatives send from distant cities. In high-income countries, increased mobility of labor has reduced family ties and also led to the decline of the extended family.

The social consequences of low education are obvious, especially in low- and middle-income countries that are facing a growing lack of security for employees as economies are reformed. Lack of secondary education may produce a diminished opportunity for persons who are depressed—especially women—to access resources to improve their situation (Patel, Araya, de Lima, Ludermir, & Todd, 1999). People living in conditions of poverty are at greater risk for physical health problems, and there is abundant evidence demonstrating the high degree of comorbidity between physical and mental illnesses.

Gender

The excess prevalence of depression for women has been demonstrated in most community-based studies in all regions of the world (Patel et al., 1999). Women are disproportionately affected by the burden of poverty, which in turn may influence their vulnerability for depression. Women are far more likely to be victims of violence in their homes; women who experience physical violence by an intimate partner are significantly more likely to suffer depression, abuse drugs, or attempt suicide (Exhibit 9-6). Women who are sexually abused as children are significantly more likely to suffer depression in adulthood, and experience of sexual and other forms of violence in youth is associated with depression in adolescence (Astbury, 2001).

Research on depression in women in low-income townships of Harare, Zimbabwe, reported that nearly 18% women had a current episode of depression, compared to only 9% of their counterparts in Camberwell, a deprived inner London district thought to have a relatively high rate of depression (Broadhead & Abas, 1998). More women in Harare had experienced a severe life event (54%) in the preceding 12 months as compared to women in Camberwell (31%). A notable finding in Harare was the high proportion of events involving humiliation and entrapment that were related to marital crises such as being deserted by husbands and left to care for children, premature death, illness of family members, and severe financial difficulties occurring in the absence of an adequate welfare safety net.

Studies in South Asia have shown that the culturally determined value placed on boys (as compared to girls) adversely influences maternal mental health. The risk for postnatal depression is elevated in mothers who have a girl child, especially if the desired sex was a boy or if the mother already had living girl children (Patel et al., 2004).

The excess prevalence of alcohol abuse for men has been demonstrated in every community-based study from every region of the world, although the disparities are greatest in low- and middle-income countries. The wide sex differences in alcohol abuse in Latin American countries and the Caribbean have been attributed to a number of gender factors (Pyne, Claeson, & Correria, 2002). Women, for example, face strict social scrutiny about many behaviors, drinking among them. Men's consumption of alcohol takes place in the public realm, whereas women's drinking more often occurs in private. Drinking among men has social meanings, such as maintaining friendships, whereas refusing a drink can imply lack of trust and denial of mutual respect. At the other extreme, intoxication of men is more socially acceptable than that of women; indeed, women often tolerate their male partners' intoxication as being a "natural" condition of manhood. Drinking and drunkenness are more often perceived to be consistent with gendered notions of masculinity; thus men who conform closely to cultural norms are more likely to drink. Drinking may also be a coping strategy when men are faced with serious life difficulties, such as unemployment, and are unable to live up to the traditional expectations.

The evidence that gender plays a role in eating disorders stems from two observations: (1) the enormous sex difference in prevalence (females with these disorder vastly outnumber men with the same conditions) and (2) the very low rates of these disorders in cultures that have been relatively immune to the media-driven creation of the ideal body image for women. Recently, a study from Fiji demonstrated that the introduction of television in a media-naïve non-Westernized population is associated with a rise in attitudes favoring thinner body image and self-induced vomiting in girls (Becker, Burwell, Gilman, Herzog, & Hamburg, 2002), adding credence to the theory that the emphasis on women's thinness by the media and fashion industries is now leading to a rise in disordered eating in societies that, through the forces of globalization, are being increasingly influenced by Western imagery and values.

Conflict and Refugees

According to the United Nations High Commissioner for Refugees (http://www.unhcr.org/4981c3dc2.html), as of 2007 an estimated 11.4 million refugees had fled their own countries, another 13.7 million were internally displaced, and 2.9 million were not considered citizens of any state. Many of these refugees have experienced enormous trauma in the form of violence, crime, or other humiliations, physical injury, economic dispossession, and disruption of family and community structures. Thus the rates of mental disorder among these people would be expected to be at least as high as and probably higher than those for migrants in general.

A recent study of more than 3,000 respondents from postconflict communities in Algeria, Cambodia, Ethiopia, and Palestine found that post-traumatic stress disorder (PTSD)—a psychiatric disorder that is considered a specific response to trauma—was the most likely MNS disorder in individuals exposed to violence associated with armed conflict (de Jong, Komproe, & Ommeren, 2003). Other mental health consequences included mood and anxiety disorders.

In addition to exposure to trauma, a number of other factors may predispose refugees and immigrants to mental disorders, such as marginalization and minority status, socioeconomic disadvantage, poor physical health, the loss of social support systems, and cultural alienation in the new society. For illegal immigrants, there is also the constant fear of being found out and repatriated; as a consequence, access to possible sources of help is severely limited.

In discussing these issues, it is relevant to note that the universal application of the concept of trauma-related mental disorders (in particular, PTSD) has been criticized because it is itself based on culturally influenced notions of how a person is supposed to react to trauma. While consensus exists that trauma does negatively affect a person's mental health, the question of whether this negative impact should be conceptualized in psychiatric terms (with the concomitant implications of diagnosis and treatment) or in social and cultural terms remains unresolved.

Indigenous Communities

As many as 370 million indigenous persons may be living in approximately 5,000 distinct groups in more than 70 countries (Horton, 2006). They exhibit a wide diversity of lifestyles, cultures, social organization, histories, and political realities. Nevertheless, they share certain historical and political realities, including being subject to violence and genocide, depopulation from infectious diseases such as smallpox and measles, dislocation from traditional lands, extreme poverty due to the destruction of their subsistence economies, and state-organized attempts to repress and eradicate their cultures. Given this history, it is not surprising that the indigenous peoples of the world are currently experiencing relatively high rates of depression, alcoholism, and suicide, as well as high rates of infectious diseases and relatively short life-expectancies (Cohen, 1999) (Exhibit 9-3).

The case of the indigenous communities of Australia serves to illustrate the confluence of these historical, political, social, and economic forces on understanding why the rates of mental disorders are higher among indigenous peoples. The indigenous peoples of Australia had a diversity of cultures dating back at least 40,000 years before the arrival of European settlers slightly more than 200 years ago. These societies had rich cultural belief systems that attributed spiritual importance to land. Social relationships were governed by codes of behavior, and local taxonomies of illness guided the treatment of health problems. The brutal history of colonization that ultimately led to the destruction and devastation of hundreds of indigenous groups, each with a distinct language and lineage, was marked by a number of severe social adversities. Notable among these were exposure to new diseases, removal from traditional lands, enslavement on white farms, imprisonment without trials, denial of basic political rights, brutal violation of human rights, sexual abuse of women, and, perhaps most tragic of all, the "stolen generations"—the children who were forcibly removed from their parents and fostered by white families in an effort to "breed" out the native population.

Among the indigenous peoples of Australia, the consequences of this history are reflected in socioeconomic, psychosocial, and health indicators of all kinds: high rates of unemployment, low levels of income, and poor educational status; age-specific mortality rates two to seven times higher, and life expectancies more than 15 years shorter, than those of the general population; and high levels of alcoholism and suicide (Cohen, 1999). It is impossible to interpret the poor mental health experienced by these communities without considering the social and historical contexts of the systematic abuse of aboriginal communities. *Ways Forward*, the Australian national inquiry into indigenous mental health conducted in the early 1990s, prioritized holistic conceptions of emotional and social well-being among these groups. From these developments, greater emphasis has been given to providing access to culturally appropriate services within mainstream healthcare settings.

Interventions

This section briefly considers the role of mental health policies, human resources for mental health care, and the evidence for the prevention and treatment of mental disorders.

Mental Health Policies and Plans

A mental health policy presents the values, principles, and objectives for improving the mental health of people and reducing the burden of mental disorders in a population. It should define a vision for the future and help to establish a model for action. A policy should be distinguished from a plan, which is a strategy for implementing actions to achieve the objectives of a policy.

In some countries, mental health policies are restricted to psychiatric services. However, a broader scope is preferable—one in which mental health services in general are addressed. These services may include primary care and specialized care, as well as all aspects of intervention (prevention, treatment, and ongoing care) (WHO, 2003). Policies need to address the coordination between mental health services themselves, as well as between mental health services and other services such as housing, education, and employment. Other key issues that policies should address include financial arrangements for the private and public sectors, expenditure prioritization, and individual and organizational capacity development (WHO, 2001b). Finally, the policy needs to provide for continuous evaluation of mental health outcomes to ensure that the policy remains appropriate to contemporary circumstances and leads to effective services.

A country's capacity to deliver appropriate mental health services to its population is seriously hampered by the absence of a mental health policy. It is thus a cause for concern that only 62% of countries have mental health policies. Low- and middle-income countries are less likely to have policies: For example, only 50% and 48% of countries in Africa and the Western Pacific, respectively, have established such policies (WHO, 2001a).

Partly in response to this shortcoming, WHO has developed the Mental Health Policy and Service Guidance Package. This package consists of a series of interrelated user-friendly modules designed to assist with policy development and service planning. One module provides a series of steps that can be taken to develop mental health policies: assess the population's needs; gather evidence for an effective policy; consult and negotiate; exchange ideas with other countries; set out the vision, values, principles, and objectives of the policy; determine areas for action; identify the roles and responsibilities of different sectors; and conduct pilot studies (WHO, 2003).

Human Resources for Mental Health Care

The implementation of mental health policies and plans depends on both the quantity and the quality of its personnel to implement interventions. There are vast differences between regions of the world in terms of the availability of mental health professionals

(Table 9-1). In almost all countries, there is a gap between the supply of personnel and the demand for their services. The deleterious consequences of the low numbers of mental health professionals are magnified when one considers that the distribution of mental health professionals is frequently uneven between countries in each region, and within countries (with the number of mental health workers per 100,000 population being considerably higher in metropolitan areas, for example). Also, the available personnel are often not used efficiently, and staff may be demoralized and demotivated (WHO, 2005).

The development of human resources should constitute a key component of an effort to improve the public mental health. WHO (2005) suggests that several steps can be taken to address this need:

- Countries need to develop policies for increasing human resources in mental health.
- They need a systematic method of calculating how many mental health staff are required and which skill mix is optimal.
- They need to develop appropriate management strategies for leadership, motivation, and deployment of scarce personnel.
- Training of mental health staff needs to be reviewed and improved, in keeping with the mental health needs of the population.
- Once professionals are qualified, continuing education, training, and supervision need to be developed for the provision of the best care.

Mental health programs require a cadre of well-trained mental heath specialists, such as psychiatrists, psychologists, social workers, mental health occupational therapists, and psychiatric nurses (Desjarlais et al., 1995). They are responsible for functions such as the management of patients with complex conditions, supervision and training of other specialists and generic health workers, research, planning, management, and consultation–liaison. It is vital that specialists stay abreast of modern international developments that are relevant for the functions they perform, including skills of evaluation, capacity building, and supervision (Patel, 2009). However, the application of such developments should be informed by local research and experience. Training efforts for specialists should occur in parallel with training for generic health workers such as doctors and nurses, who provide the majority of care in low- and middle-income countries.

One sector that is particularly important in low- and middle-income countries is the traditional health sector. In many low- and middle-income countries, the majority of people seek care from traditional healers before seeing allopathic healers. The report of the Alma-Ata International Conference on Primary Health Care concluded:

Traditional medical practitioners and birth attendants are found in most societies. They are often part of a local community, culture and tradition, and continue to have high social standing in many places, exerting considerable influence on local health practices. It is therefore well worthwhile exploring the possibilities of engaging them in primary health care and of training them accordingly. (WHO, 1978)

There are several ways in which such providers can be engaged. They can operate side by side with allopathic mental health services, perhaps even operating from the same premises; they can be trained to recognize mental disorders and refer people suffering them to allopathic services; and they can be recruited and trained to function as allopathic mental health workers. Whatever arrangements are made

Table 9-1	Median Number of Mental Health Professionals per 100,000 Population in Each WHO Region and in the World			
WHO Region	**Psychiatrists**	**Psychiatric Nurses**	**Psychologists Working in Mental Health**	**Social Workers Working in Mental Health**
Africa	0.04	0.20	0.05	0.05
Americas	2.00	2.60	2.80	1.00
Eastern Mediterranean	0.95	1.25	0.60	0.40
Europe	9.80	24.80	3.10	1.50
Southeast Asia	0.20	0.10	0.03	0.04
Western Pacific	0.32	0.50	0.03	0.05
World	1.20	2.00	0.60	0.40

Source: World Health Organization, *Mental health atlas*. Geneva, Switzerland: Author.

at an organizational level, individual mental health service providers should attempt to establish whether their patients are being subjected to any traditional interventions that are harmful. If they are, they should receive education and counseling that aim to reduce exposure to such negative interventions. Conversely, traditional practices that are helpful can be incorporated into allopathic care (Institute of Medicine, 2001).

Prevention

Prevention involves interrupting the development of a disorder by altering factors that might affect the development of mental health problems. These factors can be divided into risk and protective factors. Risk factors make it more likely that an individual will develop mental health difficulties, whereas protective factors mediate and reduce the effects of risk exposure. Risk and protective factors can exist in the biological, psychological and social domains (Table 9-2).

Preventive interventions can be indicated (where the targets are high-risk individuals who are showing evidence of early disorder), selective (where the targets are high-risk groups), or universal (where the target is the entire population). Some overlap occurs between mental health prevention and promotion, which is most evident with universal preventive interventions. Thus an activity such as providing increased opportunities for more optimal use of leisure time could be construed as both a universal preventive intervention and as a mental health-promoting activity. Other examples of interventions that straddle prevention and promotion include raising public awareness about mental disorders with a view toward reducing stigma and school-based health programs that aim to reduce substance use (Flisher, Brown, & Mukoma, 2002). The global evidence on mental health promotion, in particular related to low- and middle-income countries, has been reviewed recently (Peterson, Bhana, Flisher, Swartz, & Richter, 2010).

Table 9-2	Selected Risk and Protective Factors for Mental Health	
Domain	**Risk Factors**	**Protective Factors**
Biological	Exposure to toxins (e.g., tobacco and alcohol) during pregnancy Genetic tendency to psychiatric disorder Head trauma HIV/AIDS and other physical illnesses	Age-appropriate physical development Good physical health Services provided at mother–baby clinics
Psychological	Maladaptive personality traits Effects of emotional, sexual abuse, and neglect Difficult temperament	Ability to learn from experiences Good self-esteem High level of problem-solving ability Social skills
Social		
Family	Divorce Family conflict Poor family discipline Poor family management No family	Family attachment Opportunities for positive involvement in family Rewards for involvement in family
School or workplace	Failure to perform at the expected level Low degree of commitment to school or workplace Inadequate/inappropriate educational provision or training opportunities	Opportunities for involvement in school or occupational activities
Community	Community disorganization Effects of discrimination Exposure to violence Social conflict and migration Poverty Transitions (e.g., urbanization)	Connectedness to community Opportunities for constructive use of leisure Positive cultural experiences Positive role models Rewards for community involvement

Source: World Health Organization. (In press). *Child and adolescent mental health*. Geneva, Switzerland: Author.

An examination of Table 9-2 indicates that actions for prevention need to address factors that operate across a range of sectors—for example, labor and employment, commerce and economics, education, housing, other social welfare services, and the criminal justice system. Thus mental health input is necessary in many sectors to ensure that policies will improve the mental health of the population and not have the opposite effect. For example, mental health input in the criminal justice system can prevent the inappropriate imprisonment of people with mental disorders, make treatment for mental disorders available in prisons, and reduce the mental health sequelae of imprisonment for prisoners and their families (WHO, 2001b). Other important reasons for linking with other sectors include promoting political will for the implementation of policies and legislation that are optimal for the public mental health; exploiting the potential to meet mental health needs in a number of settings, such as schools, workplaces, and communities; increasing buy-in from other sectors; educating people as to the potential contribution of their sector to the public mental health; increasing the comprehensiveness and holism with which an issue is regarded; encouraging a continuum of care; enabling a range of different approaches to be brought to bear in addressing an issue; and increasing efficiency and cost-effectiveness through reducing duplication and enhancing synergy between sectors. It is important to keep these points in mind when engaging with other sectors so that steps can be taken to ensure that the full benefits of such linkages are realized.

The evidence base on specific strategies for the prevention of mental disorders is relatively weak, particularly in low- and middle-income countries (Patel, Araya et al., 2007). Community approaches to prevention of depression can focus on several levels:

- At the individual level, one can strengthen mood management skills, self-efficacy, and self-esteem.
- At the system level, one can focus on social support networks and increased employment.

Such interventions aim to prevent the development of depressive symptoms to the point at which they become severe enough to "cross the threshold" into a major depressive episode.

Interventions in the workplace tend to focus on stress and stress management approaches, with a secondary aim to reduce possible psychiatric symptomatology such as depression and anxiety. Some interventions target whole or part of an organization. For example, the Caregiver Support Program (CSP) for human service workers (Jané-Llopis, Muñoz, & Patel, in press) has demonstrated that improving individual skills and changing organizational processes can reduce depressive symptomatology. Effective workplace policies—ranging from worker health and safety laws to employee assistance programs for alcohol, drug, and mental health problems—are also likely to have an impact on depressive symptomatology.

Indicated prevention has focused on those persons who are suffering from chronic medical conditions or from associated depressive symptomatology. Postpartum depression prevention in the form of support provision and antenatal education has been attempted in several trials, for example. In spite of the contradictory evidence regarding the effectiveness of antenatal programs to prevent postpartum depression, they have led to improvements in other health outcomes related to children and mothers, such as mother–infant engagement (Cooper, Landman, Tomlinson, Molteno, Swartz, & Murray, 2002). Selective prevention strategies that have proved effective for adults focus on stressful life events that have a direct or indirect relation with depression and depressive symptoms. For example, a focus on providing support to unemployed persons has led to reductions in depressive symptoms. A number of randomized trials have also attempted to test whether incidence of major depressive episodes can be reduced (Muñoz, Le, Clarke, & Jaycox, 2002). In sum, while some evidence suggests that it is possible to reduce the onset of major depressive episodes in adolescents using indicated interventions, preventive interventions for adults have not yet yielded significant reduction in incidence of major depressive episodes.

At present, there are no risk factors for schizophrenia that are sufficiently sensitive and specific to serve as a screening test for schizophrenia. Even if such a test were to be developed, no interventions are available that would stop the development of schizophrenia (Institute of Medicine, 2001). There is, however, a growing evidence base on "early interventions," such as supportive psychotherapy and low-dose antipsychotic agents, that may delay or prevent progression to a first episode (McGorry et al., 2002).

Effective interventions, strategies, and policies to prevent and reduce substance use disorders can be categorized as regulatory, community based (including education), and health service based. Prohibition has been attempted for alcohol products and is currently in place in some countries; this policy is also used with classes of substances including opioids, cannabinoids, and cocaine in most countries.

Although prohibition can dramatically reduce substance use disorders in the short term, its costs in terms of civil disobedience and crime are enormous— so much so, that, in general, prohibition is not regarded as an acceptable policy option, with the exception of specific circumstances, such as drinking alcohol and driving (Anderson, Biglan, & Holder, in press). Regulatory interventions include taxation, restrictions on availability, and total bans on all forms of direct and indirect advertising. Increases in alcohol taxes, for example, have been shown to reduce both the prevalence and consumption of alcohol products. For young people, laws that raise the minimum legal drinking age reduce alcohol sales and problems among young drinkers. Reductions in the hours and days of sale, numbers of alcohol outlets, and restrictions on access to alcohol are all associated with reductions in both alcohol use and alcohol-related problems.

There is limited evidence regarding the impact of prohibition or regulatory interventions on illicit drug use. Surveys of drug users tend to show rising or constant patterns of use in many countries, and declining rates in others, even though most countries have established strong regulatory interventions for these substances. Research paints a fairly dismal picture of the results of efforts to limit the supply of illicit drugs.

Community mobilization and education have been used to prevent substance abuse in many countries (see Exhibit 9-4 for two examples). A crucial setting for prevention is in schools, where the goal of most alcohol education programs is to change the adolescent's drinking beliefs, attitudes, and drinking behaviors, or to modify factors such as general social skills and self-esteem that are assumed to underlie adolescent drinking. Scientific evaluations of school-based interventions have generally produced small effects that are short-lived unless accompanied by ongoing booster sessions.

Preventive efforts directed toward reducing the risk factors for epilepsy and developmental disabilities have focused on improving prenatal care and promoting safe delivery (Institute of Medicine, 2001; WHO, 1998). Other preventive strategies include better fever control in children; strategies aimed at reduction of the causes of brain injury, such as children's safety seats and helmets; control of infectious and parasitic diseases that infect the brain; genetic counseling; screening programs for conditions that are known to be associated with mental handicap, such as hypothyroidism; micronutrient supplementation, such as with iodine; and reductions in environmental

Exhibit 9-4	Community Mobilization and Substance Abuse in Developing Countries

Two examples from low- and middle-income countries demonstrate the impact of community interventions.

In India, a community-based approach to combating alcoholism included education and awareness building, action against drunken men, advocacy to limit the sale and distribution of alcohol in bars and shops, and mass oaths for abstinence. The program was implemented though a community movement led by young people and women and the *Darumukti Sangathana* (Liberation from Liquor) village groups. The program has led to a marked reduction in the number of alcohol outlets in the area, and a 60% reduction in alcohol consumption (Bang & Bang, 1991).

An unblinded matched community-based trial in Yunnan, China, involved multiple sectors and leaders in the community and emphasized community participation and action, education in schools, literacy improvement, and employment opportunities. This program led to a 2.7 fold greater reduction in the incidence of drug abuse (Wu, Detels, Zhang, Li, & Li, 2002).

levels of toxins such as lead (Institute of Medicine, 2001).

Treatment and Care

This section briefly reviews the evidence for the treatment of mental disorders, primary care and community-based approaches, and mechanisms for delivery of effective treatments ("packages of care").

Effective Treatments and the "Treatment Gap"

Treatment for mental disorders has progressed enormously in the past few decades, to the point that effective treatments are available for the majority of mental disorders. Treatments may involve pharmacotherapy or psychotherapy, or both. Indeed, for many disorders, the optimal approach is to provide a combination of pharmacotherapy and psychotherapy.

Examples of the pharmacotherapies include neuroleptics for schizophrenia, antidepressants, stimulants (for ADHD), mood stabilizers such as lithium (for bipolar affective disorder) and anxiolytics (for anxiety disorders). Considerable progress has been made in the development of newer psychotropic agents—for example, neuroleptics and antidepressants. In general, these newer agents may not be more effective than their older counterparts, but they have fewer side effects. However, they are generally more expensive, which means that people in low- and middle-income countries are unlikely to enjoy the benefits of the recent psychopharmacological advances.

Psychotherapy refers to planned and structured interventions aimed at influencing behavior, mood, and emotional patterns of reaction to different stimuli through verbal and nonverbal psychological means (WHO, 2001b). A range of models of psychotherapy are used, such as psychoanalysis, cognitive-behavioral therapy, and interpersonal psychotherapy. Each model can be applied in a range of individual, family, or group settings. While evidence demonstrating the effectiveness of many psychotherapies continues to emerge, we are still at an early stage in our understanding of the mechanisms through which this effect is achieved. Furthermore, brief structured psychotherapies have the strongest evidence base for effectiveness (Exhibit 9-5).

Following recovery from an episode, the treatment phase shifts to emphasizing prevention of relapse or recurrence and providing rehabilitation. Prevention generally involves a combination of pharmacotherapy and psychotherapy, whereas rehabilitation aims to facilitate optimal functioning. It involves improving both individual skills and capacities and the environment in which the person lives. This goal can be achieved by improving social competence, reducing discrimination and stigma, providing family support, providing social support (including basic needs related to housing, employment, social networks, and leisure), and facilitating consumer empowerment (WHO, 1995). The WHO Mental Health Gap (mhGAP; WHO, 2008c) initiative has issued recommendations on the use of specific treatments in primary and community healthcare settings in low- and middle-income countries (http://www.who.int/mental_health/mhGAP/en/).

Only a small proportion of people suffering from mental disorders receive effective interventions. For example, the World Mental Health surveys (WHO World Mental Health Survey Consortium, 2004), which gathered information about treatment for mental disorders, found an association between the level of severity and the likelihood of being in treatment: Persons with serious disorders were the most likely to have been in treatment, no matter where they lived. However, the proportion of people with serious disorders who received treatment never exceeded 65% in any of the countries, and was as low as 15% in Lebanon. At the same time, the survey data showed that persons with either mild disorders or no disorder accounted for approximately half of all respondents who reported being in treatment during the previous year. Together, these results indicate that (1) many people with serious disorders are not receiving treatment and (2) available resources do not always go toward the treatment of those persons most in need of care. The lack of receipt of effective treatments which has been termed as the "treatment gap," is evident in all countries, but is more marked in low- and middle-income countries (Kohn, Saxena, Levav, & Saraceno, 2004).

As mentioned earlier, few low- and middle-income countries have more than 1 psychiatrist per 100,000 people; moreover, in many countries, the bulk of the resources available for mental health services are devoted to large psychiatric hospitals and

| Exhibit 9-5 | Do Talking Treatments Work in Low-Income Countries? |

Interpersonal psychotherapy is a form of psychological treatment that has been extensively used and evaluated for the treatment of depression in high-income countries. However, the applicability and effectiveness of such "talking treatments" in non-Western settings has rarely been studied.

A team of investigators from the United States and Uganda adapted this intervention for use in a rural setting in Uganda characterized by high rates of HIV/AIDS and other communicable diseases. They chose a group setting for delivering the intervention because it allowed them to reach out to more patients and would be more cost-effective in a low-resource setting. The intervention was tested in a cluster randomized controlled trial in which 30 villages were randomized. Men received the intervention in half the villages, and women in the other half. Depression was diagnosed using locally validated questionnaires. The intervention consisted of weekly group therapy sessions lasting approximately 90 minutes each, over 16 weeks. Whereas 90% of subjects in both arms (intervention and control) met the criteria for a major depressive disorder at recruitment, only 6.5% of the subjects in the intervention villages were depressed at the end of the trial, compared to more than half of the subjects in the control villages ($p < .001$). This study demonstrated not only the effectiveness of a relatively inexpensive and safe treatment for depression in a rural setting of a poor country, but also the feasibility of undertaking complex trials for mental disorders in low-resource settings (Bolton et al., 2003).

services are concentrated in a few urban settings (WHO, 2001b). Several barriers may prevent people from accessing even those limited services that do exist: demographic factors (e.g., race/ethnicity or gender), attitudes (e.g., fear of being stigmatized, thinking that no one can help, and a belief in solving problems independently), cost (even for those with insurance, mental health coverage is frequently inferior to that for other medical conditions), and organizational factors (e.g., fragmentation of services and lack of availability of effective treatments) (Sussman, Robins, & Earls, 1987). These organizational factors are frequently more pertinent for people who are members of socially disadvantaged groups, such as minority populations (U.S. Department of Health and Human Services, 1999). The fact that effective treatments exist for the majority of mental disorders amplifies the urgency of addressing the barriers that prevent people from receiving interventions from which they would benefit.

Finally, it has been recognized for some time that an "efficacy-effectiveness gap" exists with regard to MNS disorders. This term refers to the phenomenon in which pharmacological and psychotherapeutic treatments have a greater benefit in clinical trial settings as opposed to everyday practice. Some key differences between these settings account for the differences in response to treatment. For example, in routine healthcare settings, patients are more heterogeneous and ethnically diverse, have one or more comorbid disorders, are less compliant, are less likely to be seen in specialty settings, and are less likely to have their progress carefully and objectively monitored (Dixon, Lehman, & Levine, 1995). The vast majority of efficacy studies involving psychiatric treatments have been conducted in the Western world. As great as the differences are between the clinical trial setting and the real-world setting in high-income countries, those differences are still greater in low- and middle-income countries, where evidence from clinical trials may have limited generalizability. Thus it is particularly crucial to conduct effectiveness studies in low- and middle-income countries (Institute of Medicine, 2001).

Primary Health and Community-Based Approaches to Mental Health Care

Ever since 1975 (three years before the International Conference on Primary Health Care at Alma Ata), the integration of mental health services into primary care settings has been the mantra of international psychiatry (Patel & Cohen, 2003; WHO & UNICEF, 1978; WHO & World Organization of

Family Doctors, 2008). The reasons for this emphasis are twofold. First, epidemiological research suggests that approximately one-third of patients seen in primary care settings suffer from some mental disorder, predominantly depression and anxiety (WHO & World Organization of Family Doctors, 2008). This is true in high-income countries and low- and middle-income countries alike. Second, an acute shortage of mental health professionals makes primary care settings and reliance on non-specialized health workers the only practical options for the treatment of mental disorders. Although this is reasonable, the implementation of this strategy has had limited success (Cohen, 2001), owing to three factors:

- Low- and middle-income countries' primary care systems are already overwhelmed and do not have the capacity to take on new tasks.

- Primary care workers are not sufficiently trained in the recognition and management of mental disorders, nor do they have access to adequate supervision from specialists.

- Quality psychotropic medications are not always available (Saraceno et al., 2007).

Thus each of these barriers needs to be addressed.

A carefully planned deinstitutionalization of mentally ill persons through the concurrent closure of mental hospitals and the development of community care programs is arguably one of the most impressive public mental health achievements of the latter half of the twentieth century. In high-income countries, these changes have led to vast improvements in the quality of care and, importantly, greater recognition of the rights of patients. Such sweeping changes have not been as visible in low- and middle-income countries, however. Indeed, institutional care remains the norm even in countries with relatively numerous mental health human resources, such as Brazil and India. Thus mental hospital beds account for a large proportion of psychiatric beds in most low- and middle-income countries (instead of the general hospital psychiatric units found in high-income countries), and community programs are either symbolic demonstration projects or small-scale programs run in the nongovernmental sector.

The managed closure of mental hospitals must be accompanied by a carefully planned-out strategy to ensure that mentally ill persons do not simply wind up living on the streets. Halfway and rehabilitation homes may be needed for some persons who are severely disabled by their mental illness and who do not have adequate social support networks. For other patients, community care, linked with support from a mental health professional when available, must be the goal for mental health systems in all countries. It is evident from the description of a number of models in low- and middle-income countries that community care can be implemented using locally available resources and that it can improve clinical outcomes. One such example is the Ashagram model in rural India (Exhibit 9-6).

Efforts to integrate mental health services into primary care will be aided by two developments. First, there is increasing evidence from clinical trials in low- and middle-income countries that effective interventions for the treatment of mental disorders may be delivered by nonspecialist health workers (Araya et al., 2003; Bolton et al., 2003; Patel, Araya et al., 2007; Patel, Chisholm, Rabe-Hesketh, Dias-Saxena, Andrew, & Mann, 2003; Patel et al., 2008). Second, and equally important, has been the recognition that integration is not a simple matter of training nonspecialist health workers. Primary care workers need support and supervision by psychiatric specialists, and primary care mental health services "must be supported by other levels of care including community-based and hospital services, informal services, and self-care to meet the full spectrum of mental health needs of the population" (WHO & World Organization of Family Doctors, 2008). Furthermore, primary care mental health services, although essential, cannot meet all of the mental health needs of any given population. This is especially true for people who are suffering from psychotic disorders and who need access to community mental health and rehabilitation programs, as well as emergency inpatient facilities (Chatterjee et al., 2003; Patel, Farooq, & Thara, 2007).

Delivering Effective Treatments

The evidence on delivery mechanisms for MNS disorders in low- and middle-income countries was reviewed in the *PLoS Medicine* series, "Packages of Care for Mental, Neurological, and Substance Use Disorders in Low- and Middle-Income Countries" (http://www.plosmedicine.org/article/info%3Adoi%2F10.1371%2Fjournal.pmed.1000160). Although this series identified differences in the recommendations on specific treatments among disorders, there were also many shared themes related to the delivery of these treatments. The opening editorial (Patel & Thornicroft, 2009) to the Series summarizes these findings:

> Detection and diagnosis of more common disorders (such as depression or alcohol use disorder) may be reliably carried out using brief screening questionnaires. Less common disorders (such as schizophrenia and dementia) may need a two-stage case finding procedure with probable cases being identified through com-

---

Exhibit 9-6	**Community Care for Severe Mental Disorders in Low-Resource Settings**

A community mental health program for severe mental disorders in a rural setting in India was initiated in partnership with Ashagram ("village of hope"), a nongovernmental organization (NGO) working toward the rehabilitation for people affected by leprosy. The NGO was located in Barwani, one of the poorest districts in India. Mental health care was routinely provided through an outpatient clinic that required patients to travel to the hospital to be assessed and to receive treatment.

A community-based rehabilitation (CBR) model was devised for patients with chronic schizophrenia, based on a three-tiered service delivery system. CBR relies on the active participation of the disabled and their families in rehabilitation and takes specific notice of prevailing social, economic, and cultural issues. The highest tier was outpatient (OP) care. All patients were started on antipsychotic medication. The second tier consisted of mental health workers (MHWs) drawn from the local community. After a 60-day training program, the MHWs worked with patients, families, and the local community in providing services. Each MHW served five or six contiguous villages and carried a total case load of 25 to 30 patients, including some of the study subjects. The third tier consisted of family members and other key persons in the community who formed the local village health groups (*samitis*). These groups served as a forum for the members to plan relevant rehabilitation measures and reduce social exclusion.

The evaluation of the CBR program showed that, among compliant subjects, this model was more effective than standard OP treatment as determined by a range of clinical and functional outcomes (Chatterjee, Patel, Chatterjee, & Weiss, 2003). A four-year follow-up of the cohort of persons in the CBR care arm showed that adherence with medication and participation in self-help groups predicted a favorable outcome (Chatterjee, Pillai, Jain, Cohen, & Patel, 2009). Because a lack of professional resources is a reality in low-income countries, the CBR method takes advantage of active local community participation and low levels of technical expertise to deliver services.

munity case-finding strategies followed by a diagnostic interview by an appropriately trained health worker. A combined package of pharmacological and psychosocial treatments is efficacious for the treatment of MNS disorders; however, not all persons need all treatments. The proposed packages recommend stepped care models where treatments are tailored to the needs of each individual. People with almost all of these disorders need continuing care and help to maintain regular use of medication for extended periods to achieve optimal outcomes. In these respects, MNS disorders are similar to other long term conditions, such as diabetes and cardiovascular disease (Beaglehole et al., 2008). Non-specialist health workers can deliver, safely and effectively, treatments for MNS disorders within a functioning primary healthcare system (WHO, 2008b). However, collaborative care models, in which specialists play diverse roles of capacity building, consultation, supervision and quality assurance, and providing referral pathways, greatly enhance the effectiveness and sustainability of such non-specialist health worker led care programs (Patel, 2009). These shared characteristics suggest that the packages of care for MNS disorders can be integrated at three levels: first, an integration of packages catering to individual MNS disorders with each other; second, an integration of MNS disorder packages with other long-term conditions; and finally, that packages should be integrated within the primary healthcare system by strengthening its capacity for management of long-term conditions (Beaglehole et al., 2008; Patel, Goel, & Desai, 2009). However, it is also clear that simply making care available is not sufficient to close the treatment gap; access will continue to be hampered by stigma and discrimination (Institute of Medicine, 2001). Building mental health literacy and implementing strategies for combating stigma and discrimination for the whole population are critically important. It is also clear that, as with all long-term conditions, most of the evidence is derived from high-income countries. However, it is heartening to note that where attempts to replicate effectiveness evidence have been attempted in low- and middle-income countries, the findings are consonant with those from high-income countries, suggesting that effectiveness evidence, at least, may be generalizable across cultures.

Human Rights and Mental Illness

People with mental disorders have been subjected to abuses of human rights in all spheres of their lives, perhaps most tragically when they have been in mental hospitals. The past two decades have seen increased attention to the human rights of people suffering from mental disorders (WHO, 2001b). The United Nations General Assembly Resolution, *The Protection of Persons with Mental Illness and the Improvement of Mental Health Care* (United Nations, 1991), the Declaration of Caracas (WHO, 2001b), and the Declarations of Hawaii and Madrid (Helmchen & Okasha, 2000) all set forth principles that establish basic rights for persons suffering from mental illnesses—among them, the right to the best available care, protection from exploitation and discrimination, the right to be treated in the least restrictive environment possible, and the right of confidentiality. In view of past abuses in psychiatry (Birley, 2000; Bloch, 1997), these documents have served the task of raising awareness about the need to be vigilant on behalf of persons with mental disorders. With these guidelines and legal instruments in place, it is unfortunate that many countries do not have relevant policies, programs, or legislation that protect the human rights of persons with mental disorders.

Abuses of human rights take place in all sectors of society, including in psychiatric facilities (Alem, 2000; Levav & Gonzalez Uzcategui, 2000; National Human Rights Commission, 1999). Few systematic inquiries into the conditions of care in mental hospitals have been conducted; a notable exception is the National Human Rights Commission report of 1999, which described the state of the mental hospitals of India, many which date from the colonial period. This investigation found that violations of human rights were common and included a range of forms of inhuman restraints. More generally, many psychiatric institutions are characterized by a fundamental lack of respect for the dignity of persons with mental disorders. They are vulnerable to violence, and such practices often go unreported and unpunished. Abuse may also take place in homes and in communities. Some families, who are simply unable to cope, may tie their mentally ill relatives to the bed so that they can go about their daily existence in the comfort of knowing that their relative will not come to any harm. The tragedy of Erwaddi in 2001 in south India, in which more than 20 persons with mental disorders died when a fire swept through their healing temple because they were chained to their beds, is a reflection of abuses in traditional care facilities.

One of the major reasons for this kind of human rights abuse is the pervasive stigma associated with mental illness. Stigma has been described as consisting of "problems of ignorance, prejudice, and discrimination" (Thornicroft, 2006). Discrimination is the behavioral consequence of stigma. The experiences of people living with mental disorders vividly highlight the effects of stigma and discrimination. These narratives typically testify that such experiences are even more distressing than the mental disorder itself (Thornicroft, 2006). Some people ultimately accept these negative beliefs and prejudices and lose self-esteem, which in turn may lead to feelings of shame and hopelessness. Not surprisingly, they may then withdraw from social interactions to avoid discrimination ("anticipated discrimination"). The stigma attached to mental disorders has been identified as "the main obstacle to the provision of care for people with mental disorders" (Sartorius, 2007).

Raising awareness about mental illness has been proposed as one strategy to help improve understanding about the risks to mental health, and methods of coping with these risks, thereby reducing patients' stigma in the community. One such awareness program, delivered through schools, was assessed in a controlled trial in Rawalpindi, Pakistan. The intervention was delivered in two secondary schools and the outcome measurement was based on a self-report questionnaire about various aspects of mental health and illness. The experimental group showed significantly better improvement in scores as compared to the control group (Rahman, Mubbashar, Gater, & Goldberg, 1998). More impressive was the finding that parents, friends, and even neighbors of the students in the experimental group showed significant improvements as compared to the control group. This trial indicates that delivering education regarding mental health and illness to secondary school students may be effective in raising awareness in the wider community and, therefore, may help raise mental health literacy and promote mental health at large. Well-planned public awareness and education campaigns can reduce stigma and discrimination, increase the use of mental health services, and bring mental and physical health care closer to each other (WHO, 2001b).

Such campaigns must be accompanied by strong legislative frameworks committed to implementing international human rights instruments. Legislation is essential to complement and reinforce mental health policy. It provides the legal framework for issues such as human rights, community integration of the mentally ill, links with other sectors, access to care, rehabilitation and aftercare, enhancement of the quality of care, prevention of mental disorders, and promo-

tion of mental health (WHO, 2003). Worldwide, only 78% of countries have passed any sort of mental health legislation (WHO, 2001a). However, in contrast to mental health policies, it is not the case that low- and middle-income countries are less likely to have legislation. In Africa, for example, 71% of countries have mental health legislation. A module in WHO's "Mental Health Policy and Service Guidance Package" addresses mental health legislation and human rights (WHO, 2003). This module presents a step-by-step approach to each of the phases of the legislative process: preliminary activities, the drafting process, adoption of legislation, and implementation.

Global Mental Health: A Call to Action

The World Health Report 2001 (WHO, 2001b) set out 10 key recommendations for public mental health in low- and middle-income countries (Exhibit 9-7). These guidelines remain critical strategies to achieve the call to action that has become the slogan for global mental health: to scale up services for people affected by mental disorders based on the principles of evidence and human rights. This final section discusses specific strategies not already covered elsewhere in the chapter.

Involving a range of sectors is a key aspect of achieving this call to action in all settings, and arguably even more so in low- and middle-income countries, where the formal mental healthcare system is typically inadequately developed. Previously, this chapter presented a number of examples of intersectoral,

Exhibit 9-7	Public Mental Health Priorities

1. Provide treatment in primary care
2. Make psychotropic agents available
3. Give care in the community
4. Educate the public
5. Involve communities, families, and consumers
6. Establish national policies and legislation
7. Develop human resources
8. Link with other sectors
9. Monitor community health
10. Support more research

Source: World Health Organization. (2001). *Mental health: New understanding, new hope*. Geneva, Switzerland: Author.

community action—for example, the programs to prevent alcohol and drug abuse and the community-based rehabilitation model for schizophrenia. This section highlights one specific sector that has made an important contribution to mental health care and reforms in high-income countries and has only recently achieved recognition in low- and middle-income countries: consumer- and family-led movements.

The World Fellowship for Schizophrenia and Allied Disorders and Alzheimer's Disease International are examples of NGOs that have their origins in high-income countries where strong consumer movements led by families of persons with schizophrenia and Alzheimer's disease led to their establishment. In the past decade, both NGOs have had a growing presence in low- and middle-income countries. Similarly, Befriender International, a voluntary group that provides support to persons who are suicidal, has spread to a number of low- and middle-income countries. Local NGOs led by families of persons affected by mental illness are also multiplying rapidly in low- and middle-income countries (Patel & Thara, 2003).

There are fewer examples of community movements that are led by persons who are themselves suffering from mental disorders. Perhaps the best example is Alcoholics Anonymous, which is widely represented internationally, and is one of the most well-described examples of an effective community-based intervention for a mental disorder.

All of these NGOs share many characteristics. For instance, all have a strong community orientation, with an explicit space for families and users of services to express their views and set the agenda for action. Advocacy to policy makers, the media, and other sectors in the health system is a core activity. Prominent examples of the success of these advocacy efforts include the inclusion of mental disabilities in the disability legislation passed by some countries. Many groups also provide services, usually in the form of support groups or networking for affected families, but the larger groups even support research activities and medical care.

The Movement for Global Mental Health (www.globalmentalhealth.org), which was launched in October 2008, is a coalition of individuals and institutions who are committed to taking action to improve services for people with mental disorders and promoting their human rights (Exhibit 9-8). This group takes its inspiration from global HIV/AIDS movements, which have transformed HIV/AIDS care through a massive scaling up of resources and services to provide a comprehensive continuum of care for people living with HIV (PLHIV) across the globe. Critical to the success of the global HIV/AIDS cam-

---

Exhibit 9-8	**Panel: Join the Movement!**

To join the movement, you should agree to:

1. The immediate scaling up of the coverage of services for mental disorders, especially in low- and middle-income countries, through an evidence-based package of affordable and accessible community-based services for core mental disorders

2. A new commitment to the protection of the human rights of persons with mental disorders and their families

3. Calls for new funding for mental health both as health assistance to low- and middle-income countries from international donors and lending agencies, and in budget allocations from governments

If you do, go now to www.globalmentalhealth.org.

---

paign were its specific and clear calls to action, its grounding in the evidence of treatments and human rights, and its united front of PLHIV, health practitioners, and researchers.

Research is essential to generate the evidence necessary for guiding an appropriate response by policy makers and practitioners to the large unmet needs of care for mental illnesses, particularly in low- and middle-income countries. The need for mental health research to reflect the diverse realities of the health systems and cultural factors is crucial if research is to inform local health policy and practice. As with most areas of health, the contribution of low- and middle-income countries to mental health research is very low. Surveys of high-impact journals typically reveal that less than 10% of published research originates from low- and middle-income countries, and the vast majority of journals published in low- and middle-income countries are non-indexed, limiting their impact (Patel & Sumathipala, 2001).

A major factor impeding the use of more appropriate interventions or greater prominence for mental illness in policy is the lack of evidence about treatments and the tendency for research to be focused on psychiatrists and psychiatric contexts. Perhaps if evidence demonstrated that treatments are efficacious and cost-effective, and that they are clearly linked to other community health problems, then they would be more widely advocated by health workers and health policy makers. Future research needs to be more action oriented; that is, it should take the form of actual intervention trials or studies with the explicit goal of influencing the integration of mental health care in existing community health services and public health priorities (Tomlinson, Rudan, Saxena, Swartz, Tsai, & Patel, 2009). Such research must be sensitive to local needs and encompass active participation from potential users of the findings. In selecting settings for intervention research, a variety of health systems should be considered to ensure that findings can be generalized to many regions of the world.

Perhaps the most important strategy to support mental health research in low- and middle-income countries is the need to raise skills and capacity for research in diverse regions of the world. There are some existing resources for mental health research in low- and middle-income countries, including collaborative relationships between institutions, international networks for research, a growing number of donors willing to fund mental health research, and a variety of training programs for research. However, there remains a large gap between what is available and what is needed; thus it is necessary to strengthen existing resources and develop new ones. The ultimate goals for sustainable research in low- and middle-income countries include creating a network of researchers, research centers, and forums for information exchange; making a career in research an attractive option for mental health and public health professionals in low- and middle-income countries; ensuring that research findings are taken seriously by practitioners and policy makers; and securing sufficient funding, commensurate with the global burden of mental disorders, that can support enable research in low- and middle-income countries.

While delivery research questions are a scientific and moral priority for global mental health, it is also important to recognize the limitations in our understanding of the causes of MNS disorders and their treatments. More research into the nature of mental disorders that samples populations in the global context is clearly needed, as most existing research has focused on a small and relatively homogenous fraction of the global population. Few descriptions of phenotypes in non-Western populations, and their risk and protective factors, have been published. Notably, the World Mental Health Surveys and the 10/66 Dementia Research Group program are two global, cross-national initiatives to study the prevalence, impact, and health service responses to anxiety and mood disorders and dementia, respectively. Similar initiatives are needed in other areas, such as child mental disorders and psychoses.

In addition, global mental health research could help increase the pool of efficacious treatments for mental disorders. Mindfulness-based cognitive therapy and dialectical behavior therapy are examples of treatments that have integrated "Eastern" approaches into psychological treatments. To date, there have been no systematic research initiatives to map and evaluate treatments—either pharmacological or psychosocial—used by African, Asian, and American cultures. The emergence of global mental health as a key discipline in global health offers a unique opportunity both for strengthening the scientific evidence base on prevention and treatment and for increased investment to close the treatment gap.

● ● ● Discussion Questions

1. It is difficult to place mental health high on the public health agenda of low- and middle-income countries that face an enormous burden from communicable diseases. Which evidence-based arguments might you make to challenge the notion that mental health is a luxury item on the health agenda of such countries?

2. The classification of mental disorders is mainly derived from the description of these disorders in high-income countries. Some argue that this fact limits the application of psychiatric knowledge and evidence to non-Western cultures. How valid are these concerns? In which ways has the "Western" bias been addressed in classification of mental disorders in international public health?

3. Diseases that disproportionately affect the poor are typically prioritized by governments and donors. Many people believe that disorders such as depression are problems of the middle class and affluent or represent a "medicalization of misery," and, therefore, do not deserve a share of scarce resources. What is the evidence linking poverty with mental disorders? How might poverty interact with mental health?

4. While there is now a growing evidence base on effective treatments for most mental disorders, large treatment gaps can be found in all countries, especially in low- and middle-income countries. What are the reasons for this treatment gap? How can they be addressed at the level of health policy and health service development?

5. Human rights are a major driver in global health. Even though people affected by mental disorders represent one of the most marginalized and discriminated groups in any context, their human rights are often ignored. Why is this the case, and what can be done to address this issue?

• • • References

Aben, I., Lodder, J., Honig, A., Lousberg, R., Boreas, A., & Verhey, F. (2006). Focal or generalized vascular brain damage and vulnerability to depression after stroke: A 1-year prospective follow-up study. *International Psychogeriatrics, 18,* 19–35.

Alem, A. (2000). Human rights and psychiatric care in Africa with particular reference to the Ethiopian situation. *Acta Psychiatrica Scandinavica,* 93–96.

American Psychiatric Association. (1994). *Diagnostic and statistical manual of mental disorders.* Washington, DC: Author.

Ammassari, A., Antinori, A., Aloisi, M. S., Trotta, M. P., Murri, R., Bartoli, L., et al. (2004). Depressive symptoms, neurocognitive impairment, and adherence to highly active antiretroviral therapy among HIV-infected persons. *Psychosomatics, 45,* 394–402.

Anastasi, A. (1958). Heredity, environment and the question "How"? *Psychological Review, 65,* 197–208.

Anderson, P., Biglan, A., & Holder, H. (In press). Reducing the onset of substance use disorders. In C. Hosman, E. Jané-Llopis, & S. Saxena (Eds.), *Prevention of mental disorders: An overview on evidence-based strategies and programs.* Oxford, UK: Oxford University Press.

Anderson, R. J., Freedland, K. E., Clouse, R. E., & Lustman, P. J. (2001). The prevalence of comorbid depression in adults with diabetes: A meta-analysis. *Diabetes Care, 24,* 1069–1078.

Andrews, J., Briggs, A., Porter, R., Tucker, P., & Waddington, K. (1997). *The history of Bethlem.* London: Routledge.

Araya, R., Rojas, G., Fritsch, R., Gaete, J., Simon, G., Peters, T. J., et al. (2003). Treating depression in primary care in low-income women in Santiago, Chile: A randomised controlled trial. *Lancet, 361,* 995–1000.

Astbury, J. (2001). Gender disparities in mental health. In *Mental health: A call for action by World Health Ministers* (pp. 73–92). Geneva, Switzerland: World Health Organization.

Bang, A., & Bang, R. (1991). Community participation in research and action against alcoholism. *World Health Forum, 12,* 104–109.

Beaglehole, R., Epping-Jordan, J., Patel, V., Chopra, M., Ebrahim, S., Kidd, M., et al. (2008). Improving the prevention and management of chronic disease in low-income and middle-income countries: A priority for primary health care. *Lancet, 372,* 940–949.

Becker, A. E., Burwell, R. A., Gilman, S. E., Herzog, D. B., & Hamburg, P. (2002). Disordered eating behaviors and attitudes follow prolonged exposure to television among ethnic Fijian adolescent girls. *British Journal of Psychiatry, 180,* 509–514.

Beiser, M., Cargo, M., & Woodbury, M. (1994). A comparison of psychiatric disorder in different cultures: Depressive typologies in South-East Asian refugees and resident Canadians. *International Journal of Methods in Psychiatric Research, 4,* 157–172.

Bennedsen, B. E., Mortensen, P. B., Olesen, A. V., & Henriksen, T. B. (1999). Preterm birth and intra-uterine growth retardation among children of women with schizophrenia. *British Journal of Psychiatry, 175,* 239–245.

Birbeck, G. L., & Kalichi, E. M. (2004). Epilepsy prevalence in rural Zambia: A door-to-door survey. *Tropical Medicine and International Health, 9,* 92–95.

Birley, J. L. (2000). Political abuse of psychiatry. *Acta Psychiatrica Scandinavica,* 13–15.

Blacker, D., & Tsuang, M. T. (1992). Contested boundaries of bipolar disorder and the limits of categorical diagnosis in psychiatry. *American Journal of Psychiatry, 149,* 1473–1483.

Bloch, S. (1997). Psychiatry: An impossible profession? *Australian & New Zealand Journal of Psychiatry, 31,* 172–183.

Bolton, P., Bass, J., Neugebauer, R., Verdeli, H., Clougherty, K. F., Wickramaratne, P., et al. (2003). Group interpersonal psychotherapy for depression in rural Uganda. *Journal of the American Medical Association, 289,* 3117–3124.

Broadhead, J. C., & Abas, M. A. (1998). Life events, difficulties and depression among women in an urban setting in Zimbabwe. *Psychological Medicine, 28,* 29–38.

Buitelaar, J., Barton, J., Danckaerts, M., Friedrichs, E., Gillberg, C., Hazell, P. L., et al. (2005). A comparison of North American versus non-North American ADHD study populations. *European Child and Adolescent Psychiatry 15,* 177–181.

Burneo, J. G., Tellez-Zenteno, J., & Wiebe, S. (2005). Understanding the burden of epilepsy in Latin America: A systematic review of its prevalence and incidence. *Epilepsy Research, 66,* 63–74.

Buskin, S. E., Gale, J. L., Weiss, N. S., & Nolan, C. M. (1994). Tuberculosis risk factors in adults in King County, Washington, 1988 through 1990. *American Journal of Public Health, 84,* 1750–1756.

Caetano, R., & Laranjeira, R. (2006). A "perfect storm" in developing countries: Economic growth and the alcohol industry. *Addiction (Abingdon, UK), 101,* 149–152.

Chander, G., Himelhoch, S., & Moore, R. D. (2006). Substance abuse and psychiatric disorders in HIV-positive patients: Epidemiology and impact on antiretroviral therapy. *Drugs, 66,* 769–789.

Chang, S. S., Gunnell, D., Sterne, J. A., Lu, T. H., & Cheng, A. T. (2009). Was the economic crisis 1997–1998 responsible for rising suicide rates in East/Southeast Asia? A time-trend analysis for Japan, Hong Kong, South Korea, Taiwan, Singapore and Thailand. *Social Science & Medicine, 68,* 1322–1331.

Chatterjee, S., Patel, V., Chatterjee, A., & Weiss, H. (2003). Evaluation of a community-based rehabilitation model for chronic schizophrenia in rural India. *British Journal of Psychiatry, 182,* 57–62.

Chatterjee, S., Pillai, A., Jain, S., Cohen, A., & Patel, V. (2009). Outcomes of people with psychotic disorders in a community-based rehabilitation programme in rural India. *British Journal of Psychiatry, 195,* 433–439.

Cohen, A. (1999). *The mental health of indigenous people: An international overview.* Geneva, Switzerland: World Health Organization1999.

Cohen, A. (2001). *The effectiveness of mental health services in primary care: The view from the developing world.* Geneva, Switzerland: World Health Organization.

Cook, J. A., Grey, D., Burke, J., Cohen, M., Gurtman, A. C., Richardson, J. L., et al. (2004). Depressive symptoms and AIDS-related mortality among a multisite cohort of HIV-positive women. *American Journal of Public Health, 94,* 1133–1140.

Cooper, P., Landman, M., Tomlinson, M., Molteno, C., Swartz, L., & Murray, L. (2002). The impact of a mother–infant intervention in an indigent peri-urban South African context: A pilot study. *British Journal of Psychiatry, 180,* 76–81.

Cournos, F., McKinnon, K., & Sullivan, G. (2005). Schizophrenia and comorbid human immuno-deficiency virus or hepatitis C virus. *Journal of Clinical Psychiatry, 66* (suppl 6), 27–33.

de Groot, M., Anderson, R., Freedland, K. E., Clouse, R. E., & Lustman, P. J. (2001). Association of depression and diabetes complications: A meta-analysis. *Psychosomatic Medicine, 63,* 619–630.

de Jong, J. T. V. M., Komproe, I. H., & Ommeren, M. V. (2003). Common mental disorders in postconflict settings. *Lancet, 361,* 2128–2130.

Desai, N. G., Nawamongkolwattana, B, Ranaweera, S., Shrestha, D. M., & Sobhan, M. A. (2003). *Get high on life with out alcohol.* New Delhi: World Health Organization (SEARO).

Desjarlais, R., Eisenberg, L., Good, B., & Kleinman, A. (1995). *World mental health: Problems and priorities in low-income countries.* New York: Oxford University Press.

Digby, A. (1985). Moral treatment at the Retreat, 1796–1846. In W. F. Bynum, R. Porter, & M. Shepherd (Eds.), *The anatomy of madness: Essays in the history of psychiatry* (pp. 52–72). London: Tavistock.

Dixon, L. B., Lehman, A. F., & Levine, J. (1995). Conventional antipsychotic medications for schizophrenia. *Schizophrenia Bulletin, 21,* 567–577.

Dolder, C. R., Lacro, J. P., & Jeste, D. V. (2003). Adherence to antipsychotic and nonpsychiatric medications in middle-aged and older patients with psychotic disorders. *Psychosomatic Medicine, 65,* 156–162.

Eaton, W. W., Armenian, H., Gallo, J., Pratt, L., & Ford, D. E. (1996). Depression and risk for onset of type II diabetes: A prospective population-based study. *Diabetes Care, 19,* 1097–1102.

Eisenbruch, M. (1991). From post-traumatic stress disorder to cultural bereavement: Diagnosis of Southeast Asian refugees. *Social Science & Medicine, 33,* 673–680.

Escobar, J. I., Waitzkin, H., Silver, R. C., Gara, M., & Holman, A. (1998). Abridged somatization: A study in primary care. *Psychosomatic Medicine, 60,* 466–472.

Faraone, S. V., Sergeant, J., Gillberg, C., & Biederman, J. (2003). The worldwide prevalence of ADHD: Is it an American condition? *World Psychiatry, 2,* 104–113.

Ferri, C. P., Prince, M., Brayne, C., Brodaty, H., Fratiglioni, L., Ganguli, M., et al. (2005). Global prevalence of dementia: A Delphi consensus study. *Lancet, 366,* 2112–2117.

Flisher, A. J. (1999). The management of suicidal behaviour in adolescents. *Specialist Medicine, 21,* 418–423.

Flisher, A. J., Brown, A., & Mukoma, W. (2002). Intervening through school systems. In W. R. Miller & C. M. Weisner (Eds.), *Changing substance abuse through health and social systems* (pp. 171–182). New York: Kluwer Academic/ Plenum Press.

Flisher, A. J., Hatherill, S., Dhansay, Y., & Swartz, L. (2007). Culture, ADHD and the *DSM-V* [abstract]. *Journal of Child and Adolescent Mental Health, 19,* 170.

Forsgren, L. (2008). Estimations of the prevalence of epilepsy in sub-Saharan Africa. *Lancet Neurology, 7,* 21–22.

Gajalakshmi, V., & Peto, R. (2007). Suicide rates in rural Tamil Nadu, South India: Verbal autopsy of 39,000 deaths in 1997–98. *International Journal of Epidemiology, 36,* 203–207.

Gil-Gonzalez, D., Vives-Cases, C., Alvarez-Dardet, C., & Latour-Perez, J. (2006). Alcohol and intimate partner violence: Do we have enough information to act? *European Journal of Public Health, 16,* 279–285.

Goldman, H. H. (1983). The demography of deinstitutionalization. *New Directions for Mental Health Services, 17,* 31–40.

Greenberg, P., Kessler, R., Nells, T., Finkelstein, S., & Berndt, E. (1996). Depression in the workplace: An economic perspective. In J. P. Feighner & W. F. Boyer WF (Eds.), *Selective serotonin re-uptake inhibitors: Advances in basic research and clinical practice* (pp. 327–363). New York: John Wiley & Sons.

Greenberg, P. E., Sisitsky, T., Kessler, R. C., Finkelstein, S. N., Berndt, E. R., Davidson, J. R., et al. (1999). The economic burden of anxiety disorders in the 1990s. *Journal of Clinical Psychiatry, 60,* 427–435.

Greenberg, P. E., Stiglin, L. E., Finkelstein, S. N., & Berndt, E. R. (1993). The economic burden of depression in 1990. *Journal of Clinical Psychiatry, 54,* 405–418.

Greenblatt, M. (1992). Deinstitutionalization and reinstitutionalization of the mentally ill. In M. J. Robertson & M. Greenblatt (Eds.), *Homelessness: A national perspective* (pp. 47–56). New York: Plenum Press.

Grigsby, A. B., Anderson, R. J., Freedland, K. E., Clouse, R. E., & Lustman, P. J. (2002). Prevalence of anxiety in adults with diabetes: A systematic review. *Journal of Psychosomatic Research, 53,* 1053–1060.

Grob, G. N. (1994). *The mad among us: A history of the care of America's mentally ill.* New York: Free Press.

Gureje, O., Simon, G. E., Ustun, T. B., & Goldberg, D. P. (1997). Somatization in cross-cultural perspective: A World Health Organization study in primary care. *American Journal of Psychiatry, 154,* 989–995.

Hawton, K., & van Heeringen, K. (2009). Suicide. *Lancet, 373,* 1372–1381.

Helmchen, H., & Okasha, A. (2000). From the Hawaii Declaration to the Declaration of Madrid. *Acta Psychiatrica Scandinavica*, 20–23.

Hemingway, H., & Marmot, M. (1999). Evidence based cardiology: Psychosocial factors in the aetiology and prognosis of coronary heart disease. Systematic review of prospective cohort studies. *British Medical Journal, 318*, 1460–1467.

Hendrie, H., Osuntokun, B., Hall, K., Ogunniyi, A., Hui, S., Unverzagt, F., et al. (1995). Prevalence of Alzheimer's disease and dementias in two communities: Nigerian Africans and African Americans. *American Journal of Psychiatry, 152*, 1485–1492.

Holt, R. I., Bushe, C., & Citrome, L. (2005). Diabetes and schizophrenia 2005: Are we any closer to understanding the link? *Journal of Psychopharmacology, 19*, 56–65.

Horton, R. (2006). Indigenous peoples: Time to act now for equity and health. *Lancet, 367*, 1705–1707.

Ickovics, J. R., Hamburger, M. E., Vlahov, D., Schoenbaum, E., Schuman, P., Boland, R.J., et al. (2001). Mortality, CD4 cell count decline, and depressive symptoms among HIV-seropositive women: Longitudinal analysis from the HIV Epidemiology Research Study. *Journal of the American Medical Association, 285*, 1466–1474.

Institute of Medicine. (2001). *Neurological, psychiatric and developmental disorders: Meeting the challenge in the developing world*. Washington, DC: National Academy Press.

Jablensky, A., Sartorius, N., Ernberg, G., Anker, M., Korten, A., Cooper, J. E., et al. (1992). Schizophrenia: Manifestations, incidence and course in different cultures: A World Health Organization ten-country study. In *Psychological Medicine Monograph, Supplement 20*. Cambridge, UK: Cambridge University Press.

Jackson, L. A. (1999). The place of psychiatry in colonial and early postcolonial Zimbabwe. *International Journal of Mental Health, 28*, 38–71.

Jané-Llopis, E., Muñoz, R. F., & Patel, V. (In press). Prevention of depression and depressive symptoma-tology. In C. Hosman, E. Jané-Llopis, & S. Saxena (Eds.), *Prevention of mental disorders: An overview on evidence-based strategies and programs*. Oxford, UK: Oxford University Press.

Jencks, C. (1994). *The homeless*. Cambridge, MA: Harvard University Press.

Kahn, R. S., Wise, P. H., Kennedy, B. P., & Kawachi, I. (2000). State income inequality, household income, and maternal mental and physical health: Cross-sectional national survey. *British Medical Journal, 321*, 1331–1315.

Katon, W. J., Rutter, C., Simon, G., Lin, E. H., Ludman, E., Ciechanowski, P., et al. (2005). The association of comorbid depression with mortality in patients with type 2 diabetes. *Diabetes Care, 28*, 2668–2672.

Kendler, K. S., & Gardner, C. O. Jr. (1998). Boundaries of major depression: An evaluation of *DSM-IV* criteria. *American Journal of Psychiatry, 155*, 172–177.

Kessler, R. C. (2000). Psychiatric epidemiology: Selected recent advances and future directions. *Bulletin of the World Health Organization, 78*, 464–474.

Kessler, R. C., Aguilar-Gaxiola, S., Alonso, J., Chatterji, S., Lee, S., Ormel, J., et al. (2009). The global burden of mental disorders: An update from the WHO World Mental Health (WMH) surveys. *Epidemiology and Psychiatry Society, 18*, 23–33.

Kessler, R. C., McGonagle, K. A., Zhao, S., Nelson, C. B., Hughes, M., Eshlerman, S., et al. (1994). Lifetime and 12-month prevalence of *DSM-III-R* psychiatric disorders in the United States. *Archives of General Psychiatry, 51*, 8–19.

Kleinman, A. (1988). *Rethinking psychiatry: cultural category to personal experience*. New York: Free Press.

Kleinman, A. (2004). Culture and depression. *New England Journal of Medicine, 351*, 951–953.

Knapp, M., Mangalore, R., & Simon, J. (2004). The global costs of schizophrenia. *Schizophrenia Bulletin, 30*, 279–293.

Kohn, R., Saxena, S., Levav, I., & Saraceno, B. (2004). The treatment gap in mental health care. *Bulletin of the World Health Organization, 82,* 858–866.

Kraepelin, E. (2000 [1904]). Comparative psychiatry. In R. Littlewood & S. Dein (Eds.), *Cultural psychiatry and medical anthropology: An introduction and reader* (pp. 38–42). London: Athlone Press.

Lancet Global Mental Health Group. (2007). Scaling up services for mental disorders: A call for action. *Lancet, 370,* 1241–1252.

Larson, S. L., Owens, P. L., Ford, D., & Eaton, W. (2001). Depressive disorder, dysthymia, and risk of stroke: Thirteen-year follow-up from the Baltimore epidemiologic catchment area study. *Stroke, 32,* 1979–1983.

Latthe, P., Mignini, L., Gray, R., Hills, R., & Khan, K. (2006). Factors predisposing women to chronic pelvic pain: Systematic review. *British Medical Journal, 332,* 749–755.

Lee, S. (2001). From diversity to unity: The classification of mental disorders in 21st-century China. *Psychiatric Clinics of North America, 24,* 421–431.

Levav, I., & Gonzalez Uzcategui, R. (2000). Rights of persons with mental illness in Central America. *Acta Psychiatrica Scandinavica, 83–86.*

Levy, C. J. (2002, April 28). Ingredients of a failing system: A lack of state money, a group without a voice. *New York Times.* Retrieved from http://www.nytimes.com/2002/04/28/nyregion/28SIDE.html

Lin, C. Y., Huang, A. L., Minas, H., & Cohen, A.(2009). Mental hospital reform in Asia: The case of Yuli Veterans Hospital, Taiwan. *International Journal of Mental Health Systems, 3,* 1.

Littlewood, R. (1990). From categories to contexts: A decade of the "new cross-cultural psychiatry." *British Journal of Psychiatry, 156,* 308–327.

Llibre Rodriguez, J. J., Ferri, C. P., Acosta, D., Guerra, M., Huang, Y., Jacob, K. S., et al. (2008). Prevalence of dementia in Latin America, India, and China: A population-based cross-sectional survey. *Lancet, 372,* 464–474.

Lund, C., Breen, A., Flisher, A. J., Kakuma, R., Corrigall, J., Joska, J. A., et al. (2010). Poverty and common mental disorders in low and middle income countries: A systematic review. *Social Science & Medicine 71,* 517–28.

Lustman, P. J., Anderson, R. J., Freedland, K. E., de Groot, M., Carney, R. M., & Clouse, R. E. (2000). Depression and poor glycemic control: A meta-analytic review of the literature. *Diabetes Care, 23,* 934–942.

Mac, T. L., Tran, D-S., Quet, F., Odermatt, P., Preux, P-M,, & Tan, C. T. (2007). Epidemiology, aetiology, and clinical management of epilepsy in Asia: A systematic review. *Lancet Neurology, 6,* 533–543.

Maj, M., Satz, P., Janssen, R., Zaudig, M., Satz, P., Sughondhabirom, B., et al. (1994). WHO neuro-psychiatric AIDS study, cross-sectional phase II. Neuropsychological and neurological findings. *Archives of General Psychiatry, 51,* 51–61.

Mathers, C. D., & Loncar, D. (2006). Projections of global mortality and burden of disease from 2002 to 2030. *PLoS Medicine 3,* e442.

Mbuba, C. K., & Newton, C. R. (2009). Packages of care for epilepsy in low- and middle-income countries. *PLoS Medicine, 6,* e1000162.

McGorry, P. D., Yung, A. R., Phillips, L. J., Yuen, H. P., Francey, S., Cosgrave, E. M., et al. (2002). Randomized controlled trial of interventions designed to reduce the risk of progression to first-episode psychosis in a clinical sample with subthreshold symptoms. *Archives of General Psychiatry, 59,* 921–928.

McGrath, J., Saha, S., Welham, J., El Saadi, O., MacCauley, C., & Chant, D. (2004). A systematic review of the incidence of schizophrenia: The distribution of rates and the influence of sex, urbanicity, migrant status and methodology. *BMC Medicine, 2.*

McQuistion, H. L., Colson, P., Yankowitz, R., & Susser, E. (1997). Tuberculosis infection among people with severe mental illness. *Psychiatric Services, 48,* 833–835.

Mechanic, D. (2001). The scientific foundations of community psychiatry. In G. Thornicroft & G.

Szmukler (Eds.), *Textbook of community psychiatry* (pp. 41–52). Oxford, UK: Oxford University Press.

Molero, A. E., Pino-Ramirez, G., & Maestre, G. E. (2007). High prevalence of dementia in a Caribbean population. *Neuroepidemiology*, 29, 107–112.

Molteno, C., & Westaway, J. (2001). Mental handicap. In B. Robertson, C. Allwood, & C. Gagiano (Eds.), *Textbook of psychiatry for Southern Africa* (pp. 345–357). Cape Town: Oxford University Press.

Mora, G. (1980). Historical and theoretical trends in psychiatry. In H. I. Kaplan, A. M. Freedman, & B. J. Sadock BJ (Eds.), *Comprehensive text book of psychiatry* (3rd ed., pp. 4–98). Baltimore: Williams and Wilkins.

Movement for Global Mental Health gains momentum. (2009). *Lancet*, 374, 587.

Muñoz, R. F., Le, H. N., Clarke, G., & Jaycox, L. (2002). Preventing the onset of major depression. In I. H. Gotlib & C. L. Hammen (Eds.), *Handbook of depression* (pp. 343–359). New York: Guilford.

Murdock, G.P., Wilson, S. F., & Frederick, V. (1980). World distribution of theories of illness. *Transcultural Psychiatry Research Review*, 17, 37–64.

Murray, C. J. L., & Lopez, A. D. (1996). *The global burden of disease: A comprehensive assessment of mortality and disability from diseases, injuries, and risk factors in 1990 and projected to 2020*. Cambridge, MA: Harvard School of Public Health.

Narayanan, H. S. (1981) A study of the prevalence of mental retardation in southern India. *International Journal of Mental Health*, 10, 28–36.

National Human Rights Commission. (1999). *Quality assurance in mental health*. New Delhi: Author.

Nigg, J. T. (2006). *What causes ADHD?: Understanding what goes wrong and why*. New York: Guilford Press.

Nilsson, E., Lichtenstein, P., Cnattingius, S., Murray, R. M., & Hultman, C. M. (2002). Women with schizophrenia: Pregnancy outcome and infant death among their offspring. *Schizophrenia Research*, 58, 221–229.

Osuntokun, B. O., Adeuja, A. O., Nottidge, V. A., Bademosi, O., Olumide, A., Ige, O., et al. (1987). Prevalence of the epilepsies in Nigerian Africans: A community-based study. *Epilepsia*, 28, 272–279.

Parikh, R. M., Robinson, R. G., Lipsey, J. R., Starkstein, S. E., Fedoroff, J. P., & Price, T. R. (1990). The impact of poststroke depression on recovery in activities of daily living over a 2-year follow-up. *Archives of Neurology*, 47, 785–789.

Patel, V. (In press). Alcohol and mental health in developing countries: A review. *Annals of Epidemiology*.

Patel, V. (1995). Explanatory models of mental illness in sub-Saharan Africa. *Social Science & Medicine*, 40, 1291–1298.

Patel, V. (2009). The future of psychiatry in low and middle income countries. *Psychological Medicine*, 39, 1759–1762.

Patel, V., Araya, R., Chisholm, D., Chatterjee, S., Cohen, A., De Silva, M., et al. (2007). Treatment and prevention of mental disorders in low and middle income countries. *Lancet*, 370, 991–1005.

Patel, V., Araya, R., de Lima, M., Ludermir, A., & Todd, C. (1999). Women, poverty and common mental disorders in four restructuring societies. *Social Science & Medicine*, 49, 1461–1471.

Patel, V., Chisholm, D., Kirkwood, B., & Mabey, D. (2007). Prioritising health problems in women in developing countries: Comparing the financial burden of reproductive tract infections, anaemia and depressive disorders in a community survey in India. *Tropical Medicine & International Health*, 12, 130–139.

Patel, V., Chisholm, D., Rabe-Hesketh, S., Dias-Saxena, F., Andrew, G., & Mann, A. (2003). Efficacy and cost-effectiveness of drug and psychological treatments for common mental disorders in general health care in Goa, India: A randomised, controlled trial. *Lancet*, 361, 33–39.

Patel, V., & Cohen, A. (2003). Mental health services in primary care in "developing" countries. *World Psychiatry*, 2, 163–164.

Patel, V., Farooq, S., & Thara, R. (2007). What is the best approach to treating schizophrenia in developing countries? *PLoS Medicine, 4*, e159.

Patel, V., Goel, D., & Desai, R. (2009). Scaling up services for mental and neurological disorders. *International Health, 1*, 37–44.

Patel, V., Kirkwood, B. R., Pednekar, S., Pereira, B., Barros, P., Fernandes, J., et al. (2006). Gender disadvantage and reproductive health risk factors for common mental disorders in women: A community survey in India. *Archives of General Psychiatry, 63*, 404–413.

Patel, V., Kirkwood, B. R., Pednekar, S., Araya, R., King, M., Chisholm, D., et al. (2008). Improving the outcomes of primary care attenders with common mental disorders in developing countries: A cluster randomized controlled trial of a collaborative stepped care intervention in Goa, India. *Trials, 9*, 4.

Patel, V., Rahman, A., Jacob, K. S., & Hughes, M. (2004). Effect of maternal mental health on infant growth in low income countries: New evidence from South Asia. *British Medical Journal, 328*, 820–823.

Patel, V., Simbine, A. P., Soares, I. C., Weiss, H, A., & Wheeler, E. (2007). Prevalence of severe mental and neurological disorders in Mozambique: A population-based survey. *Lancet, 370*, 1055–1060.

Patel, V., & Sumathipala, A. (2001). International representation in psychiatric literature: Survey of six leading journals. *British Journal of Psychiatry, 178*, 406–409.

Patel, V., & Thara, R. (2003). *Meeting mental health needs in developing countries*. New Delhi: Sage (India).

Patel, V., & Thornicroft, G. (2009). Packages of care for mental, neurological, and substance use disorders in low- and middle-income countries: PLoS Medicine Series. *PLoS Medicine, 6*, e1000160.

Patel, V., Weiss, H. A., Kirkwood, B. R., Pednekar, S., Nevrekar, P., Gupte, S., et al. (2006). Common genital complaints in women: The contribution of psychosocial and infectious factors in a population-based cohort study in Goa, India. *International Journal of Epidemiology, 35*, 1478–1485.

Patton, G. C., Coffey, C., Sawyer, S. M., Viner, R. M., Haller, D. M., Bose, K., et al. (2009). Global patterns of mortality in young people: A systematic analysis of population health data. *Lancet, 374*, 881–892.

Peterson, I., Bhana, A., Flisher, A., Swartz, L., & Richter, L (Eds). (2010). *Promoting mental health in scarce resource countries*. Durban: Human Sciences Research Council.

Phillips, M. R., Li, X., & Zhang, Y. (2002). Suicide rates in China, 1995–99. *Lancet, 359*, 835–340.

Pierloot, R. A. (1975). Belgium. In J. G. Howells (Ed.), *World history of psychiatry* (pp. 136–149). New York: Brunner/Mazel.

Pinel, P. (1977). A treatise on insanity. In J. C. Shershow (Ed.), *Delicate branch: The vision of moral psychiatry* (pp. 1–38). Oceanside, NY: Dabor Science.

Plomin, R., Owen, M. J., & McGuffin, P. (1994). The genetic basis of complex human behaviors. *Science, 264*, 1733–1739.

Preux, P-M., & Druet-Cabanac, M. (2005). Epidemiology and aetiology of epilepsy in sub-Saharan Africa. *Lancet Neurology, 4*, 21–31.

Prince, M. J., & Jackson, J. (2009). *Alzheimer's Disease International*. London: World Alzheimer Report.

Prince, M., Patel, V., Saxena, S., Maj, M., Maselko, J., Phillips, M. R., et al. (2007). No health without mental health. *Lancet, 370*, 859–877.

Pyne, H. H., Claeson, M., & Correia, M. (2002). *Gender dimensions of alcohol consumption and alcohol-related problems in Latin America and the Caribbean*. Washington, DC: World Bank.

Rahman, A., Mubbashar, M. H., Gater, R., & Goldberg, D. (1998). Randomised trial of impact of school mental-health programme in rural Rawalpindi, Pakistan. *Lancet, 352*, 1022–1025.

Rehm, J., Mathers, C. D., Patra, J., & Popova, S. (2009). Global burden of disease and injury and economic cost attributable to alcohol use and alcohol use disorders. *Lancet, 373*, 2223–2233.

Rehm, J. R., Mathers, C., Popova, S., Thavorncharoensap, M., Teerawattananon, Y., & Patra, J. (2009). Global burden of disease and injury and economic cost attributable to alcohol use and alcohol-use disorders. *Lancet, 373,* 2223–2233.

Rice, D. P., Kelman, S., & Miller, L. S. (1992) The economic burden of mental illness. *Hospital & Community Psychiatry, 43,* 1227–1232.

Ritchie, K., Kildea, D., & Robine, J. M. (1992). The relationship between age and the prevalence of senile dementia: A meta-analysis of recent data. *International Journal of Epidemiology, 21,* 763–769.

Rohde, L. A., Szobot, C., Polanczyk, G., Schmitz, M., Martins, S., & Tramontina, S. (2005). Attention-deficit/hyperactivity disorder in a diverse culture: Do research and clinical findings support the notion of a cultural construct for the disorder? *Biology and Psychiatry, 57,* 1436–1441.

Room, R., Babor, T., & Rehm, J. (2005). *Alcohol and public health. Lancet, 365,* 519–530.

Rwiza, H. T., Kilonzo, G. P., Haule, J., Matuja, W. B. P., Mteza, I., Mbena, P., et al. (1992). Prevalence and incidence of epilepsy in Ulanga, a rural Tanzanian district: A community-based study. *Epilepsia, 33,* 1051–1056.

Saha, S., Chant, D., Welham, J., & McGrath, J. (2005). A systematic review of the prevalence of schizophrenia. *PLoS Med, 2,* e141.

Saraceno, B., van Ommeren, M., Batniji, R., Cohen, A., Gureje, O., Mahoney, J., et al. (2007). Barriers to improvement of mental health services in low-income and middle-income countries. *Lancet, 370,* 1164–1174.

Sartorius, N. (2007). Stigma and mental health. *Lancet, 370,* 810–811.

Sartorius, N., Kaelber, C. T., Cooper, J. E., Roper, M., Rae, D. S., Gulbinat, W., et al. (1993). Progress toward achieving a common language in psychiatry. *Archives of General Psychiatry, 50,* 115–124.

Schmidt, K. E. (1967). Mental health services in a developing country in South-East Asia (Sarawak).

In H. C. Freeman & J. Farndale (Eds.), *New aspects of the mental health services* (pp. 213–236). Oxford, UK: Pergamon Press.

Scull, A. (1989). *Social order/mental disorder: Anglo-American psychiatry in historical perspective.* Berkeley, CA: University of California Press.

Scull, A. T., MacKenzie, C., & Hervey, N. (1996). *Masters of Bedlam: The transformation of the mad-doctoring trade.* Princeton, NJ: Princeton University Press.

Shah, A., & Jenkins, R. (2000). Mental health economic studies from developing countries reviewed in the context of those from developed countries. [Review] [206 refs]. *Acta Psychiatrica Scandinavica, 101,* 87–103.

Sobocki, P., Jonsson, B., Angst, J., & Rehnberg, C. (2006). Cost of depression in Europe. *Journal of Mental Health Policy and Economics, 9,* 87–98.

Srinath, S., Girimaji, S. C., Gururaj, G., Seshadri, S., Subbakrishna, D. K., Bhola, P., et al. (2005). Epidemiological study of child and adolescent psychiatric disorders in urban and rural areas of Bangalore, India. *Indian Journal of Medical Research, 122,* 67–79.

Strik, J. J., Lousberg, R., Cheriex, E. C., & Honig, A. (2004). One year cumulative incidence of depression following myocardial infarction and impact on cardiac outcome. *Journal of Psychosomatic Research, 56,* 59–66.

Sussman, L. K., Robins, L. N., & Earls, F. (1987). Treatment-seeking for depression by black and white Americans. *Social Science & Medicine, 24,* 187–196.

Swartz, S. (1999). "Work of mercy and necessity": British rule and psychiatric practice in the Cape Colony, 1891–1910. *International Journal of Mental Health, 28,* 72–90.

Szmukler, G., & Thornicroft, G. (2001). What is community psychiatry? In G. Thornicroft & G. Szmukler (Eds.), *Textbook of community psychiatry* (pp. 1–12). Oxford, UK: Oxford University Press.

Tansella, M., & Thornicroft, G. (2001). The principles underlying community care. In G. Thornicroft & G. Szmukler (Eds.), *Textbook of community psychiatry* (pp. 155–165). Oxford, UK: Oxford University Press.

Thornicroft, G. (2006). *Shunned: Discrimination against people with mental illness*. Oxford, UK: Oxford University Press.

Tomlinson, M., Rudan, I., Saxena, S., Swartz, L., Tsai, A., & Patel, V. (2009). Setting investment priorities for research in global mental health. *Bulletin of the World Health Organization, 87*, 438–446.

Tsuang, M. T., Stone, W. S., & Faraone, S. V. (2000). Toward reformulating the diagnosis of schizophrenia. *American Journal of Psychiatry, 157*, 1041–1050.

United Nations. (1991). *The protection of persons with mental illness and the improvement of mental health care, 1991*. Report No.: UN General Assembly Resolution A/RES/46.119.

U.S. Department of Health and Human Services. (1999). *Mental health: A report of the Surgeon General*. Rockville, MD: U.S. Department of Health and Human Services, Center for Mental Health Services, National Institutes of Health, & National Institute of Mental Health.

Wang, P. S., Simon, G., & Kessler, R. C. (2003) The economic burden of depression and the cost-effectiveness of treatment. *International Journal of Methods of Psychiatric Research, 12*, 22–33.

Weich, S., & Lewis, G. (1998). Poverty, unemployment and the common mental disorders: A population based cohort study. *British Medical Journal, 317*, 115–119.

Westermeyer, J. (1984). Economic losses associated with chronic mental disorder in a developing country. *British Journal of Psychiatry, 144*, 475–481.

White, D. A., Heaton, R. K., & Monsch, A. U. (1995). Neuropsychological studies of asymptomatic human immunodeficiency virus-type-1 infected individuals. The HNRC Group. HIV Neurobehavioral Research Center. *Journal of the International Neuropsychology Society, 1*, 304–315.

Whiteford, H., Buckingham, B., & Manderscheid, R. (2002). Australia's national mental health strategy. *British Journal of Psychiatry, 180*, 210–215.

World Health Organization (WHO). (1978). *Primary health care: Report of the international conference*. Geneva, Switzerland: Author.

World Health Organization (WHO). (1990). *International classification of diseases—10*. Geneva, Switzerland: Author.

World Health Organization (WHO). (1992). *The ICD-10 classification of mental and behavioural disorders*. Geneva, Switerzland: Author.

World Health Organization (WHO). (1995). *Psychosocial rehabilitation: A consensus statement*. Geneva, Switzerland: Author.

World Health Organization (WHO). (1998). *Primary prevention of mental, neurological and psychosocial disorders*. Geneva, Switzerland: Author.

World Health Organization (WHO). (2001a). *Atlas country profiles of mental health resources*. Geneva, Switzerland: Author.

World Health Organization (WHO). (2001b). *Mental health: New understanding, new hope*. Geneva, Switerzland: Author.

World Health Organization (WHO). (2001c). *World health report 2001. Mental health: New understanding, new hope*. Geneva, Switzerland: Author.

World Health Organization (WHO). (2003). *Mental health policy, plans and programmes*. Geneva, Switzerland: Author.

World Health Organization (WHO). (2005). *Human resources and training in mental health*. Geneva, Switzerland: Author.

World Health Organization (WHO). (2008a). *The global burden of disease: 2004 update*. Geneva, Switerzland: Author.

World Health Organization (WHO). (2008b). *Integrating mental health into primary care : A global perspective*. Geneva, Switzerland: WHO & World Organization of Family Doctors (Wonca).

World Health Organization (WHO). (2008c). *Mental Health Gap Action Programme (mhGAP): Scaling up care for mental, neurological and substance abuse disorders*. Geneva, Switzerland: Author.

World Health Organization (WHO). (n.d.). Suicide prevention: Live your life. Retrieved from http://www.who.int/mental_health/management/en/SUPRE_flyer1.pdf

World Health Organization (WHO) & UNICEF. (1978). *Primary health care: Report of the international conference on primary health care, Alma-Ata, USSR, 6–12 September 1978*. Geneva, Switzerland: WHO.

World Health Organization (WHO) & World Organization of Family Doctors. (2008). *Integrating mental health into primary care: A global perspective*. Geneva, Switzerland: Authors.

World Health Organization (WHO) World Mental Health Survey Consortium. (2004). Prevalence, severity, and unmet need for treatment of mental disorders in the World Health Organization World Mental Health Surveys. *Journal of the American Medical Association, 291*, 2581–2590.

Wu, Z., Detels, R., Zhang, J., Li, V., & Li, J. (2002). Community base trial to prevent drug use amongst youth in Yunnan, China. *American Journal of Public Health, 92*, 1952–1957.

Ziegelstein, R. C., Fauerbach, J. A., Stevens, S. S., Romanelli, J., Richter, D. P., & Bush, D. E. (2000). Patients with depression are less likely to follow recommendations to reduce cardiac risk during recovery from a myocardial infarction. *Archives of Internal Medicine, 160*, 1818–1823.

10

Environmental Health

TORD KJELLSTROM, ANTHONY J. MCMICHAEL, KIRK R. SMITH, AND SUDHVIR SINGH

This chapter is an update of the chapter in the second edition (by McMichael, Kjellstrom, and Smith), with the same focus on principles and health impact study methodologies. The science of environmental health has many specific features that cannot be raised here, and the reader with an interest in studying and interpreting specific situations is advised to seek out additional specialized sources of information.

This chapter first explores the definition of "environment" and its ways of affecting human health. In doing so, it takes note of several key disciplinary perspectives, the international spectrum of environmental health issues, and the ongoing emergence of larger-scale environmental problems. The main conceptual and methodological issues that relate to environmental health research and public health action are discussed. Subsequently, using a five-way subdivision of "environment" classified by scale and setting, the profiles of environmental health hazards are discussed within the household setting, in the workplace, in the community, and on regional and global scales. This consideration is important because people in low- and middle-income countries are often exposed to environmental health hazards in both their work and daily life settings. Illustrative case studies are presented to highlight these issues.

The final section considers the issues and prospects that bear on the future of environmental health research and policy. Which priorities apply in a politically and economically unequal world? What are the environmental hazards of globalization, in its several guises? How can environmental health hazards be addressed via a more integrated, "ecological" understanding of how the complex interplay between human populations and the natural "environment" affects population health?

Definition and Scope of Environment

The word "environment" is broad and elastic in scope. In this chapter, "environment" refers to those external microbiological, chemical, and physical exposures and processes that impinge upon individuals and groups and are beyond the immediate control of individuals. Within the physical category, one can include factors linked to ergonomy—that is, the links between the physical features of the human body and the environment (e.g., limitations of reach, reaction time, and ability to lift weights, all of which are associated with injury risks). This definition excludes exposures that occur largely because of individual choice, such as active cigarette smoking and personal dietary habits. It also excludes specific risk factors that arise within the sociocultural environment, such as violent crime and community stress (see Chapter 8). However, the links between the sociocultural and economic environments and the exposures and health risks due to environmental hazards need to be considered as features of "environmental health." Further, environmental conditions associated with risk of physical injury (such as traffic, workplace, and home) will be discussed only briefly (for further details, see Chapter 8).

The "environment" can be categorized several ways, including in relation to environmental media (air, water, soil, and food), the economic sector (transport, land use, and energy generation), physical scale (local, regional, global), setting (household, workplace, and urban environment), and disease outcomes (cancers, congenital anomalies, and others). A classification that comprises five categories is used here, defined jointly by physical scale and by setting. The five categories are as follows:

1. Household
2. Workplace
3. Community
4. Regional
5. Global

A sixth category, that of cross scale, should also be included. This category recognizes that the scale at which an environmental health impact eventually occurs may not be the scale at which the exposure was initiated.

Consider the hierarchy of environmental health consequences of energy use. The environmental impacts of energy production and use contribute significantly to the total human impact on the "environment" at each of the six previously mentioned levels. That is, the extraction, harvesting, processing, distribution, and use of fuels and other energy sources have major environmental impacts at all scales, from individual households to the globe itself. Combustion occurs locally, causing local air pollution, both indoors and outdoors, but it also contributes to regional acid rain and, globally, to the accumulation of carbon dioxide as a heat-trapping greenhouse gas in the lower atmosphere.

In defining the environment, there are two other points to note. First, some environmental exposures arise because of natural variation, whereas others are due to human interventions. Natural exposures arise from seasonal, latitudinal, or altitudinal gradients in solar irradiation, extremes of hot and cold weather, the occurrence of physical disasters, and local micronutrient deficiencies in soil. The usual environmental concern, however, is with exposure to human-made hazards. In high-income countries, attention has focused in recent years on the many chemical contaminants entering the air, water, soil, and food as well as on physical hazards such as ionizing radiation, urban noise, and road trauma. In low- and middle-income countries, the major environmental concerns center on the microbiological quality of drinking water and food, the physical safety of housing and work settings, indoor air pollution, and road hazards. Those hazards are kept under control in high-income countries through major investments in good-quality housing and community infrastructure (e.g., drinking water supply, sewerage, solid waste collection, and others). Natural environmental hazards, such as the 2011 earthquakes in New Zealand and Japan, and the devastating tsunami in Japan, cannot be "kept under control" even in the highest income countries.

Second, two qualitatively different dimensions of the environment are relevant to human health risks. There is the familiar local physicochemical and microbiological environment, which serves as the vehicle for various specific hazards able to cause injury, toxicity, nutritional deficiency, or infection. Less familiar are the hazards that arise from today's emerging disruptions to the biosphere's ecological and geophysical system—that is, the life-support systems that stabilize, replenish, recycle, cleanse, and produce, thereby providing climatic stability, food yields, clean freshwater, nutrient cycling, and sustained biodiversity (see also the section "Environment: Encompassing Both Hazard and Habitat," later in this chapter).

Table 10-1 provides examples of the types of environmental health hazard exposures that can occur at the different scales discussed in this chapter. Note that exposures may come via air, water, food, or other media, depending on the specific situation. Studies of environmental health impacts will, therefore, require an understanding of a number of specialized scientific disciplines.

Scale and Distribution of Environmental Risks to Health

In the last decade, a considerable amount of work has been done to estimate the global and national burden of disease attributable to environmental factors. Such estimates are difficult to construct, both because knowledge about disease etiology is incomplete and because of the latency period between environmental change and nonacute health outcomes. The complex relationships among environmental conditions, socioeconomic circumstances, demographic change, and human health present a further difficulty in estimating the environmental contribution to disease burden (Shahi, Levy, Binger, Kjellstrom, & Lawrence, 1997; World Health Organization [WHO], 1997). For example, the combination of population pressure and poverty among rural populations in low- and middle-income countries often leads to land degradation, deforestation, flooding, further impoverishment, and increased risks to health from infectious disease, food shortages, and nutritional deficiencies. The situation of sub-Saharan Africa—with its persistent poverty, environmental stresses, and marginalization in the global economy—illustrates well these complex relationships. Many of the erstwhile gains in sub-Saharan Africa's health, education, and living standards have been reversed in

Table 10-1	Examples of Sources of Unhealthy Environmental Exposures				
Scale	Household	Workplace	Community	Regional	Global
Types of Environmental Exposure					
Microbiological	Contaminated drinking water; poor sanitation and food safety	Spread of infectious diseases via air or needlesticks in health services	Contamination of local rivers and lakes from animal and human feces	Spread of contamination to major rivers	Large-scale spread of infectious diseases (e.g., malaria) due to climate change
Chemical	Exposure of children to lead from household paint	Solvents exposure from glues or paints in manufacturing industries	Urban air pollution from motor vehicles or industry	Confluence of urban air pollution into larger areas (e.g., Asian brown cloud)	Global spread of persistent organic pollutants; greenhouse gas emissions
Physical	Too-cold or too-hot indoor temperatures in households	Noisy machinery and processes; excessive workplace heat exposure.	Traffic noise	Ionizing radiation from nuclear accidents (e.g., Chernobyl, 1986)	Increased ultraviolet (UV) radiation due to ozone layer depletion
Ergonomic	Injury risks in badly designed dwellings	Heavy lifting and injury risks caused by machinery	Traffic safety risks due to bad urban design		

the past two decades: A majority of people live in absolute poverty, 42% lack safe drinking water, and 69% lack proper sanitation (United Nations, 2008). Child mortality rates in sub-Saharan African countries are more than 50% higher than those in other low- and middle-income countries, and average life expectancy is about a decade less.

In general, there is a tendency for environmental health risks to shift during the economic development process, first from the household to the community, and then to regional and global scales, as part of the "environmental risk transition" (Smith, 1997; Smith & Ezzati, 2005). Environmental risks in low- and middle-income societies are dominated by poor food, water, and air quality at the household level from inadequate sanitation, contaminated water, and low-quality fuels (McMichael et al., 2008; WHO, 1997). Some of the activities that help solve these problems act to transfer problems to the community level in the form of urban air pollution, hazardous waste, and chemical pollution. In high-income countries, where most community and household problems have come under considerable control, problems have to some extent shifted to the global scale—for example, through greenhouse gas emis-

sions; at the same time, low-income communities within these countries are often still at risk from local environmental hazards (WHO, 2008). The risk transition and the inequitable persistence of household risks have been clearly described in China (Smith, 2008).

As discussed in Chapter 1, the changes in disease patterns that are occurring during the epidemiologic transition—although their details vary substantially in different places and times—have been one of the most important features of economic development. Before there can be a shift in age-specific disease patterns, however, there needs to be a shift in the within-population pattern of risks that lead to disease. Another important characteristic that changes is the temporal scale. Many important infectious diseases—diarrhea, malaria, and measles, for example—have relatively short latency periods (hours to weeks) between exposure to risk factors and development of disease. Cancer and other chronic noninfectious diseases, by comparison, often entail time delays of several decades. Global processes such as anthropogenic climate change may involve even longer time periods. Thus the risk transition tends to involve a shift in temporal characteristics, which has important implications for research and social policy (McMichael, 2009).

Depending on definitions, assumptions, and choice of reference populations, estimates of the environmental contribution to the total avoidable global burden of disease span a wide range. In the first systematic use of a standardized metric—the disability-adjusted life-year (DALY) (Murray & Lopez, 1996), which combines morbidity and mortality data in a manner suitable for international comparisons—the World Bank (1993) attributed approximately 50% of all global DALYs to diseases associated with environmental (including microbiological) exposures in the household and an additional 30% to diseases associated with the community environment. Only a small proportion of these DALYs were deemed amenable to feasible preventive interventions, however (World Bank, 1993). Smith, Corvalan, and Kjellstrom (1999), in a more comprehensive analysis, estimated that 25% to 33% of the global burden of disease and premature death is attributable to direct environmental risk factors.

The first truly integrated comparative risk assessment of the global and regional burden of disease due to major risk factors was organized by WHO and summarized in its World Health Report 2002 (WHO, 2002). For the first time, risks from major environmental hazards were evaluated on a common basis not only among themselves, but also for comparison with such nonenvironmental hazards as smoking, unsafe sex, malnutrition, and high blood pressure. The environmental hazards identified in the 2002 report included unsafe water, sanitation, and hygiene; urban air pollution; indoor smoke from solid fuels; lead exposure; climate change; and five types of occupational risks. The results of the WHO analysis are likely to be underestimates, because the researchers used a rather conservative definition of acceptable evidence of cause–effect relationships to provide consistency across risk factors. This factor is particularly important for occupational risks in poor countries, where much work occurs in informal sectors that were not addressed by this risk assessment.

As shown in Table 10-2, in high-mortality (low-income) countries, unsafe water and indoor smoke are ranked third and fifth, respectively, among the leading risk factors for burden of disease. In low-mortality

Table 10-2	Ranking of Health Burden Due to Environmental Risk Factors in 2000 by Development Status (Percent of Total Disability-Adjusted Lost Life Years Due to Each Risk Factor)							
High-Mortality (Poor) Developing Countries (population = 2.3 billion)	% of Burden	Rank	Low-Mortality (Middle-Income) Developing Countries (pop. = 2.4 billion)	% of Burden	Rank	Developed Countries (pop. = 1.4 billion)	% of Burden	Rank
Underweight	14.7	1	Alcohol	6.3	1	Tobacco	12.2	1
Unsafe sex	10.0	2	Blood pressure	5.0	2	Blood pressure	10.9	2
Unsafe water, sanitation, and hygiene	5.5	3	Tobacco	4.0	3	Alcohol	9.2	3
Lack of vaccination for child cluster diseases	5.3	4	**Road traffic**	3.3	4	Cholesterol	7.6	4
Indoor smoke from solid fuels	3.6	5	Underweight	3.1	5	Overweight	7.4	5
Zinc deficiency	3.2	6	Overweight	2.7	6	Low fruit and vegetable intake	3.9	6
Iron deficiency	3.1	7	**Occupation**	2.4	7	Physical inactivity	3.3	7
Vitamin A deficiency	3.0	8	Cholesterol	2.1	8	**Road traffic**	1.9	8
Blood pressure	2.4	9	Low fruit and vegetable intake	1.9	9	Illicit drugs	1.8	9
Tobacco	2.0	10	**Indoor smoke**	1.9	10	**Occupation**	1.5	10
Occupational risks	1.1	14	**Unsafe water**	1.8	12	**Lead exposure**	0.65	13
Lead exposure	0.70	19	**Lead exposure**	1.4	14	**Urban air**	0.55	15
Climate change	0.61	20	**Urban air**	0.99	17	**Unsafe water**	0.39	16
Urban air pollution	0.32	23	**Climate change**	0.07	24	**Indoor smoke**	0.26	19
Road traffic accidents	0.31	24				**Climate change**	0.01	23

Environmental risks are shown in bold type.

Source: Smith & Ezzati, 2005. Source of data: WHO, 2002 and WHO's GBD Database for 2000.

(middle-income) countries, these factors are ranked twelfth and tenth, respectively. In contrast, these risks are not listed among the top 15 in high-income countries (Smith & Ezzati, 2005). Note the relative importance of occupational risks at every level of development.

The most recent assessment by the WHO in 2006 involved a country-by-country analysis of the impact of environmental factors on health. Researchers estimated that 24% of the global disease burden and 23% of all deaths can be attributed to environmental factors (Prüss-Ustün & Corvalán, 2006). The diseases with the largest attributable burden to modifiable environmental factors include diarrhea (94%), lower respiratory tract infections (42% in the low- and middle-income world) and malaria (42%). The estimated total number of healthy life-years lost per capita as a result of environmental factors is 15 times higher in low- and middle-income countries than in high-income countries. These estimates can be considered conservative, given that they are based on a limited definition of "environment."

As shown in Figure 10-1, the largest environmental health burdens occur in low- and middle-income countries with significant household-level risks, which also tend to affect young children in particular. Indeed, as a percentage of total burden as well as in absolute terms (e.g., DALYs per capita), environmental risks are most important in the poorest populations. Note that the quantitative estimates given in Figure 10-1 are just approximations, as they are often based on very limited field research in low- and middle-income countries. In recent years, global and national time trend analyses for certain environmental health hazards have been seen as becoming more feasible than in the past. This type of evaluation has been facilitated by the inclusion of several health- and environment-related indicators for the monitoring of progress toward the United Nations' Millennium Development Goals (United Nations Development Program [UNDP], 2004), agreed to in 2000 by all member states. These indicators include the proportions of the population with sustainable access to an improved water source, with access to improved sanitation, with a pattern of using solid fuels, and with access to secure residential tenure (an indicator of slum-dwelling patterns). If achieved, these targets will not only improve health but also result in profound economic benefits. For example, halving the proportion of people without sustainable access to safe drinking water and sanitation has an estimated economic benefit-to-cost ratio of 8:1 (Grimm, Harttgen, Klasen, & Misselhorn, 2006).

Environment: Encompassing Both Hazard and Habitat

Most analyses of environmental health effects focus on specific, direct-acting hazards within a localized setting. Exposure is assessed either at the individual or the group level, health outcomes are assessed, and

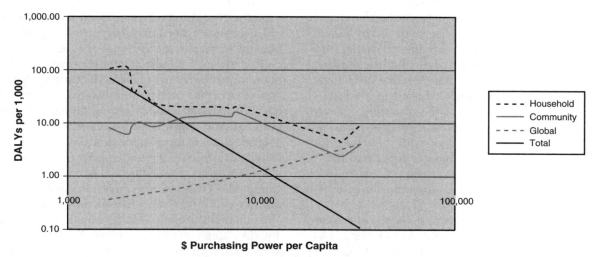

Figure 10-1 Environmental Risk Transition for Household, Community, and Imposed Global Environmental Risks in 2000. Note that household risks decline with rising income, imposed global risks rise, and community risks first rise and then fall.
Source: Adapted from Smith and Ezzati, 2005, using WHO data.

dose-response relationships are estimated, usually by fitting data to statistical models. Where data are sparse, model fitting may be guided by theoretical considerations. Once dose-response relationships have been satisfactorily estimated, and if the causal interpretation is convincing, then the results can be used to guide environmental policy. There are some caveats, however: Exposures have often been higher in workplaces than in the ambient environment, and many of the published dose-response relationships are based on occupational epidemiologic studies.

During recent decades, this mode of environmental and occupational health research, culminating in formal risk assessment (NAS, 2009; Samet, Schnatter, & Gibb, 1998), has prevailed in high-income countries. Using this system, ambient and workplace environmental exposure standards have been set for several hundred specific environmental exposure agents. There are currently more than 80,000 human-made chemical substances in commercial use worldwide, and 4,000 of these are in widespread use (United Nations, 1997). Further, thousands of naturally occurring chemicals are in general use, including many in low- and middle-income countries. There are insufficient epidemiologic and toxicologic data available to evaluate the potential health effects of most of these chemicals (NAS, 2009; Moochhala, Shahi, & Cote, 1997;).

Meanwhile, larger-scale environmental hazards to human health began to emerge in the final decades of the twentieth century. With increased emissions of greenhouse gases and various ozone-destroying gases, the basic composition of the world's lower and middle atmospheres is, for the first time, being altered by human actions. The world's great geochemical cycles of sulfur and nitrogen are also being perturbed by human actions. Human-induced environmental changes are causing worldwide depletion of soil fertility, aquifers, ocean fisheries, and—perhaps most serious—biologic diversity. These human-induced changes are beginning to weaken the world's life-supporting systems and change the conditions of the biosphere—our habitat. Various serious consequences for human health must be expected, such as changes in patterns of infectious diseases, in regional agricultural and aquatic yields, and in the effects of economic hardship or demographic displacement.

Given these considerations, the scope of the environmental health framework must be extended to include the impairment of our global habitat (McMichael & Bambrick, 2009). Meanwhile, hazard-oriented environmental health research must also be conducted. As the environmental impacts grow larger, so do the dimensions of the research, risk management, and policy development tasks.

Environmental Health Research, Risk Assessment, and Monitoring

Research Scope and Strategies

Environmental health research seeks to elucidate causal relations between environmental exposures and impaired states of health, prioritize and develop appropriate interventions to reduce risks to health, and evaluate the effectiveness of such interventions. Epidemiology is the basic quantitative science of environmental health research. In essence, epidemiologic research describes and explains variations and temporal changes in the patterns of illness and disease between and within populations. Most environmental epidemiology is observational (that is, non-experimental), which introduces some important issues in research design and data interpretation (Baker & Nieuwenhuijsen, 2008; Morgenstern & Thomas, 1993). However, where health benefit is anticipated from exposure-reducing interventions, experimental studies may be carried out.

Historically, epidemiology has played a crucial and largely self-sufficient role in identifying the environmental health hazards posed by relatively high levels of exposure—such as to severe air pollution (e.g., the "London Fog" of 1952), to heavy metals in water and food, to asbestos in workplaces, and to solar ultraviolet radiation (UVR). Those studies were mostly done in high-income countries, where research expertise existed and where technical and information resources were available. Increasingly, studies of physicochemical environmental exposures are being done in low- and middle-income countries, as well as in the former territories of the Soviet Union, where extensive environmental pollution and degradation often occurred. Meanwhile, many of the environmental health questions now being addressed in high-income countries refer to more subtle exposures, such as electromagnetic fields as a putative cancer risk and chemical exposures that mimic hormones and act cumulatively over decades on fertility and reproduction (especially via endocrine-disrupting chemicals) and on the functioning of the central nervous system and the immune system (Diamanti-Kandarakis et al., 2009). These chemicals are part of the wider concern over persistent organic pollutants (POPs) and their pervasive spread through the environment (U.S. Environmental Protection Agency [EPA], 2009).

Many environmental exposures occur at levels that are low by comparison with occupational exposures and personal habits, such as cigarette smoking. For example, in terms of the inhalation of fine particulates and various noxious gases, living in a heavily air-polluted city entails exposures equivalent to smoking several cigarettes per day. Yet most of the convincing epidemiologic studies of cigarette smoking and disease have depended on comparing persons smoking 10-plus cigarettes per day with nonsmokers. This typically lesser level of ambient environmental exposure renders difficult the task of detecting modest increments in risk. The importance of such environmental exposures is threefold:

- They typically impinge on many persons, perhaps whole populations, thereby causing a large aggregate health impact (an economic-political criterion).

- They are encountered on an essentially involuntary, and often unequal, basis (an ethical criterion).

- They are often amenable to control at the source (a practical criterion).

The epidemiologist faces two other recurrent difficulties. First, these real-world exposures are likely to be accompanied (that is, confounded) by various other exposures or risk factors—some of which may be unknown to the investigator or, indeed, to science. Second, the exposure-effect relationships often entail long-term, chronic, and sometimes subtle causal processes.

Because of these complexities, environmental health research must often be tackled in a multidisciplinary fashion so as to develop a sufficiently broad basis of evidence from which to make causal inferences. For example, causal inferences about the effect of low-level environmental lead exposure on the cognitive development of young children required the integrated consideration of the results of epidemiologic studies, animal experimental research, and neuropathological and molecular toxicological studies.

Extra leverage may be gained via interdisciplinary research in which the techniques of several disciplines are combined within one (usually epidemiologic) study. For example, the development of molecular biology over the past several decades has yielded many new techniques for measuring internal exposure, especially in relation to carcinogenesis. Molecular biological markers may also elucidate the biological mechanism, thereby strengthening the basis for causal inference. Further, these epidemiology-based research approaches, which focus on cause–effect relationships and underlying biological mechanisms, should be complemented by technical/engineering, behavioral, social/qualitative, and policy research to develop feasible interventions. In the environmental health arena, the contribution of these nonhealth disciplines may be crucial for developing effective health protection.

Causation and Other Methodological Issues

Etiologic studies examine associations between exposure and health outcome, assess the causal nature of the association, and, where possible, estimate the quantitative variation in risk as a function of variation in exposure (Baker & Nieuwenhuijsen, 2009; Bonita, Beaglehole, & Kjellstrom, 2007). The quality of the measurement of exposure and of health status is often much lower than that possible in controlled clinical trials or laboratory-based studies. The study design or analysis may also need to control for many potential confounding variables (e.g., sex, age, and smoking habits)—that is, factors that are statistically associated with the exposure variable of interest and that are also predictive of the health outcome. The sample of persons studied may not be a random sample of the source population with respect to the relationship that the sample either actually displays (selection bias) or apparently displays (classification bias) between exposure and outcome.

Over recent decades, epidemiologists have developed a set of criteria specifically suited to their predominantly non-experimental, bias-prone, confounding-rich research, with particular emphasis placed on the temporality of the relationship, its strength, the presence of a plausible dose-response relationship, the consistency of findings in diverse studies, and coherence with other disciplinary findings and biomedical theory (Bonita et al., 2007). Etiologic research in environmental epidemiology entails several distinctive methodological issues (Baker & Nieuwenhuijsen, 2009), including the following:

- Choice of the appropriate level of comparison (population, local community, or individual). Many environmental exposures (e.g., ambient air pollution or fluoride levels in drinking water) impinge on whole communities, with minimal exposure differences being noted between individuals.

- Definition of exposure and choice of the mode of exposure assessment.

- Choice of the relevant reference exposure (the theoretical minimum exposure level that a society could achieve).

- Approach to dealing with multiple coexistent, potentially interacting environmental exposures.
- Choice of study design for data collection and analysis.

These and other issues are discussed in the following sections.

Study Design Options

The same basic set of study designs that are used in general epidemiology are also used in environmental epidemiology—that is, descriptive, analytic, or experimental (Baker & Nieuwenhuijsen, 2009; Bonita et al., 2007). This section briefly introduces some of the key issues that arise with each design.

Descriptive Studies: Trends and Correlations

In descriptive studies, the pattern of variation in a population's or community's environmental exposure or health status (or both) is described, usually in relation to time, place, or category of person (e.g., age, sex, ethnicity). If the data are appropriate, the relationship between exposure factors and health status may be described. Such studies aid in identifying research priorities and in guiding the design of etiologic studies. For example, a study may show that the exposure levels are not high enough to warrant more detailed epidemiologic study. The time trend of exposure may influence how further studies are designed. Seasonal variations can be an important indicator of effects of exposures to environmental hazards that vary with season. The spatial distribution of exposure may indicate how subgroups with different exposure levels within the population should be defined.

With adequate data and sufficient variation in exposure, it is possible to examine the statistical correlation, over time or space (or both), between the descriptive population-level measure of exposure and health. Usually, such studies cannot yield definite conclusions about etiology—most often because there is inadequate information on confounding factors, uncertainty arises regarding the temporal relationship between exposure and health effects, or an association observed at the population level does not necessarily exist at the individual level (the so-called ecologic fallacy).

Time-series studies have a special role in environmental epidemiology. Some environmental exposures vary on a short-term basis, especially levels of urban air pollution and weather conditions. Intrinsically interesting questions often arise about the acute health impact of fluctuations in air pollution or temperature, such as whether asthma attacks increase on high-pollution days or whether daily death rates increase on days of extreme temperature. The statistical analytic techniques used within time-series analyses have been acquired from both econometrics and engineering research. They include sophisticated adjustments for lower-frequency (e.g., seasonal) cyclical variations, background secular trends, and autocorrelation. Time-series studies benefit from the fact that ongoing characteristics of the study population—such as age distribution, socioeconomic profile, and smoking habits—remain essentially constant over time. Further, because the comparison is made entirely within the chosen population, interpopulation confounding factors do not exist.

Analytic Studies

Analytic studies examine formal statistical associations between an exposure variable and a health outcome variable at the level of the individual or a small homogeneous exposure group (Bonita et al., 2007). Are individuals with higher exposure to indoor air pollution more likely to develop respiratory disease than those with low exposure to such pollution? Are individuals who develop diarrheal disease in a coastal city more likely to have been swimming in contaminated seawater recently than individuals without such disease? Studies to answer questions such as these can be designed to start either from exposures (cohort studies, such as the indoor air pollution example described earlier) or from the health effect (case control studies, such as the diarrheal disease example described earlier).

The study of the relationship of early-life environmental lead exposure to child cognitive-intellectual development, for example, began with various types of cross-sectional studies in the 1970s. However, it was not possible to establish from those studies the temporal relationship between occurrence of exposure and occurrence of intellectual or behavioral deficit. Cohort studies were required, in which infants and children were followed from birth, with systematic documentation of their early-life lead exposure history and cognitive-intellectual development. The largest of these investigations, which was carried out in and around the lead smelting town of Port Pirie, South Australia (Tong, Baghurst, Sawyer, Burns, & McMichael, 1998), provided the type of data necessary to resolve this important public health issue and to estimate the magnitude of the risk (Exhibit 10-1).

Exhibit 10-1	**Environmental Lead Exposure and Childhood Cognitive Development**

Lead is the most abundant heavy metal. It may have been the first metal smelted, with this kind of processing dating from 7000 to 6500 B.C. The ancient civilizations of Phoenicia, Egypt, Greece, Rome, China, and India used lead for vessels, roofs, water ducts, utensils, ornaments, and weights. There was a great resurgence in the use of this metal during the Industrial Revolution. The subsequent development of the automobile hugely increased lead usage, both in lead-acid batteries and as an antiknock additive in gasoline. All of these historical factors led to increasing amounts of lead in the environment frequented by humans: The lead content of Greenland ice layers shows a strong rise over the past 1,000 years, reaching 100 times the natural background level in the mid-1990s. The natural background (pre–Industrial Revolution) blood lead concentration of humans is estimated to be much lower than the lowest reported levels in contemporary humans living in remote regions.

Lead has adverse effects on a variety of organ systems—most importantly, the gastrointestinal tract, central nervous system, kidneys, and blood (hemoglobin synthesis). Especially high levels of exposure (leading to blood lead concentrations of 50 to 100 mg/dL) typically occur in the workplace, including through lead smelting, battery recycling, lead soldering, and various lead-based craft activities. Such exposures occurred often 50 to 150 years ago in today's high-income countries, during earlier stages of industrialization, and they remain widespread in many of today's low- and middle-income countries.

Over the past two decades, epidemiologic evidence has accrued indicating that low-level environmental lead exposure in early childhood causes a deficit in neurocognitive development (Tong et al., 1998). Evidence from animal experimental studies and neuropathologic analyses corroborates this causal interpretation. Meta-analyses estimate that a doubling in blood lead concentration from 10 to 20 mg/dL—a range of lead exposure typically found between high and low tertiles in poorly controlled urban environment—is associated with a deficit in intelligence quotient of 1 to 3 points, or 1% to 3% of the expected average IQ score of 100 (Pocock, Smith, & Baghurst, 1994). Indeed, subtle effects on IQ can result from blood lead levels as low as 5 mg/dL. A loss of IQ points will have greater impact in children with an IQ score just above 69 (mild mental retardation is defined as an IQ score of 50 to 69) than in those with a higher IQ.

Many high-income countries, including the United States and Australia, have recently set new, lower standards for environmental lead levels, in an effort to protect young children. Unfortunately, childhood lead poisoning is an increasing problem in many low- or middle-income countries. For example, the lead content of gasoline sold in Africa is the highest in the world and is associated with high lead concentrations in the atmosphere, dust, and soils. Many other exposures to lead in Africa result from industrial, cottage industry, and household sources. Surveys have shown that more than 90% of the children in Cape Province, South Africa, have blood lead levels in excess of 10 mg/dL (Nriagu, Blankson, & Ocran, 1996). In Dhaka, Bangladesh, the airborne lead concentration is one of the highest in the world, and measurements showed that the mean blood lead concentration in 93 randomly chosen rickshaw pullers was 53 mg/dL—five times higher than the acceptable limit

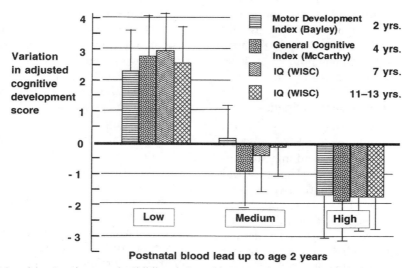

Lead Exposure and Cognitive Development in Childhood. One point approximates to a 1% change. Low, medium, and high lead exposure categories have mean blood lead concentrations of 12.5, 18.5, and 25.9 mg/dL, respectively.
Source: S. Tong et al., "Lifetime Exposure to Environmental Lead and Children's Intelligence at 11– 13 Years: The Pt. Pirie Cohort Study," 1996, British Medical Journal, 312, pp. 1569–1570. Adapted with permission.

continued

Exhibit 10-1 *continued*

in high-income countries. A recent study in six Indian cities found that more than 50% of children had blood lead concentrations higher than 10 mg/dL, and more than 12% of the children tested had concentrations higher than 20 mg/dL. In China, where industrialization and motor vehicle usage are increasing rapidly, childhood exposure to lead is becoming a significant public health issue.

Some difficulties arise in including cognitive and intellectual impairment in the risk assessment equation for evaluating and controlling environmental lead as a public health hazard. This particular functional health deficit—a subtle neurologic impairment that will have its most marked effects on the social and psychological development of children who already have a low IQ score—does not readily translate into the standard currency of deficit due to disease, disability, or death (the DALY). Hence, the burden of disease caused by relatively low but widespread exposures to lead can be readily underestimated by policy makers. Although overt lead-induced toxicity is apparent in individuals experiencing high levels of exposure, the full public health impact of widespread exposure to a range of environmental lead levels requires evaluation of more subtle health, behavioral, and developmental effects (Moore, 2003).

In developing a policy on environmental lead, and taking the evidence of cognitive impairment into account, two further questions arise. First, does the neurodevelopmental deficit persist over time? The currently available epidemiologic evidence suggests that the deficit lasts through late childhood and into early adulthood. Second, because few data are available in the very low exposure range, is there an exposure level below which no neurotoxicologic effect occurs? Overall, there is a strong case for adoption of public health measures to prevent exposure in early childhood. Because lead exposure tends to be ubiquitous within a population, even a modest health impact upon each individual would yield a substantial aggregate impact for the total population. Assessments of population-attributable burden are provided by Ostro (1994) and Schwartz (1994). Phasing out leaded gasoline is the most effective way to reduce population exposure to lead. However, a number of countries are still endangering their populations by allowing use of leaded gasoline (Moore, 2003; World Resources Institute, 1998).

An important issue in environmental epidemiology studies is how to deal with the problem of confounding factors that are statistically associated with the exposure variable, yet are independently predictive of the health outcome (Bonita et al., 2007). The issue of confounding is pervasive in epidemiologic research, reflecting the nonrandom distribution of risk factors in real-world populations. It is usually more amenable to control for this possibility in analytic individual-level studies than in population-level correlation analyses ("ecological studies").

Experimental Studies and Intervention Studies

Experimental and intervention studies begin with sets of reasonably similar populations or groups, which can then be allocated, preferably randomly, to "intervention" or "control" categories. The statistical analysis compares outcome rates in the two or more groups (the intervention may be applied at more than one level). The clinical randomized controlled trial (RCT) is the "gold standard" for this type of design, although it is best suited to studies of disease treatment or prevention in sets of individuals.

Some types of environmental epidemiologic questions can be addressed experimentally at the individual level—for example, testing whether the installation of household humidifiers reduces the prevalence of respiratory symptoms, or whether the provision of masks to reduce workplace exposure to fumes reduces headaches. However, comparisons are more usually made at the supra-individual level—for example, testing the effectiveness of the broadcasting of safety promotion advertisements on television. A well-known historical example from the 1940s was the experimental addition of fluoride to the drinking water of four towns in North America for the purpose of preventing dental caries, but not in four other similar towns, thereby allowing for subsequent comparison of dental decay prevalence in children (Fawell et al., 2006). For ethical reasons, experimental studies cannot be carried out with exposures that might be harmful to those who are exposed, although it may be ethical to test experimentally the short-term, reversible effect of annoyance factors (such as the acute effect of loud noise on blood pressure or of odors on mood).

A less rigorous approach to testing an environmental intervention is to carry out a before-and-after approach within a single group or population ("case-crossover studies"; Maclure, 1991). However, it is often difficult to ensure that nothing else of relevance changed between the timing of the two periods.

Exposure and Dose: Assessment and Definitions

Paracelsus, the sixteenth-century German physician/alchemist who is often credited with being the

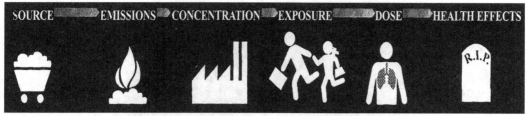

Figure 10-2 Environmental Pathway.
Source: K. R. Smith, Biofuels, Air Pollution, and Health: A Global Review (New York: Plenum Publishing, 1987). Reprinted with permission.

founder of environmental health and toxicology, wrote: "Poison is in everything, and nothing is without poison. The dosage makes it either poison or remedy" (Deishmann & Henschler, 1986). This statement lies at the heart of environmental health science, as illustrated in the environmental pathway shown in Figure 10-2.

Although some idea of the health effects of an environmental contaminant can be obtained by measuring the quantity of toxin at the source or in emissions or as environmental concentrations, these measures can be misleading, because they do not directly indicate how much of the toxin actually reaches the population. There is a huge amount of toxic mercury in the oceans, for example, but very little reaches people in normal circumstances. Volcanoes emit vast amounts of toxic gases, but fortunately few persons are usually nearby to breathe them. Far more precise for predicting health effects would be measurements of dose itself—that is, the amount of toxin that has actually reached the vulnerable parts of the body. Unfortunately, it is difficult to measure dose directly for most hazards (whether chemical or physical), either because it involves sophisticated, expensive, and invasive procedures (e.g., extracting and analyzing blood or tissue samples) or because it is beyond current scientific abilities.

For this reason, scientific and policy attention has increasingly focused on the intermediate part of the environmental pathway—exposure (see Figure 10-2), which lies directly at the interface of the "environ-

ment" and the body. Exposure is the amount of hazard actually encountered by humans in the course of their activities. More explicitly, it is the amount of material or energy in the air, water, food, and soil that reaches the body's protective barriers of the respiratory and digestive systems, skin, eyes, and ears (Figure 10-3). Exposure differs from dose in that it does not encompass any of the body's internal mechanisms for absorption, transformation, excretion, and storage of the toxin. It also differs from concentrations, in that exposure incorporates not only measures what the levels of the pollutant are in the "environment" but also who experiences them and for how long. Thus exposure integrates information about both where the pollution is and where the people are.

Total Exposure Assessment

Another important concept is that of total exposure assessment (TEA). To understand the full impact of a pollutant, it is necessary to examine all the ways it might reach people, rather than simply relying on measurements made in the most convenient places. This consideration is especially important for pollutants that can reach people through several different routes. For example, airborne lead pollution can spread through the "environment" to reach vulnerable groups, particularly children, not only through the air but also through water, soil, and food. Even though the original emissions are only to air, confining attention solely to the air route would greatly underestimate the actual total exposure (see Exhibit 10-1). It is total exposure, of course, that determines the risk to health.

The idea of TEA also applies to pollutants that contaminate only one medium. Consider, for example, the woman with the daily pattern of activities shown in Figure 10-4. What would be her health risk due to exposure to particulate air pollution? She lives in an urban slum of a low-income country where outdoor air pollution levels are fairly high. Her total exposure is even higher, however, because she spends

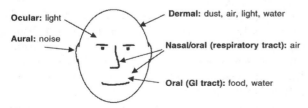

Figure 10-3 Routes of Exposure.

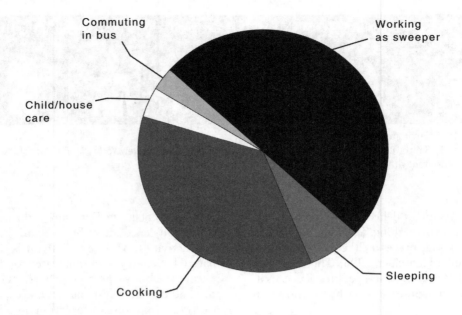

Activity	Hours/Day	Particulate Concentration (µg/m³)	Daily Exposure Equivalent (µg/m³)	Proportion of Total Exposure
Sleeping	7	100	29.2	0.07
Cooking	3	1,200	150.0	0.36
Child/house care	3	120	15.0	0.04
Commuting in bus	1	300	12.5	0.03
Working as sweeper	10	500	208.3	0.50
Total	24	mean = 415	415	1

Figure 10-4 Total Particulate Exposure for a Woman in an Urban Slum.

considerable time in locations where particulate con-centrations are higher than the outdoor levels. During the working day, she works as a sweeper on busy streets, where particulate levels are higher than the av-erage outdoor level because of proximity to traffic. In the morning and evening, she experiences even higher levels as household cook because her family can af-ford only poor-quality cooking fuels that produce large amounts of air pollution, such as briquettes made from coal dust. In the evening, she is exposed to the environmental tobacco smoke (ETS) from her husband's cigarettes. Her total exposure over the day is best estimated by the daily sum of the pollutant concentration in each major microenvironment where she spends time, weighted by the fraction of time she spends in it.

The importance of TEA derives from several con-siderations. It can change the relative importance of sources of pollution, and it can uncover important new sources of personal risk, such as ETS, that may not appreciably affect environmental concentrations. This metric also reveals a new dimension of potential control measures. For example, chimneys for house-hold stoves that would not change emissions at all— and might even increase outdoor concentrations—can lower exposures substantially by separating the people from the pollution. Laws to reduce smoking in pub-lic places can lower ETS exposure, even without mak-ing changes in total smoking emissions. In some cases, the cost-effectiveness of such exposure-control meas-ures can be much higher than exposure reduction through generalized control of outdoor sources. Although ideally all pollution sources should be con-trolled, in reality there is always a limit to the re-sources available. Choosing the most cost-effective control measures first will ensure that the most public health protection is achieved with whatever resources are available.

Biological Markers of Dose

Although not available for all situations, many types of biological markers (dose indices) are possible (WHO, 2001), such as heavy metals in hair, nails, and blood; metabolites in urine; chlorinated organic chemicals in adipose tissue; radionuclides in bone; core body temperature after excessive heat exposure; and antibody titers in relation to infectious agents. The advent of increasingly specific and sensitive laboratory assays has greatly expanded the possibilities of measuring dose. Such assays include modem fluorometric methods, atomic absorption spectroscopy, high-performance chromatography, immunosorbent assays, and the use of various molecular biological markers.

It must be remembered that a biological assay estimates the integrated outcome of a sequence of physiological and metabolic processes. There are considerable individual variations in these processes, however—and, hence, considerable individual variations in their outcomes. For this reason, assay results require careful analysis and interpretation in environmental epidemiology studies.

Consider the field of molecular epidemiology, which became prominent during the 1990s as an approach to studying the cause—especially the environmental cause—of cancer (McMichael, 1994). This same field has also become important in modern infectious disease epidemiology, particularly for the determination of environmental sources and transmission pathways for infections such as Legionnaires' disease, tuberculosis, influenza, cholera, and food-poisoning organisms. Molecular assays make use of the variation in the structures of macromolecules, particularly DNA.

One example in which DNA measurement has assisted the conventional epidemiologic study of causation has been in studies of dietary aflatoxin as a cause of liver cancer (McMichael, 1994). Aflatoxin is a biotoxin produced by the *Aspergillus flavus* mold in stored foods in warm, humid environments. Because it was not previously possible to determine directly an individual's level of aflatoxin intake, epidemiologists were limited to demonstrating ecological correlations, in eastern Africa and within China, between average aflatoxin concentrations in local diets and rates of liver cancer mortality. Today, however, they can measure the concentration of excised, excreted, aflatoxin-DNA adducts in urine and use this value as a measure of recent individual exposure. This particular measure was used successfully in a cohort study of 18,000 Chinese men in Shanghai who were followed for liver cancer incidence. The study revealed a positive association, at the individual level, between initial adduct level and cancer occurrence.

Exposure Assessment at Individual and Population Levels

In studies of the health effects of ETS, for example, it has been common practice to classify exposures according to whether an adult has a smoking spouse or a child has a smoking parent. Clearly, someone living with a smoker is more likely to experience greater ETS levels than someone who does not, but this factor does not guarantee that this is so in every case. A child with no smoking parent, for example, may have four smoking grandparents who visit every day. Another child may have smoking parents who are careful to refrain from smoking anywhere near their child. In these cases, classification of these children based on the smoking status of their parents would lead to exposure misclassification and a consequent attenuated estimate of the true effect. The risk of such exposure misclassification can be reduced by careful questionnaire design and by exposure-verification techniques, such as checking a sample of the children's urine for specific metabolites of nicotine.

The population-level classification of exposure—that is, the exposure of whole subpopulations classified according to ecological indicators such as location within a city—is often inexpensive and convenient. Nevertheless, it can yield exposure misclassification if not done carefully. It is common, for example, to conduct air pollution epidemiology studies by dividing urban populations into exposure classes according to the measurements made at the nearest outdoor air pollution monitoring station or even to use one or a few monitors to represent the exposure of an entire city for comparison with other cities. Local exposure sources can contribute to great variation between individual exposures and the estimated population average exposure. The same problem arises in studies of increasing heat exposure due to climate change. The climate data from one weather station cannot provide information about the varying heat exposures among people living in the area. Nevertheless, time-trend data from a single air pollution monitor or weather station can be very useful indicators of any changing exposures in the area (see the examples in Kjellstrom, 2009a).

Health Outcome Assessment

Many studies of the health impacts of air pollution or environmental heat have examined associations with mortality. Yet the underlying pyramid of nonfatal health effects is very broad based: Much remains to be learned about the impacts of air pollution and heat exposure on hospitalizations, primary care consultations, existence of chronic conditions, impaired organ function (which requires testing of individuals), and self-assessed symptoms.

There is a natural tendency for researchers and data-collection agencies to prefer "hard" endpoints that are well defined clinically and amenable to clear-cut counting or measurement. Yet community surveys or consultations often indicate that the main perceived health impacts of environmental factors relate to social, behavioral, and psychological disruptions, such as the mental stress of noisy environments, headaches or nausea from unpleasant odors, or under-exercised, overweight children who are constrained by traffic and lack of neighborhood facilities. As an example, the evaluation of the public health impact of road transport in Sweden (Kjellstrom, Ferguson, & Taylor, 2009) highlights the links between different exposures and effects.

Having decided on the category of health outcome to assess, a formal case definition must be constructed. For those outcomes with preexisting population-based case registration—for example, cancers and congenital anomalies—case definition is relatively simple. Conversely, when epidemiologists are starting anew from medical records, questionnaires, or test results, clear and stringent criteria must be specified. Comparison of health status between populations usually necessitates adjustments for differences in basic demographic characteristics such as age distribution, sex ratio, ethnic composition, and socioeconomic profile.

Measurement of preclinical changes may enable earlier answers to be obtained to urgent questions, including in relation to newly introduced exposures. For example, is there any form of early evidence available that can be used to determine whether there has been a change in skin cancer risk due to increased ultraviolet irradiation caused by stratospheric ozone depletion? If UVR-specific mutations in skin could be identified and assayed, this process would certainly accelerate the process of finding an answer to that question.

Data Analysis and Interpretation

The collected data are initially assembled at a group or population level, and associations are based on comparing average exposure levels and the rates or levels of health outcomes in the different groups. The comparison may involve just two groups at different exposure levels or a series of groups for which a dose-response relationship can be analyzed (e.g., see Figure 10-5; Bobak & Leon, 1992). In analytic or experimental studies, the observed association between exposure and health outcome is generally thought to be more valid because of the readier control of confounding variables, the observable intersection of exposure and health outcome at the individual level, and knowledge of the temporal relationship between those two variables.

The presentation of the results is important for effective risk communication. Suppose the statistical analysis shows that the mortality rate within a community for a particular disease has gone up by a factor of 1.3, with a 95% confidence interval of 1.1 to 1.6.

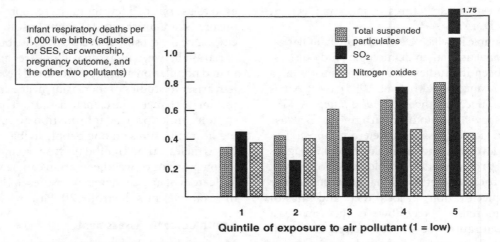

Figure 10-5 Air Pollution and Infant Respiratory Disease Mortality in Eastern Europe.
Source: Data from M. Bobak and D. Leon, "Air Pollution and Infant Mortality in the Czech Republic 1968–1988," 1992, Lancet, 340, pp. 1010–1014.

Table 10-3	Pollutants in Solid Fuel (Biomass and Coal) Smoke from Household Stoves in Poor Countries

- Small particles, carbon monoxide (CO), nitrogen dioxide (NO_2)
- Formaldehyde, acrolein, benzene, 1,3-butadiene, toluene, styrene, and many other toxic volatile organic chemicals
- Polyaromatic hydrocarbons, such as benzo(alpha)pyrene
- Coal produces all of the above, plus may emit sulfur dioxide and toxic elements, such as arsenic, lead, mercury, and fluorine
- In simple stoves, biomass and coal burning produce significant non-carbon dioxide (CO_2) greenhouse pollutants, such as methane and black carbon

Source: Smith, K. R. (1987). *Biofuels, air pollution, and health: A global review.* New York: Plenum. Reprinted with permission.

What does this relative risk of 1.3 really mean? If the disease in question is rare, the 1.3-fold increase of the absolute risk may represent a few cases per million exposed people per year. If the disease is quite common, however, a relative risk of 1.3 may imply a major public health impact. Risk estimates can also be presented in the form of the number of exposure-attributable cases per year or as the number of cases that would occur in a longer time period (e.g., a lifetime) within a community; these values are sometimes called public health impact estimates (Talbot, Haley, Dimmick, Paulu, Talbott, & Rager, 2009).

Thus it is important to consider whether the results of a study are of public health significance, in addition to being statistically significant. The analysis and presentation of the results can highlight the public health significance of that particular problem by a combination of risk estimates, as mentioned earlier, comparing the absolute risk estimates and public health impact estimates to the corresponding estimates for other health problems. This will provide an impression of the importance of the health effects identified.

A problem in making such comparisons is that it is difficult to measure the total health impact of an environmental exposure in a way that combines impacts on mortality and morbidity. In recent years, various approaches have been proposed—for example, as the loss of quality-adjusted life-years (QALYs), the loss of health expectancy (an extension of the concept of life expectancy, the latter being confined to mortality data), or the loss of DALYs. The DALY combines years of life lost from premature death and years lived with nonfatal conditions (assigned a disability weighting) (Murray & Lopez, 1996). The DALY was designed to allow for comparative risk assessment and economic impact analysis, so it can incorporate discount rates to account for the future value of healthy life. This measure has been promoted by the World Bank (1993) and WHO (2002) as a tool for priority setting in health-sector investments (see Chapter 1).

In the first published ranking of the different determinants of global burden of disease (Murray & Lopez, 1996), poor water and sanitation, occupa-

tional health hazards, and outdoor air pollutants were included in the top 10. In the more recent analyses, several environmental health hazards have been included, and poor water and sanitation as well as indoor air pollution from solid fuel burning (Table 10-3) are ranked among the top 10 global burden of disease risks (see Table 10-2). (Lopez, Mathers, Ezzati, Jamison, & Murray, 2006; WHO, 2002). An update of this comparative risk assessment was in progress in 2010, and it is likely that the ranking list will be amended as the underlying scientific evidence improves.

Environmental Health Indicators and Monitoring

Environmental health issues are increasingly being recognized as part of a broader development–environment–health perspective (WHO, 1997). To achieve a lasting, sustainable impact leading to improved public health, an intervention must address those underlying processes that created the exposure in the first place. In epidemiologic studies, the more direct the associations under study, the less likely that confounding and other complexities will cloud the interpretation. However, for effective decision making, understanding the relationships between underlying (or "upstream") factors and health outcomes may be more important than acquiring detailed information about the exposure–effect relationships. The importance of the underlying social determinants of health in determining the levels and distribution of environmental hazard exposures in different population groups has been highlighted by the report of the WHO Commission on Social Determinants of Health (WHO, 2008).

Most high-income countries have established a range of environmental performance indicators based on this approach. The most widely used scheme is that developed by the Organization of Economic Cooperation and Development (OECD, 1993): the pressure–state–response (PSR) model. To analyze human health risks of environmental conditions, an expanded framework that better represents the cause–effect relationships between human activities, environmental change, and human health has also been developed (Corvalan, Briggs, & Kjellstrom, 1996; Kjellstrom & Corvalan, 1995). Within this framework, driving forces lead to pressures; those pressures then affect the environmental quality (state), resulting in exposures (to humans) and then effects (in humans). The response to this cycle has been labeled "actions" to highlight the active role played by society, rather than any passive response. The framework was termed the DPSEEA model (Figure 10-6). (DPSEEA = the hierarchy of Driving forces, Pressures, State of environment, Exposures, Effects, Actions).

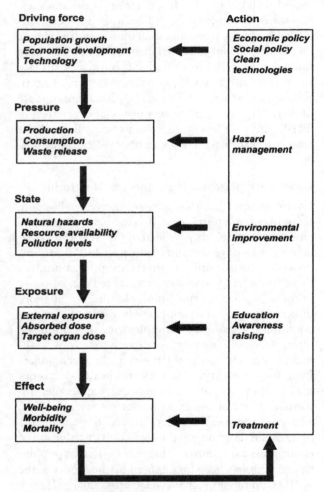

Figure 10-6 The DPSEEA Framework to Define Environmental Health Indicators.
Source: T. Kjellstrom, and C. Corvalan, "Framework for the Development of Environmental Health Indicators," 1995, World Health Statistics Quarterly, 48, pp. 144–154; and C. Corvalan, D. Briggs, and T. Kjellstrom, "Development of Environmental Health Indicators," in D. Briggs, C. Corvalan, & M. Nurminen (Eds.), Linkage Methods for Environment and Health Analysis, Document WHO/EHG/95.26 (Geneva, Switzerland: World Health Organization). Adapted with permission.

Driving force indicators are likely to be qualitative and are often expressed as yes/no answers. For example:

- Is there a policy to redirect all storm water to treatment plants?
- Are sedimentation dams in operation upstream in potentially cadmium-contaminated rivers?
- Are safety regulations for nuclear power stations adhered to?

Pressure indicators are usually quantitative. For example:

- The amount of sewage-contaminated storm water entering a beach or river after heavy rain
- The amount of cadmium transported via river water to paddy fields
- The amount of radionuclides released from a nuclear power station accident

The most common indicators are direct measurements of the environmental state—the concentration of a hazard in some environmental medium. For example:

- The enterococci concentration in beach water or drinking water
- The concentration of cadmium in rice paddy soil or rice
- The level of radioactive strontium in lichens or reindeer meat

Exposure indicators may be based on exposures calculated from state indicators, as described in "Exposure and Dose: Assessment and Definitions," earlier in this chapter. Biological indices add individual-based information and can be used to monitor both exposure (e.g., blood lead concentration, DNA-adduct level) and effects (e.g., enzyme assays for liver function, blood pressure). For example, the marked decline in human milk concentrations of dichlorodiphenyltrichloroethane (DDT) around the world is illustrated in Figure 10-7 (Smith, 1999). The materials most commonly used for these measurements are blood and urine, although hair, nails, saliva, exhaled air, human milk, and biopsy (or autopsy) materials from internal organs are also used in special circumstances.

Ideally, an indicator of health effects should identify early effects that precede irreversible health damage. Examples include free erythrocyte protoporphyrin measurements in the blood of lead-exposed people and temporary threshold shift in hearing acuity after noise exposure. The next level of indicator includes

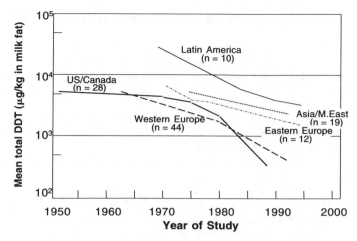

Figure 10-7 Worldwide Trends in DDT Levels in Human Breast Milk. *Note:* n = number of studies. *Source:* D. Smith, "Worldwide Trends in DDT Levels in Human Breast Milk," 1999, *International Journal of Epidemiology, 28,* pp. 179–188. Copyright 1999 by Oxford University Press, Inc. Reprinted by permission of Oxford University Press, Inc.

early pathological change that may be reversible. An example is early tubular proteinuria after cadmium exposure (WHO, 1992).

Assessment of Environmental Health Impacts and Risks

Introduction to Risk Assessment

Risk assessment is conventionally viewed as a step-wise sequence (WHO, 2002). It begins with the research-based identification of an environmental hazard. Subsequent studies then estimate, first, the exposure- or dose-response relationship between the hazard and the specified health outcome, and, second, the distribution of exposure (doses) within the population of interest. From these two sets of information, the overall risk to the population is then characterized, and risk management strategies are formulated. Although there is now some agreement about how to calculate risks, there is no completely objective way to compare alternatives with different patterns of risk. This situation is illustrated in Exhibit 10-2, which presents a choice between two ways of producing electric power with different patterns of risk and explains how reasonable consumers with different views of risk could rationally choose one over the other. This difference in risk perception is why people buy life insurance (risk aversion) and why insurance companies sell it (profits based on expected-value calculations).

Many other considerations would be included in a full assessment of alternative power plants, including various outcomes of social importance other than those directly related to health. Thus Exhibit 10-2 illustrates that a decision about how much or what kind of risk to take demands substantial scientific input but is to a considerable extent a social and political choice. The extraordinary earthquake and tsunami damage to nuclear power stations in Japan in 2011 highlights the difficulties in assessing the ultimate risks to human health and the social and economic life of communities.

Probabilistic Risk Assessment

Because nuclear power plant operation is a relatively new enterprise, few accident statistics are available, particularly for large accidents in modern plants. How, then, can overall risk be determined? For this purpose, a technique called probabilistic risk assessment (PRA) is applied to understand the potential for adverse consequences. Developed originally by NASA for assessing the risks of manned space flight, this technique basically breaks down the extremely complicated systems of large-scale technologies for which there are no overall accident information into subsystems. These subsystems may then need to be broken down even further into even smaller components until a level is reached for which failure data are available. The failure data for each subsystem are combined to predict the performance of the total system.

There is no information that would enable one to predict directly how a new type of nuclear plant will operate over time. However, such a facility is made up of thousands of components for which information is available. Information will be available, for example, about how often pumps of a certain size, switches of a certain voltage, or warning gauges of a particular

Exhibit 10-2	Risk Assessments: Additional Information for Decision Making, But No Substitute for Decision Making

Suppose a proposal has been made to build a large new power plant near your community. Everyone agrees on the need for more power and the availability of only two viable alternatives: coal and nuclear (the actual case in many parts of the world). These options are found to cost about the same. A full probabilistic risk assessment is done to compare the health implications of the two plants, and yields the results described here.

The coal plant, although of the best design, will have impacts in the form of air pollution and coal mining accidents. There is relatively little uncertainty about these factors—the probabilistic risk assessment finds that there is a 90% chance that 30 persons will die prematurely because of the operation of the plant over its lifetime. Because there might be a large accident at the coal mine or a fire at the coal plant during meteorological conditions that lead to severe local air pollution, there is a 10% likelihood of killing 60 persons.

The nuclear plant is given a 99% chance of doing very little damage (i.e., shortening only one person's life from the small amount of radiation released routinely). Unlike the coal plant, however, there is a small chance (here set at 1%) of a terrible accident in which 2,500 persons die from the radiation released.

Which plant is safer? Which would you rather live alongside? There are at least three ways to answer this question, none necessarily right or wrong, but all dependent on the set of values of the people making the decision:

- Maxi-min (maximize the chance of the minimum consequence): Because 99% of the time little damage is done and more may be learned in the future on how to reduce the chance of accidents, choose the nuclear plant.
- Mini-max (minimize the chance of the maximum consequence): Because a nuclear accident would be a tragedy (cause international headlines, go down in history, destroy the community, and so on), coal should be used so as not to have any chance of such an event.
- Expected value (calculate the odds): Because the expected number of deaths from the coal plant is 33 ($0.9 \times 30 + 0.1 \times 60$) and for nuclear, 26 ($0.99 \times 1 + 0.01 \times 2500$), choose the coal plant.

Although the numbers used here are fictional and real probabilistic risk assessments for such facilities are much more complicated (involving hundreds of branches on the risk trees shown in the figure), the overall results are often similar. Nuclear plants generally have a lower expected value of damage but carry a small probability of terrible events (much less than 1%). Coal plants produce more damage on average but do not impose anxiety about large negative events (although growing concerns about possible climate change owing to the release of carbon dioxide from coal plants may change this perception).

The fact that groups of perfectly rational people may apply different decision rules does not mean that any group is right in an absolute sense, but rather that groups start with different values. Indeed, although many other factors must be considered, the big difference in public acceptance of nuclear power between, say, France and Sweden can be partially accounted for by such differences in values.

brand are expected to fail under various conditions. Even if a new type of component is introduced, its failure rate can be experimentally determined without putting anyone at risk, unlike testing the entire power plant.

Such PRAs, of necessity, are extremely complex and difficult for even specialists to evaluate. In particular, it is hard to tell whether all possible accident scenarios have been taken into account and whether unforeseen events, such as human sabotage, might potentially circumvent many subsystems at once. A PRA also assumes that the context in which each component was originally tested is not materially different in critical respects (e.g., temperature or vibration) from the working context of the assembled plant.

Where an assessment reveals a potential or actual exposure to a chemical for which there is no human exposure history, a similar dilemma results. It would

be dangerous and unethical (not to mention time-consuming) to deliberately expose enough people to the chemical to discover its true risk. Various techniques have been developed to estimate the risks of human exposures in this situation. The most common method is to expose laboratory animals—usually rats and mice—to high enough doses of the chemical to observe effects within their relatively short life spans. When deleterious effects, such as tumors or reproductive failure, are observed, then legitimate concern arises that such effects might also be seen in humans. To quantify that risk, however, requires extrapolating from high doses in animals to (usually) low doses in humans. To do so, researchers use a mathematical model that, ideally, is based on knowledge of metabolism, tumor induction, and other often poorly understood biological processes. Frequently, alternative animal models that are equally plausible biologically will predict very different human risks for the same dose of the same chemical. (Had the antinausea drug thalidomide been tested in rats, not rabbits, the tragedy of limbless human babies would probably have been averted.) It is necessary, therefore, to establish standard conventions for which model will be used in which circumstances so that consistent risk estimates are made. At present, many of the model choices depend more on scientific intuition than on actual demonstrated knowledge. Finding more reliable and scientifically valid ways of performing such assessments is a very active research arena.

It might seem best to establish the convention of always using the most conservative model—that is, the model that predicts the largest risk. This strategy would seem to fit the classic public health dictum that, in cases of uncertainty, it is better to err on the side of caution than to underestimate potential risk. Indeed, for this reason, such a conservative approach is used in formulating official policy by some regulatory agencies. Unfortunately, and perhaps counterintuitively, if this approach is taken for each chemical independently, it can lead to the opposite effect—that is, exposing the public to unnecessary risks. The degree of conservatism (or the size of the safety factor) for specific chemicals can be quite different, depending on how well their observed effects on animals or humans actually compare with the predictions of the mathematical model employed. As a consequence, society might end up spending much to control one chemical based on a risk assessment that uses a conservative safety factor of 1,000 because it appears to be more dangerous than another that is actually more dangerous, but whose estimated risk is based on a safety factor only 10 times its true value. Because it is rarely necessary to protect the population from only one hazard at a time, it is preferable to make judgments based on the best estimate of the actual risks rather than incorporating large, but varying, safety factors into the PRA. In the real world, which is characterized by limited resources and time to deal with many possible hazards, an overly cautionary approach might be described as "too safe is unsafe."

Measures of Ill Health for Risk Assessment Purposes

As discussed in Chapter 7, various measures of ill health have been proposed to take into account, separately or in combination, the degree of prematurity of death and the time lived with nonfatal disease. Several choices must be made in such calculations—for example, whether to use different life expectancies for men and women or for different regions, how to weigh the severity of different kinds of disease, and

whether to discount the value of lost life-years in the future (as is the practice in economics). Whatever choices are made, it seems clear that measures of lost healthy life-years, due to both death and disease, are useful as a primary indicator of ill health. Such measures of forfeited healthy person-time, such as the DALY used by WHO for its burden of disease estimates, are coming into increasing use. As yet, however, few epidemiologic studies or risk assessment methods have directly applied them. More specifically, better estimates are needed of how much of the global burden of disease is attributable to environmental factors.

As the environmental risk transition progresses, and as the time between creation of a risk factor and its expression as disease tends to lengthen, the need for risk assessment increases (Smith, 1997). When evaluating measures to control diarrhea, for example, it is reasonable to monitor diarrhea rates, because the diarrhea of today is due largely to environmental exposures that occurred within a few preceding days. A similar logic can be used for increasing heat exposure due to climate change: Heat exhaustion and heat stroke are due to the exposure during the most recent hours or days (Kjellstrom, Holmer & Lemke, 2009). In contrast, for controlling environmental carcinogens or greenhouse gases, which have decades-long latency periods, waiting until ill effects start to occur would be far too late. Thus it is necessary to conduct risk assessments as best we can to make predictions well in advance of the actual events, so that appropriate measures can be taken in time.

Assessing Risk: Compared with What?

Risk assessments, when done in isolation, can be misleading. The following two examples are illustrative. Determining the risk imposed by an activity requires, explicitly or implicitly, choosing an appropriate baseline. In discussing the health effects of smoking, the appropriate baseline may be zero: It is possible for people to quit or not take up smoking. For air pollution, by comparison, the choice is not as clear. Natural sources of many air pollutants exist, and human sources are so difficult and expensive to control that a zero baseline is not feasible in many cases. Which level is then appropriate: the national standard or the WHO guideline value, or perhaps the level of the cleanest city? It is necessary to choose something, however, if we are to calculate the risk of the incremental pollution above the baseline.

Most human endeavors that are subject to risk assessment (technologies, industries, chemicals, regulations, and others) actually result in a mixture of risk-lowering and risk-raising effects. A new factory in a low-income country, for example, might impose pollution on the public and accident risk on the workers, but it may provide jobs, housing, training, security, and other benefits that could lead to substantial improvements in health. Just because these effects are less direct than the accident risk does not mean they are small. Indeed, the overall impact of industrialization must be risk lowering—otherwise, it would be the high-income countries that would be unhealthy rather than the low- and middle-income countries without industry.

Such risk lowering also occurs in high-income countries as well. Consider, for example, a pesticide residue on vegetables. Looked at in isolation, it may appear unacceptably risky. Viewed in terms of the overall impact on food cost and intake for low-income people, occupational risks to farm workers, and other factors, however, it may actually lower the overall risk compared with alternatives. This is not to say that all polluting activities will lower risks, but rather that all technologies should be judged on both their risk-lowering and risk-raising propensities. In addition, important equity and justice issues often arise in relation to who experiences the raised risk and who experiences the lowered risk. Unfortunately, our current risk assessment methods are not well developed for determining risk lowering, which is a source of potential bias in the results.

Some Special Considerations in Environmental Health Research

Several other considerations have recently assumed increasing importance in environmental health research and practice. Notably, there is a greater emphasis on seeking upstream (e.g., social, economic, political) explanations of environmental health hazards, particularly because downstream (end-of-pipe) solutions are often ineffective (see the discussion of the assessment of drivers, pressures, and environmental state changes in the earlier section, "Environmental Health Indicators and Monitoring"). The linkages between social determinants of health and environmental health hazards serve as a case in point (WHO, 2008). Meanwhile, advances in biomedical science have yielded a better understanding of how various body systems function as complex, dynamic, adaptive systems and of how their integrity might be affected, subclinically, by diverse environmental exposures. Finally, the understanding of the determinants of population and individual vulnerability to environmental stresses is improving.

Most toxicological and environmental epidemiologic studies aim to characterize effects and risks associated with specific exposure agents. When such exposures yield specific avoidable disease outcomes (e.g., bronchitis or bladder cancer), then this approach makes good sense. However, the functioning of certain organ systems can be cumulatively affected by multiple and continuing repeated exposures over time, resulting in immune system suppression, endocrine disruption, or cognitive impairment.

Both the immune system and the endocrine system entail complex interactive networks of organs, cells, and chemical messengers. Not surprisingly, many exogenous organic chemicals can cause metabolic disturbance of these systems. A growing body of evidence implicates pesticide exposures in suppression of the human immune system, for example (Repetto & Belagi, 1996). This is also the case for other environmental exposures, such as air pollution and ultraviolet radiation. There is suggestive, but inconclusive, evidence of an environmentally induced decline in human sperm count in high-income countries over the past half century, although the data sets on which this supposition is based are neither representative nor standardized. Supportive evidence comes from observations of impaired fertility and reproduction in other mammals due to endocrine-disrupting chemicals released by human societies (Colborn et al., 1993; Crain et al., 2008). Moreover, effects on specific organ systems, including the immune system, can be caused by physical factors (noise, heat, radiation) as well as by chemical factors.

Determinants of Individual and Population Vulnerability

In general, low- and middle-income populations are the most vulnerable to the health impacts of environmental degradation and change. They are typically more exposed, in terms of residential and occupational location, and have fewer resources for taking protective or adaptive action. The various social, cultural, and political influences on population vulnerability to environmental change include poverty, environmentally destructive growth, political rigidity, dependency, and isolation (Woodward, Hales, & Weinstein, 1998). Changes in the age structure of populations also affect vulnerability. For instance, as average life expectancies increase, populations become more vulnerable to many environmental stressors because of the increasing proportion of elderly persons.

Consider the more than 460 extra deaths that were attributed to the effects of an extreme heat wave in Chicago in July 1995. The rate of heat-related death was much greater in blacks than in whites, and in persons bedridden or otherwise confined to poorly ventilated inner-city housing. In the correspondingly severe 1995 heat wave in England and Wales, a 10% excess of deaths occurred in all age groups. In greater London, where daytime temperatures were higher and less cooling occurred overnight, mortality increased by approximately 15%. The excess mortality risks were generally greater in socioeconomically deprived groups. Similar patterns probably apply in low- and middle-income countries, although little such research has been done on this topic as yet.

In relation to heat exposure, it is also important to consider the additional internal heat exposure due to physical activity during work (Parsons, 2003). Working people in non-air-conditioned environments are, therefore, particularly vulnerable to climate change in places with long hot seasons (Kjellstrom et al., 2009).

The impact of regional changes in food and water availability will be greatest in potentially vulnerable regions where population growth is pronounced and food insecurity exists. Interactions between local environmental degradation and larger-scale environmental changes are likely to be important in determining the net impacts on human health. For example, local deforestation due to population pressure may directly alter the distribution of vector-borne diseases and the likelihood of flooding, both of which are also likely to increase because of global climate change.

Constitutional characteristics frequently influence an individual's susceptibility to environmental exposures. Readily seen examples include skin pigmentation modulating the risk of solar-induced skin cancer, and age modulating the efficiency of intestinal absorption of lead. Many physiological and biochemical functions of the human body—such as kidney function, liver function, eyesight, and hearing—decline with age after early adulthood. Individual variations in metabolic phenotype, which are substantially determined by genotype, are also important. Many enzyme pathways are known to be involved in the activation or deactivation of potentially carcinogenic or other toxic chemicals, such as the various oxidizing enzymes of the mitochondrial P450 system, the acetylation pathway (which yields phenotypically "fast" and "slow" acetylators), the glutathione transferase pathway, and the alpha-antitrypsin pathway.

There has been a steady accrual of epidemiologic evidence indicating that these polymorphisms modify the disease-inducing effects of an external environmental exposure; that is, a gene–environment interaction is observable at the individual level.

Discovery of such linkages opens up important opportunities for higher-resolution research. When study subjects are stratified on a metabolic polymorphic characteristic relevant to the external exposure, then the effect within the susceptible subgroup will become more evident than when the effect is diluted (averaged) across the susceptible and nonsusceptible subgroups.

Household Exposures

Because the home is where much human activity takes place, the potential for damaging exposures in households is high if pollutants are present. Unfortunately, two of the most fundamental and mundane human household activities—defecation and cooking—produce significant volumes of health-damaging waste products. When human waste is not removed completely from the household "environment" and isolated from drinking water supplies, it can lead to outbreaks of diarrhea and other water-borne diseases. When the smoke from cooking fires fueled with wood, coal, and other low-quality fuels is released into households, it can lead to respiratory diseases and other health impacts. Indeed, together these two environmental health factors account for the largest environmental burden of ill health globally; indeed, they probably account for a larger burden than any other major risk factor, environmental or not, except malnutrition. In addition to these health risks, a poorly designed or maintained home (usually due to poverty) may not provide the required shelter from extreme weather, protection from neighborhood environmental hazards, and safety in the case of natural disasters.

Sanitation and Clean Drinking Water

Ever since hunter-gatherers turned to cultivation and settled living, sanitation has been a public health problem for human societies. Further, although nearly two-thirds of the Earth's surface consists of water, only 2.5% of this is fresh water, and only 11% of this fresh water is available for human use. Political and institutional factors operate on top of this scarcity to create a global water shortage. As urban populations increase in size, the pressure on local sources of fresh drinking water increases in tandem.

Today, these two perennial difficulties remain widespread health hazards in the world, particularly in low- and middle-income countries in semiarid regions. More than 1.1 billion people in low- and middle-income countries have inadequate access to water, and 2.6 billion lack basic sanitation (WHO & UNICEF, 2010). Every year, a lack of access to clean drinking water and appropriate sanitation facilities results in more than 1.6 million deaths from diarrheal diseases around the world (Prüss-Ustün & Corvalán, 2006) (see also Chapter 5).

Two factors need to be taken into account when evaluating the relationship between health outcomes and access to clean drinking water. Most prominent are the linkages between household water availability and the health burden attributable to diarrheal diseases. In addition, intense rainfall or drought has a crucial role in facilitating water-borne outbreaks of diseases through both surface water and piped water supplies (Confalonieri et al., 2007).

Diseases related to water supply can be classified based on their route of transmission. Water-borne diseases, such as cholera and campylobacteriosis, are a result of the ingestion of contaminated water. Water-washed diseases, such as *Chlamydia* infection and scabies, are caused by a lack of hygiene secondary to a lack of water. Some classifications also include categories for water-based diseases, which include schistosomiasis, and diseases transmitted by water-related vectors, with malaria being the typical example.

A lack of sanitation may lead to the contamination of drinking water, highlighting the intertwined nature of these two problems. In Africa, 85% of the preventable burden of disease due to not being able to access clean water is caused by fecal–oral transmission of infectious disease (Cairncross et al., 2010). The costs associated with health spending, productivity losses, and labor diversions due to inadequate sanitation and clean drinking water result in sub-Saharan Africa losing approximately 5% of its GDP, or some $28.4 billion annually (Grimm et al., 2006). This figure exceeds the total aid flows and debt relief provided to the region. The main barrier to improving sanitation facilities is a lack of political will. By ensuring access to clean water and adequate sanitation facilities, the fecal–oral transmission pathway will be interrupted, resulting in an enormous flow of improvements in health, poverty reduction, and economic development.

Solid Household Fuels

The oldest of human energy technologies, the home cooking fire using wood or other biomass, remains the most prevalent fuel-using technology in the world today. Indeed, in more than 100 countries, household fuel demand makes up more than half of the total energy demand. Indoor air pollution accounted for 2.7% of the global burden of disease according to the 2002 World Health Report (WHO, 2002), and wood smoke is an important health hazard in this context (Naeher et al., 2007).

A useful framework for examining the trends and impacts of household fuel use is the "energy ladder." It ranks household fuels along a spectrum running from the simple biomass fuels (dung, crop residues, and wood), through the fossil fuels (kerosene and gas), to the most modern form (electricity). In moving up the ladder, the fuel and stove combinations that represent the higher rungs increase the desirable characteristics of cleanliness, efficiency, storability, and controllability. At the same time, capital cost and dependence on centralized fuel cycles tend to increase with upward movement on the ladder. Although local exceptions are possible, history has generally shown that when alternatives are affordable and available, populations tend to naturally move up the ladder to use of higher-quality fuel and stove combinations. Although all of humanity had its start a quarter of a million years ago at what was then the top of the energy ladder, wood, only half has since moved to higher-quality rungs. The remaining half of the world's population is either still using wood or has been forced down the ladder by local wood shortages to crop residues, animal dung, or, in some severe situations, to the poorest-quality fuels, such as shrubs and grass.

Throughout history, shortage of local wood supplies have led some populations to move to coal for household use in places where it was easily available. This occurred in the early 1800s in the United Kingdom, for example, although coal use in homes is relatively uncommon there today. In the past 150 years, such transitions also occurred in eastern Europe and China, where coal use still persists in millions of households (Figure 10-8). In the framework of the energy ladder, coal represents an upward movement in terms of efficiency and storability. Because of these characteristics as well as its higher energy density, coal can be shipped economically over longer distances than wood and can efficiently supply urban markets: In this regard, it is like other household fossil fuels. Unlike kerosene and gas, however, coal often represents a decrease in cleanliness as compared with wood.

Table 10-3 lists some of the many hundred health-damaging pollutants (HDPs) emitted as products of incomplete combustion from a range of household stoves in India. Even though biomass fuels might produce few wastes other than carbon dioxide and wa-

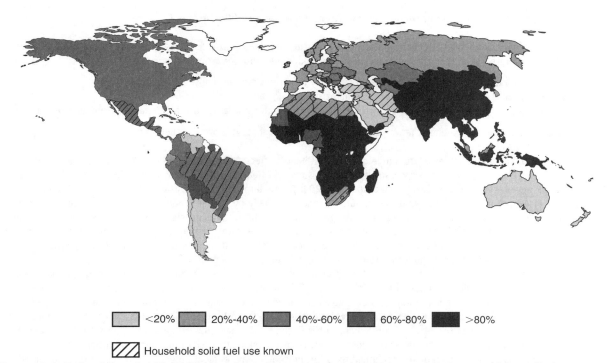

<20%   20%-40%   40%-60%   60%-80%   >80%

Household solid fuel use known

Figure 10-8 National Household Solid Fuel Use, 2000. *Source:* K. R. Smith, S. Mehta, and M. Maeusezahl-Feuz, "Indoor Smoke from Household Solid Fuels," in M. Ezzati, A. D. Rodgers, A. D. Lopez, and C. J. L. Murray (Eds.), *Comparative Quantification of Health Risks: Global and Regional Burden of Disease Due to Selected Major Risk Factors,* Vol. 2 (Geneva, Switzerland: World Health Organization, 2004). Reprinted with permission.

ter when combusted completely, in practice as much as one-fifth of the fuel carbon is diverted to products of incomplete combustion, many of which are important HDPs. Coal, by comparison, is not only difficult to burn completely because of its solid form, but also contains significant intrinsic contaminants. Most prominent among such emissions from coal, as shown in Table 10-3, are sulfur oxides. Coal in many areas also contains arsenic, fluorine, lead, mercury, or other toxic elements that lead to serious HDPs.

A practical example of the dangers of coal smoke exposure and an effective initiative to reduce this exposure has occurred in China. Since the 1980s, this country has introduced more than 180 million improved stoves with chimneys—more than in all other low- and middle-income countries combined. In Yunnan province, this strategy has led to a 50% reduction in the risk of lung cancer and chronic obstructive pulmonary disease (COPD) (Zhang & Smith, 2007).

Petroleum-based liquid and gaseous fuels, such as kerosene and liquid petroleum gas, may also contain sulfur and other contaminants, albeit in much smaller amounts than in many coals. Further, their physical

forms allow for much better premixing with air in simple devices, thereby assuring substantially higher combustion efficiencies and lower HDP emissions. In addition, kerosene and gas stoves tend to be much more energy efficient. Hence, the HDP emissions per meal from these fuels are at least an order of magnitude less than those from solid fuels.

The full story about the health risks associated with different household fuel types is still not known. A recent study (Pokhrel et al., 2010) showed that indoor air pollution from cooking fuels was associated with tuberculosis incidence in Nepal and that the greatest risk was for kerosene use for cooking and lighting.

Unfortunately, not only do solid-fuel stoves produce substantial HDPs, but a large fraction also lack chimneys for removing the emissions. Consequently, indoor HDP concentrations can reach very high levels for various important HDPs, including fine particulates and carbon monoxide. For example, fine particulate levels often reach 20 to 40 times the WHO guideline levels set to protect health. Even in households with chimneys, heavily polluting solid-fuel stoves can produce significant local outdoor pollution. This is particularly true in dense urban slums,

Exhibit 10-3	Health Impacts of Indoor Air Pollution in Low- and Middle-Income Countries

Three main categories of health effects from indoor air pollution are thought to occur, based on studies in solid-fuel households and corroborated by studies of active and passive smoking and outdoor air pollution:

- Infectious respiratory diseases, such as acute respiratory infections and, perhaps, tuberculosis
- Chronic respiratory diseases, such as chronic bronchitis and lung cancer
- Adverse pregnancy outcomes, such as stillbirth and low birth weight in infants born to women exposed during pregnancy

In addition, there is some evidence that air pollution from the household use of solid fuel increases the risks of blindness, asthma, and heart disease.

The best available estimates of the range of potential health effects within the low- and middle-income country setting come from the comparative risk assessment done by the World Health Organization, summarized in the World Health Report 2002 and in the report by Ezzati and associates (2002). This large multi-institution effort compared the burden of death and disease from more than two dozen major risk factors globally by age, sex, and region. To facilitate comparison, the studies were done under rules of "consensual discipline" in which, as much as possible, common criteria for acceptance of evidence were adopted. Under these rules, only the evidence for acute lower respiratory infections in young children and chronic obstructive pulmonary disease and lung cancer in women was deemed sufficiently robust for these conditions to be included as outcomes of indoor air pollution (Smith, Mehta, & Maeusezahl-Feuz, 2004).

This analysis yielded an estimate of 1.6 million premature deaths annually from this cause, including approximately 1 million deaths in young children. Indoor air pollution accounts for an estimated 2.6% of the total global burden of disease—larger than the contribution from all forms of tuberculosis and more than half that from all forms of cancer. In terms of mortality, indoor air pollution creates a substantially greater burden than the toll from malaria. These impacts occur largely in poor countries of South Asia (one-third), sub-Saharan Africa (one-third), and China (one-sixth). Table 10-2 compares the impact of indoor air pollution on global health compared with other risk factors, environmental and otherwise.

Although it is tempting to promote technical fixes for household environmental health problems in low- and middle-income countries, when implemented alone they often have only limited success, although in the case of China some 180 million improved stoves have been introduced (Sinton et al., 2004). Provision of improved biomass-burning cooking stoves with chimneys often fails to reduce indoor air pollution because of poor maintenance and lack of consideration of local cooking practices. Promoting the use of cleaner fuels is difficult among populations that have little disposable income but free access to local biomass resources. In general, reducing the risks related to such activities as cooking, defecation, and hygiene requires both technical and behavioral changes. Finding effective ways to achieve this goal is an important research task.

Source: Smith, K. R. (1998). *National burden of disease from indoor air pollution in India,* Mumbai: Indira Gandhi Institute of Development Research.

where such neighborhood pollution can greatly exceed the urban average levels. A study of low-income households in Guatemala (McCracken et al., 2007) showed that installing chimneys in households using open wood fires for cooking significantly reduced blood pressure in middle-aged women—a phenomenon also seen (albeit to a lesser degree) with reductions in outdoor air pollution.

Because they are usually responsible for cooking, women and their accompanying youngest children generally are the most exposed to this risk factor. Thus, although the total amount of HDP pollution released from stoves worldwide is not high compared with that from large-scale use of fossil fuels, the total human exposure to a number of important pollutants is actually much larger than the exposures created by outdoor pollution. As a result, the health effects can be expected to be higher as well.

Despite the sizes of the exposed populations and the HDP exposures involved, there has been relatively little scientific investigation of the health effects of indoor air pollution in low- and middle-income countries compared with studies of outdoor air pollution in urban populations (McMichael & Smith, 1999). Nevertheless, enough has been done to enable the magnitude of their impact to be estimated, at least for women and young children, who receive the highest HDP exposures. The impacts of the high concentrations experienced by a larger number of people with generally lower overall health status exceed those for outdoor air pollution (Exhibit 10-3).

Housing Quality

General housing quality involves such factors as ventilation, drainage, crowding, dustiness, materials that resist pests, design that limits injuries, and insulation from sun, wind, cold and heat. All of these factors have a significant influence on health. Indeed, much of the improvement in health that occurred in western Europe and North America during the latter part of the nineteenth and early part of the twentieth centuries is attributable to improved housing—although it is difficult to separate the relative benefits of improved housing from those due to concurrent changes in nutrition and personal hygiene behavior. Studies in some communities in low- and middle-income countries, however, indicate that health gains require improvements in a mix of factors, including general housing quality, rather than in just one factor at a time.

Good-quality housing for low- and middle-income communities can protect health in various ways. It provides shelter from cold, hot, or wet weather conditions. Cold indoor temperatures have been a particular problem in many countries (McMichael et al., 2008), but heat exposure is a threat as well in hot places and during heat waves in colder places. Incremental improvements of traditional designs that are basically adapted to the local conditions would be the most cost-effective means of improving shelter. An emerging feature of housing design is the protection against increasing heat exposure from the ambient environment due to climate change (Hajat, O'Connor, & Kosatsky, 2010). Another factor of importance is the structural integrity of the housing in the face of typhoons, floods, or earthquakes. In addition, the location of the house is important: The houses of many persons injured or killed in floods are in low-lying areas prone to flooding, for example.

The risk of physical injuries is another important aspect of housing quality. Children and elderly need to be protected from falls. Animals, machinery, vehicles, and cooking stoves and other sources of non-CO_2 greenhouse gases, such as methane heaters, need to be separated from areas to which small children have access.

In tropical countries, residences should be situated so that they avoid breeding sites for insect vectors of disease. Good drainage around the home and elimination of any sites where water can stagnate and mosquitoes can breed are of great importance in preventing malaria and dengue fever. In parts of Latin America, the prevention of Chagas disease (South American sleeping sickness) and the elimination of its vector, the triatomine bug, depend on the use of solid ceiling and wall materials without cracks.

The Workplace Environment

The workplace "environment" is generally more dangerous to human health than the ambient external environment. Machinery, chemicals, dusts, ergonomic hazards, and the fact that much work is carried out with the body at its peak performance are all factors that contribute to the overall level of risk. Nevertheless, many of the same specific hazards occur in the workplace and the general environment; hence there are many similarities in how their effects can be moni-

tored and managed (Rosenstock et al., 2005; Yassi & Kjellstrom, 1998).

A variety of textbooks on occupational health and occupational medicine describe the many workplace hazards to health (e.g., Levy & Wegman, 2000; Rosenstock et al., 2005; Stellman, 1998). The issues in low- and middle-income countries have been highlighted by Kjellstrom (1994), and a detailed treatise is given by Herzstein and colleagues (1998). This section summarizes several key areas of concern.

Important phenomena in the workplace "environment" of low- and middle-income countries include the problems that occur during a time of rapid industrialization. Agricultural societies are transformed during this rapid transition, but often without the infrastructure for environmental and workplace health protection that was built up in high-income countries over their many decades of industrial development. Sometimes the new industries replace existing cottage industries, and conditions may improve. In other cases industries with outmoded, dangerous technology are moved from high-income countries, creating new hazards in the receiving low- or middle-income country. The phrase "export of hazards" has been used to describe this problem (LaDou & Jeyaratnam, 1994; Moure-Eraso et al., 2007).

Agriculture

Agriculture is the most common occupation in rural areas of low- and middle-income countries, where most of the world's population lives. Most workers are engaged in subsistence agriculture, in which the boundaries between work and other aspects of daily life are fluid. Workplace hazards in this type of situation include the generally poor and unhealthy living environments, which are often characterized by unsafe drinking water, poor sanitation, and inadequate shelter.

Specific hazards may also exist in these areas, such as injury hazards from tools used in tilling the soil, vector-borne diseases related to walking in water or mud, hazardous heat exposure under extreme conditions, bites from insects and animals, and falls or drowning from working on hillsides or riversides. The health risks are further increased because subsistence farm work involves the whole family, including children and the elderly. Epidemiologic evidence of these types of health risks is scanty.

As the planting and harvesting processes become more advanced and farmers develop cash crop production, new hazards emerge. The tools involved become more mechanized, which creates new types of injury risks, particularly because the use of these tools is unfamiliar to many of the workers. Pesticides are introduced, but often without the provision of full equipment and training (WHO, 1990). As a consequence, an estimated 3 million cases of unintentional pesticide poisoning occur among agricultural workers in low- and middle-income countries each year (WHO, 2004). In addition, pesticides have been estimated to be used as a deadly poison in 30% of global suicides, with 250,000 people taking their life in this way each year (Gunnell et al., 2007); Chapter 8 discusses self-directed violence in more detail.

Agricultural work hazards are not only related to planting and harvesting food crops. An important activity is the collection of fuel wood for cooking and heating. Wood and agricultural waste is often collected in local forests by women (Sims, 1994). An analysis of time use for these activities, along with water collection and cooking, in four low-income countries showed that women spent 9 to 12 hours per day engaged in such tasks, whereas men spent 5 to 8 hours. Firewood collection may be combined with harvesting of wood for local use in construction and small-scale cottage industry manufacturing. A number of health hazards are associated with the basic conditions of the forest, including insect bites, stings from poisonous plants, cuts, falls, and drowning.

In countries with tropical heat and humidity, great physiological strain is placed on the body, whereas the cold is a potential hazard in temperate countries and the Arctic area. In countries with a high sunshine level, UVR can be another health hazard, increasing the risk of skin cancer and cataracts (Gallagher & Lee, 2006; WHO, 1994). All forestry work is hard physical labor that is associated with a risk of ergonomic damage, such as painful backs and joints as well as fatigue, which increases the risk of injuries from falls, falling trees, or equipment (Poschen, 1998). Women carrying heavy loads of firewood—and also at risk of ergonomic damage—are common in areas with subsistence forestry (Sims, 1994). Further, the living conditions of forestry workers are often poor, and workers may spend long periods in simple huts in the forest with limited protection against the weather and poor sanitary facilities.

Urbanization typically leads to the development of a commercial market for firewood and larger-scale production of firewood from logs or from smaller waste material left over after the logs have been harvested. Energy forestry then becomes more mechanized, and workers are exposed to additional hazards associated with commercial forestry (Poschen, 1998). Motorized hand tools (e.g., the chainsaw) become more commonly used—a trend that leads to high injury risk, noise-induced hearing loss, and "white finger disease" caused by vibration of the hands. In addition, fertilizer and pesticides become a part of the production system, which results in the potential for pesticide poisoning among sprayers. As the development of forestry progresses, more of the logging becomes mechanized with large machinery, reducing the direct contact between workers and materials. Workers in highly mechanized forestry have only 15% of the injury risk of highly skilled forestry workers using chainsaws (Poschen, 1998). In contrast, firewood production continues to require manual handling and, therefore, may remain a hazardous operation.

The mortality and morbidity data for occupational hazard impacts on populations are in many countries severely under-reported. However, based

Table 10-4	Occupational Injury Mortality Rates in Different Economic Sectors, 1995–2000			
	Fatality Rates			
Sector (ISIC Code)	Sweden	United States	Argentina	Zimbabwe
All occupations	2	5	15	20
Agriculture and fishing (A + B)	20	23	31	20
Mining and quarrying (C)	14	26	27	69
Manufacturing (D)	1.6	3.4	13	7.5
Electricity, gas, water supply (E)	5.6	—	28	13
Construction (F)	5.4	15	39	21
Trade and restaurants (G + H)	0.7	—	8.8	9.0
Transport (I)	4.4	13	32	65
Financial and business (J + K)	0.8	1.4	11	4.4
Administration, education, health, and other (L–O)	1.0	2	6.5	15

Note: The unit here is the number of deaths per 100,000 economically active workers in the sector.
Source: International Labor Organization statistics (Kjellstrom & Hogstedt, 2009).

on the statistics reported to the International Labor Organization (ILO), an idea of the reported mortality can be gleaned (Table 10-4). Agriculture and fishing have relatively high injury mortality rates in the four countries assessed in Table 10-4, while mining, construction, and transport have even higher rates, particularly in Argentina and Zimbabwe.

Mining and Extraction

Mining is inherently dangerous to the mine workers, as highlighted by regular media reports of severe incidents in different types of mines. Most countries, including low- and middle-income countries, have recognized this fact and developed specific legislation and systems to protect mine workers (Eisler, 2003; Ramani & Mutmanski, 1999; Stellman, 1998).

Two major types of mining exist, each with a somewhat different pattern of health hazards: underground mining and open-cast mining. Ergonomic hazards and physical (accident-inducing) hazards occur in both, but underground work includes the added hazards of being crushed by falling rock, poisoned by gas or dust buildup, or affected by heat or radiation. Each type of mine entails specific hazards associated with the rock from which the ore is excavated. Most types of rock contain high levels of silica, leading to high levels of silica dust in the air of a mine and the risk of silicosis in workers. Certain types of rock (particularly uranium ore) contain radioactive compounds that are emanated as the gas radon, which increases the risk of lung cancer. Other types of rock contain metals that are inherently poisonous (e.g., lead and cadmium) and that in certain conditions can cause dangerous exposures.

According to the United Nations' Demographic Yearbooks, miners constitute a large occupational group on a global level. They represent as much as 2% of the economically active population in some countries. Although only 1% of the global workforce is engaged in mining, this industry accounts for 8% of all fatal occupational accidents—approximately 15,000 deaths per year. A detailed review of occupational health and safety issues in mining is available in Armstrong and Menon (1998).

Mining is thus a particularly dangerous occupation. Table 10-4 highlights the high overall occupational mortality rates in selected countries. In low- and middle-income countries, coal mining employs millions of people. Coal is a major global energy source, contributing 23% of total energy consumption (Johansson & Goldernberg, 2004). It was the primary source of energy between 1900 and 1960, but subsequently has been overtaken by oil. Coal can be produced through surface mining (open cast) or un-

derground mining. Both operations are inherently dangerous to the health of the workers.

Underground coal miners are exposed to the hazards of excavating and transporting materials underground. These risks include injuries from falling rocks and falls into mine shafts, as well as injuries from machinery used in the mine. There are no reliable global data on injuries of this type from low- and middle-income countries (Jennings, 1998), but in high-income countries miners have some of the highest rates of compensation for injuries. In addition, much of the excavation involves drilling into silica-based rock, which creates high levels of silica dust inside the mine. As a consequence, pneumoconiosis silicosis is a common health effect in coal miners (Jennings, 1998). In addition, it has been shown that coal miners with silicosis have an increased risk of lung cancer.

Other health hazards specific to underground coal mining include the coal dust, which can cause "coal worker's pneumoconiosis," or anthracosis, often combined with silicosis. The coal dust is explosive, so explosions in underground coal mines are an ever-present danger for coal miners. Fires in coal mines are not uncommon, and once started may be almost impossible to extinguish. Apart from the danger of burns, the production of smoke and toxic fumes creates great health risks for the miners. Even without fires, the coal material produces toxic gases when it is disturbed—namely, carbon monoxide, carbon dioxide, and methane. Carbon monoxide binds to hemoglobin in the blood, blocking oxygen transport and causing chemical suffocation. This colorless and odorless gas gives no warning before the symptoms of drowsiness, dizziness, headache, and unconsciousness occur. Carbon dioxide displaces oxygen in the underground air and can cause suffocation.

Mines where materials other than coal are extracted (e.g. iron, copper, lead, zing, silver, gold) have similar risks of injuries, hot work environments, and exposure to silica dust. An additional health hazard is exhaust fumes from the diesel engines used in machinery or transport vehicles underground. These emissions contain very fine particles, nitrogen oxides, and carbon monoxide, all of which can create serious health problems. Underground mining may also expose the workers to extreme heat stress due to high temperature or humidity (Wyndham, 1969). The climatic conditions underground need to be assessed when scheduling work shifts and breaks.

Surface mining avoids the hazards of working underground but still involves risks from machinery, falls, and falling rocks. In addition, mining is very energy-intensive work, similar to forestry, and heat, humidity, and other weather factors can affect the worker's health. The machinery used is noisy, and hearing loss is a common effect in miners. Another health hazard is the often squalid conditions under which many coal workers in low- and middle-income countries live, which creates particular risks for the diseases of poverty.

A special type of mining is the extraction of oil and gas to supply the energy needs of societies in the midst of industrialization. Oil and gas exploration, drilling, extraction, processing, and transportation involve a number of the hazards mentioned previously: heavy workload, ergonomic hazards, injury risk, noise, vibration, and chemical exposures (Kraus, 1998). This type of work is often carried out in isolated geographic areas that are subject to inclement weather conditions. Long-distance commuting may also be involved, which increases fatigue, stress, and traffic accident risks. The ergonomic hazards have the potential to cause back pain and joint pain. Injuries may include burns and those caused by explosions. Skin damage from exposure to the oil itself and from chemicals used in the drilling processes creates a need for well-designed protective clothing. In addition, many oil and gas installations have used asbestos for heat-insulating cladding of pipes and equipment, which leads to the hazard of inhalation of asbestos dust in the installation and repair of such equipment, which in turn increases the risk of lung cancer, asbestosis, and mesothelioma (Kamp, 2009; WHO, 1998, 2006).

Much exploration and drilling for oil and gas now occur offshore. This type of mining involves underwater diving work, which is inherently dangerous. In addition, the weather-related exposures can be extreme, particularly because the work often requires continuous, around-the-clock operations (Kraus, 1998).

Construction

Construction work is another dangerous occupation with potential exposures to a variety of hazards (Weeks, 1998). Risks include injuries from falls and falling objects, and injuries from machinery or related to excavation or underground work. Because much construction work is carried out in the open, weather conditions may create hazards related to heat, cold, UVR, and dust storms. Construction work also involves heavy lifting of materials and activities in awkward body positions, leading to ergonomic hazards. Injuries, strains, and sprains are common. Many injuries are severe, leading to the high ratio of construction workers in the occupational mortality statistics (see Table 10-4).

Construction work also involves exposures to heat, cold, noise, chemicals, and biological hazards. Much of the machinery used is noisy, and this problem has only increased with the increasing mechanization of the industry. Demolition is a common aspect of construction work, and demolition activities are inherently noisy. As a consequence of these factors, noise-induced hearing loss is common among construction workers. Another aspect of the noisy "environment" is the increased safety problems caused by the masking of warning calls or other alarms.

Chemical and dust exposures are related to the composition of the building materials. Asbestos, which has long been used as insulation and as a component of asbestos-cement pipes and sheets, is a prime example of a hazardous material. Asbestosis (a form of pneumoconiosis), lung cancer, and mesothelioma (another fatal cancer) have been found in many construction workers (WHO, 1998). Mesothelioma is one of the most prominent occupational diseases in most countries where records are kept, although underreporting of asbestos-related lung cancer is common. In high-income countries, as many as 20,000 cases of lung cancer and 10,000 cases of mesothelioma occur each year due to asbestos exposures in workplaces that took place 20 to 40 years ago (Tossavainen, 2000). The use of asbestos has been reduced in most high-income countries and banned in some, but asbestos-cement building products are still widely used in low- and middle-income countries because these materials have attractive technical qualities. Alternatives to asbestos exist for almost every use, and their cost is often similar to asbestos.

The use of asbestos in low- and middle-income countries remains widespread (Kazan-Allen, 2003; Tossavainen, 2004) and, indeed, is continuing to increase (Le et al., 2010). The epidemic of serious health effects associated with exposure to asbestos takes decades to develop, so preventive actions need to be taken at an early stage. Some low- and middle-income countries have instituted bans on use of asbestos in construction, which would be the most effective means of prevention. The epidemic of asbestos-related disease is still on the ascendancy in a number of high-income countries, even though virtual bans were instituted in the 1980s—for example, in New Zealand, where the full epidemic of asbestos cancer over 40 years may kill at least 2,000 to 3,000 workers (Kjellstrom, 2004).

Other chemical and dust exposures in the construction industry include cement dust among bricklayers and concrete workers (Meo, 2004); such dust causes lung disease and dermatitis. Sand-blasting or rock drilling creates silica dust in the air, which can lead to silicosis in exposed workers. Construction work often involves welding, which adds further health hazards, such as inhalation of welding fumes that leads to bronchitis. Paint fumes often contain organic solvents that may cause neurologic disorders. The hazards of dusts and fumes are increased inside confined spaces, where these concentrations can reach extremely high levels.

Because of climate conditions, work in the construction industry is often seasonal, so contract workers may rely on other work during parts of each year. This seasonality is influenced by climate. In tropical and subtropical countries, extreme heat exposure during the hot season may cause major health and productivity issues (Kjellstrom, 2009). The intermittent character of seasonal work also creates problems in maintaining efficient prevention programs to protect workers against these hazards (Weeks, 1998), especially in low- and middle-income countries. Subcontracting or informal employment relations often reduce the responsibility taken by the main employer or contractor on a construction site. When the responsibility for health and safety is dispersed among many individuals, the protection against hazards may become insufficient. Thus, in construction work, it is important that contracts include the necessary safety provisions and that systems be in place for monitoring and enforcing these provisions.

Transport

An important industry in modern society is motorized transport of goods and people. As a country develops economically, transport occupations typically become an increasing proportion of the workforce. These jobs include drivers of trucks, buses, taxis, trains, airplanes, and other vehicles; people involved inside the vehicles (e.g., conductors, flight attendants); people involved in loading and offloading freight; and people involved in the management of the transport system (e.g., traffic police, air traffic controllers).

The motorized transport system creates several health hazards in communities as described in other sections of this chapter (e.g., air pollution, noise, injury risks). The health risks specific to the people working in the transport industry are also of importance. Table 10-4 shows the relatively high injury mortality risks for transport workers in four countries. Most of these deaths are likely to be due to "traffic accidents." Other occupational health hazards include exposures to noise, chemicals, and dusts, as well as ergonomic hazards associated with lifting heavy loads and sitting for hours in the same position driving a vehicle (Kjellstrom & Hogstedt, 2009).

Manufacturing

Manufacturing workplaces can be the sites of any of a long list of occupational hazards, some of which were mentioned in previous sections of this chapter. A review of the various hazards is included in the *Encyclopaedia of Occupational Health and Safety*, published by the International Labor Organization (Stellman, 1998). Manufacturing involves ergonomic injury hazards from improper work positions, heavy lifts, and dangerous machinery; physical hazards, such as noise, heat, poor lighting, and, occasionally, radiation; and chemical exposures of many kinds. However, as in the earlier history of today's high-income countries, the major chemical exposure problems in low- and middle-income countries today include lead, cadmium, chromium, mercury, other metals, organic solvents, and welding fumes. Increasingly, the most hazardous industries and processes are being exported from high-income countries to low- and middle-income countries (LaDou & Jeyaratnam, 1994), but without the technological improvements that have reduced workers' exposures to these risks in the high-income countries. In addition, stress and other psychosocial hazards of long work hours and shift work are common in an industry that has made large investments in machinery, from which economic benefits accrue only when the equipment is in operation.

Of the various manufacturing industries, some with particular health risks are worth highlighting. In electrical appliance manufacturing (Stellman, 1998), major risks are found in lead-acid battery manufacturing operations, which produce batteries for vehicles. Because such batteries are too heavy to transport over long distances, local production is usually established at an early stage of the "motor car society." The operation of these factories typically involves many workers who receive unacceptably high lead exposures. The usual approach is to monitor workers' blood lead levels; if the levels exceed the national standard, the worker is excused for a few weeks. Indeed, this type of risk management is enshrined in occupational health law in many countries. This approach displaces the exposure problem to the individual rather than analyzing the workplace "environment" as a whole.

Cadmium is another toxic metal of increased importance; it is used in rechargeable batteries in modern electronic equipment such as mobile phones. Unfortunately, the manufacturing of cadmium batteries involves even more risks than lead battery production. Vigilant exposure monitoring and effective protection are essential to avoid chronic poisoning in the form of kidney and lung diseases (Friberg, Elinder, Kjellstrom, T., & Nordberg, 1986).

Another manufacturing industry commonly found in high-income countries is metal processing and metal working. Smelting and refining of any metal creates a major potential for occupational exposures to many types of hazards, and a particular risk of exposure to toxic metal dusts, sulfur dioxide, and other fumes. Because these industries often involve very large-scale operations, even small concentrations of toxic compounds in the processes can yield substantial emissions into the workplace and the surrounding environment. The experience with lead smelters in many countries has produced similar results: high lead exposures for workers and contamination of the local environment. Often the workers and their families live in the vicinity of the industry, and high lead exposures from dust emissions are found in children who live in the area. These exposure situations have been studied in detail in the United States and Australia, and epidemiologic research there has produced some of the most valuable quantitative data on the health risks of lead in children and workers (see also Exhibit 10-1).

Service Occupations

Many service industries involve important occupational hazards. The services reviewed by the International Labor Organization include those characterized by specialized and sometimes severe hazards, such as emergency and security services (e.g., fire fighting and law enforcement), public and government services (e.g., garbage collection and hazardous waste disposal), and healthcare services (Stellman, 1998). Occupations that are considered likely to have less severe hazards include retail trades, banking, administrative services, telecommunications, restaurants, education, and entertainment.

Fire fighting involves exposure to carbon monoxide and toxic fumes, as well as the heat from the fire itself. Injuries from falling debris, falls, or working in awkward positions are also of concern. Protection of workers depends on protective equipment, which in low- and middle-income countries may be in short supply. Law enforcement is another high-risk occupation, as it involves hostile contacts with persons who may be armed.

Garbage collection exposes workers to risks of cuts and other injuries from the garbage itself, as well as ergonomic hazards (e.g., heavy lifting) and chemical hazards. A notable at-risk group in low- and middle-income countries is the people who scavenge on garbage dumps for recyclable materials from which to glean a meager existence. Sometimes these scavengers actually live on the garbage dump, where they are subjected to risks of infectious disease, bites from rats and dogs, and other dangers. Because hazardous wastes are not always separated out, their presence adds to the risks of the garbage collectors and scavengers. In areas where hazardous wastes are separated, the storage and handling of these materials requires sophisticated protective equipment, detailed information about the hazards, and efficient management systems; these factors are often missing even in high-income countries, however.

Healthcare workers face other hazards, such as infections from patients, transmission of HIV or hepatitis from needlesticks, and allergies to drugs given patients or to cleaning and disinfection chemicals. In reality, the most common problem faced by these workers is ergonomic hazards from lifting or moving patients, which may lead to back injuries. This type of injury creates great problems for nurses and nurse aides, and in many cases curtails their careers.

One special hazard for people in service trades that involve continuous work at computer keyboards is the development of repetitive strain injury, also known as occupational overuse syndrome (Rosenstock et al., 2005). Repetitive keyboard finger work, or repetitive fine movement of the computer mouse, may create a wear-and-tear reaction in tendons and muscles that can lead to chronic pain. As with the situation for bad backs, these painful conditions are not always accompanied by measurable anatomical or pathological changes, which has caused substantial arguments among medical practitioners as to the genuineness of the disease. However, as many people using modern computers attest, the short-term pain after intensive use of a keyboard or a mouse is real. The ergonomic design of a computer workstation and the provision of regular work breaks are essential for preventing this occupational hazard. The height of the keyboard should be adjusted to the individual user. Unfortunately, these conditions may be difficult to achieve in low- and middle-income countries.

Other Occupations

Among the other occupational exposure situations of particular importance, especially in low- and middle-income countries, are cottage industries of various types. At an early stage of industrialization, small-scale operations based on family members may be the mainstay of certain industries. They may take the form of work contracted out from a larger enterprise, or the businesses may arise directly in relation to the local market. The production of handicrafts, clothing, and consumer items for local households may be the starting point. However, more hazardous activities, such as recycling car batteries, may also develop initially as cottage industries. Such work may entail extreme exposures to toxic chemicals, with little or no protection either for the workers or for other family members. Ergonomic hazards, injuries, noise damage, and all other occupational hazards are likely to be a greater danger in these cottage industries than in larger, more organized enterprises.

Community Exposures

The community level is the level at which much environmental epidemiologic research has concentrated, particularly in relation to ambient air pollution, heat exposure during heat waves, industrial emissions, the problems associated with urban transport systems, contamination of local drinking water and local food supplies, and waste management. Difficult methodological choices often confront researchers at this level, particularly whether to attempt to measure exposures and make comparisons at the individual, small-group (microecological), or community level.

Outdoor Air Quality

Urban air pollution has, in recent decades, become recognized as a worldwide public health problem (Cohen et al., 2004; Kampa & Castanas, 2008; WHO, 1997). Substantial epidemiological research in recent years has provided clear evidence of the health risks of fine particular matter (dust) and other components of urban air pollution. For example, the studies by Pope et al. (2002, 2004) quantified the mortality impacts on the cardiopulmonary systems and lung cancer. The most recent study (Pope et al., 2009) revealed that the exposure-response relationship for cardiovascular mortality is not linear, which will have great importance for future risk assessment calculations.

In high-income countries, the industrial and household air pollution from coal burning that occurred in earlier eras has been largely replaced by pollutants from motorized transport that form photochemical smog, including ozone (a strong irritant that affects the eyes, upper airways, and lungs) in summer and a heavy haze of particulates and nitrogen oxides in winter. Although many industrialized cities do not yet meet annual standards for every pollutant, conditions are generally much better than in the past. Nevertheless, air pollution has become a renewed concern in various cities where it was once believed that the historical problems had been solved. The experience of severe air pollution incidents in the mid-twentieth century—most famously in London in 1952 (the "London Fog" incident), when the daily mortality was doubled during a two-week period—finally led to a political agreement to act against air pollution. During that episode, the daily peaks were several thousand milligrams per cubic meter (mg/m^3) for each of the pollutants. Until the first half of the twentieth century, air pollution problems were caused mainly by the industrial and household burning of coal without efficient emission controls, leading especially to high breathing zone concentrations during temperature inversions. During the subsequent decades, the annual average and daily peak levels of particulate matter and sulfur dioxide were decreased tenfold or more in most large cities in high-income countries.

In low- and middle-income countries, urban air pollution has recently reached alarming levels in many cities. In New Delhi, Beijing, and several other Indian and Chinese cities, for example, the annual average concentrations of particulates have been 5 to 10 times greater than the WHO air quality guideline (Exhibit 10-4). In China, the main source of pollution is combustion of coal. Industrial, neighborhood, and household sources all contribute to the unhealthy atmosphere, however, and emissions from automobiles are increasing sharply (Florig, 1997). The estimated morbidity and mortality in Chinese cities due to air pollution is now increasing markedly (see Exhibit 10-4). Meanwhile, in many of the cities of Central and Eastern Europe, the mix of industrial emissions and car exhausts has led to enormous increases in air pollution. In eastern Germany and in southern Poland in the late 1980s, winter concentrations of sulfur dioxide from coal burning were even higher than those in London during the infamous 1952 smog episode.

Studies relating ambient air pollution levels to health risks were, until the 1970s, largely confined to examining the health impacts of particular extreme episodes of very high outdoor air pollution levels. Subsequent studies, based on daily mortality time series, have elucidated the role of respirable particulates, including black carbon, ozone, sulfates, and nitrogen oxides in acute mortality (Schwartz, 1994; Smith et al., 2009). The advantages and attractions of daily time-series statistical analysis were discussed in the section "Study Design Options" earlier in this chapter. However, this acute component of mortality due to daily fluctuations in air pollution levels needs

---

Exhibit 10-4 | **Urban Air Pollution and Health in India and China**

The two largest countries in the world, India and China, share an unfortunate characteristic: They rely on dirty coal for large fractions of their commercial energy. In addition, as low-income countries, they have not been able to devote significant resources to either cleaning the coal before it is burned or capturing the emissions in the smokestacks before they are released into the environment. Furthermore, they have many relatively small coal-burning sources, including small factories, commercial activities such as restaurants, and, in China, boilers for heating buildings and cookstoves, from which the pollution is difficult to control. The result is high air pollution levels in many cities in both countries.

Data show, for example, that the average annual outdoor concentration of PM10 (airborne particulate matter of diameter less than 10 microns) in large Indian cities is approximately 190 mg/m^3. This concentration is six to eight times the levels in U.S. and European cities. Mean PM10 levels in large Chinese cities are similar, perhaps 180 mg/m^3. Unlike in India, however, China's coal contains significant amounts of sulfur; thus sulfur dioxide levels are sometimes markedly elevated in this country, although progress is being made to reduce them (International Scientific Oversight Committee, 2004).

Although fossil fuels dominate energy use in the urban sectors of all countries, small-scale combustion of biomass in households and small enterprises continues to make substantial contributions to pollution in many cities in India. For example, small particles from biomass combustion make up 10% to 29% of the particles in Delhi and 17% to 32% in Kolkata, depending on the season (Chowdhury, Zheng, & Russel, 2004).

Although estimations in this context are difficult, it appears that the burden of disease resulting from air pollution in each country is high. The WHO Comparative Risk Study (see Table 10-1) estimated that there were approximately 300,000 premature deaths per year in China and 110,000 such deaths in India from urban outdoor air pollution (Cohen et al., 2004). However, in addition to other uncertainties, the results of such calculations depend on which baseline is assumed—that is, how low pollution levels could realistically become. Given natural background environmental factors, a level of zero is simply not feasible.

---

to be carefully distinguished from the long-term effect of chronic exposure at an elevated level (McMichael, Anderson, Brunekreef, & Cohen, 1998). Long-term follow-up studies of populations exposed to different levels of air pollution, especially particulates, indicate that the higher the levels of exposure, the greater the mortality risk.

For example, a 16-year follow-up of 500,000 people in the United States was used to link urban air pollution exposures to mortality with appropriate control of confounding factors (Pope et al., 2002). An increased mortality in cardiopulmonary diseases was identified, and the strongest relation to air pollution (particulate matter of less than 2.5 mm diameter) was found for lung cancer. Further quantification of the exposure-response relationships based on the same cohort and other studies is now available (Pope et al., 2004, 2009).

The effects of long-term exposure can also be studied with small-scale spatial analysis within cities, taking confounding factors into account. In one such study (Scoggins, Kjellstrom, Fisher, Connor, & Gimson, 2004), a significant increase in mortality attributable to local air pollution was found in a city with relatively low air pollution levels (Auckland, New Zealand).

Asthma, whose prevalence has been increasing in high-income countries for three decades, has a still unresolved relationship to external air pollution. A recent meta-analysis found that traffic exhaust contributed to the development of asthma symptoms in healthy children (Bråbäck & Forsberg, 2009), but other studies have yielded less conclusive results. The apparent increase in the susceptibility of successive modern generations of children to asthma may well derive from changes in human ecology that have altered early-life immunological experience, such as reduced exposure to common childhood infections (due to smaller family sizes), increased allergenic household exposures (e.g., house-dust mites or fungal spores), or modern vaccination regimens.

Epidemiologists have developed a diverse and increasingly sophisticated set of methods for assessing the health impacts of air pollution. Nevertheless, the issue remains bedeviled by difficulties in exposure assessment, the uncertain differentiation of acute and chronic effects, the need to sort out independent and interactive effects between air pollutants that are often highly correlated, and the fact that the profile of air pollution keeps evolving as human activity patterns change. Although many uncertainties remain, there is general agreement that significant health effects occur at pollutant concentrations that were previously considered benign. In the case of small particulates, which can penetrate deeply into the respiratory system, there is no evidence of a threshold exposure below which no effect occurs. This absence of a safe level complicates the development of guidelines and standards, and it explains why WHO (2002) decided to publish a table of exposure-response relationship functions instead of making hard-and-fast recommendations. As a consequence, policy makers are forced to decide what level of health risk is acceptable to determine an appropriate exposure standard.

Traffic and Transport

As cities grow in size, urban transport systems expand and evolve. In particular, private car ownership and travel have increased spectacularly over the past half-century, creating new opportunities and freedoms—and new social and public health problems (Fletcher & McMichael, 1997). Currently, there seems to be no agreed-upon vision of an urban future that is not dominated by privately owned vehicles.

Transportation is one of the key polluters in the process of economic development, urbanization, and industrialization. In traditional subsistence agricultural societies, the community's basic needs could be met within a relatively localized distance. Increases in population size and density mean that specialized resources for the community, such as firewood, must be acquired from increasingly distant sources, which creates transportation needs. Modern economic development has accelerated this process through further specialization of economic tasks and dependence on resources from distant areas. Energy sources, such as coal, have had to be transported from afar to sustain local cottage industries; such was also the case with food items to sustain people in places where little could be grown or gathered for much of the year.

Initially, transportation by waterways was favored, as it required no investment in tracks (roads) for vehicles. During the twentieth century, railways and roadways dominated the transportation industry. Motor cars and trucks with internal combustion engines have subsequently had a significant impact on the "environment" and health. Combustion of petroleum fuel produces a variety of toxic emissions: particulate matter (dust), carbon monoxide, nitrogen oxides, hydrocarbon remnants from the oil, and a variety of complex hydrocarbons (as mentioned in the preceding section).

Today, the automobile has become the dominant source of air pollution in many cities (United Nations Environment Program [UNEP], 2009; World Resources Institute, 1998). Current technical solutions to this problem include making car engines more energy efficient and using pollution control devices, such as catalytic converters. The obvious, more radical solution is to reduce dependence on car traffic by encouraging people to walk and to travel by trains, buses, or bicycles. Such measures, carried out as part of a clean air implementation plan, can significantly reduce automotive air pollution, as shown in certain towns in the United States and Germany (WHO, 1997). The unprecedented action to reduce emissions that took place during the 2008 Beijing Olympics provides a profound example of the potential efficacy of clean-air implementation plans. Pollution control measures included limiting automobile usage, closing heavy industrial facilities, and pausing construction work. Collectively, these strategies resulted in a 54% reduction in particulate matter of 10 µ m or less and subsequently a 46% reduction in outpatient visits for asthma during the period of the Olympics (Li, Wang, Kan, Xu, & Chen, 2010; Zhang, Mauzerall, Zhu, Liang, Ezzati, & Remais, 2010).

In cities in low- and middle-income countries, transportation problems have grown even faster. Whereas in Europe a local transport infrastructure based on railways, trams, and buses was already in place when the car boom emerged in the 1960s, low- and middle-income countries often have negligible transport infrastructure. Hence, with increasing affluence and urbanization, the automobile is seen as the best solution for individual families. As a consequence, cities such as Mexico City experienced a rapidly deteriorating air pollution situation during the 1980s and 1990s (WHO, 1997). However, the recent experience of Mexico City also provides a case study of an effective reduction of car-generated air pollution (Exhibit 10-5).

Since the first oil crisis in the 1970s, the average fuel efficiency of the world's automobiles has increased substantially, largely through major improvements in North American car manufacturing through the mid-1990s that brought these vehicles' efficiencies nearly to European levels. Emissions of air pollutants have also been greatly reduced, partly through combustion modifications and partly through extensive application of end-of-pipe controls, in the form of catalytic converters. Nevertheless, if the number of automobiles in low- and middle-income countries continues to grow as it has in recent years, unacceptable air pollution levels will undoubtedly persist for many decades despite the application of even the best current auto technology.

Fortunately, several near-commercial technologies promise much better efficiency and lower emissions. Electric cars will probably have increasing, but still specialized, applications. However, because of the weight, capacity, cost, and lifetime limitations of batteries, they show no sign of being able to serve the main market. Hybrid cars, which are now becoming increasingly available, combine the best features of both fuel and electric drive systems and can significantly increase efficiency and lower emissions

---

Exhibit 10-5 | **Automobile Air Pollution in Mexico City: Thinking Things Through**

Mexico City has often been cited as having some of the worst urban air pollution conditions in the world, although, from a health perspective, the large Asian coal-burning cities probably create higher risk for their residents. The pollution in Mexico City has been so intense because a large population in an industrializing economy lives within a bowl-shaped valley that experiences frequent meteorological conditions that limit circulation of clean air from outside. (Having nearly 20 million persons living in such an arrangement has been termed a serious "topological error.") The rapidly growing number of automobiles in the city is a major cause not only of the pollution, but also of serious traffic congestion, with consequent negative impacts on economic and social interactions.

In the late 1980s, it was proposed to reduce vehicle pollution in the city by imposing a "day without a car" (*hoy no circula*) program, in which all cars would be prohibited from driving one weekday every week, with the prohibited day depending on the last digit on each car's license plate. The reasoning was that pollution emissions and congestion would be reduced approximately 20% by forcing people to carpool or use public transit more often.

For the first few weeks after the program's introduction, a drop in pollution and congestion was noted. The response of the population over the longer term, however, was different than anticipated. Many thousands of persons purchased second cars with a different license plate number so that they could still drive every day. Of course, once they had a second car, they tended to drive more than they would have with just one vehicle. In addition, many of these second cars were older used cars, which tend to have higher emissions levels. Thus one unintended result of the regulation was to draw older, more polluting cars into Mexico City from other parts of the country.

When proposing new pollution regulations, it is important to consider the full ramifications of the intervention. This issue is particularly critical when dealing with pollution caused by behavior at the individual level, such as use of private vehicles. Economists and other social scientists need to be involved from the start, and household surveys and pretesting are needed to gauge impacts before full implementation is attempted.

To address this issue in Mexico City, a new scheme was implemented in 1996 by the local authorities. Cars were assigned to three broad categories according to age, pollution control technology, and emission levels:

- Cars with model years of 1993 or later, all of which have a three-way catalytic converter, can obtain a verification sticker with a number 0 if they produce less than 100 parts per million (ppm) of total hydrocarbons (HC) and less than 1% carbon monoxide (CO) in their emissions. This sticker means that the cars have "zero" restrictions and can be driven every day.

- Cars without a three-way catalytic converter but with an electronic fuel injection system can obtain a sticker with the number 1 if they emit less than 200 ppm of HC and less than 2% CO, the city standards. These vehicles must comply with the "day without a car" (DWC) constraint.

- If vehicles exceed the city standard but comply with the more lenient federal standard, they receive a sticker with the number 2 and must comply with the DWC as well as with additional restrictions during high-pollution episodes. Cars without catalytic converters and without electronic fuel injection systems can obtain a sticker number 2 only if they comply with the federal limits.

The differential treatment of cars according to such criteria is probably the best approach. Such an approach offers authorities the opportunity to combine this measure with other policy instruments. For instance, the triggering point (ambient ozone levels) for the application of the episode alert can be lowered over time without changing stickers. In 2000, a car with a sticker number 1 was prohibited from being driven in Mexico City on 52 days per year, while a car with a sticker number 2 might have been prohibited 60 to 70 times. In the future, the number of days on which the more-polluting sticker number 2 cars were banned from being driven could be increased considerably by lowering the triggering point, thereby putting increasing pressure on people to move to more modern and less-polluting cars.

Such an approach recognizes the now well-demonstrated fact that most car pollution comes from a small fraction of the cars. Pollution regulations that focus on the few heavy polluters can be more effective and less economically and administratively burdensome than those that apply blanket restrictions to all cars.

---

without the changes in fuel delivery systems required by all-electric vehicles. Even more promising, although not yet commercially available, are cars powered by fuel cells. These vehicles can be extremely efficient and produce only tiny amounts of pollution when powered by clean fuels such as methane or hydrogen. Both hybrid and fuel-cell cars (especially the lat-

ter) would also reduce the emission of carbon dioxide, the main anthropogenic greenhouse gas contributing to climate change (see "Climate Change," later in this chapter).

The motor car-based transport system poses several other health risks, as detailed in a review for Sweden (Kjellstrom, Ferguson, & Taylor, 2009). Most obvious, on a global scale, is the great and increasing burden of disease due to road traffic injuries (Lopez et al., 2006). Much of the additional future health impact of this risk will occur in the currently low- and middle-income countries. Road fatality rates per 1,000 vehicles are approximately 30 times higher in Africa than in Norway, the United Kingdom, and the United States, for example. These differences highlight the injury risks at an early stage of motorization when roads are still undeveloped, pedestrians and drivers have not adjusted to one another's presence, drivers have poor driving skills, and the vehicles are not properly maintained (see Chapter 8). The dramatic public health impact of traffic crash injuries, shown in Table 10-1, has great influence on the health services sector because of the intensive and acute treatments that are required for victims; in this manner, road traffic injuries threaten services for other health problems by consuming excess amounts of scarce resources (WHO, 2004).

Car traffic also creates a major noise hazard. This by-product greatly impairs the quality of life for millions of people living close to busy roads, especially in countries with tropical climates where windows of dwellings are seldom closed. Traffic noise disturbs sleep, impairs communication (of particular importance in schools), and appears to be associated with increased blood pressure and other cardiovascular effects (Kjellstrom et al., 2009).

The proliferation of roads and highways can also disrupt social interactions within communities. Unless town planning attends to the needs of pedestrians, cars and roadways tend to dominate the built-up landscape. In Great Britain, for example, the proportion of primary school children walking to school has fallen over the past two decades from a clear majority to a shrinking minority, as traffic has become more intense and walking along roads less safe.

Another problem with the trend toward more private motor vehicle use for daily transport needs is the reduction in daily natural exercise that follows. This factor, which has been labeled an "obesogenic environment," is contributing to the global epidemic of obesity and associated disease problems (Kjellstrom, van Kerkhoff, Bammer, & McMichael, 2003).

Road building and the resultant large land area covered in tar-seal constitute yet another form of environmental hazard by greatly increasing the storm water runoff during heavy rains. Storm water drains are needed, which inevitably will be contaminated by road dust and other surface contaminants. Often the storm water drains are connected to the community sewerage system, creating sewage overflow during rains.

Industry and Manufacturing

Industrialization brings many benefits in the form of income and jobs, but, unless regulated in some fashion, can lead to significant occupational and public health hazards. The health hazards may be in the form of releases of toxic or potentially toxic material—as in the notorious cases in postwar Japan (Exhibit 10-6). Some industrial facilities carry the risk of large-scale accidental releases of toxic materials. The biggest such release in world history occurred in Bhopal, India, where an explosion at a pesticide manufacturing plant resulted in some 3,000 deaths caused by the chemical methyl-isocyanate and significant health impairment in many tens of thousands of people. The impact of this accident at the facility was exacerbated by the lack of urban zoning controls, with hundreds of households having been built directly adjacent to the plant. There was also inadequate planning for alerting and evacuating the public once the accident had occurred.

Waste Management

Few issues in environmental health have generated as much attention and controversy as the management of hazardous wastes, whether chemical or radioactive. This attention has come about through a strong sense of public outrage about numerous publicized cases in which hazardous materials have been dumped indiscriminately or clandestinely, leaving expensive and dirty waste sites for others to handle. Both industry and governments have been responsible for creating such sites, which, in high-income countries, have become very expensive to clean up. In fact, the U.S. Environmental Protection Agency (EPA) spends 20% to 25% of its entire budget on cleaning up chemically contaminated industrial sites, amounting to many tens of billions of dollars over the decades, with additional costs being incurred by industry itself. The prospects of cleaning up the chemical and radioactive contamination left as remnants of a half-century of Cold War nuclear weapons development and manufacture add significantly to this cost.

Perhaps surprisingly, in spite of the large public concern in high-income nations, as evidenced by the resources devoted to cleanup, the actual health impact of hazardous waste is not significant in most areas. Although there are certainly egregious examples of highly contaminated sites that imposed notable risks on local communities, as a societal health issue hazardous waste lies far behind more mundane forms of air and water pollution. One exception is hazardous waste from the military activities (including weapons manufacture) of the former Soviet Union; this waste

| Exhibit 10-6 | **Minamata and Itai-Itai Disease: Classic Environmental Health Disasters** |

Environmental health disasters have been important triggers for national and international action to prevent environmental pollution. The best-known such disaster may be Minamata disease, which struck the small coastal town of Minamata, Japan, in 1956 (WHO, 1990). Hundreds of people were seriously affected by methylmercury poisoning, and many victims died. This type of poisoning affects the nervous system, producing symptoms that range from slight numbness of the fingers to loss of the ability to talk and walk.

The source of the methylmercury in Minamata was a chemical production factory that used mercury as a catalyst in one of its processes. Surplus mercury was discharged via spill water into a nearby bay, and this mercury accumulated in bottom sediments. Microbes in the sediments converted the mercury to methylmercury, which eventually entered the food chain of fish and caused very high methylmercury levels in the local fish. Minamata had a substantial population of small family fisheries, and these families were the most affected.

The outbreak of the disease developed over several months, and it was initially thought that a new type of infectious disease affecting the nervous system had appeared. It took months of detailed epidemiologic research to conclude that the cause of the disease was associated with the consumption of fish. Further toxicologic and epidemiologic research over many years eventually identified the specific chemical involved. A second outbreak of similar methylmercury poisoning, in Niigata, Japan, intensified the search for a definite cause. In 1968, the Japanese government committee responsible for elucidating the cause finally incriminated methylmercury—12 years after the disease was first reported.

A similar story can be told about Itai-Itai disease, a form of chronic cadmium poisoning that developed in farmers in Toyama, Japan, at about the same time as the first outbreak of Minamata disease (Friberg et al., 1986; WHO, 1992). Painstaking research identified that the consumption of cadmium-contaminated rice and drinking water was the cause. The cadmium, which came from a mining area and a lead/zinc ore concentration plant, had reached the affected community via a river that residents used to irrigate their rice fields. The farming families in the contaminated area had small subsistence farms, providing for all of their needs. Thus, if a family's farm was contaminated, the family members ended up with very high daily cadmium intake. Cadmium is a cumulative poison that eventually damages the kidneys, indirectly leading to bone deformities and fractures because of severe osteomalacia and osteoporosis.

At the time when these two disease outbreaks occurred, Japan was a low-income country trying to recover from the disastrous economic effects of World War II. The living conditions were not dissimilar to those in today's low-income countries undergoing rapid industrialization. Rural populations consumed mainly locally produced food. Healthcare services were basic, and the environmental pollution situation was not closely monitored or managed. Local industry discharged wastes into air, rivers, or sea without much pollution control equipment. A country with similar conditions to erstwhile Japan is China, which also has lead, zinc, and copper mining; rice farming; and high local food content in the diet. Indeed, cadmium-polluted areas have been found in China (Cai, Yue, Shang, & Nordberg, 1995), and environmental epidemiologic studies have discovered exposures and effects similar to the polluted areas of Japan.

is present at such a scale that it significantly affects the health of tens of thousands of persons today. There also seem to be cases in China of widespread contamination of aquifers by chromium and other wastes, for example. Even in these countries, however, environmental health risks are dominated by more traditional water and air pollutants and by occupational hazards. In the United States, for example, it has been estimated that the current approach to hazardous waste cleanup costs more than $100 million per cancer case averted at the majority of waste sites—a huge expense when so much health improvement could be achieved in other areas at much lower cost (Mendelsohn & Olmstead, 2009).

It is interesting to speculate why hazardous wastes attract so much more attention than the actual health risk warrants. Part of their high profile is due to what

has been called the outrage factor—that is, the understandable violation felt because of the inexcusably negligent and sometimes criminal behavior of industries and governments in the past. It is also due to a natural human tendency to treat "waste" with a high degree of suspicion. In reality, people show relatively little apparent concern for exposure to the same chemicals at much higher levels while using household and agricultural chemicals, vehicle fuel, and other toxic solvents. From the perspective of the human body, there are no differences in the ill effects of, for example, benzene molecules from one source or another. Finally, and more important, by its high attention to waste, society may be expressing a type of concern not well captured by formal health risk analyses—namely, the idea that the incremental health gains and other benefits of the activities that produce the waste are no longer worth the incremental risks, even if those risks are relatively small.

Globally, the less exotic forms of waste generated by household garbage, mine tailings, and vegetation cuttings undoubtedly cause the most pervasive health damage year in and year out. Uncollected garbage breeds disease-carrying pests of many sorts, including rats and flies. Leached toxic materials and floods from unmanaged mine tailing ponds create health hazards as well. The spontaneous and purposeful burning of garbage, coal mine tailings, and vegetation cuttings is a major source of health-damaging air pollution worldwide, although it is largely controlled in high-income countries. As discussed in the following section, garbage collection is also a significant source of occupational hazards in low- and middle-income cities.

The related problem of the export of hazardous wastes, from high-income countries to their less-affluent counterparts, is addressed in "The Export of Hazard," later in this chapter.

Microbiological Contamination of Water and Food

Diarrheal disease from contaminated water and food remains one of the world's great public health problems, as discussed earlier in the section on household-related risks. Although this hazard is in a sense generated at the household level, failure to initiate community controls can lead to large-scale outbreaks.

An important example is cholera, whose incidence spread worldwide during the 1990s. The seventh, and largest ever, cholera pandemic was causing cases throughout Asia, the Middle East, Europe (occasionally), Africa (where the disease became endemic for the first time), and Latin America, where it spread widely during the 1990s, affecting more than 1 million people and causing 10,000 deaths. Meanwhile, an apparently new epidemic of cholera was detected in the early 1990s, appearing first in southern India and caused by a new strain (number 0139) of *Vibrio cholerae*. The spread of cholera has been greatly enhanced by the increasing number of slum dwellers in low- and middle-income countries, the speed and distance of modern tourism, and an apparent increase in extreme weather events, such as the massive El Niño–associated floods in Kenya in 1997 that caused epidemics of cholera in two regions of the country. In addition, the aftermaths of earthquakes, such as the one in Haiti in 2010, has lead to local epidemics of cholera because of poor water and sanitation facilities.

In the villages and slums of low- and middle-income countries, poor household water quality and sanitation often lead to food contamination. The widespread and unregulated commercial street-food sector in cities offers additional opportunities for exposure. Food contamination remains a concern even in high-income countries, where food is supplied to most of the population via long agriculture, processing, and distribution chains.

The reported rates of food poisoning have increased in high-income countries during the past two decades. The spread of the potentially lethal toxin-producing *Escherichia coli* in North America and Europe in the mid-1990s appears to have accompanied beef imported from infected cattle in Argentina. As long-distance trade expands, as commercial supply lines lengthen in large cities, and as people more frequently opt for convenience or fast foods, the opportunities for food-borne illness increase.

The intensification of meat production is another hot spot for infectious disease problems, as evidenced by these three examples: the development of mad cow disease in Great Britain and its human counterpart (a variant of Creutzfeldt-Jakob disease); the outbreak of a new strain of influenza in chickens in Hong Kong in 1997; and the surprise appearance in 1999 of the newly named (and often fatal) Nipah virus in intensively produced Malaysian pigs and in several hundred human contacts, many of whom died (Weiss & McMichael, 2004).

Chemical Contamination of Water and Food

Chemical contamination derives from three sources: (1) industrial wastes and emissions and household and agricultural chemicals (Exhibit 10-7); (2) chemicals that form during the storage and handling of food, such as the biotoxin aflatoxin; and (3) natural chemical contaminants.

Several major contamination episodes have occurred in Europe. In 1981, the toxic Spanish oil episode occurred, in which edible vegetable oil was adulterated with industrial oil, causing several hundred deaths and several thousand severe illnesses. In 1985, batches of Austrian and Italian wine were found to be adulterated with alcohol-containing antifreeze, a toxic compound. In both those episodes, the hazardous substances were added surreptitiously, for commercial gain, by persons ignorant of (or indifferent to) the potential risks to public health. In 1999 in Belgium, dioxin-contaminated fats entered the animal feed manufacturing process, leading to the contamination of pigs, poultry, and dairy cattle on 1,500 Belgian farms and to thousands of tons of contaminated food products. The potential for the rapid globalization of such environmental problems in the modern free-trading world became quickly apparent (McMichael, 1999): Countries in the Middle East,

Exhibit 10-7	**Learning from Bitter Experience: The Banning of Methylmercury Fungicides**

The infamous methylmercury poisoning catastrophe in Minamata, Japan, in 1956 highlighted the severe public health problems that could occur after environmental pollution with organic chemicals (WHO, 1990). The same chemical was used in the 1950s and 1960s as a fungicide to prevent fungal growth, which has the potential to impair crop-seed viability and cause mold damage in paper pulp. The use of this fungicide in the paper industry increased the concentrations of mercury in the factories' wastewater, which in turn led to methylmercury contamination of fish. In the late 1960s, Swedish ornithologists had identified both this source and the use of fungicide-treated seeds as a potential cause of infertility in wild birds. A major environmental pollution debate followed, and eventually these fungicides were banned—not only in Sweden, but also in most countries with functioning regulatory systems.

In 1971, Iraq received a large consignment of fungicide-treated wheat seeds from USAID. The shipments arrived when much of rural Iraq was suffering from severe drought, and farming families had little food. The seeds for planting had been dyed red to indicate that they should not be eaten, but the farmers soon found out that washing the seeds in water eliminated the dye. Unfortunately, the fungicide stayed in the seeds. The farmers then used the seeds to make bread, and about 2 months later a major epidemic of serious neurologic diseases began. Eventually 500 people died and approximately 5,000 were hospitalized from eating the tainted seeds.

The Iraqi disaster was the largest known epidemic of this type. Previously some smaller outbreaks had occurred in Africa from the same seed fungicide. After the Iraqi epidemic, a new level of awareness arose about such problems, and the use of this fungicide was subsequently banned in most countries. This intervention represents an example of successful chemical safety management, based on the scare caused by a major epidemic of toxicity.

the Americas, and Southeast and Eastern Asia quickly declared a ban on Belgian food imports. Most recently, in 2008 in China, more than 50,000 children were hospitalized and at least 6 died following the poisoning of infant formula with melamine (Ingelfinger, 2008).

Similar problems can affect the quality of drinking water. The widespread problem with arsenic in local drinking water supplies in various communities around the world, particularly in Bangladesh, Nepal, and West Bengal, India, is illustrative (Exhibit 10-8).

Urbanization

All around the globe, a spectacular shift of human populations into the world's cities is occurring. The urbanized proportion of the world's population has skyrocketed from approximately 5% to more than 50% in the past two centuries and is still rising; it is forecast to reach 70% in 20 years (UN Habitat, 2010). This urban migration reflects, to varying degrees in particular geographic areas, the advent of industrialization, the contraction of rural employment, the flight from food insecurity and other forms of insecurity, and the search for jobs, amenities, or a stimulating environment.

The urban "environment" confers various benefits upon human health and well-being. Notably, it offers better access to education and health, financial, and social services. The urban "environment" is rich with new opportunities. At the same time, big cities are often impersonal and sometimes menacing.

Noise, traffic congestion, and residential crowding are stress inducing. The air quality is poor in many cities around the world.

The mortality impact of heat waves is typically greatest in urban centers, where temperatures tend to be higher than in the leafier suburbs and the surrounding countryside, and where the relief of nighttime cooling is lessened (Hajat et al., 2010). This "heat island" effect arises because of the large heat-retaining structures and treeless asphalt expanses of inner cities and the physical obstruction of cooling breezes. Each population has a middle temperature range to which it is well adapted physiologically, behaviorally, and technically. As temperatures become colder, daily death rates gradually increase. As temperatures rise above that middle comfort zone, daily deaths increase—and they often do so rather abruptly once a certain threshold temperature is exceeded. This threshold is much more evident in some populations than in others, and it appears that the threshold is higher in places with long seasons of hot weather than in cooler places.

Urban populations play a dominant role in the mounting pressures that today jeopardize the sustainability of current human ecology—that is, cities have increasingly large "ecologic footprints" (Rees, 1996). Urbanism undoubtedly brings a wealth of ecological benefits, including economies of scale, shared use of resources, and opportunities for reuse and recycling. At the same time, urban populations depend on the natural resources of ecosystems that, in aggregate, are vastly larger in area than the city itself.

Exhibit 10-8	Arsenic in Groundwater

The concentration of various elements, such as fluorine and arsenic, varies naturally in groundwater supplies around the world. In countries such as Taiwan and Argentina, high levels of arsenic in the drinking water have been recognized as a health hazard since the mid-1900s, causing keratoses, hyperpigmentation, and skin cancer. High levels can also be found in Chile, inner Mongolia, parts of the United States, Hungary, Thailand, and China. More recently, the exposure has assumed epic proportions in Bangladesh and neighboring West Bengal, India, where several million persons in recent decades have been drinking arsenic-contaminated water obtained via tubewells, and where the number already manifesting toxic effects, especially skin lesions, is probably in the hundreds of thousands (Khan et al., 1997).

The prolonged consumption of arsenic causes a succession of toxic effects, which typically appear 5 to 10 years after first exposure. Some evidence suggests that the greatest impacts occur in low-income rural villagers with malnutrition, but this may be coincidental rather than causal. Early manifestations of arsenic poisoning include keratosis and skin pigmentation, followed by dysfunction of kidneys and liver, and, perhaps, peripheral neuropathy. With continued exposure, the arsenicosis progresses to liver failure and may cause gangrene and cancer. It is well established that arsenic in drinking water increases the incidence of cancers of the bladder, skin, lung, and kidney (Smith, Goycoleam, Haque, & Biggs, 1998); indeed, arsenic appears to be the most widespread cancer hazard in drinking water in the world. In Chile, for example, 5% to 10% of all deaths in people older than age 30 have been attributed to arsenic-induced cancers (Smith et al., 1998). A cross-sectional study in Bangladesh has compared the prevalence of diabetes mellitus in persons living in areas with high water arsenic levels and areas without arsenic contamination of drinking water (Rahman, Tondel, Ahmad, & Axelson, 1998). Diabetes prevalence was clearly higher in the exposed population. However, no historical time-trend data on water arsenic concentration were reported for either population.

West Bengal shares with Bangladesh a subterranean geologic continuity with arsenic-rich sediments. Much of the drinking water comes from the several hundred thousand tubewells sunk over the past two decades to provide villagers with safe drinking water, thereby allowing them to avoid the hazard of fecally contaminated surface water. The arsenic problem was first identified in Bangladesh in 1993. It is thought that the aeration of the deep sediment by the many bore holes associated with the tubewells leads to oxidation of the natural arsenopyrite and mobilization of arsenic into water. Many of the tubewells yield water with arsenic concentrations 10 to 50 times higher than the WHO guideline (0.01 mg/L). In the village of Samta (population 4,800), in the Jessore district on the Bangladesh and West Bengal boundary, approximately 90% of the 265 tubewells were found to have arsenic concentrations greater than 0.05 mg/L, and 10% exceeded 0.5 mg/L (Biswas et al., 1998).

Mitigation of this problem can be both complex and costly. Various chemical treatments of the water can remove arsenic by absorption onto activated salts and elements, reverse osmosis, ion exchange, or oxidation. Cheaper physical methods involve sand filtration and clarification. The simplest physical solution, where possible, is to drill the tubewells deeper, in conjunction with rapid field testing that is able to identify arsenic levels in excess of 0.05 mg/L. This approach is being used in parts of Bangladesh and West Bengal. Meanwhile, tubewells with very high contamination should be identified and, as soon as an acceptable alternative is found, closed. The practical solution includes restricting the use of arsenic-contaminated water to washing only and avoiding its use for cooking or drinking.

The highly urbanized Netherlands, for example, consumes resources from a total surface area approximately 20 times larger than itself. The estimated consumption of resources—wood, paper, fibers, and food (including seafood)—by 29 cities of the Baltic Sea region, and the absorption of their wastes, depends on a total area 200 times greater than the combined area of the 29 cities (Folke, Larsson, & Sweitzer, 1996). The scale of these externalities of urbanism is growing, and includes massive contributions to global greenhouse gas accumulation, stratospheric ozone depletion, land degradation, and coastal zone destruction. For instance, the urbanized high-income world, which is home to one-fifth of the world's population, currently contributes three-fourths of all greenhouse gas emissions (Intergovernmental Panel on Climate Change, 2001).

Regional Exposures: Transboundary Problems

As the scale of human economic activity has increased, environmental problems have increasingly spilled over beyond local community boundaries. Regional watersheds may become contaminated from multiple sources; radioactive wastes and emissions spread regionally; land-use practices affect infectious disease patterns; and the industrial emissions of sulfur and nitrogen oxides acidify the regional atmosphere. Via these larger-scale pathways, environmental changes can adversely affect human health.

Atmospheric Dispersion of Contaminants

Following the surge of industrial growth in high-income countries in the third quarter of the twentieth century, the transboundary problem of acid deposition (commonly referred to as "acid rain") became increasingly problematic. It featured prominently at the 1972 United Nations Conference on the Human Environment in Stockholm. By that time, eastern Canada was experiencing problems from acidic emissions traveling northeast from the United States, and Scandinavia was exposed to emissions from the United Kingdom and highly industrialized areas of West and East Germany. More recently, the strong increase in China's industrial production has subjected Japan to acid deposition from that source. Acid levels are also rising in other parts of Asia as energy use grows across the entire region.

The hazards to human health from this source are neither extreme nor direct. Nevertheless, the acidification of waterways and soils has demonstrably increased the mobilization of various elements—particularly heavy metals and aluminum—enabling them to enter the drinking water and the food chain. Human exposures to these elements have, therefore, increased in several regions.

Another type of regional air pollution was the release of radionuclides from the Chernobyl nuclear power plant disaster in 1986 (WHO, 1996). Much of this radioactive material was deposited within a 125-mile radius of the plant, but significant radionuclide contamination also resulted from dispersal by winds to areas several thousand miles away. Approximately 4 million persons in the most contaminated adjoining areas were significantly exposed to this contamination via the food chain or were otherwise affected by restrictions on the use of their land for farming. A large increase in the incidence of child thyroid cancer was found in the most polluted areas during the decade after the disaster. Farther afield, such as in northern Finland, Sweden, and Norway, health protection measures had major economic impacts. Reindeer farming is the major economic enterprise in these areas, and thousands of reindeer had to be slaughtered and discarded because of high radiation levels in their meat.

The impact of regional climatic variations on human well-being and health has attracted great research interest in recent years. As a consequence of these investigations, there is new understanding about the regional pattern of storms, floods, cyclones, and droughts in response to these quasi-periodic cycles. Indeed, advance warning of interannual variations in rainfall and drought conditions (with their implications for regional food production and outbreaks of certain infectious diseases) is now becoming possible.

An interesting example of a regional impact occurred in the United States, where the El Niño event of the early 1990s was associated, initially, with drought conditions in the Southwest (in the "four corners" region where Arizona, Colorado, Utah, and New Mexico meet). The dry conditions led to a decline in vegetation and in animal populations, including the natural predators of the deer mouse. When heavy rains occurred in 1993, with resultant profuse growth of piñon nuts, an uncontrolled proliferation of the deer mouse population followed. These rodents harbor a virus, transmissible to humans via dried excreta, that causes hantavirus pulmonary disease—first described at that time (Duchin et al., 1994). This disease has subsequently spread to many contiguous states and to western Canada and much of South America.

The El Niño event of 1997–1998 created unusually strong drought conditions in Southeast Asia, which exacerbated the size and duration of forest fires originally lit to clear land. The result, in addition to extensive damage to the forests, was regional air pollution in the form of wood smoke plumes that extended over thousands of miles and could easily be seen by satellites. The forest fires actually raised outdoor particulate levels to several times the acceptable upper limit in a number of large cities in the region for a period of days to weeks, apparently with significant accompanying adverse health effects. Although larger than in previous years, the same phenomenon has been occurring for decades in the region, and is likely to be repeated often unless land-use practices are modified.

Another issue of importance is the development of atmospheric "brown clouds" caused by the confluence of urban air pollution from the numerous cities and major industries in South-East Asia, India, China, and elsewhere in the world (UNEP, 2008). These high-level "clouds" result from ground-level emissions, which also cause outdoor air pollution levels to exceed air quality guidelines in large areas of Asia, even far from cities.

Land Use and Water Engineering

Regional tensions over freshwater supplies are increasing in many locations as population pressures increase and an ever larger proportion of agricultural production comes to depend on irrigation (Grimm et al., 2006). Water is essential for household hygiene, communal sanitation, and economic vitality. The problems in the West Bengal region, where freshwater availability is declining as the hydrologic cycle is perturbed by human interventions and where surface water is widely fecally contaminated, are described in Exhibit 10-8.

During the third quarter of the twentieth century, it became clear that large-scale human interventions in the natural environment—dams, irrigation schemes, land reclamation, road construction, and population resettlement programs—often affected infectious disease patterns. In particular, the composition of vector species generally changes following alterations in environmental conditions. Such large-scale developments in the eastern Mediterranean, Africa, South America, and Asia have been consistently associated with increases in vector-borne diseases, especially schistosomiasis and filariasis. In the Sudan in the 1970s, for example, schistosomiasis appeared soon after the start of the Gezira scheme, a large irrigated cotton project; the prevalence of malaria also increased markedly in this region (Fenwick, Cheesmond, & Amin, 1981; Gruenbaum, 1983). In Africa, the building of large dams in the Sudan, Egypt (the Aswan High Dam), Ghana, and Senegal caused the prevalence of schistosomiasis in the surrounding populace to increase from very low levels to more than 90% (WHO, 1997).

An example of a disastrous land-use decision, with major regional environmental health consequences, is the fate of the Aral Sea in Central Asia. This inland sea depends on the inflow of water from two major rivers. Until about 1960, the sea level was constant, and large populations in the countries surrounding the Aral Sea sustained their economies through fishing and agriculture. In the 1950s, however, large-scale cotton farming was developed along the two major rivers, with these operations relying on irrigation water diverted from those rivers. The farms also used large amounts of pesticides, which contaminated the water and the soil. Perhaps not surprisingly, signs of environmental damage began emerging in the 1960s. The level of the Aral Sea sank, the irrigated farm soils became salinated, and soil erosion by wind became an increasing problem. Since then the Aral Sea has continued to shrink, the fishing industry has collapsed, and agriculture has been increasingly impaired. Adverse health impacts in the regional population of 30 million persons have been reported—although not yet satisfactorily confirmed—apparently in association with direct toxic pesticide exposures and with the socioeconomic decline caused by the environmental disaster.

Deforestation has had variable effects on malaria mosquito vectors. In some parts of Southeast Asia, deforestation has enabled malaria-transmitting *Anopheles punctulatus* species to become established. In contrast, several *Anopheles* species, including *A. dirus* in Thailand and *A. darlingi* in South America, have disappeared following deforestation that removed the flora and fauna upon which they depended for feeding.

Forest clearance in South America during recent decades to extend agricultural land has also mobilized various viral hemorrhagic fevers that previously circulated quietly in wild animal hosts. For example, the Junin virus, which causes Argentine hemorrhagic fever, naturally infects wild rodents. In recent decades, extensive conversion of grassland to maize cultivation stimulated a proliferation of the reservoir rodent species, which in turn exposed human farmworkers to this "new" virus. In the past 35 years, the land area where this new human disease is endemic has expanded many-fold, with several hundred infected cases occurring annually, as many as one-third of whom die (Chomel, Belotto, & Meslin, 2007).

Because changes in land-use patterns are typically accompanied by changes in population density, population mobility, pesticide usage, and regional climate, it is difficult to state with authority any specific causal explanations. Indeed, many of the health outcomes result from interactions between these various change processes.

Global Environmental Change and Population Health

A major consequence of the increasing scale of the human enterprise is the potentially important health impact of global environmental changes. Humankind is now disrupting some of the biosphere's life-support systems—the natural processes of stabilization, production, cleansing, and recycling that our predecessors were able to take for granted in a less human-dominated world (Daily, 1997; McMichael, 1993; McMichael, Woodruff, & Hales, 2006). We no longer live in such a world. The composition of both the lower and middle atmospheres is changing. There is a net loss of productive soils on all continents, most ocean fisheries have been overfished, aquifers on which irrigated agriculture depends have been depleted, and whole species and many local populations are being extinguished at unprecedented speed. These large-scale environmental changes pose long-term, and unfamiliar, risks to human population health.

Climate Change

The United Nations' Intergovernmental Panel on Climate Change (IPCC, 2007) concluded that there is most likely a significant human influence on global climate. Further, trends in greenhouse gas emissions will, in the IPCC's estimation, cause an increase in average world temperature of approximately 1.8°C to

| Exhibit 10-9 | **Modeling the Future Impacts of Climate Change on Malaria Transmissibility** |

Mosquitoes—the vector organisms for malaria—are very sensitive to temperature and humidity. Further, patterns of rainfall, river flow, and surface water affect their opportunity to breed. Given these facts, scientists anticipate that a change in world climatic conditions during the twenty-first century will affect the pattern of potential transmission of malaria.

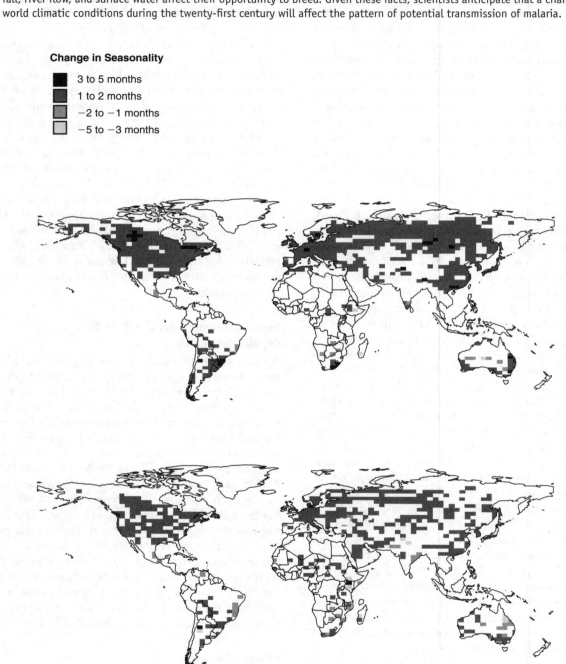

Change in Seasonality

- 3 to 5 months
- 1 to 2 months
- −2 to −1 months
- −5 to −3 months

Figure 10-9 Future Changes in Seasonality of Potential Transmission of Malaria, 2080s versus Present. (A) Change in number of transmissions per year under a future scenario of unconstrained emissions of carbon dioxide. (B) Change in number of months of potential transmission per year, under a future scenario of constrained emissions of carbon dioxide (such that atmospheric concentration stabilizes at 550 parts per million). *Source:* P. Martens et al., "Climate Change and Future Populations at Risk of Malaria," 1999, *Global Environmental Change, 9,* pp. S89–S107. Adapted with permission of Elsevier Science.

continued

| **Exhibit 10-9** | *continued* |

Both temperature and humidity affect the growth, biting rate, reproductive cycle, and longevity of the mosquito. Mosquitoes are most comfortable in a temperature range from 20°C to 30°C and at approximately 60% humidity. The malarial parasite, a single-celled sexually reproducing plasmodium, is also affected by temperature during the extrinsic phase of its complex life cycle, when sporozoites are forming within the mosquito. The two major species of plasmodia have minimum temperature requirements: For Plasmodium vivax, a minimum of 16°C is required; for the potentially fatal Plasmodium falciparum, a temperature of approximately 18°C is required. Within the previously mentioned comfort range, the higher the temperature, the more rapid the incubation—and hence the sooner the opportunity for transmission to another mosquito-bitten human.

From studies done during the 1980s and 1990s, it is clear that malaria outbreaks are closely related to inter-annual climatic variations in many countries. In Venezuela, for example, the incidence of malaria consistently surged upward throughout the twentieth century in the year following an El Niño event. This outcome was most probably due to the combination of above-average rainfall in the post–El Niño year and the drop in acquired immunity in the population because of the low malaria incidence during the dry El Niño year. Studies in India, Pakistan, and Sri Lanka all reveal similarly strong associations between malaria outbreaks and El Niño events and the associated monsoonal changes. A correspondingly strong correlation with interannual variations in temperature and rainfall has been reported for outbreaks of dengue fever (a mosquito-borne infectious disease) in Pacific island populations (Hales, Weinstein, Souares, & Woodward, 1999).

The science of forecasting climatic fluctuations three to six months in advance is steadily improving. Indeed, there is considerable economic incentive to improve the forecasting of El Niño and La Niña events, as both have global repercussions on regional agricultural yields. With sufficient advance warning, farmers can switch to more appropriate crops. The equivalent approach will soon be possible for forecasting of malaria outbreaks, thereby enabling public health interventions to be implemented prior to their occurrence (e.g., activated population-based surveillance, surface water control, insecticide-impregnated bed nets, and antimalarial prophylaxis).

Longer-term global and local forecasts are being facilitated by the collection of information about how malaria has responded to the generalized warming that has occurred since the 1970s. Forecasts on this decadal scale are relevant for inclusion in the estimation of aggregate burden of adverse health impacts that could accrue if climate change were to occur as predicted. Mathematical models are required for this type of long-range forecasting of changes in the potential transmission of malaria. Such a model integrates, for units of time (typically months) and units of surface area (e.g., 100 square kilometers), the estimated future climatic conditions (as a function of continuing excess emissions of greenhouse gases) and characteristics of the mosquito and parasite "system" and of the human population (e.g., size, age distribution, prior immunity).

Because other determinants of malaria occurrence will also inevitably change over coming decades (e.g., vaccine efficacy, human demography, land-use patterns, or parasite resistance to drugs), the modeling of climate change impacts typically indicates only changes in potential transmission (see Figure 10-9). Nevertheless, this is an important consideration in the formulation of long-term priorities and policies. In the future, more comprehensive modeling will be able to take the other salient covariables into account.

4°C over the coming century. Rainfall patterns will also likely change, as will the variability of weather patterns. All of these changes are expected to vary considerably by region (Exhibit 10-9). The health effects of climate change would encompass direct and indirect effects, as well as immediate and delayed effects (McMichael et al., 2003). Although some health outcomes in some populations would be beneficial— some tropical regions may become too hot for mosquitoes, for example, and winter cold snaps would become milder in temperate-zone countries where death rates typically peak in wintertime—most of the anticipated health effects would be adverse (Costello et al., 2009; IPCC, 2001; McMichael et al., 2003).

Direct health effects from climate change might include changes in mortality and morbidity from an altered pattern of exposure to thermal extremes, the respiratory health consequences of increased exposures to photochemical pollutants and aeroallergens, the physical hazards of the increased occurrence of storms, floods, or droughts, in at least some regions, as well as the increased direct heat exposure on people working in situations without cooling systems (Kjellstrom, 2009b). Intensified rainfall, with flooding, can overwhelm urban wastewater and sewer systems, leading to contamination of drinking water supplies. This outcome is most likely in large crowded cities where infrastructure is old or inadequate, as illustrated by an outbreak of typhoid in Tajikistan in 1994, when the city wastewater system flooded during unusual torrential rains.

Indirect health effects are likely to have a greater aggregate impact over time. They may include alterations in the range and activity of vector-borne infectious diseases (e.g., malaria, dengue fever, and leishmaniasis). These diseases are spread by vectors (e.g., mosquitoes) that are very sensitive to climatic conditions, as is the parasite's development while incubating in the vector. Scenario-based mathematical modeling has suggested that the geographic zone and seasonality of potential transmission of malaria or dengue fever will increase in many parts of the world in the coming century (IPCC, 2001; McMichael et al., 2003). In temperate Europe and North America, climate-sensitive, vector-borne infections include tick-borne encephalitis and Lyme disease. Other indirect effects may include altered transmission of person-to-person infections (especially summertime food-borne and waterborne pathogens). Of great potential importance to population health would be the adverse nutritional consequences of the likely regional declines in agricultural productivity (McMichael et al., 2007), which are forecast to reach 10% to 20% by the latter half of the twenty-first century in many already food-insecure populations in low-latitude regions. Livestock production, particularly of ruminant, digastrics, animals (sheep, cattle, buffalo, goats and others) also contributes substantial emissions of the potent green-house gas, methane, that adds significantly to the ongoing climate change (Friel et al., 2008; McMichael et al., 2007). Finally, climate change would inevitably result in adverse physical and psychological health consequences from population displacement and economic disruption due to rising sea levels (e.g., small island states, coastal Bangladesh, and the Nile Delta), declines in agroecosystems, and freshwater shortages.

Most of these negative health impacts, and heat induced reductions of the work capacity of working people (Kjellstrom, 2009b), are expected to have their greatest effects in low-income populations (Friel et al., 2008; Patz et al., 2007; Smith & Ezzati, 2005). Conversely, positive features of mitigation actions to reduce global climate change include the "co-benefits" for health (beyond the benefits related to the reduced climate change) that such actions will have (Haines et al., 2009; Smith & Haigler, 2008).

Stratospheric Ozone Depletion

Stratospheric ozone depletion is essentially a separate phenomenon from greenhouse gas accumulation in the troposphere. Ozone depletion is causing an increase in ultraviolet irradiation at Earth's surface. This increase in ultraviolet exposure is expected to peak sometime within the next two decades and then decline slowly over several decades, in response to the phasing out of the major ozone-destroying industrial and agricultural chemicals. For the first half of this century, increases are expected in the severity of sunburn and in the incidence of skin cancers in fair-skinned populations and of various disorders of the eye (especially cataracts). Some UVR-induced suppression of immune functioning may also occur, thereby increasing susceptibility to infectious diseases and perhaps reducing vaccination efficacy (UNEP, 1998; WHO, 1994).

Persistence of the ozone losses of the 1979–1992 period for several decades would cause the annual incidence of basal cell carcinoma (the dominant skin cancer type) to increase by an estimated 1% to 2% at low latitudes (5°), by 14% at 55° to 65° latitudes in the northern hemisphere (e.g., the United Kingdom), and by 25% at that latitude in the south (Madronich & de Gruijl, 1993). The estimated percentage increases in incidence of squamous cell carcinoma would be twice as great. More sophisticated mathematical modeling indicates that nonmelanoma skin cancer rates will rise to a peak excess incidence of approximately 10% in the United States and Europe around the middle of the twenty-first century (Slaper, Velders, Daniel, de Gruijl, & van der Leun, 1996).

A potentially more important—albeit much more indirect—health detriment could arise from ultraviolet-induced impairment of photosynthesis on land (terrestrial plants) and at sea (phytoplankton). Although such an effect could reduce the world's food production, few quantitative data are available for use in forecasting the magnitude and implications of this decline.

Biodiversity: Losses and Invasions

Through humankind's spectacular reproductive and technological success, the natural habitats of many other species have been occupied, damaged, or eliminated. Biologists have estimated that this fastest mass extinction might cause approximately one-third of all species alive in the 1800s to disappear before the end of the twenty-first century (Pimm, Russell, Gittleman, & Brooks, 1995). "A more recent analysis agrees with this rate of extinctions (UNEP, 2004) and states that a major reason for current extinctions is habitat loss due to human activities."

The loss of various key species would weaken whole ecosystems, with consequences that would often be adverse to human interests, such as disturbing the ecology of vector-borne infections and food-producing systems that depend on pollinators and the predation of pests, and impairing the cleansing of water and the circulation of nutrients that normally pass through ecosystems. A rich repertoire of genetic and phenotypic material would also be lost. To maintain the hybrid vigor and environmental resilience of food species, a diversity of wild species needs to be preserved as a source of genetic additives (Chivian & Bernstein, 2008). Similarly, many modern medicinal drugs in Western medicine have natural origins, and many defy synthesis in the laboratory. Scientists test thousands of novel natural chemicals each year, seeking new drugs to treat HIV, malaria, drug-resistant tuberculosis, and cancers.

The opposite side of this coin is the accelerating spread of invasive species, as long-distance trade, tourism, and migration increase in intensity. Several examples with public health consequences are given in the section "Environmental Hazards Resulting from Forms of Globalization" later in this chapter, but many others can be cited as well. For example, the vast proliferation of water hyacinth (a decorative plant from Brazil) in Lake Victoria, eastern Africa, has extended the breeding grounds for the water snail that transmits schistosomiasis. The planting of *Lantana camerata* as a garden border shrub in Uganda, and its subsequent dispersed spread, has increased the habitat for the tsetse fly, which transmits the trypanosome that causes African sleeping sickness.

Land Degradation, Food, and Malnutrition

The increase in land degradation has implications for food supplies and, therefore, for nutrition, child development, and health. During the 1980s, the combination of erosion, desiccation, and nutrient exhaustion, plus irrigation-induced water-logging and salinization, rendered unproductive one-fifteenth of the world's 1.5 billion hectares of readily arable farmland (World Resources Institute, 1998). The Green Revolution, which fed much of the expanding human population from the 1960s to the 1980s, depended on laboratory-bred, high-yield cereal grains, fertilizers, groundwater, and arable soils. In retrospect, those productivity gains appear to have come substantially from using up exhaustible ecological capital—especially topsoil and groundwater. Even as greater food yields to feed ever-more people are pursued, almost one-tenth of the world's population remains malnourished in ways that impair health. Meanwhile, at sea, many of the world's great fisheries are now on the brink of being overexploited. The Food and Agriculture Organization (FAO) of the United Nations estimates that the sustainable fish-catch limit has been neared—approximately 100 million tonnes per year (FAO, 2002).

Persistent Organic Pollutants

Various chemical pollutants, particularly the many chlorinated organic chemicals such as the polychlorinated biphenyls (PCBs), have a tendency to persist in the environment and have become globally pervasive. These substances are referred to as persistent organic pollutants (POPs) (Watson, Dixon, & Hamburg, 1998). The semivolatile members of this class of chemicals undergo a type of serial distillation process in the atmosphere as they pass from low to high latitudes, ultimately aggregating in higher concentrations in the circumpolar regions. Some of these chemicals are likely to affect neurologic, immune, and reproductive systems in humans, who feed at the top of the increasingly contaminated food chain. Weakening of ecosystems may also occur, with various additive environmental health effects in human populations (Colborn, Vom Saal, & Soto, 1993).

Pathways to the Future in an Unequal World

Sometimes low- and middle-income countries are criticized for not imposing stricter environmental and occupational standards. Too often, there are indeed situations where minimal efforts could achieve great reductions in health risks. In addition, given the likely increase in public willingness to pay for stricter standards as development continues, the early imposition of reasonable standards can often be quite cost-effective using standard economic criteria.

Despite their shortcomings, most large low- and middle-income countries today have standards that are much stricter than those found in the high-income countries when they were at the corresponding level of development. Indeed, although there are cases of the export of environmental hazard and the degradation of local environments by exploitative and destructive commercial practice (see "The Export of Hazard," later in this chapter), the overall impact of globalization may be a net export of environmental health. That is, through education, political and public pressures, technology transfer, trade agreements, and other initiatives, low- and middle-income countries have, on average, better environmental quality than would otherwise be the case.

Setting Standards: Too Safe Can Be Unsafe

Setting and enforcing environmental standards for protection of the public and workers is a difficult exercise, even in high-income countries with substantial resources. In low- and middle-income countries, which face a number of critical needs with few resources, the process is even more troublesome. Although official rhetoric about setting standards often states that the only concern is protection of health, in reality there are always economic and other trade-offs involved. It is too expensive and there are too many other demands on resources to bring every pollutant under the maximum control quickly. Politically, however, it is often difficult for governments in low- and middle-income nations to set standards that are significantly less stringent than those in high-income countries. As a result, sometimes standards are unrealistically strict and cannot be met. This disparity between the standards and the reality leads to graft, cynicism, apathy, and, too often, levels of exposures and ill health above what could be achieved by adopting more realistic approaches.

One way out of this dilemma is to emphasize environmental health protection and standard setting as dynamic and evolutionary processes rather than as static one-time-forever efforts. For example, a country might set 20-year goals for its standards that are as strict as any in the world, while establishing interim objectives that become progressively more strict. Thus pollutants and industries that pose the most risk can be emphasized first, while control over other pollutants and industries (of the kind that now attract attention in high-income countries) can be postponed until a later period. No hazard is ignored, but merely put into a rational order of priority. Industrial interests are likely to be more willing to accept stricter standards under such a scheme because they tend to have shorter-term financial goals, facilitated by clarity of the regulatory environment, whereas they are unsettled by longer-term uncertainty. A recurring problem, however, is attaining sufficient stability within governments to implement such a long-term approach.

The Export of Hazard

In recent years, concern has risen about the potential export of environmental hazard that may be occurring as part of the globalization of the world economy (LaDou, 1992; Leichenko & O'Brien, 2008). Because environmental and occupational standards and enforcement tend to be less strict in low- and middle-income countries, one might expect that polluting activities would tend to migrate to those countries, thereby imposing excess risk on workers and public.

To date, however, studies of international industrial trends have identified few cases where differences in environmental and occupational standards have been the critical determinants of such shifts, compared with labor costs, tax regimes, and other business factors. Indeed, locally owned industries tend to have higher emissions and occupational hazards than do facilities owned by multinational corporations, which often feel considerable pressure to maintain higher standards. Besides, the mere fact of a difference in standards does not necessarily mean that an injustice exists. As noted earlier, nations at different stages of development may quite rationally choose different tradeoffs between standards, job creation, and infrastructure development. The most outrageous examples of injustice arise where decisions about such tradeoffs are made by a small oligarchy without considering the needs and wishes of the population as a whole. In these cases, perhaps the only way to protect the interests of those in the low- and middle-income countries would be to establish international norms.

Flagrant examples of the problems created by the exporting of hazard exist along borders between high-income and low- and middle-income countries. On the Mexican side of the long U.S.–Mexican border, for example, one can find many highly polluting industries with poor occupational safety and health conditions relative to standards on the U.S. side of the border (Moure-Eraso et al., 2007). Because of the proximity, both the pollution and health problems tend to cross the border, frustrating attempts by U.S. border communities to maintain acceptable conditions. Attempts to impose U.S. standards on Mexican facilities understandably create friction. There have been some encouraging successes in joint efforts by neighboring Mexican–U.S. communities to address these issues in a way that takes into account the need for jobs and for clean working and living conditions on both sides.

The political and moral dilemmas are manifest. Today's high-income world followed a path to development and wealth that put economic gains ahead of human welfare and environmental conservation for most of the nineteenth century. Today's low- and middle-income countries are dissuaded, if not formally barred, from following the equivalent pathway because (1) their populations have access to more information and hence have higher expectations; (2) the high-income world has a moral obligation to assist them via the transfer of knowledge, wealth, and technology; (3) it is now clear that the integrity of the biosphere at large is jeopardized by the prospect of huge populations in these countries accruing wealth via environmentally damaging behaviors; and (4) there is pressure from public opinion in industrialized countries to achieve higher standards.

Environmental Hazards Resulting from Forms of Globalization

A dominant trend in the global economic "environment" over the past 50 years has been the rapid growth in international trade in goods, services, and human resources. The globalizing processes of the past quarter century have transformed patterns of connectedness around the world and have created new power relations among countries, international and national governance, and the public and private sectors (see Chapter 18).

In traditional agrarian-based societies that produce, consume, and trade on a local basis and with relatively low-impact technologies, the effects of those activities on the "environment" are predominantly local. Few such societies remain today, in the face of the strong and pervasive economic, technologic, and cultural influences now spanning the globe. The industrialization of the past century and the more recent globalizing processes have altered the scale of contact between societies, intensified environmental impacts, and extended the public health impacts of one society on another. In the name of economic development and free markets, low- and middle-income countries have come under pressure to grant unrestricted access to their resources, workforces, and consumer markets. This process has been associated with increasing poverty in many parts of the world, widening inequalities between and within countries, expanding pressures to reduce the power of the state, and subordinating national programs of social welfare and environmental protection to the agenda of economic growth.

Following the international debt crisis of the early 1980s, many struggling low- and middle-income countries were obliged to accept the economic stringencies mandated by the World Bank's structural adjustment program. These dictates included a reduction in spending on health throughout the 1980s and into the 1990s. Some evidence suggests that these policies adversely affected the public health capacity of those countries, with some serious health implications (Hoogvelt, 1997). In many countries, they engendered a diminished capacity to respond to the resurgence of tuberculosis, maintain environmental controls on vector-borne infectious diseases, and provide basic primary family health care. In its current

form, the world's globalizing economy operates to the general disadvantage of low- and middle-income countries. The exacerbation of land degradation, rural unemployment, food shortages, and urban crowding all contribute to health deficits for the rural dispossessed, the underfed, and the slum dweller. The health and safety conditions of working people can create particular threats to occupational health (Kjellstrom & Hogstedt, 2009).

Many features of today's globalizing world contribute to the spread of infectious diseases (Weiss & McMichael, 2004; Wilson, 1995). Human mobility has escalated dramatically, in volume and speed, between and within countries. Long-distance trade facilitates the geographic redistribution of pests and pathogens—a phenomenon well illustrated in recent years by the HIV pandemic, the worldwide dispersal of rat-borne hantaviruses, and the rapid dissemination of a new epidemic strain of bacterial meningitis along routes of travel and trade. Likewise, transport on ships has facilitated the introduction of the Asian tiger mosquito, *Aedes albopictus*—a vector for yellow fever and dengue—into South America, North America, and Africa (Morse, 1995) and of the cholera bacterium into South American coastal waters (Colwell, 1996). In an analysis of cholera outbreaks since 1817, Lee and Dodgson (2000) argue that the current (seventh) pandemic is clearly different from earlier ones, reflecting the unprecedented scale of social and environmental change in the world over recent years, the exacerbation of urban poverty, and the rapidity and intensity of intercontinental contacts.

One aspect of globalization that may have negative effects on both the "environment" and health is the harmonization of trade-related rules and legislation via the World Trade Organization (WTO). Particular attention has been paid to nontariff trade barriers, which include any national regulation or legislation that hinders trade and is not a financial levy on the trade itself. For instance, if country A legislates that the maximum level of mercury in fish sold in that country should be 0.5 mg/kg, another country B cannot sell fish with a higher mercury level to country A. If in country B, fish with levels up to 1 mg/kg can be freely sold, then country B can claim that the fish-mercury regulation of country A is a nontariff trade barrier. However, country A may have conducted a health risk assessment based on the local fish consumption patterns and decided that 0.5 mg/kg is the maximum acceptable. How should this conflict be resolved? Current WTO practice means that only internationally agreed health guidelines can be implemented in this situation. If no such guidelines exist, then country A is not allowed to have a stricter environmental health rule than country B unless country A can convince the WTO disputes committee that the trade restriction has been implemented for good reasons.

Similar situations may develop with the banning of hazardous products such as asbestos. If, for example, there is no international health guideline banning the use of asbestos, then any country taking a unilateral decision to ban asbestos use would risk trade sanctions from other countries wanting to export asbestos. If the trend in international environmental and occupational health guidelines went toward stricter prevention, this harmonization via trade rules could be good for health and the "environment." In reality, the intense lobbying from those commercial groups and countries that would benefit from lax rules makes it likely that the opposite will happen—meaning that compromises veering toward less protection will be made (LaDou, 1992).

Population Health: Index of Social and Environmental Sustainability

Current models of government reflect the compartmentalization of knowledge and policy that grew out of the classic development of scientific disciplines in the nineteenth century. To deal with a multifaceted world, our predecessors defined various sectors of knowledge, policy, and social action: environment, industry, agriculture, transport, health, social welfare, and education. Subsequently, one of the great lessons to emerge from twentieth-century science, with its origins in the realm of physics (the 1920s debate about quantum mechanics and uncertainty), was that the complexities of the real world require us to think in more integrative ways, across disciplines and topics, elevating holism (or ecological thinking) above mechanistic, reductionist thinking.

It is within this type of integrative framework that population health can be understood as part of the total social experience, a manifestation of how well the social and natural environments are being managed. Population health should be a primary criterion for all social policy making, but particularly in relation to the goal of achieving the "sustainability transition." Health is not just a type of sideshow in the policy arena, but rather is affected by the social, environmental, and (in the longer term) ecological consequences of policies in all sectors. For all these reasons, population health should be an integrating index of social policy across all sectors.

Conclusions

The perceived importance of environmental exposures as health hazards—at local, regional, and global levels—has increased steadily over the past several decades. Currently, scientists estimate that one-fourth to one-third of the global burden of disease and premature death is attributable to ambient (including household) environmental risk factors.

In high-income countries during much of the past four decades, the generally greater ease of measurement of specific exposures relating to individual lifestyle (eating, smoking, and sexual behaviors) and the workplace, compared with the more diffuse lower-concentration exposures in the external environment, resulted in the latter topic area attracting less attention and having lower credibility. More recently, improvements in exposure assessment, the harnessing of time-series analyses, the advent of spatial analytic techniques, the recognition of the legitimacy of population-level analyses, and the extra leverage afforded by molecular biological indices of exposure, susceptibility, and biological damage have all helped reveal the range and extent of ambient environmental risks to health.

Meanwhile, in low- and middle-income countries, the age-old scourges of diarrheal disease, acute respiratory infections, tuberculosis, and vector-borne infections have remained the dominant health problems. The ascendancy of specific health system interventions for those problems—sanitation, household hygiene, vaccination, pesticides, and drug treatment—has led to their wider ecological dimensions being somewhat overlooked. Many problems of environmental contamination have their origins in poverty; deficient regulation of mining, industry, and agriculture; and mismanagement of surface water and groundwater supplies. Differences in household exposure to indoor air pollution reflect the traditional division of labor (women are mostly exposed), the ongoing use of low-grade technology, and the persistence of the biomass fuels of poverty. Infectious diseases are often spread by environmental encroachments—land clearing, water damming, irrigation, and expanded trade.

The environmental health agenda is becoming ever broader. Today the burden of the growing human population and its aggregate consumption and waste generation is beginning to overload various aspects of the planet's great natural systems. The resultant global environmental changes, signifying that the biosphere's human population carrying capacity is being exceeded, pose further risks to human health. Therefore, even as environmental health scientists strive to improve their research methods for characterizing the health risks associated with local physical, chemical, and microbiological hazards, they must also extend their ideas and methods to encompass larger-scale environmental hazards and the health consequences of disrupted ecosystems. Policy makers, in many sectors, must understand the tendency of human-wrought changes in the social, built, and natural environments to affect health—if not immediately, then in the longer term, and sometimes via pathways with which we yet have little familiarity.

● ● ● **Discussion Questions**

1. What should be the scope of the term "environment"?

2. Which methodological problems are particularly characteristic of environmental epidemiology?

3. How can the differences be explained in the profile of environmental health problems between high-income countries and low- and middle-income countries? Are these differences a function of history, demography, wealth, knowledge, or something else?

4. What are the characteristics of particular environmental health problems that render them more, or less, tractable to amelioration or elimination?

5. As the scale of human impact on the global "environment" increases, people become more concerned about the consequences of disruption of our "habitat." What does this signify?

• • • References

Armstrong, J., & Menon, R. (1998). Mining and quarrying. In J. M. Stellman (Ed.), *Encyclopaedia of occupational health and safety* (4th ed., Vol. III). Geneva, Switzerland: International Labor Office.

Baker, D. & Nieuwenhuijsen, M. J. (2008). Environmental epidemiology. Study methods and application. Oxford: Oxford University Press.

Biswas, B. K., Dhar, R. K., Samanta, G., Mandal, B. K., Chakraborti, D., Faruk, I., et al. (1998). Detailed study report of Samta, one of the arsenic-affected villages of Jessore District, Bangladesh. *Current Science, 74*, 134–145.

Bobak, M., & Leon, D. A. (1992). Air pollution and infant mortality in the Czech Republic, 1986–1988. *Lancet, 340*, 1010–1014.

Bonita, R., Beaglehole, R. & Kjellstrom, T. (2007). Basic epidemiology (2nd ed.). Geneva: World Health Organization.

Bråbäck, L., & Forsberg, B. (2009). Does traffic exhaust contribute to the development of asthma and allergic sensitization in children: Findings from recent cohort studies. *Environmental Health, 8*(1), 17.

Cai, S., Yue, L., Shang, Q., & Nordberg, G. (1995). Cadmium exposure among residents in an area contaminated by irrigation water in China. *Bulletin of the World Health Organization, 73*, 359–367.

Cairncross, S., Hunt, C., Boisson, S., Bostoen, K., Curtis, V., Fung, I., et al. (2010). Water, sanitation and hygiene for the prevention of diarrhoea. *International Journal of Epidemiology, 39*, i193–i205.

Chivian, E. & Bernstein, A. (2008). Sustaining life. Oxford: Oxford University Press.

Chomel, B. B., Belotto, A. & Meslin, F.-X. (2007). Wildlife, exotic pets and emerging zoonoses. *Emerging Infectious Diseases, 13*, 6–11.

Chowdhury, Z., Zheng, M., & Russel, A. (2004). *Source apportionment and characterization of ambient fine particles in Delhi, Mumbai, Kolkata, and Chandigarh*. Washington, DC: World Bank.

Cohen, A. J., Anderson, H. R., Ostro, B., Pandey, K. D., Krzyzanowski, M., Kuenzli, N., et al. (2004). Mortality impacts of urban air pollution. In M. Ezzati, A. D. Rodgers, A. D. Lopez, & C. J. L. Murray (Eds.), *Comparative quantification of health risks: Global and regional burden of disease due to selected major risk factors* (Vol. 2, Chapter 17, pp. 1353–1434). Geneva, Switzerland: World Health Organization.

Colborn, T., Vom Saal, F., & Soto, A. (1993). Developmental effects of endocrine-disrupting chemicals in wildlife and humans. *Environmental Health Perspectives, 101*, 378–384.

Colwell, R. (1996). Global climate and infectious disease: The cholera paradigm. *Science, 274*, 2025–2031.

Confalonieri, U., Menne, B., Akhtar, R., Ebi, K.L., Hauengue, M., Kovats, R.S., et al. (2007). Human health. In Intergovernmental Panel on Climate Change, *Climate change 2007: Impacts, adaptation and vulnerability. Contribution of Working Group II to the Fourth Assessment Report of the Intergovernmental Panel on Climate Change* (pp. 391–431). Cambridge, UK: Cambridge University Press.

Corvalan, C., Briggs, D., & Kjellstrom, T. (1996). Development of environmental health indicators. In D. Briggs, C. Corvalan, & M. Nurminen (Eds.), *Linkage methods for environment and health analysis* (Document WHO/EHG/95.26). Geneva, Switzerland: World Health Organization.

Costello, A., Abbas, M., Allen, A., Ball, S., Bell, S., Bellamy, R., et al. (2009) (Lancet-University College London Institute for Global Health Commission). Managing the health effects of climate change. *Lancet, 373*, 1693–733.

Crain, D. A., Janssen, S. J., Edwards, T. M., Heindel, J., Ho, S. M., Hunt, P., et al. (2008). Female reproductive disorders: The roles of endocrine-disrupting compounds and developmental timing. *Fertility and Sterility, 90*(4), 911–940.

Daily, G. C. (Ed.). (1997). *Nature's services*. Washington, DC: Island Press.

Deishmann, W., & Henschler, D. (1986). What is there that is not poison? A study of the *Third Defense* by Paracelsus. *Archives of Toxicology, 58*(4), 207–213.

Diamanti-Kandarakis, E., Bourguignon, J. P., Guidice, L. C., Hauser, R., Prins, G. S., Soto, A. M., et al. (2009). Endocrine-disrupting chemicals: An Endocrine Society scientific statement. *Endocrine Reviews, 30*(4), 293–342.

Duchin, J. S., Koster, F. T., Peters, C. J., Simpson, G. L., Tempest, B., Zaki, S. R., et al. (1994). Hanta-virus pulmonary syndrome: A clinical description of 17 patients with a newly recognized disease. *New England Journal of Medicine, 330*, 949–955.

Eisler, R. (2003). Health risks of gold miners: A synoptic review. *Environmental and Geochemical Health, 25*(3), 325–345.

Ezzati, M., Lopez, A. D., Rodgers, A., Vander Hoorn, S., Murray, C. J. L., Lin, R. B., et al. (2002). Selected major risk factors and global and regional burden of disease. *Lancet, 360*, 1347–1360.

Fawell, J., Bailey, K., Chilton, J., Dahi, E., Fewtrell, L., & Magara, Y. (2006). Fluoride in drinking-water. London: IWA Publishing Co.

Fenwick, A., Cheesmond, A. K., & Amin, M. A. (1981). The role of field irrigation canals in the transmission of *Schistosoma mansoni* in the Gezira Scheme, Sudan. *Bulletin of the World Health Organization, 59*, 777–786.

Fletcher, T., & McMichael, A. J. (1997). *Health at the crossroads: Transport policy and urban health.* Chichester, UK: John Wiley & Sons.

Florig, K. (1997). China's air pollution risks. *Environmental Science and Technology, 31*, 276–279.

Folke, C., Larsson, J., & Sweitzer, J. (1996). Renewable resource appropriation. In R. Costanza & O. Segura (Eds.), *Getting down to Earth.* Washington, DC: Island Press.

Food and Agriculture Organization (FAO). (2002). *State of world fisheries and aquaculture.* Rome, Italy: Author.

Friberg, L., Elinder, C.-G., Kjellstrom, T., & Nordberg, G. F. (Eds.). (1986). *Cadmium and health* (Vol. 2). Boca Raton, FL: CRC Press.

Friel, S., Marmot, M., McMichael, A. J., Kjellstrom, T., & Vagero, D. (2008). Global health equity and climate stabilization: a common agenda. *Lancet, 372*, 1677–1683.

Gallagher, R. P., & Lee, T. K. (2006). Adverse effects of ultraviolet radiation: A brief review. *Progress in Biophysics and Molecular Biology, 92*(1), 119–131.

Grimm, M., Harttgen, K., Klasen, S., & Misselhorn, M. (2006). *Human development report 2006.* New York: United Nations Development Programme.

Gruenbaum, E. (1983). Struggling with the mosquito: Malaria policy and agricultural development in Sudan. *Medical Anthropology, 7*, 51–62.

Gunnell, D., Eddleston, M., Phillips, M. R., & Konradsen, F. (2007). The global distribution of fatal pesticide self-poisoning: Systematic review. *BMC Public Health, 7*, 357.

Haines, A., McMichael, A. J., Smith, K. R., Roberts, I., Woodcock, J., Markandya A., et al. (2009). Public Health Impacts of Strategies to Reduce Greenhouse Gas Emissions: Overview and Implications for Policymakers. *Lancet, 374*, 2104–2114. doi:10.1016/S0140-6736(09)61759-1.

Hajat, S., O'Connor, M. & Kosatsky, T., (2010). Health effects of hot weather: From awareness of risk factors to effective health protection. *Lancet, 375*(9717), 856–863.

Hales, S., Weinstein, P., Souares, P., & Woodward, A. (1999). El Niño and the dynamics of vector-borne disease transmission. *Environmental Health Perspectives, 107*, 99–102.

Herzstein, J. A., Bunn, W. B., Fleming, L. E., Harrington, J. M., Jeyaratnam, J., & Gardner, I. R. (1998). *International occupational and environmental medicine.* St. Louis, MO: Mosby.

Hoogvelt, A. (1997). *Globalisation and the postcolonial world.* London: Macmillan.

Ingelfinger, J. R. (2008). Melamine and the global implications of food contamination. *New England Journal of Medicine, 359*(26), 2745–2748.

Intergovernmental Panel on Climate Change (IPCC). (2001). *Third assessment report: Climate change*

2001 (Vols. I–III). New York: Cambridge University Press.

IPCC (2007). Fourth Assessment Report. Geneva, Inter-governmental Panel on Climate Change. Cambridge: Cambridge University Press, 2007. Available free on the web: www.ipcc.ch

International Scientific Oversight Committee. (2004). *Health effects of outdoor air pollution in developing countries of Asia: A literature review* (Special Report 15). Boston: Health Effects Institute. Retrieved from http://www.healtheffects.org/Pubs/SpecialReport15.pdf

Jennings, N. S. (1998). Mining: An overview. In J. M. Stellman (Ed.), *Encyclopaedia of occupational health and safety* (4th ed., Vol. III, pp. 74.2–74.4). Geneva, Switzerland: International Labor Office.

Johansson, T. & Goldernberg, J. (2004). World energy assessment overview: 2004 update. New York, New York: UNDP, UN-DESA and the World Energy Council.

Kamp, D. W. (2009). Asbestos-induced lung diseases: An update. *Translational Research*, 153(4), 143–152.

Kampa, M., & Castanas, E. (2008). Human health effects of air pollution. *Environmental Pollution*, 151(2), 362–367.

Khan, A. W., Ahmad, A., Sayed, M. H. S. U., Hadi, A., Khan, M. H., Jalil, M. A., et al. (1997). Arsenic contamination in ground water and its effect on human health with particular reference to Bangladesh. *Journal of Preventive and Social Medicine*, 16, 65–73.

Kjellstrom, T. (1994). Issues in the developing world. In L. Rosenstock & M. Cullen (Eds.), *Textbook of clinical occupational and environmental medicine* (pp. 25–31). Philadelphia: W. B. Saunders.

Kjellstrom, T. (2004). The epidemic of asbestos-related diseases in New Zealand. *International Journal of Occupational and Environmental Health*, 10, 212–219.

Kjellstrom, T. (2009a). *Climate change exposures, chronic diseases and mental health in urban populations*. Kobe: World Health Organization, Center for Health Development.

Kjellstrom T. (2009b). Climate change, direct heat exposure, health and well-being in low and middle income countries. *Global Health Action*, 2. doi: 10.3402/gha.v2i0.1958.

Kjellstrom, T., & Corvalan, C. (1995). Framework for the development of environmental health indicators. *World Health Statistics Quarterly*, 48, 144–154.

Kjellstrom, T., Ferguson, R., & Taylor, A. (2009). The total public health impact of road transport in Sweden. Technical report. Borlange: Swedish National Road Authority, 2009. Retrieved from http://publikationswebbutik.vv.se/upload/4863/2009_67_health_impact_assessment_and_public_health_costs_of_the_road_transport_sector.pdf

Kjellstrom, T. & Hogstedt, C. (2009). Global situation concerning work-related injuries and diseases. In K. Elgstrand and I. Pettersson (Eds.). *OSH for Development*. (pp. 741–761). Stockholm: Royal Institute of Technology.

Kjellstrom, T., Holmer, I. & Lemke, B. (2009). Workplace heat stress, health and productivity–an increasing challenge for low and middle-income countries during climate change. *Global Health Action*, 2, doi: 10.3402/gha.v2i0.2047.

Kjellstrom, T., van Kerkhoff, L., Bammer, G., & McMichael, T. (2003). Comparative assessment of transport risks: How it can contribute to health impact assessment of transport policies. *Bulletin of the World Health Organization*, 81, 451–458.

Kraus, R. S. (1998). Oil exploration and drilling. In J. M. Stellman (Ed.), *Encyclopaedia of occupational health and safety* (4th ed., Vol. III). Geneva, Switzerland: International Labor Office.

LaDou, J. (1992). The export of industrial hazards to developing countries. In J. Jeyaratnam (Ed.). *Occupational health in developing countries* (pp. 340–360). Oxford, UK: Oxford University Press.

LaDou, J., & Jeyaratnam, J. (1994). Transfer of hazardous industries: Issues and solutions. In J. Jeyaratnam & K. S. Chia (Eds.), *Occupational health in national development*. River Edge, NJ: World Scientific Publications.

Le, G. V., Takahashi, K., Karjalainen, A., Delgermaa, V., Hoshuyama, T., Miyamura, Y., et al. (2010). National use of asbestos in relation to economic development. *Environmental Health Perspective 118*(1), 116–119.

Lee, K., & Dodgson, R. (2000). Globalisation and cholera: Implications for global governance. *Global Governance*, 6, 213–236.

Leichenko, R., & O'Brien, K. (2008). *Environmental change and globalization: Double exposures.* New York: Oxford University Press.

Levy, B. S., & Wegman, D. H. (Eds.). (2000). *Occupational health: Recognizing and preventing work-related disease and injury* (4th ed.). Philadelphia: Lippincott, Williams and Wilkins.

Li, Y., Wang, W., Kan, H., Xu, X., & Chen, B. (2010). Air quality and outpatient visits for asthma in adults during the 2008 Summer Olympic Games in Beijing. *Science of the Total Environment, 408*(5), 1226–1227.

Lopez, A. D., Mathers, C. D., Ezzati, M., Jamison, D. T., & Murray, C. J. L. (2006). *Global burden of disease and risk factors.* New York: Oxford University Press & World Bank.

McCracken, J. P., Smith, K. R., Diaz, A., Mittleman, M. A. & Schwartz, J. (2007). Chimney stove intervention to reduce long-term wood smoke exposure lowers blood pressure among Guatemalan women. *Environmental Health Perspective, 115*, 996–1001.

Maclure, M. (1991). The case-crossover design: a method for studying transient effects on the risk of acute events. *American Journal of Epidemiology 133*, 144–153.

Madronich, S., & de Gruijl, F. R. (1993). Skin cancer and UV radiation. *Nature, 366*, 23–25.

McMichael, A. J. (1993). *Planetary overload: Global environmental change and the health of the human species.* Cambridge, UK: Cambridge University Press.

McMichael, A. J. (1994). "Molecular epidemiology": New pathway or new traveling companion? *American Journal of Epidemiology, 140*, 1–11.

McMichael, A. J. (1999). Dioxins in the Belgian food chain: Chickens and eggs. *Journal of Epidemiology and Community Health, 53*, 742–743.

McMichael, A. J. (2009). Human population health: Sentinel criterion of environmental sustainability. *Current Opinion in Environmental Sustainability, 1*(1): 101–106.

McMichael, A. J., Anderson, H. R., Brunekreef, B., & Cohen, A. (1998). Inappropriate use of daily mortality analyses for estimating the longer-term mortality effects of air pollution. *International Journal of Epidemiology, 27*, 450–453.

McMichael, A. J., & Bambrick, H. (2009). Global environmental change and health. In Detels R, Beaglehole R, Lansang MA, Gulliford R (Eds.). *Oxford Textbook of Public Health* (5th ed.). (pp. 220–237). Oxford: Oxford University Press.

McMichael, A. J., Campbell-Lendrum, D., Ebi, K., Githeko, A., Scheraga, J., & Woodward, A. (Eds.). (2003). *Climate change and human health: Risks and responses.* Geneva, Switzerland: World Health Organization.

McMichael, A. J., Powles, J., Butler, C. D. & Uauy, R. (2007). Food, livestock production, energy, climate change and health. *Lancet, 370*, 1253–1263.

McMichael, A. J., & Smith, K. R. (1999). Air pollution and health: Seeking a global perspective [Editorial]. *Epidemiology, 10*, 1–4.

McMichael, A. J., Wilkinson, P., Kovats, S. R., Pattenden, S., Shakoor, H., Armstrong, B., et al. (2008). International study of temperature, heat and urban mortality: the 'ISOTHURM' project. *International Journal of Epidemiology, 37*(5), 1121–32. doi:10.1093/ije/dyn086 [June 3 2008].

McMichael, A. J., Woodruff, R. & Hales, S. (2006). Climate change and human health: Present and future risks. *Lancet, 367*, 859–869. doi: 10.1016/S0140-6736(06)68079-3.

Mendelsohn, R., & Olmstead, S. (2009). The economic valuation of environmental amenities and disamenities: Methods and applications. *Annual Review of Environment and Resources, 34*, 325–347.

Meo, S. A. (2004). Health hazards of cement dust. *Saudi Medical Journal, 25*(9), 1153–1159.

Moochhala, S. M., Shahi, G. S., & Cote, I. L. (1997). The role of epidemiology, controlled clinical studies, and toxicology in defining environmental risks. In G. S. Shahi, B. S. Levy, A. Binger, T. Kjellstrom, & R. Lawrence (Eds.). *International perspective on environment, development and health: Toward a sustainable world* (pp. 341–352). New York: Springer.

Moore, C. F. (2003). *Silent scourge: Children, pollution and why scientists disagree*. Oxford, UK: Oxford University Press.

Morgenstern, H., & Thomas, D. (1993). Principals of study design in environmental epidemiology. *Environmental Health Perspectives Supplement, 101*, 23–38.

Morse, S. S. (1995). Factors in the emergence of infectious diseases. *Emerging Infectious Diseases, 1*, 7–15.

Moure-Eraso, R., Wilcox M., Punnett, L., Copeland, L., & Levenstein, C. (2007). Back to the future: Sweat-shop conditions on the Mexico – US border. 1. Community health impact of maquiladora industrial activity. *American Journal of Industrial Medicine, 25*, 311–324.

Murray, C. J. L., & Lopez, A. D. (1996). *The global burden of disease: A comprehensive assessment of mortality and disability from diseases, injuries, and risk factors in 1990 and projected to 2020*. Cambridge, MA: Harvard University Press.

NAS (2009). Science and decisions: advancing risk assessment. Washington, DC: National Academy of Sciences, Division on Earth and Life Studies.

Naeher, L. P., Brauer, M., Lipsett, M., Zelikoff, J.T., Simpson, C.D., Koenig, J.Q. & Smith, K.R. (2007). Woodsmoke health effects: A review. *Inhalation Toxicology, 19*, 67–106.

Nriagu, J. O., Blankson, M. L., & Ocran, K. (1996). Childhood lead poisoning in Africa: A growing public health problem. *Science of the Total Environment, 181*, 93–100.

Organization of Economic Cooperation and Development (OECD). (1993). *OECD core set of indicators for environmental performance reviews* (Environmental Monograph No. 83). Paris: Author.

Ostro, B. (1994). *Estimating the health effects of air pollutants* (Policy Research Working Paper No. 1301). Washington, DC: World Bank.

Parsons, K. (2003). Human thermal environment. *The effects of hot, moderate and cold temperatures on human health, comfort and performance* (2nd ed.). New York: CRC Press.

Patz, J. A., Gibbs, H. K., Foley, J. A., Rogers, J. V. & Smith, K. R. (2007). Climate change and global health: quantifying a growing ethical crisis. *EcoHealth, 4*, 397–405.

Pimm, S. L., Russell, G. J., Gittleman, J. L., & Brooks, T. M. (1995). The future of biodiversity. *Science, 269*, 347–354.

Pocock, S. J., Smith, M., & Baghurst, P. (1994). Environmental lead and children's intelligence: A systematic review of the epidemiological evidence. *British Medical Journal, 309*, 1189–1197.

Pokhrel, A. K., Bates, M. N., Verma, S. C., Joshi, H. S., Screeramareddy, C. T. & Smith, K. R. (2010). Tuberculosis and indoor biomass and kerosene use in Nepal: A case-control study. *Environmental Health Perspective 118*, 558–564.

Pope, C. A. III, Burnett, R. T., Thun, M. J., Calle, E. E., Krewski, D., Ito, K., et al. (2002). Lung cancer, cardiopulmonary mortality, and long-term exposure to fine particulate air pollution. *Journal of the American Medical Association, 287*, 1132–1141.

Pope, C.A. III, Burnett, R. T., Thurston, G. D., Thun, M. J., Calle, E. E., Krewski, D., et al. (2004). Cardiovascular mortality and long-term exposure to particulate air pollution: Epidemiological evidence of general pathophysiological pathways of disease. *Circulation, 109*, 71–77.

Pope, C. A., Burnett, R. T., Krewski, D., Jerrett, M., Shi, Y., Calle, E. E. & Thun, M. J. (2009). Cardiovascular mortality and exposure to air-borne fine particulate matter and cigarette smoke. *Circulation, 120*, 941–948.

Poschen, P. (1998). General profile (forestry). In J. M. Stellman (Ed.), *Encyclopaedia of occupational health and safety* (4th ed., Vol. III, pp. 68.2–68.6). Geneva, Switzerland: International Labor Office.

Prüss-Ustün, A., & Corvalán, C. (2006). *Preventing disease through healthy environments: Towards an estimate of the environmental burden of disease*. Geneva, Switzerland: World Health Organization.

Rahman, M., Tondel, M. J., Ahmad, S. A., & Axelson, O. (1998). Diabetes mellitus associated with arsenic exposure in Bangladesh. *American Journal of Epidemiology, 148*, 198–203.

Ramani, R. V., & Mutmansky, J. M. (1999). Mine health and safety at the turn of the millennium. *Mining Engineering, 51*(9), 25–30.

Rees, W. (1996). Revisiting carrying capacity: Area-based indicators of sustainability. *Population and Environment, 17*, 195–215.

Repetto, R., & Belagi, S. S. (Eds.). (1996). *Pesticides and the immune system: The public health risks*. Washington, DC: World Resources Institute.

Rosenstock, L., Cullen, M. R., Brodkin, C. A. & Redlich, C. A. (Eds.) (2005). Textbook of Clinical Occupational and Environmental Medicine. (2nd ed.) Philadelphia: W.B. Saunders.

Samet, J. M., Schnatter, R., & Gibb, H. (1998). Invited commentary: Epidemiology and risk assessment. *American Journal of Epidemiology, 148*, 929–936.

Schwartz, J. (1994). Low level lead exposure and children's IQ: A meta-analysis and search for a threshold. *Environmental Research, 65*, 42–45.

Scoggins, A., Kjellstrom, T., Fisher, G. W., Connor, J., & Gimson, N. R. (2004). Spatial analysis of annual air pollution exposure and mortality. *Science of the Total Environment, 321*, 71–85.

Shahi, G. S., Levy, B. S., Binger, A., Kjellstrom, T., & Lawrence, R. (Eds.). (1997). *International perspective on environment, development and health: Toward a sustainable world*. New York: Springer.

Sims, J. (1994). *Women, health and environment: An anthology* (Document WHO/EHG/94.11). Geneva, Switzerland: World Health Organization.

Sinton, J., Smith, K. R., Peabody, J. W., Liu, Y., Zhang, X., Edwards, R., & Gan, Q. (2004). An assessment of programs to promote improved household stoves in China. *Energy for Sustainable Development, 8*(3), 33–52.

Slaper, H., Velders, G. J. M., Daniel, J. S., de Gruijl, F. R., & van der Leun, J. C. (1996). Estimates of ozone depletion and skin cancer incidence to examine the Vienna Convention achievements. *Nature, 384*, 256–258.

Smith, A. H., Goycoleam, M., Haque, R., & Biggs, M. L. (1998). Marked increase in bladder and lung cancer mortality in a region of northern Chile due to arsenic in drinking water. *American Journal of Epidemiology, 147*, 660–669.

Smith, D. (1999). Worldwide trends in DDT levels in human milk. *International Journal of Epidemiology, 28*, 179–188.

Smith, K. R. (1997). Development, health, and the environmental risk transition. In G. Shahi, B. S. Levy, & A. Binger (Eds.), *International perspectives in environment, development, and health* (pp. 51–62). New York: Springer.

Smith, K. R. (2008). Comparative environmental assessments. A brief introduction and application in China. *Annals of the New York Academy of Sciences, 1140*, 31–39.

Smith, K. R., Corvalan, C., & Kjellstrom, T. (1999). How much global ill-health is attributable to environmental factors? *Epidemiology, 10*, 573–584.

Smith, K. R., & Ezzati, M. (2005). How environmental health risks change with development: The environmental risk and epidemiologic transitions revisited. *Annual Review of Environment and Resources, 30*, 291–333.

Smith, K. R. & Haigler, E. (2008). Co-benefits of climate mitigation and health protection in energy systems: Scoping methods. *Annual Review of public Health, 29*, 11–25.

Smith, K. R., Jerrett, M., Anderson, H. R., Burnett, R. T., Stone, V., Derwent, R., et al. (2009). Public health benefits of strategies to reduce greenhouse-gas emissions: Health implications of short-lived greenhouse pollutants. *Lancet, 374*(9707), 2091–2103.

Smith, K. R., Mehta, S., & Maeusezahl-Feuz, M. (2004). Indoor smoke from household solid fuels.

In M. Ezzati, A. D. Rodgers, A. D. Lopez, & C. J. L. Murray (Eds.), *Comparative quantification of health risks: Global and regional burden of disease due to selected major risk factors* (Vol. 2, pp. 1437–1495). Geneva, Switzerland: World Health Organization.

Stellman, J. M. (Ed.). (1998). *Encyclopaedia of occupational health and safety* (4th ed.). Geneva, Switzerland: International Labor Organization.

Talbot, T. O., Haley, V. B., Dimmick, W. F., Paulu, C., Talbott, E. O., Rager, J. (2009). Developing consistent data and methods to measure the public health Impacts of ambient air quality for environmental public health tracking: Progress to date and future directions. *Air Quality, Atmosphere, and Health, 2,* 199–206.

Tong, S., Baghurst, P. A., Sawyer, M. G., Burns, J., & McMichael, A. J. (1998). Declining blood lead levels and cognitive function during childhood: The Port Pirie Cohort Study. *Journal of the American Medical Association, 280,* 1915–1919.

Tossavainen, A. (2000). International expert meeting on new advances in the radiology and screening of asbestos-related diseases: Consensus report. *Scandinavian Journal of Work, Environment and Health, 26,* 449–454.

Tossavainen, A. (2004). Global use of asbestos and the incidence of mesothelioma. *International Journal of Occupational and Environmental Health, 10,* 22–25.

United Nations. (Annual). *United Nations demographic yearbook.* New York: United Nations.

United Nations (1997). *International action on toxic chemicals and hazardous wastes.* Earth Summit + 5 Report. New York: United Nations, Division for Sustainable Development.

United Nations (2008). *The Millennium Development Goals Report 2008.* New York: United Nations Department of Economic and Social Affairs.

United Nations Development Program (UNDP). (2004). *Human development report 2004.* New York: United Nations Development Program.

United Nations Environment Program (UNEP). (1998). *Environmental effects of ozone depletion.* Nairobi: Author.

United Nations Environment Program (UNEP). (2004) *GEO: Global environmental outlook 3.* Nairobi: Author.

UNEP. (2008). *Atmospheric brown clouds: Regional assessment report with focus on Asia.* Nairobi: United Nations Environment Program.

UNEP. (2009). *Yearbook 2009.* Nairobi: United Nations Environment Program.

UN Habitat. (2010). Urban World; a new chapter in urban development. Nairobi: United Nations Habitat Office.

U.S. EPA (2009). Persistent Organic Pollutants: a global issue, a global response. Report on website: http://www.epa.gov/oia/toxics/pop.html. Washington, DC: United States Environmental Protection Agency.

Watson, R. T., Dixon, J. A., & Hamburg, S. P. (Eds.). (1998). *Protecting our planet, securing our future: Linkages among global environmental issues and human needs.* Nairobi: UNEP, USNASA, & World Bank.

Weeks, J. L. (1998). Health and safety hazards in the construction industry. In J. M. Stellman (Ed.), *Encyclopaedia of occupational health and safety* (4th ed., Vol. III, pp. 93.2–93.8). Geneva, Switzerland: International Labor Office.

Weiss, R., & McMichael, A. J. (2004). Social and environmental risk factors in the emergence of infectious diseases. *Nature Medicine, 10,* S70–S76.

Wilson, M. E. (1995). Infectious diseases: An ecologic perspective. *British Medical Journal, 311,* 1681–1684.

Woodward, A., Hales, S., & Weinstein, P. (1998). Climate change and human health in the Asia Pacific region: Who will be the most vulnerable? *Climate Research, 11,* 31–38.

World Bank. (1993). *World development report 1993: Investing in health.* Washington, DC: Author.

World Health Organization (WHO). (1990). *Public health impact of the use of pesticides in agriculture*. Geneva, Switzerland: Author.

World Health Organization (WHO). (1992). *Cadmium* (Environmental Health Criteria No. 134). Geneva, Switzerland: Author.

World Health Organization (WHO). (1994). *Ultraviolet radiation* (Environmental Health Criteria No. 160). Geneva, Switzerland: Author.

World Health Organization (WHO). (1996). *Health effects of the Chernobyl accident* (Document WHO/EHG/96.X). Geneva, Switzerland: Author.

World Health Organization (WHO). (1997). *Health and environment in sustainable development* (Document WHO/EHG/97.8). Geneva, Switzerland: Author.

World Health Organization (WHO). (1998). *Chrysotile asbestos* (Environmental Health Criteria No. 190). Geneva, Switzerland: Author.

World Health Organization (2001). Biomarkers in risk assessment: Validity and validation (Environmental Health Criteria No. 222). Geneva, Switzerland: Author.

World Health Organization (WHO). (2002). *World health report 2002: Reducing risks, promoting healthy life*. Geneva, Switzerland: Author.

World Health Organization (WHO). (2004). *World report on road traffic injury prevention*. Geneva, Switzerland: Author.

World Health Organization (WHO). (2006). *Elimination of asbestos related diseases*. Geneva, Switzerland: Author.

World Health Organization (WHO). (2008). *Our cities, our health, our future. Acting on social determinants for health equity in urban settings*. Kobe, Japan, World Health Organization, Centre for Health Development.

World Health Organization (WHO) & UNICEF. (2010). *Progress on drinking water and sanitation: 2010 update*. Geneva, Switzerland: WHO.

World Resources Institute. (1998). *World resources 1998–99*. Oxford, UK: Oxford University Press.

Wyndham, C. H. (1969). Adaptation to heat and cold. *Environmental Research*, 2, 442–469.

Yassi, A., & Kjellstrom, T. (1998). Environmental health hazards. In J. M. Stellman (Ed.), *Encyclopaedia of occupational health and safety* (4th ed., Vol. II, pp. 53.1–53.33). Geneva, Switzerland: International Labor Office.

Zhang, J., Mauzerall, D. L., Zhu, T., Liang, S., Ezzati, M., & Remais, J. V. (2010). Environmental health in China: Progress towards clean air and safe water. *Lancet*, 375(9720), 1110–1119.

Zhang, J., & Smith, K. (2007). Household air pollution from coal and biomass fuels in China: Measurements, health impacts, and interventions. *Environmental Health Perspectives*, 115(6), 848.

Complex Emergencies

MICHAEL J. TOOLE AND RONALD J. WALDMAN

This chapter focuses on public health emergencies that arise from complex political crises but draws, in places, on lessons learned from humanitarian responses to natural disasters. Terminology changes frequently, and different definitions emphasize different aspects of a concept. The term "complex humanitarian emergencies" came into popular use following the Kurdish refugee exodus during the Gulf War in 1991. It was defined by the Centers for Disease Control and Prevention (CDC) as "a situation affecting large civilian populations which usually involves a combination of factors including war or civil strife, food shortages, and population displacement, resulting in significant excess mortality" (Burkholder & Toole, 1995). By comparison, Goodhand and Hulme (1999) defined "complex political emergencies" as conflicts that combine a number of features: They often occur within but also across state boundaries; they have political antecedents, often relating to competition for power and resources; they are protracted in duration; they are embedded in and are expressions of existing social, political, economic, and cultural structures and cleavages; and they are often characterized by predatory social formations. This latter definition clearly locates the causes and effects in the political sphere—a point echoed by numerous other writers, and one that has considerable implications for those working in these settings with a primarily public health agenda. In the new millennium, these terms have merged into "complex emergencies"

(CEs), the term that we use in this chapter to maintain simplicity and consistency.

The chapter grapples with current understanding of CEs and their political causes and considers their impact on populations and health systems.[1] It highlights current knowledge in humanitarian assistance and indicates that effective technical interventions are possible to help alleviate suffering and limit adverse effects on the health of populations. We draw attention to current efforts by the humanitarian community to improve the effectiveness, efficiency, and equity of humanitarian responses, and consider how the pattern of early responses may influence the longer-term survival of populations and systems and the nature of any postconflict society established. We are acutely aware, however, that the solutions to CEs are political and not humanitarian. Thus it is in the political sphere that both upstream and downstream responses to complex emergencies must receive priority.

Many of the public health interventions currently promoted as best practice were developed and tested during the 1970s and 1980s, when most conflict-affected populations were accessed in relatively secure refugee camps administered by the Office of the United Nations High Commissioner for Refugees

---

Acknowledgements: The authors wish to thank Anthony Zwi for his substantive contributions to this chapter in the first edition of this book.

[1] The emphasis in this chapter is on complex political emergencies and not on more traditional forms of interstate conflict and war. Furthermore, although the discussion here comments on other forms of intrastate conflict and repression, such as torture and disappearance, these forms of violence are not the focus of this chapter. Where possible, however, we have briefly highlighted these issues either through the presentation of an exhibit or through reference to the literature.

(UNHCR). Recent changes in conflicts have introduced a great deal of complexity into the emergency environment. Although the overall number of conflicts has decreased, most contemporary wars are of "protracted duration, intrastate, fought by irregular armed groups, and fuelled by economic opportunities and ethnic rivalry" (Spiegel, Checchi, Colombo, & Paik, 2010). The populations most in need are often trapped by the armed conflict, unable to flee, not residing in organized camps and, therefore, need to be accessed by relief agencies "in situ."

Although the impact of natural disasters is not the subject of this chapter, two important exceptions are made: the destructive tsunami that originated off the coast of Indonesia on December 26, 2004, and the earthquake that devastated Port-au-Prince, Haiti, and its environs on January 12, 2010. We include these catastrophic events because they had many elements of a complex emergency. The tsunami caused more than 230,000 deaths and injuries in 8 countries and displaced more than 1.5 million people from their homes (United Nations Office for the Coordination of Humanitarian Affairs, 2005). Two of the areas most severely affected (the Aceh province of Indonesia and northeast Sri Lanka) had experienced several decades of armed conflict. More than 127,000 Burmese refugees were living in the five Thai provinces affected by the tsunami; at least 1,000 perished in the disaster (United States Committee for Refugees, 2005). The massive displacement and disruption to food and water supplies, shelter, and sanitation created conditions similar to those experienced by refugees and internally displaced persons (IDPs) fleeing armed conflict.

The Haiti earthquake killed 230,000 people, injured an approximately equal number, left 604,000 people homeless in Port-au-Prince, and caused the flight of an additional 598,000 individuals from the capital city to the countryside (Office for the Coordination of Humanitarian Affairs, February 2010). Its impact on the only major city in the poorest country of the Western Hemisphere, including the government paralysis that occurred in the wake of the disaster, the massive international relief effort that included interventions by armed forces from many different nations, and the difficulty that is foreseen in returning people to their homes is, again, similar to what might be encountered in conflict setting.

In the period from the end of World War II to the end of the Cold War, most conflicts took place in the low- and middle-income regions of the world, primarily in Africa, the Middle East, Asia, and Latin America. The end of the Cold War, the breakup of the Soviet Union, and the pace and intensity of globalization led, in the 1990s, to major conflicts in Europe and the former Soviet Union, notably in Tajikistan, Chechnya, Georgia, Abkhazia, the former Yugoslavia, and Nagorno Karabakh. The number of armed conflicts globally reached a peak of 50 in 1991. Since then, there has been a significant decline to a total of 25 armed conflicts during 2008 and 20 during 2009 (Marshall, 2009). In the past 6 years, peace agreements have been signed in Southern Sudan, Angola, Liberia, Sierra Leone, Central African Republic, Chad, Sri Lanka, Nepal, and the Solomon Islands, ending, in some countries, decades of fighting (Figure 11-1). Nevertheless, in the first few months of 2011, the conflict in Cote d'Ivoire reignited and a new conflict developed in Libya.

Modern-day conflicts are increasingly internal rather than between states, and they often have as a prime objective, alongside the quest for economic and political power, the undermining of the lives and livelihoods of civilian populations associated with opposing factions. As many as 90% of those affected in recent conflicts have been civilians, with all ages and both sexes affected. The distribution of impact and health outcomes varies substantially, however, and depends on the nature of the conflict and its history, its extent and form, and prior health and health systems status.

Many CEs and major natural disasters have attracted considerable media attention and have caused people to seek to promote availability of at least a basic degree of humanitarian assistance, even if fundamental political solutions are not sought. Other ongoing crises, despite causing massive loss of life, population displacement, and infrastructure destruction, are not necessarily explicitly recognized as CEs; as a result, they attract few resources and attention. These "hidden emergencies" nevertheless pose fundamental challenges to the health and well-being of affected populations. Ongoing conflicts in Burma, Colombia, western Sudan, Uganda, and Democratic Republic of the Congo (DRC) seem to attract little attention and resources: such discrepancies are likely to result from geopolitical concerns, media interest, and economic factors. The role of the media may be particularly powerful in anointing a country as a CE worthy of attention, such as the BBC did in Ethiopia in 1984 and the *New York Times* did in Somalia in 1993, which subsequently focused world attention on these areas and brought popular demands for action.

Some wars are still fought primarily between competing armies, such as the Iran–Iraq conflict from

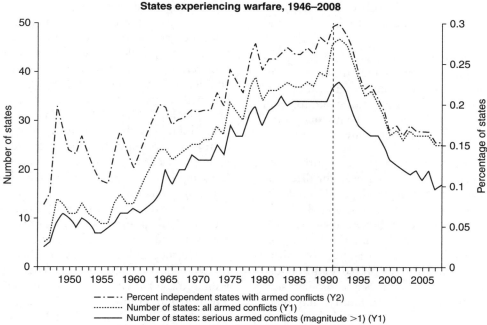

States experiencing warfare, 1946–2008

- — · — ·· Percent independent states with armed conflicts (Y2)
- ············· Number of states: all armed conflicts (Y1)
- ———— Number of states: serious armed conflicts (magnitude >1) (Y1)

Figure 11-1 States Experiencing Armed Conflict. 1946–2008.
Source: www.systemicpeace.org/conflict.htm.

1980 to 1988, in which an estimated 450,000 military personnel died (Sivard, 1996); the Gulf War of 1991; and the Eritrea–Ethiopia and India–Pakistan conflicts of 1999. The vast majority, however, now take place within states. However, in the aftermath of the September 2001 terrorist attacks on New York City and Washington, D.C., United States–led coalitions have used military force to change the regimes in Afghanistan and Iraq. These two conflicts represent a new trend in modern wars, with their huge disparities in military resources between the warring parties. These two conflicts were ongoing in 2011 with intensification of the war in Afghanistan. In addition, a coalition of governments led by the North Atlantic Treaty Organization (NATO) began bombing military installations and maintaining a no-fly zone over Libya in March 2011 to protect Libyan civilians from government forces.

During the 65 years since the Holocaust, numerous episodes of massive human rights atrocities and genocide have been committed against particular groups: Pol Pot's killing fields in Cambodia, the Guatemalan government's action against indigenous Mayan communities, and the genocide against Tutsis in Rwanda. Recent conflicts, such as that in West Darfur, Sudan, which began in 2004, highlight the

nature of internal wars, including the use of repressive techniques to evict people from their homes and to undermine their sense of security and safety, accompanied by the targeted use of force to destroy social, political, and economic structures. A particularly insidious development is the targeting of violence toward individuals and groups on the basis of their ethnicity or religion. Such conflicts have been frequent enough that the term "ethnic cleansing" has entered the vernacular. Unfortunately, opportunistic politicians have often inflamed the perceived differences between groups, especially during times of economic and political uncertainty, resulting in open armed conflict.

In the same conflicts, other key features of modern-day CEs are readily evident:

- The willingness of powerful segments of the international community to intervene in internal conflicts, and to do so in a way that minimizes their exposure to risk
- The changing nature of humanitarian assistance, which increasingly forms only one dimension of the management of conflicts, alongside political, economic, and military responses

- The changing role of the private sector, as well as the increasingly important role of local and global media
- Trends in globalization that simultaneously integrate peripheral areas within the global economy and contribute to their fragmentation, as elites compete for access to the economic and political resources associated with integration in the global political economy

One consequence of the targeting of entire communities and their livelihoods has been the dramatic rise in numbers of forcibly displaced people. Globally, in December 2008, there were an estimated 26 million IDPs and 13.6 million refugees (those seeking refuge across international borders), the vast majority fleeing conflict zones (United States Committee for Refugees, 2009). Those displaced within countries have less access to resources and services supported by the international community, may be at ongoing risk from violence perpetrated by the state and other powerful local actors, and have their needs more hidden than those persons who are displaced across borders.

Although refugee numbers are typically assessed for purposes of planning and providing relief, relatively little attention has been devoted to developing the most appropriate methods for establishing the precise composition of refugee and IDP populations, whether in terms of age, sex, religion, local geographic origin, or ethnicity. This lack of information imposes constraints given the differing needs and roles of groups within populations and may make it easier for the more complex issues of dealing with gender, equity, and ongoing intergroup rivalry to be overlooked. Particular groups, such as older adults, refugees not in camps, and IDPs, may neither be identified nor receive the required attention for their differing needs.

The changing pattern of conflict has been accompanied by significant changes in the delivery of humanitarian assistance. The number of agencies operating in these complex settings has increased dramatically; for example, more than 240 nongovernmental organizations (NGOs) worked in and around Rwanda in the aftermath of the genocide and more than 100 agencies worked with the Kosovar Albanians during 1999. Within 1 month after the 2004 Asian tsunami, more than 2,000 foreign medical personnel were working in the Indonesian province of Aceh. More than 300 organizational entities registered, at one point or another, at the World Health Organization's (WHO's) health cluster meetings during the emergency phase of the relief effort in Haiti, and literally thousands of organizations, both indigenous and foreign, were present. In contrast, lower-profile CEs may be as severe and life-threatening to large populations, such as the armed conflict in Sierra Leone in 1999, but attract much less media, intergovernmental, and humanitarian attention. New NGOs established in response to a specific conflict may be short-lived, inexperienced, and unable to cope with the challenges they face in providing services in complex political environments. Ensuring one does more good than harm must underlie all interventions.

Every conflict has winners and losers—a fact well known to the predators who identify opportunities amidst the turmoil to further enrich themselves and entrench their political position. These players may, therefore, have an interest in perpetuating the conflict. Humanitarian aid itself may become a resource over which groups compete, and such assistance and resources may directly or indirectly stoke the conflict. In some distressing circumstances, humanitarian aid was used unwittingly to attract populations who were subsequently targeted by combatants, as in the DRC and Sudan. Humanitarian workers have increasingly been directly targeted in latter-day conflicts, leading to increased efforts to work closely with the military and security sector. Despite some benefits, such as improved logistics support, this trend may bring negative consequences and additional dangers and may threaten the neutrality and impartiality to which many agencies aspire.

NGOs are not a homogeneous community. Although some are highly professional and have given considerable thought to the development of humanitarian and technical policies and programs, there have been some negative consequences of the way in which humanitarian assistance has been provided. Recognition by the humanitarian community of these problems has led to a great deal of evaluation and introspection and inspired measures to improve practice, including the development of codes of conduct for humanitarian agencies, the promotion of minimum standards for service provision, and debate regarding enhancing accountability to affected populations.

Promoting the derivation and uptake of good practice is particularly difficult in humanitarian agencies given their often rapid staff turnover, unwillingness to publicly acknowledge failures and limitations because of the possible funding consequences, and a culture of doing rather than reflecting. Interventions are often not evidence based. Also, despite most agencies valuing the concept of coordination, few wish to be coordinated. The response to the Asian tsunami in 2004 once again witnessed an almost unseemly race to be "in charge" and to dominate the relief programs. Despite the overwhelming evidence that basic needs and public health interventions were the main priority among surviving communities, many donors insisted on sending highly visible field hospitals and surgical teams well after the need for such resources had passed. Poor-quality services have significant adverse consequences: increased morbidity, mortality, and disability; further spread of communicable diseases; community dissatisfaction and breakdown; and psychosocial distress. Clear policy objectives for interventions are often lacking, and mechanisms for working with new players such as the military and the private sector remain inadequately developed. Despite recognition that the accountability of relief efforts to affected populations should be enhanced, mechanisms to assure this outcome remain in their infancy.

Ongoing humanitarian challenges include understanding how best to upgrade host population health services alongside efforts to improve those available to refugees, how to most humanely and efficiently provide good-quality services, and how to maintain the role of communities in structuring both the determination of priorities and the pattern of service provision. A key issue relates to how and whether to bolster and support resilient health and social systems and individual adaptations to conflict. The world's level of knowledge regarding these responses, and the potential to further support them, is weak. A persistent challenge to humanitarian workers is the need to institutionalize a sensitive and inclusive evidence-based culture and to build sustainable mechanisms for crystallizing policy advice from the vast and valuable foundation of field experience.

Direct Public Health Impact of War

Measuring the impact and hidden costs of conflict is complex for a variety of reasons—methodological and theoretical shortcomings, inconsistencies in definitions and terms, restricted access to areas of conflict and sources of information, the rapid evolution of many emergencies, political manipulation of data, resource constraints, and the hidden or indirect nature of the impact. One of the consequences of these data limitations is difficulty in identifying more precisely which segments of the population are at greatest risk, so that would-be helpers can develop more appropriate responses. Most poor countries lack reliable health information and vital registration systems, the absence of which increases the difficulties of determining the conflict-associated costs in terms of morbidity, mortality, and disability. Furthermore, CEs may seriously disrupt whatever surveillance and information systems do exist.

Lack of consistency in definitions used makes it difficult to make comparisons both within and across populations. Different agencies may define refugees and IDPs in different ways, case definitions for particular conditions often vary, and techniques for estimating nutritional deficiencies, for example, may vary among different agencies working with the same population. Data are at times incomplete because impartial observers who attempt to provide more accurate figures may not have access to witnesses or other reliable sources of information.

During the last 15 years, a number of expert meetings have been held in an attempt to develop more reliable methods of measuring both direct and indirect mortality resulting from CEs. Some of their proceedings have been published (Reed & Keeley, 2001). Cross-sectional retrospective mortality surveys have been increasingly employed to measure conflict-related mortality. In 2004 alone, large mortality surveys were conducted in three conflict zones: Iraq, DRC, and the West Darfur region of Sudan. All of these surveys used cluster sampling methodology.

Between 2000 and 2007, the International Rescue Committee (IRC), an international NGO, conducted a series of five mortality surveys to evaluate the humanitarian impact of conflict in DRC. The first two surveys (2000 and 2001) were confined to the five eastern provinces; the latter three (2002, 2004, and 2007) were nationwide. The 2004 study recorded a national crude mortality rate (CMR) of 2.1 deaths per 1,000 population per month, a rate more than 60% higher than that documented in the 1984 national census (Coghlan et al, 2004). Mortality was highest in the eastern provinces, where the CMR averaged 2.9 deaths per 1,000 population per month. Fewer than 10% of deaths documented in the studies were directly attributable to violence; rather, most were due to the indirect public health effects of conflict, including higher rates of infectious diseases, increased prevalence of malnutrition, and neonatal conditions. The third nationwide survey in 2007 found that the CMR in DRC remained elevated, at a level almost 70% higher than that reported in the 1984 national census and more than 55% higher than the reported baseline for sub-Saharan Africa.

The methods employed in these surveys have been subject to some criticism (Human Security Report Project, 2010); however, practical alternatives have not been proposed. The survey methods employed in DRC remain examples of best practice.

Although innovative techniques may be used to construct a picture of what transpired during a particular CE, what the needs were, and what the nature of the response was, the sources of data may be biased, as may the ways in which information has been collected. Despite these shortcomings, innovative groups—often NGOs without a political agenda linked to any of the key players in the conflict—may be able to play a valuable role in documenting precisely what occurred and what the nature of the present needs is. Médecins sans Frontières (MSF) has taken an innovative approach to documenting the impact of CEs through its MSF Speaking Out series, in which extracts from all relevant internal and external MSF documents are collated and annotated to form a compelling chronicle of a crisis and then published both in hard copy and on the "MSF-CRASH" website. For example, *A Not-so Natural Disaster* (Crombé & Jézéquel, 2009) describes the circumstances leading up to and during the famine in Niger in 2005.

Even where huge numbers of people are involved, agreement on the magnitude of impact varies. Estimates of the number of victims of the Rwandan genocide are still imprecise and vary from 500,000 to 1 million (best estimate: 800,000). Deaths during the 1991 Gulf War remain disputed; so, too, are likely to be the number of civilian deaths experienced following the invasion of Iraq by the United States–led coalition in 2003. Each party to the conflict has its own reasons for presenting data in a particular way; unless some more objective source is established, public health officials need to be extremely cautious in their use of such figures. Moreover, the term "complex emergency" has sometimes been used incorrectly by some governments to describe what in essence has been genocide (e.g., Rwanda in 1994) so as to avoid their obligations under international law.

Particular affected populations may also be difficult to assess precisely, as in the case of war orphans or unaccompanied child refugees and IDPs. Unaccompanied children may account for 2% to 5% of the refugee population in camps, although this proportion will clearly vary in different contexts. Massive population movements may occur over very short periods of time, such as the 1 million or more Hutu refugees who fled from Rwanda over a period of days. Even when the time scales are longer, considerable problems remain: For example, approximately

500,000 Liberian refugees fled to Guinea over a period of 5 years into an area that had a population of 1.2 million inhabitants (Van Damme, 1998). Such population flows present considerable challenges in terms of assessing health status, determining needs, and developing context-appropriate responses.

Political interests greatly affect which data are released, how and when such releases are made, and what accompanying analyses are provided. In the Kosovo conflict in 1999, NATO and the Yugoslav government tussled over a number of events in which civilian casualties occurred, with each side seeking to obtain maximum political and public relations benefits. Certain events, such as allegations of the use of systematic rape, appeared only at times when NATO was under pressure to justify its role and nature of engagement in the war.

Data on numbers of IDPs and refugees may be manipulated by states and organizations in an attempt to make a political point or to maximize access to resources. It has been alleged that some refugee camp administrators and refugees report fewer deaths than actually occur so as to maintain levels of international assistance—having fewer beneficiaries could result in less assistance. In Nepal, as well as elsewhere, in an attempt to encourage reporting of deaths among Bhutanese refugees, free funeral shrouds were offered to relatives of the deceased together with assurances that the reporting would not result in decreases of rations.

Physical Impact

Political conflicts in the earlier part of the twentieth century were mostly waged between armies and trained combatants. The main direct results, in the form of deaths, morbidity, and disability, reflected the nature of the conflict, the level of technology and nature of weapons used, the prior preparation and protective clothing available to military personnel, and the quality of emergency medical care and evacuation facilities (Garfield & Neugat, 1991).

In the vast majority of latter-day conflicts, however, the entire population is often targeted, both directly and with massive and sustained effort at reducing the viability and integrity of the affected community. In Mozambique, antigovernment forces killed approximately 100,000 people in 1986 and 1987 alone, a massive proportion in a relatively small country (Cliff & Noormahomed, 1988). Injuries and disabilities may follow the use of firearms, but it is notable that technology levels need not be high to achieve terrible levels of destruction. The Rwandan genocide was largely committed with a combination of guns and machetes. In Darfur (Sudan), the conflict since 2003 has caused an estimated 300,000 civilian deaths (Degomme & Guha-Sapir, 2010). In the early years of this conflict, most deaths were due to violence; since 2005, however, most deaths have been due to communicable diseases.

The numbers of war disabled and their types of disability are not well known because only a few countries—such as Zimbabwe, El Salvador, and the Tigrayan region of Ethiopia—have attempted censuses of war-related disability. In Zimbabwe in 1981–1982, 13% of all disability was assessed as being war related. In El Salvador in the mid-1990s, the census identified 12,041 war disabled, 82% of whom were combatants and the rest civilians. Approximately one-third of the 300,000 soldiers returning from the front lines at the end of the war in Ethiopia had been injured or disabled. By 1984, well before the end of the war in 1991, more than 40,000 people had lost one or more limbs in the conflict. During the bitter civil conflict in Sierra Leone between 1998 and 2002, an estimated 30,000 civilians, including children, had limbs hacked off by the rebels (Project Ploughshares, 2002).

Antipersonnel land mines are also responsible for significant population burdens, especially in a small number of heavily infested countries such as Angola, Cambodia, and Afghanistan. Estimates of mine-related disabilities are sobering: 36,000 in Cambodia (1 in every 236 persons has lost at least one limb), 20,000 in Angola, 8,000 in Mozambique, and 15,000 in Uganda. In the former Yugoslavia, more than 3 million mines were laid; in late 1994, mine laying was occurring at a rate of 50,000 per week, with many of these munitions being both unmarked and unmapped. The costs of such injuries are both physical and social, and affect all age groups. Between February 1991 and February 1992, approximately 75% of the land mine injuries treated worldwide involved children aged 5 to 15 years. Others affected may be aware of the dangers of mines but have to enter the mined areas in search of food or to continue their agricultural and pastoral activities. Many of the severely disabled will require permanent medical and social services and will strain the health resources of the affected country for many years. For years to come, the antipersonnel land mines and munitions will constitute a health hazard and contribute to thousands of deaths and severe disabilities, including those occurring in many children.

Natural Disasters

In both the Indian Ocean tsunami and in Haiti following the 2010 earthquake, the number of dead could not be precisely determined. Mass burials seemed to be the most convenient way to deal with the large numbers of dead bodies that had to be cleared.

The Haiti disaster, more than any other, was characterized by large numbers of injured; the care of those disabled by the earthquake will have to continue for years. Estimates of the numbers of amputees have varied considerably, between 2,000 and 4,000, with the lower, but still important number being considered more accurate. Severe brain trauma and spinal cord injuries have also caused permanent disabilities that will require chronic care in a country that is not well suited to provide it. These new major public health problems are added to an already overwhelming existing burden.

Sexual Violence

Rape is increasingly recognized as a feature of internal wars but has been present in many different types of conflicts. In some conflicts, rape has been used systematically as an attempt to undermine opposing groups: This policy was noted in a very high-profile way in relation to the conflict in the former Yugoslavia, where Bosnian women were systematically abused (Stiglmayer, 1994), as well as in the Rwanda, DRC, Darfur (Sudan), and Sierra Leone conflicts. It has been argued that the more extensive development of women's organizations helped to ensure that these events were made more visible and that support for survivors was mobilized. It has also been suggested, however, that some forms of sexual abuse—male rape, for example—have as a result been poorly recognized, if at all.

A study in Uganda found that despite widespread rape, few women spoke of their victimization (Bracken, Giller, & Kabaganda, 1992). In the South Kivu province of DRC, which has been affected by armed conflict since 1998, one NGO Malteser International registered, 20,517 female rape survivors in the three-year period 2005–2007, (Steiner, Benner, Sondorp, Schmitz, Mesmer, & Rosenberger, 2009). Women of all ages had been targeted by sexual violence, but only few—and many of them only after several years—sought medical care and psychological help. Sexual violence in DRC frequently led to social, especially familial, exclusion. Members of military and paramilitary groups were identified as the main perpetrators of sexual violence.

Rape, sexual violence, and exploitation may also be widespread in refugee camps, although the extent of their recognition is limited, and widely varying estimates of the numbers of victims have been reported. Violence against Somali women in refugee camps in northern Kenya attracted worldwide condemnation. Despite being relatively few in number, these incidents had a profound effect because they challenged the extent to which UN agencies, such as UNHCR, were effective in assuring the protection of refugee populations against further abuse. In the former Yugoslavia, estimates of the number of rape survivors have ranged from 10,000 to 60,000 (Swiss & Giller, 1993) and have firmly placed the issue of systematic use of rape on the international agenda. Indirectly, such events have also highlighted the need for agencies working with conflict-affected populations to more widely consider their reproductive health needs (Palmer, Lush, & Zwi, 1999).

Despite these efforts, sexual violence has continued to be a feature of recent conflicts. For example, an estimated 215,000 to 257,000 women were victims of sexual violence during the civil war in Sierra Leone (Project Ploughshares, 2002). Efforts to establish a permanent International Criminal Court, in which war crimes would be prosecuted, have clearly identified systematic use of rape in wartime as an issue to be addressed. Although sexual violence is most typically perpetrated by men against women, males and children of both sexes may also be targeted. Their plight warrants attention, especially given the additional taboos and stigma associated with these circumstances.

In addition to long-lasting mental health disorders, rapes have resulted in the transmission of human immunodeficiency virus (HIV). Wars and political conflict present high-risk situations for the transmission of sexually transmitted infections (STIs), including HIV infection (Zwi & Cabral, 1991). War predisposes victims to STI and HIV transmission in several different ways:

- Widespread population movement
- Increased crowding
- Separation of women from partners who normally provide a degree of protection
- Abuses and sexual demands by military personnel and others in positions of power
- Weakened social structures, which reduce inhibitions on aggressive behavior and violence against women

In addition, access to barrier contraceptives, to treatment for STIs, to the prerequisites for maintaining personal hygiene, and to health promotion advice are all compromised in conflict situations.

Nevertheless, studies in Africa have found that armed conflict may—at the population level—be protective against the transmission of HIV, as seems to have been the case in Angola (Spiegel et al., 2007).

This may be due to decreased mobility by the population due to the conflict.

Women who are on their own may find it more difficult to assure their safety and that of their children in a CE. They may become targets of violence from three sides: the opposing army, the armed forces in the country to which they have fled, and (sometimes) their own community (Palmer & Zwi, 1998). They may be forced to provide sex in exchange for food, shelter, or other necessities to ensure self and family survival. The experience of Afghan refugees (Amnesty International, 1995) is illustrative: "In the camps in Pakistan, most of which are controlled by one or other of the warring Afghan factions, women have been attacked, particularly those who are unaccompanied by men. If they refuse sexual favours, they are often denied access to vital rations." In Somalia, fear of rape and shooting have prevented women from leaving their homes. The trade of sex for food has also occurred following natural disasters and, in the slums of Port-au-Prince following the earthquake, rape and other forms of sexual predation were widely reported.

Women's utilization of healthcare facilities may be severely reduced if males dominate service provision. Burmese Muslim women, many of whom had been raped, who fled to Bangladesh had difficulties in accessing health care due to the predominance of male providers, highlighting the importance of a gender-sensitive analysis of conflict (UNHCR, 1992). The issue of safety of women should be carefully considered when planning camps and other facilities: The arrangement of water, sewage removal facilities, and cooking fuels should be undertaken in such a way as to reduce risks of abuse and violence.

Human Rights

Article 25 of the Universal Declaration of Human Rights, proclaimed by resolution 217 A(III) of the United Nations General Assembly on December 10, 1948, states clearly that "[e]veryone has the right to a standard of living adequate for the health and well-being of himself and of his family, including food, clothing, housing and medical care." In times of war, this declaration and other laws, covenants, declarations, and treaties that constitute the body of human rights law are complemented by international humanitarian law. The latter is "a set of rules aimed at limiting violence and protecting the fundamental rights of the individual in times of armed conflict" (Perrin, 1996). These rules are intended to govern the conduct of war by banning the use of certain weapons and by minimizing the effects of armed conflicts, whether international or internal, on noncombatants. The protection of the rights of noncombatants in wartime is based primarily on the Geneva Conventions of 1949 and the two Additional Protocols of 1977. Yet, despite the existence of both of these bodies of international law, CEs are consistently associated with serious infringements of the dignity of individuals and, more specifically, with a major impact on the health status of affected individuals and populations.

General practices that can be considered to be clear violations of international humanitarian law include the intentional targeting of civilian noncombatants, medical personnel, and civilian health facilities. Protection is also conferred upon prisoners of war, wounded and ill combatants, and military medical installations. Violations of these covenants by states and individuals occurred with great frequency during the second half of the twentieth century. Some of the most prominent included the murder of civilians by the government of Guatemala during the 1980s (Yamauchi, 1993), the intentional destruction of health facilities by RENAMO forces seeking to bring down the government of Mozambique (Cliff & Noormahomed, 1988), and the genocidal activities perpetrated upon the Tutsi population of Rwanda in 1994. In the 1990s, the governments of Serbia and Croatia pursued "ethnic cleansing" policies (more accurately termed "ethnic repression") against the populations of neighboring republics of the former Yugoslavia and, in the case of Serbia, the province of Kosovo. Members of the Arab militia in western Sudan, known as the Janjaweed, terrorized the Zaghawa, Masaalit, and Fur peoples between 2003 and 2005 with active support from the government of Sudan. This overt support led to the issuance in March 2009 of an arrest warrant by the International Criminal Court for the President of Sudan, Omar Hassan al-Bashir.

Violations of human rights law and international humanitarian law that target individuals can take many forms. Torture of civilians has been increasingly documented. More than 2,000 Bhutanese refugees in Nepal, representing approximately 2% of the total refugee population, reported having been tortured prior to their flight (Shrestha et al., 1998). Torture has also been reported as a frequently used weapon by China against Tibetans (Keller et al., 1997), and by Turkish authorities against dissenters to its regime (Iacopino et al., 1996). Sexual violence is also of increasing concern, as noted earlier in this chapter. UNHCR (1993), for example, has documented the "widespread occurrence of sexual violence in violation of the fundamental right to personal security as recognized in international human rights and humanitarian law."

The sexual abuse of Iraqi prisoners by U.S. military forces in the Abu Ghraib prison was widely reported by the international media. It is also the subject of a comprehensive report that documents the severe health consequences of systematic psychological torture of detainees by U.S. personnel in Afghanistan, Iraq, and Guantánamo (Physicians for Human Rights, 2005).

The consequences of wartime human rights violations can be enduring. The physical and psychological consequences of bodily harm to individuals do not end with the cessation of hostilities. Indeed, most societies require years of reconstruction and redevelopment to restore viable and effective health systems to serve their surviving populations. One can only speculate as to how countries such as Cambodia, Angola, Sudan, Somalia, Rwanda, Liberia, Sierra Leone, the republics of the former Yugoslavia, Timor Leste, Côte d'Ivoire, Afghanistan, and Iraq will emerge from the gross abuses of human rights that occurred on their soil.

Although violations of human rights law and international humanitarian law are crimes, the legal systems for punishing the perpetrators and compensating the victims are grossly inadequate. To date, three international tribunals have been established to prosecute war criminals from the former Yugoslavia, Rwanda, and Sierra Leone. Although these courts help to move the punishment of war criminals from theory to practice, they have been very slow to act and such proceedings are very expensive to implement. The establishment of an International Criminal Court—a permanent standing body dedicated to the trial and punishment of individuals accused and convicted of violations of human rights law—is, at least conceptually, another step toward strengthening what has in many respects been a legal system without law enforcement capability. The arrest and prosecution of alleged Serbian war criminals, including Slobodan Milosevic and Radovan Karadzic, is evidence that the Court is on the way to achieving its goals.

Reporting and responding to reports of human rights violations pose major problems. Although wars and internal conflicts have been proximate causes of most humanitarian emergencies, few of the individuals and agencies who have been involved in providing relief to the individuals affected are trained in the recognition of human rights violations or know where and how to report them. Until more widespread attention is paid to these crimes against humanity, the victims will continue to suffer from preventable acute and chronic morbidity, and the perpetrators will go largely unpunished. It would be useful to treat human rights violations as a major cause of morbidity and mortality during wars and their aftermath and to establish the epidemiologic characteristics of their distribution (Spirer & Spirer, 1993).

Indirect Public Health Impact of Civil Conflict

This section examines in detail the impact of CEs on the health of populations that is not directly the consequence of violence. Although the chapter focuses on the public health consequences of armed conflict, there is a phased evolution of public health effects as a country or region moves from political disturbances, economic deterioration, and civil strife through armed conflict, population migration, food shortages, and the collapse of governance and physical infrastructure. Thus this section attempts to frame the indirect consequences of civil conflict in the changing context of evolving humanitarian emergencies.

Food Scarcity

As political disturbances evolve in a country, they generally have significant effects on both the national and local economies. In some cases, an economic crisis may initiate political turmoil where there have been underlying tensions between political factions, ethnic or religious groups, or disadvantaged geographic areas. Under such scenarios, especially in low-income countries, one of the first health effects is undernutrition in vulnerable groups, which is in turn caused by food scarcity. Local farmers may not plant crops as extensively as usual, or they may decrease the diversity of their crops due to the uncertainty created by the economic or political situation. The cost of seeds and fertilizer may increase and government agricultural extension services may be disrupted, resulting in lower yields. Distribution and marketing systems may be adversely affected. Devaluation of the local currency may drive down the price paid for agricultural produce, and the collapse of the local food-processing industry may further diminish demand for agricultural products.

If full-scale armed conflict occurs, the fighting may damage irrigation systems, crops might be intentionally destroyed or looted by armed soldiers, distribution systems may collapse completely, and widespread theft and looting of food stores may occur. In countries that do not normally produce agricultural surpluses or that have large pastoral or nomadic communities, the impact of food deficits on the nutritional status of civilians may be severe, particularly in sub-Saharan Africa (see Exhibit 11-1). If adverse climatic factors intervene, as often happened

---

Exhibit 11-1 | **Central African Republic**

The Central African Republic (CAR), a landlocked country of just 4 million people, has the most grim human development indicators in the region. A low-income country, it is ranked 178 out of 179 countries in the 2008 UNDP Human Development Index. Repeated political and economic crises—including four coups in the last decade—have devastated the country and resulted in an overall deterioration of living conditions. The country lacks basic services, and hospitals have only the most rudimentary equipment and medicine. The security situation is precarious especially in the north, an area characterized by the flow of arms and acts of violence. An estimated 85,000 of the more than 200,000 IDPs within CAR have returned to their villages of origin or resettled elsewhere, while there are 108,000 still too scared to return.

The scarcity of food resources lies at the heart of this vicious poverty cycle. Although the country's potential agricultural output is more than adequate to feed the entire population, the incessant burning of villages, agricultural fields, and food storehouses by armed groups has terrorized local farmers to the point where agricultural production is very limited. Whereas CAR once exported meat to Europe, it now has to import meat.

A World Food Programme (WFP) assessment (May–June 2009) indicated that 30% of the population were food insecure, with the highest concentration of food-insecure households being found in the Ouham-Pende and Gribingui provinces, in the northwest part of CAR. Furthermore, insecurity in neighboring DRC at the end of 2009 led to 17,000 refugees fleeing from the Equateur province to CAR. A decline in the mining industry in southwest CAR, as a result of the economic crisis, has also led to unemployment and a loss of income, negatively affecting the affected households' purchasing power and further aggravating the already precarious food security situation. Conditions have been exacerbated by high food prices, which further restricts food access. Reports indicate that there are high levels of malnutrition in CAR.

At 6.2%, the country has one of the highest HIV prevalence rates in the African subregion. The UNDP Human Development report shows life expectancy in CAR is 39 years, and has decreased by an average of 5 months per year since 1988.

Source: Food and Agriculture Organization. (2010, March). Global Information and Early Warning System.

in drought-prone countries such as Sudan, Somalia, Mozambique, and Zimbabwe, the outcome may be catastrophic famine.

Famine may be defined as high malnutrition and mortality rates resulting from inadequate availability of food. Lack of food availability may result from either insufficient production or inadequate or inequitable distribution.

In Eastern Europe, when economic and political turmoil followed the collapse of the Soviet Union and its allies during the 1990s, currencies were devalued and the price of staple foods increased dramatically. Persons on fixed incomes, especially elderly pensioners and families with unemployed adults, found that their purchasing power was dramatically reduced. This resulted in a large proportion of the population subsisting on inadequate diets. In industrialized countries affected by armed conflict, urban residents may be at higher risk than rural communities. For example, the 380,000 citizens of besieged Sarajevo in 1992 required approximately 270 metric tons (MT) of external food aid per day. However, in late 1992, an average of 216 MT of food was delivered daily, providing approximately 2,024 kilocalories per person per day, or 75% of the minimum average winter energy requirements (Toole, Galson, & Brady, 1993). In countries subject to sanctions or blockades, such as Armenia and Iraq during the 1990s, urban families are at particularly high risk of nutritional deficiencies.

When food aid programs are established, inequitable distribution of these resources may occur due to political factors, food stores may be damaged or destroyed, food may be stolen or diverted to military forces, and the distribution of food aid may be obstructed (Macrae & Zwi, 1994). The resulting food shortages may cause prolonged hunger and eventually drive families from their homes in search of relief. There have been many examples of food aid diversion, including in Mozambique and Ethiopia in the 1980s and in Sudan and the former Yugoslavia in the 1990s and in the first years of the twenty-first century. Indeed, in latter-day CEs, targeting of relief assistance and the use of humanitarian aid as a resource that enables the warring parties to continue their violence poses an ongoing challenge for humanitarian agencies.

Population Displacement

A common response by families and communities to civil conflict is to flee the violence. Individuals may flee because they fear persecution due to their particular political beliefs, ethnicity, or religion. In some societies, migration of part of the family to a safer area may be a traditional coping mechanism, with adult males staying behind to care for their land and animals. Some of these men may also be directly involved in the conflict. Mass migration and food shortages have been responsible for most deaths following civil conflicts in Africa and Asia.

Under several international conventions, refugees are defined as persons who flee their country of origin through a well-founded fear of persecution for reasons of race, religion, social class, or political beliefs (but not for economic reasons). The number of dependent refugees under the protection and care of the UNHCR steadily increased from approximately 6 million in 38 countries in 1980 to more than 17 million in 1992. By 2003, that number had declined to approximately 12 million due to a number of large repatriations of refugees to their homelands (United States Committee for Refugees, 2004). Since 2004, however, the total number of refugees again increased to a new peak of 16 million in 2007, largely due to the war in Iraq. Table 11-1 notes major refugee populations as of December 2008.

Several of the world's largest ever mass migrations took place in the last decade of the twentieth century. For example, in 1991, as many as 1 million Kurdish refugees fled Iraq for Iran or Turkey following the Gulf War. By early 1993, there were at least 1.5 million refugees or displaced persons within the republics of the former Yugoslavia. Between April and July 1994, an estimated 2 million Rwandan refugees fled into Tanzania, eastern Zaire, and Burundi, provoking the most serious refugee crisis in 20 years. In the final years of the twentieth century and the first few years of the new millennium, major refugee flows occurred out of Kosovo, Timor Leste, Sudan, Sierra Leone, and Côte d'Ivoire. Between March and June 1999, approximately 780,000 ethnic Albanians fled the Serbian province of Kosovo in one of the most dramatic examples of ethnic cleansing in the series of Balkan conflicts. This out-migration represented more than 50% of the Albanian population of the province prior to the war.

In June 1999, approximately 400,000 Kosovars spontaneously repatriated to their homes within 2 weeks of the end of the NATO bombing campaign. During the violence and destruction that followed the August 1999 referendum on independence in Timor Leste, between 300,000 and 400,000 people were displaced (almost 50% of the population), of whom approximately 260,000 were forcibly moved into Indonesian-controlled West Timor. Other large refugee populations during this period included hundreds of thousands of Somalis in Kenyan camps and

Table 11-1	Origins of 12 Major Refugee Populations, December 2008	
Country of Origin	**Main Countries of Asylum**	**Estimated Number**
Palestinians	West Bank, Gaza, Jordan, Lebanon	3,222,000
Afghanistan	Iran, Pakistan, India, western Europe	2,739,000
Iraq	Syria, Jordan, Iran, Saudi Arabia	1,854,000
Myanmar (Burma)	Thailand, Bangladesh, India	733,000
Somalia	Kenya, Sudan, Djibouti	520,000
Sudan	Chad, Uganda, Ethiopia, Kenya	388,000
Colombia	Venezuela, Ecuador	383,000
Democratic Republic of Congo (DRC)	Congo-Brazzaville, Angola, Burundi, Central African Republic, Rwanda	361,000
Vietnam	China	319,000
Burundi	Tanzania, DRC, Rwanda, Zambia	273,000
Eritrea	Ethiopia, Saudi Arabia	212,000
Angola	DRC, Namibia, Zambia	148,000

Source: United States Committee for Refugees. (2009). *World Refugee Survey, 2009*. Washington, DC: Author.

approximately 500,000 Burmese refugees along the Thai–Burma border.

In the first decade of the twenty-first century, most of the large refugee populations were in the Middle East and Central and South Asia. The countries hosting the six largest refugee populations in 2008 were Pakistan (1.8 million), Syria (1.7 million), Gaza Strip (1 million), Iran (990,000), West Bank (760,000), and Jordan (620,000). Lebanon was hosting a further 330,000 refugees (United States Committee for Refugees, 2009).

In early 2011, two new African refugee crises occurred – in Libya and Côte d'Ivoire. In February 2011, anti-government protests erupted in Libya and soon turned violent. The conflict escalated and triggered a massive outflow of people to neighboring countries, especially Tunisia to the west and Egypt to the east. By late March, some 320,000 people had fled from Libya, mostly migrant workers from Egypt and Tunisia but included many more nationalities (UNHCR, 2011).

In Côte d'Ivoire, the main rivals in the November 2010 presidential election, incumbent Laurent Gbagbo and opposition leader Alassane Ouattara, both claimed victory. While the international community recognized Ouattra as the victor, Gbagbo refused to resign. In the first three months of 2011, fighting between supporters of the presidential rivals in the countryside and in the commercial capital,

Abidjan, accelerated forced displacement. By late March, there were an estimated 500,000 people displaced within the country. The number of Ivorian refugees in Liberia had leapt to 123,000, while other countries, such as Ghana and Togo, were accepting people fleeing Côte d'Ivoire (UNHCR, 2011).

In addition to those persons who meet the international definition of refugees, millions of people have fled their homes for the same reasons as refugees but remain internally displaced in their countries of origin. It has not proved easy to ascertain the number and location of the world's IDPs, owing not only to definitional difficulties, but also to several institutional, political, and operational obstacles. Unlike with the collection of refugee statistics, a task undertaken by UNHCR, no single UN agency has assumed responsibility for data collection related to internally displaced populations—or, for that matter, for their protection. The question of internal displacement is also a politically sensitive one. Governments are often unwilling to admit to the presence of such populations in their territory, as they may be considered an indicator of the state's failure to protect its citizens. IDPs may themselves be reluctant to report to or register with the local authorities. Indeed, some evidence suggests that a large proportion of the world's IDPs live not in highly visible camps, but rather mingled with family members and friends, often in urban areas where they can enjoy a higher degree of anonymity.

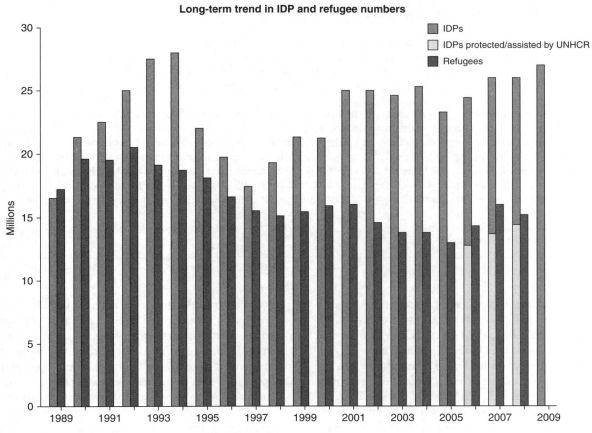

Figure 11-2 Long-Term Trend in IDP and Refugee Numbers
Source: IDMC, USCR, UNHRC, UNRWA

Finally, some very obvious obstacles to the collection of data exist in areas affected by ongoing armed conflicts. In the combat zones of Liberia, Somalia, Sierra Leone, and Darfur (Sudan), for example, the international presence was minimal or nonexistent, making it extremely difficult even to provide rough estimates of the number of people who have been displaced. Thus, in Sierra Leone, the statistics were based on food aid beneficiary lists and probably reflect only a fraction of the displaced population. In other situations, such as in Chechnya, IDPs are highly mobile, again making it very difficult to determine their exact numbers at any moment in time.

Despite all of these difficulties in data collection, there was a broad international consensus that the global population of IDPs in 2009 stood somewhere in the region of 27 million (Internal Displacement Monitoring Centre,[2] 2010): as many as 11 million

IDPs in Africa, 4 million in the Middle East, approximately 2 million each in Asia and Europe, and as many as 3 million in the Americas, almost all in Colombia. In Sudan, as of May 2010, at least 4.9 million Sudanese people were internally displaced in Darfur, the Greater Khartoum area, South Kordofan, and the 10 states of South Sudan, with unknown numbers of internally displaced people in the other northern and eastern states. The Sudanese IDPs make up one of the two largest internally displaced populations in the world, alongside that of Colombia. Some people have been displaced for more than two decades, while others were newly displaced in 2009 and 2010 (Internal Displacement Monitoring Centre, 2010). Figure 11-2 shows the trend in IDP and refugee numbers between 1989 and 2009.

The final stages of the Sri Lankan civil war created 250,000 internally displaced persons who were transferred to camps in Vavuyina District and detained against their will for many months (see Exhibit 11-2).

[2] www.internal-displacement.org

Exhibit 11-2 | **Crisis Traps IDPs in Sri Lanka**

During the first half of 2009, Sri Lanka's 26-year conflict in the north of the country intensified. Fighting between the Sri Lankan army and the Liberation Tigers of Eelam (LTTE) trapped around 70,000 civilians in a small coastal stretch of land in the north Vanni region. The UN estimated that 4,500 civilians were killed and 12,000 injured during the final stages of the conflict. The International Committee of the Red Cross (ICRC) was the only humanitarian aid agency permitted access to the area.

Eventually, LTTE forces were defeated and the fighting ceased. In the immediate aftermath, approximately 250,000 civilians were displaced and held in camps for as long as 12 months. In 5 days alone, from May 16 to 20, 2009, 77,000 people emerged from the former conflict zone in northern Sri Lanka arriving in Vavuniya District, where MSF was one of the aid agencies working with this population. MSF provided surgical and medical support to the 400-bed Vavuniya Hospital, which at one point housed 1,900 inpatients. To ease the congestion, MSF established a 100-bed field hospital. The main cause of hospitalization among the 3,000 patients admitted to the MSF hospital from June to the end of November 2009 was trauma and wounds. In total, more than 1,350 surgical procedures were performed during that time in the MSF hospital.

Source: Medical emergency in Sri Lanka [Editorial]. (2009). *Lancet*, *373*, 1399; MSF Australia. (2009, December 14). Field news. Sri Lanka: Situation update. Retrieved from www.msf.org.au

---

IDPs lack the international protection afforded by the international conventions and protocols on refugees. Nevertheless, the Geneva Conventions and certain articles of the United Nations Charter do extend some protection to IDPs. During the 1990s, the UN took some extraordinary measures to protect these populations in South Sudan, northern Iraq, the republics of the former Yugoslavia, Somalia, and Timor Leste. There have been few such UN interventions since 2000, however.

Prior to 1990, most of the world's refugees had fled countries that ranked among the poorest in the world, such as Afghanistan, Cambodia, Mozambique, and Ethiopia. However, during the following decade, an increasing number of refugees originated in relatively more developed countries, such as Kuwait, Iraq, the former Yugoslavia, Armenia, Georgia, and Azerbaijan. Despite their better economic circumstances, the reasons for the flight of these refugees generally remained the same as those for their poorer counterparts—war, civil strife, and persecution. Hunger, although sometimes a primary cause of population movements, is all too frequently only a contributing factor. For example, during 1992, although severe drought in southern Africa and the Horn of Africa affected food production in all countries in those regions, only in war-torn Mozambique and Somalia did millions of hungry inhabitants migrate in search of food.

The World Bank estimates that between 90 million and 100 million people around the world have been forcibly displaced over the past decade as a result of large-scale development initiatives such as dam construction, urban development, and transporta-

tion programs. An unknown number have also been uprooted by lower-profile forestry, mining, game park, and land-use conversion projects. The scale of such displacement seems unlikely to diminish in the future, given the processes of economic development, urbanization, and population growth that are taking place in many low- and middle-income countries.

The most common response to mass population movements, either across international boundaries or within countries, has been to establish camps or settlements. In Eastern Europe, many refugees and IDPs have been housed in hotels, resort camps, schools, and hostels, where environmental conditions have been relatively good. In contrast, in low-income countries, most refugees and displaced persons have been placed in camps located in inappropriate border areas. Exceptions include Mozambican refugees in Malawi in the 1980s, Liberian refugees in Guinea in the early 1990s, and Kosovar Albanians in Macedonia and Albania in 1999. In all three situations, at least 50% of refugees were housed in local villages.

Conditions in camps have varied enormously. In general, camps with fewer than 20,000 residents have had more favorable environmental conditions than larger camps. Camps for Rwandan refugees in eastern Zaire in 1994 contained as many as 300,000 persons; they were poorly planned and laid out, with inadequate sanitation and poor access to clean water. Relief program managers found it difficult, if not impossible, to establish equitable systems of distribution of commodities, such as food and shelter materials, and violence and other crimes ran rampant within the camps. By contrast, smaller refugee camps in Burundi were more easily managed and suffered fewer health consequences related to environmental conditions.

In addition to poor environmental conditions, crowded camps promote the spread of many communicable diseases, such as measles and acute respiratory infections. The overwhelming nature of these large camps also tends to promote a sense of loss of dignity and independence among mostly rural refugees and induces mental health disorders such as anxiety and depression.

Destruction of Public Utilities

Wars often involve the intentional or accidental destruction of public utilities, such as water and sewage systems, electricity sources and distribution grids, and fuel supplies. Although these disruptions mainly affect urban areas, local water supplies have also been destroyed in rural conflicts, such as in Somalia during the early 1990s. Moreover, land mines have sometimes intentionally been laid close to public water outlets. During the long internal conflicts in Mozambique and Angola, large cities and towns were targeted by guerrilla forces, resulting in nonfunctioning public utilities for many years. During the last two decades of the twentieth century, cities in Lebanon, Bosnia and Herzegovina, Chechnya, Somalia, Sudan, Kuwait, Iraq, Serbia, and Kosovo were perhaps the most severely affected. In September 1999, Dili, the capital of newly independent Timor Leste, was virtually destroyed in the ensuing violence.

Between 1992 and 1995, in Sarajevo (the capital) and other large cities in Bosnia and Herzegovina, municipal water supplies were destroyed by shelling; similar breakdowns in sewage systems and cross-contamination of piped water supplies led to widespread contamination of drinking water. These problems were compounded by the lack of electricity and diesel fuel needed to run generators. In the summer of 1993, residents of Sarajevo had, on average, only 5 liters of water per person per day, compared with the minimum of 15 to 20 liters recommended by WHO, UNHCR, and the Sphere Project.

Lack of electricity as a result of CEs also adversely affects urban health services—in particular, hospital and clinic curative services. During a conflict, hospital generators are often able to supply only operating rooms and emergency rooms, further promoting a concentration of services in the area of trauma management. Routine surgical procedures, inpatient medical care, and pediatric, obstetric and gynecological, and perinatal care services deteriorate. In addition, the cold chain required to maintain immunization programs is not sustainable.

Sanctions and blockades have a similar effect on public utilities, without any physical destruction. During the winter of 1992–1993, Armenian cities, such as the capital, Yerevan, were deprived of imported fuel, including gasoline, coal, kerosene, and natural gas. Consequently, practically no electricity or cooking and heating fuels were available to private homes, even though temperatures averaged well below zero Celsius (32 Fahrenheit). The cold increased the caloric requirements of individuals at a time when they faced severe food shortages. Other health effects included increased rates of acute respiratory infections.

During the first Gulf War, allied bombing damaged Iraqi sewage treatment plants and water supplies, with available potable water declining to 1.5 million cubic meters per day. Shortages of chemicals to monitor water quality contributed to outbreaks of typhoid, cholera, and gastrointestinal diseases. Later, sanctions imposed at the end of the war led to further degradation of the public health infrastructure.

Even in very poor settings, the local infrastructure may be specifically targeted by combatants. The Sudanese army, for example, deliberately destroyed hand water pumps in rebel areas, and the insurgency did likewise in government-held territory (Dodge, 1990). At the beginning of the twenty-first century, the Russian Army pounded Grozny, the capital city of Chechnya, with mortars and tanks in an attempt to defeat the separatist movement based in the territory.

Israel's three-year blockade of Gaza, commencing in 2007, led to 40% of the population being food insecure (Food and Agriculture Organization [FAO], 2009). Farmers have been unable to rebuild agricultural land or vital roads because of a lack of construction materials such as concrete and heavy equipment. Restricted access to fishing grounds has depleted catches and revenues. There are often shortages of key supplies and drugs. Delays of as long as three months occur on imports of certain types of medical equipment, such as x-ray machines and electronic devices. Clinical staff frequently lack the medical equipment they need, while medical devices are often broken, missing spare parts, or outdated.

The Effects of Armed Conflict and Political Violence on Health Services

The model presented in Figure 11-3 offers a framework for describing the health service impact of conflict and CEs. The focus here is on the health services within the countries affected by CEs; there are also related pressures and constraints on the health

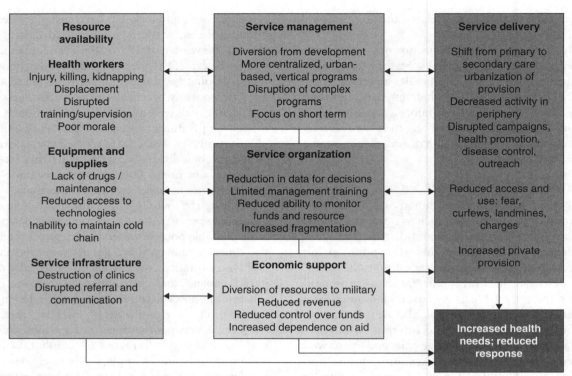

Figure 11-3 Impact of Conflict and Complex Emergencies on Health

services of host countries to which refugees may flee, however.

Access to Services

The impact of conflict on health facilities and services depends on their prior availability, distribution, and utilization patterns. Where services were originally available, as in Iraq (prior to 1991) or the former Yugoslavia (prior to 1992), the conflict may cause rapid deterioration as a result of infrastructure and distribution systems damage, resource constraints, declining health personnel availability and morale, and reductions in access. The pre-war Iraqi health system was extensive, accessible to 90% of the population, and reached 95% of the children requiring immunization (Lee & Haines, 1991). By the end of the Gulf War, many hospitals and clinics had been severely damaged or closed, those operating were overwhelmed with work, and damage to infrastructure, water supplies, electricity, and sewage disposal exacerbated problems in population health and health services activity.

Utilization is determined by geographic access (i.e., the services are not too far away), economic access (i.e., the services are affordable), and social access (i.e., no psychological or other barriers pre-

vent use of services)—all of which may be disrupted during CEs. Peripheral services may be directly targeted, as in Mozambique (Cliff & Noormahomed, 1988) or Nicaragua (Garfield & Williams, 1992) during the 1980s. Service access may be limited by fear of physical or sexual assault or by physical restrictions on access as a result of antipersonnel land mines, curfews, and, in some cases, the encirclement of areas. In Afghanistan, the Taliban imposed constraints on women accessing services that were previously available to them. In other settings, access may be restricted as a result of fear, insecurity, or lack of confidence in service providers. People injured in civil or political conflict may avoid using public services that carry a risk of security force surveillance. For example, in the Philippines and the occupied Palestinian territories, NGOs established alternative health services to allow those persons who were injured during uprisings against repressive regimes to seek care without fear of detection and detention.

Conflict may seriously disrupt links between services operating at different levels. For example, referrals may be disrupted by logistical and communication constraints, as well as physical and military barriers to access. Towns and cities may be besieged, with entry and exit controlled by militias, as in Beirut,

Sarajevo, and Juba (Sudan). Health workers may move to urban areas to seek protection, other opportunities to make a living, or opportunities to provide health services privately with greater financial returns.

Much like the situation in armed conflicts, natural disasters such as the Indian Ocean tsunami and the Haitian earthquake are often characterized by the destruction of healthcare facilities and by the need, at least in the short term, to provide care and rehabilitation for the injured. This was particularly the case in Haiti, where the need for orthopedic, neurological, and plastic surgery dominated the healthcare scene for weeks, if not months. At the same time, the need for primary health care—both preventative and curative—grew because of the large number of IDPs who were without shelter and because of the deteriorating environmental and sanitation conditions.

Health Services Adaptations

Health services may be affected in a variety of ways. For example, systems within conflict areas may shift away from primary, community-based care to secondary, hospital-based services. This trend reflects the movement of healthcare providers to urban areas, increased efforts to respond to the most serious injuries and adverse health effects, and the greater difficulty of maintaining peripheral services. Even in situations where preventive care is identified as important, such as during the struggle for liberation in the Tigrayan province of Ethiopia, priority is likely to be given to dealing with the war wounded and maintaining the health of fighters (Barnabas & Zwi, 1997).

Emphasizing care and rehabilitation for war injuries indirectly de-emphasizes longer-term health development and community-based activities, including those focusing on disease control. Malaria control activities, for example, may be seriously compromised: Vector control, house spraying, environmental programs, information and education, training, and supervision may all be disrupted. Disease treatment may become nonstandardized, haphazard, incomplete, and uncoordinated, with considerable risk of the emergence of resistant organisms. These factors are especially important in relation to malaria, STIs, and tuberculosis control. Impairment of surveillance and health information systems may undermine the ability to detect unusual or exacerbated patterns of disease occurrence and to respond to them. Public health actions such as partner notification, screening, and community education efforts may be compromised. Healthcare activities may become increasingly limited to small areas or specific districts and popula-

tions, and service provision may be increasingly organized through vertical programs that allow control over activities to assess needs, deliver services, monitor performance, and track finances. The gap between better-funded vertical programs and the general health services may widen substantially, both during and in the aftermath of major conflicts.

In this environment, adaptation occurs, with other actors likely attempting to fill the gaps caused by retreating and contracting public-sector services. Indigenous healthcare providers may become more important both in their role as healers more generally and as healthcare providers. The private healthcare sector expands, both through the provision of services by nonprofit NGOs and through the hemorrhage of public-sector workers into the private sector, whether officially or unofficially.

Infrastructure

Although direct targeting of clinics, hospitals, and ambulances may be against international humanitarian law, it has nevertheless been a fixture in latter-day conflicts. In the siege of Vukovar in eastern Slavonia during the civil war in the former Yugoslavia, the hospital was seriously damaged and much of it destroyed. Related facilities, such as those necessary for water and sanitation, sewage removal, and electricity, have been directly targeted, notably in Iraq and Serbia. In Nicaragua, the insurgency destroyed the main pharmaceutical storage facility of the country in Corinto, creating a severe shortage of medications for months.

The destruction of nonhealth physical infrastructure such as roads, electrical plants, and communication systems has indirect health consequences as well. This has often been the case in the occupied Palestinian territories, as well as in other regions of active ongoing conflict. In some Iraqi hospitals, elevators did not work during energy blackouts, with the result that patients could not be moved to surgical theaters, and emergency interventions had to be delayed or take place in suboptimal conditions. The impact on health services of the electricity supply disruption instituted by NATO bombing in Serbia and Kosovo is unknown, as are the longer-term environmental and economic consequences.

Equipment and Supplies

Access to medicines and supplies is typically disrupted during conflicts. Drug shortages, especially where the medications were previously available, may lead to an increase in medically preventable causes of death, such as asthma, diabetes, and infectious diseases. Disruption to the Ugandan Essential

Drugs Management Program, which had been organized in the early 1980s, resulted in many rural dwellers who had gained access to modern medicines and vaccines being once more deprived of basic drugs. The quality of care available may suffer greatly as a consequence. In Somalia, amputations performed without administration of intravenous antibiotics led to higher rates of infection; in the former Yugoslavia, operations were performed with inadequate anesthesia. The viability of healthcare technologies, including x-rays and laboratories, may also be undermined through lack of maintenance, spare parts, skilled personnel, chemicals, and other supplies.

Additional problems may emerge as a result of the humanitarian response. Drug donations, if poorly coordinated and standardized, may lead to a large number of expired and inappropriate drugs being off-loaded in countries experiencing CEs. These medications may not be suitable for use, yet require safe and efficient disposal, placing an additional burden on the recipient country's pharmaceutical services. Another problem that typically arises results from the poor standardization of treatments; different NGOs, host government, and other services may all treat similar problems using different drugs, often with inappropriate treatment regimes, raising the risk for emergence of multidrug-resistant organisms.

Budgetary Impact

The conflict against the Ethiopian Derg led to increases in military expenditures, whose share of the government budget rose from 11.2% in 1974–1975 to 36.5% by 1990–1991, and to declines in the health budget, whose share dwindled from 6.1% in 1973–1974 to 3.5% in 1985–1986 and 3.2% in 1990–1991 (Kloos, 1992). The deterioration of the economy typically leads to reduced public expenditures, as funds are shifted into supporting the war. In Uganda, the public health budget in 1986 was only 6.4% of what it had been in the early 1970s.

In El Salvador, the proportion of the national budget allocated to health during the civil war plummeted from 10% in 1980 to 6% in 1990, and the budget available to the ministry of health, as a percentage of the gross national product, declined from 2% to 0.9%. Prior to 1980, the El Salvadoran health budget had been higher than the defense budget, but during the first year of the civil war more funds were allocated to the military than to health. At the peak of the conflict in 1986, even the official figures indicated that the military received approximately four times more money than the health sector.

Armed conflict often takes place in areas that are rich in natural resources, such as diamonds in Sierra Leone and diamonds, coffee, and coltan (columbite-tantalite) in DRC. When the conflict disrupts these industries, it deprives central governments of tax revenue that could fund essential services.

Human Resources

Injury, killing, kidnapping, and exodus of health workers are common during CEs. In many recent conflicts, health workers have been targeted by combatants; this practice has been particularly well documented in Mozambique and Nicaragua. Even if not directly targeted, health workers may flee in search of safety and security. In Uganda, half the doctors and 80% of the pharmacists left the country between 1972 and 1985 (Dodge, 1990). In Mozambique, only 80 of the 500 doctors present before independence remained after 1975 (Walt & Cliff, 1986). In Cambodia, the dictator Pol Pot's "killing fields" were specifically directed at professional and educated people, among others, with brutal and long-lasting effects; there was some, as yet unconfirmed, evidence of professionals being similarly targeted in Kosovo.

Administrative and planning capacity related to health care may be seriously undermined in CEs by a lack of data, lack of personnel, and lack of consensus-building opportunities through which policies can be negotiated, strategies developed, and planning undertaken. In the period leading up to the referendum on independence in Timor Leste, for example, the country experienced an exodus of trained health personnel. The number of doctors in the province decreased from approximately 200 in 1998 to 69 in April 1999 (4 months before the referendum) to only 20 in February 2000.

Community Involvement

In many latter-day conflicts and those of the Cold War period, which were described as "low intensity," community leaders and social structures were frequently targeted by combatants. For example, those who waged war against the Marxist Frelimo state in Mozambique attempted to reduce access to health care and educational services, which the state had prioritized as a symbol of its commitment to promoting more equitable development. A similar process took place in Nicaragua, where opposition forces targeted health and education services, whose presence was viewed as a reflection of state commitment. Local systems of democracy and accountability are often seriously disrupted and involvement in community affairs discouraged; however, in some conflicts quite the reverse occurs—notably, in the CEs in Mozambique, Vietnam, Eritrea, and Tigray.

Organizational or political responses to conflict may be positive, facilitating opportunities for health system and societal development. In the popular conflict against the Ethiopian Derg, community-based political movements in Eritrea and Tigray promoted community participation and control in decision making and facilitated the development of multisectoral health promotion strategies. The Tigrayan People's Liberation Front trained health workers and established mobile services and innovative community financing systems. Elected local governments (*baitos*) were established, which played a significant role in mobilizing and distributing resources to ensure that drugs and adequate services were available despite considerable constraints (Barnabas & Zwi, 1997).

Policy Formulation

Violent political conflict undermines the capacity to make decisions rationally and accountably. A key problem in conflict-affected settings is the wide range of actors operating in the environment and the confused lines of accountability. In typical health systems, peripheral-level services are accountable, usually within the health sector, to district or provincial health authorities; in turn, they are responsible to central health authorities. Conflict may lead to greater degrees of centralization of decision making, even though the actual need is for increasingly decentralized decision making so as to ensure that peripheral services can respond appropriately to their local context.

The policy framework within which providers and consumers of services operate may be compromised or nonexistent during a CE, leading to an inability to control and coordinate service provision. There may be a serious lack of data upon which to base important health policy decisions. Ongoing conflict may impede learning of lessons from experience, the buildup of institutional memory, and the stimulation of ongoing critical debate regarding health and social policies, both locally and in relation to current international debates. Locally available forums for debate, such as the media and professional organizations, may be controlled or less accessible. In the postconflict setting, a key challenge is to reestablish these forums for debate and to facilitate the exchange of ideas among the range of important stakeholders operating in the health environment.

New Actors

During internal conflicts, due to scarcity of resources and government difficulties in accessing populations under the control of insurgents, NGOs usually fill part of the vacuum left by disruptions in the public sector. In recent conflict-related emergencies, various military forces have played a direct role in providing relief (e.g., in northern Iraq, 1991), as have private companies contracted by government or UN agencies (e.g., in Albania and Macedonia, 1999).

The entry of these new players has further complicated the response to CEs. The role of NGOs is extremely important both during and in the aftermath of ongoing conflict. Indigenous NGOs and church groups may be among the few service providers that continue to operate during the conflict, especially in rural areas and those more directly affected by violence. A key problem, however, is that these NGOs often provide a patchwork of services that are relatively independent of the state and do not necessarily fit in with other service provision approaches or priorities. They may communicate poorly with one another, adopt different approaches and standards of care and of health worker remuneration, and focus attention mostly at a very local level, with some impact on the equity of service availability across large regions.

Health-related peace-building initiatives may provide avenues for reconnecting people and social structures, lives, and livelihoods. Although evidence for the extent and limitations of such approaches is slowly emerging, further critical analysis and debate are needed to determine the most effective methods.

Key research challenges are to understand how health systems adapt and respond to conflict and to determine whether positive developments can be further reinforced and sustained. For example, WHO assisted the Bosnian and Croatian healthcare systems to register and respond to the needs of disabled people during the war. These efforts should then be extended in the postwar period to ensure access to rehabilitation and social support services. Likewise, surgery services developed in response to antipersonnel land mine injuries should be extended to other forms of injury surveillance and treatment. Mechanisms to protect and maintain key elements of service provision and functioning, including information systems and supplies, are crucial to assuring ongoing system functioning. How best to promote this sustainability requires further exploration.

Specific Health Outcomes

Mortality

In this section, the impact of civil conflict and humanitarian emergencies on mortality rates will be confined to indirect causes, such as food scarcity, population displacement, destruction of health facilities and public utilities, and disruption of routine curative and preventive services. Mortality directly caused by the violence of war was discussed earlier in this chapter.

The most severe health consequences of conflict—population displacement, food scarcity, and siege situations—typically occur in the acute emergency phase, during the early stage of relief efforts, and are often characterized by extremely high mortality rates. Although the quality of the international community's disaster response efforts has steadily improved, death rates associated with forced migration have generally remained high, as demonstrated by several emergencies during the 1990s.

For example, the exodus of almost 1 million Rwandan refugees into eastern Zaire in 1994 resulted in mortality rates that were more than 30 times the rates experienced prior to the conflict in Rwanda. A series of population surveys in the DRC between 2000 and 2007 found that approximately 3.8 million people had died as a result of the conflict in that country, which began in August 1998 (Coghlan et al., 2009). Death rates were highest in the eastern zones of the country, where the conflict had been most intense. Most of these excess deaths were due to easily preventable and treatable diseases; only 2% were caused by war-related injuries.

In Darfur (Sudan), death rates among civilian populations as high as 9.5 per 10,000 population per day were recorded (20 times higher than baseline mortality rates) in 2003. In contrast to the situation in DRC, between 68% and 93% of deaths in Darfur populations were due to violence (Depoortere et al., 2004). In 2004, the crude mortality rate (CMR) in three camps for IDPs in Darfur ranged between 2.0 and 3.2 per 10,000 population per day (Grandesso, Sanderson, Kruijt, Koene, & Brown, 2004). In 2008, the CMR in the same three camps ranged from 0.6 to 0.8 per 10,000 population per day (Complex Emergencies Database [CEDAT], 2008). Since 2005, most deaths have been due to communicable diseases.

Crude mortality rates have been estimated from burial site surveillance; administrative, hospital, and burial records; community-based reporting systems; and population surveys. The many problems in estimating mortality under emergency conditions have included the following:

- Poorly representative or inaccurate population sample surveys
- Failure of families to report all deaths for fear of losing food ration entitlements
- Inaccurate estimates of affected populations for the purpose of calculating mortality rates
- Lack of standard reporting procedures

In general, however, mortality rates have tended to be underestimated because deaths are usually underreported or undercounted, and population size is often exaggerated.

Early in an emergency, when mortality rates are elevated, the CMR is usually expressed as deaths per 10,000 population per day (CDC, 1992). The median annual CMR in low- and middle-income countries is approximately 9 per 1,000, corresponding to a daily rate of approximately 0.25 per 10,000 (Reed & Keeley, 2001). A threshold of 1 per 10,000 per day has been used commonly to define an elevated CMR and to characterize a situation as an emergency (CDC, 1992). In one of the most severe refugee emergencies of the 1990s, the CMR among Rwandan refugees during the first month after their arrival in eastern Zaire was between 27 and 50 per 10,000 per day (Goma Epidemiology Group, 1995).

The most reliable estimates of mortality rates have come from well-defined and secure refugee camps where there is a reasonable level of camp organization and a designated agency has assumed responsibility for the collection of data (Table 11-2). The most difficult situations in which to monitor rates have been those in which IDPs have been scattered over a wide area and where surveys could take place only in relatively secure zones (Table 11-3). These safe zones may have sometimes acted as magnets for the most severely affected elements of a population. For example, in 1998, a survey in Ajiep, southern Sudan, found that the CMR increased from 17.8 per 10,000 population per day during the period June 3 to July 11, to 69.7 per 10,000 per day between July 12 and July 20 (Brown, Moren, & Paquet, 1999). This increase may have been caused by an influx of displaced persons reaching Ajiep in a poor condition or a decrease in the food available within the town. Alternatively, it is possible that the worst-affected communities may have been in areas that were inaccessible to those performing the surveys. In either case, it has proved difficult to extrapolate the findings of surveys on mortality conducted in specific locations to broader populations in conflict-affected countries. Extensive differences in mortality survey methods have also been identified; for example, an evaluation of 23 field surveys performed in Somalia between 1991 and 1993 found wide variation in the target populations, sampling strategies, units of measurement, methods of rate calculation, and statistical analysis (Boss, Toole, & Yip, 1994).

Trends in death rates over time have varied from place to place. In refugee populations where the international response has been prompt and effective, such as was the case for Cambodians in eastern

Table 11-2	Estimated Daily Crude Mortality Rates (Deaths per 10,000 Population per Day) in Selected Refugee Populations, 1991–2009		
Period	**Country of Asylum**	**Country of Origin**	**Mean CMR for Period**
June 1991	Ethiopia	Somalia	2.3[a]
March–May 1991	Turkey	Iraq	4.7[b]
March–May 1991	Iran	Iraq	2.0[c]
March 1992	Kenya	Somalia	7.4[a]
March 1992	Nepal	Bhutan	3.0[d]
August 1992	Zimbabwe	Mozambique	3.5[e]
December 1993	Rwanda	Burundi	3.0[f]
August 1994	DRC	Rwanda	19.6–31.3[g]
May 1999	Albania	Yugoslavia (Kosovo)	0.5[h]
November 1999	Indonesia (Tuapukan Camp, West Timor)	East Timor	2.1[i]
September 2004	Chad	Darfur, Sudan	1.3[j]
July–September 2008	Chad (19 camps)	Darfur, Sudan	0.2–0.6[k]
November 2009	Syria	Iraq	0.2[l]

Note: CMR = crude mortality rate.
[a]Toole & Waldman (1993).
[b]CDC, 1991b.
[c]Babille et al., 1994.
[d]Marfin et al., 1994.
[e]CDC, 1993b.
[f]CDC, 1994.
[g]Goma Epidemiology Group, 1995.
[h]UN Administrative Committee on Coordination, Sub-Committee on Nutrition (ACC/SCN), 1999.
[i]WHO, 2000a.
[j]UN Standing Committee on Nutrition, 2004d.
[k]UN Standing Committee on Nutrition, 2009a, 2009b.
[l]UN Standing Committee on Nutrition, 2010.

Thailand (1979) and Iraqis on the Turkish border (1991), death rates declined to baseline levels within 1 month. In contrast, among refugees in Somalia (1980) and Sudan (1985), death rates remained well above baseline rates 6 to 9 months after the influx of refugees occurred (Toole & Waldman, 1990). In the case of 170,000 Somali refugees in Ethiopia in 1988–1989, death rates actually increased significantly 6 months after the influx. This increase was associated with elevated malnutrition prevalence rates, inadequate food rations, and high incidence rates of certain communicable diseases. Although initial death rates among Rwandan refugees in eastern Zaire were extremely high, they declined dramatically within 1 to 2 months (Figure 11-4). Surveys in Darfur, Sudan, in 2004 showed that mortality was higher in the pre-displacement period and generally declined once

people reached refugee or IDP camps (Depoortere et al., 2004).

Most deaths have occurred among children younger than 5 years of age. For example, 65% of deaths among Kurdish refugees on the Turkish border occurred in the 17% of the population younger than 5 years (Yip & Sharp, 1993). However, in some refugee situations, such as Goma during the first month after the refugee exodus, mortality rates were comparable in all age groups because the major cause of death was cholera, which is equally lethal at any age. Among IDPs in countries affected by severe famine, high adult mortality has been reported. For example, in the Somali town of Baidoa, 59% of the 15,105 deaths reported between August 1992 and February 1993 involved adults (Collins, 1993). In Ajiep, southern Sudan, the CMR among IDPs in

Table 11-3	Estimated Crude Mortality Rates (Deaths per 10,000 Population per Day), Internally Displaced Populations, 1991–2009	
Period	**Country (Region)**	**CMR for Period**
April 1991–March 1992	Somalia (Merca)	4.6[a]
April–November 1992	Somalia (Baidoa)	16.9[b]
April 1992–March 1993	Sudan (Ayod)	7.7[c]
April 1993	Bosnia and Herzegovina (Sarajevo)	1.0[d]
May 1995	Angola (Cafunfo)	8.3[e]
February 1996	Liberia (Bong)	5.5[f]
May 1998	Burundi (Cibitoke)	3.3[g]
June 3–July 20, 1998	Sudan (Ajiep)	26.0[h]
September 2001	Sierra Leone (Kono district)	1.4[i]
June 2002	Angola (Muacanhica, Muahimbo, Luena)	2.9–7.2[j]
February 2002	Sudan (Jonglei)	7.2[j]
April 2003	DRC (Katanga)	1.9[k]
April 2004	Sudan (Wade Saleh, Darfur)	3.6[l]
May 2008	Somalia (Afgoi and Merka)	1.0[m]
June 2008	South Darfur, Sudan (four sites)	0.75[n]
May–July 2009	North Darfur, Sudan (five sites)	0.3–0.7[o]

[a]Manoncourt et al., 1992.
[b]Moore et al., 1993.
[c]CDC, 1993c.
[d]CDC, 1993a.
[e]UN Administrative Committee on Coordination, Sub-Committee on Nutrition (ACC/SCN), 1995a.
[f]UN ACC/SCN, 1996.
[g]UN ACC/SCN, 1998.
[h]Epicentre and MSF France, in UN ACC/SCN, 1999.
[i]UN ACC/SCN, 2002a.
[j]UN ACC/SCN, 2002b
[k]UN ACC/SCN, 2003.
[l]UN Standing Committee on Nutrition, 2004b.
[m]UN Standing Committee on Nutrition, 2009a.
[n]UN Standing Committee on Nutrition, 2009b.
[o]UN Standing Committee on Nutrition, 2010.

August 1998 was equal to the under-5 mortality rate (Murphy& Salama, 1999). In most reports from refugee camps, mortality rates have not been stratified by sex; however, the surveillance system for Burmese refugees in Bangladesh did estimate sex-specific death rates, demonstrating considerably higher death rates in females. Gendered analyses that take into account differences in the sociocultural position of women have been rare in emergency settings.

The major reported causes of death among refugees and displaced populations have been diarrheal diseases, measles, acute respiratory infections, and malaria, exacerbated by high rates of malnutrition. These diseases consistently account for 60% to 95% of all reported causes of death in these populations. Measles epidemics led to high death rates among refugees during the 1980s. Epidemics of severe diarrheal disease have been increasingly common and contributed to high mortality. Cholera case fatality ratios (CFRs) in refugee camps have ranged between 3% and 30%, and dysentery CFRs have been as high as 10% among young children and the elderly.

In eastern European conflicts, much of the mortality among civilians was caused by trauma associ-

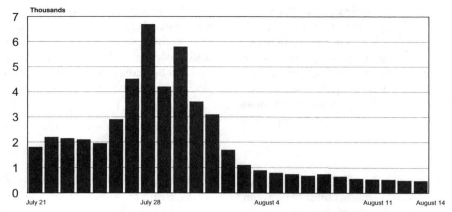

Figure 11-4 Number of Deaths per Day, July 21 to August 14, 1994, Rwandan Refugees, North Kivu Camps, Zaire.
Source: Goma Epidemiology Group, "Public Health Impact of Rwandan Refugee Crisis: What Happened in Goma, Zaire, in July 1994?" 1995, *Lancet*, 345, pp. 339–344. Reproduced with permission.

ated with the violence. Nevertheless, there was also increased mortality in these conflicts due to the collapse of the public health system. Chronic conditions, such as cardiovascular diseases, cancer, and renal conditions, were inadequately treated because the health system was focused on the management of war-related injuries. Medical services in most parts of Bosnia and Herzegovina became overwhelmed by the demands of war casualties. The major hospital in Zenica reported that the proportion of all surgical cases associated with trauma steadily increased after the beginning of the war in April 1992, reaching 78% in November 1992. Preventive health services, including childhood immunization and antenatal care, ceased in many areas. Hospitals were systematic military targets in some areas, and in Sarajevo, 38 of the original 42 ambulances were destroyed (Toole et al., 1993).

The collapse of health services in Bosnia and Herzegovina had significant public health effects. For example, perinatal mortality increased in Sarajevo from 16 deaths per 1,000 live births in 1991 to 27 per 1,000 during the first 4 months of 1993. The rate of premature births increased from 5.3% to 12.9%, the stillbirth rate increased from 7.5 per 1,000 to 12.3 per 1,000, and the average birth weight decreased from 3,700 g (8.2 lb) to 3,000 g (6.6 lb) during the same period (CDC, 1993a).

Recently, CEs have occurred without excess mortality being reported among displaced populations. For example, although mortality rates among Kosovar refugees in Albania and Macedonia remained less than 1 death per 10,000 population per day, significant threats to the health of the affected populations were present. It is important to continue to monitor

the changing epidemiology during the emergency phase and to be prepared to provide assistance targeted at the highest-priority problems.

Nutrition

Nutritional deficiencies are often the first public health effects of an evolving CE. Economic and political turmoil leads to food scarcity among vulnerable groups, as described earlier in this chapter. In many countries experiencing political and economic crises, certain ethnic groups are disadvantaged, as well as unemployed and institutionalized individuals. In Africa and Asia, nomadic communities are often forced to sell their animals and other food reserves. Among refugees and IDPs, a variety of factors might lead to high rates of nutritional deficiency disorders, including prolonged food scarcity prior to and during displacement, delays in the provision of complete rations, problems with registration and estimation of the size of an affected population, and inequitable distribution systems.

In the emergency phase, acute energy depletion is a life-threatening condition and will lead to excess mortality. A critical factor is the synergy between malnutrition and infection; thus malnutrition prevalence may be increased by high rates of infectious diseases, such as measles, diarrhea, dysentery, acute respiratory infections, malaria, and helminth infestation. Infections, by comparison, lead to decreased appetite and increased metabolic rate; thus they exacerbate acute malnutrition.

These factors may differentially affect certain demographic groups within the population. The most commonly encountered vulnerable groups include children younger than 5 years of age, pregnant and lactating women, the elderly, unaccompanied children, the disabled, the chronically ill (e.g., tuberculosis- and HIV-infected patients), households lacking an adult male, and disadvantaged ethnic or religious groups. In the later stages of famine, there may be a high prevalence of acute malnutrition among adolescents and adults. In high-income countries, the elderly are often most vulnerable, especially those living alone on fixed incomes.

Malnutrition

In estimating the prevalence of acute malnutrition in a population, the prevalence among children between 6 months and 5 years of age is typically used as a surrogate. This approach is used because the relationship between weight and height in this age group is generally similar in all ethnic groups provided those children have access to adequate food. International reference tables may be used to define various degrees of acute malnutrition.

The prevalence of moderate to severe acute malnutrition in a random sample of children between 6 months and 5 years of age (or 110 cm in height) is generally a reliable indicator of this condition in a population. Because weight is more sensitive to sudden changes in food availability than height, nutritional assessments during CEs focus on measuring weight for height. Moderate to severe acute malnutrition is defined as a weight-for-height measurement more than 2 standard deviations below the mean of the U.S. CDC, National Center for Health Statistics, and WHO reference population (Z-score less than 22) (WHO, 1995). Severe acute malnutrition is defined as a weight-for-height measurement more than 3 standard deviations below the reference mean (Z-score less than 23).

All children with edema are classified as having severe acute malnutrition. As a screening measurement, the middle upper arm circumference (MUAC) may also be used to assess acute malnutrition, although there is not complete agreement on which cutoff values should be used as indicators. Field studies indicate that a MUAC between 12.0 cm and 12.5 cm correlates with a weight-for-height Z-score of 22; the lower figure (12.0 cm) is more appropriate in children younger than 2 years of age (WHO, 2009). Acute malnutrition without edema has been termed wasting or marasmus, and acute malnutrition with edema has been termed kwashiorkor; however, a combination of the two conditions may occur in some children. Both are associated with anemia, although this complication is often more severe in children (or adults) with kwashiorkor. The anemia may be exacerbated by local conditions, such as malaria and hookworm infection.

A meeting was convened in Nairobi in 2001 by the United Nations Sub-Committee on Nutrition to review the assessment of nutritional status in adults and adolescents. The meeting recommended that assessment of adult malnutrition should be considered under the following circumstances:

- If the crude mortality rate increases in relation to the under-five mortality rate
- If many adults are present at existing supplementary feeding centers
- If very high rates of under-five malnutrition are noted in the absence of an epidemic outbreak
- If reasonable doubt exists that the child malnutrition rates do not reflect the nutritional status of the general population
- If the populations are entirely reliant on food aid and if data are required as an advocacy tool to leverage resources

The recommended indices that should be used are Cormic-adjusted body mass index (BMI) (population specific or Norgan correction) and MUAC. The Cormic index (calculated as the ratio of sitting height to standing height) may, to some extent, adjust for ethnic differences in body proportions; however, the validity of this technique has not been studied in adolescents (Woodruff & Duffield, 2000). Clinical criteria are recommended for screening adults and adolescents for severe malnutrition so as to determine the need for therapeutic feeding. In surveys of prepubertal adolescents, the extended weight-for-height chart developed by Action Contre la Faim (ACF) should be used. Moderate acute malnutrition is defined as a weight for height between 70% and 79% of the reference median (Z-scores are not used in this age group), and severe malnutrition as less than 70% of the median (Golden, 1999a).

Postpubertal adolescents and adults should be assessed using the BMI, which is the weight in kilograms divided by the height (in meters) squared (w/h^2). Genetic differences between ethnic groups are probably more significant among older age groups than among children younger than 5 years of age, so the use of an international BMI reference poses considerable problems. For example, UNHCR and CDC conducted a nutrition survey of adolescents aged 10 to 19 years in four camps in Kenya housing Sudanese and Somali refugees. Comparing the BMI of the sampled adults to the WHO BMI-for-age reference population (which is based on Americans) and using the recommended cutoff, the prevalence of acute malnutrition was estimated to be between 57% and 61%.

The morbidity and mortality data, however, did not support these high estimates. Based on this finding, the researchers strongly suggested that the WHO reference might not be appropriate for comparisons of all adolescents worldwide (Bhatia & Woodruff, 1999). As a consequence, BMI for age is not currently recommended as a screening index (Golden, 1999a). MUAC for age is also a problematic screening tool in adolescents because there are no agreed-upon cutoff points to define acute malnutrition.

MUAC is commonly used as a screening tool in adult populations. A MUAC of less than 23 cm in men and less than 22 cm in women has been proposed as indicating moderate malnutrition (corresponding to BMI values of less than 17). MUAC values of less than 20 cm in men and less than 19 cm in women have been proposed as indicators of severe wasting, corresponding to BMIs of less than 13 (Ferro-Luzzi & James, 1996). In any event, one reliable clinical sign of severe malnutrition commonly observed in adults is inability to stand.

In some settings, refugee children who were adequately nourished upon arrival in camps have developed acute malnutrition due to either inadequate food rations or severe epidemics of diarrheal disease. In early 1991, the prevalence of acute malnutrition among Kurdish refugee children aged 12 to 23 months increased from less than 5% to 13% during a 2-month period following a severe outbreak of diarrheal disease (Yip & Sharp, 1993). Surprisingly, the malnutrition prevalence among children younger than 12 months was less than 4%; however, a survey revealed that the diarrhea-associated death rate in this age group was three times higher than the death rate among children 12 to 23 months of age. It seems likely that many malnourished infants died from the diarrheal disease, resulting in deceptively low malnutrition prevalence among the survivors.

Prevalences of acute malnutrition among the internally displaced have tended to be extremely high. In southern Somalia during 1992, the prevalence of acute malnutrition among children younger than 5 years in displaced persons camps in Marka and Qorioley was 75%, compared with 43% among town residents (Manoncourt et al., 1992). Among the estimated 1 million IDPs in Darfur, Sudan, acute malnutrition prevalence ranged between 12.6% and 21.5% in March–April 2004, increasing to between 20.6% and 39% in May–June 2004. Following heightened international interest and assistance to this population, rates of malnutrition generally decreased to a range of 10.7% to 23.6% by September 2004. However, 5 years later, after many humanitarian aid agencies had been expelled from Sudan, malnutrition rates increased significantly. In northern Darfur, acute malnutrition prevalence ranged from 16.9% to 34.5% according to surveys conducted between May and July 2009 (Nutrition Information in Crisis Situations [NICS] March, 2010). (Exhibit 11-3 discusses malnutrition among Sudanese refugees.) The prevalence of acute malnutrition among children younger than 5 years of age in various displaced populations is presented in Table 11-4.

Exhibit 11-3	**Sudanese Refugees in Chad, 2004–2010**

As a result of an armed conflict in Darfur, Sudan that began in early 2003, approximately 100,000 refugees fled to Chad during that year. Initially, they lived in makeshift camps and received very little international assistance. Early nutrition surveys indicated great variation between settlements; in November 2003, rates of acute malnutrition among children ranged from 7% to 27% (UN Standing Committee on Nutrition, 2004a). By May 2004, the camps were overcrowded, water and sanitation were inadequate, and an outbreak of the waterborne viral disease hepatitis E had occurred in some camps. In June 2004, a joint agency survey found the overall acute malnutrition prevalence among children to be 35.6%, with 5.5% considered severely malnourished (UN Standing Committee on Nutrition, 2004c).

By the end of 2004, more than 200,000 Darfur refugees had fled to Chad. International media attention increasingly focused on both the conflict in Darfur and the plight of refugees and IDPs. International assistance increased, and by the end of 2004, most refugees were located in 11 camps run by UNHCR. Blanket supplementary feeding was introduced for all children younger than age 5 and all pregnant and lactating women. According to food basket monitoring, the average energy content of the food ration reached 1,967 kilocalories per person per day by October 2004 (compared with an official ration of 2,063 kilocalories). A September survey in two camps found that the prevalence of acute malnutrition had dropped to 19.6%; although this represented an improvement, it remained very high by international standards (UN Standing Committee on Nutrition, 2004d).

Five years later, the CMR in all refugee camps in Chad was less than 1 death per 10,000 population per day. The prevalence of acute malnutrition ranged between 4% and 10%. In contrast, the prevalence of acute malnutrition in IDP camps across the border in Sudan remained high; between May and July 2009, it was between 17% and 34% in six camps in North Darfur.

Table 11-4	Prevalence of Acute Malnutrition Among Children Younger Than 5 Years in Internally Displaced and Conflict-Affected Populations, 1992–2004	
Date	**Country (Region)**	**Prevalence of Acute Malnutrition (%)**
1992	Southern Somalia	47–75[a]
1994	Sudan (Bahr el Ghazal)	36.1[b]
1994	Afghanistan (Sarashahi)	18.6[c]
1995	Angola (Cafunfo)	29.2[d]
1995	Liberia (Goba town, Margibi)	11.7[e]
1995	Sierra Leone (Bo)	19.8[d]
1996	Zaire (Masisi)	31.0[f]
1998	Burundi	14[g]
1999	West Timor, Indonesia	24[h]
2002	Sierra Leone (refugee camps)	6.6–22.2[i]
2003	Bay Region, Somalia	17.2[j]
2004	Darfur, Sudan	39[k]
2008	North Darfur, Sudan	14–17[m]
2009	Bandudu Province, DRC	7–20[n]

Note: Acute malnutrition is defined either as weight for height 2 standard deviations below the reference mean or less than 80% of the reference median.

[a]Toole & Waldman, 1993.

[b]Médecins sans Frontières (MSF) Belgium, in UN ACC/SCN, 1994a.

[c]MSF Holland, in UN ACC/SCN, 1994b.

[d]Action Contre la Faim (ACF), in UN ACC/SCN, 1995.

[e]MSF Holland, in UN ACC/SCN, 1995a.

[f]MSF Holland, in UN ACC/SCN, 1996.

[g]Concern International, in UN ACC/SCN, 1998.

[h]World Health Organization, Health Information Network for Advanced Planning, 2000a, 2000b.

[i]UN ACC/SCN, 2003.

[j]UN Standing Committee on Nutrition (SCN), 2004a.

[k]UN SCN, 2004c.

[l]UN SCN, 2009a.

[m]UN SCN, 2010.

Micronutrient-Deficiency Diseases

High incidence rates of several micronutrient-deficiency diseases have been reported in many refugee camps, especially in Africa. Frequently, famine-affected and displaced populations have already experienced low levels of dietary vitamin A intake and, therefore, may have very low vitamin A reserves. Furthermore, the typical rations provided in large-scale relief operations lack vitamin A, putting these populations at high risk for deficiency. In addition, those communicable diseases that are highly incident in refugee camps, such as measles and diarrhea, are known to rapidly deplete vitamin A stores. Consequently, young refugee and displaced children are at high risk of developing vitamin A deficiency.

In 1990, more than 18,000 cases of pellagra, caused by food rations deficient in niacin, were reported among Mozambican refugees in Malawi (CDC, 1991a). Despite the increased awareness of micronutrient deficiencies among relief agencies, niacin was not a component of the general food ra-

tion for IDPs in Angola in 2000. A large outbreak of pellagra was documented, with incidence among IDPs being more than twice that in the nondisplaced population (Salama, Spiegel, & Brennan, 2001).

Numerous outbreaks of scurvy (vitamin C deficiency) were documented in refugee camps in Somalia, Ethiopia, and Sudan between 1982 and 1991. Cross-sectional surveys performed in 1986–1987 reported prevalence rates as high as 45% among females and 36% among males; prevalence increased with age (Desenclos, Berry, Padt, Farah, Segala, & Nabil, 1989). The prevalence of scurvy was highly associated with the period of residence in camps, a reflection of the time exposed to rations lacking in vitamin C. Outbreaks of scurvy and beriberi were also reported among Bhutanese refugees in Nepal during 1993 (UN Administrative Committee on Coordination, Sub-Committee on Nutrition [ACC/SCN], 1995b).

Iron-deficiency anemia has been reported in many refugee populations, affecting particularly women of childbearing age and young children. For example, a survey among IDPs in Darfur, Sudan, in 2004 found that 55% of children younger than 5 years were anemic, as well as 26.2% of women of reproductive age (UN Standing Committee on Nutrition [SCN], 2004d).

Impact of Communicable Diseases

In most CEs, the high rates of excess preventable mortality have been attributed primarily to communicable diseases. The specific causes of mortality, and their age and gender distribution, do not differ from those that prevail in nonemergency conditions. Accordingly, acute respiratory infections, diarrhea, measles, and malaria have been most frequently cited as proximate causes. Although the substandard conditions found in IDP camps do not change the diseases that account for most of the morbidity and mortality in humanitarian emergency settings, they do alter epidemiologic patterns in two important ways: (1) the incidence (i.e., attack) rates of commonly occurring and potentially fatal diseases are increased, and (2) the case fatality ratios are higher than usual.

Measles

Measles has traditionally been among the most feared of communicable diseases in emergency settings. During the 1970s and 1980s, measles epidemics were common, and it was not unusual for measles to be the major cause of mortality in large, displaced populations. High incidence rates (particularly in populations with low levels of vaccination prior to displacement), high mortality rates, and unusually high CFRs are typical of measles outbreaks in emergencies. In an epidemic that occurred in the Wad Kowli refugee camp in eastern Sudan in 1985, the overall measles-specific mortality rate was 13 deaths per 1,000 population per month, and the under-five mortality was 30 per 1,000 per month. CFRs in this outbreak reportedly reached an extraordinarily high level of 33%, probably due to a combination of underlying malnutrition, including widespread vitamin A deficiency, and inadequate medical services.

Major outbreaks of measles have been uncommon in refugee camps since the late 1980s because of the high priority accorded to mass measles vaccination campaigns in the acute phase of humanitarian emergencies. Nevertheless, major measles outbreaks, resulting in high mortality rates, were reported among IDPs in Ethiopia and DRC during 2000 and 2001 because of delays in initiating vaccination campaigns (Salama, Spiegel, & Brennan, 2001). Following a decade of political turmoil, economic ruin, and a collapsed health system, Zimbabwe experienced a major measles outbreak in early 2010, with more than 300 deaths being reported.

In well-vaccinated populations, such as Bosnian and Kosovar refugees in the Balkans, Kurds in northern Iraq (1991), and Rwandans in Tanzania and eastern Zaire (1994), measles has been a less prominent public health problem.

Diarrhea

Unlike measles, which can be easily prevented, diarrheal diseases remain one of the top three causes of mortality in humanitarian emergencies. In Somalia (1979–1981), Ethiopia (1982), Sudan (1985), Malawi (1988), northern Iraq (1991), and Goma (1994), diarrheal diseases were responsible for between 25% and 85% of all mortality and also accounted for a major share of all clinic visits (70% in northern Iraq). Although most often these conditions affect young children, cholera and dysentery—the major epidemic forms of diarrhea—affect people of all ages. Of all disease conditions, diarrhea is the most closely linked to poor sanitation, inadequate water quantity, and contaminated water.

Cholera epidemics have occurred frequently in emergency settings. Although deaths due to noncholera watery diarrhea have been far more numerous, cholera, in addition to being able to cause death rapidly from dehydration, incites fear and even panic in many populations. Its ability to affect other relief activities and to divert health personnel and supplies from other activities may even contribute to higher death tolls from other diseases. Outbreaks of cholera have occurred in all parts of the world; for example, large outbreaks were recorded in India (1971), Thailand (1979), Sudan (1985), Somalia (1985), Ethiopia (1984), Malawi (1988–1991), northern Iraq (1991), Goma (1994), and Rwanda (1996). Since 2000, there have been few large outbreaks of cholera among refugees and IDPs; however, intermittent outbreaks occurred among the internally displaced in Burundi in 2004, Afghanistan in 2005, and DRC in 2008. A major cholera outbreak began in Zimbabwe in August 2008. By end of January 2010, there had been 98,741 reported cases and 4,293 deaths from this epidemic, making it the deadliest African cholera outbreak in the previous 15 years.

In many of these settings, cholera was a recurrent problem. For example, in Malawi at least 20 separate outbreaks were recorded among Mozambican refugees during a 5-year period. Investigations of these outbreaks have documented numerous modes of transmission and risk factors, including contaminated water, shared water containers, inadequately heated leftover food, insufficient soap, and funeral gatherings for cholera victims. One of the most lethal cholera epidemics ever recorded occurred among refugees in Goma, Zaire, in 1994, when it was estimated that 45,000 people (approximately 9% of the total population) died in a 3-week period. The source of contamination is believed to have been Lake Kivu, the principal source of water on which the population depended. Epidemics due to *Shigella dysenteriae* type 1 have also been reported from a number of emergency settings and contributed to the high mortality in Goma.

Acute Respiratory Infection

Acute lower respiratory infection (ALRI), or pneumonia, has been an important cause of morbidity and mortality in emergency settings, and was identified as one of the top three causes of mortality in Thailand (1979), Somalia (1980), Sudan (1985), and Honduras (1984–1987). Risk factors for ALRI outbreaks include crowded conditions, inadequate shelter, vitamin A deficiency, and indoor air pollution, especially in societies that cook indoors (such as Nepal). ALRI is undoubtedly a major cause of morbidity and mortality in cold climates, such as northern Iraq, the Balkans, and the war-torn former Soviet republics. Even though this disease is the leading cause of death among children in low-income countries, it has been less consistently reported and investigated than many other communicable diseases in emergency settings.

Malaria

In endemic areas, including Southeast Asia, the Indian subcontinent, and most of Africa, malaria consistently ranks among the leading causes of morbidity and mortality. It has been responsible for incidence rates as high as 1,034 per 1,000 per month (Thailand, 1984) and for as many as 30% of all deaths in displaced populations (Rwanda, 1994). It was the leading cause of mortality among Cambodian refugees in Thailand in 1978, Ethiopian refugees in Sudan in the mid-1980s, and Mozambican refugees in Malawi in the 1980s. It has been well established that populations who are displaced to areas of higher malaria endemicity than their place of origin have higher incidence rates and higher mortality. Following the collapse of health services during and following the conflict in East Timor, along with mass population displacement, the incidence of malaria also increased significantly. In October 1999, approximately 30% of all morbidity was attributed to malaria, compared with 10% the previous year (WHO Health Information Network for Advanced Planning [HINAP], 2000a). The oc-

currence of epidemic malaria has also been more frequent in these circumstances. There is, however, little risk of displaced populations from areas of high malaria incidence causing increases in the diseases in areas to which they are displaced, because transmission is largely vector dependent.

Major risk factors for malaria in emergency settings include the lack of adequate housing, poor siting of refugee camps (especially when they are located in marshy areas), overcrowding, proximity to livestock (which may be the primary targets of mosquito vectors), and a general lack of competently trained health personnel. Although it has not been clearly documented in emergencies, the association of malaria with low birth weight (especially in infants of first and second pregnancies) and with iron-deficiency anemia may cause increases in incidence and CFR from a variety of causes, especially in children.

High mortality was reported during severe epidemics of malaria in Burundi, Ethiopia, and Eritrea during the first few years of the twenty-first century, though this outcome was widely blamed on the continued use of antimalarial drugs that were no longer effective. In mid-2004, an international meeting of experts recommended that most countries with endemic malaria should change their first-line treatment regimen to artemesenin-based combination therapy—a recommendation that was adopted by WHO.

Meningitis

Although not a consistent problem in emergencies, the threat of meningococcal (group A) meningitis is a formidable one. Overcrowding, especially during the drier seasons of the year, can be an important risk factor for this disease, which is transmitted via the respiratory route.

In the Sakaeo camp in Thailand in 1980, a large outbreak of group A meningococcal meningitis had an attack rate of 130 per 100,000 population and an overall CFR of 28% (50% in children younger than 5 years). Other epidemics have occurred in Sudan (1989), Ethiopia (1993), and Guinea (1993). In Goma (1994), attack rates ranged from 94 to 137 per 100,000 population over a period of 2 months.

Outbreaks of meningitis tend to be protracted, lasting from 1 to 2 months. Unless they are detected and controlled at an early stage, they can be directly responsible for high mortality. In addition, outbreaks can require resource-intensive responses, thereby pulling attention away from other high-priority health programs. In early 2005, for example, an outbreak of the emerging W135 strain of meningococcus led to the vaccination of more than 150,000 Sudanese refugees in Chad.

Hepatitis E

As with meningitis, outbreaks of hepatitis E have not been frequent occurrences in emergencies but have had major consequences when they occurred. An enterically transmitted disease, usually linked to contaminated drinking water, especially when water quantity is compromised, hepatitis E is associated with a particularly high CFR in pregnant women. Clinical attack rates appear to be higher in adults, with children relatively spared. In Somalia in 1985, an outbreak of more than 2,000 cases was associated with an overall attack rate of 8% in adults. The overall CFR of 4% was more than quadrupled in pregnant women (17%). Outbreaks of similar magnitude occurred in Ethiopia (1989) and among Somali refugees in Liboi Camp, Kenya, in 1991. In the latter scenario, the overall CFR was 3.7%, but the CFR in pregnant women was 14%.

A severe epidemic occurred in 2004 among both IDPs in Darfur, Sudan, and refugees from Darfur in Chad. Starting in West Darfur in May, a total of 2,431 cases and 41 deaths (CFR = 1.7%) of suspected hepatitis E were reported from health clinics in the Greater Darfur region. The most severely affected area was West Darfur state, with 66% of the total reported cases. A survey conducted in November 2004 found a CFR of 8.2% among pregnant women with hepatitis (Boccia, Klovstad, & Guthmann, 2004). Between June and September, a total of 1,442 cases of suspected hepatitis E and 46 deaths from this cause (CFR = 3.2%) were reported from two refugee camps and neighboring villages. Investigation of the epidemic was aided by the use of a newly licensed rapid diagnostic kit.

Tuberculosis

Tuberculosis (TB) is one of the most important communicable diseases to control in the post-emergency phase. Its reemergence as a public health problem in many parts of the world has come about largely because of its close association with immune-deficiency disorders, especially HIV infection, and with the identification of multiple-drug-resistant strains. TB can be quite common in some post-emergency situations. It is highly prevalent during the emergency as well, but because of the difficulties in developing programs to control its transmission, diagnose the disease, and reliably treat it for adequate periods, other, more acute conditions are appropriately accorded priority. In Sudan in the mid-1980s and in Pakistan throughout

the protracted displacement of Afghan refugees, TB also figured prominently as a cause of morbidity and mortality.

Other Important Communicable Diseases

HIV and AIDS and other STIs are major problems among emergency-affected populations from areas where there is a high prevalence of these conditions. Until recently, a paucity of data was available on the prevalence of HIV and AIDS in refugee populations. It has been postulated that refugees and other conflict-affected populations might be at greater risk of acquiring the HIV virus because of sexual exploitation, the breakdown of traditional societies and values, and the disruption of STI treatment and condom promotion programs. Nevertheless, some evidence suggests that conflict might actually inhibit the spread of HIV (Spiegel et al., 2007). When the 20-year conflict in Angola ended in 2002, the country had a significantly lower HIV prevalence (5% to 10% in Luanda and 1% to 3% in rural areas) than all other southern African countries (15% to 40%).

The population of Sierra Leone was thought to be highly vulnerable to HIV infection, especially given the widespread sexual violence during the civil conflict in the 1990s. Indeed, HIV prevalence among sex workers in the capital, Freetown, increased from 27% in 1995 to 71% in 1997 (a period of intense conflict); HIV prevalence among women in antenatal clinics increased from 4% to 7% in the same period; and 11% of Nigerian peacekeepers returning from Sierra Leone were found to be HIV positive, a rate that was double the Nigerian prevalence at the time. However, in 2002, a rigorous study in Sierra Leone carried out by the CDC found much lower levels of HIV prevalence (1% to 4%) among the general population. The war made movement within the country and trade difficult, and this immobility may have possibly insulated most of the population from the HIV threat. Likewise, after 4 years of war and extensive documented sexual violence in Bosnia and Herzegovina, HIV prevalence in this area remained less than 0.01% in 2004.

Between 2001 and 2003, UNHCR surveys of pregnant women in 20 refugee camps in Kenya, Rwanda, Sudan, and Tanzania found lower HIV prevalence among refugees than in the surrounding population in three of the four countries (e.g., 5% versus 18% in Kenya)—in Sudan, there was no significant difference. The UN report notes that most refugees moved to the camps from low- to high-prevalence countries, that most refugees lived in remote rural areas with restricted freedom of movement, and that NGOs had mounted HIV prevention programs targeted at easily accessible, "captive" populations.

Other communicable diseases that have occurred in emergency or post-emergency settings have had a relatively minor impact on the general population. In the individual setting in which they occur, however, they command an important allocation of resources and may be important contributors to morbidity and mortality. Yellow fever, typhoid fever, relapsing fever, Japanese B encephalitis, dengue hemorrhagic fever, typhus, and leptospirosis are all real threats. Nevertheless, morbidity and mortality in CEs have been shown time and again to be due to the same conditions that are responsible for the bulk of the disease burden in low-income countries in nonemergency settings. Important aspects of efforts to control these major communicable disease problems are presented later in this chapter.

Following the Asian tsunami in 2004, there was a significant outbreak of tetanus among wounded survivors of all ages in the Aceh province of Indonesia. Between December 31, 2004, and January 25, 2005, 91 cases of tetanus were hospitalized in Banda Aceh, Meulaboh, and Sigli (WHO, 2005). The outbreak reflected the low immunization coverage in Aceh, a likely outcome of decades of armed conflict.

Injuries

Injuries are widespread in all populations and are responsible for significant mortality, morbidity, and disability. Conflicts typically conjure up images of firearm-related morbidity and mortality, but other types of weapons—as high tech as laser-guided missiles and chemical and biological warfare agents and as low tech as machetes—can cause substantial morbidity and mortality. Injuries, aside from those that are directly war and conflict related, are typically neglected in favor of an emphasis on communicable diseases. This practice is unfortunate given the widespread occurrence of intentional (homicide, war, suicide) and unintentional (falls, traffic injuries, drowning, poisoning) injuries in many populations affected by conflict. Given their exposure to firearms and other weapons, rapid and forced population movement, poor environmental conditions, and compromised safety and security, injuries of all sorts are bound to occur in these settings. In situations where injuries are shown to be major causes of morbidity and mortality, they should be addressed as vigorously as communicable diseases.

Most global attention has been focused on land mine injuries, an area in which notable international successes have been achieved. The Ottawa process has led to the effective banning of the production and distribution of antipersonnel land mines, although a number of key countries, including the United States, have refused to sign the relevant treaties. Evidence of the harmful effects of antipersonnel land mines and their concentration in the world's poorest countries, such as Angola, Ethiopia, Cambodia, and Afghanistan, has led to a dramatic increase in press and media interest and brought about the related public policy response leading into the Ottawa process.

The spontaneous repatriation of refugees to Kosovo in mid-1999 was associated with a large number of land mine deaths and injuries. Aside from evidence of deaths and disability, the costs of caring for and supporting disabled community members through the health services and, in the longer term, within the community are considerable. The opportunity costs are similarly important: Staff and equipment devoted to war surgery and specifically the treatment of injuries resulting from antipersonnel land mines could be devoted to other activities. Indeed, extending war surgery facilities introduced by organizations such as the International Committee of the Red Cross into resource-poor countries to facilitate the provision of a much wider range of treatment and rehabilitation services that would be available to those with any sort of injury is currently being promoted by WHO.

Aside from the direct health problems associated with antipersonnel land mines, they create a wide range of other problems—fear and insecurity, as well as limited access to areas affected by mines, which consequently become unavailable for agriculture and animal husbandry. Despite community knowledge of the sites of concentration of antipersonnel land mines, community members are often forced to enter these unsafe areas to collect firewood, water, or animals that have gone astray. The widespread availability of antipersonnel land mines has also led to their use for personal security, with community members in some cases using them to protect their homes at night or when they are away. In some situations, mines have been used to assist with tasks such as fishing, and children have been known to play with them. The long-term effects of land mines are serious: High levels of surgical skill and resources are required to treat persons who are injured through contact with them, and repeated refitting and modification of prostheses are necessary if disability is to be minimized.

Reproductive Health

Unfortunately, reproductive health services for refugees and displaced persons have often been considered to be secondary priorities; however, increased attention has been paid to reproductive health issues in the past five years. Although the provision of food, water, sanitation facilities, and shelter is clearly the highest priority during a complex humanitarian emergency, steps should be taken to ensure that other critical health needs of women, men, and adolescents are met as quickly as possible. Women are a particularly vulnerable subset of the population because the gender-based discrimination that is all too common in stable societies is frequently exacerbated in times of societal stress and meager resources. Uncontrolled violence and its aftermath are characterized by a number of specific features that negatively affect reproductive health, including the breakdown of family networks, the consequent loss of protection and safety, and the blocking of channels of information to adolescents and women of reproductive age.

Loss of revenue within the family can result in a restricted ability to make appropriate reproductive health choices, and may predispose women and adolescents to risk—for example, through engaging in commercial sex work. Increased or sole responsibility for the family, as manifested by an increase in the proportion of female-headed households, also changes the way women spend their time and money as they seek increased security and well-being for their families. Finally, like all members of the affected population, women tend to pay more attention to securing health services for life-saving interventions than for nonemergency reproductive health services.

A minimum initial package of essential reproductive health services has been developed and is recommended by the major relevant international agencies. Its components are described later in this chapter. Interventions beyond this essential package require major investments of time and personnel that should not be diverted from the principal task of reducing excessive preventable mortality as rapidly as possible. In all cases, special care must be taken to ensure that female heads of household are being given equitable quantities of food and nonfood commodities for themselves and their families.

Mental Health

War and political violence have both direct and indirect mental health consequences for victims, relatives, neighbors, and communities. The severity and type of mental health problems relate to the nature, intensity, and form of the violence; the relationship of the assessed person to others affected—self, family, and community members; the cause of the conflict; and the affected person's relationship to participation, victimization, or causation of the conflict. Anxiety, uncertainty, and fear about the future and about the ability of family members and homesteads to remain alive and intact are a substantial cause of distress for affected individuals and communities. Among those who are forced to flee either as refugees or as internally displaced people, the lack of knowledge about relatives and property left behind causes stress and distress. Despite the ongoing challenges of maintaining lives and livelihoods, life as a refugee, especially in a camp situation, may be monotonous and conducive to stress, anxiety, and depression.

The extent of mental health trauma experienced during and in the aftermath of war and conflict is controversial, with some analysts identifying significant proportions of affected populations suffering from post-traumatic stress disorder (PTSD), and others arguing that this term and the response to it medicalize an essentially social phenomenon. The former school calls for large-scale counseling and mental health support structures, whereas the latter, represented by Bracken, Giller, and Summerfield (1995), argue that reconstituting a sense of community and humanity and reestablishing livelihoods and community structures are far more important interventions than establishment of mental trauma centers and counseling. What is clear, and little disputed, is that some individuals who experience particularly horrific experiences as victims of torture or gross human rights abuses during conflicts may well suffer from PTSD. The debate centers on the extent to which this label can be applied to whole populations, rather than to the minority whose experiences have been particularly extreme.

A key problem remains the difficulty of articulating the experiences suffered and of facilitating community- and individual-oriented systems of support. Women who had been raped during the civil war in Uganda, for example, benefited from opportunities to share their experiences with other women who had similarly been abused during wartime; in the absence of any health-related interventions, such experiences might have remained bottled up and been cause for continuing distress. A key issue is to learn not only from those who succumb to the stresses placed upon them but also to understand and learn from the resilience of survivors. Which mechanisms do they use to protect themselves and their mental health, and can others benefit from learning about such strategies?

Few national surveys of the mental health impact of conflicts have been published. Even if such studies could be conducted, prior measurement of the distribution of mental health status within the population would be required to assess the impact of the CE.

Although a number of small and focused studies on particular subgroups of conflict-affected populations have been conducted, their biomedical biases make their conclusions open to challenge. Little is known about the etiology of the symptoms of multiple trauma, the mental health consequences suffered by those who victimize, and the role of coping mechanisms.

Torture is a common practice in many conflicts. This was especially the case during the Cold War, when ideological factors were central to ongoing conflicts. The impact of torture has been extensively documented in Latin America and South Africa in particular. In so-called dirty wars of state-perpetrated internal repression, which were common in Latin America in the mid-1980s, torture was used systematically as a means of attempting to maintain societal structures through fear and intimidation. Mental health workers have identified disintegration as one of the consequences of torture and political repression—that is, the destruction of the person as an autonomous subject with norms and values that inspired his or her political and social activities (Barudy, 1989).

The mental conditions of persons who move to other countries or are exiled vary according to those individuals' specific circumstances. Although some political refugees and asylum seekers in high-income nations have access to comprehensive health care, even these relatively more fortunate exiles are likely to experience severe cultural and language barriers when they attempt to access those services. Uncertainty and guilt regarding relatives left behind, legal restrictions to employment, and ethnic discrimination are common causes of stress among exiles in high-income nations.

A review of mental health studies and interventions in CEs in 2004 seemed to offer some consensus on the approach to this issue. A range of social and mental health strategies and principles seem to have broad support (Van Ommeren et al., 2005).

Noncommunicable Diseases

Responses to the health needs of refugees and IDPs have traditionally emphasized the direct causes of ill health, such as firearms and other weaponry, as well as communicable diseases, which have been shown to pose a major problem in many CEs. In light of the aging of the population generally and of the changing geographic distribution of conflicts to include areas previously well served by health care, such as the former Yugoslavia, new problems are now emerging.

Noncommunicable diseases are widespread in all populations of older adults worldwide. In those situations where medical care was at some stage available, the withdrawal or destruction of medical facilities and drug distribution mechanisms, along with the withdrawal of health workers from areas of active conflict, are likely to diminish the treatment and care available for noncommunicable diseases. Examples of reductions in the quality and availability of care for noncommunicable diseases come from Iraq in the aftermath of the Gulf War, from Sarajevo during its siege in the Yugoslav civil war, and from the Kosovar Albanians, especially those internally displaced people who lost access to services and care.

Persons with conditions such as cardiovascular disease (including hypertension), diabetes, asthma, and cancer may find that their health deteriorates given the lack of access to medical care that typically occurs in conflict settings. Maintaining diagnostic and treatment services, drug supplies, and access to care is extremely difficult in an environment characterized by destruction of infrastructure, targeting of health services, disruption of logistics and supply systems, and absolute resource constraints. In some conflicts, the imposition of sanctions may play some role in reducing access to technologies and drugs necessary for the diagnosis, treatment, and care of noncommunicable disorders.

Impact of Economic Sanctions and Embargoes

The imposition of economic sanctions has become a more common means of punishing nations and is increasingly viewed as an alternative to war. The penalties and restrictions that constitute economic sanctions vary widely. Usually, trade in certain products—ranging from wheat and other agricultural products to high-technology instruments such as computers and to military equipment or items that can be used for military purposes—is limited or prohibited. At times, international travel, sporting events, and cultural exchanges can be curtailed. Assets held in foreign banks can be frozen. No matter which form the economic sanctions take, the goal of those imposing them is always to achieve political objectives while avoiding the cost and destruction of war. Sanctions tend to be used when diplomacy fails and when the costs and potential destruction that accompany military intervention are deemed to be excessive. In the first decade of the twenty-first century, international sanctions were applied against regimes as diverse as Iran, Burundi, Burma, Zimbabwe, and North Korea.

Sanctions can be imposed and administered by a single nation, a group of allied nations, or by the United Nations. The United States has used unilateral economic sanctions more than any other country; it was party to the imposition of sanctions more than

100 times during the twentieth century. More than one-third of those actions came during the 1990s. Also during that decade, the Security Council of the United Nations instituted multilateral economic sanctions against nine countries (Burundi, Haiti, Iraq, Liberia, Libya, Rwanda, Somalia, Sudan, and the former Yugoslavia) and against two nonstate parties (the Khmer Rouge in Cambodia and the National Union for the Total Independence of Angola [UNITA]).

Although economic sanctions as an instrument of foreign policy are aimed at pressuring the targeted governments, experience has usually demonstrated that they are far from a benign weapon. They are rarely successful in achieving their desired political objectives, and they frequently exact a very heavy toll on civilian populations. In fact, although the Geneva Conventions provide wartime protection to civilians by prohibiting the destruction of crops, livestock, sources of drinking water, and the like, few, if any, international standards protect civilians from the unintended consequences of broad economic sanctions imposed on their governments during peacetime. This is the case even when humanitarian exemptions are stipulated in the terms of the embargo. For example, although importation of measles vaccine intended for childhood vaccination programs in Haiti was allowed under the terms of the sanctions imposed upon that country in 1992, shipment of kerosene was not. As a result, the refrigerators required to maintain the potency of the vaccine were unable to function. In the absence of vaccination, a large epidemic of measles occurred.

Nowhere have the devastating effects of economic sanctions on a civilian population been better documented than in Iraq. The sanctions imposed on that country were associated with the deaths of as many as 200,000 children younger than 5 years between 1991 and 1997 (Garfield, 1999). Dramatic increases in rates of malnutrition and preventable infectious diseases such as childhood diarrhea occurred. The prices of basic food items such as flour, rice, oil, meat, and milk soared out of proportion to wage increases as a result of trade restrictions. Distribution systems for food and other essential commodities were severely disrupted. In addition, by 1995, 4 years after the Gulf War, national water distribution was estimated to be only 50% of prewar levels and a UNICEF survey in that year found that 50% of the population had no access to potable water. Wastewater facilities and solid waste disposal systems were also destroyed during the war, and sanctions contributed to the country's inability to restore them. Collectively, the lack of adequate quantities of food, water, and acceptable sanitation contributed to increased mortality in most segments of the population. The causes of mortality resembled those found in low- and middle-income countries more than those that had occurred prior to the sanctions, when Iraq had a relatively advanced healthcare system. Indeed, the number of deaths attributable to the imposition of economic sanctions following the 1991 war far exceeded those that occurred as a result of the war itself. Moreover, throughout it all, the government against which these severe sanctions were imposed remained in power.

Sanctions can be effective, however. For example, they are believed to have played an important role in pressuring the pro-apartheid government of South Africa to relinquish power. Nevertheless, sanctions, in the form in which they have most frequently been applied, have rarely been able to produce their desired effect and have exacted an inappropriately severe toll on the most vulnerable elements of society, including children, women (especially pregnant women), and the elderly. In this sense, the imposition of economic sanctions has been a very blunt instrument of foreign policy.

Prevention and Mitigation of Complex Emergencies

The prevention of CEs primarily entails the prevention of the conflicts that cause them; thus this task is largely political. Since 1990, most CEs have had their roots in ethnic and religious conflicts within sovereign states. Since 2001, at least two major conflicts (in Afghanistan and Iraq) have had their origins in the drive to protect the populations of Western countries.

The United Nations Charter has proved ill equipped to intervene in issues deemed to be "internal" by member states. Chapters 6 and 7 of the Charter do allow the Security Council to authorize appropriate action, including the use of force, in situations that threaten international peace and security. During the Cold War, these provisions were rarely used, because such action was likely to be vetoed by one of the five permanent members of the Security Council. Security Council resolutions did support intervention by the international community to protect civilians in conflicts in Somalia, Bosnia and Herzegovina, Haiti, Iraq, Angola, and East Timor during the 1990s. Since 2001, however, such international consensus has been rare, although one example is the UN Security Council sanctioned imposition of a no-fly zone over Libya in March 2011. The armed interventions by the United States and its allies in Afghanistan and Iraq, for example, were not conducted under the auspices of the United Nations.

In general, the international community has had little success in resolving internal conflicts. Certain private organizations, such as the Carter Center (headquartered in Atlanta, Georgia), have attempted to facilitate the resolution of conflicts in Sudan, Haiti, Somalia, Afghanistan, the former Yugoslavia, and other countries. Unfortunately, the cessation of hostilities, if attained at all, has tended to be temporary. Sometimes health campaigns have been used to seek a temporary halt to armed conflict, most commonly to implement child immunization programs. Such initiatives—for example, the Corridors of Tranquility and Health as a Bridge to Peace—have not addressed the root causes of the conflicts or led to permanent, peaceful resolution. A major victory for these efforts occurred in 2005 when the government of Sudan and the Sudan People's Liberation Front signed a peace agreement in Nairobi. Similar peace agreements have been signed since 2001 in Sri Lanka, Angola, Liberia, Sierra Leone, DRC, and Cote d'Ivoire (although the last two were still fragile in 2011).

As mentioned earlier, the United Nations has a poor record in conflict resolution. For example, the internal conflict in Somalia was allowed to evolve over 5 years into the total disintegration of the nation state. Only when famine reached appalling levels in 1992 did the Security Council authorize extraordinary action to ensure the protection and care of the civilian population. Within 6 months of their arrival, UN troops became embroiled in the conflict itself, taking sides with or against certain armed factions. This action led to heavy loss of life and the eventual withdrawal of the UN forces.

In Bosnia and Herzegovina, between 1992 and 1995, the UN mobilized peacekeeping troops to safeguard the delivery of humanitarian supplies. However, these forces were not authorized to intervene to protect civilians from the violence intentionally directed at various ethnic groups; as a result, the international community's armed representatives were forced to silently bear witness to gross abuses of human rights. This dilemma has been termed the "humanitarian trap." In one especially notable failure, approximately 7,000 Muslim men in the so-called safe haven of Srebrenica in Bosnia were massacred by Bosnian Serbs despite the presence of UN peacekeeping forces in the area.

When the genocide began in Rwanda in 1994, several Belgian peacekeepers already in the country with a UN contingent were killed by extreme Hutu nationalists. Instead of increasing the level of UN presence, the entire peacekeeping force was withdrawn, leaving civilians defenseless against these extremists. Eventually, more than 500,000 Rwandans were killed.

It is likely that this string of UN failures led to NATO taking unilateral action in the form of a massive bombing campaign against Serbia to protect ethnic Albanians in 1999. Although appearing to be well intentioned, this action seemed to accelerate the pace of atrocities and ethnic cleansing instigated by the Serbs against the Kosovar Albanians. At the time of publication of this book, it is too early to assess the effect of the "no-fly" zone over Libya.

The basis of protection of civilians in time of conflict is the Geneva Conventions of 1949 and the Additional Protocols of 1977. In addition, the 1951 Convention on the Prevention and Punishment of the Crime of Genocide was intended to protect civilians from the type of slaughters that occurred in Cambodia in the 1970s and Rwanda in 1994. General Assembly resolutions in 1971, 1985, and 1986 also elaborated on the protection of civilian populations. Of course, international human rights and humanitarian (armed conflict) laws are only as good as their enforcement.

The Office of the UN High Commissioner for Human Rights (UNCHR) in Geneva, Switzerland, is one of the official bodies that oversees this sometimes overwhelming task, relying on the documentation and testimony provided by accredited NGOs. Eleanor Roosevelt was instrumental in giving birth to the commission, along with the Frenchman Rene Cassin, who received the Nobel Peace Prize for authoring the Universal Declaration of Human Rights. Today, UNCHR passes influential resolutions on human rights abuses in member states and is the subject of intense lobbying by governments and NGOs. Thanks to the efforts of a number of human rights advocacy groups, resolutions continue to be adopted by the commission condemning human rights violators. Such resolutions occasionally lead to action by the General Assembly and Security Council, which may dispatch peacekeeping forces to a troubled region (e.g., Central America in the 1980s and East Timor in 1999) to settle the conflicts giving rise to the violations in the first place.

For example, between 2004 and 2009, a number of UN Security Council resolutions demanded that the government of Sudan abandon its support for the genocidal militia in Darfur. By the end of 2009, little progress in resolving this conflict had been achieved. In 2008, however, the Security Council authorized a United Nations/African Union Hybrid operation in Darfur (UNAMID). By February 2010, there were 21,800 uniformed personnel deployed in the region.

Unfortunately, peace and well-being for the displaced population remains elusive. After Sudan's President was targeted by an international arrest warrant issued by the International Criminal Court, most international aid agencies in Darfur were expelled by the government.

The United Nations Office for the Coordination of Humanitarian Affairs (OCHA), based in New York City and Geneva, is the UN office responsible for coordinating efforts in early warning, prevention, mitigation, and response to disasters, including CEs. One of its projects, known as Relief Web, seeks to strengthen the capacity of the humanitarian relief community through the timely dissemination of reliable information on prevention, preparedness, and disaster response. As with many other similar projects, the organization makes this information available on the Internet (www.reliefweb.int).

Given the difficulty of preventing or resolving armed conflicts, what else can be done to prevent or mitigate the worst consequences of such conflicts on civilian populations? Although not yet tested, it may be possible during the early phase of national disintegration to focus development efforts on activities that strengthen the capacity of local organizations to implement life-saving programs. Accelerated training of health workers in emergency preparedness and response, support for local food production activities, and adaptation of health information systems to the priorities of an emergency assistance program may all help to minimize the eventual impact of the CE. Given the frequency of CEs in the past decade and the likelihood that they will continue to occur, donor governments should support pilot projects to examine what can and cannot be done to prepare for such emergencies.

Early Warning and Detection

Efforts to prevent and mitigate the impact of CEs on populations must be based on accurate and timely information if they are to be effective. Given the enormous cost of military intervention (e.g., $100 million per day in Kosovo in 1999) and major relief and rehabilitation programs, it seems surprising that so little has been invested in early warning, emergency detection, preparedness, and mitigation projects. In the late 1990s, a number of systems collected, aggregated, and disseminated information on a number of indicators relevant to CEs. Most of these systems relied on information collected by other agencies, such as governments, UN agencies, and NGOs. Relief Web, a project of OCHA, has already been mentioned. The International Crisis Group also maintains an active conflict monitoring system, which provides detailed reports on countries vulnerable to complex emergencies, including Indonesia, Burma, Algeria, and Burundi.

Unlike natural disaster early warning systems and preparedness programs, efforts to monitor and detect CEs are fraught with political obstacles. The old adage that "The first casualty in war is truth" applies equally well to attempts to collect accurate data on the health outcomes of war. The existence of armed conflicts is no secret; the political response is still inadequate. What would be valuable as CEs evolve would be means to develop a more accurate picture of which health interventions need to have the highest priorities and will be most effective in preventing excess mortality and morbidity. In European wars, the most important public health priorities have been the direct effects of violence. Stopping the violence is a public health issue that can be addressed only by the world's leaders. In low-income countries, the priorities in CEs are most likely to be nutrition and communicable disease control. Thus key indicators to monitor in early warning systems would include food availability, nutritional status, immunization coverage, incidence of vaccine-preventable diseases, and antenatal program coverage.

Responses to Complex Emergencies
Primary Prevention

Primary prevention is the basic strategy of public health, and epidemiology is one of its essential tools. In situations of armed conflict, however, epidemiology can be practiced safely and reliably in very few areas. Hence, the traditional documentation, monitoring, and evaluation elements of disease prevention may be ineffective in this situation. Because war and public health are essentially incompatible pursuits, the provision of adequate food, shelter, potable water, and sanitation as well as vaccination and other primary healthcare services has proved problematic in countries disrupted by war. Primary prevention in such circumstances, therefore, means stopping the violence. More effective diplomatic and political mechanisms need to be developed that might resolve conflicts early in their evolution prior to the stage when food shortages occur, health services collapse, populations migrate, and significant adverse public health outcomes emerge.

Secondary Prevention

Secondary prevention involves the early detection of evolving conflict-related food scarcity and population movements, preparedness for interventions that mitigate their public health impact, and the development of appropriate public health skills to enable relief workers to work effectively in emergency settings. Preparedness planning needs to take place both at a coordinated international level and at the level of countries where CEs might occur. Relief agencies need resources not only to respond to emergencies when they occur, but also to implement early warning systems, maintain technical expertise, train personnel, build reserves of relief supplies, and develop their logistic capacity. At the country level, all health development programs should incorporate an emergency preparedness component, including the establishment of standard public health policies (e.g., rapid detection and management of epidemics, vaccination), treatment protocols, staff training, and the maintenance of reserves of essential drugs and vaccines for use in disasters.

Tertiary Prevention

Tertiary prevention involves prevention of excess mortality and morbidity once a disaster has occurred. Both the health problems that consistently cause most deaths and severe morbidity in CEs and those demographic groups most at risk of experiencing these outcomes have been identified. Moreover, most deaths in refugee and displaced populations are preventable using currently available and affordable technology. Relief programs, therefore, must channel all available resources toward addressing measles, diarrheal diseases, malnutrition, acute respiratory infections, and, in some cases, malaria, especially among women and young children. The challenge is to institutionalize this knowledge within the major relief organizations and to ensure that relief management and logistical systems provide the resources necessary to implement key interventions in a timely manner.

Initially, both refugees and displaced persons often find themselves in crowded, unsanitary camps in remote regions where meeting even the basic needs is highly difficult. Prolonged exposure to the violence of war and the deprivations of long journeys by refugees cause severe physical and psychological stress. Upon arrival at their destination, refugees—most of whom tend to be women and children—may suffer severe anxiety or depression, which is compounded by the loss of dignity associated with complete dependence on the generosity of others for their survival. If refugee camps are located near borders or close to areas of continuing armed conflict, the desire for security is an overriding concern. Therefore, the first priority of any relief operation is to ensure adequate protection;

camps should be placed sufficiently distant from borders to reassure refugees that they are safe (Sphere Project, 2004).

To diminish the sense of helplessness and dependency, refugees should be given an active role in the planning and implementation of relief programs. Nevertheless, giving total control of the distribution of relief items to so-called refugee leaders may be dangerous. For example, leaders of the former Hutu-controlled Rwandan government took control of the distribution system in Zairian refugee camps in July 1994, resulting in relief supplies being diverted to young male members of the former Rwandan Army. Even when their intentions are good, the priorities of communities may differ from those of international relief agencies. Whereas the latter may offer preferential treatment to children because mortality rates have been shown to be highest in younger age groups, members of the community may feel that the elderly, for example, deserve special care because they carry with them the traditions and customs of the culture. In general, the targeting of food and other supplies to communities and to vulnerable groups within those communities should be the subject of discussion between relief authorities and the communities (Jaspars & Shoham, 1999).

In the absence of conflict resolution, those communities that are totally dependent on external aid for their survival because their members have either been displaced from their homes or are living under a state of siege must be provided the basic minimum resources necessary to maintain health and well-being. The provision of adequate food, clean water, shelter, sanitation, and warmth will prevent the most severe public health consequences of CEs. The temporary location of refugees in small settlements or villages in the host country, it is suggested, would have fewer adverse public health consequences than their placement in crowded, often unsanitary camps. Where the refugees end up, public health priorities include a rapid needs assessment, the establishment of a health information system, measles vaccination, the control of diarrheal and other communicable diseases, maternal and child health services, and nutritional rehabilitation.

Critical to the success of the response is the coordination of the many agencies involved in the relief effort. Following the Goma crisis in 1994, there was recognition among the aid community that aid agencies needed to demonstrate the effectiveness of their actions. This consensus led to formation of the Sphere Project, which through a comprehensive, inclusive process developed the *Sphere Project Handbook:*

Humanitarian Charter and Minimum Standards in Disaster Response in 2000. The *Handbook* includes minimum standards for shelter, water, and sanitation, and a range of health and nutrition interventions and outcomes. It was revised in 2004, and a process of revision commenced in 2009. The English version of the third edition was published on April 14, 2011.

Rapid Assessment

Displacement is the final, desperate act of a threatened population. Whenever possible, assessments of the public health needs of the population should be conducted prior to the act of migration or resettlement, whether it is within the country of origin or beyond its borders (MSF & Epicentre, 1999). Impending disasters—even the development of CEs—can frequently be predicted. Knowing the size of the population and its age and gender distribution, having baseline data concerning its health status and the level of health services available to it, and being aware of the characteristics of the place or places to which displaced persons are most likely to move can be of immense help in knowing which relief supplies will be needed and which kinds of health programs should be implemented. Needless to say, such pre-displacement assessments have been rare.

Early assessments can be made by a variety of means. For instance, technology-dependent methods such as satellite surveillance can provide information regarding crop growth, population densities, and even troop movements, although such technology is often unavailable to those agencies that need it the most. Reviews of existing documents and other information provided by a variety of United Nations agencies, bilateral governments, NGOs, and national authorities familiar with the situation can be helpful. On-the-ground economic evaluations, including a description of trends in market prices for food and essential commodities in food-basket analyses, can be very helpful. More detailed information can frequently be obtained from visual inspection of the affected area, including mapping, key informant interviews, and observation of the affected population.

For CEs, however, political instability and increased violence are almost always compounding factors. Thus more direct means of assessment prior to displacement are often impossible. In many cases, the earliest assessment can be conducted only after the displaced population has reached a relatively safe area of resettlement.

Early, rapid assessments have multiple purposes. They can provide important information regarding the evolution of the emergency, identify groups and areas at greatest risk, evaluate the existing local response capacity, determine the magnitude of external resources required, and indicate which health programs will be required in the short and medium term. Every CE is characterized by a different set of causes and consequences, and each should be assessed for its impact on the health of the population affected.

For CEs, early assessment should include both a description of the conflict and its sequelae, in terms of the affected areas and populations, and a characterization of the health consequences of displacement. In some cases, affected populations may not have migrated to another location, but rather may be trapped in a siege-like setting, such as in Sarajevo and Beirut. For the conflict, variables of particular significance include its duration, the progress of negotiations (and the likelihood of an early return for the displaced), the patterns of violence, the size and location of inaccessible areas and populations, and the state of remaining available health services.

The highest priorities for early assessment are the availability and adequacy of drinking water, food, and shelter. The minimum standards described later in this chapter must be met. Regarding the health status of the population, perhaps the most important and most sensitive indicator is the mortality rate. Early documentation of mortality will establish an indispensable baseline and allow for monitoring of trends that attest to the overall effectiveness of the relief program. In an emergency, crude mortality rates are expressed as deaths per 10,000 population per day. A CMR of greater than 1 has been used to define the existence of a public health emergency, whereas a CMR of greater than 2 indicates a critical situation. Of course, these thresholds are gross estimates. Whenever pre-crisis mortality rates are available, they should be taken into account (Guha-Sapir & van Panhuis, 2004). In addition, age- and gender-specific mortality should be assessed to identify population groups at the highest risk.

The incidence of diseases commonly associated with high rates of preventable mortality should be assessed as early as possible. These conditions include diarrheal illnesses, acute respiratory infections, and diseases with high epidemic potential, such as cholera, dysentery, measles, and meningitis. Where appropriate, the occurrence and risk of locally endemic diseases such as malaria and dengue should be analyzed as well.

Complex emergencies are usually accompanied by food shortages that can lead to malnutrition. For this reason, assessment of protein-energy malnutrition among children should be undertaken as soon as possible, using any of a variety of methods. Although mass screening of all children is the optimal approach, an initial random sample of the population can establish the prevalence of malnutrition and indicate the need for targeted screening and feeding interventions. Vaccination coverage of children should also be assessed to determine the urgency of mounting vaccination campaigns, although in the absence of coverage data, measles vaccination should be considered a priority.

Rapid assessments require detailed planning and may fail because of the inadequacy of transportation, maps, communications equipment, and fuel. In addition, attention needs to be given to the security situation in the affected area. An assessment is of limited value unless its results are communicated in a timely and effective manner to those who can act upon them. The presentation of the findings should be organized and clear, and the recommendations of the assessment team should indicate which actions are of highest priority, what a reasonable time frame for action would be, and which resources will be required. Without these elements, the essential information required for the survival of large populations of displaced individuals may not be acted upon in time to prevent high levels of excess preventable mortality.

The potential usefulness of rapid assessment should not be underestimated. In the past, too many assessments were often done by different agencies in an uncoordinated manner. To promote efficiency, it is essential that a designated lead agency coordinate rapid assessments, ensuring that sectoral assessments (e.g., water, medical services, food) are integrated and that the findings are used to inform program policies and planning. For example, in the post-tsunami relief effort of January 2005, WHO organized teams from a number of UN and voluntary agencies, the Indonesian Ministry of Health, and the Indonesian military forces, and, using U.S. military assets for support, led a series of rapid assessments of stranded populations along the west coast of Aceh province on the island of Sumatra. These efforts proved quite helpful in identifying remote populations and their needs and in targeting appropriate relief.

In contrast, the rapid assessments attempted following the Haiti earthquake in 2010 did not yield results that guided the relief effort in a timely manner. The extent of the destruction; the need to reserve means of transport, both ground and air, for the delivery of humanitarian goods; and the lack of a clear and creditable plan for exactly what to assess and where collectively resulted in the early days of the relief effort being a data-free period. Most important in

that setting, perhaps, would have been to determine where hospital beds were available in the mostly destroyed capital city of Port-au-Prince and throughout the country. Unfortunately, identification of these assets, and especially appropriate and effective sharing of the information with those who had the greatest need for it, was not rapidly forthcoming.

Health Information Systems

Epidemiologic surveillance is the ongoing and systematic collection, analysis, and interpretation of health data. This information is used for planning, implementing, and evaluating public health interventions and programs. Surveillance data are used both to determine the need for public health action and to assess the effectiveness of programs. In CEs, after the response to an initial rapid assessment has been instituted, the development and implementation of ongoing health information systems immediately become high-priority activities. Although data on many of the subjects included in the rapid assessment will continue to be collected on a regular basis, routine use of health information systems will allow for the monitoring of a significantly larger number of other potentially important health conditions and health programs.

Characteristics of Effective Health Information Systems

To be useful, surveillance systems must be relevant, especially in CEs, where both time and other resources are frequently in short supply. Data collection should be restricted to the most important of actual and potential public health problems. Equally important, data should be collected only if the information will be useful in stimulating and guiding a response: If no intervention is feasible, there is little need to encumber the system by gathering information on the problem.

The best health information systems are the simplest. In a number of CEs, difficulties have arisen in explaining the importance of the data both to the local staff responsible for its collection and to decision makers, who frequently do not appreciate the limitations of data of variable accuracy collected under the most difficult of circumstances. Case definitions must be clear, consistent, and suited to the local capacity to make accurate diagnoses. Where no microscopes or rapid diagnostic tests are readily available, for example, malaria may have to be represented by "fever and chills." The data generated from simple systems must be acknowledged to have limitations and should not be over-interpreted. Nevertheless, good surveillance systems rely on laboratory confirmation of suspect or probable cases of diseases of public health importance. Efforts should be made to have available a basic public health laboratory, with appropriate supplies and technical expertise.

Representativeness is another essential element of health information systems that is related to the quality of the data. Careful interpretation of data collected from a surveillance system is required before extrapolations can be made to the general population. For example, in southern Sudan, nutrition and mortality assessments are difficult to interpret because health information has been collected and reported from food distribution centers to which the displaced and most severely malnourished elements of the population were drawn. As a consequence, mortality and malnutrition rates derived from these sites are not necessarily representative of the broader population of the region.

The organization and implementation of health information systems should be made the responsibility of one individual or agency, which should also be charged with ensuring widespread cooperation and coordination. If a host government is in place and guiding the response, it should establish appropriate policies and guidelines that can be implemented with help from appropriate technical partners. It is important for the interpretation and response to the data that standardized case definitions, data collection methods, and conditions of reporting be established. This strategy helps practitioners avoid the problems described earlier, in which different agencies' use of different data collection methods ruled out either collation or comparison of results.

In emergencies, both reporting and the response to it must be timely. When the goal is to prevent excess mortality, undue delays between any two links of the surveillance chain—from the peripheral data-collection level to the more central, policy-making level and back to the periphery where action needs to be taken—can result in an unnecessary loss of life. Depending on the nature of the data, especially when an epidemic illness is deemed likely or is occurring, daily reporting of select information by telephone, text messaging, or messenger is not necessarily excessive. In fact, as new technologies such as cell phones become widely available, they become the methods of choice for data transmission from more peripheral to central levels. For other conditions, data are generally reported and analyzed on a weekly basis during the emergency period and monthly during the less acute phases of the crisis.

Of course, data needs may change rapidly as an emergency evolves during a more steady state. For this reason, information systems must have a high degree of flexibility, and their response to new demands should be achieved with minimal disruption.

Methods

As long as they possess the qualities mentioned previously, surveillance systems may combine active and passive reporting mechanisms. Active reporting can include randomized population-based surveys aimed at gathering data on one or a selected few parameters, such as vaccination coverage or nutritional status. Alternatively, it can involve the hiring of personnel for the specific purpose of monitoring important health events that might occur outside the bounds of the healthcare system itself, such as hiring gravediggers to report on burials to determine mortality rates. Passive reporting generally refers to the routine collection and relaying of health statistics within the system itself, whether it is from community-based health posts, from primary care clinics, or from hospitals.

Because access to the healthcare system may be limited, and because utilization may be low owing to factors such as fear or mistrust of the healthcare providers, unfamiliarity with the system, physical destruction of facilities, and other reasons that frequently go unrecognized by relief agencies, it is especially important that emergency health information systems be regularly evaluated for the characteristics described earlier. Sometimes a combination of active and passive reporting can be used. In Haiti, for example, the system that had been previously established in 25 PEPFAR-funded hospitals that had been treating HIV and AIDS patients was adapted for use during the emergency; those reporting sites then began to report on a number of conditions for which information was required on a daily basis.

Content of Health Information Systems in Complex Emergencies

Trends in crude mortality remain an important feature of surveillance throughout the emergency phase and beyond. Sometimes mortality can be determined by means of a population-based survey, but the data derived from these surveys are subject to different sorts of bias and are frequently dated.

In many cultures, death is a family and religious matter, and deaths are not normally brought to the attention of the healthcare system. In fact, severely ill patients in hospitals are frequently taken home to die. For this reason, active surveillance is best for estimating mortality. Grave watchers—often those who dig the graves—can be hired on a 24-hour basis to report new burials and, if possible, to ascertain the age and gender of the deceased. In some cultures, the free distribution of burial shrouds or other materials used for burial or funerals can provide a useful incentive for reporting.

At times when large numbers of corpses are left unburied by families, as happened in Goma in 1994 because the ground was composed of volcanic rock that made it impossible to dig graves, or following extensive natural disasters such as the Indian Ocean tsunami of December 2004, where bodies were buried under rubble or swept away, it may be possible to ask those responsible for body collection and mass burial to keep count of the number of dead they see. In other CEs, as in Haiti, dead bodies cannot be found or are so quickly disposed of by the authorities that only gross estimates of the number of deaths can be given.

In addition to mortality data, health information systems should collect morbidity data on commonly occurring diseases and on diseases with epidemic potential. Diseases that have been prominent in all CEs include watery diarrhea, acute respiratory infections, malaria and other important endemic conditions, and malnutrition. Measles, meningitis, cholera, and shigellosis (dysentery, or bloody diarrhea) have also been responsible for major epidemics in emergency settings, and guidelines for the establishment of sensitive thresholds for the detection of each need to be followed where they already exist, or need to be developed. The detection of an epidemic should trigger an immediate and aggressive response.

In addition, at least two health programs—treatment of malnutrition and vaccination—need to be regularly monitored. Indicators of the numbers of patients in intensive or supplementary feeding programs need to be regularly tracked. Vaccination coverage rates also need to be estimated and, when deemed appropriate, measles vaccination should be offered to all children aged 6 months to 15 years regardless of prior vaccination status as soon as resources permit. Routine vaccination with the antigens available through the national Expanded Program on Immunization should be established when feasible. Other vaccines may be offered after careful consideration by public health authorities of the epidemiology of diseases and the logistical implications.

Two healthcare areas that have been relatively neglected in CEs are those of reproductive health and psychosocial health (Spiegel et al., 2010). Ample evidence has accumulated to show that in emergencies, women of reproductive age, and especially pregnant women, need special attention. Thus their health conditions, including pregnancy, should be carefully monitored by surveillance mechanisms. In terms of mental health issues, forced migration is itself a traumatic event. When it is compounded by the ethnic strife and violence that frequently accompany CEs, close attention should be paid not only to individuals who might be seriously affected by post-traumatic stress disorders, but also to the reestablishment of community structures.

Finally, when the emergency has subsided (e.g., when crude mortality rates drop to less than 1 per 10,000 per day), increased attention can be paid to dealing with more chronic or less fatal diseases, such as tuberculosis, STIs (including HIV), diabetes, hypertension, and elective surgical conditions.

The establishment of a useful health information system, with all of the characteristics described here, is an essential function of the health services. Without one, programs will be developed by guesswork and the effectiveness of program implementation will remain a matter for conjecture.

Shelter and Environment

As mentioned earlier, the placement of refugees and IDPs in small settlements or integration into local villages is preferable to the establishment of large camps. Health outcomes are probably better in these small settlements because environmental conditions are more favorable and there is less crowding. At the same time, the provision of relief assistance to a large number of scattered settlements may pose a difficult management and logistical challenge and may provoke resentment in the surrounding communities. In Guinea in the early 1990s, food aid and other relief items were provided to communities for distribution to both Liberian refugees and local inhabitants. This system may have worked well because the refugees and locals were of the same ethnic origin and many were related. In contrast, measles vaccination coverage of Mozambican refugees in Malawi who were absorbed into communities and were dependent on the national immunization program was considerably lower than that in refugee camps, where services were provided by the United Nations and international voluntary agencies.

When establishment of camps is unavoidable, three of the key determinants of location should be safety of residents, access to essentials such as adequate quantities of clean water and of fuel for cooking, and all-weather access by vehicles. In many instances, local politics determines the site of a camp, and this location is often less than desirable. For example, in 1988, the Ethiopian government placed Somali refugees in a large camp of 180,000 persons on a site that had no local supply of drinking water. The nearest source with an adequate quantity of water was situated in a town 100 km from the camp. For many years, water was delivered daily in convoys of trucks at enormous cost to the relief agencies. The Ethiopian government refused to move the refugees closer to town for fear of exacerbating political problems that it was experiencing with local ethnic Somalis. In 1981–1982, many camps for Ethiopian refugees in the central region of Somalia were flooded in the wet season, causing food trucks to be unable to reach them for weeks at a time.

Sites should be chosen with ease of water drainage in mind, although sometimes drainage systems have to be created at the time of camp construction. This consideration is critical to ensure access by vehicles, limitation of disease-vector breeding, and ease of access by refugees to services, such as health clinics and food distribution. When hundreds of thousands of refugees fled ethnic cleansing in Kosovo in 1999, spontaneous camps were established near the border of Macedonia, where as many as 45,000 refugees were camped on a muddy, snowy field sheltered only by their vehicles and makeshift tents. An added hazard was the large quantity of land mines laid by Serb forces along the border; these mines killed several refugees. In Albania, tens of thousands of refugees brought their tractors with them and created a chaotic situation in which the delivery of services and the establishment of shelters were almost impossible. In Macedonia, Kosovar refugees were forcibly removed by bus from areas where the government did not want them located.

Other inappropriate locations have included the swampy, malarious areas on the Thai border where Cambodian refugees were housed; the inhospitable mountainous area on the border between Iraq and Turkey to which the Kurdish population of Iraq fled in the wake of the 1991 Gulf War; and the volcanic, rocky ground in eastern Zaire where Rwandan refugee camps were placed, precluding both latrine construction and burial of the dead. Spontaneous settlements of displaced people can be established in urban areas as well. In Haiti following the earthquake, such camps ranged in size from a few hundred families, when church congregations, for example, stayed together, to settlements of as many as 50,000 people, as was the case on the grounds of the Petionville Golf Club. When hundreds of such settlements spring up, the delivery of humanitarian relief supplies can be problematic.

Ideally, the size of camps should be limited to 20,000 residents for reasons of security and ease of administration. Such camps should be further divided into sections of 5,000 persons for the purpose of service delivery. Shelter is an urgent priority. On average, the covered area provided per person should be 3.5 to 4.5 m^2 (Sphere Project, 2004). In warm, humid climates, shelters should have optimal ventilation and protection from direct sunlight. In cold climates, shelter material should provide adequate insulation combined with sufficient clothing, blankets, bedding, space heating, and caloric intake.

Ideally, houses should be built using a traditional design and local materials. This may pose local environmental problems such as the destruction of trees, however, so building materials should be trucked in from areas remote from the camp. Waterproofing is essential and may be achieved with plastic sheeting or tarpaulins. Tents may provide temporary shelter; however, they deteriorate in rain and wind and should be replaced with local materials as soon as possible.

To limit further environmental damage through deforestation, cooking fuel—such as charcoal, wood, oil, or kerosene—should be brought to the site from remote areas and fuel-efficient stoves provided or constructed. Camps may easily become fire hazards, and fire prevention should be an objective of proper camp design.

Water and Sanitation

When refugee camps are unavoidable, proximity to safe water sources needs to be recognized as the most important criterion for site selection. The Sphere Project minimum standard for water quantity is 15 liters of clean water per person per day for all domestic needs—cooking, drinking, and bathing. Other standards include at least one water collection point per 250 people and a maximum distance from shelter to the nearest water point of 500 meters.

Ideally, both the quantity and the quality of water provided to refugees and displaced persons should meet international standards; however, in many cases this is not possible. In general, ensuring access to adequate quantities of relatively clean water is probably more effective in preventing diarrheal disease, especially bacterial dysentery, than providing small quantities of pure microbe-free water. Nevertheless, there have been some important exceptions to this rule (see Exhibit 11-4).

The usual options for supplying water to refugees and IDPs include surface water (e.g., lakes, rivers, streams), shallow wells, springs, bore wells, and trucked water from remote sources. Although surface water is often abundant, it needs to be treated, usually through a system of sedimentation and chlorination,

---

Exhibit 11-4	Cholera in Goma, Zaire, Despite Large Quantities of Water Available

Between July 14 and 17, 1994, large numbers of ethnic Hutus fled Rwanda and sought refuge in the North Kivu region of neighboring Zaire; initial estimates of the exodus into Zaire ranged as high as 1.2 million people. Many refugees entered through the town of Goma, which is located at the northern end of a large body of deep water, Lake Kivu. Following the influx into Goma, many of the refugees were located near Lake Kivu, whose water flows very slowly, is carbonated by a volcanic bed, and is alkaline. These are favorable conditions for maintaining live *Vibrio cholerae*—pathogens that were endemic in the region. At the time, no means of purifying and transporting sufficient quantities of water to distribute to refugees were available. Although some agencies attempted to chlorinate water in containers as refugees removed it from the lake, coverage was inadequate and most refugees consumed untreated water.

After 5 to 7 days, the refugees were moved to camps that did not have any easy access to any water. Advisers to the relief program, especially the U.S. military, opted for a high-technology approach—namely, a large purification plant that was flown in after 1 week, and distribution of clean water to the camps by tankers. A few days after the refugees' arrival, a diarrhea epidemic occurred among the population and was confirmed as being due to cholera. This epidemic had already peaked before July 29, when the relief operation was able to provide an average of only 1 liter of purified water per person per day. At least 58,000 cases of symptomatic cholera occurred in this population. Given the usual high ratio of asymptomatic to symptomatic infections (up to 10:1), it is likely that most refugees in the Goma area were infected with *V. cholerae*, and that few infections were prevented (Goma Epidemiology Group, 1995). In a subsequent evaluation of the epidemic, concerns regarding failure to adopt best treatment practices and poor coordination between agencies were highlighted.

Source: Data from Goma Epidemiology Group, "Public Health Impact of Rwandan Refugee Crisis: What Happened in Goma, Zaire, in July 1994?" 1995, *Lancet, 345*, pp. 339–344.

---

and sometimes with filtration. A system of piped distribution and outlet taps needs to be developed to avoid crowding and drainage problems. Shallow wells and springs need to be protected and provided with a mechanism for drawing water, such as pumps. Although deep-bore wells provide clean water at the source, it may take some time to bring in the necessary equipment to construct the wells.

In addition, measures to prevent post-source contamination need to be implemented, including treatment at the source (e.g., "bucket chlorination"). Sufficient collection and storage containers (at least three 20-liter containers per family), especially containers with narrow openings that prevent post-collection contamination, should be made available. A study in a Malawian refugee camp in 1993 demonstrated a significant reduction in fecal contamination of water stored in such buckets compared with standard buckets. In addition, the incidence of diarrhea among children younger than 5 years of age in the households with the improved buckets was considerably lower than in control households (Roberts, Chartier, Chartier, Malenga, Toole, & Rodka, 2001). Recently, newer methods of disinfecting water at the home, including simple chlorination and/or flocculation systems, such as the Safe Water System (CDC, 2008), have been moderately successful in CEs.

Adequate sanitation is an essential element of diarrheal disease prevention and a critical component of any relief program. While the eventual goal of sanitation programs should be the construction of one latrine per family, interim measures may include the designation of separate defecation areas and the temporary provision of neighborhood latrines. The Sphere Project minimum indicator of acceptable household-level sanitation is a maximum of 20 persons per latrine. Toilets should be segregated by sex and be no more than 50 meters from dwellings for security reasons. To achieve maximal impact, these measures should be complemented by community hygiene education and regular distribution of at least 250 g of soap per person per month. Hygiene education has been shown to significantly increase the impact of sanitation programs. An analysis of data gathered in the Malawi study cited earlier demonstrated that the presence of soap in households significantly reduced the risk of diarrhea (Peterson, Roberts, Toole, & Peterson, 1998).

These sanitation goals can be difficult to achieve. In Goma, where the ground consisted of volcanic rock and digging was very difficult, sanitation remained inadequate and undoubtedly contributed to the virulence of the cholera outbreak. In Haiti, in an almost totally destroyed urban area, reconstituting even rudimentary plumbing was out of the question during the emergency period. In addition, the construction of latrines was painfully slow and greatly hampered by the prevailing conditions, even when the importance of improved sanitation was clearly recognized. The objective of post-emergency sanitation measures should be to restore the pre-disaster levels of environmental services rather than to improve on the original levels, although longer-term reconstruction efforts can certainly aim to surpass the status quo ante.

The provision of water and sanitation in emergency-affected populations in urban and rural areas of Eastern Europe has posed different challenges. For example, as mentioned earlier, the destruction of public utilities in cities such as Sarajevo and Grozny (and Beirut, a Middle Eastern city) created enormous problems. In general, the goal is to repair existing systems. For practical reasons, however, interim measures may be required, such as rehabilitating old wells, providing generators to pump water from distant sources such as rivers, and providing containers and security for residents to collect water at available sources.

Food Rations and Distribution

The quantity and quality of food rations is one of the most critical determinants of health outcomes in emergency-affected populations. During the early evolution of CEs, measures should be taken to increase access to food without forcing people to leave their homes. The establishment of "feeding camps" may act as a magnet for hungry families and lead to the spontaneous establishment of settlements and camps, with the subsequent health problems described earlier in this chapter. In addition, in conflict zones, warring parties may target areas where populations regularly congregate. Subsidized food shops; food-for-work or cash-for-work programs; emergency support for home food production, such as the distribution of fast-growing seed varieties and agricultural tools; and other measures may prove effective means of ensuring adequate nutrition prior to the onset of armed conflict.

Once armed conflict has commenced, either forcing people to flee their homes or be trapped in siege-like conditions, it is usually necessary to distribute food. General food rations should contain at least 2,100 kilocalories (kcal) of energy per person per day, plus the other nutrients listed in Table 11-5. Rations should take into consideration the demographic composition of the population, the specific needs of vulnerable groups, and access by the population to alternative sources of food and income. In cold climates, the minimum energy value of the ration should be adjusted upward. Pregnant women require, on average, an extra 285 kcal per day, and lactating women an extra 500 kcal. These extra requirements should be provided through distribution of rations within the household; however, this process may need to be monitored, perhaps indirectly via the prevalence of low-birth-weight babies.

Food should be distributed regularly as dry items to family units, taking care that socially vulnerable groups, such as female-headed households, unaccompanied minors, and the elderly, receive their fair share (see Exhibit 11-5 for an exception). Achieving this goal requires an accurate registration system listing all residents in family groups. If a refugee or displaced population is organized in well-defined communities, food may be distributed to community

Table 11-5	Minimum Nutritional Requirements of Emergency-Affected Populations (for Planning Purposes During the Initial Stage of an Emergency)	
Nutrient	**Mean Requirements (per person per day)**[a]	
Energy	2,100 kcal	
Protein	10%–12% total energy (52–63 g)	
Fat	17% of total energy (40 g)	
Vitamin A	1,666 IU	
Thiamine	0.9 mg (or 0.4 mg per 1,000 kcal intake)	
Riboflavin	1.4 mg (or 0.6 mg per 1,000 kcal intake)	
Niacin	12.0 mg (or 6.6 mg per 1,000 kcal intake)	
Vitamin C	28.0 mg	
Vitamin D	3.2–3.8 micrograms calciferol	
Iron	22 mg	
Iodine	150 micrograms	

[a]Based on standard age and sex distribution (World Food Programme/UNHCR, 1997)
Source: Sphere Project, *Humanitarian Charter and Minimum Standards in Disaster Response* (Geneva, Switzerland: The Sphere Project, 2004). Reprinted with permission.

Exhibit 11-5	Food Distribution in Somalia

During the civil conflict and famine in Somalia in 1992–1993, dry food rations distributed to families in Mogadishu were often stolen as families returned to their homes. Relief agencies were sometimes forced to establish feeding centers where cooked meals were served to people of all ages. This was an unusual exception from the general rule of providing dry food that families prepare at home, thereby enabling them to preserve some independence and dignity.

There is a widespread belief that currently available refugee rations, especially those distributed in non-European populations, are inadequate for nutrient requirements, which may be higher than the traditional recommended daily allowances. The best way to combat depletion of essential nutrients is to take active steps to increase the variety of the diet. This is not possible with relief foods that have to be capable of bulk storage and shipment—for example, cereal, pulses, sugar, oil, and salt. For this reason, recipients of international aid should be encouraged to barter food items for local produce. Market facilities should be established, supported, and controlled by camp leaders. Seeds for leaf vegetables should be distributed as part of all relief activities, even in the acute phase. Every effort should be made to provide those spices and herbs used traditionally by the population with all food baskets. There is no need to deliver a special food basket for children or pregnant and lactating women—only a sufficiently varied diet for the whole family (Golden, 1999b).

leaders, who can then divide it further to the heads of households in quantities based on the number of family members. Sometimes, as was the case during the Kurdish exodus to camps on the Iraq–Turkey border in 1991, this practice has been implemented in voluntary exchange for demographic information that allowed health authorities to enumerate the births, deaths, and other life events that were occurring. In other situations, food is distributed directly to heads of households, based on a ration card system.

In low-income countries, food rations usually comprise a staple cereal, such as rice, wheat, or maize; a source of dense fat, such as vegetable oil; a source of protein, such as beans, lentils, groundnuts, or dried fish; and extra items such as salt, tea, and spices. Experience has shown that women are fairer than men in distributing each food item in the correct quantity. Standard serving containers based on a known weight or volume of food are essential tools for distribution centers.

Guards are often necessary to maintain crowd control. In Haiti, for example, UN security forces (MENUSTAH) and the U.S. military assured security while the World Food Programme and others distributed food; there were only rare reports of violence. Because of the indignity of being counted and the fact that many refugees are afraid to have their identities known and precise locations reported, attempts at registration for the distribution of humanitarian aid should carefully take into account the security and cultural concerns of the population (Harrell-Bond, Voutira, & Leopold, 1992).

In addition to food, adequate cooking fuel, utensils, and facilities to grind whole-grain cereals need to be provided to all families. Fuel-efficient stoves, often made of mud, may lead to more efficient use of scarce fuel. In children younger than 2 years, breastfeeding

will provide considerable protection against communicable diseases, including diarrhea. Thus attempts to introduce or distribute human milk substitutes and infant feeding bottles should be strongly opposed in an emergency situation. The evidence that vitamin A deficiency is associated with increased childhood mortality and disabling blindness is now so convincing that supplements of vitamin A should be provided routinely to all refugee children younger than 5 years of age at first contact and every 3 to 6 months thereafter (Nieburg et al., 1988).

In Eastern Europe (i.e., high-income countries), the same principles have been followed; however, the types of food have varied and have included cheese, meat, powdered orange juice, and fruit. In some high-income countries experiencing economic and political instability, ration vouchers have been distributed to vulnerable persons, such as elderly pensioners, which can then be redeemed for food at designated stores.

One of the main problems in Africa, and in some parts of Asia, has been providing refugees and IDPs with foods containing adequate quantities of micronutrients, especially niacin, riboflavin, thiamin, iron, and vitamin C. Epidemics of pellagra, scurvy, and beriberi have been common in African refugee camps. For many years, micronutrient deficiencies were a blind spot in emergency food and nutrition planning; in recent years, the problem has been acknowledged, although solutions remain inadequate. In southern Africa, niacin has been added to maize flour during the milling process. However, vitamin C is water-soluble and very sensitive to heat, light, and bruising; thus the transport, storage, and distribution of large quantities of foods such as citrus fruit have proved problematic. One solution to this dilemma is to allow and encourage people to swap some of their ration items in local markets for vitamin C–containing foods, such as tomatoes, onions, potatoes, green chili peppers, and other fruits and vegetables. In addition, the provision of seeds to enable refugees to grow small amounts of vegetables in kitchen gardens is an effective measure.

The provision of fortified blended cereals has also been proposed as a vehicle for ensuring adequate micronutrient intake. Studies in Ethiopia, Nepal, and Tanzania have shown that these cereals are generally acceptable. Unfortunately, overcooking and consequent depletion of the vitamin C content may be a problem in some communities (Mears & Young, 1998). WHO has published a series of guidelines on the prevention of scurvy (WHO, 1999b), thiamine deficiency (WHO, 1999c), and pellagra (WHO, 2000d).

A food ration monitoring system is important to ensure that families receive fair and adequate quantities of food. On a food ration distribution day, monitoring teams can establish themselves at several points not far from the distribution center. They should be equipped with weighing scales and food composition tables. Families should be stopped randomly as they return to their homes and asked to participate. Each of the items in their ration should be weighed and converted to calories and other nutrients using the tables. The total weight of each food item (in grams) and the total nutrients provided should be divided by the number of family members and the number of days until the next distribution day. This monitoring allows public health workers to determine the average quantity per person per day, which may then be compared with the official ration and with standard tables of recommended daily allowances of nutrients.

Nutritional Rehabilitation

In general, the goal of an emergency feeding program is to provide adequate quantities of nutrients through the general household distribution of food rations. However, due to the many factors described earlier, some population subgroups may already be acutely malnourished or be at high risk of becoming malnourished. These groups may require targeted feeding, also known as selective feeding. Figure 11-5 demonstrates the various kinds of selective feeding; however, these programs should be seen as additions to, rather than as substitutes for, the general feeding program. They need clear objectives and criteria for opening, admission, discharge, and closure that should be based on population-based anthropometry surveys and agreed-upon nutritional indices.

During the first decade of the twenty-first century, a major change evolved in the way in which selective feeding programs are delivered—namely, there was a trend away from reliance on fixed sites to prepare and administer supplementary and therapeutic

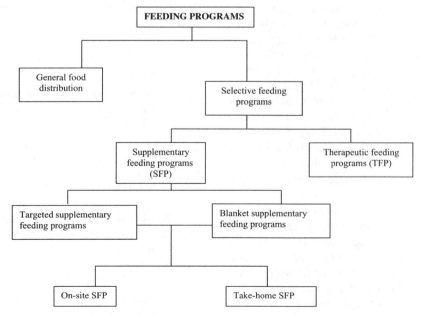

Figure 11-5 Overall Feeding Program Strategy.
Source: United Nations High Commissioner for Refugees & World Food Programme, Guidelines for Selective Feeding Programmes in Emergency Situations (Geneva, Switzerland: UNHCR, 1999). Reprinted with permission.

food. Community-based therapeutic care (CTC) programs are now the norm, except for the management of very malnourished children with complications such as dehydration, acidosis, and hypothermia. Instead of labor-intensive on-site preparation of food, ready-to-use therapeutic foods (RUTF) manufactured by commercial companies have become the most preferred products. The most commonly delivered of these foods is Plumpy'nut, which is produced by the French company Nutriset. Plumpy'nut requires no water preparation or refrigeration and has a 2-year shelf life, making it easy to deploy in difficult conditions to treat severe acute malnutrition. Its ingredients consist of peanut paste, vegetable oil, powdered milk, sugar, vitamins, and minerals combined in a foil pouch. Each 92-g pack provides 500 kcal.

RUTF has proven effective in the rehabilitation of malnourished children. In a study in Malawi, 219 children aged 1 to 5 years with severe malnutrition and edema (but without other complications) were provided with RUTF for feeding at home. More than 83% of the children recovered, while 5% died, meaning that the effectiveness of this intervention exceeded international minimum standards (Ciliberto, Manary, Ndekha, Briend, & Ashorn, 2006). The average weight gain was approximately 2.8 g/kg/day, which is less than that specified in international standards, but nonetheless resulted in good overall recovery. Research has further shown that effective RUTF can be manufactured in most settings worldwide at a very low cost using local foods and fairly common equipment.

In general, children are defined as acutely malnourished according to their weight-for-height index, although MUAC is also frequently used for this purpose. Adolescents and adults may be defined according to their MUAC, BMI, or clinical signs. Selective feeding programs should be complemented by measures to improve the food ration distribution system, provide adequate clean water and sanitation, and control measles and other communicable diseases. They should also be integrated into community health programs that offer other prevention and care services.

Supplementary feeding programs (SFPs) provide nutritious foods in addition to the general ration, with the aim of rehabilitating moderately malnourished individuals and decreasing the population prevalence of acute malnutrition. Two kinds of SFPs are possible: targeted and blanket. Each type may provide food supplements as on-site, precooked ("wet") or take-home ("dry") rations. Take-home rations are usually preferred because they require fewer resources, carry lower risks of cross-infection among recipients, and retain the family's primary responsibility for feeding. On-site feeding may be justified when the security situation is poor; when the general ration is inadequate, so that food is likely to be shared within the household; or when cooking fuel is scarce.

A targeted SFP aims to prevent the moderately malnourished from becoming severely malnourished and to rehabilitate them. Such programs generally focus on children younger than 5 years and on pregnant and lactating women. Care should be taken not to apply strict guidelines for the opening of selective feeding programs. Like all decisions taken in an emergency, establishment of such a program should be based on a review of both current public health priorities and available resources.

Current guidelines suggest that a targeted SFP should be implemented when one or more of the following situations occur:

- The prevalence of acute malnutrition among children younger than 5 years is 10% to 14%.
- The prevalence of acute malnutrition among children is 5% to 9% in the presence of aggravating factors (e.g., inadequate general food ration, CMR greater than 1 death per 10,000 population per day, epidemics of measles or pertussis, and high incidence of acute respiratory infections and diarrheal diseases).

Criteria for admission should include the following:

- Children younger than 5 years with a weight-for-height Z-score between −3 and −2
- Older children, adolescents, and adults who are moderately malnourished according to their MUAC, BMI, or clinical condition
- Referrals of children graduating from therapeutic feeding programs
- Selected pregnant women and nursing mothers

Blanket SFPs are meant to provide extra nutritious food to all members of groups at risk of malnutrition. They are started under the following conditions:

- Prior to establishment of general food distribution systems
- Problems in delivering and distributing the general ration

- Prevalence of acute malnutrition equal to or greater than 15%

- Prevalence of acute malnutrition of 10% to 14% in the presence of aggravating factors

- Anticipated increase in acute malnutrition rates due to seasonally induced epidemics

- In the case of micronutrient-deficiency disease outbreaks, to provide micronutrient-rich supplements to a target population

The primary recipients of blanket SFPs are all children younger than 5 years, pregnant women and nursing mothers (up to 6 months after delivery), and other groups such as the elderly or medically ill.

Therapeutic feeding programs (TFPs) aim to rehabilitate severely malnourished persons, the majority of whom are children with severe wasting or nutritional edema. A TFP should be initiated when the number of severely malnourished individuals cannot be treated adequately in other facilities. Although current guidelines for opening a TFP are based on population malnutrition prevalence, the decision should take into account an assessment of the public health needs and the resources available. In a large camp, the percentage of malnourished children may not be an appropriate basis for this decision. Perhaps a more practical guide would be the presence of, say, 50 potential beneficiaries in a settlement. The following criteria are used for admission (UNHCR & World Food Programme, 1999):

- Children younger than 5 years with weight-for-height Z-scores less than −3 or with edema

- Severely malnourished children older than 5 years, adolescents, or adults assessed by other means

- Low-birth-weight babies (less than 2,500 g)

- Orphans younger than 1 year of age when traditional caring practices are inadequate

- Mothers of children younger than 1 year with breastfeeding failure where relactation counseling has failed

Rehabilitation of severely malnourished individuals is a medical procedure demanding careful attention to detail; therefore, well-trained staff are essential for ensuring successful outcomes. TFPs usually have two phases:

1. The intensive care phase includes 24-hour care with medical treatment to control infection and dehydration and correct electrolyte imbalance, along with nutritional treatment. Very frequent feeds with therapeutic milk (F-75) are essential to prevent death from hypoglycemia and hypothermia. This phase usually lasts 1 week.

2. The rehabilitation phase provides at least six meals per day along with medical and psychological support, including for mothers of malnourished children. This phase usually lasts 5 weeks.

Details of the quantity and types of food recommended, discharge criteria, and reasons for stopping SFPs and TFPs are provided in two reference manuals (MSF, 1995; UNHCR & WFP, 1999). In addition, detailed information on the management of severe malnutrition is provided in WHO manuals (WHO, 1999d, 2000c).

Community Therapeutic Care

Collins et al. (2006) outline three levels of CTC: inpatient stabilization care for people with acute malnutrition and serious medical complications; outpatient therapeutic programs for people with severe acute malnutrition but no complications; and supplementary feeding for moderate acute malnutrition and no complications. Under this definition, inpatient care is provided according to WHO guidelines. Other studies have categorized CTC programs differently, however. For example, a recent review of the effectiveness of CTC separated programs into four categories: residential nutrition centers, daycare nutrition centers, clinic-based care, and domiciliary (home) care (Ashworth, 2006). Although the term CTC is frequently used in reference to slightly different models, the three-level program structure outlined here—inpatient care, outpatient care, and supplementary feeding program—is a useful one.

CTC approaches are also becoming more effective as techniques and protocols develop. In an extensive literature review, comprising 33 community-based nutrition rehabilitation programs implemented between 1980 and 2005, only one-third (33%) were considered effective, using low mortality and acceptable weight gain as indicators of success (Ashworth, 2006). In contrast, among those programs implemented between 1995 and 2005, a much greater proportion (62%) were considered effective.

Health Services: Response to Complex Emergencies

Complex emergencies severely disrupt normal health-care service activity (see Figure 11-3). In developing appropriate responses to this disruption, it is worth considering the impact on and response by at least three different sets of services:

- Service provision in the country affected by the CE
- Service provision in countries to which refugees have fled
- Service provision by multilateral agencies and NGOs

Service Provision in Countries Directly Affected by Complex Emergencies

The main challenge in these settings is to minimize the direct and indirect adverse effects of the conflict on the health services personnel and resources available. In many conflicts, as highlighted earlier, health services may be specifically targeted, as may health service providers. In such situations, it may be extremely difficult to maintain services due to absent or fleeing health personnel, lack of drugs and equipment, disruption of referral systems, and destruction of physical infrastructure, including hospitals and clinics. Even if the official health system is destroyed, however, the health workers who previously worked within it may still be present within the community (unless they have fled to safer areas) and may still be able to offer services and advice. The extent to which services can be maintained is in part dependent on earlier disaster preparedness activities, in terms of both training and the prepositioning of drugs and other supplies in areas where logistic support was predicted to be vulnerable to disruption.

In some situations, services likely to be disrupted have received stocks of drugs and equipment prior to the CE, thereby enabling them to continue to provide services despite the disruption of linkages to normal supply chains. Although this course of action might be possible with certain forms of equipment and drugs, others, such as vaccination facilities (which depend on maintaining an intact cold chain), and support activities, such as training and supervision, are invariably disrupted. Nevertheless, local-level responses are possible. In Afghanistan, despite the conflict in Kabul, the medical school was able to relocate to another city to continue its training activities.

In relation to the availability of drugs for treatment, prior distribution of necessary drugs to responsible community members, such as community and other health workers, teachers, and in some cases patients with chronic conditions, may ensure their availability despite the population having to move suddenly. Patients with chronic conditions such as leprosy or TB could be issued drug supplies sufficient for extended periods, assuming that the drugs can be procured and distributed and that patients with these conditions will be able to adhere to the treatment regimes prescribed for them.

The potential to distribute impregnated mosquito nets to populations on the move might be an option in areas of high malaria risk. Some experience in this approach has been gained among the highly mobile Burmese refugees on the Thai border.

Service Provision in Countries to Which Refugees Have Fled

When refugees flee from their country and cross borders, their normal sources of health care are no longer available to them. Therefore, they may be dependent on what they can provide for themselves, which is often desperately little if they have been forced to flee suddenly, as was the case with the Kosovar Albanians in 1999. Alternatively, they may depend on what can be provided in the host country to which they have fled, either through existing host country services or through additional services mobilized through NGOs and other organizations. Host government services may rapidly become overwhelmed if large numbers of refugees suddenly move into an area and seek to use the local health system. In addition to difficulties presented by their absolute numbers, the health condition of these refugees may be poor, especially if their journey has been traumatic and unplanned or if their prior state of health was poor.

In most cases, at least in the short term, the local host-country services will not receive additional resources and, therefore, will have to cope as best they can with the additional service load. The strain placed on the health system may disadvantage local community members who ordinarily utilize such services, because the supply of drugs and usual access to health workers may be compromised. Communities will typically be willing to accept these hardships for a time, but if the situation becomes protracted and leads to a lasting decline in services, tension may develop between the host and refugee communities. Another point of friction occurs when refugees are offered access to host services at no cost, while local community members may be required to pay user charges, both informal and formal, to obtain care. In addition, different policies may be applied to refugee and local populations. For malaria treatment, for example, international organizations providing care to the emergency-affected population might opt for more effective drugs than those designated by existing national policies. Such was the case in Burundi in 2000–2001, where disagreements between MSF and the government of Burundi over malaria treatment policies took several months to resolve (MSF, 2001). Devoting attention to issues of equity and to ensuring that host and refugee communities gain similar access to services will be in the longer-term best interests of both groups.

A key challenge to the host community is to utilize opportunities presented by the influx of refugees, along with other organizations and resources, to ensure that its services are developed further and its capacity is strengthened. Unfortunately, this outcome rarely happens, although increasing awareness of these problems has begun to highlight the need for more capacity-strengthening responses. When the Kosovar Albanians fled into Macedonia and Albania in 1999, for example, there were widespread calls for funds and other support to the health and welfare systems of these countries. This response was in stark contrast to the lack of additional support provided to Tanzania, for example, in building a more appropriate system in response to the influx of Hutu refugees following the Rwandan genocide in 1994.

Even in circumstances where the international community, through UNHCR and a wide range of international NGOs, is providing services to the refugee community, an impact on local health services may be felt. For example, these agencies' recruitment of local health workers may deplete indigenous systems of their usually already inadequate human resources. Moreover, additional burdens may be placed on other levels within the health system, such as referral, rehabilitation, and chronic disease services that the NGOs may be ill prepared for or unwilling to address. Given these potential sources of stress on the local resources, it is important to anticipate and provide support to the host health system to ensure that it is best able to respond to the increased needs without collapsing under the pressure of greater demands upon the services provided.

Service Provision by Multilateral Organizations and Nongovernmental Organizations

The key challenges for multilateral organizations and NGOs are, in the short term, to reduce excess loss of life and to reestablish an environment in which maintaining and promoting health is possible. Many of the subsequent sections of this chapter deal with the nature of the health-related interventions that are necessary in these settings. A much-debated issue is whether these interventions should focus solely on the immediate, short-term needs of CE-affected populations or whether they should also incorporate longer-term objectives. Many relief and humanitarian organizations see their primary role as saving lives that have been placed at risk as a result of extraordinary events. In such situations, doing whatever is necessary, with whatever resources are available, is deemed appropriate, even if some of what is done cannot be replicated or sustained over the longer term.

In camp settings, health services should be organized to ensure that the major causes of morbidity and mortality are addressed through fixed facilities and outreach programs. An essential drug list and standardized treatment protocols are necessary elements of a curative program. It is not necessary to develop totally new guidelines in each refugee situation, as several excellent manuals already exist, from which guidelines can be adapted to suit local conditions (WHO, 2003). Curative services should be decentralized in a camp system of community health workers, health posts, first-line outpatient clinics, and a small inpatient facility to treat severe emergency cases. Patients requiring surgery or prolonged hospitalization should be referred to a local district or provincial hospital, which will likely require assistance with drugs and other medical supplies to cope with the extra patient load.

Organizations that typically espouse a development- rather than relief-oriented approach have sought to place the issue of developmental relief onto the agenda, arguing that early attention to the difficult issues of efficiency, effectiveness, sustainability, equity, and local ownership will be beneficial in the longer term. If this approach is adopted, greater effort would be given to activities such as training, building local capacity, and keeping costs down, rather than seeing these as desirable—but not practical—goals given the acute needs faced in relation to saving lives.

An additional key concern facing the range of organizations offering services in response to humanitarian crises is the importance of coordination. Organizations need to work together very closely if they are to reinforce one another's actions, maximize the use of available resources, minimize duplication and overlap, and enhance effectiveness, equity, and efficiency. The Code of Conduct for Humanitarian Organizations highlights the need for effective coordination, usually under the aegis of a lead organization from the United Nations system, such as OCHA, UN-HCR, or, in some cases (especially for the health sector), WHO or UNICEF.

Lastly, there has been considerable unease in recent years regarding the quality of much of the service provision by NGOs operating in CEs. A key problem is the lack of transparency and accountability of such services, and the fact that even well-meaning organizations may do more harm than good. Recent initiatives, such as the Sphere Project (see Exhibit 11-7, later in this chapter), seek to establish standard and minimum indicators of acceptable performance for organizations operating in these environments. Although no enforcement mechanisms, or even effective incentives, have been developed to ensure compliance with these suggested standards, many voluntary organizations have agreed to do what they can to comply. The increasing professionalization of the field of humanitarian assistance (a topic briefly discussed toward the end of this chapter) similarly reflects these trends toward improved practice and accountability.

Refugee Health Workers

Community health workers (CHWs) were seen in many countries as the mainstay of primary healthcare promotion, although some critics have questioned their value to national primary healthcare programs (Walt, 1988). In refugee and displaced person settings, the selection and training of refugee health workers has been considered as one key mechanism by which health programs can work more closely with affected communities.

The principal advantages of refugee health workers may be related to their role as intermediaries between the affected community and the services provided by the humanitarian agencies, which are often led by expatriate staff. Refugee workers are more likely to understand the cultural, behavioral, and environmental influences on health status; to contribute to a growing potential for self-care and refugee-provided services within the community; to share the health service provision workload; to build capacity and skills that will potentially be available after repatriation; and to enhance the dignity of both the community and the healthcare providers themselves. CHWs who are relatively unskilled and trained within the community may be the mainstay of service provision. It is important to recognize that the presence of trained health workers within the affected community, whether these be midwives, nurses, doctors,

or others, represents an extremely valuable resource whose role should be promoted in whatever services are developed with expatriate agency support.

The role of CHWs in refugee settings will depend on the public health needs, the availability of host country– and NGO-provided services, the prior level of skill of the workers, and the extent and quality of training received. In many cases, refugee health workers have worked outside of health center settings and have performed a range of tasks, including the following:

- Identifying sick and malnourished community members and assisting them in obtaining assistance
- Collecting and reporting demographic data such as births and deaths
- Providing first aid and basic primary care such as oral rehydration for children with diarrhea
- Assisting in mass vaccination campaigns
- Encouraging participation in health campaigns and disease control programs
- Ensuring that the needs and perspectives of refugees are taken into account in the development of health programs

In many conflicts (notably those in Vietnam, Mozambique, Ethiopia, and Eritrea), liberation movements trained cadres of CHWs who played a valuable role in establishing core healthcare services. These workers initially focused on basic curative care, but eventually expanded their services to include preventive health and health promotion. In a number of these struggles, such health workers also played a role in community mobilization and in laying the foundations for primary care–oriented services.

One of the first refugee programs that systematically trained large numbers of CHWs as the very basis of health service delivery was established in Somalia in the early 1980s. At that time, almost 1 million refugees from Ethiopia were housed in 35 camps scattered throughout three regions of the country. The Ministry of Health's Refugee Health Unit coordinated the training of approximately 2,000 CHWs and 1,000 traditional birth attendants with the help of NGOs working in the country. The training curriculum was standardized, as were treatment protocols, essential drugs, and salaries and conditions. As NGOs gradually withdrew from the country, health services were largely provided by CHWs and traditional birth attendants, supervised by Somali Ministry of Health trainers, nurses, and doctors.

Despite the range of potential advantages to developing and working with a cadre of refugee health workers, this approach is also associated with numerous problems. It may be difficult to recruit health workers, especially in unstable settings or if potential workers have other pressing priorities, and they will require training and ongoing supervision. Their selection may be highly political, and identifying the affiliations of potential health workers may be difficult for agencies with limited knowledge of the area in which they are working. If an inappropriate mix of workers from different areas and different backgrounds is selected, this imbalance has the potential to stimulate rivalry and exacerbate perceptions of inequity. In the presence of adequately resourced host-country services, especially those that have sufficient numbers of trained staff, establishing a cadre of CHWs with more limited skills may not be seen as a priority.

Among the prerequisites for effective CHW training programs are a clear description of the tasks to be performed, an adequate level of logistic and supervisory support, a transparent system of selection and remuneration, and the consent and involvement of the affected and, where relevant, host communities.

Women's and Children's Healthcare Services

Children and women, especially pregnant women, have been repeatedly shown to be the most vulnerable members of refugee and displaced populations, especially during the emergency period. Among Rohingya refugees in Bangladesh (1992–1993), women and girl children were seen less often at health facilities than men and boys, yet had much higher mortality (Figure 11-6).

In Goma in 1994, households headed by women were found to have substantially less food and non-food commodities that had been issued at general distribution points by international relief officials than those in which an adult male was present. For these reasons, health services oriented to the specific needs of children and women are essential in reducing morbidity and mortality within a population to a minimum level. Women's and children's health (WCH) care should begin within the community, at the household level, and should not depend entirely on established health facilities. Often, as discussed earlier, community members, such as traditional birth attendants or others previously trained as CHWs, can

be recruited from within the affected population itself to provide basic services.

For children, routine screening and preventive services are important. Growth monitoring, and the referral of children whose growth is faltering to supplementary feeding programs, is an essential function of WCH services. A WCH program will also ensure that all children are vaccinated on schedule and are receiving regular supplements of vitamin A. When curative care is required, as for diarrhea and acute respiratory infection, it can be delivered within the household by trained CHWs, or the child can be referred to peripheral, first-line health facilities.

Pregnant women (who may constitute 3% of the displaced population) should be regularly monitored. At least three prenatal examinations should be conducted to identify high-risk pregnancies. All women should be vaccinated with tetanus toxoid to prevent neonatal tetanus in their newborns. Iron and folic acid supplements should be distributed (and their ingestion monitored, if possible). Insecticide-treated bed nets for the prevention of malaria should be distributed, and the presumptive treatment of malaria, if appropriate, should be undertaken when pregnant women are in their second and third trimesters. In the postnatal period, counseling services addressing a variety of issues, from family planning to child care, and especially breastfeeding, should be offered.

Finally, although many elements of WCH can be instituted in the post-emergency phase, a critical service that must be provided during the earliest stages of a relief effort is the establishment of emergency obstetrical care. Cesarean section and transfusion facilities and the ability to give parenteral antibiotics are essential if maternal mortality is to be kept low. Provisions for emergency delivery are part of an overall minimum initial service package, as discussed in the next section.

Reproductive Health

UNHCR, WHO, and the UN Population Fund (UNFPA) state that although food, water, and shelter remain priorities in an emergency assistance program, reproductive health care is among the crucial elements that accord refugees the basic human welfare and dignity that are their right (UNHCR, 1995a). The response to reproductive health problems during emergencies consists of a constellation of assessment, services, and regular monitoring that addresses the implementation of the following programs:

- A minimum initial service package (MISP)
- Safe motherhood

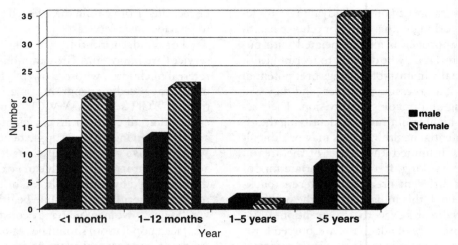

Figure 11-6 Number of Deaths Among Burmese Refugees in the Gundhum II Camp, Bangladesh, May 6 to June 26, 1992, by Age and Sex.
Source: Data from Centers for Disease Control and Prevention, "Famine Affected, Refugee, and Displaced Populations: Recommen-dations for Public Health Issues," 1992, Morbidity and Mortality Weekly Report, 41(RR-13).

- Prevention and treatment of sexual and gender-based violence
- Prevention and care for sexually transmitted diseases
- Family planning
- Reproductive health needs of adolescents

Minimum Initial Service Package

Although resources should not be diverted from attempts to control the diseases that have traditionally been the leading causes of death in CEs, five interventions related to reproductive health should be implemented even in the acute phase. In addition, a reproductive health coordinator should be designated to ensure that these measures are adequately addressed.

Emergency Contraception

Forced migration is frequently accompanied by sexual violence. To prevent unwanted pregnancies resulting from rape, emergency postcoital contraceptive supplies should be available to women who request them. Although the extent of this problem has never been adequately documented, and although it is likely to vary from one situation to the next, the current recommendation is that supplies sufficient to cover 1% of women of reproductive age should be immediately available. Two methods of emergency contraception are currently offered: the combined oral contraceptive (two formulations are used), which must be taken within 3 days of unprotected sexual in-

tercourse, or the copper intrauterine device, which must be implanted within 5 days of unprotected intercourse.

Universal Precautions

To prevent the transmission of the HIV virus, universal precautions must be respected from the very outset of an emergency. Although chaotic conditions are frequently prevalent and although health services are implemented under very stressful conditions, the threat of HIV infection can and must be minimized. Universal precautions include the following:

- Washing hands with soap and water after contact with body fluids or wounds
- Wearing gloves for procedures involving contact with blood or other body fluids
- Using protective clothing when exposure to large amounts of blood is likely
- Handling sharps safely
- Disposing of waste materials safely (burning and/or burial)
- Disinfecting or sterilizing medical equipment
- Wearing gloves when handling corpses, and washing with soap and water afterward

Availability of Contraceptives

Little is known about sexual behavior during times of emergency. To prevent unwanted pregnancies and to minimize the transmission of sexually preventable infections, including HIV, an adequate supply of condoms should be available on request to all members of the target population. Several guidelines have been developed for the prevention of HIV in refugee and post-emergency settings (Holmes, 2003; Inter-Agency Standing Committee Task Force on HIV/AIDS in Emergency Settings, 2003; Sphere Project, 2004).

Delivery Services

All populations affected by CEs are likely to include women in the later stages of pregnancy or who are at high risk for complicated deliveries. These women need services even during the acute phase of the emergency. In a population of 2,500 with a crude birth rate of about 3%, there will be approximately 5 to 8 births per month. To deal with these deliveries, simple supplies must be made available. Both simple delivery kits and midwife kits are readily available from UNICEF and other suppliers of health supplies. Skilled attendants should be present at every delivery. In addition, although it is not a formal part of the MISP, sites where complicated deliveries can be performed should be established as early during an emergency as possible. Cesarean section for obstructed delivery, transfusion for excessive hemorrhage, and parenteral antibiotics for the treatment of sepsis are the only ways to reduce maternal mortality, and these measures should be available and easily accessible from the onset of a relief operation.

Comprehensive Reproductive Health Services

The last element of the MISP is planning for the provision of comprehensive reproductive health services as rapidly as is feasible. To do so, reproductive health indicators should be included in health information systems to allow for the collection of baseline data on maternal, infant, and child mortality; prevalence of sexually transmitted diseases; and population contraceptive prevalence rates. Suitable sites for the delivery of reproductive health services should be identified, though they need not be separate from other health facilities. These areas should be secure and allow for safe passage of women between their home and the clinic. They should be easily accessible to all who wish to use them, guarantee privacy and confidentiality, and have access to clean water and latrines. In addition, an adequate referral system should be identified or established to provide care to women with obstetrical complications or other health emergencies.

Post-emergency Reproductive Health Programs

When adequate food, water, sanitation, and shelter have been provided, programs to address the initial emergency health priorities have been implemented (e.g., measles vaccination), and mortality rates have declined, the range of reproductive health services should gradually be expanded. In the post-emergency phase, health care would be quite incomplete unless the entire range of programs aimed at maintaining or improving reproductive health was included. The key to successful reproductive health programs is soliciting active participation of as many adolescents and women of reproductive age as possible. Although training female health workers (including traditional birth attendants) is usually the focus of such programs, male health workers should also be trained in the basic principles of reproductive health care. In addition, because adequate reproductive health services are frequently unavailable to the local, non-refugee population, it is a good idea to try to extend whatever programs are being made available to refugees and displaced persons by expatriate relief workers to women and adolescents in the host population.

Communicable Disease Control

Concern for the potential impact of communicable diseases has dominated the public health response in many emergency settings. As discussed previously, this attention has been frequently warranted. Although many of the technical interventions and public health programs used in emergencies draw heavily from their counterparts in stable settings, a few important differences should be considered. Key issues include addressing the needs of the local, nondisplaced, population; maintaining respect for national health policies when dealing with refugees (but not necessarily adhering to them); and promoting substantial community involvement as early as is feasible.

Measles

Because of the devastating effects that measles has had in many emergencies, it has become almost universally accepted that mass measles vaccination, regardless of vaccination history or place of provenance of the displaced, should be instituted as early during an emergency as possible. Leading reference publications (CDC, 1992; MSF, 1997; Sphere Project, 2004) accord measles vaccination the highest priority of all health-specific interventions and recommend that it be undertaken immediately after an initial rapid assessment regardless of the circumstances. If children cannot be vaccinated upon arrival or registration, a mass vaccination campaign should be undertaken. This rule should be followed unless extenuating circumstances exist, such as the cholera epidemic in

Goma in 1994 that required the full attention of the health services, although any mass vaccination program must be planned very carefully if it is to be implemented successfully. Sufficient vaccine supplies should be on hand (with a reserve in case of excess wastage) and stored in a functioning cold chain of adequate capacity. Only autodestruct syringes should be used to deliver the vaccines, and safety boxes must be available for their storage and disposal.

The target population for measles vaccination in emergencies is usually children aged 6 months to 15 years. WHO has recommended reducing the usual minimum age for measles vaccination from 9 months to 6 months because high attack rates and very high CFRs have occurred in younger children, especially in large displaced populations living in relatively crowded conditions. Because vaccine efficacy in children aged 6 to 9 months may be lower than optimal because of the persistence of passively transferred maternal antibodies to measles virus, children in this age group should then be vaccinated again at the age of 9 months. The upper age limit for mass vaccination is more flexible and depends, to a large extent, on the amount of measles vaccine, injection equipment, and health personnel available and the pressure of competing healthcare priorities. Because age and undernutrition are such important risk factors for complicated measles and for high CFRs, all children up to 15 years old who are eligible for selective feeding programs or who are hospitalized with other illnesses should be vaccinated against measles on a priority basis. Then, depending on the factors mentioned earlier, all children younger than 2 years should be considered for vaccination, followed by all children younger than 5 years. Finally, if the circumstances allow, the target population can be expanded. In any case, a mass vaccination campaign should seek to achieve at least 95% coverage of the target population.

Because a mass vaccination campaign can reach such a high proportion of the most vulnerable population, there are frequently demands to attach other services to it. Vitamin A, for example, can be offered to the same target group during the course of the campaign. Insecticide-treated bed nets can be distributed to each household in which a child resides. There have also been suggestions to provide polio vaccination along with measles vaccine, although the logistical burden of doing so must be carefully considered. In any case, a routine vaccination program for all children using the standard antigens recommended by WHO should be established during the post-emergency period. Other vaccines, such as yellow fever and meningitis, are effective in interrupting transmission after an epidemic has been detected; they should not be offered routinely at the time of measles vaccine. Cholera vaccination has also been recommended at the time of measles vaccination (a topic discussed in the following section).

The early detection of measles cases when they occur is an important feature of an effective community-based surveillance system. Measles treatment includes the administration of two doses of vitamin A and the appropriate treatment of common complications such as pneumonia, diarrhea, malnutrition, and meningoencephalitis. Children with measles should be closely monitored in regard to their nutritional status and, if indicated, should be enrolled in supplementary feeding programs during their convalescence.

Measles continues to pose an important threat to the health of children in many emergency settings. As vaccination programs in many parts of the world have progressed and as vaccination coverage levels have increased, however, the need for measles vaccination may move from center stage, to be considered alongside other priority interventions. In northern Iraq and in the Balkans, as in Goma, measles vaccination was delayed to address other, more urgent problems. Conversely, in Afghanistan (2002), in Darfur (2004), and in Aceh province, Indonesia, in the wake of the tsunami (2005), measles vaccination was among the very first interventions organized and implemented. In spite of the clear threat that measles poses to the health of populations in emergency settings, it is always appropriate to weigh the public health needs in light of the available resources and to order priorities accordingly.

Diarrheal Diseases

The importance of diarrhea as a contributor to morbidity and mortality in emergency settings cannot be overstated. The detection and reporting of diarrhea should be part of the routine surveillance system implemented in all emergencies. Both acute watery diarrhea and bloody diarrhea should be reported separately by age (younger than 5 years and older than 5 years are minimum age groups) and by gender.

All health personnel should be sensitized to the potential impact of diarrhea and should be skilled in most aspects of prevention and of treatment. The key to prevention lies in providing adequate sanitation facilities and at least the minimum recommended quantity of water of acceptable quality (see "Water and Sanitation," earlier in this chapter). The mainstay of diarrhea case management is oral rehydration therapy (ORT). Although any fluids can be used to prevent the development of dehydration, oral rehydration salts (ORS) can be used in all cases and are the treatment of choice for all levels of dehydration (see Chapter 5). In fact, the first large field trial of ORS took place in a refugee camp in West Bengal, India, where it was shown that cholera patients treated with what was the standard treatment at the time were 3.8 times as likely to die from dehydration as those treated with ORS.

Rehydration facilities should be available in all health facilities, including health posts and outreach sites within the community. Keys to the success of ORT in emergencies, where the case load can be substantial, include careful organization of ORT centers and the presence of concerned and skilled staff. Mothers or other caretakers are important contributors to ORT and must be instructed as to the quantity of fluid that their children require. Assertive administration of ORT, especially for children who are tired and reluctant to drink, is essential. Breastfeeding should be continued, and the nutritional status of children recovering from diarrhea must be carefully monitored. Rehydration of unaccompanied children should be carefully overseen and appropriate follow-up ensured (see Chapter 5).

Cholera

In populations residing in areas where cholera is a risk (e.g., if fecal culture-confirmed cholera diarrhea has occurred in three of the previous five years), WHO now recommends mass immunization with one of two available oral cholera vaccines.[3] Although all age groups are vulnerable to cholera, where resources are limited immunization should be targeted at high-risk children aged 1 year or older (Shanchol or mORCVAX) or more than 2 years (Dukoral) (WHO, 2010). Mass immunization campaigns should not disrupt or delay other critical prevention programs, such as clean water and sanitation.

Early detection of possible cases of cholera is key to the effective management of an epidemic. Although noncholera diarrhea is a far more common cause of morbidity and mortality in children, the death of an adult from dehydration should raise suspicions of cholera. Attack rates can be higher in refugee camps than in noncamp situations. Laboratory confirmation should be obtained as quickly as possible at the start of a suspected epidemic, but need not be continued. Whenever cholera is suspected, aggressive attempts to educate the community should be undertaken to limit the panic that frequently accompanies this disease. During the course of an epidemic, cases and deaths should be reported on a daily basis through the institution of an active surveillance mechanism.

The need to establish rehydration facilities at multiple sites within the community has been dramatically highlighted by the occurrence of epidemics of cholera. In an outbreak in Somalia in 1985, a new camp with only a centralized treatment facility and no trained CHWs reported a case fatality rate of 23.3%. In contrast, in seven camps in which peripheral ORT corners with trained CHWs had been established in the framework of a primary healthcare system, the CFR was limited to 2.4%. Even more dramatically, during the devastating outbreak in Goma in 1994, more than 90% of the approximately 45,000 deaths that occurred during a 3-week period occurred beyond the reach of the health system. Active case finding and rehydration therapy within the community, rather than reliance on overwhelmed and understaffed health facilities, may have averted a significant fraction of these deaths.

Although as many as 90% of patients during a cholera epidemic can be treated orally, intravenous rehydration will be required for those with the most severe disease. A referral system must be in place, and cholera treatment sites should be identified and prepared with adequate bed capacity, human resources, water, drugs and other supplies, and disposal facilities. The treatment of cholera is the same as is described in Chapter 5. In emergency settings, however, selective chemoprophylaxis is usually not indicated. Resources can be used more efficiently and effectively in other ways, such as establishing adequate water and sanitation and ensuring that all patients are identified and treated quickly and appropriately.

Dysentery Due to Shigella dysenteriae Type 1

The management of epidemics of dysentery in emergency settings is very difficult. As is true of other diarrheal diseases, ensuring adequate water and sanitation facilities is essential to minimize the risk of an epidemic. Because of the highly communicable nature of *Shigella dysenteriae* type 1, however, this measure's role in reducing transmission may be limited, especially in the crowded conditions of refugee camps. Nevertheless, the use of narrow-neck containers for water storage to reduce contamination and the distribution and use of soap for hand washing have been shown to be useful steps in preventing dysentery. Early case detection and prompt treatment are the keys to limiting spread. An epidemic of *S. dysenteriae* type 1 should be suspected whenever diarrhea with blood in the stool is reported. Laboratory confirmation and sensitivity to antibiotics should be obtained immediately, with careful attention paid to the transport of stool specimens.

---

[3] Dukoral and Shanchol or mORCVAX.

The key to dysentery case management is antibiotic therapy. Nevertheless, severe limitations to effective case management on a large scale exist, including the large case loads that may require treatment, the resistance of organisms to first-line and even second-line antibiotics, and the difficulty of ensuring patient compliance with 3- to 5-day courses of treatment. In the relatively sheltered environment of refugee or IDP camps or settlements, where an international relief effort may be instituted, access to more expensive antibiotics and better patient supervision may be possible. However, because outbreaks frequently involve the surrounding local population, careful consideration should be given to the level of care provided. During the Goma epidemic, for example, the U.S. military donated a large quantity of ciprofloxacin—then a relatively expensive antibiotic—for the treatment of refugees. The local population, which was also severely affected by the epidemic, had recourse only to nalidixic acid, an antibiotic to which many of the isolated strains of S. *dysenteriae* type 1 were resistant. This situation created tension between the local public health authorities and the international organizations working with the refugees.

In general, during epidemics of S. *dysenteriae* type 1, an effective antibiotic should be given to all patients, under close supervision of health staff. If supplies of an effective antibiotic are limited, those patients who are severely ill or most vulnerable (e.g., children, pregnant women, the elderly) should be given antibiotics, and others given supportive treatment only, consisting of nutritional support, rehydration when necessary, and other specific measures.

Malaria

Malaria control in emergencies depends to some extent on knowledge of the local vectors. In any case, site planning and selection should be done with the possibility of malaria in mind, and areas with swamps, marshes, and other characteristics that favor vector breeding should be avoided. Where mosquito density is high and immunity of the population is low, periodic residual spraying of interior walls can be undertaken, although this preventive measure is less effective where temporary and shoddy shelters are in use and where mosquitoes bite and rest outdoors. Aerial spraying should usually be avoided except in special circumstances.

Barrier protection methods can also be useful, and the impregnation of materials, including bed nets, curtains, and even clothing, has been effective. The use of impregnated plastic sheeting on dwelling units has shown promise in reducing the incidence of malaria. In all circumstances, long-lasting impregnated bed nets should be distributed (Bloland & Williams, 2003).

In emergencies where people are displaced with their livestock, periodic permethrin sponging of the animals has been shown to reduce vector density and malaria transmission.

The presumptive treatment of pregnant women with pyrimethamine/sulfadoxine in a single dose during the second and third trimesters (especially during their first and second pregnancies) is a potentially effective strategy that requires further evaluation. The presumptive treatment of children attending feeding centers can also be considered, and presumptive treatment of children for malaria at the time of measles vaccination or vaccination in routine programs may be shown to have a role in malaria control after further investigation.

Whenever feasible, the diagnosis of malaria should be confirmed, either microscopically or with one of several available colorimetric rapid diagnostic tests. If facilities are not available to do so, malaria should be treated on the basis of a presumptive diagnosis, although other causes of fever should be suspected as well.

In determining who should be treated, with which drugs, and according to what dosage schedule, it is important to consider the national guidelines of the host country, although malaria control policies may also be updated in accordance with the latest information regarding antimalarial drug sensitivities. In most parts of the world, artemesenin combination therapy is currently the most effective, and most recommended, treatment. Supplies of artemesenin-containing drugs may be low, however, and effective planning to ensure their availability is required. Strategies for uncomplicated malaria, for severe malaria, and for treatment failures should be developed and explained to all health service personnel.

Malaria may occur in epidemic form, especially when individuals are forcibly displaced into highly malarious areas from areas of low endemicity. Epidemics in Kenya (2002) and in Burundi (2000) have heightened awareness of this possibility.

Meningitis

The detection of outbreaks of meningococcal meningitis at an early stage is essential. During emergencies, a high level of suspicion should be maintained. All clinically suspicious cases should be diagnosed by either visual inspection of cerebrospinal fluid or, where available, by the appropriate microscopic, serologic, and bacteriologic analyses. Background rates of meningococcal disease vary considerably from one area to another, and the occurrence of this disease is highly seasonal. The detection of an epidemic, therefore, requires a sensitive surveillance system.

It has become customary to institute epidemic control measures when a threshold incidence rate of 15 cases per 100,000 population per week has been exceeded for 2 consecutive weeks. In small populations, or where the population has not been accurately determined, a weekly doubling of the number of cases over a 3-week period can also signal the early stages of an epidemic. WHO has established alert and response thresholds that should be reviewed and adhered to when emergencies occur in meningitis-prone areas.

Meningococcal vaccine (for group A and group C *Neisseriae meningitidis*) is effective in conferring at least short-term protection to all population groups and can contribute to reducing transmission during the course of an epidemic. More recently, a vaccine protecting against the W135 serogroup, which is becoming a more frequent cause of epidemics in Africa, has also become available. Mass vaccination campaigns are the intervention of choice in areas in which an epidemic is occurring. Such interventions have been implemented in Burundi (1992), Guinea (1993), Zaire (1994), Democratic Republic of Congo (2002), Burundi and Tanzania (2002), and Chad (2005 and again in 2010) during CEs, as well as in many other countries in other situations. Vaccination campaigns usually target the entire population aged 1 year and older, although resource limitations may require limiting the age group to be vaccinated. As is the case with *Shigella* dysentery, epidemics of meningitis usually occur in both displaced and local populations simultaneously, so arrangements should be made to provide vaccine to the host population as well.

Neither mass chemoprophylaxis nor prophylaxis of household contacts has proved to be an effective intervention during outbreaks, and neither practice should be instituted. When epidemics occur in Africa, chloramphenicol in oil is the drug of choice, especially in areas with limited health facilities, because a single dose of this long-acting formulation has been shown to be effective. Penicillin, ampicillin, and ceftriaxone are also effective in treating meningitis.

Tuberculosis

Tuberculosis control should be instituted only after mortality rates have fallen to less than 1 death per 10,000 population per day or when an emergency situation has stabilized and it is apparent that the dis-

placed population will remain in its current location for at least 6 months. From a public health standpoint, the objective of TB control is to treat patients so that they cannot infect others, while helping to restore health in infected individuals. For this reason, only sputum smear–positive individuals are usually included in TB control programs, although individuals who are severely ill with noninfectious forms of TB should also be treated if they are identified. Patients should be treated according to WHO guidelines, which stress directly observed therapy with a short course (6 to 8 months) of a combination of antituberculosis drugs. Because both infection with HIV and malnutrition are associated with TB, the presence of these conditions should be determined and dealt with appropriately.

TB programs are complicated. The decision to implement one should not be made unless clear written guidelines exist and will be followed. Laboratory facilities must be available and the regular provision of supplies ensured. Drugs must be stocked and their resupply guaranteed. Finally, a system for tracing those patients who are unable to adhere to treatment regimens must be in place so that they can be identified and assistance provided to ensure treatment completion. Successful implementation of a TB control program requires a high level of community awareness, education, and involvement. Every element of a tuberculosis control program needs to be carefully and meticulously developed and nurtured over time. Agencies that intend to implement TB control programs in post-emergency settings should have a clear commitment to continue these efforts for at least 12 to 15 months, have an adequate budget, and have the personnel and material resources necessary to run a successful program.

Role of International, National, and Nongovernmental Organizations in Complex Emergencies

The vast and complex array of organizations involved in the various stages of humanitarian emergency preparedness and response reflects the complexity of the international community itself. It is difficult to imagine any other situation that might attract such a range of players: heads of state; diplomats; celebrities; bilateral foreign assistance agencies; UN political, social, economic, and technical organizations; military forces; and a broad variety of NGOs, including an increasing number of commercial interests.

The UN Security Council plays a critical role in determining how and when the world will respond to the conflicts that lead to CEs and how emergency humanitarian assistance programs will be protected from the forces that fuel the conflicts themselves. Security Council decisions are, in turn, made by the leaders of its member states—in particular, the permanent members (the United States, Russia, France, the United Kingdom, and China). OCHA coordinates emergency preparedness and response within the UN system and is governed by an Inter-Agency Standing Committee of relevant UN agencies, including UNHCR, WHO, UNICEF, the World Food Programme (WFP), and UNFPA. OCHA launches joint appeals for funds to support coordinated UN agency response programs; however, these campaigns may sometimes compete with appeals launched by individual agencies.

UNHCR is responsible for the protection and care of all refugees who cross international borders. In some emergency situations, such as the crises in the former Yugoslavia, the UN Secretary-General has designated UNHCR as the lead relief agency. At other times, as was the case in Somalia and southern Sudan, UNICEF or WFP has been the designated lead agency in the UN system. In general, UNHCR and other lead relief agencies need to be invited to provide assistance by the government of the affected country. In situations of internal conflict, the Security Council may authorize involvement by a UN agency without the approval of the host government, as was the case concerning the displaced Kurdish population in northern Iraq in 1991. The lead UN agency is mandated to coordinate the activities of other relief agencies, including NGOs, in cooperation with the host government where that is appropriate. However, in certain chaotic emergency settings, individual NGOs have sometimes negotiated involvement directly with government authorities and ignored efforts by the lead agency to coordinate activities.

United Nations Reforms

Between 2005 and 2010, the United Nations instituted a set of Humanitarian Reforms. The three major points of the reforms, which are intended to improve the coordination of humanitarian relief efforts and to streamline the chaotic funding streams, are summarized here.

First, a Humanitarian Coordinator will be appointed in every situation from which an appeal for emergency funds will emanate. Every UN agency, as well as those NGOs that wish to participate in the response, can submit an estimate of its financial needs to the Humanitarian Coordinator, who is charged with aggregating these requests into one consolidated appeal. Ideally, this system will reduce the level of competition between the individual UN agencies, and between the UN agencies and the NGO community, and provide the donors with a clear and agreed-upon approximation of financial needs for the relief effort.

Second, the UN has established the Central Emergency Response Fund (CERF). CERF was created by the United Nations General Assembly in 2005 and is, essentially, a bank account to which donors deposit and from which the Emergency Relief Coordinator (ERC) of the UN can withdraw to provide funds to UN agencies in a timely and efficient manner when humanitarian relief needs arise. In 2008, more than 80 countries pledged more than $400 million to the CERF, and more than $250 million was spent in more than 40 countries for emergency relief. In addition, CERF funds can be used, at the discretion of the ERC, to provide funds to "chronically underfunded" or "silent" emergencies, such as those that have plagued central Africa for most of the past decade.

Third, a system of technical "clusters" has been developed to bring a systematic approach to a previously cluttered humanitarian scene. For a range of technical areas, a UN agency has been assigned to function as the "lead agency" to bring together donors, NGOs, other UN agencies, and other responders to develop and review policy, formulate plans for coordinated responses, and review and evaluate past performance. The current global clusters include, but are not restricted to, health (WHO lead), logistics (World Food Programme), shelter (UNHCR), water and sanitation (UNICEF), nutrition (UNICEF), and food security (WFP). In the field, each cluster is cochaired by an NGO that, together with the appropriate UN agency, works in cooperation with and under the guidance of the host country government. The performance of the clusters has varied widely to date. External evaluation, it is hoped, will bring about improvements to what appears a promising system, albeit one that is difficult to implement.

Host Country Role

In many emergencies, especially those involving large refugee populations, the host government has granted temporary asylum to the refugees and has become actively engaged in the relief effort. Many countries have coordinating bodies, such as relief commissions, that take a lead role in mobilizing, organizing, and delivering relief services. For example, in Somalia in the early 1980s, the Ministry of Health formed the Refugee Health Unit (RHU), which coordinated public health and nutrition assistance to the 800,000 Ethiopian refugees scattered in 35 camps throughout the country. NGOs wishing to provide assistance to refugees had to agree to follow technical guidelines developed by the unit and signed a tripartite agreement with the RHU and UNHCR. In contrast, in areas such as southern Sudan, where rebel forces are largely in control, relief programs are implemented with little or no involvement by the national government.

During the tsunami relief effort of 2004–2005, the picture was mixed regarding host country involvement. In India and Thailand, most of the relief effort was run entirely by national authorities. In Indonesia and Sri Lanka, a combination of national and international organizations collaborated on policy development and on the day-to-day implementation of relief services.

The International Committee of the Red Cross (ICRC), based in Geneva, is mandated to carry out the protection and care of civilian populations during armed conflict as outlined in the Geneva Conventions. The ICRC relies on low-key and confidential negotiations with all parties to a conflict to allow it to carry out its humanitarian assistance. This organization is committed to carrying out its mission with independence, impartiality, and neutrality.

Although the ICRC was once the only organization to operate within areas affected by conflict, in recent years many other NGOs have joined the ICRC in taking on this challenge. Some of these NGOs, while providing relief impartially to all those in need, believe that they should also speak out in the face of gross human rights abuses and have become advocates for more effective international responses. This action may sometimes jeopardize their ability to remain in the affected area and, therefore, is not taken lightly. One of the most hotly debated issues within NGOs is whether to provide humanitarian relief and remain silent about human rights abuses and the diversion of relief resources or to speak out and risk having to leave the area.

Many NGOs are engaged in providing humanitarian assistance in emergencies, including national Red Cross and Red Crescent societies, international secular and religious agencies, and local churches and community-based organizations in the affected country. Specialized public health agencies such as the CDC, a U.S. government agency, and the Paris-based Epicentre, a private organization closely linked to Médecins Sans Frontières, provide technical advice to a range of bilateral, UN, and nongovernmental operational agencies. The level of technical skills, experience, management, and logistics capacity of NGOs varies enormously.

A number of initiatives have been undertaken in an effort to promote coordination and the implementation of best practices among NGOs. These include the Code of Conduct for the International Red Cross and Red Crescent Movement and NGOs in Disaster Response and the Humanitarian Charter and Minimum Standards in Disaster Response (Sphere Project, 2004), which has been referred to frequently in this chapter. Most professional relief NGOs have signed on to these initiatives, and their adherence to these codes is being monitored and evaluated (Van Dyke & Waldman, 2004). In addition to relief NGOs, an increasing number of human rights advocacy NGOs have been active in CE responses in recent years, including Amnesty International, Human Rights Watch, Physicians for Human Rights, and Africa Watch.

Funding for international humanitarian assistance programs generally comes from the governments of high-income countries, such as the United States, Japan, members of the European Union, and other OECD states. The generosity of such governments varies enormously and often depends more on the perceived geopolitical importance of the conflict than on the actual needs of the affected populations. High-profile media, such as CNN, the *New York Times,* and the BBC, often play an influential role in determining the size of the response to an emergency. For example, the blanket media coverage of emergencies in northern Iraq and Kosovo ensured that relief programs were adequately funded. In contrast, the conflict in Somalia was largely ignored prior to late 1992, when then President George H. W. Bush decided to promote a highly visible humanitarian relief operation in the waning months of his presidency.

The outpouring of support for the relief efforts that were implemented in response to the Indian Ocean tsunami in December 2004 from both public and private sectors is perhaps unprecedented. Why natural disasters seem to attract a more generous funding response than the silent tsunamis that plague areas in conflict for years and that usually take a much larger toll in human life is a matter of speculation. What is certain is that until a consistent response to conflict-related emergencies around the world is realized, the quality and timeliness of humanitarian responses will be unpredictable.

Rehabilitation, Repatriation, and Recovery

In countries emerging from conflict, the costs of reconstruction may be staggering. In the immediate aftermath of the first Gulf War, it was estimated that

Iraq would require $110 billion to $200 billion and Kuwait $60 billion to $95 billion to repair the war damage inflicted by the United States–led coalition (Lee & Haines, 1991). Initial estimates for the reconstruction of Afghanistan were on the order of $1 billion to $2 billion per year for at least a decade.

Within 2 weeks of the December 2004 tsunami in the Indian Ocean, $4 billion had been pledged by donor countries for relief and reconstruction. In comparison, implementing worldwide the goals adopted by the World Summit for Children in 1991 would require $20 billion.

Estimates of the cost of rehabilitation and recovery in countries affected by the Kosovo crisis show that many billions of dollars will be required annually for a considerable period of time, not only for Kosovo, but for the entire subregion if ongoing conflict is to be averted. Notably, the entire annual budget of the UN Authority in postconflict Kosovo was less than 50% of the daily cost of the NATO bombing campaign.

A particularly important issue for those engaged in dealing with the aftermath of conflicts is to determine the extent to which the prior health system will be simply reestablished along the lines of how it previously existed, or whether it will be reformed in an effort to improve efficiency, effectiveness, and equity. The usual response is to seek to reconstruct what has been destroyed in the conflict, although the mantra for the reconstruction of Haiti (a natural disaster) has been "build it back better."

This apparently logical response may be deeply flawed, however. One key impediment is that the resource base available for reconstructing and operating the health system may be vastly inferior to that existing prior to the CE. In Uganda, the postconflict resource base was less than 10% of that prior to the civil war, making simple reestablishment of previously available services totally unfeasible. Furthermore, much changes during the period of ongoing conflict: the range of providers operating, the role of the state, the attitude and demands of the community that uses services, and the approach of the international community and key donor organizations. Outside contributors, for example, may seek to promote a radically different state—one that functions as a steward of the health system, running the civil service, setting policies, establishing evaluation frameworks, and so on, but not providing services, and that places cost-effectiveness and value for money at the core of the system. This has been the case in Afghanistan, since 2003. All health services, except those in Kabul, are contracted out to NGOs within a standard basic package of health services. During the postconflict

phase, international financial institutions and donor governments may greatly influence policy direction, and frequently do so in favor of reducing state expenditures and enhancing the role of the private sector.

In the period between the onset of periods of conflict and their resolution (which may last for decades), approaches to the nature of health services, along with the purchasers and providers of those services, have changed. In many conflicts, other providers may fill the gap left by retreating and undermined state-provided health services—these include for-profit and not-for-profit providers, as well as the indigenous and traditional sector. Little documentation of how and why the private sector emerges to play an important role in these settings exists, nor is there any clarity about how best to control and regulate such activities in the interests of ensuring that minimum standards are met and that the medical treatment offered by different providers does not compromise public health goals and objectives. The emergence and changing roles of members of the nonprofit, nongovernmental sector are easier to appreciate. Such entities fill gaps resulting from withering state services, and their initiatives are often supported by donor country funds that ensure humanitarian relief services are provided in acute emergencies and development-oriented services are offered where suitable funding and partner organizations, including the government, can be identified.

A major weakness of NGO-provided services is that they are often poorly coordinated, act in parallel with the state systems, have a different vision of the system they are seeking to bolster or reestablish, and compete for partners, resources, and publicity. It is not too far-fetched to consider NGOs to be competitors with the state for funds from the donor community. Failing to support indigenous capacity may increase the risk of little being left behind when humanitarian agencies withdraw from the area; increasingly, debate is focusing on how such services can best interface with host government services and policy and reinforce the limited capacity often present in the host country.

A particularly important and difficult challenge is to establish the policy framework within which health services and the health system will operate. Different stakeholders (politicians, professionals, donors, multilateral organizations, private sector) inevitably have their own agendas. A key role of government, when it functions effectively, is to provide a framework within which the different actors can operate. In many settings, including those countries emerging from major periods of conflict, this policy framework may be lacking or challenged, given its often uncertain legitimacy. In the presence of challenges to a government's legitimacy, as in Cambodia after the overthrow of Pol Pot by a Vietnamese-backed party, international donors may withdraw development funding and assistance or, where they do provide such relief and development support, may choose to channel it outside of government structures (Lanjouw, Macrae, & Zwi, 1999). Such actions may simultaneously undermine local capacity and reinforce fragmentation.

At the same time, it is important to recognize that NGO-supported interventions may be extremely effective and may facilitate the emergence of good—or at least better—practice. Moreover, NGOs generally promote more genuine participation by local communities in development activities.

Thus an important role for policy makers, both locally and internationally, is to facilitate the development of consensus about broad health system direction and the policy framework within which service provision will be undertaken. Exhibit 11-6 discusses the case of postconflict authority in East Timor.

Key issues to be debated in the aftermath of periods of conflict include the financing of health services, the extent to which these services can and should be decentralized, the role of the private sector, and the priority to be accorded to issues of equity. These issues need to be placed within the broader context of promoting and consolidating the peace, reestablishing the economy, facilitating the demobilization of troops and their absorption into the economy, and facilitating the return of refugees and internally displaced people. Other key priorities include determining and establishing accountable systems of governance.

Ensuring that, to as great an extent as possible, existing inequities in distribution and access to health services are resolved in the aftermath of conflict may assist in lowering tensions between rival groups. Such inequities are often significant contributors to conflict between communities and different social groups in civil society. In the postconflict period, a fundamental challenge is to understand and seek to address those factors that contributed to the conflict. Promoting the development of a more equitable health and social system may provide an important opportunity for bringing together different groups within affected populations, and may provide early opportunities to stimulate debate, exchange ideas, and rekindle trust. The concept of health as a bridge to peace is relatively untested, however, and it is apparent that in some circumstances health-related interventions, if insensitively or differentially applied, may reinforce tensions and conflicts within and between communities.

Identifying opportunities to increase the availability of funds for responding to basic needs in rural, urban, and periurban poor areas will be important to ensure a degree of public health control. Likewise,

---

| Exhibit 11-6 | **Transitional Authority in East Timor** |

The violence following the August 1999 independence referendum was stopped by a United Nations–authorized international force in East Timor (INTERFET). In February 2000, responsibility for the administration of the territory was assumed by the UN Transitional Authority in East Timor (UNTAET), headed by a special representative of the UN Secretary-General, for a period of 2 years leading up to elections and full independence for the new nation. Security was maintained by UN peacekeepers from 41 member nations.

The development of public policies and services, including health, was conducted within the framework of a National Consultative Council, which comprised three senior UNTAET officials, seven members of the major East Timorese political coalition (CNRT), and seven non-CNRT East Timorese representatives (e.g., churches, human rights organizations). Given the shortage of skilled local specialists, much of the policy direction was driven by consultants from various specialized technical agencies, such as WHO and UNICEF. Although the UN was reluctant to work closely with CNRT, the World Bank promptly consulted with the coalition, and a $20 million trust fund was established for "community empowerment" projects that were to be implemented through local community structures.

In that country of 800,000 people, 60 international NGOs and 68 locally registered NGOs were active in the postconflict phase; however, very few had a commitment to capacity building and long-term national development. Various sectoral committees (e.g., health, education, police) were formed with representation by the various players mentioned earlier. The role of the National Consultative Council was to consider policy recommendations made by these committees and to provide approval when appropriate and in the longer-term national interest.

enhancing the quality of both publicly and privately provided services and identifying new partnerships between state and nonstate actors will be important in developing more sustainable systems for the future.

Gender inequalities permeate many societies. In the postconflict environment, it may be possible to address these disparities given that the conflict itself may have changed gender relations and modified the traditional roles of men and women. Conflict often leads to women taking on a more important role in relation to making household decisions and controlling household resources—even in patriarchal societies, men will often be absent during periods of conflict, such that women will, of necessity, absorb a multitude of usually male-dominated roles. Certain countries, notably Eritrea, Ethiopia, and South Africa, have clearly positioned gender issues as part of the postconflict dispensation sought by many. The Palestinian conflict drew extensively on women as a major force within the political struggle. Post-conflict development of civil society and good governance may reflect opportunities for positive change; if inadequate support is given to such groups, however, such as in the former Yugoslavia, opportunities to promote a more accountable state that seeks negotiated (rather than violent) means of resolving conflict may be missed.

The reorganization of health services to promote preventive and primary care should receive at least as much attention as physical reconstruction of the infrastructure. In many settings, however, emphasis appears to be mistakenly placed largely on the rehabilitation and construction of hospitals and clinics, with little attention being devoted to the more difficult tasks of improving the policy process, expanding management capacity, consolidating human resources, developing preventive care programs, and extending services to the poor. Major international donors often play a significant role in undermining more effective policy development in this areas, as such donors typically seek high-visibility inputs, often dominated by infrastructure support, or support tightly controlled vertical programs.

An initiative to focus on the health system challenges facing countries emerging from conflict identified a number of key priorities for intervention (Zwi, Ugalde, & Richards, 2005):

- Maximizing the contribution of both government and donors to the formulation and development of health policy
- Developing a clear conceptual framework, informed by multidisciplinary approaches, to guide health system development

- Establishing inclusive processes that involve a range of stakeholders in a participatory and transparent process of identifying needs and priorities and agreeing on models and approaches to health system development
- Appreciating the limitations and constraints operating upon the range of different stakeholders (e.g., government at central and local levels, UN agencies, NGOs, traditional public and private sector providers) in financing, providing, and overseeing health services
- Promoting evidence-based policy and planning to ensure that more good than harm results from interventions and that resources are used as equitably and efficiently as possible

Donor Assistance and Coordination

As mentioned earlier, considerable confusion surrounds the different roles played by donors and implementing agencies in relief and development contexts, and little clarity exists regarding how these roles change in relation to the financing and provision of services during periods of postconflict reconstruction, rehabilitation, and development. The provision of relief is dominated by attempts to secure survival with the input of materials and support, often using NGOs as the key providers. In longer-term development projects, equity and reform are key objectives, human resources and institutional capacity development are key inputs, and partnership with government dominates the form of interaction with government. The transition from one phase to another is often uncertain, contested, and marked by competition and self-interest.

Since the end of the Cold War, the funds allocated to global emergencies have generally increased, though they appear to have peaked around the midpoint of the 1990s. At the same time, development assistance has declined, in part because of budgetary pressure, but also reflecting the changing geopolitical situation in the absence of two clear superpowers.

Improving Donor Coordination

Donor coordination is, at the best of times, highly contentious and disputed. Although enhanced donor coordination is clearly desirable, the mechanisms to achieve this feat in the highly politicized and contested postconflict settings are unclear. Although postconflict settings have heightened needs for policy coordination, they may be particularly unstable and complex, thus lessening government capacity to manage and direct the process. Innovative approaches and sector-wide approaches based on the identification of a common basket of funds and agreement on the key features of reform and development to be promoted may facilitate coordination, although experience of these mechanisms in weak countries emerging from conflict is poor.

Recognizing the problems outlined previously, a group of donors have launched a Good Humanitarian Donorship initiative. Establishing principles and good practices of humanitarian donorship, this group agreed, among other things:

- To strive to ensure that funding of humanitarian action in new crises does not adversely affect meeting the needs in ongoing crises
- To recognize the necessity of a dynamic and flexible response to changing needs in humanitarian crises
- To allocate humanitarian funding in proportion to needs and on the basis of needs assessments
- To request that humanitarian organizations ensure adequate involvement of beneficiaries in the design and implementation of humanitarian response
- To provide humanitarian assistance in ways that are supportive of recovery and long-term development
- To support the central and unique role of the United Nations in providing leadership and coordination of international humanitarian action

This initiative has the potential to bring order to what has been a chaotic area. Only time will tell if the actions of the donors will live up to these lofty principles, however.

Conceptual Framework for Health System Development

Having a clear conceptual framework for how the health system will operate is fundamental. The process of establishing this structure needs to be inclusive, involving a wide range of stakeholders in an open and transparent policy debate. Inputs to such processes include making available relevant literature, reports, and studies to all parties; sponsoring health-related media work; promoting policy forums in which participants from different institutions and organizations can exchange views and develop trust; and developing the roles of professional organiza-

tions to promote peace building and more equitable services.

The definition of a clear policy framework is often contested by different parties and groups, as any proposed structure will inevitably have winners and losers. In the presence of a functional state, the government at the central and especially at local levels should play a key role in policy formulation and implementation. Analysis to inform the development of appropriate frameworks needs to be conducted by credible groups that can assist in supporting the state's capacity to manage the period of negotiation and policy formulation.

Experience from Mozambique highlights the value of early preparation and commitment to postwar health system development. Such plans need to be flexible and adaptable to new conditions. Nevertheless, in Mozambique, the existence of a broad policy framework for planning was valuable in guiding human resources development and capital and recurrent expenditure decisions in the immediate postwar period.

Decentralization and Participation

The need to promote more widespread participation in highlighting needs and influencing policy decisions regarding health matters was discussed earlier in this chapter. In particular, local civil society organizations and local government structures can play valuable roles in contributing to policy debates. Working closely with decentralized systems may help ensure more effective targeting of health services—the directing of resources to what and where they are most needed—and facilitate intersectoral planning and decision making.

Development of Human Resources

The maintenance and development of human resources is a fundamental challenge in postconflict settings. A lack of staff (numbers and quality), an inability to retain staff, difficulty attracting longer-term funding to support an appropriate human resources strategy, and a shortage of skills due to the lack of continuity and decline in infrastructure are all key impediments to effective delivery of health services. Attention to these issues needs to be devoted to both public and private sectors, at local and central levels, and in relation to management and technical functions. Improving standards of care and developing a range of training approaches sensitive to different constraints and capacities, including short courses, distance-based learning, and on-the-job training, may be valuable; facilitating ongoing commitment to local institutions and their development is a key pillar of such health services interventions.

These challenges, of course, are taking place in the context of a global crisis in the health workforce. Nearly all low-income countries now face problems with worker shortages, skill-mix imbalances, maldistribution, negative work environments, and weak knowledge bases. Especially in the poorest countries, the workforce is under assault by HIV and AIDS, out-migration, and inadequate investment (Chen et al., 2004).

Promoting Evidence-Based Policy

Key inputs to the promotion of evidence-based policy are information about needs and about the perspectives of different actors, especially affected communities, concerning the nature and form of the future health system. Health policy should be based on evidence not only of effectiveness and efficiency, but also of equity, sustainability, satisfaction, and local ownership and leadership.

Information needs include assessments of human, material, and financial resources; donor aid flows and activities; private contributions to health-sector activity; the distribution and condition of health facilities and logistic supports; the capacity and quality of available human resources; and the availability of drugs and equipment. Assessing health needs requires examination and analysis of baseline information on mortality, morbidity, and disability. Routine surveys such as the Demographic and Health Surveys or UNICEF's Multiple Indicator Cluster Surveys, which are conducted regularly in some countries, could provide useful data. Qualitative data on community perceptions and priorities are similarly extremely important, albeit often lacking. Making more data available would help promote accountability, transparency, and democracy. The collected data should routinely be made available in the public domain. Data-gathering measures should clearly be undertaken within a framework that seeks to build local capacity to undertake and further develop their applied research and information system management capabilities.

Attention to Particular Disease Burdens

Specific disease burdens may be exacerbated by conflict and demand attention. STIs, HIV, and AIDS may be exacerbated, for example, as may other communicable diseases such as malaria, tuberculosis, and a variety of water-related conditions. Psychological distress may be widespread, demanding efforts to reestablish communities and their livelihoods. Injuries, violence, and specifically violence against women may be widespread and require attention and collaboration across and between different sectors.

Current Issues

With each new CE, new problems arise that must be addressed. In addition, the response to each emergency has led to reconsideration of previously encountered problems. Although countless issues might be considered to be at the forefront of contemporary thought in this field, three are consistently debated and are deserving of special attention: the role of new humanitarian actors, efforts to improve the quality of NGO programs, and the role of research in developing more effective responses.

The Role of the Military and Other Humanitarian Actors

Traditionally the domain of international agencies and not-for-profit nongovernmental humanitarian organizations, CEs have evolved into major geopolitical theaters in which many diverse and disparate actors have sought to carve out new roles for themselves. Because an increasing number of CEs have been precipitated by armed conflict within and between nations, third-party military forces, especially those of Western nations, have been prominently involved in recent relief operations.

Following the Gulf War of 1991, an extensive international humanitarian effort for the Kurdish population of northern Iraq was coordinated by the U.S. military, which operated under the auspices, but not the command, of the United Nations. For almost the first time, NGOs were to a large degree dependent on Western military forces (including those from Germany, the United Kingdom, France, and the Netherlands, in addition to the United States) for security, transportation, and logistics. The establishment of a secure operational area and the delegation of the delivery of relief services to the humanitarian community were important elements in bringing about a rapid response to the plight of the internally displaced Kurds. However, many NGOs, including the ICRC, were uncomfortable with working closely with the military and were forced to confront and reassess their notions of political neutrality. In addition, although their presence was positive in a number of ways, the military authorities proved to be novices when it came to humanitarian relief. They were ignorant of its basic principles, unfamiliar with appropriate relief services, and unable to promptly deliver essential supplies, such as measles vaccine, to meet the public health needs of a civilian population where maternal and child health problems were the main priority.

The military intervention in Somalia by Allied armed forces, including those of the United States, in 1992 was launched for humanitarian reasons, with the assent of the UN Security Council. In this chaotic situation characterized by generalized lawlessness, severe factional combat, and the total collapse of governance, compounded by crop failure and ensuing famine, the only way to secure the delivery of essential relief was with the protection of armed forces. From a military standpoint, the intervention was deemed a fiasco. In contrast, many humanitarian organizations suggested that the military operation contributed to decreasing the high mortality rate, at least initially. Prior to this episode, military forces had steadfastly maintained that their role should be limited to providing security for humanitarian supplies; following the Somali experience, they began to review in earnest the broader role of the military in humanitarian relief.

The war over Kosovo, which was fought between NATO and Serbia, was associated with a CE in which military forces exercised control over the relief operation. A general lack of coordination between UN organizations, NGOs, and the military commanders resulted in information gaps, confusion regarding roles and responsibilities, and a generally chaotic situation. Fortunately, morbidity and mortality levels among the refugees in Macedonia and Albania remained low, but the potential for a humanitarian disaster in the face of a military victory was clearly present.

Following the invasion of Iraq by the United States in 2003 and the overthrow of the Saddam Hussein regime, much of the relief and reconstruction effort was contracted by the U.S. Department of Defense to private contractors. For the first time, NGOs were for the most part sidelined from the CE response. This event has been the subject of intense debate in the humanitarian community, and it is not clear whether this episode is an exceptional one or whether the entire nature of humanitarian relief is in the process of tumultuous change.

Important lessons for current and future peace and stability operations can be found in the experiences of Provincial Reconstruction Teams (PRTs) in Afghanistan. PRTs are small, joint civilian–military organizations whose mission is to promote governance, security, and reconstruction throughout the country.

They are managed by the United States and other members of the International Security Assistance Force (e.g., the United Kingdom, Italy, Germany, France, Australia, the Netherlands). The U.S. PRTs have stressed governance, force protection, and quick-impact development projects to "win hearts and minds." Their contribution to long-term health development is dubious, however.

The role of armed forces in the relief efforts that follow natural disasters may be less controversial. The United States, Germany, Australia, Singapore, and many other countries used their armed forces to provide humanitarian services in Aceh province, Indonesia, following the December 2004 tsunami. A large Indonesian Army contingent was also present. These forces provided transport, logistic, and hospital support both within the provincial capital of Banda Aceh and along the west coast of Aceh province, where small groups of people would have gone entirely without relief were it not for the ability of military forces to access the area by helicopter and ship.

In Haiti, the United States dispatched a large contingent of armed forces to join the United Nations peacekeeping forces who were already stationed on the ground for security purposes. In addition to bolstering security, providing unparalleled "lift" capacity for humanitarian supplies, and donating labor for search and rescue operations, clearing of rubble, and initiation of reconstruction, the U.S. military was very active in providing health services. The United States Naval Ship *Comfort,* a floating tertiary care hospital with a capacity of almost 1,000 beds, became an important and very visible addition to the medical relief effort. Its use had some important disadvantages, however: It was forced to remain offshore, which greatly hampered transportation to and from the ship; many of its beds, which were built bunk-style, could not be used by the orthopedic patients; and, most importantly, its presence artificially raised the level of care that had been available in Haiti prior to the earthquake to such a large extent that it became difficult to find appropriate placements for postoperative care of patients treated on the *Comfort.*

The increasingly constant presence of armed forces in CEs has raised a number of issues within the relief community. Currently, there is a need to reconsider whether the fundamental principles of neutrality and impartiality held so dearly by most humanitarian agencies are compatible with such close involvement with military forces, who are trained to wage war. On the one hand, at a time when deaths of civilian relief workers outnumber those of peacekeeping forces, a need for increased personal security in areas where conflict is occurring is obvious. On the other hand, the aversion of many civilian NGOs to the presence of the military in humanitarian crises should be considered in light of the assistance that these forces may be able to bring to populations in need.

In sum, a serious review of the roles and responsibilities of the military, the United Nations, bilateral governmental agencies, and private humanitarian organizations should be undertaken. All of these players should strive to develop a mode of operating in CEs that will work to relieve, and not to prolong, the suffering of those in greatest need of humanitarian relief. For military involvement to be useful, however, commanders may have to relinquish certain decision-making roles to those more experienced in the effective delivery of public health services.

In addition to the military and other participants listed earlier in this chapter, other important agencies have emerged in recent years as players in CE response. Organizations that specialize in monitoring, detecting, and publicizing human rights abuses and prosecuting their perpetrators, for example, have become increasingly active during CEs. These include the Office of the UN High Commissioner for Human Rights; regional organizations such as the Office for Security and Cooperation in Europe; private organizations such as Amnesty International, Human Rights Watch, and Physicians for Human Rights; and national committees supporting the international war crimes tribunals. In some situations where human rights abuses were extremely common, such as in Rwanda in 1994 and Kosovo in 1999, these organizations have helped ensure that public health assistance programs addressed the sequelae of these abuses.

Finally, criticism of existing relief organizations has increased in recent years because of their perceived inability to implement relief programs on the scale that is frequently necessary. Some have suggested that the rapid construction, maintenance, and management of large refugee camps, global logistical support, organization of healthcare services to large populations, and even the provision of security services might be done more effectively, rapidly, and efficiently by commercial companies contracted by governments or the UN. This challenge to the existing relief mechanisms, based as they are on the humanitarian motive, has yet to be resolved. If such an approach is widely adopted, it could lead to the transformation of humanitarian relief into a business enterprise—one that might inevitably become more closely linked to the donor agencies and used by them as agents of foreign policy. This has been the experience of bilateral development programs, for example.

Professionalization

Partly to stave off this challenge, and partly to correct perceptions of incompetence and amateurism, efforts have been made to establish certain minimum standards of performance for relief workers (see Exhibit 11-7). Due to the transient nature of NGO relief programs and the high turnover of personnel both in the field and at NGO headquarters, experiences are not easily institutionalized and lessons need to be learned repeatedly. Limited field experience, a poor understanding of the public health priorities of emergencies, and inadequate skills to carry out the most essential tasks, such as organizing large-scale vaccination and ORT programs, have frequently led to problems in NGO operations. After what is widely regarded as an

---

Exhibit 11-7	The Sphere Project

Perhaps the largest single effort to establish minimum standards of care in emergency settings has been the Sphere Project (www.sphereproject.org). Launched in 1997 by a group of private humanitarian agencies, Sphere recognized that humanitarian relief would be increasingly required for many years and that the existing capacity to respond with high-quality interventions was, for the most part, lacking. To address this situation, a large consortium (including more than 228 private humanitarian organizations) from around the world participated in the development of the Sphere Humanitarian Charter and Minimum Standards in Disaster Response. First published in 1999, and substantially revised in 2004, these standards are intended to govern the overall conduct of relief NGOs and to provide benchmark levels of performance in the areas of water supply and sanitation, food security, nutrition, food aid, shelter and site management, and health services. The Sphere Project does not intend to establish new standards. Instead, it seeks to consolidate and reach agreement based on existing information. Standards will continue to be developed and existing standards will be modified in accordance with new findings, both from research and from experience gained in the field, following the initial dissemination in the field. During 2010, a consultative process of review was undertaken with stakeholders, and the third edition of the Sphere Manual was published on April 14, 2011.

initially ineffective relief effort in Goma in 1994, major efforts were undertaken to improve the technical abilities of relief workers in the public health sector.

A number of short-term training courses have been developed and implemented by schools of public health, government disaster relief agencies, and the NGOs themselves. Master of public health (MPH) programs in humanitarian assistance and public health in CEs have been established in schools of public health in the United States and Europe. Although emergency public health workers are not yet required to have accredited qualifications, the quality of health care may improve as more of these training courses become available.

Research

The acquisition of new knowledge relevant to public health practice in displaced populations has been scant. Although most emergency public health programs rely on the safe and effective interventions that already exist (e.g., vaccines, ORS, water purification, essential drugs, and the like), their implementation in emergency settings may be affected by the size of the populations and the urgency of the circumstances. Little is known about the impact of rapid, forced migration on human behavior, disease transmission, and the delivery of effective services in emergency settings. For many years, it had been considered unethical to conduct research of any kind among emergency-affected populations, who could be characterized as the most vulnerable members of the world's population. However, it is increasingly acknowledged that without applied research studies designed specifically to address operational issues in the context of emergencies, it will be difficult to reduce morbidity and mortality levels from their current, excessively high levels.

Existing standards are largely based on field experience; few reflect findings from rigorously designed and evaluated observational field trials. Although policies in some areas, such as measles vaccination and aspects of food and nutrition, are based on field research, for example, this is not the case in other important public health areas, such as reproductive health and the control of sexually transmitted diseases. Conversely, little reliable information is available on which to base policies and programs to promote psychosocial health, despite its rapid emergence as a consistent major public health problem. Of course, research is truly useful only where there is genuine concern for improving performance. Unfortunately, emergency relief has been largely guided by short-term concerns.

Many of the lessons learned in humanitarian response are rapidly lost in the fever to deal with the next crisis. Of the many people who have worked in the field, few forge careers in humanitarian assistance. Data that are collected and reported by field workers are often either discarded or filed in internal agency reports and never seen again. There is no professional society for humanitarian public health workers, and no peer-reviewed journal in which the results of high-quality studies can be published. Although the number of people affected by CEs continues to grow, a solid body of research on which to base policy and practice remains sadly lacking. Without such a database, relief policies will remain relatively uninformed, and mistakes will continue to be made.

Conclusion

Significant progress has been made during the past two decades toward the provision of effective, focused, needs-based humanitarian assistance to conflict-affected populations. Greater emphasis is now placed on the impact, including health outcomes, of international aid. The quantity of aid delivered is no longer considered a valid indicator of effectiveness; its relevance, quality, coverage, and equitable distribution are now accepted as more pertinent concerns. As public health in emergency settings has developed as a specialized technical field, a number of relief agencies, especially NGOs, have developed technical manuals, field guidelines, and targeted training courses. Ability to meet the standard performance indicators developed recently by the Sphere Project and adherence to the international NGO code of ethics are now widely perceived as valid criteria against which to assess the quality of specific agencies.

Although a considerable body of knowledge has accumulated specifically relating to the health needs of emergency-affected populations, many areas require further development. Donor agencies should acknowledge the need to support applied health research in emergency settings if more effective interventions are to be developed against old problems, such as cholera, and emerging issues such as HIV, AIDS, TB, mental health, and reproductive health. The recent process of identifying applied health research priorities in emergencies, sponsored by WHO, and the creation of research and ethical advisory committees represent steps in the right direction.

In planning for responses to future humanitarian emergencies, public health workers need to recognize that improving the technical and management capacity of operational agencies will not be good enough. Recent experience has dramatically demonstrated that those in need will not benefit unless the international community ensures that mechanisms to permit secure access by those agencies are available. The means by which this access is provided is critical, and will most likely be the central focus of international policy dialogue. The varied nature of the responses to emergencies in northern Iraq, Somalia, Bosnia, Rwanda, Kosovo, Sierra Leone, East Timor, and Darfur demonstrates the lack of consistency and predictability in CE-focused operations.

Finally, there remains the issue of primary prevention. The perceived differences between communities are generally tolerated in prosperous societies, whereas conflict and all its consequences generally arise in times of economic distress and political instability. Although programs in good governance proliferate, the reality is that governments everywhere today are perceived as having failed to provide for the basic needs of their peoples. Unless these root causes of conflict are seriously addressed, all that will be accomplished is the perpetuation of a perennial relief industry that inevitably will experience only patchy success.

● ● ● Discussion Questions

1. What are the major objectives in the initial management of a refugee emergency?

2. What does the word "complex" as used in the term "complex emergency" imply?

3. What is the best indicator of the general health of a refugee population during an emergency?

4. Why are female-headed households in refugee camps at special risk of food scarcity?

5. What are the minimum standards in emergency relief operations for the provision of water and latrines?

6. What roles do general rations, supplementary feeding programs, and therapeutic feeding programs play in maintaining population nutrition?

7. At what age should children in emergency-affected populations be vaccinated against measles?

8. What are the immediate measures that can be taken in an emergency-affected population to prevent HIV and AIDS?

9. How adequate are the existing international legal statutes in protecting internally displaced persons?

10. Which roles may community health workers play in an emergency public health program?

11. What are the immediate interventions that should be in place to address the reproductive health needs of women and men in a public emergency?

12. What population-based interventions have been developed to address the mental health needs of emergency-affected populations?

• • • References

Ashworth, A. (2006). Efficacy and effectiveness of community-based treatment of severe malnutrition. *Food and Nutrition Bulletin, 27*(3), S24–S48.

Amnesty International. (1995). *Women in Afghanistan: A human rights catastrophe.* London: Author.

Babille, M., de Colombani, P., Guerra R., Zagaria, N. & Zanetti, C. (1994). Post-emergency epidemiological surveillance in Iraqi-Kurdish refugee camps in Iran. *Disasters, 18,* 58–75.

Barnabas, G. A., & Zwi, A. B. (1997). Health policy development in wartime: Establishing the Baito health system in Tigray, Ethiopia. *Health Policy and Planning, 12*(1), 38–49.

Barudy, J. (1989). A programme of mental health for political refugees: Dealing with the invisible pain of political exile. *Social Science and Medicine, 28,* 715–727.

Bhatia, R., & Woodruff. B. (1999, February 11). Ngonut Internet discussion group (ngonut@abdn.ac.uk).

Bloland, P. B., & Williams, H. A. (Eds.). (2003). *Malaria control during mass population movements and natural disasters.* National Research Council. Washington, DC: National Academies Press.

Boccia D., Klovstad, H., & Guthmann, J. P. (2004, December). *Outbreak of hepatitis E in Mornay IDP Camp, Western Darfur, Sudan.* Paris, France: Epicentre.

Boss, L. P., Toole, M. J., & Yip, R. (1994). Assessments of mortality, morbidity, and nutritional status in Somalia during the 1991–1992 famine. *Journal of the American Medical Association, 272,* 371–376.

Bracken, P. J., Giller, J. E., & Kabaganda, S. (1992). Helping victims of violence in Uganda. *Medicine and War, 8*(3), 155–63.

Bracken, P. J., Giller, J. E., & Summerfield, D. (1995). Psychological responses to war and atrocity: The limitations of current concepts. *Social Science and Medicine, 40*(8), 1073–1082.

Brown, V., Moren, A., & Paquet, C. (1999). *Rapid health assessment of refugee or displaced populations. Annex 3.* Paris: Epicentre & Médecins sans Frontières.

Burkholder, B. T., & Toole, M. J. (1995). Evolution of complex disasters. *Lancet, 346,* 1012–1015.

Centers for Disease Control and Prevention (CDC). (1991a). Outbreak of pellagra among Mozambican refugees—Malawi, 1990. *Morbidity and Mortality Weekly Report, 40,* 209–213.

Centers for Disease Control and Prevention (CDC). (1991b). Public health consequences of acute displacement of Iraqi citizens: March–May. *Morbidity and Mortality Weekly Report, 40,* 443–446.

Centers for Disease Control and Prevention (CDC). (1992). Famine affected, refugee, and displaced populations: Recommendations for public health issues. *Morbidity and Mortality Weekly Report, 41,* RR-13.

Centers for Disease Control and Prevention (CDC). (1993a). Status of public health—Bosnia and Herze-govina, August–September 1993. *Morbidity and Mortality Weekly Report, 42,* 973, 979–982.

Centers for Disease Control and Prevention (CDC). (1993b). Mortality among newly arrived Mozambican refugees, Zimbabwe and Malawi, 1992. *Morbidity and Mortality Weekly Report, 42,* 468–469, 475–477.

Centers for Disease Control and Prevention (CDC). (1993c).Nutrition and mortality assessment—Southern Sudan, March 1993. *Morbidity and Mortality Weekly Report, 42,* 304–308.

Centers for Disease Control and Prevention (CDC). (1994). Health status of displaced persons following civil war—Burundi, December 1993–January 1994. *Morbidity and Mortality Weekly Report, 43*(38), 701–703.

Centers for Disease Control and Prevention(CDC). (2008). Safe water systems. Retrieved from www.cdc.gov/safewater

Chen, L., Evans, T., Anand, S., Boufford, J. I., Brown, H., et al. (2004). Human resources for health: Overcoming the crisis. *Lancet, 364,* 1984–1990.

Ciliberto, M. A., Manary, M. J., Ndekha, M. J., Briend, A., & Ashorn, P. (2006). Home-based therapy for edematous malnutrition with ready-to-use therapeutic food. *Acta Paediatrica, 95,* 1012–1015.

Cliff, J., & Noormahomed, A.R. (1988). Health as a target: South Africa's destabilization of Mozambique. *Social Science and Medicine, 27*(7), 717–722.

Coghlan, B., Brennan, R., Ngoy, P., Dofara, D., Otto, B., & Stewart, T. (2004). *Mortality in the Democratic Republic of Congo: Results from a nationwide survey conducted April–July 2004.* New York: International Rescue Committee and Burnet Institute.

Coghlan, B., Ngoy, P., Mulumba, F., Hardy, C., Nkamgang Bemo, V., Stewart, T., et al. (2009). Update on mortality in the Democratic Republic of Congo: Results from a third nationwide survey. *Disaster Medicine and Public Health Preparedness, 3,* 88–96.

Collins, S. (1993, August). The need for adult therapeutic care in emergency feeding programs. *Journal of the American Medical Association,* 637–638.

Collins, S., Sadler, K., Dent, N., Khara ,T., Guerrero, S., Myatt, M., et al. (2006). Key issues in the success of community-based management of severe malnutrition. *Food and Nutrition Bulletin, 27*(3), S49–S82.

Complex Emergencies Database (CEDAT). (2008). What do health indicators tell us about humanitarian crises in 2008? Retrieved from http://www.cedat.be/what-do-health-indicators-tell-us-about-humanitarian-crises-2008

Crombé, X., & Jézéquel, J. H. (2009, June 16). *A not-so natural disaster.* London: Hurst.

Desenclos, J. C., Berry, A. M., Padt, R., Farah, B., Segala, C., & Nabil, A. M. (1989). Epidemiologic patterns of scurvy among Ethiopian refugees. *Bulletin of the World Health Organisation, 67,* 309–316.

Dodge, C. P. (1990). Health implications of war in Uganda and Sudan. *Social Science and Medicine, 31,* 691–698.

Degomme, O., & Guha-Sapir, D. (2010). Patterns of mortality rates in Darfur conflict. *Lancet, 375,* 294–300.

Depoortere, E., Checchi, F., Broillet, F., Gerstl, S., Minetti, A., Gayraud, O., et al. (2004). Violence and mortality in West Darfur, Sudan (2003–2004): Epide-miological evidence from four surveys. *Lancet, 364,* 1315–1320.

Ferro-Luzzi, A., & James, W.P. (1996). Adult malnutrition: Simple assessment techniques for use in emergencies. *British Journal of Nutrition, 75*(1), 3–10.

Food and Agriculture Organization (2009). FAO's emergency role in the West Bank and Gaza Strip. http://www.fao.org/emergencies/country_information/list/middleeast/westbankandgazastrip/en/

Garfield, R., & Neugat, A. I. (1991). Epidemiologic analysis of warfare: A historical review. *Journal of the American Medical Association, 226,* 688–692.

Garfield, R., & Williams, G. (1992). *Health care in Nicaragua: Primary care under changing regimes.* Oxford, UK/ New York: Oxford University Press.

Garfield, R. Morbidity and Mortality Among Iraqi Children from 1990 Through 1998: Assessing the Impact of the Gulf War and Economic Sanctions. CASI Internet version published July 1999. http://www.casi.org.uk/info/garfield/dr-garfield.html

Golden, M. (1999a, June 22). Indicators for adolescent malnutrition. Ngonut Internet discussion group (ngonut@abdn.ac.uk).

Golden, M. H. (1999b). *Preventing nutritional deficiency in emergencies.* Presentation at Enhancing the Nutritional Status of Relief Diets, Washington, DC, April 28–30, 1999.

Goma Epidemiology Group. (1995). Public health impact of Rwandan refugee crisis. What happened in Goma, Zaire, in July 1994? *Lancet, 345,* 339–344.

Goodhand, J., & Hulme, D. (1999). From wars to complex political emergencies: Understanding conflict and peace building in the new world disorder. *Third World Quarterly, 20*(1), 13–26.

Grandesso, F., Sanderson, F., Kruijt, J., Koene, T., & Brown, V. (2004, September). Mortality and malnutrition among populations living in South Darfur, Sudan: Results of 3 surveys. *Journal of the American Medical Association, 293,* 1490–1494.

Guha-Sapir, D., & van Panhuis, W. (2004). Conflict-related mortality: An analysis of 37 Datasets. *Disasters, 28*(4), 418–428.

Harrell-Bond, B. E., Voutira, E., & Leopold, M. (1992). Counting the refugees: Gifts, givers, patrons and clients. *Journal of Refugee Studies, 5*(3/4), 205–225.

Holmes, W. (2003). *Protecting the future: HIV prevention, care, and support among displaced and war-affected populations.* New York: International Rescue Committee & Kumarian Press.

Human Security Report Project. (2010, January). *The shrinking costs of war.* Vancouver: Oxford University Press.

Iacopino, V., Heisler, M., Pishevar, S., & Kirschner, R. (1996). Physician complicity in misrepresentation and omission of evidence of torture in post-detention medical examinations in Turkey. *Journal of the American Medical Association, 276*(5), 396–402.

Inter-Agency Standing Committee Task Force on HIV/AIDS in Emergency Settings. (2003). *Guidelines for HIV/AIDS interventions in emergency settings.* Geneva, Switzerland/New York: Author.

Jaspars, S., & Shoham, J. (1999). Targeting the vulnerable: A review of the necessity and feasibility of targeting vulnerable households. *Disasters, 23*(4), 359–372.

Keller, A., Eisenman, D., Saul, J., Kim, G., Connell, J., & Holtz, T. (1997). *Striking hard: Torture in Tibet.* Boston, MA: Physicians for Human Rights.

Kloos, H. (1992). Health impacts of war in Ethiopia. *Disasters, 16,* 347–354.

Lanjouw, S., Macrae, J., & Zwi, A.B. (1999). Rehabilitating Health Services in Cambodia: The challenge of coordination in chronic political emergencies. *Health Policy and Planning 14*(3), 229–242.

Lee, I., & Haines, A. (1991). Health costs of the Gulf War. *British Medical Journal, 303,* 303–306.

Macrae, J., & Zwi, A. (Eds.). (1994). *War and hunger: Rethinking international responses to complex emergencies.* London: Zed Books.

Manoncourt, S., Doppler, B., Enten, F., Nur, A., Mohamed, A., Vial, P., et al. (1992). Public health consequences of civil war in Somalia, April 1992. *Lancet, 340,* 176–177.

Marfin, A. A., Moore, J., Collins, C., Bielik, R., Kattel, U., Toole, M., et al. (1994). Infectious disease surveillance during emergency relief to Bhutanese refugees in Nepal. *Journal of the American Medical Association, 272,* 377–381.

Marshall, M. G. (2009). Major episodes of political violence 1946–2009. Center for Systemic Peace. Retrieved from http://www.systemicpeace.org/warlist.htm

Mears, C., & Young, H. (1998). *Acceptability and use of cereal-based foods in refugee camps: Case studies from Nepal, Ethiopia, and Tanzania.* Oxford, UK: Oxfam, UK.

Médecins sans Frontières (MSF). (1995). *Nutrition guidelines.* Paris: Author.

Médecins sans Frontières (MSF). (1997). *Refugee health: An approach to emergency situations.* London: Macmillan.

Médecins sans Frontières (MSF). (2001). *Activity report 2000–2001. Burundi: Fever, hunger, and war.* Retrieved from www.msf.org

Médecins sans Frontières (MSF) & Epicentre. (1999). *Rapid health assessment of refugee or displaced populations.* Paris: MSF.

Moore, P. S., Marfin, A. A., Quenemoen, L. E., Gessner, B. D., Ayub, X. X., Miller, D. S., et al. (1993). Mortality rates in displaced and resident populations of Central Somalia during the famine of 1992. *Lancet, 341,* 935–938.

Murphy, P., & Salama, P. Coordinating a Humanitarian Response in Sudan. *Field Exchange.* Issue 6. February 1999. Retrieved from http://fex.ennonline.net/6/coordinating.aspx

Nieburg, P., Waldman, R. J., Leavell, R., Sommer, A., & DeMaeyer, E. (1988). Vitamin A supplementation for refugees and famine victims. *Bulletin of the World Health Organisation, 66,* 689–697.

Nutrition Information in Crisis Situations (2010). Report Number XXI. United Nations Standing Committee on Nutrition. New York. March 2010.

Office for the Coordination of Humanitarian Affairs, Haiti Earthquake Situation Report #20, New York, February 10, 2010.

Palmer, C. A., Lush, L., & Zwi, A. B. (1999). The emerging international policy agenda for reproductive health services in conflict settings. *Social Science and Medicine, 49,* 1689–1703.

Palmer, C. A., & Zwi, A. B. (1998). Women, health and humanitarian aid in conflict. *Disasters, 22*(3), 236–249.

Perrin, P. (1996). *War and public health.* Geneva, Switzerland: International Committee of the Red Cross (p. 381).

Peterson, E. A., Roberts, L., Toole, M. J., & Peterson, D. E. (1998). Soap use effect on diarrhea: Nyamithutu refugee camp. *International Journal of Epidemiology, 27,* 520–524.

Physicians for Human Rights. (2005). *Break them down: Systematic use of psychological torture by US forces.* Cambridge MA: Author.

Project Ploughshares. (2002). Retrieved from www.ploughshares.ca/

Reed, H. E., & Keeley, C. B. (Eds.). (2001). *Forced migration and mortality.* National Research Council. Washington, DC: National Academies Press.

Roberts, L., Chartier, Y., Chartier, O., Malenga, G., Toole, M. J., & Rodka, H. (2001). Keeping clean water clean in a Malawi refugee camp: A randomized intervention trial. *Bulletin of the World Health Organization, 79,* 280–287.

Salama, P., Spiegel, P., & Brennan, R. (2001). No less vulnerable: The internally displaced in humanitarian emergencies. *Lancet, 357,* 1430–1432.

Shrestha, N. M., Sharma, B., Ommeren, M. V., Regini, S., Makaja, R., Komproe, I., et al. (1998). Impact of torture on refugees displaced within the developing world: Symptomatology among Bhutanese refugees in Nepal. *Journal of the American Medical Association, 280*(5), 443–448.

Sivard, R. L. (1996). *World military and social expenditure 1996* (16th ed.). Washington, DC: World Priority Review.

Sphere Project. (2004). *Humanitarian charter and minimum standards in disaster response.* Geneva, Switzerland: Author.

Spiegel, P. B., Bennedsen, A. R., Claass, J., Bruns, L., Patterson, N., Yiweza, D., & Schilperoord, M. (2007). Prevalence of HIV infection in conflict-affected and displaced people in seven sub-Saharan African countries: A systematic review. *Lancet, 369,* 2187–2195.

Spiegel, P. B., Checchi, F., Colombo, S., & Paik, E. (2010). Health-care needs of people affected by conflict: Future trends and changing frameworks. *Lancet, 375,* 341–345.

Spirer, H. F., & Spirer, L. (1993). *Data analysis for monitoring human rights.* Washington, DC: American Association for the Advancement of Science.

Steiner, B., Benner, M. T., Sondorp, E., Schmitz, K. P., Mesmer, U., & Rosenberger, S. (2009). Sexual violence in the protracted conflict of DRC: Programming for rape survivors in South Kivu. *Conflict and Health, 3,* 3 (open access).

Stiglmayer, A. (Ed.). (1994). *Mass rape. The war against women in Bosnia-Herzegovina.* Lincoln, NE/London: University of Nebraska Press.

Swiss, S., & Giller, J. E. (1993). Rape as a crime of war. *Journal of the American Medical Association, 270,* 612–615.

Toole, M. J., Galson, S., & Brady, W. (1993). Are war and public health compatible? Report from Bosnia-Herzegovina. *Lancet, 341,* 1193–1196.

Toole, M. J., & Waldman, R. J. (1990). Prevention of excess mortality in refugee and displaced populations in developing countries. *Journal of the American Medical Association, 263,* 3296–3302.

Toole, M. J., & Waldman, R. J. (1993). Refugees and displaced persons: War, hunger, and public health. *Journal of the American Medical Association, 270,* 600–605.

United Nations Administrative Committee on Coordination, Sub-Committee on Nutrition (ACC/SCN). (1994a, August). *Refugee nutrition information system* (Vol. 6). Geneva, Switzerland: Author.

United Nations Administrative Committee on Coordination, Sub-Committee on Nutrition (ACC/SCN). (1994b, October). *Refugee nutrition information system* (Vol. 7). Geneva, Switzerland: Author.

United Nations Administrative Committee on Coordination, Sub-Committee on Nutrition (ACC/SCN). (1995a, July). *Refugee nutrition information system* (Vol. 11). Geneva, Switzerland: Author.

United Nations Administrative Committee on Coordination, Sub-Committee on Nutrition (ACC/SCN). (1995b, November). *Report of a Workshop on the Improvement of the Nutrition of Refugees and Displaced People in Africa, Machakos, Kenya, 5–7 December 1994*. Geneva, Switzerland: Author.

United Nations Administrative Committee on Coordination, Sub-Committee on Nutrition (ACC/SCN). (1996, April). *Refugee nutrition information system* (Vol. 15). Geneva, Switzerland: Author.

United Nations Administrative Committee on Coordination, Sub-Committee on Nutrition (ACC/SCN). (1998, June 15). *Refugee nutrition information system* (Vol. 24). Geneva, Switzerland: Author.

United Nations Administrative Committee on Coordination, Sub-Committee on Nutrition (ACC/SCN). (1999, March). *Refugee nutrition information system* (Vol. 26). Geneva, Switzerland: Author.

United Nations Administrative Committee on Coordination, Sub-Committee on Nutrition (ACC/SCN). (2002a, April). *Refugee nutrition information system* (No. 36/37). Geneva, Switzerland: Author.

United Nations Administrative Committee on Coordination, Sub-Committee on Nutrition (ACC/SCN). (2002b, October). *Refugee nutrition information system* (No. 39). Geneva, Switzerland: Author.

United Nations Administrative Committee on Coordination, Sub-Committee on Nutrition (ACC/SCN). (2003, November). *Refugee nutrition information system* (No. 43). Geneva, Switzerland: Author.

United Nations High Commission for Refugees (UNHCR). (1992). *Bangladesh social services mission 22–31 March 1992*. UNHCR Program and Technical Support Section. Geneva, Switzerland: Author.

United Nations High Commissioner for Refugees (UNHCR). (1993). *Refugee protection and sexual violence: Executive Committee Conclusion No. 73 (XLIV), Preamble*. Geneva, Switzerland: Author.

United Nations High Commissioner for Refugees (UNHCR). (1995a). *Reproductive health in refugee situations: An inter-agency field manual*. Geneva, Switzerland: Author.

United Nations High Commissioner for Refugees (UNHCR). (2011) Responding to the Libya Crisis. http://www.unhcr.org/pages/4d7755246.html

United Nations High Commissioner for Refugees (UNHCR) &World Food Programme (WFP). (1999, February). *Guidelines for selective feeding programmes in emergency situations*. Geneva, Switzerland: UNHCR.

United Nations Standing Committee on Nutrition (SCN). (2004a, February). *Nutrition information in crisis situations*. Report Number I. Geneva, Switzerland: Author.

United Nations Standing Committee on Nutrition (SCN). (2004b, May). *Nutrition information in crisis situations*. Report Number II. Geneva, Switzerland: Author.

United Nations Standing Committee on Nutrition (SCN). (2004c, August). *Nutrition information in crisis situations*. Report Number III. Geneva, Switzerland: Author.

United Nations Standing Committee on Nutrition (SCN). (2004d, November). *Nutrition information in crisis situations*. Report Number IV. Geneva, Switzerland: Author.

United Nations Standing Committee on Nutrition (SCN). (2009a, March). *Nutrition information in crisis situations*. Report Number XXI. Geneva, Switzerland: Author.

United Nations Standing Committee on Nutrition (SCN). (2009b, June). *Nutrition information in crisis situations*. Report Number XXI. Geneva, Switzerland: Author.

United Nations Standing Committee on Nutrition (SCN). (2010, March). *Nutrition information in crisis situations*. Report Number XXI. Geneva, Switzerland: Author.

United States Committee for Refugees. (2004). *World refugee survey, 2003*. Washington, DC: Author.

United States Committee for Refugees. (2005). Update on Asian tsunami. Retrieved from http://www.refugees.org/

United States Committee for Refugees. (2009). *World refugee survey, 2009*. Washington, DC: Author.

Van Damme, W. (1998). *Medical assistance o self-settled refugees: Guinea 1990–96*. Antwerp, Belgium: ITG Press.

Van Dyke, M., & Waldman, R. (2004). *The Sphere Project evaluation report*. Columbia University, New York: Mailman School of Public Health.

Van Ommeren, M., Saxena, S., Saraceno, B. (2005). Mental and social health during and after acute emergencies: Emerging consensus? *Bulletin of the World Health Organization, 83*, 71–75.

Walt, G., & Cliff, J. (1986). The dynamics of health policies in Mozambique 1975–1985. *Health Policy and Planning, 1*(2), 148–157.

Walt, G. (1988). CHWs: Are national programs in crisis? *Health Policy and Planning, 3*, 1–21.

Woodruff, B. A., & Duffield, A. (2000). *Adults and adolescents: Assessment of nutritional status in emergency-affected populations*. Geneva, Switzerland: United Nations Standing Committee on Nutrition.

World Food Programme (WFP) & United Nations High Commissioner for Refugees (UNHCR). (1997). *Joint WFP/UNHCR guidelines for estimating food and nutritional needs in emergencies*. Rome, Italy/Geneva, Switzerland: Authors.

World Health Organization (WHO). (1995). *Physical status: The use and interpretation of anthropometry. Report of a World Health Organization expert committee* (Technical Report No. 854). Geneva, Switzerland: Author.

World Health Organization (WHO). (1999b). *Scurvy and its prevention and control in major emergencies*. WHO/NHD/99.11. Geneva, Switzerland: Author.

World Health Organization (WHO). (1999c). *Thiamine deficiency and its prevention and control in major emergencies*. WHO/NHD/99.13. Geneva, Switzerland: Author.

World Health Organization (WHO). (1999d). *Management of severe malnutrition: A manual for physicians and other senior health workers*. Geneva, Switzerland: Author.

World Health Organization (WHO). (2000a). *Health Information Network for Advanced Planning (HINAP): Health situation report—West Timor, December 8, 1999*. Geneva, Switzerland: Author.

World Health Organization. (2000b). *Health Information Network for Advanced Planning (HINAP): Health situation report—West Timor, January 5, 2000*. Geneva, Switzerland: Author.

World Health Organization (WHO). (2000c). *The management of nutrition in major emergencies*. Geneva, Switzerland: Author.

World Health Organization (WHO). (2000d). *Pellagra and its prevention and control in major emergencies*. WHO/NHD/00.10. Geneva, Switzerland: Author.

World Health Organization (WHO). (2003). *Communicable disease control in emergencies: A field manual*. Connolly, M. A. (Ed.). Geneva, Switzerland: Author.

World Health Organization (WHO). (2009). *WHO child growth standards and the identification of severe acute malnutrition in infants and children: A joint statement by the World Health Organization and the United Nations Children's Fund*. Geneva, Switzerland: Author.

World Health Organization (2010). Cholera vaccines: WHO position paper. Recommendations. *Vaccine*. July 5, 2010. *28*(30), 4687–8.

Yamauchi, P. E. (1993) Patterns of death: Descriptions of geographic and temporal patterns of rural state terror in Guatemala, 1978–1985. *PSR Quarterly, 3*(2), 67–78.

Yip, R., & Sharp, T. W. (1993). Acute malnutrition and high childhood mortality related to diarrhea. *Journal of the American Medical Association, 270,* 587–590.

Zwi, A. B., & Cabral, A. J. (1991). Identifying "high risk situations" for preventing AIDS. *British Medical Journal, 303,* 1527–1529.

Zwi, A., Ugalde, A., & Richards, P. (2005). The effects of war and political violence on health services. In L. Kurtz (Ed.), *Encyclopaedia of violence.* New York: Academic Press.

12

The Design of Health Systems

ANNE J. MILLS AND M. KENT RANSON

Health systems are the means whereby many of the programs and interventions discussed in earlier chapters of this book are planned and delivered. They are a crucial influence on the extent to which countries are able to address their disease burden and improve overall levels of health and the health of particular groups in the population.

A health system comprises all organizations, institutions, and resources that produce actions whose primary purpose is to improve health (World Health Organization [WHO], 2000). The health system consists of those organizations, institutions, and resources that deliver health care to individuals. Health systems vary greatly from country to country. Unlike the study of disease, there is only limited standardized terminology or methodology for studying and understanding health systems. Each country's health system is the product of a complex range of factors, especially its historical patterns of development and the power of different interest groups. Nonetheless, it is possible to identify common features, and knowledge is increasing regarding which design features are associated with which outcomes, thereby facilitating cross-country learning.

It is essential to study and understand how health systems function and how they can be changed, in part because they are a large and expanding sector of the world economy. Total expenditure on health care grew from 3% of world gross domestic product (GDP) in 1948 to 8.7% in 2006 (WHO, 2009). Health tends to consume a rising share of GDP as income increases: WHO figures show the percentage of GDP absorbed by health care to be 4.3% in low-income countries, 4.5% in lower middle-income countries, 6.3% in up-per middle-income countries and 11.2% in high-income countries.

Nevertheless, countries at similar income levels differ greatly in how effectively they look after the health of their populations. The health-related differences between countries of similar income can be enormous. For example, Bangladesh, with a 2008 gross national income (GNI) per capita of $520, has an under-five mortality rate of 61 deaths per 1,000 live births and a maternal mortality rate of 570 deaths per 100,000 live births, whereas for Chad, with 2008 GNI per capita of $530, these rates are 209 infant deaths and 1,500 maternal deaths, respectively (World Bank, 2010a). To take two somewhat richer countries, Thailand (GNI per capita of $2840) has an under-five mortality rate of 7 per 1,000 and a maternal mortality rate of 110 per 100,000, while Turkmenistan, with the same GNI per capita, has rates of 50 infant deaths and 130 maternal deaths, respectively. Although a variety of factors affect health, it is clear that the health system is an important determinant.

The recent global attention being given to achieving the health-related Millennium Development Goals (MDGs) has focused attention on the state of the health systems of many low- and middle-income countries. Disease and program-specific initiatives such as the GAVI Alliance (supporting immunization) and the Global Fund to Fight AIDS, TB and Malaria have realized that the achievement and maintenance of their disease-focused goals is not possible in countries with weak and fragile health systems. Research has pointed to the multiple problems affecting the health systems of low-income and many middle-income countries, and analyzed the multiple constraints they face in scaling up needed interventions to achieve high levels of coverage (Mills & Hanson, 2003).

Understanding health systems, including how they can be changed, is an endeavor that can benefit from the insights of a number of disciplines—most notably, economics, sociology, anthropology, history, political science, and management science. In recent years, not least because concerns regarding resource scarcity, cost inflation, and efficiency have been uppermost in policy makers' minds, the discipline of economics has had a dominant influence on the study of health systems. This chapter, therefore, draws primarily on economics to review key features of the design of health systems. Of course, it is also important to acknowledge other perspectives on health systems—see, for example, the report of the health systems knowledge network of the Commission on Social Determinants of Health for a somewhat broader perspective (Gilson, Doherty, Loewenson, & Francis, 2007).

The section that follows provides a conceptual map of the health system and its key elements. The historical development of health systems is then briefly reviewed, followed by a section addressing the fundamental and controversial question of the role of the state. Subsequent sections then consider each of the key functions of health systems in turn: regulation, financing, resource allocation, and provision. Current trends in health system reform and the lessons that have emerged from reform policies are then reviewed. Throughout, the text is illustrated by country examples, but a core set of illustrations is drawn from Tanzania, India, Mexico, and Thailand, which have been chosen to illuminate key differences in health systems across the world.

Conceptual Maps of the Health System

Since the seminal study carried out by Kohn and White (1976), an expanding body of literature has attempted to systematize the discussion of the various elements of health systems, categorize health systems into a limited number of different types, and develop performance indicators (e.g., McPake & Machray, 1997; Roemer, 1991; WHO, 2000). These three issues are discussed in the following subsections.

Elements of Health Systems

Roemer (1991) identified five major categories that enable a comprehensive description of a country's health system to be made (Figure 12-1):

- Production of resources (trained staff, commodities such as drugs, facilities, knowledge)
- Organization of programs (by government ministries, private providers, voluntary agencies)
- Economic support mechanisms (sources of funds, such as tax, insurance, and user fees)
- Management methods (planning, administration, regulation, legislation)
- Delivery of services (preventive and curative personal health services; primary, secondary, and tertiary services; public health services; services for specific population groups, such as children, or for specific conditions, such as mental illness)

More recently, WHO (2007) has developed a system for describing and categorizing health systems based on six "building blocks":

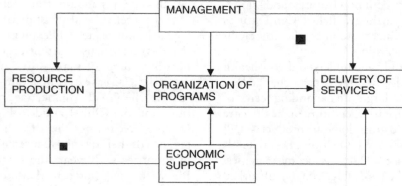

Figure 12-1 The Elements of Health Systems.
Source: M. I. Roemer, National Health Systems of the World: Vol. 1. The Countries (Oxford: Oxford University Press, 1991). Copyright 1991 by Oxford University Press, Inc. Reprinted by permission of Oxford University Press, Inc.

- Service delivery
- Health workforce
- Information
- Medical products, vaccines, and technologies
- Financing
- Leadership and governance (stewardship)

These types of categorization are helpful for describing health systems; indeed, Roemer (1991, 1993) applied his approach to a very large number of countries. Unfortunately, the categorizations are less helpful for understanding how well health systems perform. This assessment would require much more detailed subcategories and greater elaboration of the relationships, not just within each category but particularly between categories (e.g., between economic support mechanisms and organization of programs).

Typologies of Health Systems

To make comparisons of how different types of health systems perform, it is necessary to group countries and their health systems into distinct types. Numerous attempts to do so have been made. For example, countries can be classified according to the following criteria:

- The dominant method of financing (e.g., tax, social insurance, private insurance, out-of-pocket payments)
- The underlying political philosophy (e.g., capitalist, socialist)
- The nature of state intervention (e.g., to cover the whole population or only the poor)
- The level of gross national product (GNP) (e.g., low, middle, high)

- Historical or cultural attributes (e.g., industrialized, non-industrialized, transitional)

A key difficulty, however, is that countries do not fit neatly into these categories. Roemer (1991), for example, used two dimensions:

- Economic level (with four categories: affluent and industrialized, developing and transitional, very poor, resource rich)
- Health system policies (with four categories: entrepreneurial and permissive, welfare orientated, universal and comprehensive, socialist and centrally planned)

Although some of these categories are less relevant today than they were at the time of their formulation (e.g., centrally planned health system policies), it is also the case that the second dimension does not classify well the health systems of low- and middle-income countries, which tend to be fragmented, with different arrangements for different population groups (McPake & Machray, 1997). For example, Roemer (1991) classified Thailand as "entrepreneurial and permissive," and Mexico and India as "welfare orientated." Yet, as shown in Exhibit 12-1, which summarizes the structure of the health systems in these three countries plus Tanzania, these countries cannot be clearly placed into such neat categories.

The Organization for Economic Cooperation and Development (OECD, 1992) has developed a typology that is helpful for categorizing not only the economic dimensions of health systems in OECD countries, but also the directions in which reforms are taking them. The key categories are as follows:

- Whether the prime funding source consists of payments that are made voluntarily (as in

---

Exhibit 12-1	**Illustrations of the Structure of Health Systems**

Tanzania (GNI per capita = $440)

   The public sector plays a leading role in the Tanzanian health system, with the government owning approximately 64% of all health facilities and covering all levels of health care, from primary to tertiary (Mtei, Mulligan, Palmer, Kaumuzora, Ally, & Mills, 2007). Relative to neighboring countries, the public system is quite decentralized, with public services managed at the district level. Mission (church) services are a very important source of care outside the main towns, providing the same number of hospitals as the government, and are subsidized by the state. Private doctors practice in the main cities, and there is a large informal sector of traditional practitioners and drug sellers. The majority of health expenditure flows through government; most of the remainder consists of out-of-pocket expenditure. A national health insurance fund provides health insurance coverage to government workers, a parallel scheme covers formal-sector employees, and a number of community-based insurance schemes also exist. Nevertheless, the coverage of insurance schemes is still limited.

continued

Exhibit 12-1   *continued*

India (GNI per capita = $1,070)

The public-sector health system in India is large in absolute terms, providing all levels of care. Health care is, in general, a state-level function, with central government involved mainly in overall policy and specific disease control programs. There is also a very large formal private sector, providing both ambulatory and inpatient care, and an even larger informal sector consisting of unlicensed and unqualified practitioners and drug sellers. A compulsory state insurance system covers lower-paid, formal-sector workers, and another scheme covers government workers. Numerous community-based health schemes exist, some with an insurance component. A new health insurance scheme was launched by the government of India in 2008, covering first level hospital care for the 300 million people who live below the poverty line. By the end of 2009, only a small percentage of the target population had been reached (Ministry of Labour & Employment, Government of India, n.d.), but the scheme is now expanding rapidly. Several new state insurance schemes are offering access to tertiary level care for the poor.

Mexico (GNI per capita =$9,980)

Both the public and private sectors play an important role in financing and provision of health care in Mexico. Formal-sector employees are covered by various social insurance institutions, whereas the poor receive care through government facilities or private providers (allopathic and traditional). There is very little interaction between public and private sectors, in the form of either regulation or contracting for service delivery. Concern about duplication and waste of resources between the three subsystems—social security, other government, and private—and lack of protection against increasing healthcare costs (especially for the poor) has led to reforms based on decentralization, managed market principles, and a new voluntary insurance scheme for the uninsured, which over time is gradually extending its population and service coverage (Frenk, Sepúlveda Gómez-Dantés, & Knaul, 2003). In 2007, 27% of the Mexican population remained uninsured.

Thailand (GNI per capita = $2,840)

Both the public and private sectors have major roles in the Thai health system, providing all levels of care. There is widespread use of the private sector, especially for outpatient care. Compulsory social insurance covers those in formal employment and finances care provided by public and private hospitals (chosen by the insured). Civil servants have their own medical benefit scheme, which pays for care at public and private hospitals. The remaining part of the population—who formerly could get a low-income card exempting them from fees if they were poor, purchase a voluntary health insurance card, or pay out of pocket for care—are now part of a universal coverage arrangement in which they register at a local facility and can then access a wide range of free healthcare benefits (Towse, Mills, & Tangcharoensathien, 2004).

Note: Gross national income (GNI) is in 2008 dollars.

---

private insurance or payment of user fees) or are compulsory (as in taxation or social insurance)

- Whether services are provided by direct ownership (termed the integrated pattern, where a ministry of health or social insurance agency provides services itself), by contractual arrangements (where a ministry of health or social insurance agency contracts with providers to deliver services), or simply by private providers (paid by direct out-of-pocket payments)

- How services are paid for (prospectively, where financial risk is transferred to providers, or retrospectively, where the cost of care is reimbursed)

This framework is most relevant to countries at a relatively advanced stage of development, where the coverage of the health system is universal or consists of a limited number of arrangements. As with the Roemer classification, it does not allow for the diversity of arrangements seen in practice in poorer countries.

Because a typology suitable for low- and middle-income countries has yet to be developed, the content of this chapter is based on a simple framework (shown in Figure 12-2) that identifies four key actors and four key functions required in any health system. The actors are as follows:

- The government or professional body that structures and regulates the system

- The population, including patients, who as individuals and households ultimately pay for the health system and receive services

- The financing agents, who collect funds and allocate them to providers or purchase services at national or lower levels

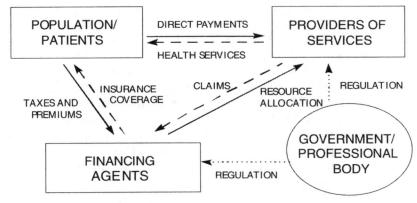

Figure 12-2 A Map of the Health System.
Source: A. Mills, "Reforming Health Sectors: Fashions, Passions and Common Sense," in A. Mills (Ed.), Reforming Health Sectors (London: Kegan Paul International, 2000b), pp. 1–24. Adapted with permission.

- The providers of services, who themselves can be categorized in various ways, such as by level (primary, secondary, tertiary), function (curative, preventive), ownership (public; private, for-profit; private, not-for-profit), degree of organization (formal, informal), or medical system (allopathic, Ayurvedic)

The functions are as follows:

- Regulation
- Financing (through taxes, premiums, and direct payments)
- Resource allocation
- Provision of services

Evaluation of Health Systems

WHO (2000) argues that the health system has three main objectives, which are intrinsically valuable:

- Good health (both its absolute level and its distribution across the population)
- Fairness in financial contribution
- Responsiveness to peoples' expectations (both level and distribution)

In assessing actual performance of health systems, criteria of efficiency and equity are frequently applied, so it is important to understand their various meanings. Efficiency has a number of different dimensions:

- *Macroeconomic efficiency* refers to the total costs of the health system in relation to overall health status; countries differ in how efficiently their health systems convert resources used into health gains.
- *Microeconomic efficiency* refers to the scope for achieving greater efficiency from existing resources. It is of two types:

  Allocative efficiency: devoting resources to that mix of activities that will have the greatest effect on health (i.e., is most cost-effective)

  Technical efficiency: using only the minimum necessary resources to finance, purchase, and deliver a particular activity or set of activities (i.e., avoiding waste)

Equity refers to the fair distribution of the costs of health services and the benefits obtained from their use among different groups in the population. It is inherently a question of values, and views differ as to what constitutes fairness of financing or access to health care. However, indicators of who pays for health services and who receives benefits provide evidence on the basis of which judgments can be made on the degree of equity achieved by particular health systems.

Equity is commonly expressed in two different ways:

- *Horizontal equity* refers to the equal treatment of equals. With respect to financing and resource allocation, it is taken to imply that the charge levied by all agents or providers for a particular good or service should be the same for households with equal ability to pay (regardless of gender, marital status, and so on). Horizontal equity is, therefore, assessed by the extent to which contribution levels are similar among those with similar ability to pay. With respect to provision of services, horizontal equity means that individuals with the same health condition should have equal access to health services.

- *Vertical equity* is based on the principle that individuals who are unequal in society should be treated differently. Vertical equity in the financing and purchasing of health services means that consumers should be charged for the same good or service according to their ability to pay.

Table 12-1 demonstrates how equity and efficiency criteria can be used to guide the financing, allocation of resources, and provision of health services and to evaluate performance.

In the *World Health Report 2000*, a conceptual framework, based on the goals and functions listed earlier, was applied to country data to assess and understand country health system performance (WHO, 2000). Countries were ranked in relation to their attainment of the individual goals, in relation to overall goal attainment, and in terms of performance on level of health and the functioning of the overall health system. Although the conceptual framework and new databases have proved useful, the ranking was extremely controversial (e.g., see Almeida et al., 2001; Coyne & Hilsenrath, 2002) and has not been continued in subsequent World Health Reports.

Historical Development of Health Systems

As indicated by archaeological evidence, medicine has had its role in all cultures and civilizations (e.g., in ancient Mesopotamia and Egypt). It has also been a concern of the state—the law code of Hammurabi (1792–1750 BC) specified the fees for an operation to be paid to a healer on a sliding scale, depending on the status of the patient, and also specified penalties for failure. The Romans built hospitals for domestic slaves and soldiers in permanent forts in occupied

Table 12-1	Equity and Efficiency Criteria Applied to Financing, Resource Allocation, and Provision of Health Care			
	Efficiency		**Equity**	
Functions	**Allocative**	**Technical**	**Horizontal**	**Vertical**
Financing	—	Maximize the proportion of resources raised that are actually available for purchasing health care (e.g., reduce the overhead costs of collecting taxes)	Equal payment by those with equal ability to pay (e.g., same insurance premium for same income group)	Payment in relation to ability to pay (e.g., progressive income tax rates)
Allocating resources	Purchase that mix of interventions that provides the greatest health gains	Maximize the proportion of resources spent by agents that are actually available for providing health care	Services purchased for similar groups (e.g., the elderly) should be the same in different geographical areas	Services purchased should reflect the different needs of different groups (e.g., the elderly versus children)
Providing services	Provide those interventions that return the greatest value for money (e.g., in a poor country, antenatal care should be provided before radiotherapy for cancer)	Make the best use of resources in providing interventions deemed worthwhile (e.g., have nurses as opposed to doctors provide most antenatal care)	Equal access for equal need (e.g., equal waiting times for treatment for patients with similar conditions)	Unequal treatment for unequal need (e.g., unequal treatment of those with trivial versus serious conditions)

Source: Donaldson, C., & Gerard, K. (1993). *Economics of Health Care Financing: The Visible Hand.* London: Macmillan Press. Reprinted with permission.

territories such as England. However, the real development of the hospital derived from the spread of Christianity and of ideas of Christian charity and caring for all who might be in need after the conversion of Constantine (died AD 337) made Christianity an official imperial religion (Porter, 1996a). Hospitals were founded in the main cities of the Christian world, often associated with churches or monasteries. The Islamic world also developed hospitals, and by the eleventh century large hospitals could be found in every major Muslim town. Hospitals were for the sick who lacked families or servants to care for them—the poor, travelers, and those working away from home (Abel-Smith, 1994).

In Europe, by the Middle Ages, a multiplicity of institutions and organizations had developed with pretensions to authority over medicine: the church, guilds, medical colleges, town councils, and powerful individuals. In Brussels, for example, a board of clergy, doctors, and midwives licensed midwives in the fifteenth century. The arrival of the plague—the Black Death—which in its first wave killed around 25% of Europe's population, stimulated growing state involvement to protect health through measures such as imposing quarantine and isolating the sick.

From the early nineteenth century, the scientific basis of medicine was increasingly established, with scientific training becoming essential for the practice of medicine (Porter, 1996b). The eighteenth and nineteenth centuries saw a vast expansion of hospitals in Europe and the United States, supported by philanthropy as well as by public funds, especially for hospitals for infectious diseases and the mentally ill (Porter, 1996a). As medicine became more elaborate and expensive, however, the reliance on charitable and voluntary funding of hospitals in many countries led to a crisis. The enormous increase in the number of surgical procedures and the development of technology led both to much greater numbers of patients and much higher costs per patient.

As voluntary hospitals ran into financial difficulties, they sought new ways to assure their financial stability. In the United States, hospitals developed business strategies based on insurance that could attract affluent patients. In the United Kingdom, where insurance was much less well developed, hospitals were eventually brought into public ownership. In Scandinavia, local authorities had had responsibility for providing hospital services since the late nineteenth century, so they developed largely as a public service (Abel-Smith, 1994).

The strong development of the discipline of public health in the nineteenth century was a response to the disease hazards of the urban environment. In England and Germany, public health measures focused on safe water supply and drains.

Over the eighteenth and nineteenth centuries, modern forms of medical regulation developed. Countries in which medicine was dominated by free markets (such as the United States) converged with countries in Europe with strong state control (such as Germany) to produce the closely regulated medical markets that exist today. However, the degree of state involvement in the provision of health services varied enormously between countries—a source of disparities that persists even today.

A key development was the increase in collective arrangements for funding health services. State services developed in all Western countries to provide health services for those who could not afford to purchase them themselves. In addition, mutual insurance schemes emerged in Europe and the United States as means to protect workers against financial losses, and these often included medical care (Abel-Smith, 1994). Such schemes were encouraged by the German states and developed into a national program of health insurance. In the United Kingdom, in contrast, they were nationalized as part of the expansion of state welfare. Other European countries also saw the development and expansion of compulsory financial arrangements for health services, whether through the extension of insurance arrangements for medical care (the Bismarck model, named after the German chancellor who introduced the first compulsory insurance scheme) or through general taxation (the Beveridge model, named after the British minister of health who is regarded as the founder of the United Kingdom National Health Service). Since World War II, all high-income countries, with the exception of the United States, have extended mechanisms for protection against the financial risks of ill health to the point where they can be said to have achieved universal coverage.

Another key development in the creation of the modern health system was the development of organized systems of medical care, as opposed to fragmented and competing individual doctors and hospitals. World War I marked a turning point in Europe, when the need to organize medical care on a massive scale highlighted the advantages of a large, coordinated system. In the United Kingdom, the Dawson report in 1920 designed a system of district health services based on general practitioners and health centers, with referral upward to hospitals (WHO, 1999). The later development of the philosophy of national economic plans and of a strong government role in many sectors of the economy also supported the development of organized health systems. Even in those countries with less of a tradition of a strong state role in health services, cost escalation in recent decades has forced greater state involvement.

In the late nineteenth century Western medicine spread around the world, often as part of the process of colonial expansion (Zwi & Mills, 1995). Medicine acted in part as an agency of Western imperialism, and organized health services were a component of British, French, German, and Belgian colonization efforts. These services were initially intended for the military, settler, and civil service communities, but it rapidly became apparent that protecting the health of expatriates required addressing health needs among the colonized peoples. In addition, health services were introduced by commercial interests that believed their economic returns would improve as a result of this step, and by churches as part of their missionary activities. To a much greater extent than was the case in the home countries of the colonizers, the provision of health services became associated with the state.

This relationship was accentuated in the postcolonial era by the prevalent ideologies of state-led growth and state responsibility for the welfare of all inhabitants. In its most extreme form in socialist countries such as Tanzania, China, and Vietnam, this policy banned private practice. However, more generally in Africa and Asia, the attention of policy makers focused on publicly financed and provided services, neglecting the often large private sector. The aim was to extend public services to cover the whole population, even if the reality was very different.

Developments in Latin America were somewhat different. As in Africa, the earliest Western health services were developed by the colonists, especially for the armed forces and the police. Major employers provided health services, particularly where enterprises were remote from urban centers. Some religious hospitals were built to care for the poor (Abel-Smith, 1994). These hospitals were later supplemented by government hospitals and clinics, especially in areas without charitable hospitals. A key difference from most of Africa and Asia was the early development of compulsory insurance arrangements for workers in the formal sector in Latin America. Because medical care infrastructure was lacking, the insurance agencies often built and ran their own services, thereby contributing to the emergence of the parallel health systems seen today in many Latin American countries.

The historical development of health services in many countries resulted in a health infrastructure that was biased toward hospitals. Attempts to reorient services culminated in 1978 in the Declaration of Alma Ata, which emphasized the importance of primary health care, involving the delivery of curative and preventive services at the community level. This Declaration encouraged strong emphasis on the building up of integrated health services, involving community-based health workers. Nonetheless, a rival approach argued in favor of selective primary health care, to include those interventions that addressed the greatest disease burden and were most cost-effective (Walsh & Warren, 1979). Services for children were a key priority in this approach, and, together with the emphasis on family planning that resulted from the preoccupation of many donors with world population growth, meant that peripheral health services in many low-income countries were targeted primarily at women and children. Only recently has there been greater emphasis on achieving a more integrated approach to the delivery of health services at peripheral levels, and on the health of adolescents and adults.

A marked development in the 1980s and 1990s was the increasing questioning of the government's role in health systems. The most radical changes occurred in countries formerly under strict communist rule, where a market economy was introduced and market forces allowed to influence health services (see Saltman & Figueras, 1997, for discussion of such developments in Eastern and Central Europe). Social insurance arrangements were introduced for individuals in formal employment, health professionals were permitted to have private practices, private markets were encouraged in pharmaceuticals, and much greater costs have fallen directly on household budgets. In China, for example, in 1981, approximately 71% of the population—including 48% of the rural population—had some insurance protection; by 1993, the overall insurance coverage rate had dropped to 21%, with 7% coverage of the rural population (WHO, 1999). Although less radical changes occurred in other parts of the world, most governments were forced by economic crises in the 1980s and 1990s to consider how they could best prioritize their care goals and ration services to those most in need. In response, many introduced revenue generation schemes, such as user fees. This reconsideration was also forced by rapidly growing private markets in medical care.

Most recently, in the early years of the twenty-first century, there has been a marked increase in development assistance for health, in part associated with the movement surrounding the MDGs but also driven by the international response to the HIV/AIDS pandemic, and the introduction of new sources of funding such as the Bill and Melinda Gates Foundation and new funding mechanisms such as the Global Fund for HIV, TB and Malaria. Funding streams have become increasingly stratified by disease or health program, in marked contrast to the primary healthcare ethos of earlier decades. By 2009, this approach was producing a strong reaction, with analyses highlighting how the success of disease-specific programs have been hampered by weak health systems (Travis et al., 2004), and calling for much greater investment in health system strengthening (Taskforce on Innovative International Financing for Health Systems, 2009).

The Role of the State

This brief historical review indicates that one of the key issues in the design of health systems is the role assigned to the state. This section examines the economic arguments commonly put forward to specify the state's role in health and then considers other explanations for the roles observed in practice.

The first main economic justification lies in explanations of market failure. The efficient outcomes of private markets depend on a number of conditions being met. Because of the particular characteristics of health and health services, these criteria may not be satisfied in the health sector.

First, the presence of externalities means that the optimal amount would not be produced or consumed. Externalities are costs or benefits that are not taken into account in the transactions of producers or consumers. For example, an individual's decision on whether to be immunized will be related to the value of the protection to that individual, not to the protection that may be accorded to others by reducing the pool of susceptible individuals.

Second, the market may fail to produce public goods. Public goods are those for which consumption is characterized as nonrival (consumption by one person does not reduce the consumption of another) and nonexcludable (a consumer cannot be prevented from benefiting from the good—for example, through requiring payment). Control of mosquito breeding sites to reduce malaria transmission is an obvious example—everyone living in the area will benefit from this intervention regardless of whether they have paid for it. Information can also be seen as a public good because it is nonrival; it is not nonexcludable, but the cost of providing information to extra people is often very low. This description applies to knowledge gained through research, for example.

Third, monopoly power can lead to market failure, because it enables the provider to charge more than if the market were competitive. Monopoly power may be held by a hospital in a particular geographic area, by a pharmaceutical firm, or even by a profession as a whole (such as the medical profession).

These arguments provide a rather weak justification for state intervention in the entire health system because the range of services to which they apply is quite limited. They are most relevant to public health services and preventive care, and less relevant to the bulk of curative services. Moreover, problems such as monopoly are not unique to health and are commonly dealt with by regulation rather than state provision. A more powerful argument for a large state role lies in the asymmetry of information between provider and consumer. Medical consultations are often sought precisely because patients do not know what is wrong with them—thus they are ill informed, in contrast to the normal assumption made in economics of perfectly informed consumers. Hence, in medical care, providers are in an unusually strong position. Although they may act as perfect agents for the consumer, it is also possible—especially when income is related to care provided—that the personal interests of the providers may enter into decisions made on treatment. The poor and less well educated are particularly vulnerable to unscrupulous profit seeking by private providers.

Another characteristic of health care is its uncertain nature, and the potential for very high costs. This possibility makes it an obvious candidate for insurance, but it is generally accepted that private insurance markets do not work well (World Bank, 1997). Individuals who purchase insurance may indulge in activities that put their health more at risk than if they were not insured, or once ill may consume more health care. This phenomenon, which is known as moral hazard, tends to raise the cost of insurance, making it unaffordable for some. Another problem is that those who are at greatest risk of needing care will be more likely to seek insurance, but due to asymmetries of information between insurer and insured, it is often difficult for the insurer to tailor the premium charged to the nature of the risk. This process, which is known as adverse selection, means that the insurer ends up with a more costly risk pool, premiums rise, and the more healthy individuals opt out. In addition, insurance becomes more expensive, so that many who cannot afford the increased premiums are excluded from coverage. Although the result is clearly inequitable, it is also inefficient because there will be people unprotected who would be willing and able to purchase insurance if the market worked well.

Other arguments in favor of state involvement focus on issues other than market failure. For example, one argument notes that some types of health services are merit goods—that is, goods that society believes should be provided, but that individuals, if left to themselves, might underconsume because they are not the best judge of what is in their own or the public's interest. This argument is strongest for health services for children and the mentally ill.

Another argument is founded on equity principles—even with perfectly operating private markets for health services and health insurance, there will inevitably be some individuals too poor to afford to access them. Although this problem could potentially be taken care of by income redistribution policies, equitable access to health services is of concern; hence it can be argued that providing benefits in kind is appropriate.

Although these points are the standard arguments used to explore the appropriate role of the state in health services, the judgment on their significance differs greatly among economists, leading to radically different policy prescriptions. Even though much of this debate has focused on the relative merits of the U.S. health system versus the Canadian or U.K. health systems, it has also influenced the nature of the debate concerning the reform of health systems in low- and middle-income countries, as noted later in discussion of health reform trends. Underlying this debate are alternative views on the ethical basis of a health system. One view sees access to health services as similar to access to other goods and services, and dependent on an individual's success in gaining or inheriting income. The other sees access to health services as a right of citizenship that should not depend on individual income or wealth. According to the first view, the state's role in health should be confined to regulation of the market, public health measures, and public welfare for the poor to provide a minimum acceptable level of service, but nothing like the level of service available to those better off. According to the second view, the role of the state should be to ensure equal access to health services that does not differ depending on individuals' economic or social status.

Although these kinds of economic arguments provide justification for state involvement in health systems, they provide little guidance on the precise nature of intervention. In particular, they do not necessarily imply that the state should itself provide health services (as opposed to purchasing services from others). A key change in recent decades in thinking about public management has been the recognition that the state need not provide services itself directly, but instead can play an enabling role (Walsh, 1995).

An important influence on this position is recognition that in many countries the state has failed in its policies to provide good-quality public services, including health services, for everyone. These arguments derive from a number of strands of economic thinking, notable among which are public choice theory and property rights theories. The former is concerned with the nature of decision making in government. It argues that government officials are no different from anyone else in pursuing their own interests. Thus politicians will be concerned to maximize their chances of being reelected, and bureaucrats will serve their own interests (e.g., maximizing their budgets because their own rewards [salary, status] are related to that achievement). The result is that the public sector is wasteful because politicians and bureaucrats have no incentive to promote allocative or technical efficiency.

Property rights theorists argue that the source of inefficiency in the public sector is the weakening of property rights. In the private sector, it can be argued that entrepreneurs or shareholders have a strong interest in the efficient use of resources. In contrast, in the public sector, there is little obvious threat to an enterprise if staff perform poorly; hence, incentives for efficient performance are weak.

These theories underlie what has been termed the "new public management," which seeks to expose public services to market pressures, without necessarily privatizing them (Walsh, 1995). Such approaches change the nature of state involvement, through policies of opening up services to competitive tender or putting services out to contract on a competitive basis, introducing internal markets where public providers have to compete for contracts from public purchasers, devolving financial control to organizations such as individual hospitals, spinning off parts of government into separate public agencies (such as an agency to manage government health services), and increasing the choice and influence of consumers by giving them resources in cash or kind (e.g., vouchers for treating sexually transmitted diseases)—termed demand-side financing—to purchase healthcare services from their chosen (usually accredited) provider.

Although theories justifying particular roles of the state feature prominently in the literature on health systems, in practice the actual role of the state in any particular country is shaped by a wide variety of influences. Most notable are the history of state involvement in health services and the rationale for its involvement over time, the extent to which private providers and insurers developed early in the history of the health system and thus were able to play a prominent role, and the attitude of the medical profession to an increased state role in the health system (Mills et al., 2001). One key issue has been the extent to which the state takes on itself the responsibility for providing services to the whole population versus concerning itself only with the poor and indigent.

Exhibit 12-2 summarizes the role of the state in four countries. In Tanzania and India, the state's aims have historically been to provide services free at the point of use to the whole population. In contrast, both Mexico and Thailand have had specific schemes that cater to the poor and indigent, although recently Thailand has extended financial protection to the whole population through its "universal coverage" policy (Towse et al., 2004).

Regulation

Regulation is a role that all governments must carry out, regardless of their degree of involvement in health services provision. Regulation occurs when government exerts control over the activities of individuals and firms (Roemer, 1993). The traditional rationale for this role relates to the arguments of market failure outlined previously as well as to the desire of governments to meet other social objectives, such as equity. Market failure creates the need to regulate either to make the market work better (e.g., to limit the control any one pharmaceutical firm may have over the market) or to prevent harmful effects (e.g., to ensure minimum quality standards for private clinics).

Although regulation is often thought of as action involving control, sanctions, and penalties, it can also take the form of incentives to encourage appropriate behavior. In health services, where outcomes are difficult to observe (i.e., it can be difficult to relate treatment to change in health), it can be argued that

---

Exhibit 12-2	**Illustrations of the Role of the State**

Tanzania

    Health services for the whole population have traditionally been seen as the responsibility of the state in Tanzania. Government spending on health accounts for 3.7% of GDP and 58% of total health expenditures. While 40% of hospitals are government owned, a further 40% are provided by churches. Independence brought in a government that was anti-private sector and, until recently, the for-profit private health sector was ignored in government policy. Public-sector reforms have decentralized public management and introduced fees for public services. The poor are reliant mainly on state and church services and the informal private sector for health services.

India

    In India, historically the emphasis was on a strong state role, but resources were never provided to make this goal a reality (public expenditure accounts for 0.9% of GDP and 25% of total health expenditures; 65% of total hospital beds are public). Public services are often of poor quality and are adversely affected by the private practice of government doctors. In general, people distrust the state. The policies for charging for use of public facilities vary by state, but income from fees is very small. There is very widespread use of the private sector by all sections of the population, including the poor.

Mexico

    In Mexico, the public health sector consumes 2.9% of GDP and 44.2% of total health expenditures, and provides 80% of hospital beds. The government's primary role is as owner of social security institutions, which account for some 67% of general government expenditures on health. The Ministry of Health and municipalities play a residual role in caring for the poor and uninsured. There is dissatisfaction with the quality of both Ministry of Health and social security services, with those who can afford it preferring to use private services.

Thailand

    In Thailand, the public health sector consumes 2.3% of GDP and 64.5% of total health expenditures; 76% of total hospital beds were in the public sector in 2005 (Ministry of Public Health, n.d.). Thailand has a tradition of strong central government and laissez-faire economic policies. Historically, government policies have encouraged the private sector to grow through tax exemptions and public funding for private care for specific groups. With the introduction of the recent universal coverage policy, the government has strengthened its commitment to inclusive social policies. Public services are of generally good quality; their main problem is considered to be a lack of consumer orientation.

Note: Expenditure data were retrieved January 11, 2010, from http://www.who.int/nha/country/en/.

incentives are particularly appropriate, although they can be complicated to design and predicting response can be difficult (Baldwin & Cave, 1999). In low- and middle-income countries, where capacity and resources for enforcement are typically not as strong as in high-income countries, incentives in combination with other tools such as consumer information, contracting, accreditation, and use of other actors such as consumer groups or NGOs can offer policy makers a wider and softer approach to enforcement (Ensor & Weinzierl, 2007).

In practice, regulatory action seeks to influence the following aspects of the market:

- Market entry and exit
- Remuneration of providers
- Quality and distribution of services
- Standards and quality

Key mechanisms used in the health system to regulate the provision of health services are summarized in Table 12-2. Controls over market entry and exit are not shown separately because they also serve to influence quantities and quality.

Licensing of professionals to provide services is one of the key forms of regulation, with professional councils usually being empowered to carry out this function. As new professions arise or become more important, eventually they are brought within the scope of laws. Although such laws dictate entry into the market, their prime rationale from a government perspective is to maintain quality and protect the consumer. Actual experience, however, demonstrates that licensing on its own is not adequate to ensure quality.

A second key type of regulation is licensing or registration of facilities, which is required before they can open. Legislation often specifies the requirements for particular categories of facilities, covering such aspects as trained staff, availability of equipment and supplies, and buildings. Because of the cost-enhancing capabilities of high technology, some countries have an approval process for the purchase of major items

Table 12-2	Examples of Regulatory Mechanisms for Healthcare Provision	
Variable	**Mechanism**	**Examples from Low- and Middle-Income Countries**
Quantities/distribution	• Licensing of providers	• Universal for main professional groups
	• Licensing of facilities	• Increasingly common for hospitals and clinics
	• Controls on number and size of medical schools	• Common in many countries (e.g., in Latin America)
	• Controls on practicing in over-provided areas	• South Africa: private hospitals
	• Controls on introduction of high technology	• Being considered by Malaysia and Thailand
	• Incentives to practice in under-served areas and specialties	• In many countries for doctors, often in the form of compulsory rural service
	• Requirement of capitation or case-based payment to control the supply of services	• Social insurance in South Korea (case payment) and Thailand (capitation)
Prices	• Negotiation of salary scales	• Zimbabwe: nursing salaries; Argentina: doctors
	• Fixing of charges (e.g., for lab tests, drug price markup)	• South Africa: drug price markups for reimbursement by medical schemes
	• Negotiation of reimbursement rates	• Many social insurance schemes (e.g., Chile)
Quality	• Licensing of practitioners	• Universal for the major healthcare professions
	• Registration of facilities	• Increasingly common; specifies structural standards
	• Control of the nature of services provided	• Restrictions on drug dispensing by general practitioners (e.g., Zimbabwe); range of procedures (clinical officers—Kenya)
	• Accessibility	• Hospitals legally obliged to provide emergency care irrespective of patient financial status (Thailand, Malaysia)
	• Required complaints procedures	• Consumer laws applicable (India)
	• Required provision of information for monitoring quality	• Many countries
	• Control of training curricula	• Many countries
	• Requirements for continuing education	• Increasingly being introduced
	• Accreditation	• Increasingly being introduced; used in Taiwan, and pilot schemes launched in Brazil and Thailand

Sources: Bennett, S., et al. (1994). *Public and private roles in health: A review and analysis of experience in sub-Saharan Africa.* Geneva, Switzerland: World Health Organization; and Kumaranayake, L. (1998). *Economic aspects of health sector regulation: Strategic choices for low and middle income countries.* London: London School of Hygiene and Tropical Medicine, Health Policy Unit, Department of Public Health and Policy.

of equipment. Entry to medical school may also be controlled with the same aim—that is, controlling costs by limiting supply. In a normal market, such action might be expected to raise costs, but it is considered justified in health because of the power physicians have to generate their own income or to prevail on government to employ greater numbers of workers or more expensive technology than the country can really afford.

Often countries are concerned about the geographic distribution of providers, and controls and incentives are used to influence where new providers can set up. For example, South African provinces can control the creation and expansion of private hospitals, depending on the number of private beds already existing in their areas. Certificate-of-need legislation has been used for many years to control the construction of new buildings and investment in new equipment in the United States.

Control of prices and reimbursement levels may have several purposes: to restrict incomes in the private sector so that remuneration differences between public and private professionals do not get too great; to ensure that health services remain affordable for the not-so-wealthy; and to restrict the financial burden placed on risk-pooling arrangements, such as social insurance or employer medical benefit schemes. Nevertheless, given the power of the medical profession, there is always a risk that price control will operate more in the interests of the profession than the public; in addition, it can be difficult to enforce or monitor.

Control of quality is one of the prime concerns of regulation. Licensing and registration have it as an aim, as well as control of quantity. For example, in Kenya a private clinic must be kept in good order and state of repair, not be a residential building, and keep essential drugs on hand and accurate drug records.

Regulations often seek to control the nature of services provided, thereby ensuring that services are within the competence of a particular type of provider and limiting the potential for excessive service provision. Regulations usually lay down which type of health professional can prescribe which type of drug—limiting, for example, the range of drugs that can be given by low-level health workers. It is quite common for private practitioners to be allowed to dispense medicines only if no pharmacy is located nearby. Where this rule does not exist, drug dispensing is often a major source of the income of private doctors, leading to predictable concerns about overprescribing.

Control of training curricula is fundamental to ensuring quality, and is often one of the functions given by law to professional bodies. A trend in high-income countries, which is also becoming apparent elsewhere, is the requirement for professionals to receive regular refresher training if they are to continue to be licensed. Such a provision places high demands on regulatory bodies, however, because it requires the introduction of monitoring procedures, training programs, and relicensing arrangements.

Accreditation is a process of certifying that a facility meets a certain standard, and is usually applied as a self-regulating procedure that is voluntary and managed by an independent body. In practice, it may act more as a regulatory device than as a peer review process, especially when accreditation is required for hospitals to be eligible for reimbursement from a social insurance scheme, as in Taiwan.

Governments also regulate other markets with considerable relevance to health services, including the health insurance and pharmaceutical markets. Both have features unique to themselves. In the case of insurance, regulations may impose a particular approach to risk pooling (e.g., requiring schemes to give lifetime coverage or to use community rather than risk rating). In the case of pharmaceuticals, regulations may establish which drugs can be imported and which can be sold over the counter or require a doctor's prescription; they may also specify quality control procedures for both imported and locally made drugs.

Separate consideration may also be given in regulatory structures to not-for-profit providers. On the one hand, they may be treated more strictly. For example, their fee structures may be regulated, they may be required to provide a certain amount of free care to the poor, and requirements to provide information may be stricter. On the other hand, they may benefit from their not-for-profit status. For example, tax exemptions are often available to these entities.

In practice, a number of key problems are associated with regulation, as highlighted in Exhibit 12-3 (Mills et al., 2001). Notably, laws are frequently outdated and are difficult to change. For example, many low-income countries have laws they inherited from colonial regimes that have not kept pace with the development of the private sector, resulting in whole categories of facilities that may be completely unregulated. Private laboratories are often a case in point.

Another problem is that regulation requires substantial knowledge on the part of the regulatory bodies. Unfortunately, it is all too common in low- and middle-income countries for even basic information, such as lists of providers and facilities, to be incomplete. Moreover, the poorer the country, the greater the proportion of providers who are small and informally organized, making it difficult to require any regular provision of information.

Exhibit 12-3 | **Key Regulatory Problems in Selected Countries**

Zambia[a]

- The state relies on legal instruments rather than complementing them with other approaches to regulation.
- The country has limited capacity to enforce regulations, especially with respect to drug prescribing and sales.
- Regulations related to private providers permits the Health Minister to set maximum prices for medical treatment; in reality, private hospitals are free to charge what they like.
- The registrar of private hospitals has a mandate to inspect private facilities but such inspections are rarely performed.

India

- Few states require any registration and inspection of private hospitals.
- Practice by unqualified personnel is widespread.
- Unethical practices (e.g., payments between hospitals and general practitioners to encourage referrals) are widespread.
- No database of private providers exists.
- There is little ability to enforce regulations.
- Regulatory bodies lack resources.

Mexico[b]

- Private hospitals are not subject to a strict process of accreditation that verifies their capacity to provide an acceptable standard of care.
- There is a lack of control over pharmacists prescribing and selling most drugs.
- Public facilities are used for treating private patients.
- The private sector resists providing epidemiologic and other information.

Thailand[c]

- The regulatory framework is largely complete, but its application is weak.
- Regulatory bodies lack resources for enforcement.
- There is insufficient information on activity in the private sector.
- It is difficult to control unethical practices (e.g., turning away emergency cases).
- Professional council regulation is largely ineffective.

Sources:
a. Mtei et al., 2007.
b. Miguel Betancourt, personal communication.
c. Teerawattananon, Tangcharoensathien, Tantivess, & Mills, 2003.

A third problem relates to regulatory capture—that is, the situation in which the body meant to be doing the regulating in practice operates in the interests of those being regulated, not in the public interest. This is a common problem in the case of regulation of professional groups, which is often done by the profession itself, leading to very slow processing of complaints and concerns of professional negligence. India has had the interesting experience of introducing a consumer rights law, which the courts have ruled applies to government health services as well as those that are privately provided. This legislation provides an alternative channel for pursuing complaints against healthcare providers. However, India is also a country where the overlap of public and private interests makes it extremely difficult to introduce new regulations or change existing laws. In India, as in a number of countries, it is common to find government-employed doctors with private practices—with or without legal sanction—and senior Ministry of Health officials, as well as politicians, having financial interests in private-sector health services (Mills et al., 2001). Thus there is no clear distinction between the regulators and those being regulated.

A fourth problem is the inadequacy of the resources provided to the regulatory bodies to apply the laws effectively. Quality monitoring, in particular, requires regular inspection to ensure laws are being followed. This practice places great demands on the limited staff capacity of regulatory agencies, especially for drugs and clinics, where outlets are numerous and widely dispersed. A further problem may be that low-paid staff seek illicit payments in lieu of carrying out their job effectively. An extreme form of this has been found in China, where government subsidies to public health activities were severely cut, making environmental health units dependent on revenue generation for much of their income. As a consequence, regulators tended to inspect those firms that were more able to pay their fees (Liu & Mills,

2002). Those that were less profitable, and hence likely to have worse safety and hygiene practices, went uninspected.

A final problem is a lack of institutional structures to back up the regulatory process. Strong consumer groups, media, professional associations, and insurance agencies all have important roles to play in oversight of health systems (Kumaranayake, 1998). The consumer role is particularly important because consumers can both identify problems through complaint procedures and legal action and levy pressure more broadly through consumer groups. However, the common imbalance in power and access to resources between consumers and professionals suggests that complementary pressures are also important. One source of such leverage can be the purchasing agencies considered later in this chapter.

Financing

This section establishes a conceptual model for describing the system for financing health services, defines and evaluates the major sources of health financing in developing countries, describes trends in health financing across countries, and presents the national health account methodology that is increasingly being used to collect health financing data.

Conceptual Model

Financing refers here to the raising or collection of revenue to pay for the operation of the system. The term is, therefore, used in a narrower way than has become common practice by WHO, for example, where the financing building block is considered to encompass raising money, pooling funds, and paying providers. *Financing agents* are those entities that collect money to pay providers on behalf of consumers. Financing agents may be publicly or privately owned, and may provide health services directly (e.g., the ministry of health through public hospitals and health centers) or purchase health services from providers (e.g., a private insurer that purchases inpatient care from a variety of hospitals).

There is some disagreement in the literature as to the definition of sources of financing. *Sources* may be defined as those entities that provide funds to financing agents (Berman, 1997). Individuals and firms can be thought of as the primary sources of funds. Individuals generate income in the form of wages or salaries, while businesses may earn profit on capital investments or rent on properties owned. Resources may pass through several levels of sources before reaching the agents. For example, the ministry of finance can be thought of as a secondary-level source insofar as it generates funds by taxing the incomes of households and businesses and then transfers these resources to other government agencies to purchase health services. A single entity may act both as a source and an agent of financing. For example, households commonly pay for health services both indirectly (through taxation, contributions to social and private insurance, donations to charities, and so on) and directly (through out-of-pocket payments).

More often, however, the term "source" is applied to the method whereby an agent mobilizes or collects resources. For example, the sources of financing for the ministry of health include personal and business taxes, and donations, loans, and grants from domestic and foreign agencies. The sources of financing for private insurance agencies are premiums paid by the enrollees in these schemes. In this chapter, the term "source" is used with this definition in mind unless otherwise indicated.

Description and Evaluation of Predominant Sources

This section defines the most commonly used sources of financing and briefly discusses the efficiency, equity, and revenue-generating ability of each source. Table 12-3 summarizes the relative merits of each source. The relative advantages of differing sources in pooling financial risks are dealt with in detail in Chapter 13, which provides a more detailed review of evidence on their efficiency and equity implications.

Efficiency with respect to a source of financing involves a number of elements, including administrative (or technical) efficiency, stability, and flexibility. Administrative efficiency relates to the cost of the management of the system and is the difference between gross yield (all funds that are collected) and net yield (that portion of the gross yield that is actually available for the purposes of health service delivery). This difference results from the costs of revenue collection, allocation, and distribution; advertising and promotion; and funds lost to corruption and fraud as well as the cost of fighting corruption and fraud. The stability of an agent is determined by the degree to which revenue raising varies with changes in economic or political conditions. Finally, for a financing agent to be efficient, there must be flexibility in terms of the allocation of funds to different expenditure categories. Least flexible are those sources of financing pledged to a specific activity. Public-sector sources tend to be less flexible than private-sector sources due to the stringent rules and regulations that

Table 12-3	Evaluation of Health Financing Sources					
	Efficiency			Equity		
	Administrative Efficiency	Stability	Flexibility	Horizontal	Vertical	Revenue Generation
Public Sources						
General tax revenues	High	Low	Low	High	Progressive	High
Retail sales taxes	High	High	Low	High	Regressive	Low
Lotteries and betting	Low	High	Low	High	Regressive	Low
Deficit financing	Low	Low	Low	Depends	Depends	Depends
External grants	Low	Low	Low	High	Progressive	Low
Social insurance	Low	High	Low	High	Regressive	Depends on size of formal sector
Private Sources						
Households	Low	High	High	Low	Regressive	High
Employers	Low to medium	High	Variable	Low	Depends	Low
Private insurance	Low	High	High	Low	Regressive	Low
Voluntary organizations	High	Variable	Variable	High	Progressive	Medium

are often applied to government spending as well as the political constraints on reallocation.

The concepts of horizontal and vertical equity of financing were introduced earlier in this chapter. With respect to vertical equity, a progressive system is one in which lower-income groups pay a lower proportion of their income for services compared to higher-income groups. A regressive system is one in which lower-income groups pay a higher share of income for services compared to higher-income groups. A proportional or neutral system is one in which all income groups pay the same percentage of their income for services.

Apart from problems of inefficiency and inequity, health systems in many low- and middle-income countries face the difficulty of simply not being able to generate sufficient funds to ensure that the entire population has access to a minimal package of health services. Thus a goal of the financing function of health systems is to increase the availability of funds for the purchase and provision of health services. As countries become richer and the demand for high-technology, hospital-based interventions increases, the goal generally shifts from generating funds to constraining the financial flow through the health system (i.e., cost containment).

Public Sources of Financing

Direct taxes are paid directly by individuals or organizations to government and include personal income tax, property and land taxes, taxes on domestic business transactions and profits, duties on imports and exports, and property taxes. Some portion of these resources may then be allocated to the annual budget for health services. The best-known examples of general tax financing for health services are in the United Kingdom and other Commonwealth nations (Hsiao, 1995).

Direct tax revenues should have relatively high net yields, but this will depend on the overhead costs of the government bureaucracy needed to collect, allocate, and disburse them. They may not be a particularly reliable or stable source of funds for the health system, because the health sector must compete directly with other social and economic programs for a portion of the government's budget; as such, this source may fluctuate depending on the economic and political climate. Furthermore, this source of financing is likely to be inflexible because it is controlled by public-sector agents that are constrained by rules and regulations and the political feasibility of reallocations.

Direct taxation achieves horizontal equity insofar as taxes on individuals are generally not related to characteristics other than income. Income tax is generally the most progressive form of revenue raising, because income tax rates usually rise as a person's taxable income increases (Doorslaer, Wagstaff, & Rutten, 1993; Wagstaff et al., 1999). Direct taxes are very progressive, for example, in Bangladesh, the Philippines, Sri Lanka, and Thailand, where direct taxes are almost exclusively paid by the better-off (O'Donnell et al., 2008). The ability of taxation to redistribute resources from the rich to the poor is hindered when the wealthy are able to evade the payment of taxes.

Ability to mobilize resources is another strength of direct taxation. Although most low- and middle-income countries are restricted in their ability to collect income taxes and indirect taxes (due to limited infrastructure and small formal sectors), the government has many other options for generating tax revenue, including property, business, and import and export taxes. For example, taxes on international trade in 2007 accounted for 27% of central government revenues in Bangladesh, 23% in Russia, and 27% in Niger (World Bank, 2009).

Indirect taxes pass through an intermediary en route to government coffers. Such taxes are incorporated into the selling price of a good or service; they include sales and value-added taxes (taxes on a broad variety of items) and excise duties (imposed on the sale of specific items, such as tobacco products, beer, and liquor). Revenues generated in this manner are often allocated to finance specific programs. Taxes that are pledged to a specific sector or activity are termed hypothecated, and the practice is known as earmarking.

As with direct sales taxes, the net yield of indirect taxes will vary depending on the efficiency of the government agency responsible for collecting them. Indirect taxes are likely to be reliable when they are earmarked for the health sector, or even specific projects within the health sector. The flexibility of this source may be constrained by the government rules and regulations that guide revenue allocation.

Indirect taxation, and excise duties in particular, are generally regressive, because poorer households often spend a higher percentage of their income on the goods being taxed (e.g., alcohol and cigarettes). A study of healthcare financing in OECD countries, using data from the 1980s and 1990s, found that indirect taxes were regressive in all countries except Spain (Wagstaff et al., 1999).

Lotteries and betting may also serve as sources of earmarked income for health services, although these methods are not often used. They have low net yields because they are costly to administer. As with indirect taxes, the resulting revenues are likely to be reliable because they are earmarked, but inflexible because they are administered by public agents. As with retail sales taxes, lotteries and betting tend to impose a particularly heavy burden on the earnings of the poor (because of their popularity among lower-income groups).

National authorities can augment general tax revenues through domestic and international deficit financing (loans) and through grants. Deficit financing means that funds are borrowed for a specific project or activity and must be paid back to the source over some future period of time. Domestic deficit financing is usually achieved through the issue of debt certificates, or bonds, with guaranteed interest rates. International borrowing typically takes the form of loans from bilateral and multilateral organizations. External grants are transfers to governments made in cash, goods, or services by foreign governments or organizations; they do not have to be repaid.

More than 100 international entities provide development assistance for health (World Bank, 2008). Total development assistance for health reached nearly $17 billion in 2006, up from 6.8 billion in 2000 (World Bank, 2008). Major sources of grants include the bilateral donor agencies—such as the United Kingdom's Department for International Development (DFID) and the U.S. Agency for International Development (USAID)—as well as the Bill and Melinda Gates Foundation and the Global Fund to Fight AIDS, Tuberculosis, and Malaria. One of the largest financiers of health services in low- and middle-income countries is the World Bank, which provides two different types of loans (World Bank, 2010b). The first type is for low- and middle-income countries that are able to pay near-market interest rates. The second type of loan goes to the 79 poorest countries in the world, 39 of which are in Africa. These loans carry little or no interest, and are very long term (generally 40 years, including 10 years' grace). Loans that bear an interest rate substantially below market interest rates are termed "soft loans."

The costs of processing and administering donor assistance in the health sector can be quite high, particularly when the aid to a country is fragmented into a large number of donor projects. Fragmentation is common—according to the World Bank (2004), a typical recipient country in 2000 received aid from about 15 bilateral donor agencies and 10 multilateral agencies—and results in officials spending a large amount of their time meeting donors' requirements. Stability of funding is limited, insofar as external funds are typically of short duration, with no guarantee of renewal.

The flexibility of loan and grant financing is variable. At one time, it was common for external funds to be made for specific, free-standing health projects; decisions on expenditure were usually made prior to disbursement. Increasingly, in recent years, donor assistance has been made to sector investment programs (SIPs), whereby government and donors agree to a public-expenditure program that incorporates both domestic and foreign resources. The International Health Partnership Plus (IHP+) is one such initiative (International Health Partnership, 2010). Donor countries and development partners commit to supporting a single national health plan. Intended benefits include improved coordination between country governments and development partners, reduced transaction costs (including the costs of accounting and reporting), and improved long-term stability of financing for health systems strengthening.

The equity of deficit financing will depend entirely on how the loan is ultimately paid back. If, for example, funds generated through direct taxation are used to pay back a loan, then their impact may be progressive.

External grants should be equitable because they are provided by wealthy nations and should be used to establish and run projects in remote or underserved areas (although this aim is by no means always the case). Ultimately, the extent to which they actually achieve a progressive redistribution of resources will depend on the extent to which the government shifts spending as the result of the grants. Only limited resources are generated through external loans and grants except in the very poorest countries—low-income countries spend on average $25 per capita on health; of this only $6 comes from development assistance (Taskforce on Innovative International Financing for Health Systems, 2009). In specific countries, however, the share of external funding in total health expenditures can be as high as 57%, as in Mozambique.

Social insurance premiums are mandatory insurance payments made by employers and employees in the formal sector, usually as a percentage of wages, and hence are often termed payroll taxes. Social insurance payments can have relatively low net yields due to the cost of processing claims. According to WHO (1993), administrative costs in Western European insurance funds amount to approximately 5%, compared with an upper limit of 28% among social insurance schemes in Latin America, and potentially higher costs in Africa. The monies generated through such schemes are likely to be stable because they are earmarked for the health sector; however, they may not be flexible, again related to government restrictions and requirements.

While the value of social insurance premiums is generally based on income, social insurance contributions tend to be regressive in countries with universal systems, such as France, Japan, the Netherlands, Spain, and South Korea (O'Donnell et al., 2008; Wagstaff et al., 1999). This situation arises because contributions are typically subject to a ceiling. Social insurance premiums may be progressive if ceilings can be eliminated or if low-income groups are exempt from contributions. In low- and middle-income countries, where social insurance tends to include only wealthier, formal-sector workers, contributions are progressive. This is the case, for example, in China, Indonesia, and the Philippines (O'Donnell et al., 2008). In these countries, however, the insurance coverage is largely restricted to the better-off.

Coverage achieved by social insurance schemes in many low- and middle-income countries has been limited, because premiums can only easily be collected from formal-sector employees. This limitation has given rise to much criticism of the equity of social insurance arrangements, because a relatively small proportion of the population has access to better services than much of the rest of the population, and in addition sometimes benefits from government subsidies to the social insurance program. Some countries, including Costa Rica, the Republic of Korea, and Taiwan, have achieved universal or near-universal coverage through combining funds from social insurance with general tax revenues, thereby ensuring that all population groups have access to similar types and levels of care (Mills, 2000a).

Private Sources of Financing

Direct household expenditure includes all out-of-pocket payments or user fees paid by the consumer of health services directly to the provider (including private practitioners, traditional healers, and private pharmacists). Even services provided by the government or an insurance program may include some element of copayment, which may take a variety of forms. Coinsurance means that the consumer is responsible for paying for a certain percentage of all services received. Limited indemnity means that the insurer covers health service costs only up to a pre-specified absolute amount (or ceiling), above which the consumer is responsible for paying the remainder of costs. A deductible is a specific amount that must be paid by the consumer, above which reimbursement starts.

The administrative efficiency of direct household expenditure is low, due to the labor-intensive task of collecting fees from individuals. Household spending on health will vary according to household income, but it is likely to be fairly stable unless economic crisis causes widespread poverty. Household spending is extremely flexible and will be allocated to the most pressing health needs as they are perceived by members of the household. It is horizontally inequitable, because it varies according to factors such as distance lived from health facilities and individual preferences. Out-of-pocket payment is the most regressive modality of financing (Doorslaer et al., 1993).

User fees can be made more equitable by implementing any of several schemes. Abel-Smith (1994) provides the following examples:

- Full-cost charges can be levied on patients who bypass the referral system by going directly to hospitals without being referred or being a genuine emergency.

- Charges can be levied for private rooms at government hospitals that charge for the full costs.

- Clinics at government facilities can be opened outside normal working hours for those patients who are willing to pay and want to avoid queues.

Direct employer financing occurs when firms pay for, or directly provide, health services for their employees. Employers as agents are likely to be more efficient than households, albeit less efficient than compulsory purchasers of care (such as social insurance schemes) due to the former's fragmentation. Employer financing is likely to be reliable (in the absence of economic crisis) but relatively inflexible, because employers are biased toward specific types of health services (e.g., curative care). Direct payment by employers contributes to horizontal inequity in the health system as a whole, in that employed workers are disproportionately young and healthy. Because the benefits of employer financing are generally restricted to employees of the formal sector, this approach is likely to have little impact on the redistribution of resources among different income groups. The quantity of resources mobilized by employees is high in some countries; for example, in Zambia, financing provided by parastatal copper mines accounted for roughly 13% of all health resources (Department of Economics, University of Zambia & Swedish Institute for Health Economics, 1996). As governments implement social insurance schemes, these arrangements replace employer financing of health services.

Private health insurance premiums are regular, voluntary payments to private insurance companies in return for coverage of prespecified health service costs. Private insurance typically does not cover the costs of frequent, predictable events (such as pregnancies). Experience rating means that premiums are based on an individual's actuarially determined likelihood of illness. Community rating means that the premium is based on the pooled risk of a defined group of people (e.g., inhabitants of a geographic area or employees of a firm).

Private health insurance tends not to be an efficient method of mobilizing funds for the health sector. Its net yield is low because of the costs of assessing risk, setting premiums, designing benefit packages, distributing the insurance, marketing, processing claims, reinsuring, and detecting fraud. The administrative costs of private insurers in OECD countries vary from 5% to almost 30% of revenues collected through premiums (Thomson & Mossialos, 2004). In unregulated markets, administrative costs plus profits may account for 35% to 45% of the premiums. Private health insurance is a stable agent of financing because it is not subject to political allocation processes, and it must be flexible to respond to consumers' needs and to attract clientele.

Private health insurance premiums are a perfect example of a horizontally inequitable source. Experience rating means that premiums will vary according to factors that are considered by the insurer to be related to risk of illness, such as age, sex, and occupation. Private insurance tends to be regressive because rates are adjusted for risk, and the poor are at highest risk of falling ill. The ability to mobilize resources through private insurance is limited in poorer countries because these schemes are targeted at a very small (albeit affluent) segment of the population—less than 2% of the population in most cases.

Charitable contributions are contributions made in cash or in kind. Examples include cash contributions from wealthy families, business enterprises, or religious organizations; community labor for construction and maintenance of local health facilities, including clinics as well as environmental sanitation projects; and local help in specific disease eradication campaigns. Voluntary organizations or NGOs have high net yields, although they may be unpredictable in their ability to generate funds. The flexibility will vary from one voluntary organization to another, but generally these sources prefer to fund specific types of health services, not necessarily those most suitable for the community being served. Voluntary organization funding should be progressive in that such organizations raise revenue from the better-off, although their ability to mobilize resources is limited.

Mixes of Financing Sources

No one source of financing stands out as being superior in terms of all the outcomes considered, nor is there an optimal mix of sources that can be prescribed for all countries. Countries vary in terms of the number of financing agents and methods that are used, and the mix can change over time within a country. The mix of sources used will depend in part on the relative importance that policy makers assign to the various objectives described previously and in part on the mix of sources historically used in that country. Most low- and middle-income countries have more pluralistic health financing structures than are found in high-income countries. Low-income countries typically finance the bulk of their healthcare expenditures from (1) direct household expenditure, (2) taxation, and (3) external financing. The most important financing agents are typically the ministry of health (and other government agencies), households, and firms.

Although using a variety of sources may increase the resources available for health care and may allow better adaptation to the diverse social and economic conditions that may exist within a country, it makes the pursuit of health policy goals more complex than in a single-source system (WHO, 1993). The greatest risks in a pluralistic health financing system are those of "duplication and overlap in function and coverage" (WHO, 1993). According to Mach and Abel-Smith (1983), "In many countries the different financial sectors of the national health effort operate in water-tight compartments even when there are monetary flows between them." This adversely affects both efficiency, because of duplication, and equity, because of limited risk pooling and cross-subsidies between income groups.

Another complex but important issue relates to the displacement effect that one source of finance may have on others (termed fungibility). The introduction or expansion of one source of financing may alter the efficiency, equity, or revenue-generating ability of other sources. This consideration may be especially important when large external grants or loans are introduced into a health sector. For example, it might seem that a large external grant earmarked for the treatment of tuberculosis among the rural poor would be equitable. However, in response to such a grant, the ministry of health may shift resources that would have been spent on this activity toward high-technology, hospital-based services. Thus the positive effect that the new source of funding has on equity might be counterbalanced by the negative equity effect of displacement. Fungibility is one of the rationales for sector investment programs and general budgetary support.

Compiling Financing Data: National Health Accounts

The development of improved financing policies is affected by the limited availability of good information on financial flows. This constraint affects both national analysis and cross-country comparisons, the latter of which is often hampered by the lack of reliable data on out-of-pocket expenditures. Where they exist at all, estimates are often incomplete and prone to measurement errors. Furthermore, private health expenditures are rarely disaggregated into different forms of payments, such as direct fees for service, insurance premiums or other forms of prepayments, and cost-sharing payments (Bos, Hon, Maeda, Chellaraj, & Preker, 1998).

In recent years, emphasis has been placed on creating a national health account (NHA), which is a statement that provides information about the flow of health funds between sources (here referring to the entities that provide funds), agents, and uses in a country (Berman, 1997). The NHA is intended to give a comprehensive picture of both public and private health spending and requires calculation and presentation of national estimates through a "sources and uses" matrix, which shows the sources of health financing and what those funds are spent on.

The main objective of an NHA is to provide the key pieces of information required by decision makers. By systematically bringing together data on sources, agents, and uses of health funds, the NHA can provide answers to many different questions. Data contained in the NHA include the following:

- Total health expenditures
- Proportion of funds from different sources, including out-of-pocket payments
- Health expenditure by level of care and type of program

An NHA enables concrete answers to be given to questions such as the extent to which expenditure is biased in favor of hospitals, and the extent to which the burden of paying for care falls on out-of-pocket payment by households. In addition, the NHA provides a framework for modeling reforms and monitoring the effects of changes in financing and provision.

Resource Allocation

The significance of processes of resource allocation in a health system has been clearly acknowledged only in the past two decades or so. Financing agents, such as government bodies at various levels (ministries of health and provincial offices), social insurance agencies, and private insurers, have always been one of the components of a health system, channeling funds from sources (taxpayers, payers of insurance premiums) to providers. What is new is the emphasis on their role as active purchasers of services rather than as passive allocators of funds. For government bodies, such as ministries of health, this shift in activity has demanded the creation of a clear distinction between their role as purchasers of health services and their role as providers of health services. For other financing agents, this trend requires them to take a much more active role in decisions on which services should be paid for and how they should be paid for.

The Purchasing Role

An emphasis on the purchasing role has arisen for a number of reasons:

- Integrated systems of purchasing and provision, such as those created in 1948 in the United Kingdom's National Health Service and existing in many similar public systems across the world, are thought to operate more in the interests of providers than in the interest of the general public and to lack incentives to be technically efficient. Highlighting purchasing as a separate function helps redress the balance and strengthen the power of managers.

- Patients, who in markets for other goods and services would be the purchasers, are believed—for the reasons laid out earlier—to be in a weak position to be active purchasers.

- In health systems such as the United States, where there is third-party payment (i.e., insurance agencies pay providers), cost escalation has been a major problem because patients choose their health provider, who is then reimbursed by the insurer. Although the insurers fund a large volume of services, traditionally they did not use this power to influence either the quantity or the price of services provided. The development of managed care has led to an emphasis on the role of the purchaser as managing the provision of health services and ensuring that there are incentives for efficiency and cost containment (and for equity, where the purchaser has public responsibilities). "Strategic purchasing" has included, for example, strict control over utilization, especially of specialists and of inpatient care; controlling drug costs by creating drug formularies and using generic medications; and disease prevention and management programs.

Purchasers may be of different types and sizes. The most limited role would be that assumed by an insurance agency, whose concerns are solely the patient group it cares for and ensuring it maintains its position in the marketplace. The most extensive role occurs when a purchaser has responsibilities for the health services of the population of a defined geographic area and, therefore, can plan services on a

population basis. This position is now occupied by some public purchasers in health systems that were previously integrated but in which the roles of purchaser and provider have now been separated.

The purchasing process is essentially a planning cycle; what marks it as different from a traditional planning process is that the concern of the purchaser is not to maintain a network of services, but rather to purchase services to meet the needs of its population (Witter, 1997). The contracts that are agreed on with providers may be formal legal contracts (a necessity where providers are private bodies) or may simply be management agreements. As discussed in "Health System Reform" later in this chapter, contractual relationships have become one of the key features of health reform plans in a number of countries.

An important issue in the design of a purchasing role is whether there should be a single purchaser or a number of purchasers who compete with one another for clients. Private insurance agencies compete for clients, and it can be argued that this approach pressures them to demonstrate efficiency and develop services that meet client preferences. In contrast, for tax-funded and social insurance-funded health systems, it remains an open question whether a single purchaser or multiple purchasers is desirable. Reasons for caution about encouraging competition among purchasers include the following:

- If the system of allocating funds does not provide adequate compensation for meeting the costs of the health risks covered, the purchaser will have an incentive to avoid enrolling the more expensive risks; this problem is known as cream skimming. In reality, it is difficult to predict the health service needs of a given population and compensate purchasers appropriately.

- It can be difficult for individuals to choose between competing purchasers—the more superficial aspects of the promised package of health services may influence them, rather than technical quality, which is more difficult to judge. As a consequence, purchasers may be encouraged to compete on the superficial aspects.

- If economies of scale in purchasing are possible, they may be lost in a competitive environment.

- Transactions costs—the costs of agreeing on arrangements for purchasing services—may be higher.

Whatever the number of purchasers, information systems are crucial in enabling them to carry out their role. Government health systems traditionally have poor information on cost and quality, such that new systems have to be developed to underpin the purchasing function. Insurance agencies often have much information because they are paying for services, but commonly do not exploit these data to monitor providers. Purchasers need information to act as active purchasers, including information on provider performance (e.g., waiting times, specific health outcomes where they can clearly be related to services provided) and adherence to standard treatment protocols (e.g., with respect to use of antibiotics).

Payment Mechanisms

A key influence on the extent to which the purchasing role is carried out successfully is the method chosen to pay providers, whether these be bodies responsible for services for specific populations, individual providers, or specific facilities. Although financial remuneration is not the only influence on provider performance, it is certainly a powerful one.

Authorities responsible for the provision of services to a specific population can be provided with a global budget. A key issue is how that budget is determined. Use of a resource allocation formula to calculate the budget appropriate to the populations of different geographic areas has attracted increasing attention in recent years. The most well-known example is found in the United Kingdom, where funds have been allocated from the national level to regions using a formula that reflects the need for health services of each region, as proxied by indicators such as size of population and standardized mortality ratios (Department of Health and Social Security, 1976). Similar formulas are being used in South Africa and Zambia to allocate funds geographically. This approach is combined with various means of paying individual providers and facilities within each geographic area.

Individual providers can be paid by salary, fee-for-service, or capitation schemes. Salary represents a fixed annual payment unrelated to workload. Salary scales allow an individual's remuneration over time to be increased. Although in theory "raises" can be based on performance, in practice it is common for years of service alone to determine pay increases and promotions, thereby undermining incentives to work hard. Another problem with salary payment that is not inherent in the method is the level of the salary. In low-income countries, such remuneration is often very low, further weakening the incentive to work hard or to work the required number of hours, and encouraging staff to find additional ways of generating income, such as demanding informal payments from patients.

Additional elements can be added to salary payments to encourage good performance. These can be financial, as when an element of performance-related pay is included (e.g., a pay increase or end-of-year bonus can be based on a performance assessment), or nonfinancial (e.g., award of certificates or other ways of giving recognition to high performers).

Salary is the basis for remuneration in public systems, especially in hospitals and in privately owned facilities for nonmedical staff and even for physicians in some high-income countries. Although evidence is scanty, it is probably not uncommon in low- and middle-income countries for at least some of the physicians in private hospitals to be salaried.

Fee-for-service has traditionally been the payment method for general physicians and specialists in a number of countries in continental Europe and in North America and Japan. This mechanism has also been adopted in some new social insurance schemes in Asia and eastern Europe. Fee-for-service is usually the method of payment that physicians prefer because it does not involve an employer–employee relationship, which explains its persistence despite known problems. Where a financial agent pays the bill, there will be agreement on the fee schedule, which is usually negotiated with the medical association.

From a patient's perspective—particularly a patient covered by insurance—fee-for-service is attractive. It readily permits free choice of doctors, because payment can follow the patient. It encourages the doctor to be responsive to the patient, and there is no incentive to underprovide services. From the purchaser's perspective, however, fee-for-service payment encourages doctors to provide more consultations and more expensive procedures. Visit rates in countries using fee-for-service payment are often double those in countries that use capitation, and more tests and drugs are prescribed with the former mechanism (Ensor, Witter, & Sheiman, 1997). Surgical rates are also often higher (Abel-Smith, 1994). Administrative costs are higher with fee-for-service because of the need to monitor claims, and some degree of fraudulent claims is inevitable. When financing agents try to hold down costs by not increasing fee rates, there is good evidence that doctors respond by increasing the volume of service, as occurred in Taiwan.

Some adjustments can be made to fee-for-service methods of payment to address these problems. For example, the overall budget can be fixed, as in Germany, so that volume of services in excess of that budgeted for will cause the fee per item of service to decline. In addition, copayments can be required from patients, although there is little good evidence that these fees act as a constraint on physicians' behavior, and they may simply render care unaffordable for lower-income groups in the population.

Capitation, which is most commonly used for reimbursement of primary care services, involves a fixed payment per year per person registered with the provider. The amount provided may differ depending on the nature of the patient—for example, the elderly and children may be allocated higher payments, reflecting their greater needs for health services. Capitation payment has been the traditional form of payment for general physicians in much of Europe, sometimes supplemented by extra payments to encourage particular aspects of primary care services (such as primary care teams) or priority services (such as preventive care).

This payment system supports continuity of care and an emphasis on preventive services, not just curative care; it makes the general physician a gatekeeper for hospital care, thereby encouraging the provision of services at the lowest possible level. It leaves the doctor substantially free to practice medicine and to organize the primary care service with little interference and with minimal administrative requirements. From the patient's point of view, capitation can ensure a personal relationship with a doctor and a personal medical record, although changing doctors may be difficult. However, because payment does not depend on the number of times a patient is seen, capitation can encourage doctors to minimize the volume of services given to patients and to refer patients to the hospital unnecessarily, subject only to the need to keep patients sufficiently satisfied that they do not change doctors. Doctors may also try to avoid registering more demanding and expensive patients. The extent to which this is a problem will depend on how much of the cost of services is covered by the capitation fee (e.g., whether drugs are paid for separately) and to what degree the capitation fee is risk adjusted.

Hospitals may be paid a fixed annual budget (often called a global budget) or in a variety of ways that reflect their workload. Fixed budgets have traditionally been paid to public hospitals, but some countries have introduced them even for private hospitals that are paid by an insurance fund. Budgets are a highly effective means of cost containment and can provide a manager with great flexibility if discretion is allowed on line-item expenditures. Unfortunately, with this payment mechanism, there can be little incentive to have a high turnover of patients (which increases costs) or to provide good-quality service. These problems can be addressed by implementation of good monitoring systems.

Payments to hospitals that reflect workload can be based on itemized bills, a daily rate (including all recurrent costs), the average cost per patient, case ad-

justed for diagnosis, types of services, or block and volume contracts. The options are listed here ordered from the most detailed—and therefore the most demanding and costly to administer—to the least detailed and the simplest to administer. All have their own particular advantages and disadvantages.

Payment by itemized bill has the same inherent problems as fee-for-service for doctors—it encourages excessive procedures and hospital stays. Per diem rates discourage excessive procedures but encourage unnecessary stays. Average cost per patient discourages long length of stay but does not encourage technical efficiency. Case-based payment, particularly as developed in the United States with the diagnosis-related group (DRG) approach, reimburses hospitals for the "average" case but provides an incentive to classify patients within more expensive groups or to shift patients out of the hospital earlier. Case-based payment is also information intensive and, therefore, costly to administer.

The introduction of contracts into the United Kingdom health system was accompanied in the early years mainly by block and volume contracts. In the former approach, a provider is contracted to deliver one or more services (e.g., acute hospital services) to a given population for a fixed sum—it is, in effect, a capitation payment. Such a payment mechanism transfers financial risk to the provider, so it may encourage cream skimming and the provision of too few services. This type of payment, which is often risk adjusted to a certain extent, is increasingly being used in managed care arrangements and between social insurance agencies and providers, as in Thailand. Volume contracts, by comparison, are appropriate where the purchaser wishes to limit the number of procedures paid for (e.g., elective surgery). Purchasers can use these contracts to take advantage of economies of scale that can be achieved by larger units with high volume.

This list of payment methods provides a confusing range of options. The key issues relate to which incentives each payment method creates for providers (summarized in Table 12-4). In particular, important questions include the following:

- What are the incentives to overprovide or underprovide services to patients within the facility? A key issue is who bears the financial risk—purchaser or provider.
- What are the incentives to be technically efficient?
- What are the incentives to exclude altogether certain types of patients?

Table 12-4	Healthcare Payment Methods and Their Incentives to Providers	
Payment Method	**Unit of Services Reimbursed**	**Financial Incentives for Providers**
Salary	Usually one month's work	Restrict the number of patients and services provided
Fee-for-service	Individual acts or visits	Expand the number of cases seen and service intensity; provide more expensive services and drugs
Capitation/block contract	All relevant services (e.g., primary care, hospital care) for a patient in a given time period	Attract more registered patients (especially healthier individuals); minimize contacts per patient and service intensity
Fixed budget	All services provided by a facility in a given time period	Reduce the number of patients and services provided; keep patients in hospital longer
Daily rate	Patient day	Expand the number of bed days (through longer stays or more admissions)
Case payment	Cases of different types	Expand the number of cases seen (especially the less serious); decrease service intensity; provide less expensive services

Source: Bennett, S. (1997a). Health-care markets: Defining characteristics. In S. Bennett, B. McPake, & A. Mills (Eds.), *Private health providers in developing countries.* London: Zed Books, p. 92. Adapted with permission.

- Given these incentives, what are the administrative costs of the payment system together with the monitoring required to prevent abuse?

This provides a rather crude basis for evaluating methods, however, not least because financial remuneration—although important—is not the only factor affecting the behavior of providers. The effects of a method in practice will also depend on the system and context within which it is introduced:

- The extent to which purchasers or patients can change providers
- Whether strict ethical standards are adhered to and monitored by the medical profession (thus limiting cream skimming and both underprovision and overprovision)
- Whether the media are active in publicizing cases of medical negligence
- The extent to which consumers are well informed and able to exercise their freedom of choice effectively

Because each payment approach has both advantages and disadvantages, which depend also on the context in which it is introduced, it is difficult to be prescriptive. In practice, some of the problems with any one method are addressed by combining methods (e.g., using capitation payment but with additional fees for certain procedures). Perhaps the strongest conclusion that can be drawn is that fee-for-service payment should be avoided as the main payment approach. Studies have suggested that providing care on a fee-for-service basis costs one-third more than using capitation, without substantial differences in health outcomes, and that fee-for-service payment for outpatient care is associated with 11% higher expenditures in OECD countries (Ensor et al., 1997). A further conclusion is that no payment method will work well if providers think they are seriously underpaid.

Provision of Services

Health service providers in low- and middle-income countries can be categorized into seven main groups:

1. Government-run health services for the general public (these include the services of the ministry of health and those services coming under other government ministries, such as local government and education).

2. Services run by social insurance agencies for the insured and their dependents.

3. NGO services, including those run by church organizations and charitable groups.

4. Occupational healthcare providers (medical services provided by employers for their employees). This group includes providers of services for the armed forces and police, which come under government ministries. Universities may also run services for their own staff.

5. Private, for-profit allopathic providers, both individuals and facilities.

6. Traditional systems of medicine, such as Ayurveda, homeopathy, and Chinese medicine; and traditional healers of various types, including traditional birth attendants.

7. The informal sector of drug peddlers and unqualified practitioners.

In general, the richer a country, the more organized and structured and the less diverse the system of health service provision. For example, over time government-run services may be brought within a single structure, as they were in the United Kingdom under successive rounds of reorganization; services of the ministry of health and social insurance agency may be amalgamated, as they were in Costa Rica. As government services and services for the insured improve, there is less reason for occupational health services to provide general medical care. Moreover, as regulatory structures strengthen, the informal sector becomes much smaller.

Information on the supply of health services in low- and middle-income countries is sorely lacking, and indeed is much weaker than information on the demand side. Hence it is difficult to summarize the relative significance of these different sources of services. Most studies focus on what is called the public–private mix—that is, the relative numbers of providers in public and private sectors.

McPake (1997) suggested that there may be at least three different patterns. Among the lowest-income countries, the formal private, for-profit sector is small, but especially in Africa there is a rather larger NGO sector. The informal sector is large, consisting of unregistered allopathic providers, drug sellers, and a variety of traditional practitioners. For example, in Zambia 0.2% of beds are available in the private, for-profit sector and 25% in the NGO sector, and 73% of private expenditure is on drugs.

In other low-income countries, especially in Asia, the private, for-profit sector plays a much more important role; this constitutes the second pattern. For example, in India, 75% of total health expenditures are from private sources; of this amount, 91% comes from out-of-pocket payments (WHO, 2009). An estimated 93% of hospitals and 63% of hospital beds are privately owned, mainly by individual physicians (Peters, Yazbeck, Sharma, Ramana, Pritchett, & Wagstaff, 2002). Large and concentrated populations may be one explanation for the appearance of this pattern; another may be a longer history of Western health services and training of professionals, together with government health services that have never ex-

tended to provide coverage for the whole population. However, even in countries with this pattern of healthcare services, private provision remains concentrated at lower levels of the health system. For example, in India, until recently, there has been very little presence of the private sector at the tertiary care level, and the private sector provides 79% of outpatient care for those below the poverty line, much of it of low quality and provided by untrained providers including drug sellers.

McPake (1997) identifies a third pattern of provision, in countries with rather higher per capita GNP. This pattern usually includes a major role for social insurance (funding services either through its own facilities, as is common in Latin America, or through mixed public and private providers, as is more common in Asia) and a private sector that is playing an increasingly important role (certainly at the secondary level and sometimes also at the tertiary level).

Hanson and Berman (1998) assembled what data they could find on private physicians and hospital beds to see if any general patterns emerged. These authors found extreme variability in both absolute numbers and public/private shares. The supply of both private physicians and for-profit beds is income elastic (i.e., they increase at a rate that is higher than the growth rate of income). In contrast, the number of public beds increases much more slowly than the rate of growth of income. Thus, although it is well established that the public role in financing increases with rising income, it seems that the public share of provision (measured in this study as beds and physicians) decreases.

Because the relative roles of public and private sectors have been a key policy question, there has been much interest in whether private providers are more efficient. Those who believe in the virtues of private markets claim this to be the case, but information supporting this contention is scanty, of poor quality, and equivocal. A review by Bennett (1997b) found that private providers were more efficient, but she pointed out that all the studies referred to not-for-profit providers, suggesting that differences in efficiency are not due to the profit motive. In addition, comparisons are problematic because an increasing number of studies have noted that the patients seen by private, for-profit hospitals differ in important ways from those dealt with by public hospitals. In particular, the illness of patients in the former setting may be less severe and require only a short length of stay. Moreover, the structure of the payment method for their patients will affect whether these facilities have an incentive to be efficient. For example, in South Africa, medical benefit schemes pay private hospitals a fixed per diem for hotel-type services, which encourages hospitals to organize these services as efficiently as possible. Conversely, drugs and supplies are reimbursed with a percentage markup, encouraging use of the most expensive drugs.

Another difficulty in drawing conclusions stems from the fact that there is a tendency to make an overall judgment that is then applied to all private providers. However, ample evidence indicates that these providers are highly diverse. In India, for example, at one end of the spectrum there are private hospitals delivering services of international standard; at the other end are unlicensed and unqualified practitioners using Western prescription drugs. In between, there exist trained physicians and Western-style hospitals whose quality of care can be extremely poor (Bennett, 1997a). Private clinics, although in theory run by doctors, in practice often depend on staff with little training; this approach arises because, in many countries, doctors also have public posts where they spend at least some part of their time, as well as working in several clinics. Financial relationships between different types of facilities are also a concern in a number of countries—hospitals, laboratories, and diagnostic centers may pay general practitioners to refer patients to them or may pass them a share of their fees.

Absolute lack of resources can place a limit on the costliness of public facilities. Nevertheless, there is ample evidence of poor resource use, such as very low staff productivity and waste of drugs and supplies (Mills, 1997). This evidence is by no means conclusive—it comes from a relatively small number of country-specific studies, and the evidence of greatest inefficiency comes from the lowest-income countries in Africa, making it difficult to know to what extent the conclusions of these studies can be generalized. In addition, examples of highly efficient public health centers and hospitals can be cited (World Bank, 2003).

As in the case of private facilities, a variety of explanations have been put forth for observed public provider inefficiencies, some of which do not relate to ownership per se (Mills, 1997). In particular, decision making may be centralized and staff at the hospital level given little power to control resource use. Very low salaries also contribute to poor performance, because they reduce staff motivation, and staff may need to spend time generating income in other ways to ensure an income adequate for survival.

The clearest area where private facilities outperform public ones is in their acceptability to patients. Patients commonly complain that the staff of public services are rude and unhelpful, in contrast to private providers. The latter are also open longer hours, especially in the evening, and do not run short of complementary resources, such as drugs. However, people generally make shrewd judgments of the motivations of providers. Patients may use private providers for the convenience and the available resources, but they are aware that the profit motive may drive the private providers' behavior and influence the care given, rather than a humanitarian ethic (Mills et al., 2001).

Performance of Different Types of Systems

The previous sections have demonstrated that the design of health systems varies greatly between countries, particularly with respect to the following aspects:

- The sources of funding (e.g., balance between tax, insurance, and out-of-pocket payment)
- The degree of integration of financing agents and providers (Are there large numbers of financing agents or one major one, such as a ministry of health or single social insurance agency? Are financing agents and providers integrated or separated?)
- The ownership of providers (public; private, not-for-profit; private, for profit)
- The extent to which the whole population of a country has access to the same services, or different groups in the population have different entitlements and use different providers

Perhaps not surprisingly, these marked differences have led to intense debate over whether any one design can be shown to perform better, in terms of criteria such as efficiency and equity, than any other. Attention has particularly focused on differences between the U.S., Canadian, and U.K. systems. The United States has relied heavily on voluntary insurance organized largely through employers, plus publicly funded programs for low-income patients and older adults; Canada has a compulsory national insurance system; and the United Kingdom relies largely on general tax revenues to fund its health system. Whereas most services in the United Kingdom are publicly owned, privately owned services play an important role in Canada and especially in the United States.

Table 12-5 shows some key comparative indicators for the United States and Canada for 2006 or nearby years (Folland, Goodman, & Stano, 2010). Canada had substantially lower per capita spending

Table 12-5	Comparative Data on U.S. and Canadian Health Systems	
Indicators	**Canada**	**United States**
Population, 2007 (in millions)	33.4	301.1
GDP per capita, 2008 (in 2008 dollars)	38,200.0	46,000.0
Per capita health expenditure, 2006	3,678.0	6,714.0
Health spending, 2006 (as a percentage of GDP)	10.0	15.3
Percentage of health spending, 2006		
• Public expenditures	70.4	45.8
• Inpatient care	28.4	25.9
• Outpatient care	25.0	44.8
• Pharmaceuticals	18.2	12.8
Acute care inpatient beds per 1,000 population, 2005 (Canada) 2006 (United States)	2.8	2.7
Average length of stay in days, 2005	7.2	4.8
Percentage of population with no insurance, 2007	0.0	14.6
Out-of-pocket payments per capita, 2006	532.0	856.0
Private insurance as a percentage of expenditure on health, 2006	12.6	36.0
Life expectancy (in years) at birth: females, 2005	82.7	79.8
Life expectancy (in years) at birth: males, 2005	80.4	75.2

Note: Financial data are denoted in U.S. dollars.

Source: Folland, S., Goodman, A. C., & Stano, M. (2010). *The economics of health and health care* (6th ed.). Upper Saddle River, NJ: Prentice Hall, p. 501. Reprinted with permission.

on health and size of the GDP share devoted to health services than the United States, despite a bed per population ratio that was greater than that in the United States. The United States spent approximately 83% more per capita on health than Canada, even though 15% of its population had no health insurance. Health status indicators such as life expectancy were better in Canada. Studies of waiting times and physician practice patterns show that in some instances Canadians got less health care or had to wait longer, but these differences had few observable effects on mortality and other outcome indicators.

Analysis of explanations as to why Canada spent less highlights two key differences (Folland et al., 2010). First, physician fees and hospital costs were significantly lower in Canada, no doubt because these payments are regulated. Physician fees are negotiated between physician associations and provinces, and hospital budgets are set by the provinces. Second, the Canadian system has substantially lower administrative costs. Administration was estimated to account for approximately 31% of total healthcare spending in the United States in 1999, as compared to 16.7% in Canada. Studies comparing expenditures in a larger number of high-income countries have found that countries in which health services are financed primarily by private payments have the highest expenditures, and that there is no evidence that this greater spending level is reflected in better health status. Health systems where there is comprehensive risk

pooling based on compulsory insurance or tax finance and covering the whole population appear to be more cost-effective (WHO, 1999).

Similar, detailed comparisons have not been done for low- and middle-income countries. They can take two key lessons from richer countries:

• A significant public share in financing enables greater control over expenditures, meaning that higher population coverage can be achieved at lower cost.

• The greater the fragmentation of the health system and the greater the reliance on private insurance, the greater the proportion of total health expenditures taken up by administrative costs.

Nevertheless, high-income countries demonstrate that there are a variety of ways in which a strong public role and coordinated health system can be achieved, and that the traditional model prevalent in many low- and middle-income countries of an integrated public system financed from general taxation is only one approach to providing health services.

Health System Reform

Widespread dissatisfaction with the performance of health systems in rich and poor countries alike has encouraged what can be seen as a worldwide movement of health-sector reform (Roberts, Hsiao, Berman, & Reich, 2004). The term "reform" is used deliberately here, in the sense of "a sustained process of fundamental change in policy and institutional arrangements, guided by government, designed to improve the functioning and performance of the health sector, and ultimately the health status of the population" (Sikosana, Dlamini, & Issakov, 1997).

Most recently, vigorous policy debate on reforms has been encouraged by two key events. First, the report of the Commission on Macroeconomics and Health emphasized the contribution of health to economic growth, and argued that much greater sums of external funding should be made available to the health systems of low-income countries (WHO, 2001). Second, the Millennium Development Goals (MDGs), established at the UN Millennium Summit in 2000, are having an important influence on the focus of external assistance for health. A number of the MDGs concern health—for example, reduced child mortality—and slow progress toward some of the goals, especially in sub-Saharan Africa, is focusing attention on health system deficiencies and means to rectify them (Taskforce on Innovative International Financing for Health Systems, 2009).

The key problems that reforms are designed to address have been referenced at various points in this chapter and can be summarized as follows:

- In many low-income countries, resources and funds are grossly inadequate to provide even a basic level of care for the population, with many governments spending less than $10 per capita on health services.

- Levels of health produced by health systems are often lower than what is technically possible.

- Many activities funded by the public sector are not very cost-effective, and coverage of interventions that are highly cost-effective is inadequate (World Bank, 1993). Conversely, too high a share of the budget is spent on hospital care, especially higher levels of hospital care.

- Health systems operate with low or very variable levels of technical efficiency. Studies of facility costs invariably show great variation in costs across similar types of services, to an extent that is not easily explained by differences in quality but is more likely to be due to problems of managing resources (Mills, 1997).

- Quality of services is poor in public facilities, especially in the poorer countries where funds are very limited, health service inputs are in short supply, equipment is poorly maintained, and staff are poorly paid and hence poorly motivated; staff are often criticized for their lack of courtesy to patients and lack of responsiveness to their needs. Many private services are also often of very low quality and almost completely unregulated.

- The possibilities for health interventions created by technological developments place ever-increasing demands on limited funds, accentuating the need for governments to consider ways of setting priorities and defining limits to what can be provided.

- New problems, such as HIV/AIDS and the growing importance of chronic diseases, are putting even greater pressure on services.

- The number of healthcare workers is grossly inadequate in most countries, and their unequal distribution means that rural services are even more poorly staffed.

- Most low- and middle-income countries fare poorly in terms of both equity of access to health services and equity of payment for services, with a few notable exceptions. Poorer households commonly use health services less frequently, especially in rural areas where access is more difficult and expensive, and spend a much higher proportion of their income on health services, partly because public subsidies do not meet their needs well.

The objectives of health-sector reform follow from this list of key problems—namely, increased use of services in the poorest countries and especially improved equity of access, better efficiency, and greater consumer satisfaction. The means of reform have been significantly influenced by shifts in beliefs about the appropriate role of the state and the appropriate means for the delivery of public services. Current ideologies favor a slimmed-down state; increased efficiency in the provision of public services through mechanisms such as decentralization, contracting out, and competition; and an extension of the role of the private sector. While these ideas are being applied to the government's role in general, they are influencing reforms in the health sector to a major degree. Current thinking emphasizes the following key roles of the state:

- Setting and enforcing standards, including minimum quality standards
- Monitoring the behavior and performance of providers and insurers (where they exist), including ensuring information is available to do so
- Defining an appropriate package of services and benefits
- Regulating the health system to encourage efficient and equitable financing and delivery of services and to constrain cost inflation
- Ensuring financing of health services through taxation or compulsory insurance arrangements in better-off countries, and targeting public funding at the poorest sections of the population in poorer countries

Reforms are considered here following the same headings of the key health system functions used earlier—namely, regulation, financing, resource allocation, and provision. Table 12-6 lists the key reform areas under each heading.

Table 12-6	The Main Areas of Health-Sector Reform

Regulation

Liberalizing laws on the private health sector and introducing incentives for improved efficiency and equity
Updating regulatory structures

Financing

User fees, exemptions, and targeting
Community financing, including community-based insurance
Social health insurance

Resource Allocation

Creation of purchasing agencies
Introduction of contractual relationships and management agreements
Reforming payment systems
Specification of essential packages

Provision

Decentralization of health services and hospital management
Encouraging competition and diversity of ownership
Organization of service delivery
Strengthening primary care
Evidence-based health care
Quality improvement measures
Improved accountability to service users and population

Regulation

As part of health-sector reforms, many countries have been amending out-of-date legislation and seeking to ensure that new private activities are brought within the scope of the law. Countries that previously banned or strictly controlled the private sector, such as countries in Eastern and Central Europe, some countries in Africa, and Vietnam and China, now allow, and even in some cases, encourage its development through tax subsidies. However, much of the expansion of the private sector has taken place without deliberate planning, and often with little regulation.

These changes have increased the need to strengthen regulations, but attempts to tighten regulations are frequently opposed by powerful interest groups. Moreover, regulation of a private sector that consists of numerous small-scale providers is inherently difficult, and few countries have the administrative capacity to do so effectively. Few lessons are yet available on the success of different approaches to strengthening the regulatory role of the state.

Sources of Financing

Reform of health financing has been at the top of the policy agenda in many countries. In the 1990s, the introduction (or raising) of user fees was advocated, on the grounds that they offered a significant source of additional revenue, with their harmful effects on access countered by exemption policies. Expectations are now less sanguine and opposition to user fees are widespread for the following reasons: administrative difficulties associated with fee collection have proved formidable; ability to pay has been a significant barrier to use, and exemption schemes have not been effective in alleviating this barrier; and even if there is ability to pay, people have been unwilling to pay if service quality does not improve. As a consequence, interest has grown in other avenues to ensure that public funds are targeted to the poorest people (considered later in this section in the discussion of resource allocation).

Partly because of the increased concern over the equity effects of user fees, attention has shifted to the possibilities for expansion of locally based insurance schemes. Although a number of such schemes exist in various countries, there is as yet limited experience to suggest how they can be encouraged to grow in size and scope. Historically, local plans were an important stage in the development of universal coverage of health services in Europe and Japan, but few low- and middle-income countries have schemes that are yet sufficiently developed to offer this sort of promise in the near future. Exceptions are Rwanda, where voluntary health insurance had reached coverage of approximately 85% of the population by 2008, and Ghana, where a combination of compulsory insurance for those in the formal sector, voluntary insurance for others, and free cover for the poorest, brought coverage to 38% of the population by 2006. The limited depth of coverage in Rwanda and the very limited coverage of the poor in Ghana mean that these schemes are still very much evolving and lessons for other countries are as yet unclear (Taskforce on Innovative International Financing for Health Systems, 2009).

The introduction of compulsory insurance has been a component of reform policies in the rapidly industrializing countries of Southeast Asia and in Central and Eastern Europe. Compulsory insurance has also been of considerable interest in a number of African countries and in the Caribbean, and a number of Latin American countries have sought to reform their existing schemes. According to Mills (2000a), key issues have included the following:

- Should compulsory insurance be introduced when the proportion of the population in formal employment is still rather small?

- Should the insured have a choice of competing schemes or should there be a single fund?

- Is there any role for private insurers?

- What should be the relationship between the insurance agency and providers—which form of contract and which payment method?

- As schemes cover a higher proportion of the population, how can they be integrated with arrangements for other groups of the population so as to eliminate the two-tier arrangement in which those in the scheme have access to much better services than those outside the scheme?

These questions concern the nature of the purchaser and the provider, rather than of the funding source itself. They are discussed further in subsequent sections of this chapter.

Resource Allocation

One of the most common features of sector-wide reforms has been the introduction of a purchaser–provider split in public systems that were previously integrated. Planned management reforms in South Africa, Zimbabwe, and Zambia all envisaged a purchasing role for local health authorities. In Thailand, the social security office acts as a purchaser on behalf of the

insured and accredits and monitors the hospitals that they use.

Along with the specification of the purchaser's role has come an emphasis on contractual arrangements between purchasers and providers. At one extreme, these arrangements may be seen as no more than the formalization of a management relationship, as where annual contracts are agreed upon between the ministry of health and a regional health authority (Trinidad), or between a province and a district (South Africa, Zambia, Zimbabwe). At the other extreme, the contracts may be awarded on a competitive basis and may be legally binding (as was the case in New Zealand).

Despite the popularity of this reform, its value has not been well established. Such reforms have experienced considerable implementation difficulties, especially where they were accompanied by a policy to decentralize employment contracts of health workers.

A more recent development has been the use of contracts with NGOs to reform or expand service provision in contexts where governments function poorly or have very limited capacity. The experiments with contracting district health services in Cambodia are widely cited in this regard (World Bank, 2003), and similar arrangements are being tried in Afghanistan and Rwanda, for example. Contracting with NGOs is also being increasingly used to expand availability of HIV/AIDS prevention.

A vital element of the relationship between purchaser and provider is the payment mechanism—that is, the basis on which funds are allocated from purchasers to providers. Health-sector reforms commonly involve changes to traditional modes of payment, although the nature of the reforms depends on the starting point and is severely constrained by powerful interest groups; hence, a great variety of reforms are apparent in practice. Although, in general, fee-for-service methods of payment are seen to be undesirable, countries such as those in Eastern and Central Europe that previously provided salaries to primary care providers have sought to raise remuneration levels and encourage greater productivity by using a mix of salary, fee-for-service, and capitation. Indeed, capitation appears to be one of the areas where there is the most experimentation worldwide. Traditionally an approach for paying primary care providers, capitation has been extended to pay for hospital services as well (e.g., in Thailand) and is the basis for payment in many managed care arrangements.

Global budgets for hospitals have been a feature in Europe under different funding regimes. Concern that they do not provide incentives to efficiency has led to the introduction of mechanisms that relate payment to measures of hospital activity, such as bed days or cases, or even specific services. Some similar reform trends can be seen elsewhere; Thailand, Taiwan, and Korea have all tried case-based payments, with Thailand adopting the approach nationwide.

"Pay for performance" (P4P), to both individual workers and facilities, has also attracted considerable interest and has the potential to improve public-sector performance. It can be distinguished from fee-for-service or case-based payment by its aim to use measures of performance rather than merely activity as the basis for remuneration, though in practice this distinction may not be very clear. In Rwanda, for example, performance incentives to facilities (used mainly to increase staff salaries) were based on their overall quality, as reflected in an index of both structural and process measures of quality of care for various types of services. A prospective quasi-experimental evaluation found that the P4P scheme had a large and significant positive impact on institutional deliveries and preventive care visits by young children, and improved quality of prenatal care (Basinga, Gertler, Binagwaho, Soucat, Sturdy, & Vermeersch, 2010). At the same time, P4P raises many concerns, including those of effective monitoring of performance, management capacity to channel funding in relation to performance, effects on nontargeted services, and cost-effectiveness relative to other ways of improving performance (Taskforce on Innovative International Financing for Health Systems, 2009).

Concern that the poorest often do not benefit from public funding has led to the use of various approaches to improve targeting, including geographic targeting through resource allocation formulae, additional funding for specific programs targeted at populations with the least access, equity funds that reimburse health facilities for exemptions, social funds that often involve local communities in decisions on spending (World Bank, 2003, 2004), and vouchers or cash payments that channel purchasing power directly to those in need, such as vouchers for pregnant women that reduce the price of an insecticide-treated mosquito net, or cash to pregnant women to help cover the costs of accessing safe delivery services. Conditional cash transfer schemes, such as the Opportunidades program in Mexico, involve making a welfare payment to poor households dependent on regular use of services such as preventive care.

In those countries introducing compulsory insurance and those engaged in reforming existing systems, a key and controversial issue has been whether to encourage competition between insurance funds and to encourage choice of insurer. In Western Europe, countries have proceeded very cautiously in this area. In contrast, active exploration of arrangements that would permit competitive pressures to be felt by financing agents is under way in some countries in Latin America and in Central and Eastern Europe. A model of reform has been proposed for Latin America that involves the social insurance agencies competing with private insurers to enroll individuals and being compensated by a risk-adjusted capitation payment (Londono & Frenk, 1997). This approach has, for example, been implemented in Colombia and Argentina. A study in Colombia found some evidence of sickness fund selection based on health status, confirming fears that cream-skimming can be a problem in the presence of competitive pressures on insurers (Trujillo & McCalla, 2004).

A trend for the future is the increasing prominence of healthcare companies anxious to break into low- and middle-income markets. Latin America already has a large number of people enrolled in managed care arrangements, and U.S. companies, keen to expand, have been actively exploring markets in Latin America, South Africa, and Asia. Options for involvement include contracting with governments or social insurance agencies to manage health programs for particular population groups, or covering groups allowed to opt out of social insurance arrangements. These possibilities require a strong regulatory framework to be put in place.

The specification of essential packages of health services, which purchasers require providers to make available, has been a key feature of many reform programs. The *World Development Report 1993*, on the basis of analyzing the burden of disease and the cost-effectiveness of interventions, proposed a package of essential health services that governments should ensure are universally available (World Bank, 1993). In low-income countries, this package would comprise the following:

- Public health services for children, such as immunization and school health services; tobacco and alcohol control; health, nutrition, and family planning information; vector control; sexually transmitted infection (STI) prevention; and monitoring and surveillance
- Clinical services, such as tuberculosis treatment, treatment for sick children, prenatal and delivery care, family planning, STI treatment, treatment of infection and minor trauma, and pain relief

The initial global analysis has been followed by many country studies, to identify country-specific packages. However, ensuring reallocation of public subsidies away from lower-priority services such as tertiary hospital care has proved politically difficult, and there is as yet inadequate evidence of the successful implementation of this approach to priority setting. There is, however, increasing recognition of the need to involve the general public in priority-setting processes to ensure acceptability and use of the package.

Provision of Services

Key reform themes affecting providers have been decentralization, competition and diversity of ownership, strengthening primary care services, evidence-based medicine, and quality improvement.

Even in health systems that maintain a strong public role in provision, decentralization has been an almost universal theme. At the national level, decentralization has taken the form of restructuring the role and functions of the ministry of health, with some countries creating executive agencies to take over management responsibility at the national level (e.g., Ghana), leaving the ministry to concentrate on regulation, policy, and monitoring. Some form of decentralization to intermediate and local levels is also a common theme, with most countries choosing to decentralize services within a hierarchical structure with the ministry of health at the top, although there are a few notable examples of devolution of health to local government (e.g., the Philippines). Finally, decentralization even further, to the hospital level, is a common trend in countries with centrally funded, public systems of health provision (Mills et al., 2001). In the lowest-income countries, because of limits on management capacity, this reform may be confined to teaching hospitals. In other countries, such as Indonesia, a wider range of hospitals have been made "autonomous" or "corporatized."

Competition between providers is similarly being widely promoted as a means to encourage efficiency, although with more caution and stronger doubts about its effects than in the case of decentralization. Diversity of ownership is also promoted as a means to increase competitive pressures, especially on poorly performing public systems of provision. African governments, for example, have been urged to give greater emphasis to NGOs. In a number of Southeast Asian countries, tax incentives have been provided for the construction of private hospitals (e.g., India, Philippines, Thailand), although from the perspective of the health sector as a whole there are considerable doubts about the desirability of this policy (Mills et al., 2001).

Strengthening the role of primary care has long been a theme in reforms in many countries, albeit often without substantial changes in resource allocation patterns. Reforms in the United Kingdom, which gave funds to primary care doctors to purchase other services, have aroused much interest. Nevertheless, efforts to create high-quality primary care services, with a gatekeeper role for the primary care provider, do not as yet appear to feature strongly in reforms in most low- and middle-income countries, with the exception of Thailand.

Included in many reform packages have been measures to improve the quality of the services provided. In high-income countries, a range of approaches is being used, including evidence-based medicine, technology assessment, clinical guidelines, medical audits, quality assurance methods, and payment incentives. These strategies are beginning to be featured in less wealthy countries. In the lowest-income countries, more basic problems have been addressed, such as availability of drugs and supplies, improvement of staff skills, and maintenance of equipment.

Increasingly, human resources is being highlighted as the key area where reforms are needed. In many of the poorest countries, the number of trained health providers is grossly inadequate to provide even a basic package of services to the whole population. HIV/AIDS has made this imbalance far worse in heavily affected countries—for example, in Mozambique, 20% of student nurses died from HIV/AIDS in 2000 (World Bank, 2004). The international "brain drain" is also having a devastating effect on some countries. In Ghana, an estimated 31% of trained health personnel left the country between 1993 and 2002. Brain drain is one symptom of a widespread problem in many countries of low financial remuneration of health workers, low motivation, and poor performance, which has to be tackled by action on a number of fronts. Although only limited experience with reforms has accrued as yet (see the Taskforce on Innovative International Finance Working Group 1 report [2009] for a recent summary), policy options include greater use of community-based workers, improved remuneration and conditions of service, performance-related pay, and reform of management cultures and systems to put greater emphasis on results and ensure merit-based promotion.

Reforms may also seek to increase the influence of users and communities over health providers—to hold them accountable for good performance—but there are few well-evaluated examples to prove the value of this approach. In many of the poorest countries, local government structures are weak, ruling them out as an immediate means for ensuring local representation. Some reforms include the introduction of health or hospital boards with citizen representation. Often community involvement is seen to occur via NGOs rather than government health services. Little attention has been paid to patient rights, and patients tend to appear as the object of reforms, rather than as the subject.

Conclusion

This chapter has outlined the main components of health systems in low- and middle-income countries. It has focused mainly on the healthcare system, with little attention (due to lack of space) being given to the sectors that supply resources to the health system (such as education and training institutions, and the pharmaceutical, medical supplies, and medical equipment industries) or to broader influences on health, such as government policies on smoking, alcohol consumption, and transport—all of which have major effects on health.

For the health system, its key functions include regulation, financing, resource allocation, and provision, and the key actors are the government, populations, financing agents, and providers. Although these core elements can be identified in all systems, the number of bodies involved in each one, and the way they relate to one another, differ enormously in practice, making it difficult to draw clear conclusions on whether any one arrangement of functions and actors is better than any other.

This chapter has also reviewed the most common reforms being proposed and implemented to deal with weaknesses of current health systems. A number of agencies are suggesting that reform policies are converging to include the following features (Mills, 2000b):

- An emphasis on the regulatory and enabling role of the state
- An emphasis on increasing public control over sources of funding and increasing risk pooling (although not necessarily increasing funding from general taxation, except in countries that devote very little public money to health)
- More explicit prioritization of which services can be financed and provided, especially by the public sector (it is often argued that this process should be driven by considerations of cost-effectiveness)
- Greater targeting of public subsidies to those most in need

- Greater involvement of the private sector, especially in the provision of health services
- Greater decentralization of the management of provision within the public sector
- Creation of arrangements that encourage competition between providers, so as to improve efficiency and quality
- Greater emphasis on the role of consumers, both as informed purchasers and as citizens to whom providers should be accountable

Currently, there is a tendency for ideology—rather than good empirical evidence—to serve as the driving force for these reform policies. Such types of reforms are much reviewed and discussed, but little strong empirical evidence exists to indicate how well they work and whether systems reformed along these lines will perform better than unreformed ones. Because country health systems differ greatly, so should reform policies, and there is no ideal blueprint for reform (Roberts et al., 2004). Evidence from countries suggests that reform is often more rhetorical than real, not least because it uses the fashionable language of current reform ideology. Reforms affect the position of powerful interest groups, which mobilize to block change. Far greater understanding is needed of the best ways to introduce reforms and manage these various interests.

• • • Discussion Questions

1. How can the concepts of efficiency and equity be used to assess the performance of a health system?

2. Access to health care can be viewed as similar to access to other goods and services—that is, as dependent on an individual's success in gaining or inheriting income, or as a right of citizenship that should not depend on individual income or wealth. Debate the relative merits of these two positions.

3. What should be the respective roles of the government and the private sector in the health systems of low- and middle-income countries?

4. Imagine that you live in a formerly socialist country and that the health system is soon to be opened to private investment. Which kinds of regulatory mechanisms might be put in place to optimize efficiency and equity?

5. What are the relative strengths and weaknesses of the main financing sources in a low- and middle-income country context?

• • • References

Abel-Smith, B. (1994). *An introduction to health: Policy, planning and financing*. London: Addison Wesley Longman.

Almeida, C., Braveman, P., Gold, M. R., Szwarcwald, C. L., Mendes Ribeiro, J., Miglionico, A., et al. (2001). Methodological concerns and recommendations on policy consequences of the World Health Report 2000. *Lancet, 357*, 1692–1697.

Baldwin, R., & Cave, M. (1999). *Understanding regulation: Theory, strategy, and practice*. Oxford, UK: Oxford University Press.

Basinga, P., Gertler, P. J., Binagwaho, A., Soucat A. L. B., Sturdy J. R., & Vermeersch, C. M. J., (2010, January). *Paying primary health care centers for performance in Rwanda*. Policy Research Working Paper 5190. World Bank Human Development Network Chief Economist's Office & Africa Region Health, Nutrition & Population Unit. Washington DC: The World Bank.

Bennett, S. (1997a). Health-care markets: Defining characteristics. In S. Bennett, B. McPake, & A. Mills (Eds.), *Private health providers in developing countries* (pp. 85–101). London: Zed Books.

Bennett, S. (1997b). Private health care and public policy objectives. In C. Colclough (Ed.), *Marketizing health and education in developing countries: Miracle or mirage?* (pp. 93–123). Oxford, UK: Clarendon Press.

Bennett, S., & Ngalande-Banda, E. (1994). *Public and private roles in health: A review and analysis of experience in sub-Saharan Africa*. Geneva, Switzerland: World Health Organization.

Berman, P. A. (1997). National health accounts in developing countries: Appropriate methods and recent applications. *Health Economics, 6*, 11–30.

Bos, E., Hon, V., Maeda, A., Chellaraj, G., & Preker, A. (1998). *Health, nutrition, and population indicators: A statistical handbook*. Washington, DC: World Bank.

Coyne, S. C., & Hilsenrath, P. (2002). The World Health Report 2000: Can health care systems be compared using a single measure of performance? *American Journal of Public Health, 92*, 30–33.

Department of Economics, University of Zambia, & Swedish Institute for Health Economics. (1996). *Zambia health sector expenditure review, 1995*. Lusaka: University of Zambia.

Department of Health and Social Security. (1976). *Sharing resources for health in England*. Report of the Resource Allocation Working Party. London: Her Majesty's Stationery Office.

Donaldson, C., & Gerard, K. (1993). *Economics of health care financing: The visible hand*. London: Macmillan Press.

Doorslaer, E., Wagstaff, A., & Rutten, F. (Eds.). (1993). *Equity in the finance and delivery of health care: An international perspective*. CEC Health Services Research Series. Oxford, UK: Oxford University Press.

Ensor, T., & Weinzierl, S. (2007). Regulating health care in low- and middle-income countries: Broadening the policy response in resource constrained environments. *Social Science & Medicine, 65*(2), 355–366.

Ensor, T., Witter, S., & Sheiman, I. (1997). Methods of payment to medical care providers. In S. Witter & T. Ensor (Eds.), *An introduction to health economics for Eastern Europe and the former Soviet Union* (pp. 97–114). Chichester, UK: John Wiley & Sons.

Folland, S., Goodman, A. C., & Stano, M. (2010). *The economics of health and health care* (6th ed.). Upper Saddle River, NJ: Prentice Hall.

Frenk, J., Sepúlveda, J., Gómez-Dantés, O., & Knaul, F. (2003). Evidence-based health policy: Three generations of reform in Mexico. *Lancet, 362*(9396), 1667–1671.

Gilson, L., Doherty, J., Loewenson, R., & Francis, V. (2007). *Challenging inequity through health systems: Final report*. Knowledge Network on Health Systems. WHO Commission on Social Determinants of Health. Geneva, Switzerland: World Health Organization.

Hanson, K., & Berman, P. (1998). Private health care provision in developing countries: A preliminary analysis of levels and composition. *Health Policy and Planning, 13*(3), 195–211.

Hsiao, W. C. (1995). A framework for assessing health financing strategies and the role of health insurance. In D. W. Dunlop & J. M. Martins (Eds.), *An international assessment of health care financing*. Washington, DC: World Bank.

International Health Partnership. (2010). Retrieved March 1, 2010, from http://www.international healthpartnership.net/en/home

Kohn, R., & White, K. L. (1976). *Health care: An international study*. London: Oxford University Press.

Kumaranayake, L. (1998). *Economic aspects of health sector regulation: Strategic choices for low and middle income countries*. London: London School of Hygiene and Tropical Medicine, Health Policy Unit, Department of Public Health and Policy.

Liu, X., & Mills, A. (2002). Financing reforms of public health services in China: Lessons for other nations. *Social Science and Medicine, 54*, 1691–1698.

Londono, J. L., & Frenk, J. (1997). Structured pluralism: Towards an innovative model for health system reform in Latin America. *Health Policy, 41*, 1–36.

Mach, E. P., & Abel-Smith, B. (1983). *Planning the finances of the health sector*. Geneva, Switzerland: World Health Organization.

McPake, B. (1997). The role of the private sector in health service provision. In S. Bennett, B. McPake, & A. Mills (Eds.), *Private health providers in developing countries* (pp. 21–39). London: Zed Books.

McPake, B., & Machray, C. (1997). International comparisons of health sector reform: Towards a comparative framework for developing countries. *Journal of International Development, 9*(4), 621–629.

Mills, A. (1997). Improving the efficiency of public sector health services in developing countries: Bureaucratic versus market approaches. In C. Colclough (Ed.), *Marketizing education and health in developing countries: Miracle or mirage?* (pp. 245–274). Oxford, UK: Clarendon Press.

Mills, A. (2000a). The route to universal coverage. In S. Nitayarumphong & A. Mills (Eds.), *Achieving universal coverage of health care: Experiences from middle and upper income countries* (pp. 283–299). Thailand: Ministry of Public Health, Office of Health Care Reform.

Mills, A. (2000b). Reforming health sectors: Fashions, passions and common sense. In A. Mills (Ed.), *Reforming health sectors* (pp. 1–24). London: Kegan Paul International.

Mills, A., Bennett, S., Russell, S., Attanayake, N., Hongoro, C., Muraleedharan, V. R., & Smithson, P. (2001). *The challenge of health sector reform: What must governments do?* Basingstoke, UK: Macmillan.

Mills, A., & Hanson, K. (Eds.). (2003). Expanding access to health interventions in low and middle-income countries: Constraints and opportunities for scaling-up. *Journal of International Development, 15*(1), 1–131.

Ministry of Labour & Employment, Government of India. (n.d.). Rashtriya Swasthya Bima Yojna. Retrieved January 4, 2010, from http://www.rsby.in/

Ministry of Public Health. (n.d.). *Thailand health profile report 2005–7*. Bangkok: Ministry of Public Health.

Mtei G, Mulligan J, Ally M, Palmer N, Mills A. (2007). *An Assessment of the Health Financing System in Tanzania*. Report on SHIELD Work Package 1, SHIELD. Cape Town: Heath Economics Unit, University of Cape Town.

O'Donnell, O., van Doorslaer, E., Rannan-Eliya, R. P., Somanathan, A., Adhikari, S. R., Akkazieva, B., et al. (2008). Who pays for health care in Asia? *Journal of Health Economics, 27*, 460–475.

Organization for Economic Cooperation and Development (OECD). (1992). Sub-systems of financing and delivery of health care. In *The reform of health care* (pp. 19–29). Paris: Author.

Peters, D. H., Yazbeck, A. S., Sharma, R., Ramana, G. N. V., Pritchett, L., & Wagstaff, A. (2002). *Better health systems for India's poor: Findings, analysis, and options*. Washington, DC: World Bank.

Porter, R. (1996a). Hospitals and surgery. In *The Cambridge illustrated history of medicine* (pp. 202–205). Cambridge, UK: Cambridge University Press.

Porter, R. (1996b). Medical science. In *The Cambridge illustrated history of medicine* (pp. 154–201). Cambridge, UK: Cambridge University Press.

Roberts, M. J., Hsiao, W., Berman, P., & Reich, M. (2004). *Getting health reform right*. Oxford, UK: Oxford University Press.

Roemer, M. I. (1991). *National health systems of the world: Vol. 1. The countries*. Oxford, UK: Oxford University Press.

Roemer, M. I. (1993). *National health systems of the world: Vol. 2. The issues*. Oxford, UK: Oxford University Press.

Saltman, R. B., & Figueras, J. (1997). *European health care reform: Analysis of current strategies*. Copenhagen: WHO Regional Office for Europe.

Sikosana, P. L. N., Dlamini, Q. Q. D., & Issakov, A. (1997). *Health sector reform in sub-Saharan Africa. A review of experiences, information gaps and research needs*. Geneva, Switzerland: World Health Organization.

Taskforce on Innovative International Financing for Health Systems. (2009) *Constraints to scaling up and costs*. Working Group 1 Report. Geneva, Switzerland: World Health Organization.

Teerawattananon, Y., Tangcharoensathien, V., Tantivess, S., & Mills, A. (2003). Health sector regulation in Thailand: Recent progress and the future agenda. *Health Policy, 63*, 323–338.

Thomson, S., & Mossialos, E. (2004). Private health insurance and access to health care in the European Union. *Euro Observer, 6*(1), 1–4.

Towse, A., Mills, A., & Tangcharoensathien, V. (2004). Lessons from the introduction of universal access to subsidised health care in Thailand. *British Medical Journal, 328*, 103–105.

Travis, P., Bennett, S., Haines, A., Pang, T., Bhutta, Z., Hyder, A., et al. (2004). Overcoming health-systems constraints to achieve the Millennium Development Goals. *Lancet, 364*(9437), 900–906.

Trujillo, A. J., & McCalla, D. C. (2004). Are Colombian sickness funds cream skimming enrollees? An analysis with suggestions for policy improvement. *Journal of Policy Analysis and Management, 23*(4), 873–888.

Wagstaff, A., van Doorslaer, E., van der Burg, H., Calonge, S., Christiansen, T., Citoni, G., et al. (1999). Equity in the finance of health care: Some further international comparisons. *Journal of Health Economics, 18*, 263–290.

Walsh, J. A., & Warren, K. S. (1979). Selective public health care: An interim disease control strategy in developing countries. *New England Journal of Medicine, 301*, 967–974.

Walsh, K. (1995). *Public services and market mechanisms: Competition, contracting and the new public management*. London: Macmillan Press.

Witter, S. (1997). Purchasing health care. In S. Witter & T. Ensor (Eds.), *An introduction to health economics for eastern Europe and the former Soviet Union* (pp. 81–94). Chichester, UK: John Wiley & Sons.

World Bank. (1993). *World development report 1993: Investing in health*. Oxford, UK: Oxford University Press.

World Bank. (1997). *Sector strategy: Health, nutrition and population*. Washington, DC: World Bank Group.

World Bank. (2003). *World development report 2004: Making services work for poor people*. Oxford, UK: Oxford University Press.

World Bank. (2004). *The Millennium Development Goals for health: Rising to the challenges*. Washington, DC: Author.

World Bank. (2008). *Global monitoring report*. Washington, DC: Author.

World Bank. (2009). *2009 world development indicators*. Washington, DC: Author.

World Bank. (2010a). *World Development report 2010: Development and climate change*. Washington, DC: Author.

World Bank. (2010b). Retrieved February 28, 2010, from International Development Association website: http://web.worldbank.org/WBSITE/

EXTERNAL/NEWS/0,,contentMDK:20040630~
menuPK:34480~pagePK:34370~theSitePK:4607,0
0.html

World Health Organization (WHO). (1993).
*Evaluation of recent changes in the financing of
health services*. Geneva, Switzerland: Author.

World Health Organization (WHO). (1999). *The
world health report 1999: Making a difference.*
Geneva, Switzerland: Author.

World Health Organization (WHO). (2000). *The
world health report 2000: Health systems—
improving performance.* Geneva, Switzerland:
Author.

World Health Organization (WHO). (2001).
Macroeconomics and health: Investing in health for
economic development. Report of the Commission
on Macroeconomics and Health. Geneva,
Switzerland: Author.

World Health Organization (WHO). (2007).
*Everybody's business: Strengthening health systems
to improve health outcomes. WHO's framework
for action.* Geneva, Switzerland: Author.

World Health Organization (WHO). (2009). WHO
statistics 2009: Health expenditure. Retrieved April
18, 2010, from http://www.who.int/whosis/whostat/
EN_WHS09_Table7.pdf

Zwi, A., & Mills, A. (1995). Health policy in less
developed countries: Past trends and future directions. *Journal of International Development, 7*(3),
299–328.

13

Management and Planning for Global Health

ANDREW GREEN, CHARLES COLLINS, AND TOLIB MIRZOEV

What Is Management?

This chapter focuses on an area essential within global health for all parts of public health—management. We focus particularly on management at the national level and below. Management in the health field has an unfortunate reputation. It is often regarded as an unnecessary activity that at best diverts resources from the real front-line activities of providing health care or preventing ill health. At worst, it is seen as interfering in these activities in an unhelpful and bureaucratic manner. When working well, its presence is not noticed; when malfunctioning, it is a likely scapegoat. In this chapter, a more balanced perspective on management is sought, beginning by asking what management really is.

The key to understanding management is the relationship between resources and objectives. Management is a process of making decisions about how resources will be generated, developed, allocated, combined, and used in pursuit of particular organizational objectives.[1] It is difficult to deny the need for such decisions, given the fact that resources (financial, staff, medical supplies, and transport) are limited.

How these limited resources are deployed is critical. Decisions are needed at a macro level within a health service regarding how resources are to be allocated among different areas of activity, and at a more operational level among different approaches to the delivery of the service. Management is concerned with improving the allocation of such resources. For example, there may be an imbalance between the resources targeted at curative activities versus public health, between levels of care (primary versus secondary versus tertiary), between disease control programs, between geographic areas, between social or ethnic groups, between spending on different items such as personnel versus medicines, and between allocations of different personnel such as physicians versus nurses.

How such decisions are made is critical, and this process in part relates to the question of who manages. Management functions are best carried out as a shared responsibility between staff whose only activity is management and those whose prime function is working as health workers. One important role of specialist managers is to provide health professionals with the space and resources they require to carry out their roles.

Although the discussion presented here so far has focused on limited resources and managers' key role in responding to this major constraint, it is important to recognize other constraints that managers have to work with, including political ones (in the widest sense). Managers may respond in different ways to such constraints—accepting, challenging, or looking for ways of maneuvering around them. Indeed, the success of management is often a function of the ability of a manager to work creatively with, rather than passively accept, constraints. This key attribute of management is one way in which it is different to administration, which is more related to routine implementation of existing rules and procedures.

The earlier definition of management may suggest it comprises a technocratic mechanical process. In reality, effective management is as much an art as a

---

[1] This definition builds on the work of Keeling (1972), as do the differences between management and administration discussed in this chapter.

science. One particular aspect of management often forgotten is its role in dealing with contradictions (discussed later in this chapter). To be effective, managers have to recognize the context within which they operate and adapt their approach accordingly. Such contextual factors could include the health situation, the degree of political stability, the general attitude toward public-sector reforms, the level of the country's economic growth, and international influences. Solutions that are appropriate in one situation may not work in another. One key message of this chapter, therefore, is to exercise caution against adopting blueprint approaches to management.

Management occurs at different levels of a country's health system, including at organizational (for example, within a ministry of health), sectoral (health sector), and health system (across the social sectors) levels. Management at sectoral and system levels can also be interpreted as a reflection of approaches to, and principles of, governance within the health system.

The political character of management also needs to be emphasized. It is expressed in two ways. First, although management requires certain technical skills, it inevitably deals with change, which can be threatening to affected groups and, therefore, stimulates opposition. For management to succeed requires political analysis as well as technical skills. Various techniques have been developed to map attitudes to particular interventions, of which the best known is stakeholder analysis (Brugha & Varvasovszky, 2000). How different groups are involved in management is likely to affect the quality of the management process, the speed of decision making, and the ownership of the resultant decisions and action. For example, consultation may occur at different points in the management process—with different implications. It can be seen as the following types of engagement:

- Seeking views as to priorities and strategies at the beginning of decision making

- Seeking views on alternative options once these choices have been formulated

- Seeking views on a formulated plan of action

The later in the process that consultation takes place, the more it may be viewed as a formal and even tokenistic process. The earlier it takes place, the more likely it is to influence the thinking behind the development of management. Consultation can take place in a variety of ways, including directly with the stakeholders (e.g., through surveys or focus groups) or indirectly through representative organizations. It can take place through special one-off mechanisms or

through ongoing management processes. Each approach has both advantages and disadvantages in terms of the resources and time required and the robustness of the information gathered.

Another key point regarding management is this: Management is not value free. One determinant affecting the particular choice of management approach is the values underpinning the health sector, which could include the following:

- Equity, including its different interpretations
- Efficiency
- Choice
- Gender sensitivity
- Transparency and accountability of decision processes
- Market values, including the pursuit of profits
- Broad participation in decision making
- Solidarity

The pursuit and realization of these values through management is political in that it affects the interests and views of different groups in society. Furthermore, managers themselves are not value neutral, but rather bring to the job their own political perspectives and positions.

A health sector committed to the pursuit of accountability and transparency is bound to approach its decision-making processes and consultation differently from one that assigns less importance to this value. Closely related to this are differences between approaches to management and planning within the public and private sectors.[2] Although the main difference between these two sectors is often suggested to be the freedom of maneuvering enjoyed by a manager, a more salient difference stems from the values and principles that underpin the public and private sectors, and in particular their organizational motives. The private (for-profit) sector is aimed at profit generation for its owners. This stance contrasts with the social goals of the public sector, whose formal objectives are health promotion and protection, equity and accountability, and, increasingly, efficiency and cost containment. This difference in motivation should suggest different styles of management in the public and private sectors, with the former emphasizing longer-term sustainability, collaborative as opposed to competitive strategies, and political debate

---

[2] Particular aspects of the analysis in this chapter referring to the public sector and its characteristics and contradictions draw on and develop points raised by Stewart and Ranson (1994).

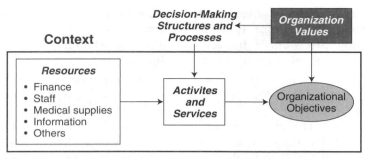

Figure 13-1 Key Elements in Management and Planning.

and negotiation regarding social values. This chapter focuses primarily on public-sector management.

Figure 13-1 depicts a framework for management and the approach taken in this chapter. The chapter follows this schema. It first draws out the important aspects of context, making particular reference to low- and middle-income countries. This consideration is followed by a discussion of the structures within which health care may be organized. We then look at planning as a key activity in management that determines the pattern of activities and services to be developed to meet an organization's objectives. Next, the chapter examines issues in the management of resources, focusing on finance, staff, transport, and information. It concludes by discussing some cross-cutting themes in management. Because the area of management is very wide, the analysis in this chapter cannot be exhaustive and is, in parts, necessarily selective.

Health Management and Context

Management is a social process of relations that differs according to the social situation in which it is found. One would not expect the process of management of a public health service in Mali to be the same as the process of management of a multinational corporation based in the United States, for example.

This potential for variation poses dilemmas for a manager, who needs to recognize that the management process does not occur in a vacuum. The way in which managers relate resources to objectives needs to adapt to the environment in which that management takes place. However, the manager faces two difficult issues in ensuring this flexibility. First, he or she must confront what is called universalism—the idea that there is one best way for management to work, irrespective of time, place, or condition (the content of this "one best way" is often similar to an idealized

version of how private enterprise is supposed to operate). Second, the relationship between the management process and the context is not easy to understand and respond to. On the one hand, the context strongly influences the management process. Management cannot be simply transplanted from one situation to another; rather, the manager must read the changing context and assess the most appropriate response. The economic, social, and political context determines the social well-being of communities and the health needs they express, together with the pressures on healthcare organizations. The context affects the feasibility and effectiveness of the options available to managers. On the other hand, the influences do not just flow in a single direction: Managers can (and indeed are expected to) have an impact on the environment.

This section analyzes the complex relationship between the management process and the context in which it operates. For organizational purposes, the context is broken down into different areas, such as political, social, and economic. However, these are analytical constructs and do not represent real-life boundaries. In reality, such boundaries are overlapping, permeable, and flexible. As Tesch (1990, p. 136) points out, "the entire idea of categorisation as a mental overlay on our world becomes more comfortable when we can think of it as stretchable and soft."

Economic Context

The economic circumstances of a society will condition employment and income and the extent to which individuals and groups can meet their basic needs. These macroeconomic circumstances provide the fundamental backdrop to social well-being—or the lack of it—to which management needs to respond.

The management process is also conditioned by the amount and type of resources available to managers. The flow of resources to, and within, the health sector reflects the country's economic circumstances (e.g., economic growth and amount of government taxation) and resource allocation decisions. The flow of resources has important effects on the freedom with which managers are able to work through various options.

Social Context

The broader processes of social change set the scene for the health context in which managers work. For example, unemployment, aging of the population, and migration all raise social and health issues, placing new demands on the health sector. At the same time, social factors condition the feasibility and effectiveness of options. For example, although managers may seek to develop community participation, the feasibility of this endeavor will depend on factors such as past experiences with community participation, geographic settlement patterns, and the degree of social homogeneity. Exhibit 13-1 provides two examples from Nepal and Brazil that illustrate the contextual impact on health management.

Political Context and Public Sector

The political framework in which the public sector operates is also important. Four key issues are explored in the following subsections.

Public Service Orientation, Corruption, and Patronage

The management process should be concerned with health and healthcare objectives for the public. Defining these objectives is difficult enough given the contradictory interests of social and political groups in society—yet public-sector managers constantly face an even further challenge, related to the contra-diction between this public service role and the opportunities for private gain through the public sector that arise in four interrelated ways (Green & Collins, 2003):

- *Corporate gain*: Private companies often profit from the public sector. Obvious examples include pharmaceutical, construction, and information technology companies. Tax concessions or public-sector training for the private sector may subsidize the private medical industry. The private sector may also be able to capture those public agencies designed to regulate it.

- *Corruption*: Illegal and unethical use of public resources for private gain can take many forms, ranging from bribes to theft, and can have an adverse effect on government activities. It is important to note that corruption is not solely the preserve of low- and middle-income countries. As Szeftel (1998) points out, "those looting the African State can only envy the size of the 'pot' available to those in other countries."

- *Patronage*: Public resources may be used to strengthen the political position of a patron or political leader. Complex networks of patronage can emerge and sustain themselves, particularly through the manipulation of employment (Collins, Omar, & Hurst, 2000).

- *Professionalism*: Although its contribution to standards and the quality of care can be positive, professionalism can also lead to factionalism and the manipulation of public resources to favor the interests of particular professional groups to the detriment of the public interest.

Exhibit 13-1   Social Context and Health Management

Case 1: Community Involvement and Resource Flows in Nepal

In Nepal, legislation stipulated an increased health role for village development committees (VDCs). Research in two rural VDCs showed a correlation between the extent to which lower-caste members were represented on the VDCs and community contributions to health centers (Bishai, Niessen, & Shresha, 2002). This finding suggests that an option for managers is to look for greater community involvement as a way to increase resources. However, the possible interaction between management and context suggests that a manager's capacity to increase community involvement is socially conditioned.

Case 2: Local Context and Decentralized Health Management in Brazil

Research analyzed the factors that condition the effectiveness of decentralized health management in three Brazilian municipalities. The study identified a variety of contextual factors, including political patronage, different ethical notions of acceptable practices, and differing commitments of staff to the localities. While showing the effects of context on the management process, the study also highlighted the role of managers in influencing that context by referring to the "space for the formal health system to influence local social organisation and political culture and offer a potential for change" (Atkinson, Medeiros, Oliveira, & de Almeida, 2000, p. 632).

Integrity and Cohesion of the Public Sector

Public-sector management takes place within a system that is not always cohesive. Such discontinuities are a particularly problematic issue in some low- and middle-income countries. The impact of neocolonial domination, economic crises, political conflict, famine, and national disasters can lead to disintegration and fragmentation of state authority. These interrelated factors affect the public sector's capacity to generate and use resources to meet health needs.

Structural Change of the Public Sector

The public sector in many countries is undergoing significant change. Health-sector management and planning has been part of that change, as witnessed by the two major waves of international health reform affecting low- and middle-income countries—the Alma Ata Primary Health Care (PHC) movement and the more recent market-based reforms (discussed in Chapter 12). Table 13-1 identifies potential implications these broader changes have had on the role and operation of health-sector management in low- and middle-income countries.

The management changes outlined in Table 13-1 have been mediated by other factors and have had different impacts both between and within country health systems. First, alternative health-sector approaches, drawing their inspiration from the PHC approach, have continued to emphasize, for example, the importance of citizenship, equity, and social justice, and have focused on community participation in health systems decision making. This multiplicity of aims can generate contradictions for management (Flynn, 1997). For example, market-based strategies of service delivery emphasizing individual customer choice may clash with more citizen-based strategies based on community participation and collaborative relations within the public sector.

Second, and quite different from the first point, capacity for the type of management changes outlined in Table 13-1 is constrained in many low- and middle-income countries by the prevalence of informal

Table 13-1	Health-Sector Change and Management
Management Change	**Examples**
New management responsibilities	The introduction of competitive relations, contracting, voucher systems for service users, and market research to assess customer responses generates new responsibilities for managers.
New management skills	The introduction of the above responsibilities can require new skills in areas such as contracting, customer relations, and quality assurance techniques.
New management boundaries	The introduction of public–private joint ventures, contracting out to the private sector, and the use of competitive markets have led to a blurring of the distinction between the public and private sectors. This evolution suggests new boundaries for public-sector managers, with implications for management values and relations.
Changing management actors	Reforms can lead to greater diversity within the health system as public-sector facilities gain semiautonomous status and private-sector facilities (both nonprofit and for profit) become involved in health care. Managers need to take note of this diversity in developing a range of relations, from collaboration to competition.
Changing management objectives and values	Efficiency and health facility financial survival and growth can eclipse objectives and values based more on social justice and equity. For some, the generation of profit or financial surplus becomes an accepted objective of management action.
Changing management structures, systems, and processes	Management structures, processes, and systems associated with the private sector have been introduced into the public sector—for example, performance-based incentives in pay structures and competition between health facilities.
New management options	Reforms in many countries have opened up the option of contracting out service provision to the private sector, as opposed to relying on internal service provision.
Dealing with new challenges and contradictions	Decentralization has been associated in some countries with the requirement that health facilities be financially self-sufficient. Managers face the challenge of simultaneously ensuring the continuity of healthcare provision, meeting equity objectives, and generating resources for institutional survival.

arrangements in the economy and public sector and the scarcity of general administrative and managerial skills and systems (Schick, 1998). Corruption and patronage frequently maintain a stranglehold on health management and planning, thereby limiting systems' capacity for change. The result is often a changing blend of different approaches, providing a muddled, confused, and contradictory character to public-sector management. At times, a thin veneer of reform fails to disguise a cumbersome bureaucracy bent on corruption and patronage. At other times, purposive action by dedicated health staff overcomes strong constraints to provide health care to communities.

Increasing Role of the Private Sector

The private sector consists of for-profit and not-for-profit institutions, each with a different set of objectives. The primary objective of the for-profit private sector is to benefit financially (e.g., through the provision of expensive curative services), whereas the objectives of not-for-profit private health sector are closer to the social objectives of the public sector. The private sector can include in-country institutions (such as private hospitals or private insurance companies), international agencies (e.g., international pharmaceutical companies) and global institutions (e.g., Global Fund Against AIDS, TB and Malaria). The distinction between private and public sectors is often blurred—for example, many public-sector health staff may have private practices in addition to fulfilling their public-sector jobs.

The role of the private sector differs significantly across different countries, but typically includes different engagements in the areas of policy making, financing, provision of services and regulation. Depending on the degree of the private sector's involvement in these functions, the shape of the health sector can range from a "free market" system to a state-dominated system.

The main roles of the private health sector entail financing of health care (e.g., through establishing and managing private health insurance schemes), provision of health services, production and supply of pharmaceuticals, training of professionals, and contracting of support services. The last task may include contracting with the public sector as well as direct provision of services independently by the private sector. Outsourcing through contracts with the private sector is seen as a way of benefiting from economies of scale and the technical expertise of specialist contractors in areas unfamiliar to the central responsibilities of healthcare organizations. Some also argue that the private sector's perceived efficiency

and the control and accountability through contracts are further advantages associated with this model. Concerns raised by outsourcing of these responsibilities include the transaction costs of contracting out; questions about whether lower costs are merely the result of lower salary costs; the lack of sustainability and management learning in contracts; potential problems with poor quality, collusion, and corruption; and the lack of contracting skills in purchasing organizations (McPake & Banda, 1994; Mills, 1998; Stewart, 1993; Walsh, 1995).

The private sector—especially the for-profit segment—is often involved in the delivery of expensive tertiary (and thus profitable) health care. Similarly, private health insurance can be very selective and often contributes to health inequalities. Other areas of the private sector's involvement in the health sector include regulation of health care (e.g., in licensing and accreditation) and advocacy and lobbying for policy change.

The public and private sectors can engage in different interrelationships, referred to by many as the public–private mix (PPM) or public–private partnerships (PPPs). The underlying assumptions for the PPM model are its perceived greater efficiency in service delivery; a recognition that the public sector alone may be unable to ensure comprehensive coverage of, and access to, health services; and the complementary nature of the public and private sectors in achieving this aim.

The role of the private health sector (both the for-profit and nonprofit segments) was widely promoted in the mid-1990s through, for example, incentives to the private sector (e.g., tax concessions on capital invested or on private health insurance), public-sector contracting with the private sector (e.g., in Brazil), outright privatization and outsourcing in the private sector (e.g., support services in a public-sector hospital; see McPake & Banda, 1994). There are numerous examples of successful PPPs, for example, in tuberculosis (TB) control (Karki, Mirzoev, Green, Newell, & Baral, 2007). Nevertheless, the uncontrolled growth of the private sector as part of health reforms in many countries has led to concerns about the quality and coverage of many health services delivered through private-sector companies (Mills, Brugha, Hanson, & McPake, 2002), leading to further health inequalities. This result has led to calls for better regulation of the private sector (Bennett et al., 1994; Kumaranayake, 1997), as discussed in Chapter 12.

Private-sector money and influence is on the rise. Significant funding is provided by the Global Fund to

Fight Aids, TB and Malaria, the Bill and Melinda Gates Foundation, and other philanthropic institutions for health systems development in low- and middle-income countries. These initiatives are known as global public–private partnerships (GPPPs) (Reich, 2002) or Global Health Initiatives. Apart from increased funding to the health sector, the GPPPs may pose challenges related to management, including

> . . . skewing national priorities by imposing external ones; depriving specific stakeholders a voice in decision-making; inadequate governance practices; misguided assumptions of the efficiency of the public and private sectors; insufficient resources to implement partnership activities and pay for alliance costs; wasting resources through inadequate use of recipient country systems and poor harmonisation; and inappropriate incentives for staff engaging in partnerships. (Buse & Harmer, 2007, p. 259)

These changes in the public–private mix pose new challenges for public-sector managers in understanding the new range of providers and negotiating new relationships through, for example, contracts, leasing, and concessions. The growing private sector also brings specific challenges for the public manager who must devise strategies to retain staff in the light of potentially more attractive alternative employment. In addition, the public sector faces pressure to incorporate the style and techniques of private-sector management into the workings of public agencies through, for example, performance-related pay, generating a surplus through self-funding, and market-based competition.

International Context

The international economic and political context has an important effect on the national and local economic, social, and political processes of a country through, for example, investment, interest rates on debt repayments, and trade. The growth of the international policy presence of the World Bank during the 1980s and 1990s had an important impact on health management reform in low-income countries. The powerful financial presence of international donors can leave health ministries in a dependent relationship. The development of budget support, Poverty Reduction Strategy Papers (PRSPs), and sector-wide approaches (SWAps) has also engendered changes in the relationship between national governments and international agencies. More recently, the global financial crisis in 2008 affected the availability of resources for health sectors at both the national and international levels (Bednarz, 2010; NEPAD Secretariat, 2010). The general concern that underfunded and weak health systems are hindering the achievement of health-related Millennium Development Goals (MDGs) also spurred an exploration of alternative health financing mechanisms, as shown by the establishment of a High-Level Taskforce on Innovative International Financing for Health Systems (Fryatt, Mills, & Nordstrom, 2010).

The general point raised by this section is the importance of understanding the interrelationship between context and management action. Managers need to interpret the wide range of changing and complex contextual factors that influence the way in which management is actually conducted in the health system. At the same time, managers can be proactive; they are not powerless (Atkinson et al., 2000, Grindle, 1997). There is a margin of maneuverability in which they can operate, which varies in time but allows purposive action to be developed. One example of this flexibility can be seen in the different forms of sector-wide approaches that have emerged in response to different country contexts (World Health Organization [WHO], 2006a). Another example is related to the changing role of governments in regulating and managing the private sector in the context of emerging market realities in Tanzania and Zimbabwe (Kumaranayake et al., 2000).

Organizing

An important management function is developing the organizational structure—that is, the way work is assigned, both vertically and horizontally, together with the formal framework of links with other organizations and groups. Managers usually inherit an established structure. Recognizing this fact, this section takes the form of a review of organizational structure, indicating the key issues and the options available to managers to address those issues.

In reviewing this organizing function, several points need to be emphasized. First, health managers need to review the full range of structural changes open to the organization. For this purpose, this section presents a framework setting out the dimensions of a review of the organizational structure. For purposes of illustration, it refers to ministries of health, although the framework could be adapted to decentralized health authorities or health facilities. The role of managers in structuring an organization will depend on their authority within the organization and the significance of the structural issue to the organization.

Second, in deciding on organizational structure, managers need to take into account contextual factors, such as the staff capacity, the health policy, and the overall government structure.

Third, there is a need to secure a balance between two factors. On the one hand, managers have to keep the organizational structure under review and implement necessary changes. Structural changes are not the only component of change, however; they are just one factor to be considered and balanced against changes in resources, systems, values, and skills. On the other hand, managers need to recognize that structural changes can be both expensive in terms of resource use and disruptive to staff motivation and service delivery. Change should also not be used to mask more difficult and controversial issues of resource availability or health policy content.

Three overlapping dimensions of the organizational structure are reviewed here:

- Center–periphery relations
- Relationships with other organizations and groups
- Internal hierarchy and division of labor

These dimensions relate system-level issues to more micro-level issues. Reference may be made to Chapter 12 on health systems to understand the issues in greater depth.

Center–Periphery Relations

A ministry of health (MOH) is organized according to relations that link the center to the periphery. This raises important dimensions of geographic decentralization, purchaser–provider relations, and delegated semiautonomy.

Decentralization

Decentralization is "a transfer of authority to make decisions, to carry out management functions and use resources. Focusing on the public sector, it means the passing of these from central government authorities to such bodies in the periphery as local government, field administration, subordinate units of government, specialised authorities and semiautonomous public corporations" (Collins, 1994).[3]

_____

[3] These definitions of decentralization and its forms are based on the work of Cheema & Rondinelli (1983).

Authority, resources, and responsibilities may be deconcentrated to lower administrative offices over which the center maintains line management control. In contrast, the same transfer can be made to a devolved level of government over which the center has no line management authority. In this case, the local or regional government is usually multifunctional and will have its own form of appointment or election and its own sources of revenue. One would normally expect devolved governments to have more decision space than local administrative offices, although this is not always the case (Bossert, 1998).

Purchaser-Provider Relations

As explained in Chapter 12, health-sector reforms have encouraged a shift from organizationally integrated and hierarchically structured systems to a separation between the purchaser organization, which has the finance and interprets the needs, and the provider, which is responsible for service provision. This separation is intended to contain costs, improve efficiency, and remove decisions on service provision from political and professional self-interest. It allows for the introduction of contracts and quasi-markets into health care—which are supposed to improve effectiveness and efficiency—and the introduction of the private sector through public funding and private-sector provision.

Delegated Semiautonomy

Delegated semiautonomy, as a form of decentralization, involves the transfer of semiautonomous authority to manage an organization. In health care, its most common form involves hospitals organizationally attached to a health ministry. These facilities may be managed by a board that is only partly appointed by the ministry; staff may be hospital (not ministry) employees, while the hospital has powers of staff appointment, revenue generation, determination of salaries, and purchasing authority. This delegation can take the form of a purchaser–provider separation and be executed through a contract that formalizes the hospital's responsibilities and the ministry budget allocations to the hospital.

Another form in which purchaser–provider separation is combined with delegated semiautonomy occurs when the whole operational side of health care is taken out of the MOH and located in a separate health service structure. This is the case formally in the Ghana Health Service, illustrated in Figure 13-2. The MOH contracts with the provider organization, the Ghana Health Service, which is internally deconcentrated through regional and district levels. Outside

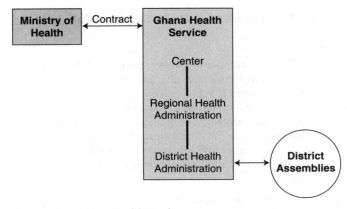

Figure 13-2 Ghana Health Service.

this system is the devolved system of elected district assemblies, although these entities do not have principal provider roles.

Managers should have a responsibility for developing the center–periphery relations, or at least be consulted as important stakeholders in the process of organizational change. These sorts of change are linked to important changes in organizations and the managerial process, as suggested in Exhibit 13-2.

Relationships with Other Organizations and Groups

The public sector—in our example, the MOH—needs to have clear and defined relations with a variety of external organizations and groups. Private-sector growth requires organizational links with government such as joint ventures, contracting out, and policy consultation. Community participation raises issues of how the community will be organizationally integrated into the health system. Many low- and middle-income countries depend on international organizations, both bilateral and multilateral, for significant financing of the health sector and develop important relations around health policy formulation and implementation. This organizational relation can take the form of aid agencies developing links with parts of the healthcare system when they take responsibility for financing particular disease control programs or particular geographic zones. Notably, the more recent development of the SWAp has led to organizational linkages between international donors and the MOH to develop health policy frameworks.

The MOH also relates to other government agencies—an interaction typically required as part of the cross-governmental process of management in relating to ministries such as finance, social affairs, and labor. An important aspect of this interagency cooperation is the development of a multisectoral approach to health development. Structuring relationships with special interests, such as the private, for-profit healthcare sector, forms an important part of consultation. At the same time, the MOH is required to exercise regulatory powers over the same special interests.

Internal Structure[4]

Related to the two dimensions of center–periphery and external relations is the organization's own internal relations and assignment of roles. These consist of four interrelated factors:

- Hierarchy and spans of control
- Relations of authority
- Horizontal divisions
- Internal linking

Hierarchy and Spans of Control

Organizations usually adopt some form of hierarchical shape consisting of different levels of management. These recognized levels of authority have a specific depth of authority and span of vision over the organization: The higher up the hierarchy, the greater the authority and the broader the vision. An organization can adopt different hierarchical shapes, although it is often thought that a flatter organizational shape is more appropriate for effective communication and decision making (Child, 1984).

Health ministries often suffer from overextended and overly tall hierarchies. This structure can result from bloated bureaucracies and the tendency to confuse public service grading systems with management

---

[4] This section draws on the work of Collins (1994).

Exhibit 13-2	Center–Periphery Relations and Examples of Management Change

Decentralization and Management

It might be thought that decentralization would lead to improved local health staff motivation through, for example, an improved sense of ownership, greater links with the community, and the general satisfaction from greater authority at the local level. However, a number of studies suggest that the situation is more complex. A review of health-sector decentralization in the Philippines and Zambia by Bossert and Beauvais (2002) noted both positive and negative effects on staff morale. Similarly, McIntyre and Klugman (2003) identified problems of staff morale in the area of reproductive health services and decentralization in South Africa; these included the "uncertainty created by the ongoing health sector restructuring" (p. 116), lack of being valued, and confused lines of accountability. Lakshminarayanan (2003) sees devolution in the Philippines as leading to lower salaries and limited career paths, thereby resulting in staff demotivation, poor morale, and declines in the quality of care.

Purchaser–Provider Separation, Contracting, and Management

The introduction of purchaser–provider separation and contracting requires the development of new skills and systems, such as contract monitoring and evaluation. According to Mather (1989), contracting "strengthens opportunities for quality control and concentration of resources on supervision and compliance" (cited in Walsh, 1995, p. 112). Whether purchasers in low- and middle-income countries have this capacity is another matter. For example, Abramson's (2001) study of the Costa Rican Social Security Fund's monitoring and evaluation of a contract with a health provider cooperative described an unsophisticated system of rating and a deficient relationship between indicators and contract objectives. Mills and Broomberg (1998, p. 25) note "fairly extensive evidence of very weak government capacity to monitor the performance of both for-profit and not-for-profit contractors." Using formal and elaborate contract procedures can lead to greater transaction costs and be considered inappropriate to contracting of primary care activities in low- and middle-income countries. Not only may purchasers have a low capacity for developing contracts in detail, but primary care activities can also be more difficult to specify and monitor (Palmer, 2000).

Delegated Autonomy and Management

Semiautonomy means that the hospital becomes a delegated institution within the organizational scope of the ministry, while having responsibilities in a number of key management areas:

- In human resources management, this might include the hospital determining its own staff establishment, with some measure of autonomy in recruitment, selection, appointment, conditions of service, rewards, and disciplinary system.
- In financial management, the hospital might possess the right to formulate and submit its own budget to central government for approval, receive a fixed global budget, obtain grants and loans, raise its own income (e.g., through user fees or billing private health insurance, and income from nonhospital ventures, such as the hospital cafeteria), retain surpluses for use in the hospital, and be responsible for its own internal financial management. (Teaching hospitals may receive additional allocations from the ministry of education or its equivalent.)
- The hospital may be free to make and submit plans for capital developments, run its own tendering process, and establish its own arrangements for internal management and organization.
- In logistics management, the hospital may be allowed to maintain (service and repair) its own infrastructure internally or through contract.

This is an extensive range of authority. Although direct control by the MOH might well have stifled the practice of management within the hospital, it cannot be assumed that the mere act of delegating authority will automatically generate the skills and systems to make it work.

---

levels (the number of management levels increases to accommodate new grades). Hierarchies can be made flatter by allowing several grades to occupy the same management levels and by increasing the average spans of control, leading to a reduction in management levels (Child, 1984). However desirable it may seem to widen the spans of control, this endeavor can be difficult. Attention has to be paid, for example, to the capacity of both managers and subordinates in

dealing with widened spans of control as well as to the nature of the work and environment (Child, 1984).

Relations of Authority

Relations of authority are important in binding the organization together. Healthcare organizations, depending on the type of decentralization, typically exhibit different forms of overlapping authority, such as strategic, main line managerial, technical, profes-

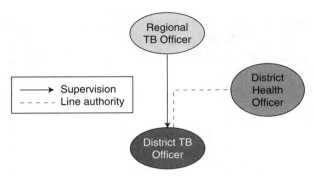

Figure 13-3 Dual Authority Relations
Source: R. Rowbottom and D. Billis, *Organisational Design: The Work Level Approach* (Aldershot, England: Gower, 1987), p. 16. Adapted with permission.

sional, and supervisory (Rowbottom & Billis, 1987). Strategic authority is fundamental to a MOH and involves decision making with implications for the direction in which the whole or a significant part of the organization is working.

One feature of healthcare organizations is the existence of dual authority relations in which staff have more than one relation of authority (Rowbottom & Billis, 1987). In Figure 13-3, for example, the district TB officer is under the managerial authority of the district health officer but under the technical authority of the TB regional officer.

Dual authority relations can be used to widen spans of control (Rowbottom & Billis, 1987). Figure 13-4 shows how a health manager can increase his or her span of control by appointing a supervisor or support staff to help in the management of staff. The supervisor falls under the main line management con-

trol of the health manager, as do the subordinates. Each subordinate, however, is under the joint authority of both the supervisor and the main line manager. Because the pressure of direct supervision has been taken off the main line manager, his or her span of control can be widened.

Although dual authority relations may appear strange and confusing, they are commonplace in health systems. Increasing health system decentralization through devolution to local government presents challenges for authority relations, however. Technical and hierarchical relations with the center need to be balanced with the strengthened horizontal relations within the local government authority.

Managers need to design authority relations in such a way as to avoid potential confusion. There are two complementary ways of clarifying dual authority situations. First, the different forms of authority in operation should be clarified and explained to the staff. For example, the relationship in Figure 13-3 between the regional TB officer, the district TB officer, and the district health officer might be clarified by identifying one superior, the district health officer, as possessing main line managerial authority and the other as holding another form of authority, such as technical supervisory, monitoring, coordinating, or prescribing. A second method of clarifying the dual authority structure is to specify the areas of management for the exercise of authority. Table 13-2 provides a checklist of key areas of authority to be allocated among the authority holders. Both methods require a clear specification of authority and responsibilities and a culture of understanding between the persons involved.

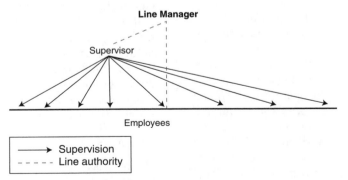

Figure 13-4 Reducing the Burden of Wide Spans of Control on a Main Line Manager Through the Creation of Supervisory Staff.
Source: R. Rowbottom and D. Billis, *Organisational Design: The Work Level Approach* (Aldershot, England: Gower, 1987), p. 62. Adapted with permission.

Table 13-2	Checklist for Determining the Split of Management Functions in Dual Authority Situations		
		Exercised by	
Management Functions	**District Health Officer**	**Regional TB Officer**	**Others**
Appointment			
Induction and training			
Performance review			
Pay and grading			
Dismissal, suspension, transfer			
Responsibilities and organization			
Methods and standards			
Policies and programs			
Resources and budgets			

Source: R. Rowbottom and D. Billis, *Organisational Design: The Work Level Approach* (Aldershot, England: Gower, 1987), p. 16. Adapted with permission.

Horizontal Grouping

At each managerial level, work has to be assigned to staff within different groupings, such as divisions, departments, and units. This division of work may be based on criteria such as geography (e.g., in a decentralized system), functions (as in planning or national disease control programs), or occupational groupings (as in a nursing department) (Child, 1984). The MOH could be based on a simple logic of planning, doing, and supporting, with directorates of planning (including aid coordination and information systems), health services (including primary healthcare services, national health programs, and hospital services), and support services (including human resources and financial administration) (Collins, 1994). This sort of arrangement has drawbacks, however: Notably, it can lead to a lack of horizontal links between the directorates and to imbalances, with one directorate being the most powerful.

Internal Linking

The previous discussion focused on the application of internal structures to divide work, which runs the risk of fragmenting the organization. The health organization needs to be brought together and act as an integrated whole (Child, 1984). In part, such cohesiveness is ensured through the operation of strategic authority. Strategic policy authority and resource allocation flow downward, maintaining vertical integration. At the same time, horizontal collaborative links are developed between the various divisions, departments, and units in the organization. Several structural arrangements may be employed to accomplish this goal:

- Job descriptions to specify lines of authority in the particular job in addition to job liaison responsibilities and membership of teams

- Organizational devices, such as interdepartmental committees and task groups, in addition to specific linking responsibilities assigned to staff

- Matrix systems (e.g., staff may belong to the basic departments in the organization in addition to specific task units and projects)

Planning

Like the more general management function, planning does not have a good reputation in many parts of the health sector.[5] Its record is not good, with plans often not being implemented or implemented ineffectively. The reasons for this failure vary, but frequently include top-down, rigid, and often bureaucratic centralist processes; a failure to integrate planning processes with other decision-making processes such as budgeting; and a failure to involve key groups, including health service managers, professional groups, and users in planning. These criticisms should not, however, be interpreted as pointing to the inevitable failure of planning, but rather as recognizing the need to develop systems appropriate to the particular healthcare needs and context of a country. This section looks at various background planning issues and provides an overview of the planning cycle.

Why Plan?

Planning is an essential element of management that is concerned with making decisions today to influence the future. It is a response to the dilemma that faces organizations, of an inevitable shortfall in re-

---

[5] This section draws on the work of Green (2007).

sources compared with health needs and hence the need to make choices between competing uses for the resources—that is, to set priorities.

Three other critical issues underpin the importance of planning. First is the changing nature of health and health care. Decisions on resource usage need to take account of likely future changes to health needs, resources, and potential health service strategies and technologies. Health need changes include both new diseases—such as HIV/AIDS or, more recently, severe acute respiratory syndrome (SARS) and avian influenza—and changes in the relative prevalence of particular problems as a result of epidemiologic or demographic transition. Variations on this theme include, for example, the growth of multidrug-resistant strains of TB. Resource changes that require consideration include both financial forecasts and the availability of key resources—in particular, health professionals. In many countries, the international migration of key staff such as doctors and nurses may lead to critical future shortages unless appropriate policies are developed now. The last area of forecasting relates to future technology developments and their impact on the health sector.

Second, as noted earlier in this chapter, decisions about priorities take place within a social and political context that will vary between countries and within countries over time. Health planning, therefore, can be seen as means of identifying and responding to the context-specificity of different health systems.

The third issue is the recognition that the current allocation of resources within the health sector is not optimal, as discussed earlier. As a consequence, planning is concerned not just with dealing with changes in the future, but also with addressing current problems in a way that will have effects in the future (e.g., effects of distribution of human resources on availability and quality of services and, ultimately, on health status). Shifts in resources could lead to a more effective and efficient use of resources.

What Is Planning?

The discussion so far has assumed a general understanding of what is meant by planning. A formal definition is given by Green (2007, p. 3):

> A systematic method of trying to attain explicit objectives for the future through the efficient and appropriate use of resources, available now and in the future.

The important components of this and other similar definitions are as follows:

- Where one is going (objectives)

- With what (resources)
- How (efficient and appropriate implementation)
- When (future)
- The degree of formalization (explicitness, systematic, and method) about the process.

There are, however, different approaches to, and types of, planning. In particular, we can contrast strategic (or allocative) and operational planning. *Strategic planning*, which closely resembles policy making, aims to provide an open and formalized process for making these difficult decisions as to which health needs will be met by the limited resources and how. Thus it attempts to provide a broad direction of travel for the health sector. In contrast, *operational planning* (also known as activity planning) focuses on the detail of implementation by setting out time frames for activities in the short term. In practice, the two types of planning should be linked, and often there will be elements of both within any particular plan document. Highlighting the conceptual difference between the two is helpful, however.

Health planning also involves a chain of interrelated processes at different levels of a country's health system. The following levels of planning can be distinguished: country (e.g., PRSPs), sector (e.g., SWAps, policy and strategy), and program and project (e.g., Maternal and Child Health (MCH) (Green & Mirzoev, 2008).

One criticism of planning is that it is seen as being unfeasible during periods of uncertainty or instability. However, the reverse can also be argued—that planning is itself a means of dealing with uncertainty, while retaining a strategic direction. However, it needs to be sufficiently flexible to achieve this aim.

Several common misperceptions about planning need to be addressed. Table 13-3 sets these out along with the counter-views.

How Would Decisions Be Made Without a Planning System?

In all organizations, decisions are made as to how resources will be used for the future. However, they are not necessarily made in an open, explicit, and planned way. There are four potential ways in which decisions may be unsatisfactorily approached.

First, they may be avoided, resulting in the status quo prevailing. This failure to face up to the challenge of making decisions is frequently encountered—and unsatisfactory.

In a second approach, a small, elite group makes decisions, but in a closed and non-accessible manner. Such decisions are likely to be suboptimal because they fail to consult a wide group of people, which

Table 13-3	Misperceptions About Planning
Misperception: Planning Is . . .	**But . . .**
About the production of plans	Planning is concerned with change, not documents
About capital budgets	Planning should also focus on recurrent budgets
Only concerned with projects	Projects are simply one way of achieving change
A highly technical and specialist activity	Much planning is common sense
Carried out by specialist planners	Planning needs to be shared by a wide group of actors
An objective and neutral activity	Planning involves value judgments

Source: A. Green, *An Introduction to Health Planning in Developing Health Systems*, 3rd ed. (Oxford, England: Oxford University Press, 2007), pp. 378–379.

would lead to the advantages of better information and ownership of resultant decisions.

In the third approach, which is common in the health sector, the professionals who deliver the services effectively force decisions through their current actions and their power base. The difficulty with this approach is that currently popular specialties may be able to attract funding at the expense of other services. Public health, geriatrics, and mental health are likely to be disadvantaged at the expense of specialties such as surgery, even though this outcome may not reflect the health needs or priorities of a country.

The last unsatisfactory alternative is when decisions are made by donor agencies in the absence of adequate national processes.

None of these approaches is satisfactory, though all of them may coexist within a single institution. In this circumstance, planning as an open, formal process is needed. We turn now to the structures and processes by which this type of planning can be ensured.

Planning for Health and the Health Sector

The arguments for a government lead in planning hinge on whether health care is viewed as a special good for which the normal market mechanisms are not appropriate (e.g., because of equity implications or because of their public-good nature). The following discussion takes the widely held position that (1) at a minimum the state has a responsibility to set and regulate policies, and (2) the state will continue to provide certain key healthcare services for the foreseeable future.

Historically, planning in the public sector has tended to focus on the state's own healthcare services. More recently, it has become more widely recognized that planning by government needs to recognize the actual and potential inputs (both positive and negative) of other healthcare agencies, such as those in the private for-profit sector and nongovernmental organizations (NGOs). This expanded reach calls for the

development of new policy and planning tools to implement such strategies (see, for example, Bennett et al., 1994). It is also of increasing importance given the development of strategic plans for SWAps (Green & Mirzoev, 2008).

In addition, although we tend to label plans in the health sector as health plans, in reality they tend to focus on health care, with little recognition of the positive and negative effects of other (non-healthcare) agencies on health. Genuine health plans need to broaden their scope and incorporate appropriate actions related to other sectors.

The changes in the structure and roles of government that have been taking place in many health sectors in recent years often require corresponding changes in the government planning approach. In particular, the increasing number of healthcare providers that are not directly managed or controlled by one government agency and the decentralization of authority mean that governments need to develop new ways of achieving change in providers other than those whom they directly manage. New forms of incentives and regulatory powers are needed, in contrast to the traditional managerial command-and-control approaches. This trend also implies that a greater onus is placed on the lead government agency to provide overall policy frameworks for the health sector that specify appropriate roles for other agencies.

Approaches to Planning and Relationship to the Context Within Which It Occurs

Various different approaches to planning are possible. Following are descriptions of two contrasting approaches, although it is important to note that they are not mutually exclusive.

Problem-solving reactive approaches versus longer-term needs assessment. Planning can focus on, and try to identify solutions to, existing problems. A well-known example of such an approach was that used in Ghana (Cassels & Janovsky, 1995). A variety of techniques have been developed to assist planners and managers in problem identification and solving, including problem tree and fish-bone analysis (Thunhurst & Barker, 1999). One danger with such an approach, however, is that its focus on current problems may detract from longer-term needs assessment and timely responses to emerging needs.

Structured logical frameworks versus looser strategic directional approaches. In recent years, a number of organizations, and in particular donor agencies, have adopted an approach to planning (generally projects) using logical frameworks (logframes) that set out in a very structured manner a hierarchy of objectives and activities, together with means of identifying whether they have been achieved, and the potential future risks or assumptions (Nancholas, 1998). Such an approach can be contrasted with a looser narrative strategic plan.

Plans can also have a different focus. Plans may focus on any of the following:

- An organization such as a hospital
- An administrative geographical level such as a district and its population
- Particular programs (such as reproductive health or TB)
- At the most focused level, specific projects that incorporate time-bound interventions

The appropriate approach to and focus of planning will depend on the context in which the planning occurs. As an extreme example, the presence of conflict or an emergency situation will affect planning. For example, in Sierra Leone during the recent civil war, quarterly plans were set, in recognition of planners' inability to take a longer-term strategic view during this period.

Planning and Organizational Levels

Planning occurs—or should occur—at all levels in the health system, as illustrated in Figure 13-5. As decentralization policies are implemented, it is important that they incorporate a clear expression of the relative planning responsibilities of the different levels of the health system. Table 13-4 gives an example of the division of responsibilities in a two-level system.

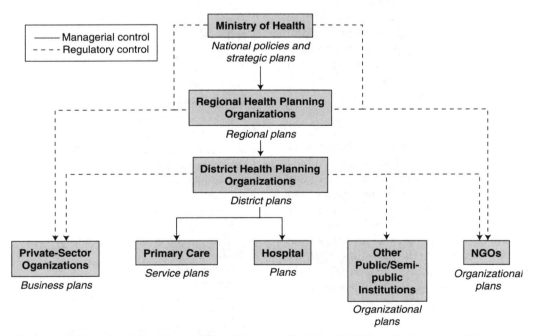

Figure 13-5 Examples of Planning at Different Organizational Levels Within a Deconcentrated System.
Source: A. Green, *An Introduction to Health Planning in Developing Health Systems*, 3rd ed. (Oxford, England: Oxford University Press, 2007), p. 44. Adapted with permission.

Table 13-4	Example of the Division of Responsibilities Between Center and Periphery		
Central Functions	**Joint Activities**		**Local Functions**
Broad policy leadership	Monitoring and evaluation jointly with central level		Local needs assessment
Resource generation and allocation			Development of local plans
Donor coordination			Implementation of local plans
Liaison with central ministries			
Coordination of local plans			
Planning of central specialist services			
Human resources planning			
Technical planning support			
Legislation			

Source: A. Green, *An Introduction to Health Planning in Developing Health Systems*, 3rd ed. (Oxford, England: Oxford University Press, 2007), p. 364. Reprinted with permission.

Types of Planning Time Scales

Planning, as we have seen, focuses on actions related to the future. However, decisions have to be made as to the time scale. For many planning systems, a period of five years has been taken as the standard time frame. Other health systems have found this practice too rigid and have adopted a rolling process of planning, as exemplified in Figure 13-6, where each year the plan period (in this example, three years) is rolled on by a year. To maintain an overall set of strategic direction, this type of plan is often combined with a long-term perspective plan that sets out a very broad set of policies or direction of strategic travel.

Planning timetables need to take account of both the need for wide consultation at different stages of planning and the fact that planning at each level (e.g., district) must link to planning both at higher and lower levels and other parts of the overall system (e.g., local government plans).

Elements of Planning

Figure 13-7 sets out diagrammatically the health planning spiral, which shows the various stages involved in planning. Two general points need to be made. First, conceptually, this process is a spiral rather than a cycle—suggesting movement in a direction rather than a repetitive cycle. Second, planning refers to a process rather than a chronological sequence. Several activities may be occurring at the same time, together with various iterations within, and across, the six stages of the planning process. Each of these stages in planning is briefly introduced here.

Situational Analysis

The situational analysis step assesses the current situation and projected future changes to it. It also represents a useful mechanism for getting a planning team working well together early in the planning process and for opening up the process to a wider group of agencies and individuals. Table 13-5 sets

Table 13-5	Key Components of a Situational Analysis

Population Characteristics

Demographic information
Religious, educational, and cultural characteristics

Area Characteristics and Infrastructure

Geographic and topographic situation
Infrastructure
Socioeconomic situation
Public- and private-sector structures

Policy and Political Environment

Overall national policies
Existing health policies
Political and ideological environment

Health Needs

Medically perceived health needs
Community perceived health needs

Services Provided by, and Plans of, the Nonhealth Sector

Health services
    Service facilities
    Service utilization
    Service gaps
    Health service organizational arrangements
Resources
    Financial resources
    Personnel
    Buildings, land, equipment, and vehicles
    Other supplies

Efficiency, Effectiveness, Equity, and Quality of Current Services

Source: A. Green, *An Introduction to Health Planning in Developing Health Systems*, 3rd ed. (Oxford, England: Oxford University Press, 2007), p. 186. Reprinted with permission.

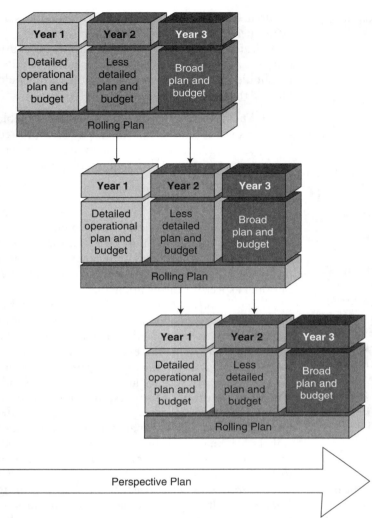

Figure 13-6 Three-Year Rolling Plan and Long-Term Perspective Plan.

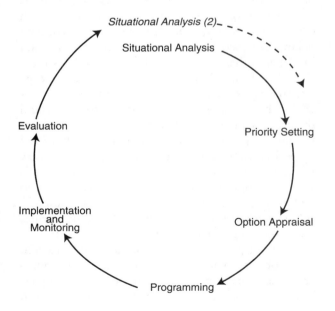

Figure 13-7 The Planning Spiral. *Source:* A. Green, *An Introduction to Health Planning in Developing Health Systems,* 3rd ed. (Oxford, England: Oxford University Press, 2007), p. 36. Reprinted with permission.

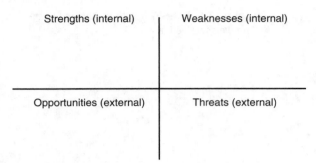

Strengths (internal)	Weaknesses (internal)
Opportunities (external)	Threats (external)

Figure 13-8 SWOT Analysis Framework.

out key information needs related to both the current situation and likely future trends.

A SWOT (strengths, weaknesses, opportunities, and threats) analysis may also be used during situational analysis (see Figure 13-8). This technique directs attention toward internal and external aspects of institutions and is generally better suited to assessing an institution such as a commercial firm, but there may be occasions when it provides a useful format for health-sector organizations.

The end product of the situational analysis stage should be usually a focused overview of the current situation with identification of specific areas requiring actions.

Priority Setting

The second stage of planning sets priorities for the organization, in the light of competing needs and limited resources. Setting priorities is perhaps the most critical and most difficult planning stage—but a part of the planning process that cannot be avoided. Priority setting has become one of the areas on which health-sector reform has focused through development of essential or minimum packages.

For the state providing an overall strategic plan, its priorities need to be sufficiently broad to allow for local variations as a result of differing needs. Underpinning all of the issues regarding how priorities are set is a tension between attempts to make decisions on priorities as rigorous as possible and recognition of the essentially political or value-laden nature of such decisions.

What Should Priorities Be Based On? At one level, the most obvious answer to the question of the basis for prioritization is that priorities should be set on the basis of greatest health need. However, this response in itself raises various further questions, such as how health need is perceived. In particular, is a broad or a narrow view of health taken, how is

health need measured, and should priorities focus on health needs or healthcare needs?

Clear criteria are needed so that the process of priority setting can be as open as possible. These criteria should be derived from overall policy and could include the following:

- The maximum health gain given the available resources (efficiency), which may be expressed as a combination of the magnitude of the potential impact of different interventions
- The equity effects
- Public demands

These criteria may sometimes work against one another. For example, there may be a tradeoff between equity and efficiency unless efficiency is seen as a means to achieve objectives that include the distributional aspects of the health gain.

Who Should Set Priorities? A critical issue within the planning process relates to who has the right or responsibility to set priorities at which level in the national health system. For example, good arguments may be made for any of the following groups to be involved in priority setting: health professionals, administrators, users of services, and, more widely, communities or politicians. The priorities set will depend significantly on who makes them. Techniques of stakeholder analysis (Brugha & Varvasovszky, 2000) are useful in assessing the strengths of different groups in society.

Establishing Priorities Within a Planning Framework. It is important that the planning process makes explicit how priorities are to be set. This process needs to satisfy various criteria. First, it needs to allow a broad view of health, rather than health care alone. Second, it needs to find an appropriate balance between decision making at the national and local levels that reflects the degree of decentralization. Third, the planning process itself needs to be transparent; stakeholders with an interest in influencing the priorities set need to be able to understand the process and recognize where their legitimate entry into the process can occur. Finally, it needs to end up with objectives that are feasible. A common flaw in the priority-setting process is that everything is viewed as high priority, meaning effectively that no real priorities have been set. Indeed, a good test of a robust priority-setting system is whether it clarifies those areas that are not viewed as high priority.

Various processes and techniques can be used to set priorities, including economic appraisal, multivariable decision matrices, and Delphi techniques. The resource allocation processes from the center to

Allocated Score	Criteria			
	Cost per DALY	**Public Demands**	**Mortality Rates**	**Disability Rates**
4	Measles	AIDS	AIDS	Polio
3	TB	Alcoholism	TB	Alcoholism
2	Malaria		Malaria	
1			Gastroenteritis	

Scoring		
	AIDS	8
	Alcoholism	6
	TB	6
	Measles	4
	Malaria	4
	Polio	4
	Gastroenteritis	1

Figure 13-9 Hypothetical Example of a Multivariable Decision Matrix.

lower health service levels are also an important vehicle for ensuring that broad priorities (and particularly those of equity) are reflected in the budgets allocated for service delivery.

Economic appraisal is frequently suggested as an important technique for setting priorities, in that it has the potential for combining consideration of health gain and resources. The 1993 World Development Report (World Bank, 1993) suggested that priorities should be set using cost per disability-adjusted life-year (DALY) as the basis for measurement. Arguments against the narrow use of such techniques include the lack of appropriate data and the potentially disempowering nature of economic appraisal (see, for example, Barker & Green, 1996). Furthermore, there is a danger in assuming that economic appraisal is value free, when it actually incorporates a number of implicit values, such as the weighting between disability and life gain (in a DALY), the weighting given to years of life at different ages, and the choice of discount rates.

Multivariable decision matrices offer an alternative approach in which any number of criteria can be incorporated and the information used either quantitatively or qualitatively. Figure 13-9 provides an example. Caution is needed when such tools are used, however, because they can easily mask implicit value judgments such as relative weightings between the criteria.

The end result of a priority-setting process should be a set of clear objectives for an organization. Although different terms are often used by different organizations for objectives (e.g., goals, purpose, aims, objectives, targets), the important feature is that they are structured in a hierarchy, such as the following:

- Broad overall health goals achieved through x
- Specific health aims related to particular health problems to be achieved by x
- Health-sector activity objectives to be monitored by x
- Targets that are milestones along the way to achieving aims and objectives

Figure 13-10 sets out an example of a hierarchy of objectives. The mnemonic SMART is often applied to objectives to suggest that they should be

- Specific
- Measurable
- Attainable
- Relevant
- Time bound

Option Appraisal

For each priority area, there may be various strategies that can be followed to realize those aims. The third stage in planning appraises each of the alternatives to determine which is most appropriate according to various criteria. These criteria should include those that underpin economic appraisal techniques (cost and effectiveness) as well as others such as equity, feasibility, and acceptability.

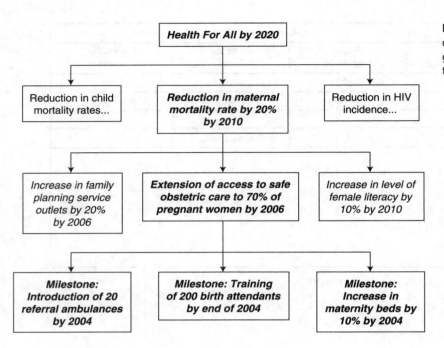

Figure 13-10 Example of the Hierarchy of Objectives. *Note:* Acknowledgment is given to Dr. Nancy Gerein for help with this figure.

A variety of options are available to any organization, but are particularly feasible for use by the state, which has various "carrots and sticks" that it can deploy to encourage or require action by other organizations (see, for example, Bennett et al., 1994). In traditional command-and-control planning systems, plans were expected to be implemented through managerial commands and compliance, rather than through incentives and creation of an enabling environment for better performance. With the recognition of the importance of other sectors and providers, a wider range of tools has become necessary. Thus the state may see, as one of the options to be appraised, the contracting out of services to other, nonstate organizations. Table 13-6 provides some examples of these planning tools.

Table 13-6	Examples of Planning Mechanisms and Tools
Resource Related	**Regulation**
Budgeting	Incentives and controls
Resource allocation	Legislation
Health financing flows	Norms and standards of care
Human resource plans	Regulation and licensing of supply of health facilities
Other input planning (e.g., medicines)	Regulation and licensing of health professions
Tax, pricing, subsidy policies	
External funding support	
Organization and Management	**Public/Private Interrelationships**
Development of healthcare packages	Managed markets
Organizational restructuring	Contracting of services and outsourcing
Health systems research	Privatization of public-sector assets
Plan statements	Nationalization of private-sector assets
Projects	
Wider Society	
Policies in health-related sectors	
Development of quasi-public bodies	
Advocacy	
Use of the media	

Source: Based on work done by Jane Shaw, to whom acknowledgment is given.

The end product of the option appraisal stage should usually be a detailed record of alternative options considered, along with clear framework for assessment and justifications for the chosen planning option.

Plans, Programs, Projects, and Services

The next stage encompasses programming. The aims and agreed-upon approaches to meeting the organization's objectives are brought together in a document that sets out these mechanisms, along with a time frame and financial plan. The level of detail, particularly regarding the budget and time frame, will depend on whether the plan is primarily strategic or more operational. Table 13-7 outlines the components of a typical plan document.

Logframes (logical frameworks) are often advocated as a means of both ensuring that a logical approach to project design is followed and providing a means of monitoring progress (Nancholas, 1998). Figure 13-11 gives an example of a logframe layout.

The end product of the programming stage should be a detailed plan of action identifying clearly the resource implications, time frame, and distribution of responsibilities.

Table 13-7	Possible Outline for a Plan

- Situational analysis, including the health needs or problem being tackled
- Objectives of the plan
- Strategies to meet these objectives
- Resources required, including finance to provide the services and sources of these resources
- Timetable
- Foreseeable constraints or risks

Implementation and Monitoring

Planning is useful only if it ends up in implementable action. Unfortunately, planning has a poor implementation record, with failure being possible for a variety of reasons:

- Lack of funds
- Lack of relevant resources
- Poor timing of inputs
- Resistance to change
- Neglect of institutional or legal requirements
- Unexpected results

Objectives	Objectively Verifiable Indicators	Means of Verification	Assumptions/Risks
Goal			
Purpose/Objectives			
Outputs			
Activities	Inputs		

Figure 13-11 Example of a Logframe Layout. *Note:* See Nancholas (1998) for a description of the process.

- Poor coordination
- Unforeseen circumstances

Frequently, the root cause is poor planning design, often as a result of a failure to recognize the political nature of planning at the design stage and development of overly optimistic and infeasible objectives.

A key activity that can improve implementation is monitoring. It requires an explicit time frame for well-specified activities and a clear understanding of who is responsible both for implementation and for monitoring of the activities. Monitoring techniques such as GANTT charts set out, in tabular form, activities by expected date of completion. In addition, planners must ensure that monitoring does not end up being viewed as an end in itself, but rather as a means of achieving the set objectives. As such, it is important that only the minimum number of monitoring indicators are chosen and *used*, and that monitoring is seen as a supportive (rather than punitive) activity. This understanding is closely linked to the concept of performance management of an organization, which seeks to identify the progress toward the organization's objectives and any barriers to this advancement.

The end product of this stage should be a record of implementation (e.g., services provided) including the challenges faced and any deviations from, or changes to, the original plan.

Evaluation

The final stage of planning involves the evaluation of the plan. Similar to monitoring, evaluation seeks to establish whether and to what degree the objectives have been achieved. Such evaluations may be formative (process evaluation) or summative (end evaluation). Evaluation is also regarded by many as a separate activity in itself, involving a series of stages that are similar to those occurring in research (i.e., identification of questions to answer, methodology design, data collection, analysis of findings, and report writing). The key areas that an evaluation is likely to focus on are the following:

Inputs

- Did the resources planned arrive?
- Were they sufficient for the services provided?
- Were the resources turned into services?

Processes

- How were resources allocated, and by whom?
- How were services provided, and how was quality assurance performed?

Outputs

- Were the services provided?
- Were the services appropriate, relevant, and adequate?

Outcomes

- What were the objectives of the activity being evaluated? Were they appropriate?
- Were the objectives set achieved? If not, why not?
- Did any health improvements occur as the direct result of the activity?
- Were there any other effects of the activity?

The results of the evaluations should be fed into the next round of the situational analysis, hence completing one round of the planning spiral.

Political Aspects of Planning

The preceding discussion outlined a number of techniques used in developing plans. It is important, however, to recognize that at all of these stages there is a need to consider the political dimension of planning, which is inevitable in a process that is designed to determine who gets what in the health sector (Table 13-8). There are two levels at which planners need to

Table 13-8	Examples of Political Decisions in Planning

Situational Analysis

Who chooses the information (e.g., in determining health needs)?
Whose view is taken, and which analysis is undertaken (e.g., which groups are taken as the denominator)?
What emphasis is placed on the different information?

Priority Setting

Whose views are taken?
Which view of health is chosen, and by whom?
Which criteria for priorities are chosen (e.g., equity versus efficiency)?

Option Appraisal

Who chooses, and how, the original options that are appraised?
What criteria are chosen, and by whom, for the option appraisal?

Programming

How are resources distributed, and by whom?
Who is responsible for the different tasks?

Evaluation

Who is involved in the evaluation?
What are the criteria for evaluation?

be aware of the political nature of planning as a process. First, they need to recognize that techniques are rarely completely value free. Second, they need to understand that techniques such as stakeholder analysis and political mapping may be used at different points in the planning cycle to analyze levels of support for different strategies.

Management of Resources

Management, as we have seen, is about resources—how they are generated and developed; allocated; and combined and used with a view to achieving objectives. Management of resources can be either direct or indirect (for example, through contracting out this function to the private sector or other agencies within the public sector). Resources of particular importance in the health sector include financial, human, information, supplies including pharmaceuticals, and transport.

This section first presents an overview of the main issues related to resource generation, allocation, and use; it is followed by a more detailed discussion of how the principal resources—money and staff—are managed. This is followed by brief comments on the management of supplies, transport, and information. In most countries, management of specific resources is undertaken by separate subsystems that have their own staff, organizational rules, and objectives (e.g., health management information system).

Resource generation and development relates to the different processes for production and enhancement of various types of health resources. Examples of these processes include preservice training of health staff, manufacturing of pharmaceuticals and medical supplies, different types of health financing (e.g., taxation, insurance, user fees), and procurement of transport and technology. Given the complementarity of such resources in their eventual use, it is important that the generation of these resources is planned in a coordinated way. Unfortunately, this is not always the case—there may, for example, be an imbalance between the number of health workers trained and the health facilities in which they are to work.

A broad interpretation of the concept of resource allocation defines it as "the process by which available resources are distributed between competing uses" (Pearson, 2002, p. 7). This definition suggests that there are links between resource allocation and priority setting or rationing (Martin & Singer, 2003). A well-known example of the result of prioritization of resources within the health sector is a minimum/essential package of healthcare services. Although some systems of resource allocation focus on nonfinancial resources, such as the distribution of staff (Munga & Maestad, 2009), the most common interpretation of the term "resource allocation" relates to financial resources.

Different classifications of *approaches to resource allocation* exist in the literature, including a distinction between normative and empirical approaches (Martin & Singer, 2003) as well as negotiation and political compromise, incremental budgeting, and allocation according to health needs (Pearson, 2002). Some authors also relate these approaches to various underlying values and theories such as theories of justice or organizational ethics (Martin & Singer, 2003). Approaches to resource allocation rarely exist in isolation; for example, the allocation of financial resources for health in Mexico, Nicaragua, and Peru is done through a combination of legal, political, and technical approaches (Arredondo, Orozco, & De Icaza, 2005).

The *types of resource allocation* can be described using two continua: (1) the allocation of resources across different levels (for example, between the center and decentralized levels) and (2) the allocation of resources within a single level (for example, within a district health system).

The types of resource allocation also reflect the underlying *methods for allocating health resources*. Resource allocation may include different combinations of (1) *input-based models* (for example, based on numbers of facilities or staff) and (2) *needs-based models* (for example, based on identified health needs requiring specific types of health services). Other principles in allocating resources include continuation of historical trends and patterns in utilization of health services.

A variety of economic tools and techniques are available to support allocation of resources, with the most commonly used tools including cost-effectiveness, cost-utility, and cost-benefit analyses, plus the use of disability-adjusted life-years (DALYs) and quality-adjusted life-years (QALYs) (Arnesen & Kapiriri, 2004; Eichler, Kong, Gerth, Mavros, & Jönsson, 2004; Hutubessy, Chisholm, Edejer, & WHO, 2003; Kapiriri, Norheim, & Heggenhougen, 2003; Robinson, 1999).

From a management perspective, the use of different resources refers to the most efficient and effective combination of available resources to provide services. Where different management subsystems are set up to manage different resources, a particular challenge is ensuring the coordinated and complementary deployment of these resources.

Financial Management

A key resource for any organization is, self-evidently, finance, and this section looks at the main elements of good financial management.[6] Finance is, of course, only important in that it allows the hiring of staff and the purchase of goods and services. Good financial management supports the health organization in the achievement of its objectives. As such, it must be closely linked to other key decision processes and, in particular, to planning. Financial management, like general management, must be viewed as a means rather than an end in itself. The elements of financial management are described next.

Resource Generation

Various sources of finance are available to a health service organization, and it is important to recognize the interrelationships between these different sources and consider them as a whole in planning. These sources are explored in Chapter 12.

Financial Resource Allocation and Budgeting

Financial resource allocation refers to the distribution of block financial resources from a higher level to a lower level in an organization (a vertical process). Budgeting refers to the allocation of financial resources within an organization.

Within the public health sector, financial resource allocation from the center is a common feature. Its importance will depend on the health financing system and the degree of decentralization of resource generation within the health system (Green et al., 2000).

Frequently, financial resource allocation is based (explicitly or implicitly) on one or more of the following factors:

- Previous allocations
- Service or facility patterns and norms
- Capital developments and associated recurrent implications
- Political profile and compromise

These approaches, although potentially nonthreatening to existing budget holders, fail to address issues of efficiency and equity. In contrast, an equity-focused strategy bases its resource allocation on an assessment of the needs of particular areas or population groups. Figure 13-12 sets out a conceptual model for

such a process. The potential components for allocation are as follows:

- The population's size, composition, and health needs
- The costs of providing services
- Variations in costs between different areas
- The costs of activities other than health care, such as research or teaching
- Flows of patients across administrative boundaries

"Health need" is the most significant and most difficult element to measure, as its ingredients include demographic factors; morbidity, mortality, and disability; and indicators of deprivation.

Formulae to allocate resources on the basis of needs have been developed in a number of health systems; the U.K. RAWP (Resources Allocation Working Party) model is a well-known example (Carr-Hill, 1989). A number of issues arise regarding the implementation of such formulae, however—most importantly, the choice of indicators, and the availability of information. Other issues affecting the introduction and implementation of resource allocation formulae include the absorptive capacity of areas receiving significant additional funding and the political resistance of "losing" areas. In many countries, it may be necessary to start with very basic allocative formulae based on population before developing more sophisticated approaches. One particular challenge that managers often face is to balance resource allocation of core funding with other types of budgets such as pooled funds in SWAps or program-specific budgets, such as those funded by the Global Health Initiatives.

Budgets refer to the allocation of financial resources within an organization. These statements of intended expenditure are required in the implementation of planned activities, and should reflect the plans of an institution or service. Thus budgets are vital management tools. Two major forms of budgets are distinguished:

- *Capital/development*: for buildings, large equipment, and vehicles
- *Recurrent/revenue*: for running expenses, including salaries and supplies

In addition, an organization may develop separate project budgets, which may combine both of these forms.

A budget consists of three components: what it is spent on (line items such as personnel, medicines, and equipment), for what purpose (service or institution or geographic area), and when. Within health organ-

---

[6] Acknowledgment is given to Jane Shaw for her input into this section.

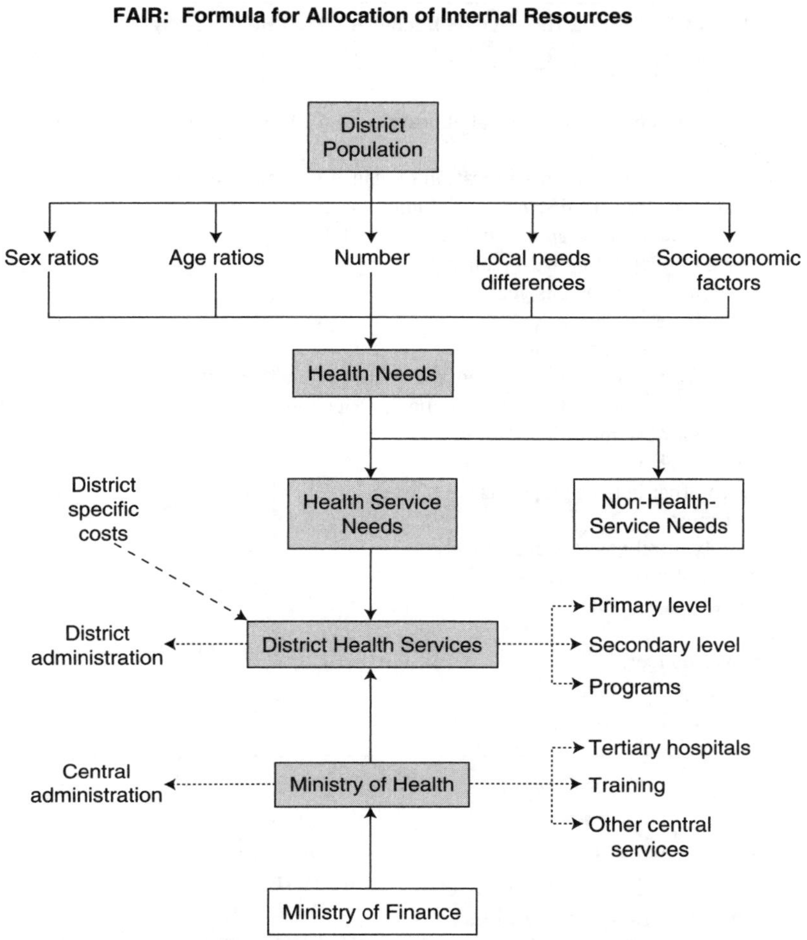

FAIR: Formula for Allocation of Internal Resources

Figure 13-12 Conceptual Model for Needs-Based Resource Allocation. *Source*: Derived from A. Green, *An Introduction to Health Planning in Developing Health Systems*, 3rd ed. (Oxford, England: Oxford University Press, 2007), p. 285.

izations, budgets may also be set up on the basis of programs (such as maternal health) that cover all aspects of care irrespective of where it takes place. Such program budgets are better aids in planning because they allow for programs to have different priorities; however, they are much more difficult to manage.

Budgets may be set in various ways. The most commonly used practice is historical incrementalism, whereby the previous period budget is increased across the board. Such an approach is easy to administer and nonthreatening, but it does not reflect major changes in priorities or new developments. A common variant on this approach involves additional increases to a budget (over and above the historical increment) arising from capital developments such as a new building and its associated service.

A contrasting method is activity-based budgeting, whereby the budget is set based on predicted activity levels. This technique allows for a clear link between the budget and the service objectives. An extreme example is zero-based budgeting, in which no prior assumptions are made, and every item in the budget for each year has to be fully justified.

Zero-based budgeting is more time-consuming and generally more politically sensitive compared to historical incrementalism, as it requires information on both the level of activity and the costs of a unit of activity. The costs may, of course, change depending on the level of activity and on the relationship between fixed and variable costs.

A possible timetable for budgeting is given in Table 13-9.

Table 13-9	Annual Budget Cycle for a Three-Level Deconcentrated Health System
Month	**Activity**
1	Financial year begins.
5	Ministry of health receives provisional annual allocation from central government, together with any special constraints or conditions.
6	Ministry of health issues broad resource allocation guidance to regions on the basis of provisional allocation.
7	Regions issue broad allocations to districts on a similar basis.
8	Budget holders develop and return proposals showing the following: • Review of service targets in line with plan • Estimated expenditure for previous year • Estimated expenditure for current year • Reasons for under- or over-spending • Budget proposals for following year, costed and showing how they will meet planned service targets
8	Budgets are totaled and reconciled first at the regional level and then at the ministry of health.
9	Adjustments are made for the following reasons: • To reflect national policy • To reconcile with other budget proposals • To reflect constraints • To reconcile with central government allocations
9	Discussions with central government.
10	Adjustments with service managers.
11	Informal approval.
12	Government approves budget.
1	Budgets issued to budget holders.

Source: Green, 2007, Box 11.3. Adapted with permission.

Expenditure Drawing and Disbursement

The next element is that of expenditure against a set budget. Each financial management system will have mechanisms to authorize named officials to incur expenditures, within certain predefined limits and conditions, that reflect the level of decentralized authority.

Expenditure Monitoring and Control

Monitoring of expenditures against the budget throughout the year is an important management function. Critical to this process is a good information system. Each management system will have its own set of accounting methods. Such a system needs to be able to give the manager up-to-date information not only on past expenditures, but also on any commitments already made. For managers to understand the real implications of such information, they also need to have an indication of the likely expected profile of expenditures throughout the year so that they can discover any variance from the budget early enough that they can take the necessary remedial action. Some resources (such as staff salaries) may be evenly spread out throughout the years; others, such as medicine purchases, may occur more sporadically (in batches) and may reflect within-year differences in usage due, for example, to seasonal disease incidence. Capital equipment is even more lumpy in terms of expenditure patterns.

A manager needs to be able to compare actual expenditure against such expected profiles and understand the likely reasons for possible differences. An example of a simple monitoring tool appears in Table 13-10. It shows a monthly management statement after nine months of the year. The "Budget to Date" column shows what might be expected to have been spent three-fourths of the way through the year. It is assumed here that spending will be equal each month (which is unlikely, of course); more sophisticated estimates could be made. The variance columns show the relative (not actual) over- or under-spending.

Once managers have identified a projected over-expenditure (or under-expenditure), they need to consider the various options open to them to prevent this departure from the budget. Potential actions include the following:

- Seeking additional funds
- Instituting cost-control mechanisms, such as freezing expenditures
- Revising service objectives
- Reallocating funds from one budget (line item) to another

Table 13-10	Monitoring Tool Example						
Month: 9	Full-Year Budget ($000)	Expenditure to Date ($000)	Budget to Date ($000)	Variance from Budget to Date (+, underexpenditure; −, overexpenditure) Amount ($000)	Percentage	Projected Year-End Expenditure Projected to Estimated ($000)	Comment
Personnel	600	400	450	+50	+11.1	500	Underspending is due to recruitment difficulties
Medical supplies	150	140	112.5	−28	−24.4	160	Earlier epidemic, likely to result in final overspending
Transport	80	75	60	−15	−25.0	95	Earlier epidemic
Utilities	50	10	37.5	+28	+73.3	50	Delays in invoicing
Other	120	100	90	−10	−11.1	100	
Total	1,000	725	750	+25	+3.3	905	Overall underspending projected

To select the appropriate option, the manager needs to have a clear understanding of the reasons for the over-spending or under-spending, as they are likely to suggest the best remedial strategy. It is also important that the implications of any remedial actions be weighed against their effects on the organization's objectives. Cost-control mechanisms, for example, will affect services in terms of either the quantity deliverable, the quality, or the efficiency with which the services are delivered. The first two of these factors will be related to the service objectives.

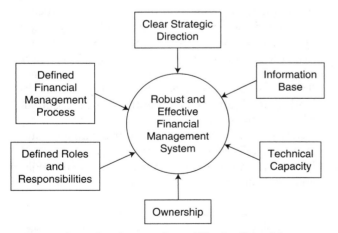

Figure 13-13 Requirements for an Effective Financial Management System.

Auditing (Internal and External)

The last element of the financial management process is auditing. An internal audit is a process of testing and validating the financial control and accountability systems to ensure that they are working correctly. This task is performed by a special department of the organization, which is separate from the normal accountancy group. In external auditing, the accounts of an organization are subjected to independent external scrutiny to confirm that they do not contain errors or hide fraud. For any organization, auditing is an important part of its governance.

Requirements for an Effective and Appropriate Financial Management System

Figure 13-13 identifies a number of critical features of an effective financial management system. If these aspects are lacking, there is a real danger that the system will not perform its expected task—that is, to ensure that the desired strategic direction is followed.

Management of Staff

The management of health staff has been a neglected issue,[7] and only recently have international policy makers explicitly turned their attention to human resources

---

[7] Acknowledgment is given to Tim Martineau for his input into this section.

Table 13-11	Decentralization and Options for Civil Service Structure
Civil Service Option	**Commentary**
Centrally controlled system	Terms for the civil service are centrally controlled and staff are seconded or transferred to local units, as in Papua New Guinea and the Philippines.
Health-sector centrally controlled system	Health-sector staff are taken out of the national civil service and included in a national system exclusively for health staff, as in Ghana.
A national local government system	All local government units operate under the terms and conditions of a national system that is specifically designed for local government staff.
Local public service commissions	In Uganda, local public service commissions are created, and some form of non-national local service commissions are foreseen in Nepal.
Decentralized unit	The decentralized unit determines the terms and conditions and employs its own staff.
Mixed system	Following decentralization, existing staff are kept as part of the national civil service, while new staff are employed under the new decentralized system, as in Jamaica.

Sources: Kolehmainen-Aitken, 2004; Collins, 1994.

for health (WHO, 2006b). In the past, attention largely focused on reforming health systems through new financing arrangements or organizational changes, such as decentralization. Yet staff costs are a major part of the health budget, and the quality of staff is vital to ensure the effectiveness of health care (Buchan, 2004; Rondeau & Wager, 2001). Furthermore, the development of staff management systems and skills throughout the health system increases in importance as decentralization and hospital autonomy spread out the management responsibility throughout the health system. This issue is also becoming increasingly important as international migration and the effects of the HIV/AIDS pandemic lead to major staff shortages of key personnel in a number of health systems.

In developing staff management, several important factors must be considered.[8] First, the inequitable distribution of health staff must be addressed. It is often difficult to persuade health staff to work in poorer areas, where incentives such as good living conditions and the possibility of private practice are lacking. Second, health systems are undergoing important changes, such as decentralization, that are affecting how health staff are managed (Kolehmainen-Aitken, 2004; Wang, Collins, Tang, & Martineau, 2002). This transformation can mean important changes in civil service arrangements, for example, as shown in Table 13-11. Two other influences on how staff are

managed, mentioned earlier in this chapter, are professional authority and power, and corruption and patronage.

There are many systems and skills for managing staff, ranging from defining staffing needs and jobs to employing people and developing their performance. The discussion here focuses on a number of key issues and functions.[9]

Staffing Review

An important issue is how the labor force can be used to improve performance in meeting health needs. A review may be undertaken, with key questions focusing on the number of staff employed, possible substitution by technology, and changes in the skill mix and grades currently employed (Strike, 1995). A simple technique for defining staffing needs of a healthcare unit is provided by Kolehmainen-Aitken and Shipp (1990); it involves the definition of job responsibilities and calculation of a "standard workload" for each person (e.g., number of outpatients attended per day). This value is compared with projected workloads in the health facility to estimate staff required. The possibility of using such planning tools is restricted by the degree of autonomy managers are given, the existence of patronage, the availability of information, the capacity of managers to use the tools, and the willingness of staff to move.

---

[8] Useful studies of health human resources are provided by Martineau and Martinez (1997) and Martinez and Martineau (1998).

[9] A more comprehensive and in-depth analysis would cover issues such as employee relations, change management, staff communication, and conflict management.

Table 13-12	Steps in the Employing Process
Step	**Commentary**
Job analysis	The job analysis consists of a review of a job to determine the context in which it is performed, relationship with higher-level objectives, job responsibilities, skills required, standards required, and relationship with other jobs. Data are collected, reviewed, and recorded, and managers can use the data for various purposes, including planning for staffing need, performance management, writing a job description, recruitment and selection, and defining training and development needs (Schmidt, Riggar, Crimando, & Bordieri, 1992).
Job description	The job description document identifies the character of a job through a job summary, basic duties, relations with other jobs (accountability, supervision, team membership, and liaison), work conditions (e.g., traveling), background of job holder (e.g., qualifications, experience), training and development in the job, and processes for the review of the job holder's performance (McMahon, Barton, & Piot, 1992; Schmidt et al., 1992). The job description is important as a link between staff management functions and in gaining clarity for more effective performance.
Person specification	The person specification links the job analysis and description to the characteristics required of a job holder. It can include physical characteristics (e.g., health history), educational characteristics (e.g., training), skills (e.g., language), and personal characteristics (e.g., motivation). Among its uses are preparing for recruitment and selection and definition of training and promotion exercises.
Recruitment	Through recruitment, managers seek to identify candidates for a particular job. In this step, managers must perform tasks such as deciding whether to look inside or outside the organization, ensuring employment legislation is respected, conducting initial screening, and drawing up a short list of candidates.
Selection	The most appropriate person for the job should be selected for employment, although both recruitment and selection can be affected by patronage and corruption. Those involved in selection need to be explicit about their decision-making process. Criteria for selection need to be determined, and selection techniques (e.g., interviews, aptitude tests, group tests) defined. The selected candidates need to be informed of the process.
Posting	The new employee needs to be posted to a workplace.
Induction	It is necessary to plan the way in which the new employee is inducted into the post, so that he or she has an understanding of the organization, work unit (and particularly the work team), and the particulars of the job (Schmidt et al., 1992).

Defining Jobs and Employment

The defining of jobs and staff employment may be viewed as a set of logical steps (Table 13-12). Systematic bias—whether based on gender, family, politics, race, or ethnicity—can stifle the employment process. The definition and use of clear principles and rules and an open and transparent process can make it more difficult for such bias to occur.

Staff Payment

The issue of payment is related to the staff grading system and form of public service system (see the earlier discussion). Changes in health systems, such as decentralization, can lead to corresponding changes in the source and level of pay. The form of payment may be based on time spent working, physical results produced, individually assessed performance, or a com-

bination of these factors (Brown & Walsh, 1994). Payment by time is simple, whereas performance-related pay is both complicated and controversial (Alimo-Metcalfe, 1994; Kessler, 1994). The latter approach assumes that staff will work more, and will perform better, if their earnings are related to their performance. In addition to practical difficulties in measuring performance, drawbacks of this strategy include its potential to introduce conflict between staff and counteract a teamwork approach.

Reliance on material incentives downplays the important motivation that public health staff may derive from the inherent usefulness of their jobs and public service. In fact, the extent to which pay actually acts as a motivator will vary according to the context and the type of staff concerned. For many staff, poor and inequitable pay can be more of a demotivator than a motivator, although low-paid staff may well value more pay. Another source of controversy is the extent to which health staff are allowed to earn additional income through practicing privately and the way in such activity affects their public-sector work.

Delegation

Delegation involves transfer, trust, responsibility, tasks, and authority. Delegation is a transfer of authority and tasks between two people or groups of people (Kempner, 1980). It entails entrusting part of your own authority to someone else (French & Saward, 1983). Although the person receiving the delegation has the responsibility or obligation "to perform tasks and account for their satisfactory completion" (Mescon, Albert, & Khedouri, 1985), the person doing the delegating does not lose responsibility for that task (Kempner, 1980). Rather, he or she retains "responsibility for that person's exercise of authority" (French & Saward, 1983, p. 122). This responsibility can also involve authority over resources—an issue that is important to recognize in the act of delegation.

The purpose behind the delegation is likely to affect its form and should be clear. For example, delegation might be used to overcome work overload or underload, to motivate staff, to bring decisions nearer the point of service delivery, or to gain a better understanding of service needs and achieve more timely decisions and increased flexibility and adaptability. Greater ownership among staff may also be achieved with a more participative management style.

Delegation is not easy, however, and potential constraints on its effectiveness can prove problematic (see Exhibit 13-3). In a setting of limited resources, for example, delegation may not transfer authority over those resources. Managers may resist losing authority and control; staff may lack the knowledge, skills, and values to practice delegation. They may also lack motivation where the delegation has no additional incentives and a culture of blame exists in the organization that is not conducive to delegation.

It is important to identify the objectives involved to communicate them to staff, monitor the effectiveness of the delegation, and design the means of delegation. An ongoing concern is that managers may delegate certain responsibilities because they simply do not like (or are unable) to do a task themselves, they consider the task to be impossible, or they are displaying favoritism.

The delegation needs to be clearly identifiable in terms of tasks, authority, control over resources, and its limits. A particular issue is the capacity (e.g., skills and experience), support, and motivation of the person receiving the delegation. Is that person equipped to receive the delegation? A useful concept is that of staff "maturity" (Hersey, Blanchard, & LaMonica (1978), which encompasses the skills, experience, and willingness to take on new responsibility.

Performance Management

In the field of staff management, performance management is frequently associated with annual confidential reviews or appraisals that are bureaucratic and routine, and do little to develop performance. Effective performance management requires not only reinvigoration of such yearly events, but also a broader approach of continuous performance management (Table 13-13).

Performance can be improved by focusing on its various aspects. Grindle (1997), for example, has examined organizational culture and identified which aspects of an organization lead to good performance. These elements include an organizational mission and a strong sense of attachment to it among staff; good management relations, such as fairness and teamwork; positive expectations concerning staff performance; and institutional autonomy in staff management.

Incentives and Motivation

Incentives and motivation represent an area in which there has been considerable theoretical debate and that has provided useful indications about possible

---

Exhibit 13-3	Staff Interest in Delegated Responsibilities in the Middle East

Research on bureaucracy in Egypt found that "most senior officials did attempt to concentrate as much authority as possible in their own hands; most subordinates did seek to avoid responsibility" (Palmer, Leila, & Yassin, 1989, pp. 149–150). Similar results emerged from interviews conducted in the Ministry of Health in Bahrain (Benjamin, Ahmed, & Al-Darazi, 1997). The research confirmed that lack of delegation was perceived by both managers and their subordinates as a key ingredient for efficiency and effectiveness, and its lack as a major problem.

Table 13-13	Steps in Performance Management
Steps	**Commentary**
1. Explain and reinforce the logic of performance management.	Managers explain to staff the organization's performance management and supervision practice.
2. Understand job context, content, and relations.	Performance management needs to be based on appreciation of the job content and the often complex relations of authority it involves. When they understand the job context, managers and staff should recognize the various factors that affect performance.
3. Agree on performance criteria.	Managers and staff develop a joint understanding about the meaning of "effective work." This agreed-upon standard accompanies an understanding of the conditions that need to be in place (e.g., logistics support, flow of funds, skills) for actual performance to meet these standards.
4. Compare actual performance with standards.	Managers and staff monitor performance using the agreed-upon performance indicators (both quantitative and qualitative).
5. Discuss and agree on action.	This step involves both feedback on performance with dialogue and agreement on the causes of this performance and possible changes required (including agreement on training needs).
6. Take action and monitor.	Action may need to be taken in areas, such as job context, content, and support. The effects of this action need to be monitored.

Sources: Bacal, 1999; McMahon et al., 1992; Weightman, 1996.

causes of staff motivation. Unfortunately, theories on motivation often fall short of providing health managers with a comprehensive framework that would allow them to understand fully the wide range of factors that can motivate or demotivate staff. Furthermore, the list of such factors can be so long as to render it useless as a managerial guide.

Another problem associated with attempts to explain motivation is that different individuals and groups of health staff respond to different factors (Weightman, 1996). Attempts to generalize across groups are not easy, although a general distinction may be made between "satisfiers" and "dissatisfiers" (Herzberg, Mausner, & Snyderman, 1959).[10] Dissatisfiers are those factors that in themselves do not necessarily motivate workers, but whose absence can demotivate individuals; they are related primarily to attracting people into jobs and ensuring their retention. Typical examples are pay and security. In contrast, the presence of satisfiers does lead to improved motivation and performance; typical examples are career development and job achievement. The following factors can have a bearing on staff motivation (Henderson & Tulloch, 2008; Willis-Shattuck, Bidwell, Thomas, Wyness, Blaauw, & Ditlopo, 2008):

- Career development
- Job characteristics
- Working and living conditions
- Managerial style and organizational culture
- Job rewards

In using such a checklist, managers need to distinguish between the satisfiers and the dissatisfiers. Job characteristics, for example, can be the cause of demotivation for staff if too many duties are imposed on the job holder; if the job lacks variety, scope, and delegated authority; and if the job is badly defined and, therefore, the object of conflict. Job holders may, however, feel that the job is meaningful and contributes to social welfare and solidarity. Staff working in the poorer areas of a country may feel that they have inadequate working conditions (e.g., office accommodation, information technology) and living conditions (e.g., schools)—also dissatisfiers.

In contrast, transparent and open management, showing an interest in good supervision and communication, staff involvement in policy making and problem solving, good teamwork, and reinforcement of ethical standards can be positive forces (satisfiers). The pattern of rewards and incentives is important and can include the extent to which the basic needs of the health worker are met and are considered equitable, the regularity and security of payment, and nonfinancial rewards such as stability and status of

---

[10] For a brief description of Herzberg's approach and its application to a low- and middle-income country context, see Dieleman et al. (2003).

employment. The possibility of career development can also be important.

Supervising

Like the other management functions, supervision is a process and not an end in itself. Supervision supports staff through a process of continuous professional improvement, includes all levels of the organization, and uses information from the staff, service users, and the community. It is defined as "A range of measures to ensure that personnel carry out their activities effectively through direct, personal supervisory contact on a regular basis to guide, support and assist designated staff to become more competent in their work" (Management Sciences for Health [MSH], 2003, p. 3).

Among the roles of the supervisor are the following (Collins, 1994; Schmidt et al., 1992):

- Defining tasks to be carried out and planning their implementation
- Providing professional and technical advice
- Problem solving and decision making
- Ensuring performance standards (technical, ethical, and legal) and providing feedback
- Personal counseling and employee motivation
- Providing referral, broker, and advocate services
- Ensuring appropriate support for the job
- Providing training and development support

A distinction may be made between line management authority and supervisory authority (see Figure 13-3). In particular, the two may be separated to allow the line manager to widen his or her span of control (Rowbottom & Billis, 1987). Depending on the relation between supervisor and line manager, the supervisor can also be involved in disciplinary actions and career development.

Despite its importance, the value of good supervision is often overlooked. Pressures on time and the demoralizing lack of incentives and overall support to managers and health workers may shunt supervision aside, such that it is perceived as a peripheral activity. Yet the importance of effective supervision is well recognized. For example, Trap and associates (2001) recorded the effect of supervision on pharmaceutical management in Zimbabwe and concluded that it had a positive impact, emphasizing the importance of training in supervision.

Managers have a variety of options at their disposal with which to improve the supervisory process.

Individual or group supervisory techniques may be considered (Collins, 1994; Jacobson et al., 1987), and a combination of formal and informal methods may be implemented (Collins, 1994; MacMahon et al., 1992). For example, Loevinsohn, Guerrero, and Gregorio (1995) examined the use of systematic supervision schedules in a controlled field trial in the Philippines. A correlation was found between the use of supervision schedules, frequency of supervision, and staff performance.

The style of supervision is also important. The concept of supportive supervision is emphasized by Management Sciences for Health as one of the most effective ways of supporting improvements in staff performance (MSH, 2003). A distinction can be made between supervision that focuses on the supervisee's performance and supervision that focuses on the more personal relationship factors. Thus the style of supervision may be contingent on a variety of factors, some of which are discussed later in this chapter.

Finally, the supervisory process may be formalized. A three-stage scheme for such a process is presented by Flahault, Piot, and Franklin (1988), consisting of preparation, supervision, and follow-up.

Teamwork

Teams are widely recognized as a positive influence in the health sector and can improve decision making, problem solving, and innovation; motivate team members; improve communication, collaboration, and support; and allow for training. Teams are used in a variety of health-sector settings and for a variety of reasons (Exhibit 13-4).

Although Exhibit 13-4 suggests reasons for developing health teams, such groups do have the potential to be associated with problems. Accountability within the team may be dispersed and lost, and team meetings can put pressure on time. Moreover, teams may result in indecision, cover up domination and power (Finlay, 2000), generate conflict, and lead to what has been referred to as groupthink (Janis, 1972), whereby diversity and debate are exchanged for the dominant and blinkered ideology of the team.

The effectiveness of teams will depend on factors such as definition of the objectives and tasks of the team, team members' willingness to modify their working styles to fit it, good motivation among team members and leadership, effective team meeting skills, getting team size and members' characteristics right, understanding the changing nature of teams, good team action planning, and achieving a balance between team cohesion and diversity (Noakes, 1992; Pheysey, 1993).

Exhibit 13-4	The Importance of Teams for Health and Health Care

In the United Kingdom, Noakes (1992) recognized the importance of teams in primary care, Stead and Leonard (1995) referred to the use of a multidisciplinary team in developing change within a healthcare unit, Firth-Cozens (1992) analyzed the use of teams in the audit process, and Finlay (2000) looked at the mixed experiences of occupational therapists in multidisciplinary teams. In Zimbabwe, Tumwine (1993) analyzed the use of ward health teams in developing community involvement.

Teams are an essential component of a multisectoral approach to health development (Aminu, 1985). They represent a break from the traditional, bureaucratic, and top-down form of organization that tended to individualize and isolate employees. By comparison, teams represent a shift to a more organic, less hierarchical form of organization that is interested in flexibility, multipurpose roles, and innovation. Although most organizations utilize a combination of these mechanistic and organic features, the importance of effectively operating teams in shifting organizational balance needs to be recognized.

Managing Staff Development

Staff development is an important factor affecting motivation and performance of staff. It can be done through various combinations of training, delegation of tasks, and supportive supervision. Although training is often associated with off-work courses, there is scope for incorporating staff development into the management process. We have already noted the importance of induction for new recruits. Table 13-14 looks beyond this step, suggesting informal processes that allow training to become an integral part of the management process. Many of these mechanisms avoid taking workers out of their environment and disrupting service delivery. At the same time, learning in the workplace can be more relevant and realistic.

Unfortunately, interest in these mechanisms may arise for the wrong reasons, such as cost cutting or the ineffectiveness of poorly managed training courses. Learning environments are not easily created at work, where employees face strong pressures to ensure service delivery. Furthermore, when carried out properly, on-the-job training is not a cheap option.

Personnel Administration

Most of the staff management functions outlined previously may be performed by either line managers (and supervisors) or personnel specialists or administrators. Personnel specialists can take on strategic, advisory, and operational roles (Cole, 1988). The last category encompasses the mostly routine administrative and procedural activities associated with functions such as recruitment, selection, pay administration, staff contracts, staff grading, promotion, transfer, staff communication, health, safety, and welfare in addition to maintaining a human resources information system (Strike, 1995).

Supplies Management

The management of supplies includes those resources related to health technologies such as medicines and diagnostics, and nonmedical items (such as food, fuel, and cleaning materials). This section focuses mainly on medicines, although many of the principles apply to other supplies.[11]

As much as one-third of the national budget for health care is spent on medicines and, as Reich (1995) shows, this is an area of political interest (see Chapter 14). It is also a complex area requiring, among other things, the choice of new health technologies at global, national, and local levels (Frost & Reich, 2008), and a process of procurement (including international and national tendering) characterized by complicated technical specifications and strict quality assurance throughout the process. Effective management of pharmaceuticals requires international-, national-, and local-level management processes. At the international level, standards of quality, safety, and efficacy need to be set and monitored. An example of such a system is the WHO prequalification project, which since 2001 has monitored the compliance of selected HIV/AIDS, tuberculosis, and malaria medicines with unified standards of quality, safety, and efficacy (WHO, 2010). Another important global public health task is the control of counterfeit medicines in international trade (International Medical Products Anti-Counterfeiting Taskforce [IMPACT], 2010). At the national level, in addition to robust systems for ensuring quality, safety, and efficacy of medicines, the

---

[11] Acknowledgment is given to Mayeh Omar and Reinhard Huss for their input in this section.

Table 13-14	Forms of Training Within Management
Form of Training	**Commentary**
Self-development	A learning agreement may be used in which the conditions are provided for staff to take the initiative in planning their own training. This experience can be isolating, however, and those workers who are less able and more in need of training may be less able to achieve self-development. Also, there is no guarantee that the staff view of self-development will coincide with the interests of the service.
Shadowing	A worker learns from another employee through observation. Potential drawbacks are that the "shadower" may be exploited as a "free helper," observation may not be systematically recorded, and the "shadowed" individual may be unconvinced of the usefulness of the procedure. Care needs to be taken that the experience is relevant.
Mentoring	Mentoring may involve an experienced colleague (not the worker's manager or supervisor) taking on roles such as providing advice, setting specific learning tasks, and suggesting new work options. Recognizing the problems that can occur within the context of this relationship, Jackson and Donovan (1999) stress the following points: Roles should be clear; mentoring should be voluntary; the relationship should be confidential; and it is not an element in promotion or discipline.
Supervision	Although there is a danger of overloading this important relationship, there are opportunities for supervisor and supervisee to agree upon and implement plans for skills development and problem solving.
Delegation	Delegation may provide an opportunity for developing staff, although the worker receiving the delegated task should have sufficient capacity to perform it. Good supervision is necessary to take full advantage of the possibilities inherent in delegation.
Secondment	Staff can gain from the experience of temporarily working in another unit or organization. Care needs to be taken to ensure that the secondment experience is relevant to the responsibilities of the original job and that opportunities are given for learning.
Job rotation	Staff may undergo a planned movement about the organization to develop new knowledge and experience.
Action learning	Learning through participation in completing tasks in a challenging environment may be useful. Such learning must be carefully planned and should not disrupt service delivery. This strategy is particularly useful to ensure deep approach to learning (Kolb, 1984).
Group-based work	Such work can involve a range of activities such as study circles, support groups, professional and occupational groups for developing quality standards, and specific group meetings.

Sources: Kerrigan & Luke, 1987; Storey, 1994.

appropriate mechanisms for licensing of medicines and regulating costs are important. Local challenges concern the storage and distribution of medicines in often inhospitable climatic and inaccessible geographic conditions with limited resources.

Problems with the availability of medicines in many services can be a major source of community complaints and irritation for health staff. In part, this issue arises because of the scarcity of material resources and the economic context. Other challenges relate to the existence of an underpaid and insufficient workforce with inadequate training, which may lead to poor management and corrupt practices. Poor management, for example, may include poor determination of need and demand, inappropriate selection, long delays in procurement, weak distribution

systems, inadequate systems for medicine storage, and unsuitable use.

Supplies management is sensitive to changes in health systems and health policies. Reorganization of this system, for example, may result in separation of the regulator, purchaser, and provider functions. Decentralization requires new definitions of responsibilities in supplies management. Potential economies of scale in central purchasing must be reconciled with the forms of local supplies management and accountability and their associated responses to local needs and flexibility. National medicine policies should include key issues such as the pricing and taxing of essential medicines, the development of legislation and regulatory capacity, the training of health workers and education of the public, and implemen-

Exhibit 13-5	**Stages of the Supplies System**

Selection

Selection should consider the needs of the health units and programs in addition to understanding the health situation of the particular communities concerned, their unmet needs, and the way in which these factors affect medicine requirements. Among the key considerations are the medicine requirements of the different levels of health care, priorities set, targeting of specific groups (e.g., children younger than 5 years), the use of an essential medicines list and generic medicines, and the design and implementation of quality assurance specifications.

The quantities required need to be estimated. Such estimates can be constructed via methods that use (1) population-based data on morbidity and mortality complemented by norms, (2) service-based data on diagnoses (and frequency) complemented by standard treatment norms, or (3) historical consumption data. Each of these methods has both pros and cons. For example, the second method fails to take into account unmet demand, and the third method may be the easiest to use but fails to account for changes. Adequate supplies have to be maintained over time; thus attention needs to be paid to issues such as consumption patterns over time, lead time for procurement, safety stocks, and reconciliation of medicine needs with available resources.

Procurement

Medicines are obtained through a procurement process, which involves actions such as following purchase procedures (e.g., tendering, negotiating), selecting the supplier (according to criteria such as price and quality through inspections), clarifying the terms of supply and supply periods (fixed or variable intervals), monitoring order status, and receiving and checking the medicines.

Distribution

Distribution can be based on either a "push" (kits) system or a "pull" (inventory) system. In the former system, quantities of medicines are sent at regular intervals, based on estimates of anticipated usage. The latter system requires the health unit to order medicines according to need. Use of this approach assumes, for example, the existence of an adequate stock control system and good communications for ordering and delivering. Among the issues to be considered are the simplicity, regularity, and reliability of the push system, in addition to how it compares with the greater sophistication and adaptability of a pull system.

Use

The use stage involves "diagnosis," "prescribing," "dispensing," and "patient compliance." A variety of indicators can be developed to monitor and evaluate medicine use.

Source: Courtesy of Mayeh Omar.

tation of international policy initiatives such as those developed by the Global Fund (Anderson et al., 2004).

The supplies management system for pharmaceuticals can be seen as comprising four basic stages: selection, procurement, distribution, and use (MSH & WHO, 1997). These four stages, which are linked and cyclical, need to be made operational to ensure that the right quantity and quality of medicines are located and used at the right time and right place. Exhibit 13-5 outlines each of the four stages and identifies some of the key issues and techniques involved in this process. A more detailed description of management of medicines is provided in Chapter 14.

An important feature of supplies management is the coordination of the various resources such as health technologies, information, money, staff, transport, and nonmedical items. Several functional subsystems are required for good supplies management, such as health management information, regulation,

financial/budget management, and transport management. For example, the supplies process must be linked to budget profiling. Also, efficient supplies management relies on a good management information system to monitor items such as stocks and treatment supplies. Exhibit 13-6 illustrates this coordination function by showing the important relationship between effective supplies system, training, and staff supervision in Zimbabwe.

Transport Management

The importance of managing an effective transport system should not be underestimated. Transport is central to ensuring access of patients to health services and the effective working of the referral system through both the emergency ambulance service and the transport of nonemergency patients. Health policies based on improved access and the principle of equity should take full note of transport systems.

Exhibit 13-6	Supplies, Training, and Supervision in Zimbabwe

Staff training was conducted in Zimbabwe to improve stock management and rational medicine use in the 1980s and 1990s. Although the training led to improvements in the health system, these gains were not sustainable. A new strategy was implemented that focused on improving supervision. A randomized controlled trial was conducted in three types of health facilities to assess the impact of supervision on stock management and the level of adherence to standard treatment guidelines. The study showed, in general, improvements in both variables, although supervisors needed to be trained and confounding interventions had to be taken into account. The authors concluded that "allocating resources to supervision is likely to result in improved performance of health workers with regard to the rational use of medicines, resulting in improved efficiency and effectiveness" (Trap et al., 2001, p. 273).

For example, Okonofua, Abejide, and Makanjuola (1992, p. 323) highlighted the impact of transport on equity and maternal mortality in Nigeria: In their study, transportation problems were seen to be "an important cause of delay in the case of maternal deaths;" Campbell and Sham (1995) drew attention to transport problems in the referral of pregnant women in Sudan.

The management and operation of primary healthcare units and the implementation of community health programs require transport. MacKenzie and colleagues (1995) pointed out the importance of good and careful transport for equipment in an otology and audiology study in Kenyan schools, while a study in Tanzania (Ahmed, Mung'Ong'O, & Massawe, 1991) found that poor transport was the second most important health management problem in urban areas, and the first problem in rural areas.

Community work that involves nonresident health workers relies heavily on good transport. In Zimbabwe, poor transport hindered outreach programs in maternal and child health, supplementary food production, and immunization (Woelk, 1994). Mobility and transport are also vital for effective management such as supervision and the running of a supplies system. Finally, transport takes up an important part of the health service budget.

Although there are undoubtedly areas of good transport practice, problems in transport management are also commonplace, including lack of man-

agement skills and systems. For example, there may be an insufficient number of drivers, inappropriate or poorly maintained vehicles, no supervision, no vehicle scheduling or usage information, or poor maintenance. A tendency to treat transport as a free good may be one cause of a lack of cost-consciousness. Donor involvement may lead to a multiplicity of vehicle makes, making it difficult to maintain an effective capacity for spare parts and repairs. Corruption and the appropriation of transport for private use may also diminish the effectiveness of the transport function. Table 13-15 outlines measures to improve transport management and planning.

Attempts to develop a comprehensive policy for transport management have been made in countries such as Ghana (Ministry of Health, Ghana, 1993) and South Africa (Department of Health and Developmental Social Welfare, 1999). Transaid (a transport international NGO working in the health sector in low- to middle-income countries) has developed a transport management system geared toward service delivery organizations. Two key elements within its system are "operational vehicle planning" and using information (Transaid, 2008).

Ideally, the operational planning of transport will be coordinated by a transport officer. The discussion here assumes that transport in the organization is pooled and that appropriate decisions are made on how to use it best. Users of transport, such as health programs and units, identify their transport needs, and subsequent decisions are made based on, for example, service delivery and urgency. Vehicles are programmed, with every effort being made to meet needs and priorities, effectively monitor the process, and ensure the transparency of the process.

Table 13-15	Measures to Improve Transport Management

Include transport in the health policy, planning, and programming process
Determine the organizational arrangements and responsibilities for transport management and planning
Ensure financial management arrangements for transport
Develop vehicle programming
Develop fleet management, including vehicle maintenance and repair and operational norms for transport use
Manage and develop human resources for transport
Use information for improving transport performance
Clarify the contribution made by donors to transport management and planning

Sources: Collins, Myers, & Nicholson, 1992; Transaid, 2001.

The use of information for improving performance is a theme throughout resource management and is particularly evident in transport. Managers responsible for transport need to pay attention to developing, for example, log sheets, vehicle maintenance records, fuel consumption reports, budget management instruments, and reports on accidents and incidents. Key indicators on performance need to be developed relating to the distance traveled (per vehicle), utilization of fuel, vehicle running costs, vehicle availability, and utilization, together with information on the safety of each vehicle and the extent to which the vehicle meets service needs.

A particular issue relevant to areas such as facilities, supplies, and transport management is the extent to which these functions rely on commercial lines or are semi-autonomous, self-funding operations within healthcare organizations. In addition, the extent to which the public sector contracts them out to the private sector, as discussed earlier in this chapter, must be addressed.

Information for Management and Management of Information

One resource that the manager is both responsible for and relies heavily on is information. The next section discusses issues related to the development of an organizational culture of evidence-based management. Information systems provide "information support to the decision-making process at each level of an organization" (WHO, 2004, p. 3). A health management information system (HMIS) is "an information system specially designed to assist in the management and planning of health programmes, as opposed to delivery of care" (WHO, 2004, p. 3). This section looks at issues related to the management of information.

Types of Information

Managers are constantly bombarded with, and attempting to make sense of, information. Most tend to consider information for use in management as that which is explicit, and often the information gold standard is seen as quantified information. In practice, however, most managers continuously use a considerable amount of information without being aware of it—often information derived from their own experience and frequently of a qualitative nature. It is important to recognize and value this type of input, while at the same time being aware that such information may be difficult to validate, in part because of its implicit nature. Managers need to identify points at which decisions are sensitive to critical information

and, where necessary, triangulate the information. Data collection and analysis also carries substantial costs; thus a characteristic of a good manager is someone who is able to request and use only the minimal amount of information at the minimal level of accuracy required for that decision.

Information, therefore, may be of many types and describe a wide range of issues of importance to a manager. Indeed, a number of examples of information systems were described in the preceding sections, including those dealing with budgetary information, information on transport usage, and personnel information. Within these health information systems, three domains of information can be distinguished: information on determinants of health (e.g., socioeconomic factors), information on a population's health status (e.g., mortality, morbidity, wellbeing), and information related to the functioning of a health system (inputs, processes, and outputs—for example, health services) (Health Metrics Network [HMN], 2008).

Sources of Information

The sources of health-related information can be classified into six broad categories (HMN, 2008; Stanfield, Walsh, Prata, & Evans, 2006):

- National census
- Population surveys
- Public health surveillance
- Vital events monitoring (civil registration)
- Health service records (statistics)
- Resource tracking subsystem

The following four categories are particularly important from the management perspective:

- Routine ongoing data collection (such as immunization records or resource tracking)
- Specific periodic or one-off surveys (such as community health surveys)
- Comparative information from other health systems

Each source has both strengths and weaknesses in terms of accuracy, costs, and relevance to decision processes. A weakness of some management information systems (MISs) is that too much emphasis is placed on routine data collection systems when less frequent data collection would suffice. There is a temptation to institutionalize all data requirements, which can lead to an unwieldy formal MIS and may lead to a devaluing of the overall system.

Users and Providers of Information

Information systems include a number of components, with the information process being the central element. It comprises the following stages (HMN, 2008; Lippeveld, Sauerborn, & Bodart, 2000):

- Identification of information needs
- Collection of relevant data
- Analysis of data to provide information
- Use of information
- Timely feedback to providers of information

Other important elements of information systems include the organizational and systems procedures and rules (e.g., the frequency of reporting) and the availability of resources (e.g., human resources, software and hardware, consumables).

Weaknesses can occur in an MIS at any stage of the information process. In some cases, data collected may not be relevant. For example, a manager seeking to understand why there is low utilization of health care is unlikely to get answers from service-based information. One frequent failing in information systems is a lack of feedback to data providers, which can lead to a downward information spiral in which the accuracy of data collected declines due to poor motivation and, as a result, is used even less.

Sometimes, inappropriate amounts and types of information may be found at different levels in the management system. Figure 13-14 illustrates a common failing in which a similar amount of data flows up all levels of the system; ideally, the higher management levels should operate on increasingly selective amounts of key data.

Analysis of data and its transformation into information also raise issues in terms of the level at which these tasks are best done and by whom. A gen-

eral rule of thumb is the closer to the collection of the data, the better.

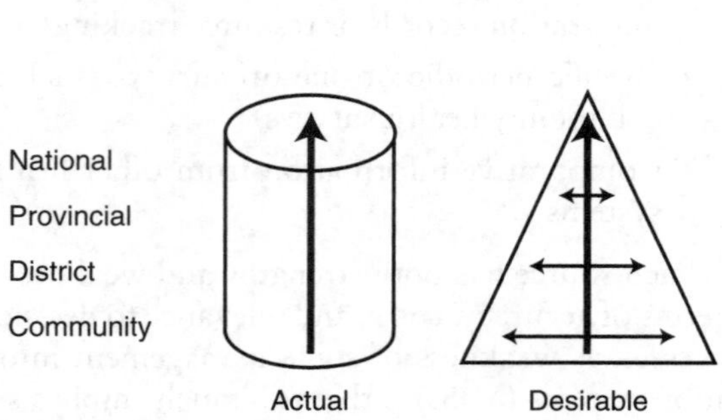

Typically, HMIS represents the mainstream information system, covering all services. However, individual programs and projects may establish vertical information systems (e.g., MCH or Mental Health Information System), which may contribute to fragmentation of the health information system.

Finally, the rapid development of information technology provides both opportunities and challenges in this area.

Management Themes

The previous sections reviewed three key management activities: organizing, planning, and resource management. Permeating these activities are various themes. How these broader concepts are approached will have an impact on the way management is carried out. This section focuses on the following issues, which in many respects also apply to health planning:

- Styles of leadership in management
- Accountability
- Evidence-based management
- Systems approach
- Linking and working together
- Sustainability
- Contradictions, tensions, and change

Styles of Leadership in Management

Many of the issues related to leadership have been mentioned earlier in connection with supervision. Leadership is understood as a process of "providing direction to, and gaining commitment from, partners and staff, facilitating change and achieving better health services through efficient, creative and responsible deployment of people and other resources" (WHO, 2007 p. 1). More than 400 definitions of leadership exist in the literature (King & Cunningham, 1995), and numerous frameworks have been developed for understanding leadership styles and approaches. Examples include a four-way typology of leadership styles denoting the distinction between high and low degrees of political and business orientations (Goodwin, 2000) as well as the various underlying theories of leadership (King & Cunningham, 1995). One framework of particular relevance to management is based on the distinction between the two broad leadership styles: *transformational leadership*,

Figure 13-14 Data Flow.
Source: R. G. Wilson, B. F. Echols, J. H. Bryant, and A. Abrantes (Eds.), *Management Information Systems and Microcomputers in Primary Health Care* (Geneva, Switzerland: Aga Khan Foundation, 1988). Reprinted with permission.

which inspires and motivates followers, and *transactional leadership*, which is based more on reinforcement and exchanges (Aarons, 2006; Hater & Bass, 1988; Stordeur, Vandenberghe, & D'hoore, 2000).

Table 13-16 presents one view of the functions of a leader. How managers practice effective leadership will depend on various factors. Personal qualities are important—for example, one would expect a good leader to show personal understanding, confidence, and principled conduct. These personal qualities are difficult to be precise about and measure. Styles of leadership are also important. They can be viewed as varying, for example, from authoritarian to democratic, and from technically based to more personal-based leadership. However, leadership style needs to be adapted to the circumstances in which it is practiced, including the nature of the task. For example, problems with open-ended solutions may require a more flexible leadership style than more closed or finite problems; problems requiring immediate solution may lead to a tighter style of leadership.

The category of staff over which leadership is exercised is also important. As noted earlier in this chapter, Hersey, Blanchard, and LaMonica (1978) identified task and relationship behavior as key variables of leadership activities. Four combinations of these variables have been identified related to the maturity of staff: "capacity to set high but attainable goals (achievement–motivation), willingness to take responsibility, and the education and the experience of an individual or group." Managers adapt their style of supervision according to the level of maturity of their staff. For example, staff with a low level of maturity need a high level of task leadership exercised over them. As the maturity of the staff increases, the level of task leadership can decrease and relationship behavior can increase.

Table 13-16	Functions of a Leader

- Structuring the situation: making it clear where the group is going and what has to be done
- Controlling group behavior: creating and enforcing appropriate rules for guiding the behavior of group members
- Speaking for the group: sensing and articulating (both internally and externally) the objectives and feelings of the group
- Helping the group achieve its goals and potential: mobilizing and coordinating group resources and decision making

Sources: Coleman (1969), as quoted in Smith et al., 1982.

The various styles of leadership in management are outlined in the following subsections. Note that these styles are not mutually exclusive, but rather can coexist within a single organization.

Proactive

A proactive approach reflects a difference between management and administration and lies at the heart of the pursuit of objectives. When this style is applied, management performance should not be measured based on adherence to rules and regulations, as in administration, but rather on the extent of movement toward objectives. Such movement requires a proactive approach and reflects the ability to predict constraints and new opportunities, influence the environment, develop coalitions of support, foresee future problems and take early preventive action, and monitor performance so as to take corrective action.

There is a potential danger that managers' performance may be (perceived to be) judged on their proactive appearance. This circumstance can lead to shows of being proactive, such as the appearance of haste, workaholic behavior, and constant change. In some contexts, the necessity to demonstrate a proactive approach may lead to "change for change's sake," with little consideration of the underlying rationale. This is not good management.

Risk Taking

Risk taking reflects another important difference between administration and management. It expresses the inventiveness of managers, reflecting an approach that does not accept that existing ways of doing things are the only way. New methods and approaches involve an element of risk, however, and hence represent danger for managers. There are necessary limits to the extent to which managers should take risks; this point is particularly evident in the field of health. The notion of reasonable and acceptable risk needs to be understood.

How staff performance is managed is also related to risk. For example, if staff are routinely criticized for failure and not praised or rewarded for success, then few staff will be willing to take reasonable and acceptable risks. Effective and supportive communication and supervision, together with the existence of clear and agreed-upon ethical and technical work standards, can create a more conducive environment of acceptable risk taking.

Problem Solving

One function of management is to seek solutions to problems arising from unforeseen changes in circumstances either within the organization or externally. An attribute of good management is the ability to deal creatively with new issues. One danger of paying too much attention to "problems," however, is neglect of future emerging issues at the expense of current fire fighting. Problem-solving management needs to be balanced with a more long-term set of considerations.

Accountability

Accountability refers to "the means by which individuals and organisations report to a recognised authority, or authorities, and are held responsible for their actions" (Edwards & Hulme, 2002, p. 183). Accountability can be interpreted as a value as well as a principle of good governance (Siddiqi et al., 2009; Travis, Egger, Davies, & Mechbal, 2002), and its importance permeates the health system. It is essential to performance management, underlines the seriousness of health and health care and the concern for people's lives, and is crucial to exercising checks and balances on the use of resources. Networks of different (but overlapping) and changing forms of accountability run through the management of the health system, as illustrated in Table 13-17.

Managers need to recognize and respond to each form of accountability. In some cases, they are reporting to authorities; in others, they are themselves the authority. Each form of accountability imposes rights and obligations on the management process. At the same time, individuals involved in management take part in the design of accountability relations and need to balance the network of complex, changing, and overlapping relations. In so doing, they will be influenced by the values in the health system and by demands for new forms of accountability. The PHC approach, for example, puts the onus on community-based accountability, whereas the contemporary reform of health systems toward devolution emphasizes politically devolved forms of accountability. Exhibit 13-7 indicates the thinking outlined in the World Bank's *World Development Report 2004*, which emphasizes more market-based forms of accountability.

Evidence-Based Management

As stressed earlier in this chapter, management differs from administration in that it requires individual initiative rather than reliance on preexisting rules and regulations. The success of a manager in exercising such initiative is based on a combination of factors, including his or her technical skills and his or her judgment. Both of these rely also on the ability of the manager to draw on existing evidence (from HMIS, research, and other sources) in making managerial decisions. Different models have been proposed for utilization of evidence in decision-making processes, including knowledge-driven, problem-solving, inter-

Table 13-17	Different and Changing Forms of Accountability
Form of Accountability	**Commentary**
Managerial	Managerial authority sees subordinates as managerially accountable to the hierarchically superior manager. This perspective is typically expressed in the main line managerial relations in the organizational chart.
Professional	Professions are hierarchically structured, so that junior staff are technically accountable to those higher up on the professional ladder. Members of the profession may also be accountable to a professional body for their actions and behavior.
Political	Political representatives can hold staff accountable for their actions and behavior—for example, under devolution, where health staff are accountable to an elected local council.
Community	Health staff may be formally accountable to the community through mechanisms that monitor areas such as availability of medicines, personal relations with health staff, and punctuality of staff.
User	User accountability differs from the community form in that health staff are accountable to users of a particular service, who could take on similar roles.
Market	Users are viewed as consumers of a particular service, for which they pay. Health staff are accountable to the consumers of the service through the market. Consumers who are dissatisfied with the service may go elsewhere.

Exhibit 13-7	Accountability and the 2004 World Development Report

The *World Development Report* 2004 (World Bank, 2004) recognizes the existence of different forms of accountability and arrangements for service delivery. The most appropriate mix of these arrangements will depend on the nature of politics, the ease of monitoring, and the type and voice of citizens. The report identifies "long" accountability routes, such as through pro-poor politics and an accountable public service. The term "long" reflects the idea that governments will assume the responsibility to finance and regulate provision of services and, therefore, play the role of intermediaries between clients and service providers. Because these features are not always present or effective, "shorter" routes of accountability may sometimes be appropriate, based on the power of clients and their direct relationship with service providers. They could be achieved through such means as increasing choice for clients, using voucher schemes, or increasing competition among providers.

The introduction of these shorter routes has been controversial. Critics point to various disadvantages associated with their use, such as the lack of enough providers to allow for true competition, the impact of payment schemes on access and equity, the asymmetry of information in health care, and the negative impact of competition on collaborative strategies for health.

active, political, tactical, and enlightenment models (Bowen & Zwi, 2005; Hanney, Gonzalez-Block, Buxton, & Kogan, M. (2003). Most health systems comprise a combination of those models.

For the use of evidence to occur, various preconditions need to be met. First, there needs to be an organizational culture that seeks, generates, and accepts the use of evidence in its decision making. A major concern of many organizations relates to their failure to use evidence. This omission may result from either a genuine lack of evidence or a resistance to research-generated evidence that is not perceived as relevant—the "know–do" gap (Campbell, Redman, Jorm, Cooke, Zwi, & Rychetnik, 2009; Hanney et al., 2003). In addition, some of this resistance may be generated by stakeholders with a vested interest in maintaining a particular position that evidence might challenge. Managers have a responsibility to generate an organizational culture that respects such evidence-based approaches.

Second, a level of accuracy of evidence is needed that is appropriate to the decisions being made. As noted earlier, there are clearly costs involved in seeking evidence, and these costs are directly related to the level of validity and accuracy required. A manager needs to request only the minimum level of accuracy necessary for any particular decision.

Third, a manager needs to set up, and adequately resource, information systems that will provide the appropriate evidence.

In the end, we return to the theme of a manager as a practitioner of an art rather than a science. An indefinable quality of a good manager, which in part results from experience, is the ability to sift through information, select the appropriate information, and act appropriately on it. Judgment is the necessary counterpart to good evidence.

Systems Approach

The advantages of the division of labor lead to organizations and health staff adopting specialized tasks. Although understandable, this approach runs the danger of producing fragmentation, narrow perspectives, and inflexible working patterns. In the management process, staff need to complement their own specialized responsibilities with a broader, more flexible approach—that is, with a *systems approach*.

First, embrace of the systems approach means that staff, in addition to their own specialized tasks in management (such as human resources or logistics management), need to adopt a broad range of knowledge, skills, and aptitudes. This wide scope is important for the management process because managers need to combine and use different resources. It is also important in that it allows for more flexible working patterns, allowing staff to be more multifunctional to take into account short-term changes in the organization's work.

Second, it means that staff are clear in relating their own positions in the organization to the overall organizational objectives. Thus the TB manager is not just concerned with a reduction in TB morbidity and mortality, but also with how overall community morbidity and mortality can be reduced. In this case, staff appreciate how their own actions relate to other parts of the organization. Perhaps extra resources for one department or program are taking resources away from an area of greater priority. Or maybe extra staff for a health center located in a high-income area may mean staff not being assigned to health centers in poorer areas. The systems approach means appreciating the opportunity costs of managerial action. The concept of systems thinking is recognized by the WHO Alliance for Health Policy and Systems Research in its flagship publication with identification of 10 steps in the process (De Savigny & Adam, 2009).

Linking and Working Together

The need for more collaboration is a frequent recommendation in management reports. Collaboration, however, remains an elusive feature of management, although attempts have been made to define its different manifestations such as coordination and cooperation (e.g., Wang, Collins, Vergis, Gerein, & Macq, 2007). The forces behind individualism, exclusive group interests, and group interorganizational and intraorganizational conflicts are difficult to overcome. Yet the health system, if it is to provide improved health care, needs to push collaborative strategies to the front of managerial action. Health staff, in their various organizations, need to work together. This includes the development of integrated management of patient care, team approaches within an organization, interdepartmental cooperation, public–private partnerships, and interorganizational and intersectoral linkages.

The importance of working together through a multisectoral approach has long been advocated. Health depends on a wide range of non-healthcare factors. The challenge for management is to devise approaches, actions, mechanisms, structures, and attitudes that can lead to greater ability of healthcare personnel to work together. The following subsections set out key strategies to realize this goal.

Coordinating

Coordination involves two or more units agreeing on joint objectives, dedicating resources, and developing a joint organization and program (Rogers & Whetten, 1982). For example, educational and healthcare organizations might develop a joint program for control of sexually transmitted diseases and the use of condoms in communities.

Cooperating

Cooperation occurs when two or more organizations keep their own separate but compatible objectives and agree to help each other when possible and, at the least, to avoid actions that would hinder the other organization in achieving its objectives (Rogers & Whetten, 1982). For example, health and agricultural organizations might agree to support the cultivation of subsistence crops and to protect fish-bearing rivers to ensure adequate nutrition of rural workers.

Community Supporting

Communities can also view needs from a more integrated perspective than that of the public sector. In this case, health and health-related government organizations might support policies designed to strengthen community involvement in decision making and planning. In turn, this endeavor would lead to more community-based demands and support for integrated action by the public sector.

Nesting

Nesting involves locating or allocating resources or linking to initiatives in other organizations that support a multisectoral approach (Wang et al., 2007). For example, the MOH might strategically support initiatives of a multisectoral character in local governments, community associations, and NGOs by locating or nesting support to strategic points in these locations. In return for action of a multisectoral nature, these bodies would receive resources and technical support.

Advocating

The MOH takes on the role of advocating for a health perspective to be used across the various sectors of the public sector—for example, through control over tobacco consumption, the use of car seat belts and motorcycle helmets, and elimination of fire hazards. Fulfilling this role requires, among other things, that the MOH takes on the challenge of intellectual policy leadership for health; effectively disseminates research on the causes of ill health and policy analysis on new initiatives; creates a dialogue concerning health and compatible social, political, and economic objectives; participates in policy forums throughout the different sectors; and develops a wide network of links with policy makers from other sectors.

Regulating

As discussed in Chapter 12, the MOH has authority to ensure compliance from other individuals and organizations. A particular challenge arises from the significant growth of the private sector, as doubts often arise about its contribution toward addressing health inequalities in many low- and middle-income countries. As an extension of the examples given in the prior discussion of advocacy, the MOH and other health-related organizations may be invested with legitimate regulatory authority to demand certain behaviors leading to health improvement. This role requires the development of legal expertise within the MOH, the focus of regulatory action on health objectives, the creation of regulatory mechanisms to require certain behavior, and the development of a sustainable administrative structure to implement regulations. As in the case of advocacy, it requires a proactive stance in relation to health, including willingness to develop a dialogue and intellectual leadership geared toward meeting health objectives. At the same time, this role needs to rest on a political commitment to back up the regulatory authority. Having said this, a wide range of constraints have the potential to limit the capacity of regulatory authorities, such as a lack of state legitimacy; a shortage of resources for regulation, such as trained inspectors; and political capture of the regulatory authority by vested interests.

Shifting Authority Upward or Downward

Authority for setting a cross-cutting strategic direction can be shifted upward in the hierarchy of government, moving above the organizational and sectoral divisions. A powerful cross-governmental commission for social development involving related ministries, for example, could provide multisectoral decision making and national planning and resource allocation.

Authority can also be shifted downward to multifunctional devolved units at the local level. As a form of decentralization, devolution opens up the potential for a multisectoral approach between healthcare systems and other departments such as education and social services, although the divisions between departments within local government can still constitute strong constraints.

Developing Collaborative Skills and Techniques

Collaborative skills and techniques need to be fostered among staff to develop collaboration.

- Trust is an essential component of effective collaboration, although it is difficult to develop. Hudson and associates (1999) suggest that organizations seeking to build trust calculate the risk involved in trusting and begin with small ventures to build up confidence; keep to "principled conduct"; and develop personal and more stable relations.

- Support has to be given to those persons in the organization responsible for interorganizational collaboration (Hudson et al., 1999; Hunter, 1990). Particular skills and tensions are associated with occupying these roles, and staff require strong support to carry them out. A particular problem can be that of dual accountability—that is, the situation in which health staff owe allegiance both to their parent

organization and to any new coordinating body (Hudson et al., 1999).

- Effective collaboration must be based on broad ownership in all the agencies concerned. It cannot be based solely on agreements made by top managers, but rather requires a more generalized ownership in the agencies concerned.

- Organizational learning (Hardy, Turrell, & Wistow, 1992) is important. Organizations have to learn from the process of collaboration for future ventures.

Management Systems

Collaboration can be built into the management systems of organizations related to how they use resources. Agreements on consultation and use of information, for example, could be integrated into the system of district health planning and other sector planning. Information systems can also take on a multisectoral character (de Kadt, 1988).

Contracting

Contracts between organizations can be a useful means for developing collaboration.[12] A contract is "an agreement between one or more economic agents through which they undertake to assume or relinquish, do or not do, certain things. A contract is therefore a voluntary alliance of independent parties" (Perrot, Carrin, & Sergent, 1997, p. 17). The existence of a contract assumes some form of separation between the purchaser or commissioner (who has the funds and is the prime agent for determining the needs to be met by the contract) and the provider. The distinction between the two agents is "a contract in which one person (the principal) employs another (the agent) to carry out on his behalf a given task, whereby a degree of decision-making power is delegated to the agent" (Perrot et al., 1997, p. 26). As shown in Figure 13-15, this relationship involves a commissioning body or purchaser, the contract, and the provider. The contract itself can include issues relating to services, object, and payment, and can take place in a competitive or noncompetitive environment.

---

[12] The sections on contracting and sustainability draw on and reproduce parts of a research report (Collins & Green, 2002) written by two of the authors for a European Union–supported work on contracting and primary care in Central America (Contract ICA4-CT-2001-10011). The European Union holds no responsibility for the content, while the authors take full responsibility for the content reproduced.

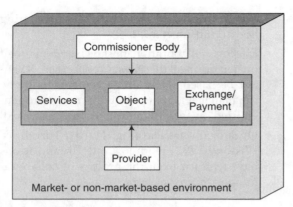

Figure 13-15 Elements in Contracting.

The elements involved in the contracting process suggest that variations in these components can lead to a number of different contractual forms (Table 13-18). The different types of contracting may be appropriate to different environments.

For example, one can distinguish between a time-based and lump-sum nature of payments in contracts. Walsh (1995) distinguishes between performance-based contracts and methods-based contracts in addition to sanction-based contracts and cooperative contracts. Flynn (1997, p. 141) differentiates an obligational contracting relationship from an adversarial contracting relationship: In the former, "the two parties trust each other, work together for mutual benefit, share risk and do things for each other which go beyond the details of the contract"; in the latter, the relationship "is based on low trust, the expectation that each side wishes to gain at the expense of the other and contracts are used to protect each side from the other."

Palmer (2000, p. 823) highlights an existing distinction between classical contracts ("discrete transactions between people who will never see each other again"), neoclassical contracts ("less discrete and therefore contain techniques for flexibility within the terms of the contract, such as third party determination of performance"), and relational contracts (the terms of the contract are not the key element; rather, the whole relationship between the parties over time is key, and importance is put on harmony and keeping the relationship). She suggests that contracting in low- to middle-income countries is often justified in terms of classical and neoclassical contracting, despite the possibility that relational contracting might well be more promising.

Sustainability

An important theme in management is that of the sustainability of services. Lafond (1995, p. 63) sees sustainability as "the capacity of the health sector to function effectively over time, with a minimum of external input." The mention of "external input" is of particular relevance to poor countries that are heavily reliant on funds from international agencies. Olsen's (1998) definition emphasizes the longer term: "A health service is sustainable when operated by an organisational system with the long-term ability to mobilize and allocate sufficient and appropriate resources (manpower, technology, information and finance) for activities that meet individual or public health needs/demands" (p. 289).

The relevance of sustainability to health management rests on two key points. First, health care is rarely time limited. Disease control, for example, requires continued interventions over time. The continuity of action in TB control is important to limit the spread of disease. In particular, continued medicine

Table 13-18	Variables in the Analysis of Contracting Primary Care Services
Variable	**Comment**
Object of the contract	Ranging from type of service to geographic coverage
Type of contracting	Ranging from formal and legalistic to more flexible contracting
Type of commissioner	Could include central or decentralized agencies with different degrees of organizational autonomy and financing (e.g., taxes, insurance systems, fee-based)
Type of provider	Public-sector organization, NGO, or private for-profit organization, each with its own variations
Type of exchange or payment	Based on a definition of services and payment system, which could be, for example, performance-based
Market or non-market based	Contracts can be based on competitive tendering, with services provided in a market environment, or without competitive tendering, with service providers operating in a noncompetitive environment

supply and continued treatment are important to avoid drug-resistant TB.

Second, the importance of sustainability draws on four problematic and interrelated features of the public sector, particularly in low- and middle-income countries:

- The extremely limited resource base of poor societies, coupled with the limited authority of national governments, leads to intense resource scarcity in the public sector. It is this limitation that underlies the problem of maintaining a secure and constant flow of resources to finance government programs and produces high levels of dependence on international aid.

- The historical focus of international aid to low- and middle-income countries on capital investment, with less support being given to recurrent expenditure, leads to difficult problems of maintaining programs of action. This issue is compounded by the vertical and cyclical nature of foreign aid projects.

- Corruption has a marked impact on the continuity and effectiveness of government given the high level of resource scarcity.

- High staff turnover may lead to limited effectiveness and reduced sustainability of government programs (Collins et al., 2000).

Sustainability is not actually an end in itself, but rather a means to a wider end. It is colored by the policy objectives held by the stakeholders. This influence introduces two possibilities:

- *Appropriate sustainability* occurs when a particular activity has continuity over time and has outputs that continue to be valued. For example, policy objectives typically may consist of the achievement of improved and equitable health care, with certain types of action essential to achieve this outcome.

- *Inappropriate sustainability* occurs when programs and activities need to be stopped at a particular point, but continue. For example, as the incidence of a particular health problem declines, related interventions may need to be reduced. Smallpox vaccination is a classic example.

Of course, what is seen as appropriate sustainability by one stakeholder may be viewed as inappropriate by another. Stakeholders in a particular government activity will have different interpretations of a program, largely determined by how it affects their own particular interests. Table 13-19 illustrates the possible interests of different stakeholders in sustainability.

To capture the determining features of sustainability, the analysis of the health system needs to recognize the broad-ranging character of sustainability and its multiple determinants. The factors influencing sustainability not only will be wide ranging, but also will vary between situations.

Contradictions, Tensions, and Change

The introduction to this chapter briefly acknowledged the political character of health management. In itself, this factor places the health management process at the center of contradictions, tensions, and change. The importance of context and its impact on management were then examined. Three areas of tension are of particular relevance to the contemporary management process in low- and middle-income countries. First, the contradiction between public interest and private gain may be manifested through corruption, patronage, professional self-interest, and corporate gain. Second, many healthcare systems are undergoing change along pro-market and neoliberal lines, which have tended to respond more to an internationally driven ideology than the health needs of poor communities. For the manager, this shift places

Table 13-19	Stakeholders' Potential Interests in Sustainability
Stakeholder	**Potential Interests in Sustainability**
Donors	Shifting resource dependence away from donors and increasing local contributions
Ministry of health	Ensuring regularity of donor resources and/or shifting resource dependence away from donors and increasing local contributions
Staff	Ensuring continuity in employment and career progression
Users	Ensuring continuity of improved service delivery
Nonusers	Expansion of service on a regular basis to cover their needs
Private-sector contractors	Shift to public financing and private provision under favorable conditions

an onus on change management and raises issues of mediating between competing values, using evidence-informed decision making to direct change, programming change on the basis of logical sequencing, and consulting and negotiating with affected interests (Green & Collins, 2003). Third, managers sometimes need to reconcile the organizational objectives with broader system goals in the translation of policies into operational plans—for example, national health programs may be based on country-level averages of morbidity and mortality and, therefore, do not always fully reflect the health needs of each specific district.

The challenge for the management process is how to deal with these contradictions, which is the focus of the concluding section.

Conclusion and Challenges for Managers

Management is fundamentally concerned with the relationship between resources and objectives. It deals with scarce resources, operates within various technical and political constraints, is strongly influenced by values, can operate in a political manner, and has a strong interrelationship with the social, political, economic, and international context. Three interrelated functions of management have been emphasized in this chapter: planning, organizing, and management of resources. Themes permeating these management activities have been summarized as styles of management; accountability; systems approach; linking and working together; sustainability; and contradictions, tensions, and change.

The future direction of health management in low- and middle-income countries is far from clear. Certainly, health systems development will require significant improvements in health management and planning. However, such a process cannot be divorced from some challenging questions.

What Is the Future of Public-Sector Management?

Criticisms of the state and public-sector management have ranged from simple market orthodoxy to a more nuanced approach that recognizes its needs and social responsibilities. However, a prevailing portrayal of corruption, bureaucratic expansion, administrative fragmentation, and patronage has made it easy for many to levy such criticisms. Nevertheless, two points need to be recognized.

First, public-sector management operates in a context of low funding, intense need, and unstable environment. We return to this point later in this section.

Second, there is a need to recognize the specific characteristics of public-sector management. Public-

sector and private-sector management have much to learn from each other. Yet all good learning takes into account specific circumstances and requirements in an effort to assess appropriateness (Stewart & Ranson, 1994). The future development of management, and the values that underpin it, need to take into account three factors:[13]

- The public sector seeks to meet public needs and interests, although different social and political groups have different interpretations of these needs and interest. This demand requires open and transparent participation and negotiation regarding the definition of public interest. Public-sector bodies need to define their objectives in relation to those public needs and interests.

- The multifaceted nature of public needs means that public-sector organizations can achieve their objectives only by engaging in collaborative strategies with other bodies, whether public-sector organizations, NGOs, or private for-profit organizations. It also requires collaborative strategies between the public sector and communities.

- Social needs are not ephemeral in nature but rather are long-term issues, and they require public-sector management to recognize their persistence. Planning, sustainability, continuity of service provision, capacity building, systems development, and planning for professional development are among some of the key features of public management.

Are Managers Being Asked to Manage the Unmanageable?

That managers have to deal with contradictions, tensions, and change is nothing new. The immensity of these challenges becomes evident as we consider the paucity of resources available and the scale of the health needs stressed elsewhere in this book. In dealing with these challenges, there is a gap, which varies from one country to another, between the existing capacity of management to meet those challenges and the potential that exists to do so through management strengthening. It is a matter of concern, however, that an already difficult situation is being made worse through sharpening contradictions and weakened means to respond.

---

[13] These three points draw on the work of Stewart and Ranson (1994).

First, the tension between public interests and private gain is increasing as a result of the growth of public–private partnerships and the trend toward self-funding public bodies. Second, the public sector faces threats because of the poor rewards for public servants, the downgrading of the role of the public sector, and a hollowing out of its rationale and process. The culture of individualism, internal markets, and self-funding of health units and programs all stand in opposition to the public sector's perspective of social interests, collaborative strategy, longer-term framework, and public ethos. In the words of Flynn (1997, p. 232):

> What is needed is a change in attitude towards the public sector. If spending could be based on need and a realistic assessment of what is affordable rather than a constant state of crisis and if management arrangements could be based less on distrust and fear and more on co-operation, then public services could make a valuable contribution to the economic health and quality of life of society.

What Are the Challenges Facing Public-Sector Health Managers?

This chapter has given what can only be considered a brief overview of the key issues that a manager working in the public health sector needs to address. Management, we have argued, is a key, but often undervalued, component of a health system. As managers seek to establish the structures, resources, and processes necessary for meeting the Millennium Development Goals, what are the emerging challenges that they will face?

First, public health managers will need to grapple with the increasingly diverse structures of the health system and new approaches to funding. The ever-more-intertwined public and private institutional complexity and changing relations between the center and the local levels, combined with new funding flows through SWAps and public–private partnerships, suggest that managers need to seek new ways to meet these challenges.

Second, although low- and middle-income countries continue to face major financial resource constraints, the emerging crisis of the health professional gap must be seen, for many countries, as an even greater constraint. This trend, coupled with the low staff morale in many health systems, presents major challenges for managers, who will need to seek new ways to cope with shortages of healthcare workers.

Third, managers face an increasingly vocal and empowered citizenry, conscious of a rights agenda.

This trend will—and rightly so—place greater demands for accountability on the part of the health system; managers will represent the front line in meeting this demand.

Fourth, new technology is continually emerging and being increasingly used in various aspects of health systems, including provision of health services, planning, and management. Its utility is often counterbalanced by the high costs of the new technology, with managers being called upon to respond to and manage the potential of the technology.

The nature, and indeed excitement, of management, lies in identifying and responding to such emerging challenges. Management as a scientific art must continuously develop new approaches and tools to accomplish this feat. It is hoped this chapter has provided a platform from which such new approaches can be built.

• • • Discussion Questions

1. Which approaches to health management exist in a country known to you? Which factors affect any differences in approaches to health management at different levels of the country's health system, and why?

2. Consider which kind of health planning takes place in a country known to you. How successful is it? Which major health needs exist that are not met? Can you identify an expenditure that is of lower priority than these unmet identified needs? How could health planning be improved?

3. How are healthcare priorities decided within the health sector of a country known to you? What is the role of the manager in this process?

4. Describe the financial management system of a country known to you. How are resources allocated to lower levels? Are there any differences in allocation between different types of resources? How is resource allocation linked to the planning process?

5. Which system of decentralization exists in your country? What are its strengths and weaknesses for the health sector?

6. Which practical steps could be taken to improve intersectoral collaboration for health in your country?

7. Consider the way in which local-level health staff are managed. Which steps could be taken to improve the way in which these staff are managed?

• • • References

Aarons, G. A. (2006). Transformational and transactional leadership: Association with attitudes toward evidence-based practice. *Psychiatric Services*, 57(8), 1162–1169.

Abramson, W. B. (2001). Monitoring and evaluation of contracts for health service delivery in Costa Rica. *Health Policy and Planning*, 16(4), 404–411.

Ahmed, A. M., Mung'Ong'O, E., & Massawe, E. (1991). Tackling obstacles to health care delivery at district level. *World Health Forum*, 12(4), 483–489.

Alimo-Metcalfe, B. (1994, October 20). The poverty of PRP. *Health Services Journal*, 22–23.

Aminu, J. (1985). Teaming up for better health. *Social Science and Medicine*, 21(12), 1349–1353.

Anderson, S., Huss, R., Summers, R., & Wiedenmayer, K. (2004). *Managing pharmaceuticals in international health*. Basel: Birkhaeuser Verlag.

Arnesen, T., & Kapiriri, L. (2004) Can the value choices in DALYs influence global priority-setting? *Health Policy*, 70(2), 137–149.

Arredondo, A., Orozco, E., & De Icaza, E. (2005). Evidence on weaknesses and strengths from health financing after decentralization: Lessons from Latin American countries. *International Journal of Health Planning and Management*, 20(2), 181–204.

Atkinson, S., Medeiros, R. L., Oliveira, P. H., & de Almeida, R. D. (2000). Going down to the local: Incorporating social organisation and political culture into assessments of decentralised health care. *Social Science and Medicine*, 51, 619–636.

Bacal, R. (1999). *Performance management*. New York: McGraw-Hill.

Barker, C., & Green, A. (1996). Opening the debate on DALYs. *Health Policy and Planning*, 11(2), 179–183.

Bednarz, D. (2010). Impacts of the economic crisis on public health, part II: Paradigms and the right questions. *Energy Bulletin*. Retrieved from http://www.energybulletin.net/node/52172

Benjamin, S., Ahmed, A. A., & Al-Darazi, F. (1997). Management in the ministry of health: What are the vital signs? *World Hospitals and Health Services*, 33(1), 2–12.

Bennett, S., Dakpallah, G., Garner, P., Gilson, L., Nittayaramphong, S., Zurita, B., & Zwi, A. (1994). Carrot and stick: State mechanisms to influence private provider behaviour. *Health Policy and Planning*, 9(1), 1–13.

Bishai, D., Niessen, L. W., & Shrestha, M. (2002). Local governance and community financing of primary care: Evidence from Nepal. *Health Policy and Planning*, 17(2), 202–206.

Bossert, T. (1998). Analysing the decentralisation of health systems in developing countries: Decision space, innovation and performance. *Social Science and Medicine*, 47(10), 1513–1527.

Bossert, T. J., & Beauvais, J. C. (2002). Decentralisation of health systems in Ghana, Zambia, Uganda and the Philippines: A comparative analysis of decision space. *Social Science and Medicine*, 17(1), 14–31.

Bowen, S., & Zwi, A. B. (2005) Pathways to "evidence-informed" policy and practice: A framework for action. *PLoS Medicine*, 2(7), e166.

Brown, W., & Walsh, J. (1994). *Managing pay in Britain*. In K. Sisson (Ed.), *Personnel management: A comprehensive guide to theory and practice in Britain* (pp. 437–464). Oxford, UK: Blackwell Business.

Brugha, R., & Varvasovszky, Z. (2000). Stakeholder analysis: A review. *Health Policy and Planning*, 15(3), 239–246.

Buchan, J. (2004). What difference does ("good") HRM make? *Human Resources for Health*, 2, 6.

Buse, K., & Harmer, A. M. (2007). Seven habits of highly effective global public–private health partnerships: Practice and potential. *Social Science & Medicine*, 64(2), 259–271.

Campbell, M., & Sham, Z. A. (1995). Sudan: Situational analysis of maternal health in Bara District, North Kordofan. *World Health Statistics Quarterly*, 48, 60–66.

Campbell, D., Redman, S., Jorm, L., Cooke, M., Zwi, A., & Rychetnik, L. (2009). Increasing the use of evidence in health policy: Practice and views of policy makers and researchers. *Australia and New Zealand Health Policy*, 6(1), 21.

Carr-Hill, R. (1989). Allocating resources for health care: RAWP is dead—long live RAWP. *Health Policy*, 13(2), 144.

Cassels, A., & Janovsky, K. (1995). *Strengthening health management in districts and provinces*. Geneva, Switzerland: World Health Organization.

Cheema, G. S., & Rondinelli, D. A. (Eds.). (1983). *Decentralisation and development*. Beverly Hills, CA: Sage.

Child, J. (1984). *Organization: A guide to problems and practice*. London: Harper and Row.

Cole, G. A. (1988). *Personnel management: Theory and practice*. London: DP Publications.

Collins, C. (1994). *Management and organisation of developing health systems*. Oxford, UK: Oxford University Press.

Collins, C., & Green, A. (2002). *Public contracting of private providers for primary health care services: Context, sustainability and accountability*. CAPUBPRUV, UE ICA4CT-2001-10011.

Collins, C. D., Myers, G., & Nicholson, N. (1992). A successful transport scenario for the health sector in developing countries. *World Hospitals*, 28(3), 9–14.

Collins, C., Omar, M., & Hurst, K. (2000). Staff transfer and management in the government health sector in Balochistan, Pakistan: Problems and context. *Public Administration and Development*, 20, 207–220.

de Kadt, E. (1988). Making health policy management intersectoral: Issues of information analysis and use in less developed countries. *Social Science and Medicine*, 29(4), 503–514.

De Savigny, D., & Adam, T. (Eds.). (2009). *Systems thinking for health systems strengthening*. Geneva, Switzerland: Alliance for Health Policy and Systems Research, World Health Organization.

Department of Health and Developmental Social Welfare (DHDSW). (1999). *Transport management manual*. South Africa: DHDSW, Save the Children (UK), & Transaid.

Dieleman, M., Cuong, P. V., Anh, L. V., & Martineau, T. (2003). Identifying factors for job motivation of rural health workers in North Viet Nam. *Human Resources for Health*, 1, 10.

Edwards, M., & Hulme, D. (2002). NGO performance and accountability: Introduction and overview. In M. Edwards & A. Fowler (Eds.), *The Earthscan reader on NGO management* (pp. 187–203). London: Earthscan.

Eichler, H.-G., Kong, S. X., Gerth, W. C., Mavros, P., & Jönsson, B. (2004). Use of cost-effectiveness analysis in health-care resource allocation decision-making: How are cost-effectiveness thresholds expected to emerge? *Value Health*, 7, 518–528.

Finlay, L. (2000). Safe haven and battleground: Collaboration and conflict within the treatment team. In C. Davies, L. Finlay, & A. Bullman (Eds.), *Changing practice in health and social care* (pp. 155–162). London: Sage.

Firth-Cozens, J. (1992). Building teams for effective audit. *Quality in Care*, 1, 252–255.

Flahault, D., Piot, M., & Franklin, A. (1988). *Supervision of health personnel at district level*. Geneva, Switzerland: World Health Organization.

Flynn, N. (1997). *Public sector management* (3rd ed.). London: Harvester Wheatsheaf.

French, D., & Saward, H. (1983). *A dictionary of management*. London: Pan.

Frost, L. J., & Reich, M. R. (2008). *Access: How do good health technologies get to poor people in poor countries?* Cambridge, MA: Harvard University Press.

Fryatt, R., Mills, A., & Nordstrom, A. (2010). Financing of health systems to achieve the health Millennium Development Goals in low-income countries. *Lancet*, 375(9712), 419–426.

Goodwin, N. (2000). Leadership and the UK health service. *Health Policy*, 51(1), 49–60.

Green, A. (2007). *An introduction to health planning in developing health systems* (3rd ed.). Oxford, UK: Oxford University Press.

Green, A., Ali, B., Naeem, A., & Ross, D. (2000). The allocation and budgetary mechanisms for decentralized health systems: Experiences from Balochistan, Pakistan. *Bulletin of the World Health Organization, 78*(8), 1024–1035.

Green, A., & Collins, C. (2003). Health systems in developing countries: Public sector managers and the management of contradiction and change. *International Journal of Health Planning and Management, 18,* 67–78.

Green, A. T., & Mirzoev, T. N. (2008) Planning for public health policy. In K. Heggenhougen & S. Quah (Eds.), *International encyclopedia of public health.* (pp. 121–132). San Diego, CA: Academic Press.

Grindle, M. S. (1997). Divergent cultures? When public organisations perform well in developing countries. *World Development, 25*(4), 481–495.

Hanney, S., Gonzalez-Block, M., Buxton, M., & Kogan, M. (2003). The utilisation of health research in policy-making: Concepts, examples and methods of assessment. *Health Research Policy and Systems, 1*(1), 2.

Hardy, B., Turrell, A., & Wistow, G. (1992). *Innovation in community care management: Minimising vulnerability.* Aldershot, UK: Avebury.

Hater, J. J., & Bass, B. M. (1988). Superiors' evaluations and subordinates' perceptions of transformational and transactional leadership. *Journal of Applied Psychology, 73,* 695–702.

Health Metrics Network (HMN). (2008). *Framework and standards for country health information systems* (2nd ed.). Geneva, Switzerland: HMN, World Health Organization.

Henderson, L., & Tulloch, J. (2008). Incentives for retaining and motivating health workers in Pacific and Asian countries. *Human Resources for Health, 6*(1), 18.

Hersey, P., Blanchard, K. H., & LaMonica, E. L. (1978). A situational response to supervision: Leadership theory and the supervising nurse. In Rackich J. S., & Darr K., (Eds.), *Hospital organization and management: Text and readings* (pp.184–191). New York: Spectrum.

Herzberg, F., Mausner, B., & Snyderman, B. B. (1959). *The motivation to work.* New York: John Wiley & Sons.

Hudson, B., Hardy, B., Henwood, M., & Wistow, G. (1999). In pursuit of inter-agency collaboration in the public sector: What is the contribution of theory and research? *Public Management, 1*(2), 235–260.

Hunter, D. (1990). "Managing the cracks": Management development for health care interfaces. *International Journal of Health Care Planning and Management, 5,* 7–14.

Hutubessy, R., Chisholm, D., Edejer, T., & World Health Organization (WHO). (2003). Generalized cost-effectiveness analysis for national-level priority-setting in the health sector. *Cost Effectiveness and Resource Allocation, 1,* 8.

International Medical Products Anti-Counterfeiting Taskforce (IMPACT). (2010). Retrieved from http://www.who.int/impact/about/en/

Jackson, A. C., & Donovan, F. (1999). *Managing to survive: Managerial practice in not-for-profit organisations.* Buckingham, UK: Open University Press.

Jacobson, M. L., Labbok, M. H., Murage, A. N., & Parker, R. (1987). Individual and group supervision of community health workers: A comparison. *Journal of Health Administration Education, 5*(1), 83–94.

Janis, I. L. (1972). *Victims of groupthink.* Boston: Houghton-Mifflin.

Kapiriri, L., Norheim, O. F., & Heggenhougen, K. (2003). Using burden of disease information for health planning in developing countries: The experience from Uganda. *Social Science & Medicine, 56*(12), 2433–2441.

Karki, D., Mirzoev, T., Green, A., Newell, J., & Baral, S. (2007). Costs of a successful public–private partnership for TB control in an urban setting in Nepal. *BMC Public Health, 7*(1), 84.

Keeling, D. (1972). *Management in government.* London: Allen & Unwin.

Kempner, T. (Ed.). (1980). *A handbook of management*. Harmondsworth, UK: Penguin.

Kerrigan, J. E., & Luke, J. S. (1987). *Management training strategies for developing countries*. Boulder, CO: Lynne Rienner Publishers.

Kessler, I. (1994). Performance pay. In K. Sisson (Ed.), *Personnel management: A comprehensive guide to theory and practice in Britain* (pp. 465–494). Oxford, UK: Blackwell Business.

King, K., & Cunningham, G. (1995). Leadership in nursing: More than one way. *Nursing Standard*, *10*(12–14), 3–14.

Kolb, D. A. (1984). *Experimental learning: Experience as a source of learning and development*. Upper Saddle River, NJ: Prentice Hall.

Kolehmainen-Aitken, R.-L. (2004). Decentralisation's impact on the health workforce: Perspectives of managers, workers and national leaders. *Human Resources for Health*, *2*, 5.

Kolehmainen-Aitken, R.-L., & Shipp, P. (1990). "Indicators of staffing need": Assessing health staffing and equity in Papua New Guinea. *Health Policy and Planning*, *5*(2), 167–176.

Kumaranayake, L. (1997). The role of regulation: Influencing private sector activity within health sector reform. *Journal of International Development*, *9*(4), 641–649.

Kumaranayake, L., Lake, S., Mujinja, P., Hongoro, C. & Mpembeni, R. (2000). How do countries regulate the health sector? Evidence from Tanzania and Zimbabwe. *Health Policy and Planning*, *15*(4), 357-367.

Lafond, A. K. (1995). Improving the quality of investment in health: Lessons on sustainability. *Health Policy and Planning*, *10*, 63–76.

Lakshminarayanan, R. (2003). Decentralisation and its implications for reproductive health: The Philippines experience. *Reproductive Health Matters*, *11*(21), 96–107.

Lippeveld, T., Sauerborn, R., & Bodart, C. (2000). *Design and implementation of health information systems*. Geneva, Switzerland: World Health Organization

Loevinsohn, B. P., Guerrero, E. T., & Gregorio, S. P. (1995). Improving primary health care through systematic supervision: A controlled field trial. *Health Policy and Planning*, *10*(2), 144–153.

MacKenzie, I., Thompson, S., Smith, A., Bal, I. S., & Hatcher, J. (1995). Practical advice on field studies into hearing impairment in a developing country. *Tropical Doctor*, *25*(1), 25–28.

Management Sciences for Health (MSH). (2003). *Supervision guidelines*. Boston: Author. Retrieved May 18, 2009, from http://erc.msh.org/documents/hr/HCD9a.doc

Management Sciences for Health (MSH) & World Health Organization (WHO). (1997). *Managing drug supply* (2nd ed.). West Hartford, CT: Kumarian Press.

Martin, D., & Singer, P. (2003). A strategy to improve priority setting in health care institutions. *Health Care Analysis*, *11*, 59–68.

Martineau, T., & Martinez, J. (1997). *Human resources in the health sector: Guidelines for appraisal and strategic development (Health and Development Series, Working Paper No. 1)*. Brussels, Belgium: European Commission.

Martinez, J., & Martineau, T. (1998). Rethinking human resources: An agenda for the millennium. *Health Policy and Planning*, *13*(4), 345–358.

McIntyre, D., & Klugman, B. (2003). The human face of decentralisation and integration of health services: Experiences from South Africa. *Reproductive Health Matters*, *11*(21), 108–119.

McMahon, R., Barton, E., & Piot, M. (1992). *On being in charge: A guide to management in primary health care* (2nd ed.). Geneva, Switzerland: World Health Organization.

McPake, B., & Banda, E. E. N. (1994). Contracting out of health services in developing countries. *Health Policy and Planning*, *9*(1), 25–30.

Mescon, M. H., Albert, M., & Khedouri, F. (1985). *Management: Individual and organisational effectiveness*. New York: Harper and Row.

Mills, A. (1998). To contract or not to contract? Issues for low and middle income countries. *Health Policy and Planning*, *13*(1), 32–40.

Mills, A., & Broomberg, J. (1998). *Experiences of contracting: An overview of the literature (Macroeconomics and Health and Development Theory No. 33)*. Geneva, Switzerland: World Health Organization.

Mills, A., Brugha, R., Hanson, K., & McPake, B. (2002). What can be done about the private health sector in low-income countries? *Bulletin of the World Health Organization*, *80*, 325–330.

Ministry of Health, Ghana. (1993). *Transport management handbook*. Prepared by Save the Children Fund (UK).

Munga, M., & Maestad, O. (2009). Measuring inequalities in the distribution of health workers: The case of Tanzania. *Human Resources for Health*, *7*(1), 4.

Nancholas, S. (1998). How to do or not to do a logical framework. *Health Policy and Planning*, *13*(2), 189–193.

NEPAD Secretariat. (2010). *The impact of financial crisis on health*. Document discussion during Session 4 on the Impact of The Crisis on Health at the 13th Meeting of the Africa Partnership Forum, January 25, 2010, Addis Ababa, Ethiopia.

Noakes, J. (1992, June 18). Team spirit. *Health Service Journal*, 26.

Okonofua, F. E., Abejide, A., & Makanjuola, R. A. (1992). Maternal mortality in Ile-Ife, Nigeria: A study of risk factors. *Studies in Family Planning*, *23*(5), 319–324.

Olsen, I. T. (1998). Sustainability of health care: A framework for analysis. *Health Policy and Planning*, *13*(1), 287–295.

Palmer, M., Leila, A., & Yassin, E. S. (1989). *The Egyptian bureaucracy*. Cairo, Egypt: American University in Cairo Press.

Palmer, N. (2000). The use of private-sector contracts for primary health care: Theory, evidence and lessons for low-income and middle-income countries. *Bulletin of the World Health Organization*, *78*(6), 821–829.

Pearson, M. (2002). *Allocating public resources for health: Developing pro-poor approaches*. London: DFID Health Systems Resource Centre.

Perrot, J., Carrin, G., & Sergent, F. (1997). *The contractual approach: New partnerships for health in developing countries (Macroeconomics, Health and Development Series No. 24)*. Geneva, Switzerland: World Health Organization.

Pheysey, D. C. (1993). *Organizational cultures: Types and transformations*. New York: Routledge.

Reich, M. (1995). The politics of health sector reform in developing countries: Three cases of pharmaceutical policy. *Health Policy*, *32*, 47–77.

Reich, M. R. (Ed.). (2002). *Public–private partnerships for public health*. Cambridge, MA: Harvard University Press.

Robinson, R. (1999) Limits to rationality: Economics, economists and priority setting. *Health Policy*, *49*(1–2), 13–26.

Rogers, D. L., & Whetten, D. A. (1982). *Interorganizational coordination: Theory, research, and implementation*. Ames, IA: Iowa State University Press.

Rondeau, K. V., & Wager, T. H. (2001). Impact of human resource management practices on nursing home performance. *Health Service Management Research*, *14*(3), 192–202.

Rowbottom, R., & Billis, D. (1987). *Organisational design: The work level approach*. Aldershot, UK: Gower.

Schick, A. (1998). Why most developing countries should not try New Zealand's reforms. *World Bank Research Observer*, *13*(1), 123–131.

Schmidt, M. J., Riggar, T. F., Crimando, W., & Bordieri, J. E. (1992). *Staffing for success: A guide for health and human service professionals*. London: Sage.

Siddiqi, S., Masud, T. I., Nishtar, S., Peters, D. H., Sabri, B., Bile, K. M., & Jama, M. A. (2009). Framework for assessing governance of the health system in developing countries: Gateway to good governance. *Health Policy*, *90*(1), 13–25.

Smith, M., Beck, J., Cooper, C., Cox, C., Ottaway, D. & Talbot, R. (1982). *Introducing organisational behaviour*. London: Macmillan Education.

Stanfield, S., Walsh, J., Prata, N., & Evans, T. (2006). Information to improve decision making for health. In D. Jamison, J. Breman, A. Measham, G. Alleyne, M. Claeson, D. Evans, et al. (Eds.), *Disease control priorities in developing countries* (2nd ed.) (pp. 1017–1030). Washington, DC/New York: World Bank & Oxford University Press.

Stead, A., & Leonard, M. C. (1995). Changing to a client-focused quality service through more effective team work. *Health Manpower Management, 21*(4), 23–27.

Stewart, J. (1993). The limitations of government by contract. *Public Money and Management, 13*(3), 7–12.

Stewart, J., & Ranson, S. (1994). Management in the public domain. In D. McKevitt & A. Lawton (Eds.), *Public sector management theory, critique and practice* (pp. 54–70). London: Sage.

Stordeur, S., Vandenberghe, C., & D'hoore, W. (2000). Leadership styles across hierarchical levels in nursing departments. *Nursing Research, 49*(1), 37–43.

Storey, J. (1994). Management development. In K. Sisson (Ed.), *Personnel management: A comprehensive guide to theory and practice in Britain* (pp. 365–396). Oxford, UK: Blackwell Business.

Strike, A. J. (1995). *Human resources in health care: A manager's guide*. Oxford, UK: Blackwell Science.

Szeftel, M. (1998). Misunderstanding African politics: Corruption and the governance agenda. *Review of African Political Economy, 25*, 221–240.

Tesch, R. (1990). *Qualitative research: Analysis types and software tools*. New York: Falmer Press.

Thunhurst, C., & Barker, C. (1999). Using problem structuring methods in strategic planning. *Health Policy and Planning, 14*(2), 127–134.

Transaid. (2001). *Transport management manual*. London: Transaid Worldwide.

Transaid. (2008). Introduction to Transaid's transport management system manual. Draft 3: August 2008. Retrieved from http://www.transaid.org/images/resources/TMS%20Consolidated%20Manual%20Revised%20Aug08.pdf

Trap, B., Todd, C. H., Moore, H., & Laing, R. (2001). The impact of supervision on stock management and adherence to treatment guidelines: A randomised control trial. *Health Policy and Planning, 16*(3), 273–280.

Travis, P., Egger, D., Davies, P., & Mechbal, A. (2002). *Towards better stewardship: Concepts and critical issues*. Geneva, Switzerland: World Health Organization.

Tumwine, J. (1993, March–May). Health centres: Involving the community. *Health Action, 4*, 8.

Walsh, K. (1995). *Public services and market mechanisms: Competition, contracting and the new public management*. London: Macmillan.

Wang, Y., Collins, C., Tang, S., & Martineau, T. (2002). Health system decentralisation and human resources management in low and middle income countries. *Public Administration and Development, 22*, 439–453.

Wang, Y., Collins, C., Vergis, M., Gerein, N., & Macq, J. (2007). HIV/AIDS and TB: Contextual issues and policy choice in programme relationships. *Tropical Medicine & International Health, 12*(2), 183–194.

Weightman, J. (1996). *Managing people in the health service*. London: Institute of Personnel and Development.

Willis-Shattuck, M., Bidwell, P., Thomas, S., Wyness, L., Blaauw, D., & Ditlopo, P. (2008). Motivation and retention of health workers in developing countries: A systematic review. *BMC Health Services Research, 8*(1), 247.

Woelk, G. B. (1994). Primary health care in Zimbabwe: Can it survive? *Social Science and Medicine, 39*(8), 1027–1035.

World Bank. (1993). *World development report 1993: Investing in health*. New York: Oxford University Press.

World Bank. (2004). *World development report 2004: Making services work for poor people*. New York: World Bank & Oxford University Press.

World Health Organization (WHO). (2004). *Developing health management information systems: A practical guide for developing countries*.

Manila, Philippines: Author. Retrieved from http://whqlibdoc.who.int/publications/2004/9290611650.pdf

World Health Organization (WHO). (2006a). *A guide to WHO's role in sector-wide approaches to health development*. Geneva, Switzerland: Author.

World Health Organization (WHO). (2006b). *The world health report 2006: Working together for health*. Geneva, Switzerland: Author.

World Health Organization (WHO). (2007). *Building leadership and management capacity in health*. Geneva, Switzerland: Author.

World Health Organization (WHO). (2010). The WHO prequalification project. Retrieved March 23, 2010, from http://www.who.int/mediacentre/factsheets/fs278/en/index.html

Pharmaceuticals

KARA HANSON, BENJAMIN PALAFOX, STUART ANDERSON, JAVIER GUZMAN, MARY MORAN, RIMA SHRETTA, AND TANA WULIJI

Introduction

Pharmaceuticals are a critical element of the health system. They consume a large share of total health spending, estimated by the World Health Organization (WHO, 2004b) to be 15.2% of the total spent globally on health in 2000 and amounting to $440 billion, and are a potent symbol of effective health system functioning. When medicines and vaccines are not available in health facilities, the confidence of both patients and providers is undermined. Pharmaceuticals also play a vital role in global development, as they are identified as key inputs to a number of the Millennium Development Goals (MDG), including MDG 4 (reduce under-five mortality), MDG 6 (halt progress of malaria and other diseases), and MDG 8 (provide access to affordable essential drugs in low- and middle-income countries).

Yet, according to WHO (2000b), an estimated 30% of the world's population lacks regular access to existing drugs, with this figure rising to more than 50% in the poorest parts of Africa and Asia. Within these populations, it is the poorest socioeconomic groups who disproportionately suffer from a lack of access to existing medicines. Combined with their greater exposure to disease risk, this lack of access contributes to the immense health inequities that persist between the rich and the poor (Victora et al., 2003).

Improving access to pharmaceuticals is, therefore, a global public health priority, as evidenced by the number of international health movements that have included it as part of their central goals. Among these are the Bamako Initiative of 1987, which committed to implementing strategies to improve the availability of essential medicines across sub-Saharan

Africa; the Abuja Declaration from the 2000 African Summit on Roll Back Malaria, which set a target of providing prompt access to effective treatment to at least 60% of those persons suffering from malaria; the Doha Declaration on the Agreement on Trade-Related Aspects of Intellectual Property Rights (TRIPS) and Public Health of 2001, which affirmed the supremacy of the public's need to access medicines over the protection of intellectual property rights; and the United Nations' MDGs.

Yet improving access in low- and middle-income countries continues to be a complex challenge, as economic reforms and the globalizing world have greatly increased the number and range of actors involved in the field of medicines supply. Moreover, the epidemiologic and demographic transition taking place in these countries has increased the chronic disease burden, with a corresponding increase in the costs of treatment. Pharmaceutical access is influenced by all of the core health system "building blocks" (deSavigny & Adams, 2009). In particular, it requires adequate funding, used to purchase supplies efficiently and equitably; a workforce that is sufficient in number and appropriately distributed and trained; strong information systems and the ability to use the resulting information to inform purchasing decisions and broader pharmaceutical policy; and an effective governance system capable of regulating the introduction of new products, ensuring the safety and appropriate distribution of existing products, and providing transparent procurement. Addressing the challenge of pharmaceutical access, therefore, is strongly linked to the broader health systems strengthening agenda (see Chapter 12 on the design of health systems).

The conceptual organization of this chapter is adapted from a framework developed by Frost and

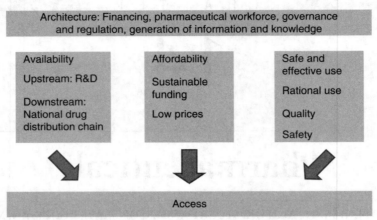

Figure 14-1 Access to Pharmaceuticals Framework.
Source: Adapted from Frost L, Reich M. *Access: How do good health technologies get to poor people in poor countries?* Cambridge: Harvard Centre for Population and Development Studies; 2008.

Reich (2008) to describe the components of access to new health technologies. Three key components of improved access are addressed here: availability (addressing both "upstream" issues of product discovery and development and "downstream" challenges of national pharmaceutical supply systems), affordability, and safe and effective medicines use. In addition, the chapter explores the broader "architecture" of the pharmaceuticals system, which includes the key health system building blocks of the pharmaceutical workforce as well as the generation of information and knowledge about medicines and their use. The influence of these building blocks on the ultimate goal of improved access to pharmaceuticals is shown in Figure 14-1.

Throughout the chapter, we strive to maintain consistency in terminology, while recognizing that the preferred names of the products that are discussed have changed over time. Currently, *medicine* is the preferred term over *drug* for any substance that is used to modify physiological systems or pathological states for the benefit of the recipient, as the latter is now widely regarded as referring to illicit substances; *pharmaceutical* is a broader term that generally encompasses both medicines (prescription and over-the-counter) and vaccines in their finished form. Although *medicine* and *pharmaceutical* are often used interchangeably, the latter may also encompass other products of the pharmaceutical industry. These products may include the active pharmacological ingredients used in production (API), other biologicals such as

blood products and insulin, veterinary medicines, and diagnostic products such as those used for blood typing and test kits for the HIV and malaria viruses (Anderson & Huss, 2004; WHO, 2002a).

Other important definitions and concepts germane to the discussion presented here include *essential medicines*, which are defined as the medicines that satisfy the priority healthcare needs of the population, and that are selected based on public health relevance, evidence on efficacy and safety, and comparative cost-effectiveness; and *generics*, which are pharmaceutical products that are intended to be interchangeable with the original innovative product and are marketed after the expiry of original product's patent or other exclusivity rights. Generic products may be marketed either unbranded ("commodity generics") or under a new brand name ("branded generics") (Anderson & Huss, 2004; WHO, 2010b).

Pharmaceutical Availability: Upstream Issues

Ensuring the existence and availability of safe and effective products that address the major causes of disease burden is a critical element of pharmaceutical access. This section considers the "upstream" issues related to the development and introduction of new pharmaceuticals. We explore the reasons why "market failure" (the failure of unregulated markets to reach efficient and equitable social outcomes) arises in the development of pharmaceuticals to address the health problems of the world's poor, and examine some of the solutions that have been developed to increase investment in research and development (R&D) in this area.

Market Failure and the Concept of Neglected Diseases

In today's world, the development of new pharmaceuticals is largely the responsibility of the large multinational companies that bring the majority of new medicines to market. These firms invest resources raised from capital markets into their R&D activities with the expectation that this investment will be recouped once successful products are sold in the market. Companies focus their R&D on areas of high market demand that offer a high potential return on investment, and in which monopoly intellectual property rights allow them to charge higher prices so as to recoup their R&D costs, recover losses from products terminated during development, and make a reasonable profit.

The interests of the community and of health providers are fed into this system in several ways, with the most important being their purchasing power—in other words, their ability and intention to purchase the new products. The public sector can also influence the direction of product development by funding research in areas that are deemed public health priorities. Indeed, much research begins in publicly funded laboratories and universities, where researchers identify promising compounds and technologies that are then taken up, developed, and registered by multinational pharmaceutical companies. Companies will take on this burden only if the first proviso is met, however—that is, if they estimate market demand will be sufficiently high to provide adequate returns on their development investment.

Governments in high-income countries may also encourage the pharmaceutical industry to invest in R&D by tipping the balance of investment and returns in its favor through policies such as R&D subsidies or incentives that increase profit. These measures are used, for example, to encourage investment into treatments for rare ("orphan") diseases in high-income countries, where too few patients are affected to constitute a viable market for companies.

Even this brief overview makes it clear that a market-driven system is unsuited to addressing the diseases that disproportionately affect the low- and middle-income world. The governments and patients in these regions have neither sufficient revenues to fund large-scale R&D incentives nor sufficient collective purchasing power to offer the returns that the pharmaceutical industry seeks and can make by investing in areas such as hypertension, cancer, and depression that afflict both wealthy and poor countries.

The result of this market failure is a range of "neglected diseases" for which R&D investment is well below the level required by health needs, and where decades can elapse before new products are developed. A typical example is tuberculosis (TB), for which the most commonly used diagnostic tool is the AFB test developed in 1882, and for which standard therapy still relies on 6- to 8-month regimens using drugs developed during the 1950s and 1960s. The net effect of this market failure was recognized in a 1999 study showing that of the 1,223 new drugs commercialized from 1975 to 1997, only 13 (1%) were specifically developed for tropical diseases such as malaria, African trypanosomiasis, leishmaniasis, and tuberculosis, even though these diseases collectively affect millions of (mostly poor) patients per year (Pecoul et al., 1999).

At first glance, this problem might appear to be irresolvable. In reality, the paradigm of high costs and poor patients is not a single intractable problem, but rather a complex and varied set of issues, many of which are amenable to solutions.

The R&D Process and Opportunities for Neglected Diseases

Historically, the development of a new pharmaceutical has been reported to take more than a decade and cost approximately $800 million to $1 billion if the cost of capital is included (DiMasi, Hansen, & Grabowski, 2003). In fact, the cost, time, and risk of making new pharmaceuticals vary dramatically depending on the type of product (Table 14-1).

Where costs are smaller, development times shorter, and risks lower, even small markets can be attractive to developers, thereby stimulating R&D in an underserved area. This is particularly so for smaller companies and companies in the low- and middle-income world, which generally have lower cost structures than multinational pharmaceutical companies.

The degree of market failure is also determined by the existence, or absence, of related commercial markets that can cross-subsidize investment into products for poor countries, as described by the 2001 Commission of Macroeconomics and Health (WHO, 2001d):

- Type I diseases are prevalent in both high- and low-income countries. Their substantial commercial markets in high-income countries

Table 14-1	Development Times and Costs by Type of Product		
Type of Product	**Development Times**	**Development Costs (Excluding Cost of Capital)**	**Risk**
Diagnostics	3–5 years (Foundation for Innovative New Diagnostics, 2009)	$1 million to $10 million (Foundation for Innovative New Diagnostics & Special Programme for Research & Training in Tropical Diseases, 2006)	Lower scientific and financial risk
Drugs	More than 7–10 years (Moran et al., 2005)	$115 million (Pekar, 2001) to $250 million (RBM Partnership, 2008; Pekar, 2001) (including cost of failure)	High scientific and financial risk
Vaccines	11–15 years (Moran et al., 2007)	$200 million to $500 million (Serdobova & Kieny, 2006) (including cost of failure)	Very high scientific and financial risk

drive R&D activity, so there is no product shortfall. Affordability is often an issue, however. Examples include noncommunicable diseases such as diabetes, cardiovascular diseases, and tobacco-related illnesses, as well as infectious diseases such as pneumonia, hepatitis B, and *Haemophilus influenzae* type b (Hib).

- Type II diseases are "incident in both rich and poor countries, but with a substantial proportion of the cases in the poor countries"—for example, HIV/AIDS and tuberculosis. These diseases have modest markets in wealthy countries; thus some R&D activity exists, although it is often targeted to high-income groups rather than the poor (e.g., short-term courses of antimalarial agents for travelers and members of the military, or complex high-priced antiretroviral drugs).

- Type III diseases occur overwhelmingly or exclusively in low- and middle-income countries and have no commercial market to drive R&D—for example, Chagas' disease, Buruli ulcer, and African sleeping sickness (trypanosomiasis). There are often limited or no treatments for these diseases.

Type II diseases are often termed "neglected diseases" and Type III "very neglected diseases" (Morel et al., 2009).

The 2000 Watershed

Prior to 1999, the lack of treatments and R&D for neglected diseases went largely unremarked in the health policy literature. Health professionals working in low- and middle-income countries had long been accustomed to using older diagnostics and therapies, such as chloroquine for malaria or lengthy treatment regimens for TB, even when these interventions were not appropriate or development of resistance was evident. For many diseases, there were no safe, effective treatments—for example, for Buruli ulcer, late-stage human African trypanosomiasis (sleeping sickness), and Chagas' disease. Some organizations continued to work toward development of new treatments, such as the WHO-based Special Programme for Research and Training in Tropical Diseases (TDR); however, their funding and political support were often limited. For instance, the total annual budget for TDR to develop medicines for the 10 neglected diseases in its remit, as well as to carry out capacity-building activities, was only $20 million in 1975 (Special Programme for Research & TDR, 2007).

This situation changed dramatically in the late 1990s, with the advent of a civil society campaign led by Médecins Sans Frontières and Oxfam to improve access to essential medicines. Although it initially focused on securing access to existing medicines—in particular, affordable HIV/AIDS drugs—the campaign also began to call for development of new safer and more effective medicines for neglected diseases.

This campaign coincided with several seminal developments in pharmaceutical development. Groups such as the Bill and Melinda Gates Foundation and the Rockefeller Foundation—and some governments, such as those in the United Kingdom, the Netherlands, and Switzerland—also began to take an interest in R&D of new pharmaceuticals for the low- and middle-income world. Philanthropic groups in particular were willing to provide levels of funding well beyond those seen previously, and to take risks in supporting new and unproven R&D models that promised both greater efficiency and delivery of products that were better suited to and more affordable for patients and health systems in the low- and middle-income world.

The earliest of these new models was the public–private partnership, or product development partnership (PDP) as they are now more commonly known. These ventures include the International AIDS Vaccine Initiative (IAVI), established in 1996; the Medicines for Malaria Venture (MMV; see Exhibit 14-1) and PATH Malaria Vaccine Initiative (MVI), both established in

---

| Exhibit 14-1 | Medicines for Malaria Venture |

Medicines for Malaria Venture (MMV) is a not-for-profit product development partnership established as a foundation in Switzerland in 1999 to discover and develop new, effective and affordable antimalarial drugs. So far, it has delivered on its initial goal to develop a single new drug by 2010 and is making progress on its goal to produce an additional antimalarial every five years thereafter. In 2006, MMV broadened its mission to include access and delivery activities, aiming to increase the uptake and health impact of its products.

Portfolio

MMV registered its first product in 2008: Coartem Dispersible, the first high-quality artemisinin combination therapy especially formulated for children. The organization currently oversees a portfolio of more than 50 projects, including two new antimalarials, Eurartesim and Pyramax, that are expected to be registered by 2012.

Partners

MMV works in partnership with more than 150 research institutions and companies across the world, including multinational pharmaceutical companies such as GlaxoSmithKline, Novartis, and Merck & Company; small pharmaceutical and biotechnology companies such as BioCryst Pharmaceuticals, Magellan Biosciences, and Mycosynthetix; universities such as the University of Bamako, University of Cape Town, University of Nebraska, and the London School of Hygiene & Tropical Medicine; and research centers such as the Kintampo Health Research Centre, Manhiça Research Centre, and Ifakara Health Institute (all in Africa).

Funding

MMV raised $480 million in past and forward commitments from public, private, and philanthropic sources for the period from 2000 to 2015 (MMV, 2010), and had spent $310 million by the end of 2009 (MMV, 2009). The Bill and Melinda Gates Foundation has provided 66% of MMV's total funds, while development agencies from the United Kingdom, Netherlands, United States, Ireland, Spain, and Switzerland have contributed 25% of total funding received and pledged. Funding was also received from other sources, such as the U.S. National Institutes of Health (NIH), Wellcome Trust, and World Bank (Figure 14-2).

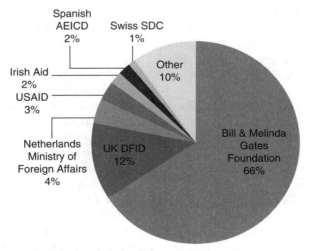

Figure 14-2 MMV Funding Sources (Received and Pledged) from 2000 to 2015.
Source: Modified from Medicines for Malaria Venture. (2010). "MMV funding and expenditure." Retrieved 30 June 2010, from http://www.mmv.org/invest-us/mmv-funding-and-expenditure.

Table 14-2	Examples of Product Development Partnerships		
PDP	**Setup Date**	**Disease Area**	**Product**
Aeras Global TB Vaccine Foundation (Aeras)	1997	TB	Vaccines
Drugs for Neglected Diseases Initiative (DNDi)	2003	Malaria, kinetoplastids	Drugs
European Malaria Vaccine Initiative (EMVI)	1998	Malaria	Vaccines
Foundation for Innovative New Diagnostics (FIND)	2003	TB, malaria, sleeping sickness	Diagnostics
Global Alliance for TB Drug Development (TB Alliance)	2000	TB	Drugs
Infectious Disease Research Institute (IDRI)	1993	HIV, TB, leishmaniasis, leprosy	Vaccines, diagnostics
Institute for One World Health (iOWH)	2000	Malaria, leishmaniasis, diarrheal diseases	Drugs
International AIDS Vaccine Initiative (IAVI)	1996	HIV/AIDS	Vaccines
International Partnership for Microbicides (IPM)	2002	HIV/AIDS	Microbicides
International Vaccine Institute (IVI) (including the Pediatric Dengue Vaccine Initiative, Diseases of the Most Impoverished Program, Rotavirus Program, Cholera Vaccine Initiative)	1993	Diarrheal diseases, dengue, bacterial pneumonia and meningitis, typhoid and paratyphoid fever	Vaccines
Medicines for Malaria Venture (MMV)	1999	Malaria	Drugs
Program for Appropriate Technology in Health (PATH; including Malaria Vaccine Initiative, Meningitis Vaccine Project, Rotavirus Vaccine Program, Pneumococcal Vaccine Project, and other programs)	1979	HIV, malaria, meningitis, rotavirus and other diarrheal diseases	Vaccines, microbicides, diagnostics
Sabin Vaccine Institute (including Human Hookworm Vaccine Initiative [HHVI] and Schistosomiasis Vaccine Initiative [SVI])	1993	Helminth diseases (hookworm and schistosomiasis)	Vaccines
Special Programme for Research and Training in Tropical Diseases hosted by the World Health Organization (WHO-TDR)	1975	TB, malaria, kinetoplastids, helminth diseases, dengue	Diagnostics, drugs

1999; and the Global Alliance for TB Drug Development (TB Alliance), established in 2000 (Table 14-2).[1] PDPs offered a crucial link between industry skills in making medicines and public health interest in addressing diseases disproportionately affecting the low- and middle-income world by providing a platform that allowed public-sector researchers, public and philanthropic funders, and private companies to work together.

The final catalyst was the decision of the pharmaceutical industry to take legal action against the South African government, led by Nelson Mandela, for its efforts to import cheaper HIV/AIDS medicines for its population—a move the industry described as an attack on TRIPS, the intellectual property (IP) system governing pharmaceuticals (see Chapter 18 on globalization and health, as well as the discussion of safe and effective medicines use later in this chapter). The victory for South Africa in 2001 had severe negative repercussions for the pharmaceutical industry. The move against South Africa, which involved legal action specifically naming Nelson Mandela, and the attempt to block access to cheaper HIV/AIDS drugs for Africa, proved (perhaps unsurprisingly) to be a spectacular public relations disaster. It also brought into question the IP system that underpinned industry profits, and shone a spotlight on industry's failure to address R&D for diseases disproportionately affecting the low- and middle-income world.

While companies responded to the criticism by energetically defending the IP system, some sought to repair their global standing and address their corporate social responsibilities through drug donation campaigns or initiation of R&D programs for neglected diseases. For instance, GlaxoSmithKline set up the Tres Cantos Institute in Spain and Novartis set up the Novartis Institute for Tropical Diseases (NITD), both of which focus on neglected disease R&D. As

---

[1] Although TDR was the first PDP-type partnering model, it is a department within an international organization rather than a formal PDP in the sense of an independent, free-standing, not-for-profit organization.

mentioned earlier, it is extremely expensive and risky for a private company to invest shareholder funds into R&D of products that can never make a profit, but these developments make this prospect more feasible, in particular the advent of PDP partners and new funding.

Product Development Partnerships

Although each PDP differs in its approach, all share some common features. All are not-for-profit public health–focused organizations that drive neglected disease product development in conjunction with partners from both the public and private sectors, including in both low- and middle-income and high-income countries. Although some PDPs conduct R&D themselves, their predominant role is in identifying, facilitating, managing, and funding the research and development of products suitable for use in low- and middle-income countries in conjunction with external partners. Their ability to do so is predicated on their ability to access promising leads from multiple sources—both public and private—and to identify and secure funds to advance products in their chosen field. As they mature, PDPs typically manage larger portfolios, allowing them to select high-performing projects and drop low-performing ones. Virtually all PDPs play a role in advocating for their target disease area, and some also conduct capacity-building activities in those low- and middle-income countries where their target disease is endemic.

Since the late 1990s, seed funding to PDPs from the Rockefeller Foundation, the Bill and Melinda Gates Foundation, and a handful of governments has grown into substantial revenue streams as the PDP model has become more widely accepted. In 2008, PDPs received a total of $580 million, accounting for 25% of total global grants for neglected disease R&D, and for approximately 40% of government grant funding for neglected disease R&D, excluding the funding for the NIH (Moran et al., 2009).

An important factor in PDPs' credibility—and thus their funding—has been their ability to deliver new products for neglected diseases at investment levels well below those associated with the pharmaceutical industry (see Table 14-3). Note, however, that PDPs are not the "holy grail" of product development. Rather, they play a more prominent role in some disease areas than in others, and performance between PDPs varies depending on their in-house skills, management quality, level of funding, and ability to sustain the wide range of partnerships needed to create a broad portfolio of new products and leads.

Other Sources of New Neglected Disease Products

For some neglected diseases, PDPs are not the only source—or even the main source—of R&D activity. Many public and academic research groups now work in the neglected disease field, particularly in the area of basic research and early identification of leads. In addition, WHO recently set up the African Network

Table 14-3	Sample of Novel Neglected Disease Products Registered or in Late Stage Trials
Product (Disease)	**Status**
β-Arteether (malaria)	Approved in 2000
Miltefosine (visceral leishmaniasis)	Approved by Drugs Controller General of India (2002)
Artemether/lumefantrine pediatric label extension (malaria)	Approved by Swissmedic (2004)
Intramuscular paromomycin (visceral leishmaniasis)	Approved by Drugs Controller General of India (August 2006)
ASAQ (malaria)	Approved by Moroccan medicines regulatory authority (February 2007)
Artemether/lumefantrine dispersible (malaria)	Approved by Swissmedic (December 2008)
ASMQ (malaria)	Approved by Brazilian National Health Surveillance Agency (ANVISA) (April 2008)
Eurartesim (malaria)	Submitted to European Medicines Agency (EMEA) for approval (July 2009)
Arterolate/PQP (malaria)	Clinical development
AZCQ (malaria)	Clinical development
Conjugate meningitis A vaccine (meningitis)	Clinical development
Fexinidazole (sleeping sickness)	Clinical development
Moxifloxacin (TB)	Clinical development
PA-824 (TB)	Clinical development
RTS,S vaccine (malaria)	Clinical development

for Drugs and Diagnostics Innovation (ANDI) to catalyze and facilitate drug discovery conducted by African researchers.

Independent pharmaceutical company activity in neglected diseases also exists, although it is very rare for a company to develop a product targeting such a disease on its own. Instead, most seek and need public funding and skills to conduct large-scale clinical trials in low- and middle-income countries, to secure buy-in of public health groups internationally and at the country level, and to facilitate regulatory and policy processes. The exception is the private sector in low- and middle-income countries such as India, where firms can find low- and middle-income country and domestic markets sufficiently attractive to incentivize them to conduct development alone, particularly for Type II diseases such as HIV/AIDS and TB.

The Global Portfolio

The result of civil society pressure, increased public and philanthropic funding, revitalized industry interest, and new models for product development has been a transformation of the neglected disease R&D landscape in the past decade. After decades of failure to address these areas, in 2010 there were 143 candidates in PDP neglected disease product pipelines (Strub-Wourgraft, 2010), with members of the pharmaceutical industry being responsible for 67 leads and products (many as part of PDP portfolios) (Greenidge, 2009). New products are already registered, with many more in late-stage clinical trials (Table 14-3).

Funding levels have also increased dramatically. Total global investment in neglected disease R&D amounted to $2.9 billion in 2009. Nevertheless, it is clear from Table 14-4 that many diseases and product areas remain underfunded—in particular, the aptly named "most neglected diseases."

New Challenges

All change brings unexpected consequences, and the renewed investment in neglected disease R&D is no exception. The rapid increase in discovery and development of new products for neglected diseases has largely caught policy makers unawares, with the re-

Table 14-4	Total R&D Funding by Disease in 2008				
Disease	FY2007 (US$)*	FY2008 (US$)*	FY2008 Nominal (US$)†	FY2007(%)	FY2008(%)
HIV/AIDS	1,083,018,193	1,164,882,551	1,215,841,708	42.3	39.4
Malaria	468,449,438	541,746,356	565,985,827	18.3	18.3
Tuberculosis	410,428,697	445,927,582	467,538,635	16.0	15.1
Kinetoplastids	125,122,839	139,207,962	145,676,517	4.9	4.7
Diarrheal diseases	113,889,118	132,198,981	138,159,527	4.4	4.5
Dengue	82,013,895	126,752,203	132,470,770	3.2	4.3
Bacterial pneumonia and meningitis	32,517,311	90,844,284	96,071,934	1.3	3.1
Helminth infections (worms and flukes)	51,591,838	66,837,827	69,518,274	2.0	2.3
Salmonella infections	9,117,212	39,486,243	41,079,293	0.4	1.3
Leprosy	5,619,475	9,769,250	10,073,184	0.2	0.3
Rheumatic fever	1,670,089	2,179,609	2,268,099	0.1	0.1
Trachoma	1,679,711	2,073,659	2,225,330	0.1	0.1
Buruli ulcer	2,412,950	1,954,465	2,140,303	0.1	0.1
Platform technologies	9,997,190	16,298,026	16,569,978	0.4	0.6
Core funding of a multidisease R&D organization	110,921,673	101,097,348	110,403,054	4.3	3.4
Unspecified disease	51,619,120	74,707,997	78,179,894	2.0	2.5
Total	**2,560,068,749**	**2,955,964,344**	**3,094,202,328**	**100**	**100**

* Figures are adjusted for inflation and reported in 2007 U.S. dollars.
† Figures are in 2008 U.S. dollars.
Notes: Fiscal year (FY) 2007 figures include only typhoid and paratyphoid fever R&D investments. In FY2008, the scope of the survey was broadened to include other *Salmonella* infections, specifically non-typhoidal *Salmonella enterica* (NTS) and multiple *Salmonella* infections.
   Platform technologies are technologies that can be applied to a range of diseases and products—for example, a slow-release technology that could be used to deliver different drugs.
   Core funding refers to organisational grants that are not tied to specific disease projects.
Source: Moran et al., 2009.

sult that potential products are now outpacing the policies and funding needed to finalize, register, and implement them. Key areas of tension relate to R&D financing, medicines regulation, product procurement, and overall prioritization and coordination of R&D and funding.

Financing and Incentives

Currently, R&D funding relies on a handful of donors, with 10 organizations providing 75% of global funds for neglected disease R&D in 2008. Notably, two organizations—the U.S.-based NIH and the Bill and Melinda Gates Foundation—provided a striking 60% of the global total. The remaining 25% came from the pharmaceutical industry (12% of global investment) and other public (12 %) and philanthropic donors (1%) (Moran et al., 2009).

It is unlikely that this reliance on so few funders can continue. Since 2008, several key public funders have substantially scaled back their neglected disease R&D investments in response to the global financial crisis. At the same time, funding demand has increased exponentially due to the rapid progression of successful new neglected disease drug and vaccine candidates from lower-cost early research stages into the large, expensive late-stage field trials that precede product registration and rollout. As an example, PATH MVI received a $183 million grant from the Bill and Melinda Gates Foundation in 2009 to support the large-scale clinical trials needed for the late development of the new RTS,S malaria vaccine; in these studies, 16,000 children and infants will be enrolled in 11 sites in Africa. Additionally, almost all of the "most neglected diseases" will require significantly increased investment in all research areas if new products are to be delivered (see Table 14-4).

Regulating the Introduction of New Medicines

For many decades, low- and middle-income countries have managed with older medicines—in particular, lower-cost generic versions of medicines that have already been approved by stringent medicines regulators in the high-income world, such as the U.S. Food and Drug Administration (FDA) and the European Medicines Agency (EMEA). As a result, many medicines regulatory authorities (MRAs) in low- and middle-income countries have limited experience with the process of assessing the safety and efficacy of novel medicines for their populations.

The advent of new products for neglected diseases, however, has highlighted the problem of relying on Western regulators to approve medicines that will largely be used by patients in low- and middle-income countries. Western regulatory authorities, while highly experienced in assessing safety, efficacy, and quality of medicines for their own populations and diseases, generally have limited experience with medicines for tropical and neglected diseases, and little knowledge of the circumstances in which they will be used in low- and middle-income countries. A further difficulty is that Western medicines regulations are aimed at local needs, and are neither intended nor designed to address safety or efficacy in other countries or settings. For instance, they may omit data requirements vital for safe large-scale use in Africa (e.g., trials assessing the safe interaction of HIV/AIDS and malaria drugs, or the safe use of drugs in malnourished patients).

The relative risk–benefit tradeoffs for neglected disease drugs are also dramatically different in Africa and the West, with the result that regulatory analysis against the same criteria can lead to completely different conclusions in different countries. For instance, RotaShield, the first rotavirus vaccine, was registered in the United States in 1998 but withdrawn in 1999 due to a 1 in 10,000 risk of intussusception in U.S. children. In the U.S. setting, where rotavirus causes fewer than 60 deaths per year, this risk–benefit ratio was unacceptable. In contrast, the same risk–benefit calculation leads to a very different result in low- and middle-income countries, where rotavirus is responsible for approximately 5% of deaths in children younger than the age of five (mortality rate of 183 deaths per 100,000 population). In other words, in low- and middle-income countries, the risk of childhood death from rotavirus infection is approximately 18 times greater than the risk of intussusception associated with the vaccine. Unfortunately, the negative FDA finding led to withdrawal of RotaShield from the market, making it unavailable for use in low- and middle-income countries.

In response to these shortcomings, policy makers have developed a range of regulatory pathways specifically tailored to assessing new neglected disease products:

- The EMEA's Article 58 assesses new neglected disease products that will be used outside Europe, providing an "opinion" that low- and middle-income country MRAs can use to support their own deliberations. This provision is rarely used (four products assessed from 2004 to 2009 [EMEA, 2005]), however. Instead, most product developers prefer to use other regulatory options that offer greater incentives and benefits—in particular, those that provide

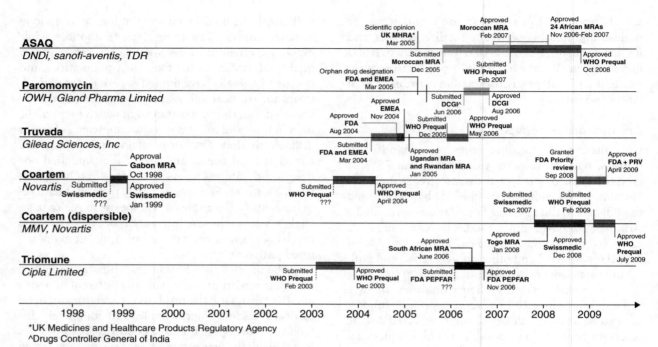

*UK Medicines and Healthcare Products Regulatory Agency
^Drugs Controller General of India

Figure 14-3 Neglected Disease Drug Registration Timeline.

access to Western markets where financial returns can be made, such as "orphan drug" legislation.

- The FDA's "tentative approval" gives regulatory approval to HIV/AIDS drugs that will be used outside the United States in U.S. government-sponsored HIV/AIDS programs. Although this practice allows new HIV/AIDS generic medications and formulations to be rapidly approved and introduced into AIDS programs in low- and middle-income countries, the HIV/AIDS focus means it has limited impact on the overall problem of how to regulate new neglected disease products.

- WHO assesses and "prequalifies" drugs and vaccines on an ongoing basis for use in low- and middle-income countries and on behalf of international procurement groups such as UNICEF and the Global Fund to Fight AIDS, Tuberculosis and Malaria (Global Fund or GFATM). The WHO "stamp of approval" allows low- and middle-income countries to access safe, effective, quality medicines, even if they may not have sufficient in-house regulatory capacity to conduct assessments themselves. The drug prequalification program focuses on only a handful of diseases: 99% of prequalified drugs are for HIV/AIDS (86%),

TB (7%), and malaria (6%). The vaccine prequalification program chiefly focuses on vaccines used in Expanded Programme on Immunization (EPI) programs. Neither program is designed to conduct first assessment of novel products for use in the low- and middle-income world; instead, both primarily assess generic products or new combinations or formulations of existing medicines.

A further problem is the lack of coordination between these regulatory initiatives. All too often, new neglected disease products are assessed and reviewed by one regulatory body after another, adding expense and delaying patient access in the low- and middle-income world (Figure 14-3).[2]

In recent years, there has been some progress on this front. Groups developing TB drugs, for example, have worked with regulators to develop a more streamlined system to cut back on the time needed to test combination TB products in clinical trials. In ad-

---

[2] FDA tentative approval is linked to WHO drug prequalification, so that HIV/AIDS drugs approved under the FDA scheme receive automatic prequalification approval by WHO. The EMEA is also working with WHO to seek automatic WHO prequalification of medicines approved under Article 58.

dition, the FDA and the EMEA are now collaborating on measures to align "orphan drug" approvals. Finally, several groups are now examining how to streamline and better integrate the disparate national, regional, and multilateral mechanisms (Burki, 2010; Kaiser Family Foundation, 2010; Moran et al., 2010; Torres, 2010).

Procurement of New Products

Development of new products for neglected diseases immediately raises the issue of how these products will be paid for and rolled out, given that countries in which neglected diseases are endemic rarely have the resources to do so unaided.

Central procurement agencies do exist, including well-known groups such as UNICEF (which provides childhood EPI vaccines) and the Global Drug Facility (which provides drugs for TB). Regional groupings of low- and middle-income countries have also banded together to develop procurement mechanisms to serve their own needs—for example, the Pan American Health Organization (PAHO), the Southern African Development Community (SADC), and the East African Community (EAC) (WHO, 2007). These initiatives play a key role in selecting and procuring safe, effective medicines at affordable prices for low- and middle-income countries, and in securing continuity of supply.

Unfortunately, these centralized procurement agencies and mechanisms have neither the remit nor the funding capacity to undertake large-scale purchases of novel medicines as they come online. This problem was highlighted by the introduction of antiretroviral drugs (ARVs) for HIV/AIDS. Even at generic prices, these medications proved to be beyond the reach of many sub-Saharan African countries with substantial HIV/AIDS burdens. The same challenge remains an issue for all new neglected disease medicines. In the past decade, several new centralized procurement or funding streams have been created and linked to global health initiatives (discussed later in this chapter) in an effort to respond to demand for new medicines, including the following measures:

- The Global Fund to Fight AIDS, TB and Malaria, set up in 2002, has a remit that includes funding for purchase of ARVs and novel antimalarials (artemisinin combination therapies [ACTs]).
- Bilateral programs include the U.S. President's Emergency Plan for AIDS Relief (PEPFAR) for

ARV procurement and the U.S. President's Malaria Initiative (PMI) for antimalarials.
- The Global Alliance for Vaccines and Immunization (GAVI), set up in 2000, has recently added several novel products to the list of vaccines it will provide at subsidized prices, including rotavirus vaccines and pneumonia vaccines (still in development under an advance market commitment agreement, as discussed later in this chapter).
- The Affordable Medicines Facility—Malaria (AMFm) was set up in 2009 specifically to fund purchase of novel antimalarial agents, aiming to keep their prices competitive with those of older, less effective products, such as chloroquine (discussed later in this chapter).

Each of these mechanisms was set up, or extended, only after years of lobbying and negotiations, and all must regularly seek renewed commitments from donors to refill their purchase fund coffers. They may also contribute to the creation of parallel procurement systems (discussed later in this chapter). There is no systematic approach to assessing future (often competing) demand for access to novel products emerging from the development pipeline, nor is there a dedicated long-term funding stream to support their timely purchase and delivery to low- and middle-income countries.

Prioritization and Coordination (Including of the New Philanthropy)

The rapid increase in new product development for neglected diseases raises similar issues for both donors and low- and middle-income countries in the field of R&D. There is a plethora of actors and organizations in all arenas, including R&D, funding, procurement, and policy; the range of participants encompasses multilateral organizations, governments, philanthropists, and companies. The work of each of these entities, while highly valuable, is often uncoordinated with others, and their choice of target area can reflect their own understandings rather than the needs and demands of low- and middle-income countries themselves. For instance, research and development of HIV/AIDS-related products receives 39.4% of global R&D funding, and procurement mechanisms for new medicines are also heavily focused on HIV/AIDS drugs. While important and necessary, given that the HIV/AIDS pandemic is a problem of global significance, it nevertheless remains the case that HIV/AIDS is not the number one cause of morbidity and mortality in any low- or middle-income region. Instead, this dubious honor goes to pneumonia and diarrheal illnesses in sub-Saharan Africa and to noncommunicable diseases in middle-income countries. However, both of these unmet needs have until recently received little attention and even less funding for R&D of relevant products, although this situation is beginning to change in some areas.

Finally, low- and middle-income countries and central and regional procurement agencies now face the daunting task of determining which new products they should purchase and implement first, given that resources are insufficient to take up all of them. A degree of prioritization occurs in this area, with the WHO Strategic Advisory Group of Experts (SAGE) reviewing current and upcoming vaccines to determine which to focus on, and the GAVI Alliance also conducting internal analysis to guide its procurement priorities. These measures do not extend to other medicines such as drugs and diagnostics, however, nor do they take these products into account in making their own decisions. The work of the WHO Drug Prequalification unit provides a degree of de facto prioritization in the drug field, given that WHO prequalified drugs are more likely to be purchased and have rapid take-up by low- and middle-income countries. Nevertheless, this unit focuses primarily on drugs for HIV, TB, and malaria, with products for other tropical diseases not being factored into the equation.

Lack of coordination and prioritization invariably results in gaps in funding and distorted priorities in both R&D and procurement, leaving low- and middle-income countries in the position of having to accept the net result of multiple uncoordinated decisions rather than benefiting from careful planning and investment. Finding new approaches to coordination and harmonization is clearly a priority for the future, and is an issue that spans the entire spectrum from R&D through to national procurement and distribution.

New Financing Mechanisms for R&D

Public funding is generally provided in the form of either "push" or "pull" incentives (Table 14-5). Push funding is provided *during* the R&D process to subsidize development costs. It can take the form of either direct public grants to academic researchers and PDPs working in nonprofit areas, or tax breaks or R&D subsidies to companies.

The vast majority of current R&D funding is in the form of push grants. Push grants are particularly suitable for groups that do not have the capacity to self-fund product development (which, as noted earlier, can cost hundreds of millions of dollars and span

10 to 15 years), such as small companies, biotechnology firms, public groups, and PDPs. Public push funding is generally cheaper than pull funding, because it does not borrow money from capital markets and usually pays only for the cost of research—that is, it does not include profit margins. It is also considered to be a higher risk, because a high proportion of the funded research will inevitably fail.

A second potential source of push funding is private venture capital. Venture capital is normally raised in the stock market and invested with the aim of reaping large profits if the product is successful. Clearly, this practice has limited application in the low- or no-profit neglected disease area. Nevertheless, double-bottom-line venture capital investment in neglected disease R&D is possible, with private investors putting up development cash alongside public or philanthropic investors and accepting lower returns in exchange for lower financial risk and a high public health impact in the form of new neglected disease products.

By contrast, pull funding is provided as a reward or incentive at the *end* of the R&D process, thereby motivating developers by not only retrospectively reimbursing their R&D costs, but also providing profit margins that are theoretically comparable to commercial returns. The financial rewards often take the form of extended market life, in which either the product is allowed to be registered earlier (thereby extending its monopoly sales life) or a monopoly marketing period is provided during which competitors cannot sell their products (e.g., through orphan drug legislation). For neglected diseases where an extended monopoly market would still be largely valueless, the reward is sometimes "swapped" or transferred to a commercial product. For example, the developer of a new antimalarial drug can receive a priority review voucher, which allows it early registration on the commercial product of its choice. More recently, governments have put together a large cash pull fund, known as the advance market commitment, for pneumonia vaccines. New ideas for publicly funded pull funds are also being encouraged, including large prizes for development of new neglected disease products and a Health Impact Fund, under which government funding would be used to pay companies based on the health impact of their product, rather than requiring them to seek returns by selling them at commercial prices (Hollis & Pogge, 2008).

Pull funding has the advantage of being paid only upon delivery of a successful product—that is, it does not pay for failures. It is appropriate for only a limited range of activities, however, because few product developers can finance themselves for the 7 to 15

Table 14-5	Push and Pull Mechanisms for Financing Neglected Disease R&D
Financing Mechanisms	**Description**
Push Mechanisms	
Research and business grants	Direct public funding to conduct research.
R&D tax breaks	Providing tax breaks to companies for their neglected disease R&D investment (e.g., U.K. Vaccine Research Relief).
Product development partnerships (PDPs)	Public health–oriented, not-for-profit organizations that drive product development for neglected diseases in conjunction with external partners. They develop products that are specifically suitable for use in low- and middle-income countries using private-sector management practices, including portfolio management and industrial project management in their R&D activities.
Pull Mechanisms	
Longer patents (e.g., pediatric extensions)	Patent extension awarded to a company in return for evaluating the product in pediatric populations.
Transferable intellectual property rights (TIPR)	Patent extension awarded to a company on a product of its choice in exchange for developing a neglected disease product.
Advance market commitments (AMCs)	Legally binding fund to subsidize purchase of an as-yet-unavailable vaccine at a price that includes a profit margin to allow product developers to recoup their R&D costs. The product profile and the price are agreed upon prior to the R&D being undertaken.
Priority review voucher (PRV)	Offers FDA priority regulatory review on a commercial product in return for registration of a neglected disease product.
Mixed Mechanisms	
Orphan drug legislation	Incentive package aiming to encourage R&D into rare diseases. Includes research grants, an accelerated regulatory pathway, and market exclusivity for the finished product for 7 years (United States) or 10 years (European Union).

years needed to develop a new product and reach the final reward. In theory, pull funding is best suited to multinational drug companies, which can sustain long-term investment from in-house reserves; for low-cost or shorter-term R&D (e.g., development of simpler adaptive products such as new formulations or combinations of existing drugs); or for the final stages of clinical development. In practice, pull prizes would need to be very large to compete with comparative commercial investments. Thus smaller pull funds (e.g., the advance market commitment of $1.3 billion for pneumonia vaccines) are more likely to be used in conjunction with push funding for the earlier stages of R&D.

In addition to push and pull funding, a number of novel approaches have been devised to reduce the cost of neglected disease product development and reduce barriers to creation of new products by promoting a more open, collaborative approach to product development. Leading approaches include open-source drug discovery, in which researchers share information and promising chemical leads to al-

low low-cost rapid development of early drug candidates, and patent pools, which allow researchers free and open access to patented compounds owned by members of the pool (including companies and public researchers). In both cases, funding for further development of these leads would need to be provided through either push or pull mechanisms if no commercial drivers exist.

Availability: Country-Level Distribution Systems and Pharmaceutical Management

Pharmaceutical Supply Chain Systems: Introduction and Scope

Access to pharmaceuticals, as outlined in the framework introduced earlier in this chapter, depends on strong pharmaceutical supply systems to ensure the consistent availability of affordable and high-quality diagnostic and treatment commodities at the places where the target population seeks care. Furthermore, the supply chain is responsible for transferring information on supply and demand back to the central level where planners and policy and decision makers handle financial flows, so that the system is adequately resourced and replenished.

Recent global initiatives have greatly increased the resources flowing into low- and middle-income countries for the procurement of medicines as well as for their development. These resources are expected to increase the value of donor financed health commodities to more than $10 billion by 2011 (Ballou-Aares et al., 2008). While these resources are greatly welcomed as a means to improve the availability of essential commodities, they also have the potential to place considerable pressure on already weak supply chain management systems in low- and middle-income countries.

The pharmaceutical management framework (Figure 14-4) provides the foundation for improving access to medicines. It illustrates four basic pharmaceutical management functions: selection, procurement, distribution, and use, all of which are interrelated, with each major function building on the previous one and leading logically to the next (Management Sciences for Health [MSH], 1997).

- *Selection* involves reviewing the prevalent health problems, identifying treatments of choice, choosing individual medicines and dosage forms, and deciding which medicines will be available at each level of health care.
- *Procurement* includes quantifying medicine requirements, selecting procurement methods,

managing tenders, establishing contract terms, assuring pharmaceutical quality, and ensuring adherence to contract terms.

- *Distribution* includes clearing customs, controlling stock, managing stores, and delivering to drug depots and health facilities.
- *Use* includes diagnosing, prescribing, dispensing, and proper consuming by the patient.

A breakdown in one part of the framework leads to failure of the whole pharmaceutical management process and compromises access.

At the center of the pharmaceutical management framework is a core of *management support* systems: organization, financing and sustainability, information management, and human resources management. Finally, the entire framework relies on *policies, laws, and regulations* which, when supported by good governance, establish and support the public commitment to essential medicine supply.

This section focuses specifically on the supply chain components of the framework, including selection, procurement, and distribution. Medicine use is covered in the next section. In addition, the final section of this chapter discusses the challenges associated with human resources essential for the operation of the pharmaceutical system.

Selection

Essential medicines are those that satisfy the priority healthcare needs of the majority of the population. Essential medicines are intended to be available within

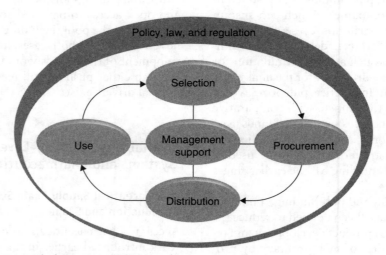

Figure 14-4 The Pharmaceutical Management Framework.
Source: From MSH. *Managing Drug Supply*. 2nd ed. West Hartford, CT: Management Sciences for Health in collaboration with the World Health Organization. 1997. Reproduced with permission from the Centre for Pharmaceutical Management, Management Sciences for Health

the context of functioning health systems at all times in adequate amounts, in the appropriate dosage forms, with assured quality and adequate information, and at a price the individual and the community can afford. Medicines should be selected on the following bases:

- Relevance to the pattern of diseases
- Proven efficacy and safety
- Evidence of performance in a variety of settings
- Quality
- Cost-effectiveness
- Pharmacokinetics
- Acceptability

In 1977, WHO defined the first Model List of Essential Drugs. The rationale for creating this list was that having a limited list of medicines would result in lower costs, better supply, and more rational use. This list has since been updated 14 times, and many countries have used it as the basis for developing their own lists.

Procurement

Effective procurement ensures the availability of the right medicines of appropriate quality in the right quantities at reasonable prices with timely delivery to avoid stock-outs. Effective procurement is a collaborative process between the procurement department of the Ministry of Health and the technical committees or disease control programs (e.g., HIV/AIDS or malaria). These committees often make the final decision on which medicines to buy and in which quan-

tities. Procurement can be annual, scheduled, or perpetual. Different models may be used at different levels or for different medicines. In most cases in the public sector, a form of group purchasing is used in which a central procurement department (e.g., a central medical store) negotiates contracts for its members.

The procurement process involves the following steps:

1. Review the drug selections
2. Determine the quantities needed, using either quantification or forecasting (based on consumption information collected)
3. Reconcile needs and funds
4. Choose the procurement method
5. Locate and select suppliers
6. Specify the contract terms
7. Monitor the order status
8. Receive and check the medicine
9. Make payment

Challenges can arise at any point in this process (Exhibit 14-2).

Four main methods of procurement are used: open tender, restricted tender with performance monitoring, negotiated procurement, and direct procurement. Some countries and donors may opt for some form of direct procurement from nonprofit suppliers such as UNICEF or the International Dispensary Association. Since January 2005, the Global Fund and most major donors have required that tenders for the procurement of HIV/AIDS, malaria, and tuberculosis commodities be restricted to WHO-prequalified

Exhibit 14-2	**Common Procurement Challenges**

- Absence of a comprehensive procurement policy
- Inadequate rules, regulations, and structures
- Public-sector staff with little experience and training to respond to market situations
- Government or donor funding that is insufficient or released at irregular intervals
- Donor agencies with conflicting procurement regulations
- Fragmented medicine procurement at the provincial or district level
- Lack of unbiased market information
- Currency fluctuations
- Limited number of prequalified suppliers
- Long procurement lead times
- Insufficient product specifications
- Insufficient capacity and data for forecasting
- Poor planning
- Corruption and lack of transparency

products, wherever possible, to facilitate access to medicines that meet high standards of quality, safety, and efficacy (International Dispensary Association, 2004; UNICEF, 2004).

A number of tools are available to facilitate pharmaceutical procurement. For example, the Global Fund Secretariat developed the Price and Quality Reporting system as a means to gather information about product prices, product quality, and supplier performance. This system represents a source of information that purchasers can use during negotiation of price and delivery conditions (GFATM, 2010c). Management Sciences for Health (MSH, 2004) publishes an annual international drug price indicator guide that reports procurement prices from multiple international sources. In addition, Stop TB's global drug facility was established to enable health ministries in low- and middle-income countries to procure quality medicines at competitive prices (Matiru & Ryan, 2007).

Competitive tenders are recommended for most public-sector procurement. A formal tender process includes drug selection, quantification, preparation of tender documents and contracts, notification and invitation to bid, receipt, formal opening and collation of bids and supplier selection, award of contracts, performance monitoring of suppliers and clients, and enforcement of contract terms when necessary. Supplier selection should be based on formal written criteria.

Quantification and Forecasting

Three main methods for estimating medicine requirements exist. The *consumption method* uses historical data on drug consumption. If these data are available from a reliable system of reporting, this technique provides the most accurate prediction of future needs. New programs or new treatments will not have historical data on consumption, however. Thus, in such cases, purchasers must rely on the *morbidity method*, which estimates future drug demand based on estimates of disease burden using data on incidence, cases (from attendance at health facilities) or episodes, and standard treatment guidelines. If there are no data on consumption or morbidity, it may be possible to use *proxy consumption*—that is, extrapolation of data from proxy facilities, regions, or countries—as a means of estimating need. Table 14-6 summarizes the main methods for quantification and forecasting, including their use, data needed, and limitations.

Distribution

Effective and efficient drug distribution relies on good management and system design. An efficient distribution system should have the following characteristics:

- Maintain an uninterrupted supply of medicines
- Provide appropriate storage
- Keep medicines in good condition throughout the distribution process
- Minimize losses due to damage and expiry
- Maintain accurate inventory management records
- Use available transportation efficiently
- Reduce pilferage
- Provide accurate information for quantification and forecasting

Table 14-6	Comparison of the Various Quantification Methods		
Method	**Consumption**	**Morbidity**	**Proxy Consumption**
Uses	First choice if historical consumption data are available	Used when no consumption data exist, particularly in new programs or new treatments	Used when other methods are unreliable Uses data from other areas/supply systems
Data	Reliable inventory/consumption records of medicines Complete knowledge of supply pipeline	Number of episodes of disease at health facilities Incidence of disease in population Incidence of disease in facilities and patient attendance Standard treatments (ideal, actual)	Data from a comparison area or system with good per-capita data on consumption, patient attendance, service level, and morbidity
Limitations	Need accurate consumption data Can perpetuate irrational use	Morbidity data are not available for all diseases Standard treatments may not really be used Accurate attendance is difficult to predict	Questionable comparability of patient populations, morbidity, and treatment practices

Source: Adapted from MSH, 2010.

A distribution system consists of four main elements (MSH, 1997):

- *System design:* geographic or population coverage, number of levels in the system, push versus pull system, degree of decentralization
- *Information system:* inventory control, records, consumption reports, information flow
- *Storage:* selection of storage sites, building design, handling systems, order picking
- *Delivery:* collection versus delivery, choice of transport, vehicle procurement and maintenance, delivery schedules and routes

Distribution systems face a number of challenges (Exhibit 14-3), all of which can lead to problems of stock-outs. Stock-outs have serious implications for the implementation of programs, as they undermine the ability of health workers to follow treatment protocols. When a first-line medicine is not available, patients are either sent away to buy the medicine in the private sector, which leads to a progressive lack of confidence in the public health system, or treatment is adapted based on the availability of other medicines with a similar effect. Stock-outs can be prevented through efficient procurement and financial planning, accurate forecasting, and good inventory management. Several initiatives are under way to prevent stock-outs in health facilities, including the Stop Stock-outs Campaign (http://stopstockouts.org/) and the use of mobile phone and information technology to track commodities (Roll Back Malaria, 2010).

Storage and distribution costs represent a significant component of the health budget, and adequate resources must be allocated to these functions to ensure that the medicines get to their point of use. In fact, transport costs can be more than the value of the medicines themselves, especially when pharmaceuticals must be moved to remote, sparsely populated areas.

At least five alternatives have traditionally existed for supplying medicines and supplies to governmental and nongovernmental health services:

- *Central medical stores (CMS):* This is the classic public-sector pharmaceutical supply system, in which medicines are procured and distributed by a centralized government unit. The state is the owner and funder (using national or donor resources) for the entire supply system. This approach has been employed in a number of countries in Africa (e.g., South Africa and Ghana), Asia, Europe, and Latin America. In Ghana, the CMS distributes products to 10 regional medical stores, which in turn distribute those supplies to roughly 2,200 service delivery points. In Zambia, the CMS distributes products to 72 district medical stores, which then distribute the supplies to roughly 1,500 service delivery points.
- *Autonomous supply agency:* In this alternative to the CMS system, distribution is managed by an autonomous or semiautonomous pharmaceutical supply agency. This strategy has been used in Tanzania and Benin (see Exhibit 14-4).
- *Direct delivery system:* In this decentralized, non-CMS approach, medicines are delivered directly by suppliers to districts and major facilities. The government pharmaceutical procurement office selects the supplier and establishes the price for each item, but the government does not store and distribute medicines. This approach has been used in the Caribbean.

Exhibit 14-3	Commonly Encountered Distribution Challenges

- Vertical and fragmented supply systems
- Insufficient funding for storage, distribution, and inventory management systems
- Poor planning
- Poor security and leakage
- Short shelf life of medicine
- Limited geographic reach
- Insufficient warehousing and transport
- Poor information management systems to monitor stocks for planning and forecasting
- Stock-outs and expiry
- Poor cold chain
- Vertical and parallel distribution chains

- *Primary distributor (or prime vendor) system:* In this non-CMS system, the government pharmaceutical procurement office establishes a contract with one or more primary distributors, as well as separate contracts with pharmaceutical suppliers. The contracted primary distributor receives medicines from the suppliers and stores, and distributes them to districts and major facilities. Thus private channels are used to supply publicly funded medicines to government operated health facilities. This strategy is used in the United States.

- *Primarily or fully private supply:* In some countries, medicines for public-sector patients are provided by private pharmacies in or near government health facilities. With such an approach, measures are required to ensure equity of access for poor and other vulnerable populations. This approach is used in Canada and Australia.

These systems vary considerably with respect to the role of the government, the role of the private sector, and incentives for efficiency. Mixed systems in which different categories of pharmaceuticals are supplied through different mechanisms are frequently seen, and countries that take advantage of the capacities in both the public and private sectors usually have systems that are more effective and efficient.

Management of Donated Medicines

Unwanted or inappropriate donations take up storage space, require tracking, and may incur costs such as customs clearance. This problem may be exacerbated with multiple drug donations as in emergency situations. Three core principles for useful donations have been established:

- Donations should be intended to assist the recipient.
- Donations should be given with full respect for the authority of the recipient, including national drug policies.
- There should not be double standards in product quality: Items that are unacceptable in the donor country are unacceptable for the recipient country.

Exhibit 14-4	An Autonomous Medical Supply Service: Medical Stores Department in Tanzania

Prior to 1994, Tanzania employed a traditional CMS model for procurement, storage, and distribution of medicines. Due to operational and financial sustainability issues and ineffective CMS management throughout the 1980s, the Ministry of Health then made reforming the CMS a priority. The reforms resulted in the development of an autonomous Medical Stores Department (MSD) to procure, store, distribute, and sell health commodities to the public sector and authorized private organizations. Its mandate was to make available essential medicines and supplies on a nationwide basis, be financially self-sustaining, and base decision making on sound commercial principles.

MSD is currently the predominant (and single) distributor of pharmaceuticals and medical supplies in Tanzania. It creates its own rules, regulations, and procedures, and operates a self-sustaining revolving drug fund with eight zonal stores. MSD serves national referral hospitals, regional and district health facilities, health centers and dispensaries, faith-based health facilities, and approved nongovernmental organizations.

Although MSD improved the supply of essential medicines and health commodities to the public sector, major increases in its workload in recent years have stretched MSD's physical and managerial capacity. Previously, MSD had a virtual monopoly over the distribution of medical supplies to all public sector and faith-based health facilities. Now, because of decentralization, districts and health facilities have control over their own budgets and can procure medicines and supplies from other sources. A 2007 survey showed that only 33% of health facilities procured products exclusively from MSD, with the remainder obtaining medicines and supplies from private pharmaceutical wholesalers and pharmacies. Nevertheless, MSD sales turnover has been steadily increasing.

Storage space and general stock availability from MSD have been ongoing problems. In a 2001 assessment, MSD was able to supply fewer than 80% of items requested. In 2003, its facilities had an average of 49% of essential medicines available—far short of the target of 100% availability for these medicines. MSD reported product delivery delays and insufficient forecasting to be the main problems resulting in stock-outs. The assessment did find good practices for storage and stock management at the central and regional stores. Stocks were secure, protected from light in properly ventilated areas, and well organized, and the information technology stock management system was functioning. A more recent assessment in 2007 looking at the availability of 20 essential medicines found that these products were available in 83% of MSD zonal stores and in 89% of health facilities assessed.

Source: MOHSW, 2008; MSH, 2010; Strategies for Enhancing Access to Medicines (SEAM)

Exhibit 14-5	Tsunami-Related Donations of Medicines and Supplies

On December 26, 2004, a massive earthquake in the Indian Ocean triggered a tsunami that devastated 11 countries in South Asia. Although international donors were quick to respond with aid, the lack of coordination and knowledge about the actual needs of the population decreased this effort's effectiveness and generated additional challenges for the public health response.

In Indonesia, although the government asked for no medicines, more than 4,000 tons of pharmaceuticals were received for a population of 2 million, according to an assessment conducted by Pharmaciens Sans Frontières Comité International. Of these donations, most were deemed inappropriate: 60% of the medicines were not on the Indonesian national list of essential medicines, 70% were labeled in a foreign language, and 25% had an inadequate expiry date. Of the medicines that were appropriate, some arrived in extremely large quantities that would not likely be used before they expired. Approximately 661 tonnes of the donated medicine needed to be destroyed at an estimated cost of U.S. $2.93 million.

In Sri Lanka, relief workers requested a donation from a pharmaceutical manufacturer of intravenous antibiotics to treat infected wounds. Although the manufacturer shipped the antibiotics quickly to a nonprofit consolidator working in Colombo, the shipment was initially delayed by bureaucratic procedures at the airport. Furthermore, it took additional time to get the medicines to those in need. By the time any of the shipment made it into the affected regions, the antibiotics were no longer needed—either because patients had died already or because of the difficulty in assessing the need in the midst of the chaos. Sri Lankan officials were concerned about the stockpile expiring before it was used (Chase & Barta, 2005).

The Pharmaciens Sans Frontières assessors in Banda Aceh, Indonesia, concluded that in the 10 years after the first publication of the WHO's *Guidelines for Drug Donations* in 1996, the quality of pharmaceutical donations in emergency situations had not improved.

Sources: Chase & Barta, 2005; Mason, 2005; Pharmaciens Sans Frontières Comité International, 2005.

In 1996, WHO issued guidelines for drug donations to avoid the adverse effects sometimes associated with unwanted donations. Unfortunately, many donations still present problems to the recipient (WHO, 1999b). Exhibit 14-5 describes some of these challenges.

Private-Sector Supply of Pharmaceuticals

The (for-profit) private sector includes manufacturers at the international and local levels, importers and wholesalers, distributors, and private prescribers, pharmacies, retail outlets, and itinerant medicine vendors. It can play four roles in support of one or more channels within the health system (Ballou-Aares et al., 2008):

- Selling medicines, supplies, and equipment (e.g., manufacturers, wholesalers).

- Selling supply chain services, such as procurement, transportation, warehousing, and information and financial services to one or more channels. Services may include supply chain design, needs quantification, or logistics management and information system design.

- Providing a distribution channel (e.g., pharmacy, private health clinic, franchise network).

- Assisting in implementation of supply chain best practices, such as scheduled delivery

networks, integrated supply chains, pay-for-performance systems, or cash-to-cash cycle time management approaches (e.g., consultants, trainers, educators, change agents).

Private pharmaceutical outlets are often more numerous than their government counterparts and play an important role in the provision of health services in many countries, particularly in rural and underserved communities (Abuya et al., 2007; Marsh et al., 1999; McCombie, 1996). Many countries also have thriving illegal markets that offer pharmaceuticals at retail and sometimes wholesale levels. Understanding the systems that supply these providers is critical to designing effective interventions to improve quality and affordability in this sector (see Exhibit 14-6).

Several strategies have recently been developed and tested to engage the private sector—particularly retail shop owners, so as to increase access to essential medicines—including training (Marsh et al., 1999, 2004; Okeke & Uzochukwu, 2009; Patouillard et al., 2010; Sabot et al., 2009), franchising (Chiguzo et al., 2008), and accreditation (SEAM), with some success. Exhibit 14-7 describes how Tanzania has used accredited drug dispensing outlets to increase access to artemisinin-based combination therapies for malaria.

Exhibit 14-6	The Private-Sector Distribution Chain for Antimalarial Drugs

In many low- and middle-income countries, the retail sector plays an important role in the treatment of malaria. Retailers are perceived as being more accessible and responsive than other providers and are often argued to respond to public-sector failures. A wide range of retail outlets exist, including pharmacies, drug shops, general stores, market stalls, and itinerant hawkers, and the availability of antimalarial medicines is generally high. Yet important concerns arise regarding the performance of retailers in providing quality and affordable malaria treatment: Highly effective, but more expensive drugs are rarely available, especially in more remote and less formal outlets, and antimalarial medicines are often substandard or even fake.

A number of studies have explored the retail-sector distribution chain for antimalarial medicines, with a view toward understanding how retailers decide which drugs to stock and what prices to charge. Key findings have been that the number of levels within the chain varies across countries; within countries, there are generally more levels in the distribution chains serving more remote outlets and employing less qualified staff. As one would expect, fewer suppliers operate at the top of the chain than at the bottom, and some operate at more than one level, creating considerable overlap across chain levels. Another finding has been that different types of wholesalers supply different types of retail outlets. For example, in Tanzania and Kenya, wholesalers that supply drugs alongside other commodities serve general shops, whereas wholesalers that specialize in handling drugs serve pharmacies and drug shops. Overall, wholesale markets tend to be relatively concentrated, especially at the top of the chain, where a relatively small number of importers account for most of the antimalarial volumes sold.

Wholesale price markups play a key role in determining affordability at the retail level. Markups vary significantly across chain levels, ranging from 2% to 67% at the level supplying retailers directly, and from 8% to 99% at those supplying higher levels. Retail markups tend to be higher, ranging from 3% to 566% in pharmacies, 29% to 669% in drug shops, and 100% to 233% in general shops.

Source: Patouillard, Hanson, & Goodman, 2010.

Exhibit 14-7	Increasing Access to Malaria Treatment in Tanzania Through Accredited Drug Dispensing Outlets

When Tanzania shifted its recommended first-line treatment to an artemisinin-based combination therapy (ACT), the National Malaria Control Program (NMCP) recognized that a public sector–focused program alone would not benefit the majority of Tanzanians who treat malaria at home. Nevertheless, providing malaria therapy through the private sector in this country has its challenges: Registered pharmacies are scarce and charge unaffordably high prices for ACT, while retail drug sellers are untrained and largely unregulated.

With funding from the U.S. President's Malaria Initiative and technical support from the MSH's Rational Pharmaceutical Management Plus Program, the Tanzania Food and Drug Authority and NMCP designed a plan to make subsidized ACTs available through accredited drug dispensing outlets (ADDOs) in the Morogoro and Ruvuma regions. The ADDO program is an innovative public–private initiative that uses accreditation, inspection, incentives, and training to increase access to essential medicines. Its design included allowing prescription ACTs to be sold in ADDOs, training ADDO dispensers on the new treatment, and collaborating with stakeholders to determine the price at which ADDOs will sell subsidized ACTs.

The pilot program covered approximately 2.9 million people, an estimated 8.4% of the population of Tanzania. In the Ruvuma and Morogoro regions, 1,363 ADDO dispensers from 650 ADDOs have been accredited and trained and are now identifying and treating uncomplicated malaria with ACTs. In comparison, only 600 pharmacists exist in the public and private sectors in the entire country. One year after the pilot program was initiated, a review of records from 448 ADDOs indicated that the percentage of ADDOs that dispensed at least one course of ACT rose from 26.2% during July–September 2007 to 72.6% during April–June 2008, and that ADDOs dispensed more than 300,000 treatments over that period. For the five districts in Ruvuma that reported data for July–September 2008, this percentage increased to 81.5%. These results illustrate the enormous potential of ADDOs to improve community access to recommended malaria medicines through the private sector.

Sources: Center for Pharmaceutical Management, 2008; Rutta et al., 2009; SEAM.

Mixed Systems and Interconnectedness Between Public and Private Sectors

Most countries have mixed public and private financing and delivery of care, such that the public sector may supply public health facilities, while the private sector supplies the public sector, private hospitals, clinics, and retail outlets. In many instances, there is a great deal of interaction between the two sectors, with both being involved in procurement, importation, financing, service delivery networks, and market and product information. In Ghana, the CMS procures a large percentage of its products on the local market from private-sector suppliers. Similarly, as much as one-fifth of CMS sales are directed to non-public-sector entities. In addition, health facilities commonly buy products directly from the private sector, with some regional medical stores procuring more

than 85% of their products from this source (Ballou-Aares et al., 2008). In many countries, illicit flows may also occur within and between the sectors due to leakage from public-sector facilities, diversions from the port, and donations by NGOs. Figure 14-5 illustrates the potential flow of medicines in the public and private sectors, highlighting interactions among the various sectors and stakeholders. Understanding these systems, and the connections between the public and private sectors, is critical to intervening to improve access and quality.

The Effect of Global Health Initiatives on the Pharmaceutical Distribution Chain

Since 2000, the emergence of several large disease-specific global health initiatives (GHIs) has contributed to an unprecedented increase in the resources available

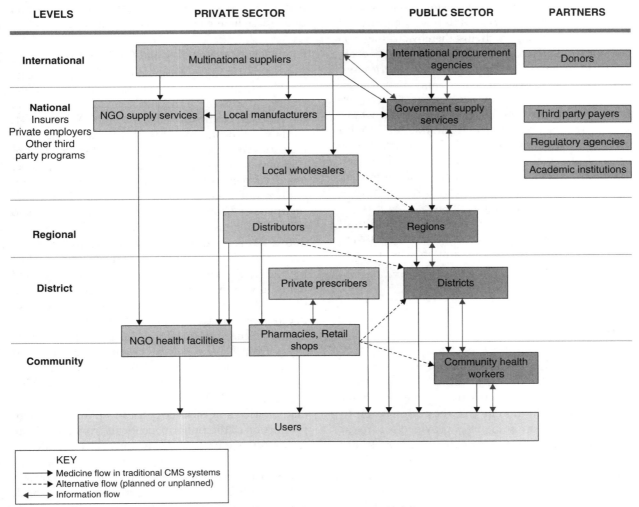

Figure 14-5 Flow of Medicines in the Public and Private Sectors and Potential Interactions.
Source: Adapted from MSH (1997). Managing Drug Supply, 2nd ed. J. Quick, J. Rankin, R. Laing, et al. West Hartford, CT.

for programs. Establishment of GHIs has led to large increases in the supply of and demand for medicines, vaccines, insecticide-treated bed nets, and diagnostic and laboratory materials, and has been associated with improvements in the quality, availability, and affordability of many of these commodities, particularly in relation to vaccines and antiretroviral medicines for HIV/AIDS (Chauveau et al., 2008; Gupta et al., 2002; Hagmann, 2001; Laing & McGoldrick, 2000; Samb et al., 2009; Sharma, 2003; WHO, UNAIDS, & UNICEF, 2008).

In some instances, countries and GHIs have worked together to strengthen national procurement and distribution networks (Mtonya & Chizimbi, 2006; Oomman, Bernstein, & Rosenzweig, 2008; Stillman & Bennett, 2005). However, although alignment with country procurement systems is included as one of the indicators of aid effectiveness in the Paris Declaration on Aid Effectiveness (2005) and the Accra Agenda for Action (2008), such synergy has not always occurred. In some instances, GHIs have duplicated or displaced country supply chains, thereby creating parallel systems (Laing & McGoldrick, 2000; Smith et al., 2005). Poor harmonization between countries and GHIs has resulted in elevated costs and inefficiencies, and opportunities to strengthen country-level capacity for procurement and supply management have been missed (Samb et al., 2009; Shretta, 2007; Smith et al., 2005; Stillman & Bennett, 2005). Furthermore, although the availability of specific medicines such as antiretroviral medicines and vaccines has improved, other essential medicines distributed through the public system are frequently out of stock (Samb et al., 2009). While recent efforts have focused on integrating the distribution systems for medicines, vaccines, and contraceptives, in some places separate systems continue to operate (Samb et al., 2009).

Affordability

As outlined in the introduction to this chapter, affordability is a key factor affecting access to pharmaceuticals. It relates the price that a patient must pay for a product to the amount that the person is able to pay. While drugs are sometimes provided for free at public health facilities, patients frequently seek care outside the public sector—for example, in private drug shops, clinics, or pharmacies. Even where drugs are officially free in the public sector, stock-outs and informal charges may mean that patients still incur payments for their receipt. Medicines are often in-

cluded in insurance benefit packages, but they may nonetheless require a copayment. Thus, in many cases, patients are required to make out-of-pocket payments to purchase drugs at the time they are ill.

Affordability is commonly measured as the number of days' wages (e.g., of the lowest-paid, unskilled government worker in a given setting) required to purchase a treatment course. To illustrate, the affordability of salbutamol inhaler, a medicine commonly used for the treatment of asthma, purchased in the private sector is given in Table 14-7. As this example demonstrates, the significant variation in affordability for the same treatment is not only pronounced across countries, but also within countries between originator and generic brands (WHO & Health Action International [HAI], 2008).

This section examines some of the factors that have reduced the affordability of pharmaceuticals in low- and middle-income countries, and the strategies that have been devised both to reduce the prices of and to increase financing for pharmaceuticals.

Pharmaceutical Spending and Affordability

In low- and middle-income countries, governments fund less than 30% of total pharmaceutical spending, compared with more than 40% of such spending in high-income countries (WHO, 2004b). While the affordability of pharmaceuticals is a key issue in all countries regardless of income, it is of particular importance in low- and middle-income countries, where less developed health systems and lower wages generally result in a greater share of personal income being spent on health, thereby exposing households to the risk of catastrophic health expenditure (WHO, 2004a). This situation has arisen for a number of reasons. Notably, worsening economic conditions during the latter part of the twentieth century required many low- and middle-income countries to reform their health sectors. This process often resulted in reduced public funds available for health and greater reliance on mechanisms for raising complementary funds from private sources, such as user fees and health insurance (Gilson & Mills, 1995). The situation is compounded by the chronically low public-sector availability of pharmaceuticals, which forces many patients in these countries to purchase a high proportion of their pharmaceuticals from the private sector, often at greater cost (Cameron et al., 2009).

Global trade agreements—most notably those related to intellectual property rights—also pose a threat to the affordability of pharmaceuticals. Such agreements may restrict low- and middle-income countries' access to more competitively priced generic

Table 14-7	Affordability of One Salbutamol Inhaler 0.1 mg/Dose Purchased from the Private Sector in Selected Countries, 2004	
Country (Date of Survey)	**Originator Brand**	**Lowest-Priced Generic Brand**
Uganda (April 2004)	5.6 days	2.0 days
Ghana (October 2004)	8.0 days	4.6 days
Mali (March 2004)	4.2 days	2.7 days
Pakistan (July 2004)	1.4 days	1.4 days

Source: Adapted from WHO & HAI, 2008.

versions of patented products (see Chapter 18 on globalization and health).

Price is yet another critical factor that affects the affordability of pharmaceuticals. In the public sector, the efficiency of the procurement process is an important determinant of both the affordability and the availability of public-sector pharmaceuticals. A 2009 study that examined the government procurement prices of 15 commonly purchased medicines in 36 countries revealed that although the median government procurement prices for those medicines were only 1.11 times the international reference prices from open international procurements for generic products (indicating a relatively good level of procurement efficiency on average), the range of procurement prices varied widely, from 0.1 to more than 5 times the international reference prices, indicating that the procurement process often did not secure the best value (Cameron et al., 2009).

In the private sector, the retail price of pharmaceuticals can present a serious barrier to access and affect rational use of medicines. In November 2009, Health Action International (HAI) took a global "snapshot" of the private-sector retail price of the antibiotic ciprofloxacin, comparing the price of the originator brand product to the lowest-priced generic equivalent across 93 countries. The results of its study showed that the price for a 7-day treatment course of ciprofloxacin varied widely both between and within countries, ranging from \$0.42 to \$131, and that a significant difference between the lowest-priced generic and the originator brand (the "brand premium") persisted in many countries despite the fact that the patent on ciprofloxacin expired a number of years ago (HAI Global, 2010).

To understand why prices vary or may become unreasonably high, it is important to understand their many components. These elements differ by country, by sector of the health system, and by type of pharmaceutical, but generally include the manufacturer's selling price; insurance, freight, port charges, inspection charges, and duties for imported products; the markups added by importers, wholesalers, and retail distributors; various taxes; and fees associated with dispensing. A more comprehensive list and description of pharmaceutical price components appears in Exhibit 14-8.

Exhibit 14-8	Components That May Contribute to the Price of Pharmaceuticals

A five-stage supply chain approach has been used by the WHO and HAI in their medicines surveys to identify and compare the cumulative price components of pharmaceuticals as they move from manufacturer to patient across healthcare sectors and across countries.

Stage 1: Manufacturer's Selling Price + Insurance and Freight

- The *manufacturer's selling price* (MSP) is affected by whether the product is novel, requires a complex manufacturing process, is intensively marketed, or is produced in relatively small quantities. The MSP of locally produced goods may be affected if tariffs (see stage 2) are applied for the importation of materials used for manufacture or packaging.
- *Insurance* and *freight* charges are added during the shipping of imported goods. Fluctuation in the price of fuel is an important consideration in the value of these charges.
- *Drug registration fees* are typically one-off charges imposed by national drug regulatory authorities (NDRAs) to register a product for use in the country and are often incorporated into the MSP.

continued

Exhibit 14-8 continued

Stage 2: Landed Price

- *Finance/banking fees* are usually incurred during a procurement process involving large tenders. These fees may include the transaction costs for obtaining letters of credit, the purchase of foreign exchange, commissions, and special licenses for importation.
- *Inspections* to verify the quality, quantity, value, and eligibility of the imported goods are conducted either prior to shipment or upon the goods' arrival in the receiving country. The fees charged for these inspections may be a flat fee or a rate applied to the order value.
- *Port* and *clearance charges* may be collected to cover temporary storage, stamp duty, handling, and insurance while the goods are in port. Governments may also charge for documentation, such as data collection for statistical purposes.
- The *pharmacy board fee* or *national drug authority fee* is a percentage or fixed charge collected in some countries that goes to the pharmacy board (or similar body), or the national medicines regulatory authority. In some countries, this fee is applied to all pharmaceuticals; in other countries, it is applied only to imported or locally manufactured products.
- *Tariffs* are fees that may be collected by governments and may be calculated either as rates applied to the value order or as fixed fees. Depending on how the fees are structured, they may be intended to raise government revenues and to give the local pharmaceutical industry an advantage over foreign exports. The level of the tariff may vary by product, and exemptions may apply depending on the products, sector, or program. (Tariffs on pharmaceuticals are discussed later in this section in more detail.)
- Some countries collect *national, state, and/or local taxes* on the procurement of pharmaceuticals at this and at later stages.
- The *import markup* accounts for the profit gained and costs incurred by the importer, including rent, utilities, staff, security, local transport, packaging, and marketing. In some countries, governments regulate the maximum markup that may be applied to pharmaceuticals at different stages of the supply chain, with the rate varying by product. This practice may be poorly enforced, however. (See Exhibit 14-6 on the distribution chain for antimalarial drugs.)

Stage 3: Wholesale Selling Price or Central Medical Stores Price

- The *wholesale markup*, like the markup at the import level, covers the operating costs of the wholesaler (private sector) or the CMS (public sector) and any profit margins that may be added by private-, public-, and mission-sector wholesalers. In the low- and middle-income countries for which data are available, these markups range from 2% to 380%. (See Exhibit 14-6 on the distribution chain for antimalarial drugs.)
- *Transport costs* may be incurred for moving goods from the warehouse (wholesaler) to the point of delivery (retailer) or, in the public sector, from the central or regional medical stores to the hospital pharmacies/dispensaries or health post.

Stage 4: Retail Price (Private Sector) or Dispensary Price (Public Sector)

- The *retail markup* is similar to the other markups added at higher levels of the supply chain. At the retail level, however, there may be great variation in markups (ranging from 10% to 55%), particularly in settings where there is no regulation. This variation may be more pronounced in the informal sector.

Stage 5: Dispensed Price

- A *value-added tax* (VAT) and *goods and services tax* (GST) may be levied on pharmaceutical sales, with their rates varying both across and within countries. In many countries, medicines or certain sectors are exempted from the VAT or GST; in other countries, the VAT is collected at each stage of the supply chain. In the low- and middle-income countries for which data are available, the VAT varies from 4% to 15%. In some countries, a GST is also charged on medicines.
- Pharmacies may be allowed to charge a *dispensing fee* per item dispensed or per prescription filled. This fee is intended to reflect the work involved in handling a prescription and can take various forms: a percentage markup, a fee per item, or a fee per prescription. Dispensing fees can also vary for originator brand and generic formulations.

Sources: Adapted from WHO & HAI (2008) and MDG Gap Task Force (2009).

Strategies to Improve Sustainable Funding for Pharmaceuticals

Increasing the amount of sustainable funding available for pharmaceuticals is one of the pillars of WHO's campaign to improve equitable access to medicines.

The key actions recommended to policy makers include increasing public funding for health; expanding health insurance through national, local, and employer schemes; targeting external funding from grants, loans, and donations at specific diseases with high public health impact; reducing out-of-pocket spending, especially by the poor; and exploring other innovative financing mechanisms (WHO, 2004a).

Increasing public funding to improve delivery of pharmaceuticals through the national health system presents the most direct route to improving equitable access by optimizing consumption of products that have a high degree of public benefit, such as vaccines, and by subsidizing medicines for the poor (Madrid, Velázquez, & Fefer, 1998). However, this does not mean that resources should be taken away from other important health programs; rather, the extra funds should be raised from additional domestic or external sources (WHO, 2004a). For the past decade or so, the proportion of pharmaceuticals procured for the public sector using external funding through donor and development assistance has increased substantially. As of 2008, 37% of the $5.1 billion disbursed by the Global Fund went directly to ministries of health, much of which was spent on pharmaceuticals and strengthening the supply chain; another 35% of Global Fund disbursements went to civil society organizations, many of which run pharmaceuticals-related programs that complement those in the public sector (GFATM, 2010b). The GAVI Alliance (2010) has been co-financing country procurement of vaccines for immunization programs based on each country's ability to pay since 2007.

External funding has also been used in innovative financing mechanisms for pharmaceuticals, including targeted use of debt relief funds, in-kind funding in the form of medicine donations, solidarity funds, and revolving drug funds (WHO, 2004a). A recent initiative designed to increase the provision of affordable antimalarial drugs through the public, private, and NGO sectors is the Affordable Medicines Facility—Malaria (AMFm). This Global Fund–managed program will use external funding to reduce the manufacturer sales price of quality-assured artemisinin-based combination therapy (ACT) for buyers in the public, private, and not-for-profit sectors to approximately $0.05 for each course of ACT. It will do so by negotiating a lower price for the medicines and then paying a large proportion of this price directly to manufacturers on behalf of buyers (a buyer "copayment"). This approach is expected to result in a significant reduction in the patient price of ACTs, from $6 to $10 per treatment to $0.20 to $0.50 per treatment (GFATM, 2010a).

Financial protection to help patients cope with rising pharmaceutical costs and increased out-of-pocket payments is another important action to improve affordability. Universal and comprehensive health insurance can significantly improve access,

particularly in the case of newer, more expensive treatments; but also has the ability to improve equity by pooling risks between those who are sick and those who are healthy, and by allowing for income-related cross-subsidies. Nevertheless, despite this emphasis on promoting health insurance, coverage in low- and middle-income countries remains low: 35% in Latin America, 10% in Asia, and less than 8% in Africa (WHO, 2004a). Expanding health insurance to those employed in the informal sector is particularly challenging. For these populations, consideration should be given to community-based insurance schemes (Madrid, Velázquez, & Fefer, 1998) and to mobilization of additional domestic funds through taxation (MDG Gap Task Force, 2009). (See Chapter 12 on design of health systems for more detail.)

Strategies to Improve Affordability by Reducing Pharmaceutical Prices

More affordable pharmaceutical prices can be pursued through a number of mechanisms. The guidelines listed in Exhibit 14-9 are the key actions recommended by WHO (2004a) to policy makers in this area.

Two of the price-reduction mechanisms in Exhibit 14-9 have been more recently debated: the reduction of taxes and tariffs and the use of the public health safeguards incorporated into the World Trade Organization's (WTO) Agreement on Trade-Related Intellectual Property Rights (TRIPS).

A recent study showed that although the global average for import tariffs on pharmaceuticals in 2009 had dropped to 3.5%, down from 5% in 2005, many low- and middle-income countries with very high burdens of infectious diseases still imposed import duties as high as 15% on antibiotics and 40 countries continued to impose tariffs on imported vaccines (Stevens & Linfield, 2010). Tariffs on medicines are widely regarded as regressive taxes that disproportionately affect the poor, who are more likely to purchase their treatment in the private sector. Nevertheless, it has been argued that such measures foster the growth of the local pharmaceutical industry by protecting it from international competition and generate government revenues. Another study showed that the majority of tariffs did not achieve these objectives, as 59% of countries continued to levy import tariffs on the ingredients used to manufacture pharmaceuticals locally and pharmaceutical tariffs in general raised little revenue for governments. Both studies concluded that removing pharmaceutical tariffs would not be detrimental to either local industry or government revenues (Olcay & Laing, 2005; Stevens & Linfield, 2010).

Exhibit 14-9	Key Actions Recommended by WHO to Pursue More Affordable Prices

1. *Use available and impartial price information* to obtain the best price during the procurement process and price negotiations, to locate new supply sources, and to assess procurement efficiency. Several international and regional price information services, such as those offered by MSH, WHO, UNICEF, are publicly available.
2. *Allow price competition in the local market* through the tendering of generic products and therapeutic competition (i.e., competition between products belonging to the same therapeutic class).
3. *Promote bulk procurement* by pooling together pharmaceutical orders, focusing on a list of priority products, and minimizing duplication within therapeutic categories. This can be done not just across organizations or facilities within a country, but also between countries.
4. *Implement policies to expand the use of generic products* at all levels of the supply chain, such as regulations supporting the local registration and manufacture of generic products of assured quality, laws requiring prescriptions to be written using generic names, and laws permitting generic substitution.
5. *Negotiate prices for newly registered products, particularly for those that target priority diseases* and are still protected by patents. Equitable pricing (also known as tiered, differential, or preferential pricing) is one such mechanism whereby the prices charged are adapted to reflect countries' ability to pay as measured by their level of income. Widespread equitable pricing is economically feasible provided that low-priced medicines do not leak back to high-income countries.
6. *Encourage local production of essential medicines of assured quality* when economically feasible and where it follows good manufacturing practices.
7. *Reduce or eliminate duties, tariffs, and taxes* for both generic and patented essential medicines (see the discussion in the text) and *reduce markups through more efficient distribution and dispensing systems.*
8. *Include World Trade Organization (WTO)/TRIPS-compatible safeguards for public health in national legislation.* (See the further discussion in the text and Chapter 18 on globalization and health.)

Sources: Adapted from WHO, 2001c, 2004a.

The TRIPS agreement was negotiated between 1986 and 1994 during the Uruguay Round of the WTO's trade negotiations. This agreement set the minimum standards for intellectual property protection that all WTO member countries must respect, some of which did not provide patent protection for pharmaceuticals prior to the agreement. TRIPS states that all pharmaceutical patents shall be available for at least 20 years from the filing date for all products "invented" after January 1, 1995. To abide by the agreement, WTO members have to modify their intellectual property legislation to make them consistent with the new WTO standards, although countries at different levels of economic development were given different deadlines to comply with this mandate (Boulet et al., 2000). Health-sector advocates argued that these standards should take protection of public health into account, so a provision to allow circumvention of the patent requirement in the event of "public health emergencies" was included in the agreement (WHO, 2001b). To further clarify this provision, and after much pressure from the international health community, the WTO produced the Declaration on the TRIPS Agreement and Public Health, also known as the Doha Declaration of 2001,

and a subsequent Decision on the Interpretation of Paragraph 6 of the TRIPS Agreement was reached in 2003. These clarifications affirmed the flexibilities available to member states seeking to protect public health (Kerry & Lee, 2007), allowing countries to issue a compulsory license to manufacture generic versions of patented products for either domestic use or export, or to import generic versions, on the basis of public health need.

Although TRIPS and its successors were hailed as a "watershed in international trade," fully realizing the potential to improve access to affordable medicines offered by these flexibilities has proved difficult in practice. A number of studies have cited a lack of country-level capacity to fully integrate these provisions into relevant legislation and the increasingly common inclusion of so-called TRIPS-plus measures in bilateral trade agreements between powerful trading nations and low- and middle-income countries. These agreements include intellectual property rights (IPR) obligations that go well beyond the TRIPS minimum standards and supersede them in these jurisdictions (Haakonsson & Richey, 2007; Kerry & Lee, 2007; Oliveira et al., 2004; Roffe & Spennemann, 2006).

Safe and Effective Medicines Use

Even when the right medicines are in the right place and are affordable, many challenges remain in ensuring safe and effective therapy. Are the medicines of appropriate quality? Are they being used appropriately? What must be done to ensure their continued safety? These are the questions to which we now turn.

Rational Use of Medicines

The concept of rational medicine use has been adopted by many countries. WHO defines it as follows: The rational use of medicines requires that "patients receive medications appropriate to their clinical needs, in doses that meet their own individual requirements, for an adequate period of time, and at the lowest cost to them and their community" (WHO, 2002b). This definition is expressed mainly in medical and financial terms. However, patients have their own rationale for taking medicines; thus what may be seen as irrational from a medical perspective may be perceived as entirely rational from the consumer's point of view (Wiedenmayer, 2004b).

Nature of Nonrational Use

Irrational use of medicines takes many forms and can occur at the prescribing, dispensing, and patient administration stages. Studies in both high-income and low- and middle-income countries describe numerous examples of nonrational medicine use (Exhibit 14-10).

The extent of irrational use of medicines worldwide is enormous. For example, as many as 75% of antibiotics are prescribed inappropriately. WHO also estimates that only 50% of patients worldwide take their medicines correctly. There is often little rela-

tionship between medicines use and sound therapeutic principles.

In an effort to stem this tide of nonrational use, governments are increasingly using evidence-based approaches to inform their decisions about therapeutic options. The WHO Model List of Essential Medicines (sixteenth edition, updated March 2010) provides a mechanism for aligning medicines use with therapeutic principles. It consists of a core list of the minimum medicine needs for a basic healthcare system, and a complementary list presenting essential medicines for priority diseases in which specialist support is needed (WHO, 2010c).

Consequences of Nonrational Medicine Use

The nonrational use of medicine carries enormous costs and impacts. In addition to inefficient use of limited resources, such use may lead to adverse clinical consequences and unnecessary suffering by patients. Wasting resources in this way may lead to increased costs later and the need to use more expensive medicines. In addition, nonrational use of medicines can lead to increased morbidity and mortality, along with increased risks of adverse drug reactions and the emergence of antibacterial resistance. Inappropriate use of medicines may also lead patients to believe that there is "a pill for every ill."

Medicine Use Behaviour

The use of medicines has to be viewed in both biomedical and social contexts. A number of actors are involved in this process (principally prescribers, dispensers, and patients), which involves a number of steps:

Exhibit 14-10	Examples of Nonrational Medicine Use

- Polypharmacy (multiple or over-prescription)
- Use of medicines that are not related to diagnosis
- Unnecessarily costly medicines
- Inappropriate prescription and use of antibiotics
- Indiscriminate use of injections
- Irrational self-medication with under-dosing and over-dosing
- Incorrect administration, dosages, and timing, formulation, or duration
- The use of medicines when no medicine therapy is indicated
- Failure to prescribe available, safe, and effective medicines
- Poor adherence to tuberculosis treatment
- Underuse of effective medicines for hypertension and depression
- Hospital medicine use problems such as antibiotic misuse for surgical prophylaxis

Source: Wiedenmayer, 2004b.

- Diagnosis: identification of what is wrong

- Therapy: development of a therapeutic objective and plan

- Prescribing: information, instructions, warnings, and prescription writing

- Dispensing: supply, advice, counseling, instructions, and warnings

- Adherence by the patient: understanding of the therapy, patient responsibility, and valuing of treatment

The factors that determine individual medicine use patterns are complex. The medicine use system in which they occur is part of a larger healthcare system, which is itself shaped by the social, cultural, economic, and political contexts of the country concerned. Furthermore, both the prescriber and the patient bring a host of beliefs and motivations to their interaction (Horne & Weinman, 1999). A number of tools are now available to examine patients' cognitive beliefs about medicines (Horne, Weinman, & Hankins, 1999). The concept of concordance, where the aim is agreement about medication action, has been suggested to be more helpful in ensuring correct medicine use than compliance (Horne, 2006; WHO, 2003a). Medicine use encounters take place in many different locations, such as the hospital, private practice, a pharmacy, at home, health center, dispensary, at the traditional healer, with a medicine seller, or in the marketplace. Once a medicine is prescribed, the psychosocial setting in which it is given or taken may further influence the patient's response to it.

The importance of cultural factors has been demonstrated in anthropological studies of medicine use in low- and middle-income countries (see Exhibit 14-11) (van Der Geest & Reynolds Whyte, 1988). These investigations have illustrated how people base their actions on what they believe and have shown that Western medicines often need to be reinterpreted within a local cultural perspective. Failure to understand the local cultural context is a common cause of inappropriate medicine use (Wiedenmayer, 2004b).

Strategies to Improve Medicine Use

The problem of nonrational use of medicines has been recognized for many years, and many suggestions have been made about how to improve matters. Improving the use of medicines by health workers and the general public is crucial to reducing morbidity and mortality from both communicable and noncommunicable diseases, preventing and minimizing

---

Exhibit 14-11	How Beliefs Influence Use

In Sierra Leone, medicines' efficacy is linked to color symbolism. Red medicines, for example, are thought to be good for the blood (Bledsoe & Goubaud, 1985).

In Uganda, one study described reasons for the popularity of injections. People in this country believe that medicine injected into the bloodstream does not leave the body as quickly as that administered orally. Oral medicine is compared to food, which enters the digestive system and eventually leaves the body through defecation (Birungi et al., 1994).

An investigation in Ghana described how people consider heat to be the main cause of measles. In this belief system, heat causes constipation and stomach sores in children. To treat measles, people give Septrin (co-trimoxazole) syrup, Multivite syrup, calamine lotion, akpeteshie (local gin), and a herbal concoction given as an enema to "flush out" the heat (Senah, 1997).

---

drug resistance, and containing drug expenditure. Therapeutically sound and cost-effective use of medicines by health professionals and consumers needs to be achieved at all levels of the health system, in both the public and private sectors. According to WHO, a sound rational-use program in any country has three elements (Exhibit 14-12), which are formulated in such a way as to reflect the main responsibilities of a national essential medicines program.

WHO and the International Network for Rational Use of Drugs (INRUD) have developed extensive resources and literature on the promotion of rational medicine use. The INRUD Drug Use Bibliography is an annotated bibliography of published and unpub-

---

Exhibit 14-12	Elements of Rational Medicines Use Programs

- *Rational use of medicines strategy and monitoring:* Advocating rational medicines use, identifying and promoting successful strategies, and securing responsible medicines promotion.

- *Rational use of medicines by health professionals:* Working with countries to develop and update treatment guidelines, national essential medicines lists, and formularies, and supporting training programs on rational use of medicines.

- *Rational use of medicines by consumers:* Supporting creation of effective systems of medicines information, and empowering consumers to take responsible decisions about their treatment.

Source: WHO, 2010g.

lished articles, books, reports, and other documents related to medicine use, with a special focus on low- and middle-income countries.

Effectiveness of Interventions to Improve Medicine Use

In general, medicine use can best be improved through interventions targeted at specific problems with an identifiable audience, or by a system change such as preventing the unnecessary prescribing of expensive branded medicines through use of nationally accepted clinical practice guidelines. The most effective medicine use intervention is one that is participatory, interactive, problem based, and focused (Wiedenmayer, 2004b). In general, it is more efficient and effective to combine a number of strategies into a multifaceted intervention to improve medicine use. Some strategies have proved more successful than others. A review by Laing et al. (2001) identified 10 key initiatives that have been shown to make a difference (Exhibit 14-13).

Medicines Quality

A prerequisite for the rational use of medicines is that they should be of good quality, both at the time of manufacture and at the time of consumption by the patient. Unfortunately, a wide variety of potential hazards may emerge between manufacture and end use of these products. Substandard and counterfeit medicines are major problems, as are smuggling and the illegal importation of medicines. These activities present major challenges to national authorities and seriously undermine initiatives aimed at rational medicine use.

Defining Quality of Medicines

WHO (2010h) defines substandard medicines (also called out-of-specification [OOS] products) as "genuine medicines produced by manufacturers, authorized by the NMRA (National Medicines Regulatory Authority) which do not meet quality specifications set for them by national standards." Normally, medicines produced by manufacturers have to comply with a set of quality specifications, and NMRAs review products against these criteria before they are authorized for marketing. The quality of medicines reaching the patient can be affected by the manufacturing process, packaging, transportation and storage conditions, handling, and other factors (Wiedenmayer, 2004a). Moreover, these influences can be cumulative. Loss of activity due to the instability of the drug itself is unusual; poor initial quality of the medicine is a more serious problem. Examples of substandard medicines include those with a loss of potency due to poor bioavailability, expiry, or poor storage conditions;

Exhibit 14-13	**Ten Recommendations to Improve Use of Medicines in Low- and Middle-Income Countries**

1. Establish procedures for developing, disseminating, utilizing, and revising national (or hospital-specific) standard treatment deadlines
2. Establish procedures for developing and revising an essential drug list (or hospital formulary) based on treatments of choice
3. Request hospitals to establish representative Pharmacy and Therapeutics Committees with defined responsibilities for monitoring and promoting quality use of medicines
4. Implement problem-based training in pharmacotherapy in undergraduate medical and paramedical education based on national standard treatment guidelines
5. Encourage development of targeted, problem-based in-service educational programs by professional societies, universities, and the ministry of health, and require regular continuing education for licensure of health professionals
6. Stimulate an interactive group process among health providers or consumers to review and apply information about appropriate use of medicines
7. Train pharmacists and drug sellers to be active members of the healthcare team and to offer useful advice to consumers about health and drugs
8. Encourage active involvement by consumer organizations in public education about drugs, and devote government resources to support these efforts
9. Develop a strategic approach to improve prescribing in the private sector through appropriate regulation and long-term collaborations with professional associations
10. Establish systems to monitor key pharmaceutical indicators routinely to track the effects of health-sector reform and regulatory changes

Source: Laing et al., 2001.

those with too low or too high concentration of active ingredients due to manufacturing or compounding error and counterfeiting; those that have degraded into toxic substances; those producing adverse reactions; and injectables, creams, syrups and eye drops that have been contaminated with bacteria or fungi.

Two other concepts need to be distinguished. Quality assurance (QA) is the whole process of assuring quality from manufacturer to end user. Quality control (QC) involves testing key characteristics of the final product—namely, the identity and potency of the active ingredient, the content range (with acceptable range usually set at 95% to 110%), purity (involving checks to exclude contaminating substances or microorganisms), uniformity (in terms of color, shape, and size), bioavailability (the rate and extent of absorption of a medicine into the body), and stability (adequate shelf life and expiry).

Detailed descriptions of medicine characteristics and of analytical techniques to verify them are usually laid down in national pharmacopoeias, such as the United States Pharmacopoeia (USP) and the British Pharmacopoeia (BP). WHO (2010d) publishes an International Pharmacopoeia that is more suitable for low- and middle-income countries, as it is based on standard chemical tests that can be carried out without sophisticated equipment.

Quality Assurance Programs

The three main activities involved in assuring the quality of medicines are registration of medicines with the NMRA, inspection of manufacturing plants to ensure compliance with Good Pharmaceutical Manufacturing Practice (GMP), and testing of medicines based on product types and characteristics. GMP covers all aspects of production, with its guidelines focusing on personnel, facilities, equipment, sanitation, raw materials, manufacturing processes, labeling and packaging, quality control systems, self inspection, distribution, documents and records, and complaints and adverse medicine reaction systems.

Quality assurance programs must include training and supervision of staff involved at all stages of the process. Effective information systems are essential for following up and documenting quality problems. Although the foundation of QA consists of regulations and standards, it is the people who enforce the regulations or work to comply with the standards who make the difference between QA and the lack of it (WHO, 1997). WHO's prequalification program (discussed earlier in this chapter) is another mechanism for ensuring pharmaceutical quality, including the quality of new products (WHO, 2010i).

Role of Regulatory Agencies

An important determinant of both QA and medicine quality is effective medicine regulation. Of the 190 WHO member states, only some 20% have well-developed medicine regulation (International Medical Products Anti-Counterfeiting Taskforce [IMPACT], 2006). Approximately 50% have partially developed regulatory systems, and the remaining 30% have no or very limited capacity in this area. When enforcement is weak or lacking, pharmaceutical manufacturers, importers, and distributors may ignore regulatory requirements and the quality, safety, and efficacy of both imported and locally manufactured medicines may be compromised.

Both NMRAs and WHO play an important part in ensuring the quality of medicines. Regulatory decisions on medicines have been compiled in the *UN Consolidated List of Products Whose Consumption and/or Sale Have Been Banned, Withdrawn, Severely Restricted or Not Approved by Governments*. WHO (1975) has published two updates to this list entitled *Pharmaceuticals: Restrictions in Use and Availability*.

Counterfeit Medicines

A separate and distinct issue from substandard drugs is the proliferation of counterfeit medicines; however, the absence of a universally accepted definition makes it difficult to exchange information between countries and measure the size of this problem. WHO has established its own definition: "A counterfeit medicine is one which is deliberately and fraudulently mislabeled with respect to identity and/or source. Counterfeiting can apply to both branded and generic products and counterfeit products may include products with the correct ingredients or with the wrong ingredients, without active ingredients, with insufficient active ingredients or with fake packaging" (IMPACT, 2006).

The counterfeiting of pharmaceuticals constitutes a serious health risk for the world's population. Trade in counterfeit medicines is a serious crime. In recent years, increasing international trade of pharmaceuticals and sales via the Internet have facilitated the entry of counterfeit products into the distribution chain. In areas in some low- and middle-income countries, more than 30% of medicines sold are counterfeit. Counterfeiting of medicines is on the rise, and it is estimated that more than 70% of this practice occurs in low-income countries (IMPACT, 2006).

The problem of counterfeit medicines was first addressed at the international level in 1985 at the Conference of Experts on the Rational Use of Drugs in Nairobi. A number of initiatives have since been taken. In 2006, WHO launched the International

Medical Products Anti-Counterfeiting Taskforce as part of the Declaration of Rome; this entity has remained the main conduit for WHO's work against counterfeiting operations.

Factors Contributing to Counterfeiting of Medicines

Medicines are attractive to counterfeiters for a number of reasons. They are high-value items for which demand exceeds supply, and ingredient costs can be very low. Moreover, production can often be undertaken using simple equipment, and overhead costs are minimal. Finally, patients are rarely in a position to judge the quality of a medicine.

The majority of counterfeit cases involve tablets and capsules. Antibiotics, hormones, analgesics, antihistamines, and steroids account for almost 60% of reported cases of counterfeit medicines. In approximately one-third of cases, products contain no active ingredient, and 20% contain an incorrect quantity. A further 20% contain the wrong ingredient, and almost 10% contain high levels of impurities and contaminants (Deisingh, 2005). Counterfeit medicines pose a serious health risk to patients and are a major cause of waste of both public and private funds.

A wide range of methods are now available for the detection of counterfeit medicines (WHO, 1999a). Although some require the use of expensive equipment, simple chemical approaches have also been developed. An initiative of pharmaceutical companies in Germany, the German Pharma Health Fund (GPHF), has also developed a mini-laboratory of simple tests to detect a wide range of counterfeit products. More than 300 mini-labs are currently in use, mainly in Africa and Asia.

Counteracting Counterfeit Medicines

The problem of counterfeit medicines is a global one; thus a global response is required to address it. Guidelines for the development of measures to combat counterfeit drugs have been published by WHO (1999a). Exhibit 14-14 lists the steps that should be taken to curb medicines counterfeiting.

Many countries are stepping up their offensives against the counterfeiting problem, but the results have so far been mixed. In Nigeria, intensive action has led to the proportion of fake or adulterated drugs in circulation being reduced from 70% to 16%; in contrast, in India, the share of spurious drugs has grown from 10 to 20% of the market (IMPACT, 2006). Further global action will be necessary if this problem is to be contained (Cockburn, Newton, et al., 2005).

Medicines Safety Issues

The availability of medicines of appropriate quality presents its own problems, as the use of any medicine brings with it the possibility of unintended consequences. When harmful, these effects are referred to as adverse drug reactions (ADRs). ADRs can be either predictable or unpredictable. A range of approaches are used to report and analyze ADRs, including pharmacovigilance and postmarketing surveillance.

Exhibit 14-14   WHO-Recommended Steps to Curb Medicines Counterfeiting

- National laws should regulate the manufacture, trade, distribution, and sale of medicines effectively, with severe penalties being imposed for manufacturing, supplying, or selling counterfeit medicines.
- The NMRAs responsible for the registration and inspection of locally manufactured and imported medicines should be strengthened.
- NMRAs should develop standard operating procedures and guidelines for the inspection of suspected counterfeits, and should initiate widespread screening tests for the detection of counterfeits.
- Adequate training and powers of enforcement against counterfeits should be given to personnel from NMRAs, the judiciary, customs personnel, and police.
- Partnerships should be established between health professionals, importers, industry, and local authorities to combat counterfeits.
- Countries should systematically use the WHO Certificate Scheme on the Quality of Pharmaceutical Products Moving in International Commerce. Countries in the same region should work toward harmonization of their marketing authorization procedures.
- Countries should exchange experience and expertise in areas related to quality control, medicine detection, and enforcement.

Source: WHO, 1999a.

Adverse Drug Reactions

An adverse drug reaction may be defined as "any response to a medicine which is noxious, unintended and occurs at doses normally used for prophylaxis, diagnosis or therapy" (Kanjanarat et al., 2003). ADRs are unwanted effects of a medicine, including idiosyncratic ones, that occur during its proper use. They should be distinguished from accidental or deliberate excessive dosage and administration errors. The costs associated with ADRs are considerable, although the literature includes few reports about their impact in low- and middle-income or transitional countries (Moore et al., 1998).

Two main types of ADRs are distinguished. In Type A reactions, the effects are directly linked to the pharmacological properties of the medicine. Examples include hypoglycemia induced by an antidiabetic medicine. In Type B reactions, the effects are unrelated to the known pharmacology of the medicine. Examples include anaphylactic shock induced by penicillin. A serious adverse event is one that is fatal, life threatening, or permanently or significantly disabling; requires or prolongs hospitalization; causes a congenital anomaly; or requires intervention to prevent permanent impairment or damage (Wiedenmayer, 2004a).

Patients respond differently to the same treatment, so their risk of ADRs likewise varies. Genetic makeup and concurrent disease, for example, can make a patient more prone to ADRs. The very old and very young are more susceptible. Drug–drug interactions are some of the most common causes of adverse effects. Interactions can also occur with alcohol and traditional medicines. In medical literature and package inserts for patients, incidence and frequency of ADRs are usually listed according to international standards. ADRs occurring in more than 1 in 10 patients are described as very common; between 1 in 10 and 1 in 100 as common (or frequent); between 1 in 100 and 1 in 1,000 as uncommon (infrequent); between 1 in 1,000 and 1 in 10,000 as rare; and fewer than 1 in 10,000 as very rare (Lazarou et al., 1998).

ADRs may be easily confused with outcomes of disease processes and are sometimes difficult to distinguish from other causes. WHO (2002c) has proposed a stepwise approach to assess possible ADRs.

Pharmacovigilance

WHO defines pharmacovigilance as "the science and activities relating to the detection, assessment, understanding and prevention of adverse effects or any other possible drug-related problems" (Cobert & Biron, 2002). In recent years, pharmacovigilance has extended its remit to include herbals, traditional and complementary medicines, blood products, biologicals, medical devices, and vaccines. The major source of new information about ADRs is spontaneous reporting.

Once limited to the high-income world, pharmacovigilance has developed rapidly. Reliable systems of pharmacovigilance are now recognized as a prerequisite for the rational, safe, and cost-effective use of medicines in all countries. In addition, pharmacovigilance extends to the regulatory measures required to prevent future ADRs and improve the benefit–risk ratio of pharmaceuticals. It supports effective decision making by NMRAs and facilitates the exchange of drug safety information between countries and the monitoring of global trends in ADRs. A regional pharmacovigilance network and training center for West Africa is currently under development, and similar collaborations are planned on an international scale.

Postmarketing Surveillance

Premarketing trials of drugs are undertaken on relatively small numbers of patients and lack the power to detect important but less common ADRs, to detect ADRs that occur some time after the original use of the medicine, or to detect consequences associated with long-term medicine administration. Type A ADRs with a frequency of less than 1 in 1,000 will not usually be detected in such trials, nor will more serious Type B ADRs. Premarketing trials often do not include special populations such as pregnant women, the elderly, or children, all of whom may be at risk from unique ADRs or from an increased frequency of ADRs compared with the general population. For these reasons, postmarketing surveillance is an important tool to detect less common but sometimes serious ADRs (Brewer et al., 1999). WHO (2002c) publishes a *Guide to Detecting and Reporting Adverse Drug Reactions*.

The spontaneous reporting of ADRs is the cornerstone of postmarketing safety surveillance. Such reports can be made to the NMRA or to the pharmaceutical company concerned. Companies may also have to submit international reports, giving details of ADRs reported in other countries to the national authority. In certain countries, only doctors are allowed to report suspected ADRs; in others, reports from a wider group of health professionals—sometimes including pharmacists and nurses—are accepted (International Drugs Surveillance Department, 1991). The frequency of reporting varies considerably between countries, and it is estimated that only 1% to 10% of all cases are actually reported to the authorities.

All suspected ADRs considered of clinical importance need to be reported. Arrangements for reporting vary from country to country. Many countries have standardized forms that need to be completed and sent to the relevant authority. Case report forms usually include patient information, a description of the adverse event and outcome, the suspect medicine, its manufacturer, the indication, the dosing, and the patient's concurrent diseases and medicines.

Many countries have established drug monitoring systems for early detection and prevention of medicine-related problems. Postmarketing surveillance is mainly coordinated by national pharmacovigilance centers, which collect and analyze case reports of ADRs, distinguish signals from background noise, make regulatory decisions based on strengthened signals, and alert prescribers, manufacturers, and the public to new risks of ADRs (WHO, 2002a). The number of national centers participating in WHO's International Drug Monitoring Program increased from 10 in 1968 to 67 in 2002.

Antimicrobial Resistance

The development of antimicrobial resistance means diseases that until recently were close to being controlled, contained, and curable are now difficult to treat and likely to reemerge. Underuse and misuse of antimicrobials have led to countless deaths from preventable and curable conditions (WHO, 2002a). A penicillin-resistant strain of *Staphylococcus aureus* first emerged in the 1950s. Resistant strains of *Gonorrhoea*, *Shigella*, and *Salmonella* followed. In addition, multiple-drug-resistant tuberculosis (MDR-TB) has spread to several locations around the world.

Many factors have led to the emergence of resistance to antibiotics. One key practice is the treatment of viral infections of the respiratory tract with antibiotics, which may be inappropriately prescribed or available without prescription. In many countries, the free availability of antibiotics leads to unqualified self-diagnosis and overuse. Where antimicrobials are available, patients may buy enough for a few days' treatment, or resort to substandard or counterfeit medicines. Resistance emerges whenever antibiotics are used at doses lower than indicated. Misdiagnosis by poorly trained health staff, who often must deal with inadequate diagnostic facilities to test for culture and sensitivity, often leads to inappropriate prescribing.

Antimicrobial resistance has become a serious and global public health concern whose economic, social, and political implications cross borders (WHO, 2000a). The consequences of antimicrobial resistance are extensive. Resistant infections are more often fa-

tal, and they result in prolonged illness with a greater chance of resistant organisms spreading to other people. Their emergence is also associated with increased costs of care owing to the need to use newer, more expensive medicines.

Strategies to Contain Antimicrobial Resistance

The development of effective policies and programs to address inappropriate antibiotic use must include a proper understanding of factors that influence antibiotic use. WHO (2001a) has called for international action aimed at improving antibiotic use and containing antimicrobial resistance. A number of studies have examined the perceptions of decision makers and stakeholders regarding the inappropriate use of antibiotics and policy options to address the issue. Exhibit 14-15 summarizes a case study from Mexico.

| **Exhibit 14-15** | **Antibiotics in Mexico** |

In this study, 52 interviews were conducted with government officials, NGOs, pharmaceutical-sector representatives, researchers, and health professionals to analyze their perceptions about inappropriate use of antibiotics and policy options available to address the problem.

Most interviewees perceived inappropriate antibiotic use as a less important problem than access to medicines. Researchers stressed the urgency of the problem, whereas government officials highlighted the lack of indicators with which to formally assess its importance. The problem was framed around three themes: as an aspect of national culture; as secondary to lack of access to health care; and as a feature of how appointments are made to government positions. In exploring policy options, respondents highlighted obstacles rather than enablers—namely, the scarcity of resources to implement programs and conflicts between vested interests. Only one interviewee referred to relevant WHO recommendations.

A number of key factors were identified as important in explaining current inaction in this area: low problem recognition and awareness; the framing of the problem in complex cultural and structural contexts, making them difficult to act on; the lack of awareness of international policy recommendations in this area, resulting from lack of expertise and high staff turnover; and lack of recognition of responsibility for the problem and its solutions. These factors illuminate possible barriers to action, and should be considered when bringing inappropriate antibiotic use to the policy agenda in low- and middle-income countries.

Source: Dreser et al., 2009.

Exhibit 14-16	Action Necessary to Control Antibacterial Resistance

- Adoption of international policies and strategies to prevent, treat, and control infectious disease. This includes vaccination, treatment guidelines such as the Integrated Management of Childhood Illness (IMCI), and the Directly Observed Treatment, Short-course (DOTS) strategy for tuberculosis and surveillance systems.
- Education of health staff and the public on rational use of medicines.
- Containment of resistance in hospitals by better hygiene and hand washing.
- Reductions in the use of antimicrobials in livestock and food.
- Increased research into new medicines and vaccines.
- Partnerships to increase access particularly for poor populations.

Source: WHO, 2010a.

Substantial investment of resources is needed to contain antimicrobial resistance. Approaches include training for health staff, more appropriate treatment regimens, community education, immunization programs, improved hygiene, improved nutrition, and enhanced vector control (Radyowijati & Haak, 2003). Concerted action is required by all parties involved—patients, prescribers and dispensers, hospital managers, governments, the pharmaceutical industry, international agencies, NGOs, and professional organizations. Exhibit 14-16 summarizes an action plan to control antibacterial resistance proposed by WHO.

Resistance can be effectively approached and treated by rational medicine use, in which the correct medicine is administered by the best route, in the right dose, and at the optimal intervals for the appropriate period after an accurate diagnosis. Prescribers should be advised not to prescribe antibiotics for simple coughs and colds or for virally caused sore throats, to limit prescribing antibiotics for uncomplicated cystitis to three days in otherwise fit young women, and to not prescribe antibiotics over the phone other than in exceptional cases.

Pharmaceutical System Architecture

As noted in the introduction to this chapter, the challenge of securing access to pharmaceuticals reflects the challenges facing the broader health system. Pharmaceuticals are a key component of both the "technology" and the "service delivery" building blocks, but also have links to the financing, human resources, information, and governance functions (deSavigny & Adam, 2009). Many of these topics have been addressed in previous sections; here we focus particularly on the pharmaceutical workforce and the methods for generating new knowledge about medicine use.

The Role of the Pharmaceutical Workforce

Pharmaceutical human resources (HR) form the major component of the infrastructure or architecture in a pharmaceutical system (Frost & Reich, 2008). They are required to operationalize the mechanisms and institutions that manage the availability, affordability, and safe and effective use of medicines upstream and downstream. Across the pharmaceutical sector and throughout the medicines use process, they perform diverse functions such as research and development, manufacturing, distribution, procurement, regulation, dispensing, pharmacovigilance, and improving adherence. In many countries, particularly in sub-Saharan Africa, pharmaceutical HR are limited and inequitably distributed. In some high-income countries, the number of pharmacists per capita is more than 100 times that in low- and middle-income countries (International Pharmaceutical Federation [FIP], 2009).

The International Labour Organization (ILO, 2009) defines three main cadres or professional classifications of pharmacy worker: pharmacists (high level), pharmaceutical technicians and assistants (mid-level), and pharmacy aides (lower level). Pharmaceutical technicians and assistants usually undergo formal training and generally perform roles related to dispensing and stock management under the supervision of pharmacists, although they may work independently in some countries. Pharmacy aides have little or no formal training and provide basic support for dispensing and storage of medicines. Pharmacists complete 4 to 6 years of higher education in addition to internships; their roles are described further in this section. Other health cadres and community health workers, particularly in countries that lack a pharmaceutical workforce, may also be responsible for providing pharmaceutical services.

Pharmaceutical Workers' Roles and Impact on Health Outcomes

A growing body of evidence, including some from low- and middle-income countries (Benrimoj et al., 2000; Blenkinsopp, Anderson, & Armstron, 2003;

Bokyo et al., 1997; Bond, Raehl, & Franke, 1999, 2000; Bond, Raehl, & Patry, 2004; Hourihan, Krass, & Chen, 2003; Howard et al., 2003; Kritikos et al., 2005; Leape et al., 1999; Mayhew et al., 2001; McMullin et al., 1999; Ritzenthaler, 2005; Tuladhar et al., 1998; Ward et al., 2003), demonstrates the impact of pharmacists and their services on improving health outcomes, ensuring access to and rational use of medicines, and reducing hospital admissions and medicines-related adverse events. Reductions in hospital mortality and drug expenditures in U.S. hospitals have been associated with the provision of clinical pharmacy services such as in-service education, drug information, ADR management, drug protocol management, attendance on ward rounds, and taking drug histories upon patient admission (Bond, Raehl, & Patry, 2004). Several studies have established a correlation between clinical pharmacist staffing in hospitals and reduced mortality (Bond & Raehl, 2007; Borja-Lopetegi, Webb, Bates, & Sharott, 2008). In many countries, pharmaceutical cadres constitute the first point of contact for patients with a healthcare professional, with private pharmacies often identified as preferred healthcare providers due to their accessibility and confidentiality of advice and treatment, as in the case of managing sexually transmitted diseases (Ward et al., 2003).

Shortages and Imbalances

The shortage of pharmaceutical HR, particularly in sub-Saharan Africa, has been cited as a key capacity limitation to the delivery of pharmaceutical services and access to medicines, including HIV/AIDS programs (Hirschhorn et al., 2006; Muula et al., 2007; Waako et al., 2009; UN Millennium Project, 2005). The severity of the shortage is illustrated in Figure 14-6, in which the size of countries is shown proportional to their share of global pharmaceutical HR. In this map, sub-Saharan Africa is barely visible, despite its 25% share of the global disease burden.

The negative impacts of these shortages will be magnified as the level of medicines consumption increases with economic development, necessitating more HR to support this growing demand (Wuliji et al., 2010). Therefore, the challenge for those countries hardest hit by the HR crisis is twofold: to scale up pharmaceutical HR to meet current demands and then to further amplify these efforts to meet the likely increasing demands in the long term.

The causes of this shortage are complex but are mainly due to the inadequate capacity of countries to train and retain sufficient HR (Chan & Wuliji, 2006; FIP, 2009; Wuliji, 2009). Pharmaceutical education capacity is absent or limited in most countries in sub-Saharan Africa, although there has been a recent expansion with the scale-up of existing training institutions and establishment of new facilities. The private sector is an important source of pharmaceuticals, and the shortage of pharmacists also has implications for the density of pharmacies. Sub-Saharan African countries have been observed to lack not only pharmacists, but also pharmacies—both of which are concentrated in urban areas (FIP, 2009). Countries such as Nepal, Pakistan, and Vietnam have 5 to 10

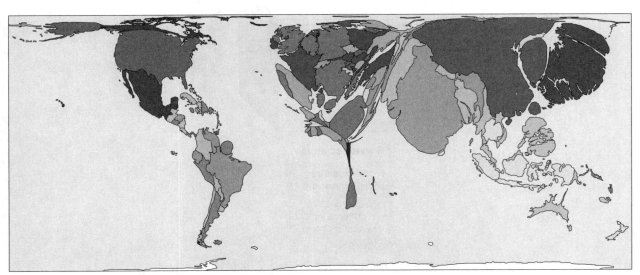

Figure 14-6 Share of Global Pharmaceutical Human Resources.
Source: From WorldMapper, 2008. Data source: Global atlas of the health workforce, WHO, 2006; Copyright 2006 SASI Group (University of Sheffield) and Mark Newman (University of Michigan). Reproduced with permission.

times more premises where medicines can be accessed than the number of trained pharmaceutical human resources (FIP, 2009). The distribution of pharmacists by sector of practice also varies greatly between regions, with as many as 55% working in the pharmaceutical industry in Southeast Asia compared to fewer than 5% working in this sector in Africa.

Strategies for Human Resources Development

Given that pharmaceutical HR forms the architecture of pharmaceutical systems, dimensions of HR development can be linked to different aspects of pharmaceutical services (Figure 14-7) (Wuliji, 2009). This conceptual framework can be used to guide the development of targeted interventions for specific capacity limitations. Service level—defined as the technical level at which services are provided—is determined by workforce competency. Service coverage (i.e., hours, facilities) is linked to the workforce size and distribution. Service scope (range of specialized services) is dependent on workforce capacity (skill mix, supervision, working environment).

Key strategies to strengthen the pharmaceutical workforce are summarized in Exhibit 14-17 (Borja-Lopetegi et al., 2008).

Generating Knowledge About Medicines Use

Access to information about medicines is a prerequisite for their appropriate use, accessibility, availability, and affordability. Rational use requires good information about the action and uses of drugs; information about their costs is vital in considering affordability; and information about supply chain issues is important when considering availability.

Information about the actions and uses of medicines comes from many sources. Primary sources include scientific journals reporting clinical trials and official health statistics on medicines use. Secondary sources include review articles in scientific journals and meta-analyses such as Cochrane Collaboration reports. Tertiary sources include essential medicine lists and standard treatment guidelines. Information from all of these sources needs to be interpreted with care to avoid problems of bias.

Although a wide range of information about medicines and their uses is available, from manufacturers and other sources, a fundamental requirement for the more rational use of medicines is the collection of key information about which policies are in place and how medicines are being used, by whom, and where in a consistent way. This effort requires effective management information systems for pharmaceuticals. At the country level, a mechanism for monitoring the extent to which these systems are in place is available in WHO's *Operational Package for Monitoring and Assessing Country Pharmaceutical Situations*. A range of methodological approaches have been developed to provide the essential information required, including drug utilization studies, pharmacoepidemiology, and pharmacoeconomics.

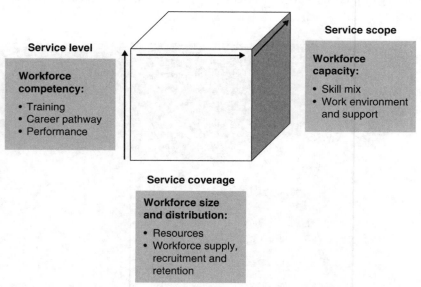

Figure 14-7 Dimensions of Pharmaceutical Service and HR Development.
Source: Originally published in Wuliji, 2009. ©2009, American Society of Health-System Pharmacists, Inc. All rights reserved. Distributed with permission. (R1013)

Exhibit 14-17	Key Strategies to Strengthen Pharmaceutical Human Resources

Workforce Competency (Service Level)

- *Development of competency frameworks*: Such frameworks are used on a policy level to guide the planning of curriculum and scopes of practice for each cadre and at an HR management level to guide continuing education and performance assessment.
- *Needs-based education development and reform*: Pharmaceutical service needs should be assessed against the competencies required to provide these services defined and, in turn, matched with learning objectives in the curriculum to support the development of these competencies (Anderson et al., 2009).
- *Career pathways*: Career pathways for all cadres can improve motivation and retention as well as define the competencies required to provide pharmaceutical services at each level.

Workforce Size and Distribution (Service Coverage)

- *Resources*: Sustainable funding is required in the mid- to long term (5 to 10 years) to invest in building training infrastructure, expand the labor market through the creation of required positions or posts in both the public and private sectors, improve human resources management, and implement retention schemes.
- *Workforce supply*: Encouraging the establishment and growth of private-sector training institutions has been successful in many countries, as has scaling up pharmaceutical technologist training in Kenya and pharmacist training in Sudan (Mandour & Salih, 2009; Thoithi & Okalebo, 2009). Investment should be made in building teaching capacity.
- *Workforce recruitment*: Rural recruitment strategies should provide a package of financial and nonfinancial incentives to attract workforce into underserved areas (Dolea et al., 2009; Mathauer & Imhoff, 2006; Vujicic et al., 2004). The use of external agencies to expedite the recruitment process in the public sector has been effective in Namibia (Frelick & Mameja, 2006).
- *Workforce retention*: Retention strategies are more effective when they include a package of both financial and nonfinancial incentives, rather than only one type of incentive (Mathauer & Imhoff, 2006; Vujicic et al., 2004).

Workforce Capacity (Service Scope)

- *Skill mix*: A competency framework may aid the development of the required skill mix.
- *Supervision and support*: Remote service provision and supervisory systems may be a valuable tool in redressing skill mix imbalances, particularly in remote or rural areas (Poulson, Nissen, & Coombes, 2010).
- *Work environment*: Work environments should be equipped appropriately for the scope of service (e.g., sterile cabinet, computers, counseling room, cytotoxic waste disposal). Good Pharmacy Practice (GPP) policies may provide guidelines for basic requirements.

Drug Utilization Studies

Drug utilization research was defined by WHO in 1977 as research addressing "the marketing, distribution, prescription, dispensing, and use of drugs in a society, with special emphasis on the resulting medical and social consequences" (WHO, 2003b). Drug utilization studies are a vitally important approach to establishing which medicines are used and how. They can be implemented at the facility, regional, subsector, sector, or international level. Such studies address key questions including why drugs are prescribed; who the prescribers are; for whom the prescribers prescribe; whether patients take their medicines correctly; and what the benefits and risks of the drugs are. The ultimate goal of drug utilization research is to assess whether drug therapy is rational.

Drug utilization studies have four principal objectives: (1) to measure the use of pharmaceuticals;

(2) to understand the reasons for their use; (3) to educate health professionals; and (4) to design, monitor, and evaluate interventions aimed at improving the use of medicines. Both quantitative and qualitative methods are used to achieve these objectives. Quantitative methods include recording of WHO indicators on medicines use, collection of aggregate data on medicines consumption, case record reviews, and prescription audits in health facilities. Qualitative methods include focus-group discussions with users or providers, in-depth interviews of key informants, structured observations of medicines use encounters (defined as the "contact period" between the healthcare provider and the user), questionnaires, and simulated patient surveys (Huss, 2004). Mixed-method studies, which combine quantitative and qualitative methods, can be used to address both the "what is happening" and "why" questions at the same time.

Drug utilization studies can help identify specific problems of medicines use, but they also allow the follow-up of interventions to compare the medicines use situation in different facilities or healthcare systems. In the case of interventions, it is important to have baseline data, to have a control group whose members have not received the intervention, and to follow up on changes over time, especially after the intervention is administered. When facilities or systems are compared, it is important to take into account variations in staffing, equipment, epidemiology, socioeconomic and cultural situation, and other features of the context that may help explain any differences identified by the comparison.

Medicine Use Indicators

WHO (2010f) has developed a core indicator package to monitor and evaluate country pharmaceutical situations. Ministries of health (MOHs) are responsible for assessing the current pharmaceutical situation in their country—an evaluation that can easily be repeated at regular intervals. MOHs use the information as a guide for determining priority areas for intervention, tracking progress, planning programs, assessing program effectiveness, coordinating donors, and raising funds. WHO uses the data to target its expertise to individual country needs. Medicines use indicators are usually measured as part of drug utilization studies. As mentioned earlier, WHO has also published an operational package for monitoring and assessing country pharmaceutical situations (Department of Technical Cooperation for Essential Drugs, 2007).

Pharmacoepidemiology

Pharmacoepidemiology can be defined as "the application of epidemiological knowledge, methods, and reasoning to the study of the effects (both beneficial and adverse) and uses of drugs in human populations" (Walley, Haycox, & Boland, 2009). Its objectives are to describe, explain, control, and predict the effects and uses of pharmacological treatments in a defined time, space, and population. Epidemiology studies the distribution of health and disease in human populations. Medicines use can be a key influence on such distribution, which explains the importance of pharmacoepidemiological studies. Pharmacovigilance represents one application of pharmacoepidemiology, as demonstrated in postmarketing surveillance.

Other epidemiological methods applied to the safety of medicines include case reports and case-control studies. These techniques offer the advantage

that rare ADRs can be detected at low cost and relatively high speed in comparison to cohort studies. They do have some disadvantages, however: They are prone to biases, cannot determine causation unless the adverse event is very rare, and do not permit measurement of the incidence of an ADR. An example of a pharmacoepidemiological study of self-medication in adults visiting pharmacies in Alexandria, Egypt, is shown in Exhibit 14-18.

Pharmacoeconomics

Pharmacoeconomics can be defined as "the discipline that describes and analyses the costs and benefits of pharmaceutical and alternative therapies to the healthcare system, the different stakeholders, and society as a whole" (Department of Technical Cooperation for Essential Drugs, 2007). A number of high-income countries have introduced the requirement that all new drugs (and many procedures and medical devices) be subjected to a pharmacoeconomic assessment before they can be included on the national drug formulary (e.g., Australia) or be funded through the public health system (e.g., the United Kingdom). Some middle-income countries, such as Thailand, have introduced similar requirements. For example, Thailand's Health Intervention and Technology Assessment Programme (HITAP, 2008) recently reviewed evidence related to the vaccine for humanpapilloma virus (HPV—the virus responsible for cervical cancers) and concluded that the intervention was unaffordable at the current vaccine price level.

Exhibit 14-18   Pharmacoepidemiological Case Study

A cross-sectional study was conducted to determine the extent and pattern of self-medication among adults, to identify their knowledge and practice concerning the purchased drugs, and to calculate prescribing and purchaser care indicators. Following WHO methods, 35 pharmacies were randomly selected from districts in Alexandria City, Egypt. Of 1,294 clients interviewed at these pharmacies, 1,050 (81.1%) purchased self-medication; the most common reason given was a belief that the condition was minor. The most frequently dispensed drugs were those for the respiratory system. The mean number of drugs per encounter was 1.10, the mean cost was $1.30 (LE 7.29), and the mean dispensing time was 2.53 minutes. Purchasers' knowledge and practice regarding the purchased drugs were poor.

Source: Sallam et al., 2009.

In pharmacoeconomic assessment, the costs include all necessary resources that are usually measured in monetary terms. Cost and benefits can be either medical or nonmedical, such as transportation. They can encompass employment and productivity, and intangibles such as well-being and suffering. Not only are different types of costs involved, but different perspectives are as well. Transport costs, for example, are a real cost from the patient's perspective, but may not be seen as a cost from the provider's point of view. Given that benefits and costs also occur at different points in time, economists have developed a technique to calculate them at present prices by applying a discount rate to benefits and costs incurred in the future.

Several other factors need to be considered in a pharmacoeconomic evaluation, including the time horizon, the alternative (or comparator) therapy, the need for a sensitivity analysis for the different assumptions made in the study, and the need for an incremental analysis to assess the relative economic attractiveness in comparison to alternative therapies. Such considerations serve to underline the tension that exists in pharmacoeconomics between methodologies (which try to take into account all factors) and transparent and robust approaches (which are simplified models of reality). The latter are more easily understood by potential users and less prone to manipulation by vested interests.

Conclusion

This chapter has identified a number of challenges to ensuring access to pharmaceuticals. These issues include the need to finance R&D for new medicines and vaccines for neglected diseases; the drive to strengthen national pharmaceutical distribution and management to ensure that the right pharmaceutical products are consistently available throughout the health system; the problems of affordability and the need to generate sustainable financing for medicines that are reasonably priced; the challenges of ensuring safe and rational drug use; and the need to secure a pharmaceutical workforce whose members are appropriately trained and deployed to support the delivery of pharmaceuticals to those in need.

In many ways, these unmet needs are "old" problems that have challenged pharmaceutical systems in low- and middle-income settings for decades. In addition, a number of new challenges will demand further flexibility and responsiveness from these systems in the future. These factors include the epidemiologic transition away from infectious diseases and toward more chronic diseases, issues around the adoption and supply of new pharmaceutical tools, and the challenges of coordination and priority setting in an increasingly complex global environment.

In the case of chronic disease management, the challenge will be to ensure that appropriate and affordable medicines are available to support the changes in health service delivery models needed to provide greater continuity of care. These demands will include adapting supply chains to reach community-based care settings. The convergence in health needs between the rich and poor worlds will help to ensure that new and effective products are available for use in the low- and middle-income world (because of the greater share of disease burden that will fall into Type I category); however, it will be essential that these new products are both affordable and appropriate for low-income healthcare delivery systems.

It is clear that the environment within which pharmaceuticals are developed, procured, and distributed is becoming increasingly more complex, with a plethora of new actors playing roles in this sometimes chaotic environment. At the national level, insurance funds and regulators will increasingly exert influence over pharmaceutical decisions that once were the main responsibility of national health ministries. At the international level, new actors include new corporate and philanthropic funding sources, new funding mechanisms and intermediaries, multinational pharmaceutical firms based in the global South, and regional and international regulatory bodies. These agents may have different incentives for their engagement and sometimes face conflicting priorities. While this new environment has had a generally positive impact on the availability of pharmaceuticals to meet the needs of the low- and middle-income world, it also poses clear risks to the strength and stability of national pharmaceutical systems, and the new initiatives have at times created duplication, inefficiency, and resulting inequities.

From the material presented in this chapter, it should be clear that the functioning of the pharmaceutical system provides a snapshot of the performance of the health system as a whole. The measures that are needed to strengthen health systems in low- and middle-income settings—such as improved governance, universal coverage of equitable healthcare financing mechanisms, and an adequate, high-performing and appropriately distributed workforce—will all have positive repercussions for the pharmaceutical system and represent an important step toward ensuring access to pharmaceuticals for all.

Acknowledgments

We are grateful to Edith Patouillard for providing the text for Exhibit 14-6. All of the authors of this chapter are members of the London International Development Centre, which facilitated the planning meeting for the chapter.

Discussion Questions

1. Availability, affordability and safe and effective use are the main challenges to improving pharmaceutical access. Define what is meant by each, and explain how they can be addressed.

2. What are "neglected diseases" and why are they neglected? Which policy interventions are available to stimulate investment in pharmaceuticals to address these conditions?

3. Describe three approaches to improving affordability of medicines, and some of the challenges in implementing them.

4. Which strategies can be employed to improve supply chain management?

5. How can quality assurance be maintained throughout the supply chain?

6. How have global health initiatives challenged national pharmaceutical systems? How can they improve their synergy with national programs?

7. Define a counterfeit medicine. Which factors contribute to counterfeiting, what are the consequences of taking counterfeit medicines, and which measures can be taken to curb the proliferation of these products?

8. Describe how the use of drug utilization studies, pharmacoepidemiology, and pharmacoeconomics can contribute to the more rational use of medicines.

9. Explain the implications of antimicrobial resistance. Which strategies can be used to contain the problem?

10. Define an adverse drug reaction and describe the roles of postmarketing surveillance and pharmacovigilance in promoting the safe use of medicines.

11. Which strategies can be used to strengthen the pharmaceutical workforce?

••• References

Abuya, T. O., Mutemi, W., Karisa, B., Ochola, S. A., Fegan, G. & Marsh, V. (2007). Use of over-the-counter malaria medicines in children and adults in three districts in Kenya: Implications for private medicine retailer interventions. *Malaria Journal*, 6, 57.

Anderson, C., Bates, I., Beck, D., Brock, T. P., Futter, B., Mercer, H., et al. (2009). The WHO UNESCO FIP Pharmacy Education Taskforce. *Human Resources for Health*, 7(45).

Anderson, S., & Huss, R. (2004). Issues in the management of pharmaceuticals in international health. In H. R. Anderson, R. Summers, & K. Wiedenmayer (Eds.), *Managing pharmaceuticals in international health*. 1, 1–18. Basel: Birkhauser Verlag.

Ballou-Aares, D., Freitas, A., Kopczak, L. R., Kraiselburd, S., Laverty, M., Macharia, E., et al. (2008). *The private sector's role in health supply chains: Review of the role and potential for private sector engagement in developing country health supply chains. Technical partner paper 13*. Dalberg Global Development Advisors, MIT—Zaragoza International Logistics Program, & Rockefeller Foundation. Retrived from http://www.dalberg .com/PDFs/Health_Supply_Chains.pdf

Benrimoj, S., Langford, J., Berry, G., Collins, D., Lauchlan, R., Stewart, K., et al. (2000). Economic impact of increased clinical intervention rates in community pharmacy: A randomised trial of the effect of education and a professional allowance. *Pharmacoeconomics*, 18(5), 459–468.

Birungi, H., Asiimwe, D. & Reynolds Whyte, S. (1994). *Injection use and practices in Uganda*. WHO/DAP/94.18. Geneva, Switzerland: World Health Organization.

Bledsoe, C., & Goubaud, M. (1985). The reinterpretation of Western pharmaceuticals among the Mende of Sierre Leone. *Social Science and Medicine*, 21(3), 275–282.

Blenkinsopp, A., Anderson, C., & Armstrong, M. (2003). Systematic review of the effectiveness of community pharmacy-based interventions to reduce risk behaviours and risk factors for coronary heart disease. *Journal of Public Health Medicine*, 25, 144–a53.

Bokyo, W., Yurkowski, P. J., Ivey, M. F., Armitstead, J. A. & Roberts, B. L. (1997). Pharmacist influence on economic and morbidity outcomes in a tertiary care teaching hospital. *American Journal of Health-System Pharmacy*, 54(14), 1591–1595.

Bond, C., & Raehl, C. (2007). Clinical pharmacy services, pharmacy staffing, and hospital mortality rates. *Pharmacotherapy*, 27(4), 481–493.

Bond, C., Raehl, C., & Franke, T. (1999). Clinical pharmacy services, pharmacist staffing, and drug costs in United States hospitals. *Pharmacotherapy*, 19(12), 1354–1362.

Bond, C., Raehl, C., & Franke, T. (2000). Clinical pharmacy services, pharmacy staffing, and the total cost of care in United States hospitals. *Pharmacotherapy*, 20(6), 609–621.

Bond, C. A., Raehl, C. L., & Patry, R. (2004). Evidence-based core clinical pharmacy services in United States hospitals in 2020: Services and staffing. *Pharmacotherapy*, 24(4), 427–440.

Borja-Lopetegi, A., Webb, D. G., Bates, I., & Sharott, P. (2008). Association between clinical medicines management services, pharmacy workforce and patient outcomes. *Pharmacy World & Science*, 30(4), 418–420.

Boulet, P., Perriens, J., Renaud-Théry, F. & Velasquez, G. (2000). *Pharmaceuticals and the WTO TRIPS Agreement: Questions and answers*. Geneva, Switzerland: UNAIDS & World Health Organization.

Brewer, T., & Colditz, G. A. (1999). Postmarketing surveillance and adverse drug reactions. *Journal of the American Medical Association*, 281(9), 824–829.

Burki, T. (2010). Building medical regulatory authorities in Africa. *Lancet*, 10, 222.

Cameron, A., Ewin, M., Ross-Degnan, D., Ball, D. & Laing, R. (2009). Medicine prices, availability, and affordability in 36 developing and middle-income countries: A secondary analysis. *Lancet*, 373(9659), 240–249.

Center for Pharmaceutical Management. (2008). *Accredited Drug Dispensing Outlets in Tanzania*

Strategies for Enhancing Access to Medicines Program . Arlington, VA: Management Sciences for Health. Retrieved from http://www.msh.org/seam/reports/TANZANIA_Final_ADDO.pdf

Chan, X. H., & Wuliji, T. (2006). *2006 FIP global pharmacy workforce and migration report.* The Hague: International Phamaceutical Federation (FIP).

Chase, M., & Barta, P. (2005). Antibiotics without patients: Drug shipment's long road to treating tsunami victims illustrates obstacles to aid. *Wall Street Journal.* 2 February 2005, p. B1.

Chauveau, J., Meiners, C. M., Luchini, S. & Moatti, J.-P. (2008). Evolution of prices and quantities of ARV drugs in African countries: From emerging to strategic markets. In B. E. Coriat (Ed.), *The political economy of HIV/AIDS in developing countries: TRIPS, public health systems and free access* (pp. 78–100). Cheltenham, UK/Northampton, MA: Elgar.

Chiguzo, A. N., Mugo, R. W., Wacira, D. G., Mwenda, J. M. & Njuguna, E. W. (2008). Delivering new malaria drugs through grassroots private sector. *East African Medical Journal, 85*(9), 425–431.

Cipla. (2007). Once-daily dosage lamivudine another ARV first for Cipla Medpro. Retrieved March 16, 2010, from http://www.ciplamedpro.co.za/news.php?nid=26

Cobert, B. L., & Biron, P. (2002). *Pharmacovigilance from A to Z: Adverse medicines event surveillance.* Oxford, UK: Blackwell Science.

Cockburn, R., Newton, P. N., Agyarko, E. K., Akunyili, D. & White, N. J. (2005). The global threat of counterfeit drugs: Why industry and governments must communicate the dangers. *Public Library of Science Medicine, 2*(4). Retrieved from e100.1371/journal.pmed.0020100

Deisingh, A. K. (2005). Pharmaceutical counterfeiting. *Analyst, 130,* 271–279.

Department of Technical Cooperation for Essential Drugs. (2007). *Operational package for monitoring and assessing country pharmaceutical situations.* Geneva, Switzerland: World Health Organization.

deSavigny, D., & Adam, T. (Eds.). (2009). *Systems thinking for health systems strengthening.* Geneva, Switzerland: Alliance for Health Policy and Systems Research, World Health Organization.

DiMasi, J., Hansen, R., & Grabowski, H. (2003). The price of innovation: New estimates of drug development costs. *Journal of Health Economics, 22,* 151–185.

Dolea, C., Stormont, L., Shaw, D., Zurn, P. & Braichet, J. M. (2009). *Increasing access to health workers in remote and rural areas through improved retention: Background paper for the first expert consultations on developing global recommendations on increasing access to health workers in remote and rural areas through improved retention.* Geneva, Switzerland: World Health Organization.

Dreser, A. (2009). *Inappropriate antibiotic use and the health policy agenda in Mexico.* Presentation at the Twelfth World Congress on Public Health, Istanbul, Turkey.

European Medicines Agency (EMEA). (2005). Background information on the procedure. Retrieved from http://www.ema.europa.eu/humandocs/PDFs/EPAR/truvada/2832505en7.pdf

Foundation for Innovative New Diagnostics and Special Programme for Research & Training in Tropical Diseases. (2006). *Diagnostics for tuberculosis: Global demand and market potential.* Geneva, Switzerland: World Health Organization.

Foundation for Innovative New Diagnostics. (2009). Product pipeline. Retrieved February 23, 2010, from http://www.finddiagnostics.org/programs/tb/pipeline.html

Frelick, G., & Mameja, J. (2006). *Strategy for the rapid start-up of the HIV/AIDS program in Namibia: Outsourcing the recruitment and management of human resources for health.* Capacity Project, USAID Global Health/HIV/AIDS, & the Africa Bureau Office of Sustainable Development. Retrieved from http://www.capacityproject.org/images/stories/files/promising_practices_namibia.pdf

Frost, L., & Reich, M. (2008). *Access: How do good health technologies get to poor people in poor countries?* Cambridge, MA: Harvard Center for Population and Development Studies.

GAVI. (2010). GAVI Alliance: 10 years of saving lives. Retrieved April 20, 2010, from http://www.gavialliance.org/index.php

Gilson, L., & Mills, A. (1995). Health sector reforms in sub-Saharan Africa: Lessons of the last 10 years. *Health Policy, 32*(1–3), 215–243.

Global Fund to Fight AIDS, TB and Malaria (GFATM). (2010a). Affordable Medicines Facility—Malaria (AMFm). Retrieved April 22, 2010, from http://www.theglobalfund.org/en/amfm/

Global Fund to Fight AIDS, TB and Malaria (GFATM). (2010b). The Global Fund 2010: Innovation and impact. Retrieved from http://www.the globalfund.org/documents/replenishment/2010/Global_Fund_2010_Innovation_and_Impact_en.pdf

Global Fund to Fight AIDS, TB and Malaria (GFATM). (2010c). Price and quality reporting. Retrieved from http://pqr.theglobalfund.org/PQRWeb/Screens/PQRLogin.aspx

Greenidge, A. (2009). *Funding R&D for diseases of the developing world (DDW)*. IFPMA Presentation to WHO Expert Working Group on Funding R&D for Diseases of the Developing World (DDW) given by Alicia D. Greenidge, Director General, IFPMA to WHO Expert Working Group, Geneva, 12 Jan 2009. Retrieved from http://www.ifpma.org/fileadmin/pdfs/2009_01_16_IFPMA_DG-EWG_120109_FINAL.pdf

Gupta, R., Cegielski, J. P., Espinal, M. A., Henkens, M., Kim, J. M., Lambregts-van Weezenbeek, C. S. B., et al. (2002). Increasing transparency in partnerships for health: Introducing the Green Light Committee. *Tropical Medicine and International Health, 7*(11), 970–976.

Haakonsson, S. J., & Richey, L. A. (2007). TRIPs and public health: The Doha Declaration and Africa. *Development Policy Review, 25*(1), 71–90.

Hagmann, M. (2001). TB drug prices slashed for poor countries. *Bulletin of the World Health Organization, 79*(9), 904–905.

Health Action International (HAI) Global. (2010). Global pill price "snapshot" reveals large differences in the price of ciprofloxacin. Retrieved January 11, 2010, from http://www.haiweb.org/medicineprices/05012010/PressRelease.pdf

Hirschhorn, L., Oguda, L., Fullem, A., Dreesch, N. & Wilson, P. (2006). Estimating health workforce needs for antiretroviral therapy in resource-limited settings. *Human Resources for Health, 4*(1), 1.

Hollis, A., & Pogge, T. (2008). *The Health Impact Fund: Making new medicines accessible for all.* Incentives for Global Health. Retrieved from http://www.yale.edu/macmillan/igh/hif_book.pdf

Horne, R. (2006). Compliance, adherence, and concordance: Implications for asthma treatment. *Chest, 130*(1), 65S–72S.

Horne, R., & Weinman, J. (1999). Patients' beliefs about prescribed medicines and their role in adherence to treatment in chronic physical illness. *Journal of Psychosomatic Research, 47*(6), 555–567.

Horne, R., Weinman, J., & Hankins, M. (1999). The Beliefs about Medicines Questionnaire: The development and evaluation of a new method for assessing the cognitive representation of medication. *Psychology & Health, 14*(1), 1–24.

Hourihan, F., Krass, I., & Chen, T. (2003). Rural community pharmacy: A feasible site for a health promotion and screening service for cardiovascular risk factors. *Australian Journal of Rural Health, 11*(1), 28–35.

Howard, R., Avery, A. J., Howard, P. D. & Partridge, M. (2003). Investigation into the reasons for preventable drug related admissions to a medical admissions unit: Observational study. *Quality and Safety of Health Care, 12*, 280–285.

Huss, R. (2004). Investigating the use of medicines. In S. C. Anderson, R. Summers, & K. Wiedenmayer (Eds.), *Managing pharmaceuticals in international health. 12*, 191–206. Basel: Birkhauser Verlag.

Institute for One World Health. (2009). Visceral leishmaniasis. Retrieved March 7, 2010, from http://www.oneworldhealth.org/leishmaniasis

International Dispensary Association. (2004). E-catalogue of products. Retrieved from http://www.ida.nl/en-us/content.aspx?cid=42

International Drugs Surveillance Department (Ed.). (1991). *Drug safety: A shared responsibility.* Edinburgh: Churchill Livingstone.

International Health Policy Program & Health Intervention and Technology Assessment Program (HITAP). (2008). *Research for development of an optimal policy strategy for prevention and control of cervical cancer in Thailand.* Bangkok: Ministry of Public Health, Thailand.

International Labour Organization (ILO). (2009). International Standard Classification of Occupations (ISCO-08). In *ISCO-08 Group definitions - Final draft.* Retrieved from http://www.ilo.org/public/english/bureau/stat/isco/isco08/index.htm

International Medical Products Anti-Counterfeiting Taskforce (IMPACT). (2006). *Counterfeit medicines: An update on estimates.* Geneva, Switzerland: IMPACT, World Health Organization.

International Network for Rational Use of Drugs (INRUD). (n.d.). INRUD bibliography. Retrieved March 12, 2010, from http://www.inrud.org/Bibliographies/INRUD-Bibliography.cfm

International Pharmaceutical Federation (FIP). (2009). *FIP global pharmacy workforce report.* The Hague: Author.

Kaiser Family Foundation. (2010). FDA drafts new rules for testing, approving drug cocktails; public–private partnership for TB treatment development launched. Retrived from http://globalhealth.kff.org/Daily-Reports/2010/March/18/GH-031810-FDA.aspx

Kanjanarat, P., Winterstein, A. G., Johns, T. E., Hatton, R. C., Gonzalez-Rothi, R. & Segal, R. (2003). Nature of preventable adverse drug events in hospitals: A literature review. *American Journal of Health-System Pharmacy, 60*(14), 1750.

Kerry, V. B., & Lee, K. (2007). TRIPS, the Doha declaration and paragraph 6 decision: What are the remaining steps for protecting access to medicines? *Global Health, 3,* 3.

Kritikos, V., Saini, B., Bosnic-Anticevich, S. Z., Krass, I., Shah, S., Taylor, S. & Armour, C. L. (2005). Innovative asthma health promotion by rural community pharmacists: A feasibility study. *Health Promotion Journal of Australia, 16*(1), 69–73.

Laing, R., Hogerzeil, H., & Ross-Degnan, D. (2001). Ten recommendations to improve use of medicines in developing countries. *Health Policy Plan, 16*(1), 13–20.

Laing, R. O., & McGoldrick, K. M. (2000). Tuberculosis drug issues: Prices, fixed-dose combination products and second-line drugs. *International Journal of Tuberculosis and Lung Disease, 4*(12 suppl 2), S194–207.

Lazarou, J., Pomeranz, B. H. & Corey, P. N. (1998). Incidence of ADRs in hospitalized patients: A meta-analysis of prospective studies. *Journal of the American Medical Association, 279*(15), 1000–1005.

Leape, L., Cullen, D. J., Clapp, M. D., Burdick, E., Demonaco, H. J., Erickson, J. I., et al. (1999). Pharmacist participation on physician rounds and adverse drug events in the intensive care unit. *Journal of the American Medical Association, 282,* 267–270.

Madrid, I., Velázquez, G., & Fefer, E. (1998). *Pharmaceuticals and health sector reform in the Americas: An economic perspective.* Washington, DC: World Health Organization.

Management Sciences for Health (MSH). (1997). *Managing drug supply* (2nd ed.), J. Quick et al. (Eds.). West Hartford, CT: MSH & World Health Organization.

Management Sciences for Health (MSH). (2004). *International drug price indicator guide.* Arlington, VA: Management Sciences for Health, Inc.

Management Sciences for Health (MSH). (2010). (In press) *MDS-3: Managing access to medicines and other health technologies.* Arlington, VA: Author.

Mandour, M. E., & Salih, N. (2009). Country case study: Sudan. In T. Wuliji (Ed.), *FIP global pharmacy workforce report* (pp. 54–61). The Hague: International Pharmaceutical Federation.

Marsh, V. M., Mutemi, W. M., Muturi, J., Haaland, A., Watkins, W. M., Otieno, G., et al. (1999). Changing home treatment of childhood fevers by training shop keepers in rural Kenya. *Tropical Medicine and International Health, 4*(5), 383–389.

Marsh, V. M., Mutemi, W. M., Willetts, A., Bayah, K., Were, S., Ross, A., et al. (2004). Improving malaria home treatment by training drug retailers in rural Kenya. *Tropical Medicine and International Health, 9*(4), 451–60.

Mason, P. (2005). Tsunami relief: Same mistakes repeated. *Pharmaceutical Journal, 274,* 7335.

Mathauer, I., & Imhoff, I. (2006). Health worker motivation in Africa: The role of non-financial incentives and human resource management tools. *Human Resources for Health, 4*(1), 24.

Matiru, R., & Ryan, T. (2007). The Global Drug Facility: A unique, holistic and pioneering approach to drug procurement and management. *Bulletin of the World Health Organization, 85*(5), 348–353.

Mayhew, S., Nzambi, K., Pépin, J. & Adjei, S. (2001). Pharmacists' role in managing sexually transmitted infections: Policy Issues and options for Ghana. *Health Policy Plan, 16*(2), 152–160.

McCombie, S. C. (1996). Treatment seeking for malaria: A review of recent research. *Social Sciences and Medicine, 43*(6), 933–945.

McMullin, S., Hennenfent, J. A., Ritchie, D. J., Huey, W. Y., Lonergan, T. P., Schaiff, R. A., et al. (1999). A prospective, randomized trial to assess the cost impact of pharmacist-initiated interventions. *Archives of Internal Medicine, 159,* 2306–2309.

MDG Gap Task Force. (2009). *Millennium Development Goal 8: Strengthening the global partnership for development in a time of crisis.* New York: United Nations.

Medicines for Malaria Venture (MMV). (2009). Medicines for Malaria Venture: Annual report 2009. Retrieved from http://www.mmv.org/newsroom/publications/mmv-annual-report-2009

Medicines for Malaria Venture (MMV). (2010). MMV funding and expenditure. Retrieved from http://www.mmv.org/invest-us/mmv-funding-and-expenditure

Ministry of Health and Social Welfare, Tanzania (MOHSW). (2008) *In-depth assessment of the medicines supply system in Tanzania.* Dar er salaam: Author.

Moore, N., Lecointre, D., Noblet, C. & Mabille, M. (1998). Frequency and cost of serious adverse drug reactions in a department of general medicine. *British Journal of Clinical Pharmacology, 45*(3), 301–308.

Moran, M., Ropars, A.-L., Guzman, J., Diaz, J. & Garrison, C. (2005). *The new landscape of neglected disease drug development.* London: Wellcome Trust.

Moran, M., Guzman, J., Ropars, A.-L., Jorgensen, M., McDonald, A., Potter, S., et al. (2007), *The malaria product pipeline: Planning for the ruture.* London/Sydney: George Institute for International Health.

Moran, M., Guzman, J., Henderson, K., Ropars, A.-L., McDonald, A., McSherry, L., et al. (2009). *Neglected disease research and development: New times, new trends.* London: George Institute for International Health.

Moran, M., Guzman, J., McDonald, A., Wu, L., & Omune, B. (2010). *Registering new drugs: The African context.* London: George Institute for International Health.

Morel, C. M., Serruya, S. J., Penna, G. O. & Guimaraes, R. (2009). Co-authorship Network analysis: A powerful tool for strategic planning of research, development and capacity building programs on neglected diseases. *Public Library of Science Neglected Tropical Diseases, 3*(8), e501.

Mtonya, B., & Chizimbi, S. (2006). *Systemwide effects of the Global Fund in Malawi: Final report. The Partners for Health Reformplus Project.* Bethesda, MD: Abt Associates.

Muula, A. S., Chipeta, J., Siziya, S., Rudatsikira, E., Mataya, R. H. & Kataika, E. (2007). Human resources requirements for highly active antiretroviral therapy scale-up in Malawi. *BMC Health Services Research, 7.*

Okeke, T. A., & Uzochukwu, B. S. (2009). Improving childhood malaria treatment and referral practices by training patent medicine vendors in rural southeast Nigeria. *Malaria Journal, 8,* 260.

Olcay, M., & Laing, R. (2005). *Pharmaceutical tariffs: What is their effect on prices, protection of local industry and revenue generation?* World Health Organization & Commission on Intellectual Property Rights, Innovation and Public Health.

Retrieved from http://www.who.int/intellectual property/studies/TariffsOnEssentialMedicines.pdf

Oliveira, M. A., Bermudez, J. A. Z., Chaves, G. C. & Velasquez, G. (2004). Has the implementation of the TRIPS Agreement in Latin America and the Caribbean produced intellectual property legislation that favours public health? *Bulletin of the World Health Organization*, 82(11), 815–821.

Oomman, N., Bernstein, M., & Rosenzweig, S. (2008). *Seizing the opportunity on AIDS and health systems*. Washington, DC: Center for Global Development.

Patouillard, E., Hanson, K. G., & Goodman, C. A. (2010). Retail sector distribution chains for malaria treatment in the developing world: A review of the literature. *Malaria Journal*, 9, 50.

Pecoul, B., Chirac, P., Trouiller, P. & Pinel, J. (1999). Access to essential drugs in poor countries: A lost battle? *Journal of the American Medical Association*, 281, 361–367.

Pekar, N. (2001). *The economics of TB drug development*. New York: Alliance for TB Drug Development.

Pharmaciens Sans Frontières Comité International (PSFCI). (2005). *Study on drug donations in the province of Aceh in Indonesia: Synthesis*. Clermont-Ferrand, France: Author.

Poulson, L., Nissen, L., & Coombes, I. (2010). Pharmaceutical review using telemedicine: A before and after feasibility study. *Journal of Telemedicine and Telecare*, 16(2), 95–99.

Radyowijati, A., & Haak, H. (2003). Improving antibiotic use in low-income countries: An overview of evidence on determinants. *Social Science and Medicine*, 57(4), 733–744.

Ritzenthaler, R. (2005). *Delivering antiretroviral therapy in resource-constrained settings: lessons from Ghana, Kenya and Rwanda*. Retrieved from http://www.fhi.org/NR/rdonlyres/ej5r3pyybpgewqtq tinm6qlso4lhave7bvceqlqvxwxjldycjhlhu5bg7z2ur7 3q2rczwt5tfqw7tp/ARTLessonsLearned083106.pdf

Roffe, P., & Spennemann, C. (2006). The impact of FTAs on public health policies and TRIPS

flexibilities. *International Journal of Intellectual Property Management*, 1(1–2), 75–93.

Roll Back Malaria Partnership (RBM). (2008). *The global malaria action plan*. Geneva, Switzerland: World Health Organization.

Roll Back Malaria Partnership (RBM). (2010). SMS for life 2010. Retrieved from http://www.roll backmalaria.org/psm/smsWhatIsIt.html

Rutta, E., Senauer, K., Johnson, K., Adeya, G., Mbwasi, R., Liana, J., et al. (2009). Creating a new class of pharmaceutical services provider for underserved areas: The Tanzania accredited drug dispensing outlet experience. *Progress in Community Health Partnerships: Research, Education, and Action*, 3(2), 145–153.

Sabot, O. J., Mwita, A., Cohen, J.M., Ipuge, Y., Gordon, M. & Bishop, D., et al. (2009). Piloting the global subsidy: The impact of subsidized artemisinin-based combination therapies distributed through private drug shops in rural Tanzania. *PLoS One*, 4(9), e6857.

Sallam, S. A., Khallafallah, N. M., Ibrahim, N. K. & Okasha, A. O. (2009). Pharmacoepidemiological study of self-medication in adults attending pharmacies in Alexandria, Egypt. *Eastern Mediterranean Health Journal*, 15(3), 683–691.

Samb, B., & World Health Organization Maximizing Positive Synergies Collaborative Group. (2009). An assessment of interactions between global health initiatives and country health systems. *Lancet*, 373(9681), 2137–2169.

Senah, K. (1997). Money be man: The popularity of medicines in a rural Ghanaian community. In *Community drug use studies*. Amsterdam: Het Spinhuis.

Serdobova, I., & Kieny, M. P. (2006). Assembling a global vaccine development pipeline for infectious diseases in the developing world. *American Journal of Public Health*, 22(9), 1554–1559.

Sharma, D. C. (2003). ARV prices nosedive after Clinton brokering. *Lancet*, 362(9394), 1467.

Shretta, R. (2007). *Global Fund Grants for Malaria: Summary of lessons learned in the implementation* of ACTs in Ghana, Nigeria, and Guinea-Bissau. Submitted to the U.S. Agency for International Development by the Rational Pharmaceutical Management Plus Program. Arlington, VA: Management Sciences for Health.

Smith, O., Gbangbade, S., Hounsa, A. & Miller-Franco, L. (2005). Benin: System-wide effects of the Global Fund: Interim findings. Bethesda, MD: Partners for Health Reformplus Project, Abt Associates.

Special Programme for Research & Training in Tropical Diseases (TDR). (2007). Making a difference: 30 years of research and capacity building in tropical diseases. Geneva, Switzerland: World Health Organization.

Stevens, P., & Linfield, H. (2010). Death and taxes: Government mark-ups on the price of drugs. London: International Policy Network.

Stillman, K., & Bennett, S. (2005). Systemwide effects of the Global Fund: Interim findings from three country studies. Bethesda, MD: Partners for Health Reformplus Project, Abt Associates.

Strategies for Enhancing Access to Medicines (SEAM). (n.d.). Tanzania: Accredited drug dispensing outlets—Duka la Dawa Muhimu. Arlington, VA: Management Sciences for Health. Retrieved from http://www.msh.org/seam/reports/SEAM_Final_Report_Summary-Tanzania_ADDOs.pdf

Strub-Wourgaft, N. (2010). Strengthening pharmaceutical innovation in Africa. Pretoria. Retrieved from http://www.dfid.gov.uk/r4d/PDF/Outputs/DNDI/strub_dndi_cohred-nepad_plenarysession_feb2010.pdf

Thoithi, G., & Okalebo, F. (2009). Country case study: Kenya. In T. Wuliji (Ed.), FIP global pharmacy workforce report (pp. 49–53). The Hague: International Pharmaceutical Federation.

Torres, C. (2010). Rare opportunities appear on the horizon to treat rare diseases. Nature Medicine. 16(3), 241.

Tuladhar, S. M., Mills, S., Acharya, S., Pradhan, M., Pollock, J. & Dallabetta, G. (1998). The role of pharmacists in HIV/STD prevention: Evaluation of an STD syndromic management intervention in Nepal. AIDS, 12(suppl 2), S81–S87.

UNICEF. (2004). Supply catalogue. Retrieved from http://www.supply.unicef.dk/catalogue/index.htm

van Der Geest, S., & Reynolds Whyte, S. (1988). The context of medicines in developing countries: An introduction to pharmaceutical anthropology. Dordrecht: Kluwer Academic Press.

Victora, C. G., Wagstaff, A., Schellenberg, J. A., Gwatkin, D., Claeson, M. & Habicht, J.-P. (2003). Applying an equity lens to child health and mortality: More of the same is not enough. Lancet, 362(9379), 233–241.

Vujicic, M., Zurn, P., Diallo, K., Adams, O. & Dal Poz, M. R. (2004). The role of wages in the migration of health care professionals from developing countries. Human Resources for Health, 2(1), 3.

Waako, P., Odoi-adome, R., Obua, C., Owino, E., Tumwikirize, W., Ogwal-okeng, J., et al. (2009). Existing capacity to manage pharmaceuticals and related commodities in East Africa: An assessment with specific reference to antiretroviral therapy. Human Resources for Health, 7(1), 21.

Walley, T., Haycox, A., & Boland, A. (2009). Pharmacoeconomics. London: Elsevier.

Ward, K., Butler, N., Mugabo, P., Klausner, J., McFarland, W., Chen, S., et al. (2003). Provision of syndromic treatment of sexually transmitted infections by community pharmacists: A potentially underutilized HIV prevention strategy. Sexually Transmitted Diseases. 30(8), 609–613.

Wiedenmayer, K. (2004a). Medicine quality, adverse reactions and antimicrobial resistance. In S. C. Anderson, R. Summers, & K. Wiedenmayer (Eds.), Managing pharmaceuticals in international health. (pp. 153–174). Basel: Birkhauser Verlag.

Wiedenmayer, K. (2004b). Rational use of medicines. In S. C. Anderson, R. Summers, & K. Wiedenmayer (Eds.), Managing pharmaceuticals in international health. (pp. 141–152). Basel: Birkhauser Verlag.

UN Millennium Project. (2005). Prescription for healthy development: Increasing access to medicines. Report of the Task Force on HIV/AIDS, Malaria, TB and Access to Essential Medicines, Working Group on Access to Essential Medicines. Sterling, VA: Earthcscan.

World Health Organization (WHO). (1975). Certification scheme on the quality of pharmaceutical products moving in international commerce. In *Twenty-eighth World Health Assembly, Geneva, 13–30 May 1975. Part 1: Resolutions and decisions, annexes. Official records of the World Health Organization* (pp. 94–95). Geneva, Switzerland: Author.

World Health Organization (WHO). (1977). *The selection of essential drugs: Report of a WHO expert committee. WHO Technical Report Series 615*. Geneva, Switzerland: Author.

World Health Organization (WHO). (1997). *Quality assurance of pharmaceuticals: A compendium of guidelines and related materials*. Geneva, Switzerland: Author.

World Health Organization (WHO). (1999a). *Guidelines for the development of measures to combat counterfeit drugs*. Geneva, Switzerland: Author.

World Health Organization (WHO). (1999b). *Guidelines for drug donations*. WHO/EDM/PAR/99.4. Geneva, Switzerland: Author.

World Health Organization (WHO). (2000a). *Overcoming antimicrobial resistance*. Geneva, Switzerland: Author.

World Health Organization (WHO). (2000b). *WHO medicines strategy 2000–2003: Framework for action in essential drugs and medicines policy*. Geneva, Switzerland: Author.

World Health Organization (WHO). (2001a). *Global strategy for containment of antimicrobial resistance*. Geneva, Switzerland: Author.

World Health Organization (WHO). (2001b). Globalization, TRIPS and access to pharmaceuticals. In *WHO policy perspectives on medicines*, 3 (pp. 1–6). Geneva, Switzerland: Author.

World Health Organization (WHO). (2001c). *How to develop and implement a national drug policy*. Geneva, Switzerland: Author.

World Health Organization (WHO). (2001d). *Macroeconomics and health: Investing in health for economic development*. Geneva, Switzerland: Author.

World Health Organization (WHO). (2002a). *The importance of pharmacovigilance: Safety monitoring of medicinal products*. Geneva, Switzerland: Author.

World Health Organization (WHO). (2002b). Promoting rational use of medicines: Core components. In *WHO policy perspectives on medicines*, 5. Geneva, Switzerland: Author.

World Health Organization (WHO). (2002c). *Safety of medicines: A guide to detecting and reporting adverse drug reactions*. Geneva, Switzerland: Author.

World Health Organization (WHO). (2003a). *Adherence to long-term therapies: Evidence for action*. Geneva, Switzerland: Author.

World Health Organization (WHO). (2003b). *Introduction to drug utilization research*. Geneva, Switzerland: Author.

World Health Organization (WHO). (2004a). Equitable access to essential medicines: A framework for collective action. In *WHO policy perspectives on medicines*, 8 (pp. 1–6). Geneva, Switzerland: Author.

World Health Organization (WHO). (2004b). *The world medicines situation*. Geneva, Switzerland: Author.

World Health Organization (WHO). (2006). Declaration of Rome. In *WHO International Conference on "Combating Counterfeit Drugs: Building Effective International Collaboration," 18 February 2006*. Rome: Author.

World Health Organization (WHO). (2007). *Multi-country regional pooled procurement of medicines: Identifying key principles for enabling regional pooled procurement and a framework for inter-regional collaboration in the African, Caribbean and Pacific Island countries*. Geneva, Switzerland: Author.

World Health Organization (WHO). (2008). *Global atlas of the health workforce*. Geneva, Switzerland: Author.

World Health Organization (WHO). (2010a). Antimicrobial use. Retrieved from http://www.who.int/drugresistance/use/Antimicrobial_Use/en/index.html

World Health Organization (WHO). (2010b). Essential medicines. Retrieved from http://www.who.int/medicines/services/essmedicines_def/en/index.html

World Health Organization (WHO). (2010c). Essential medicines list and WHO model formulary. Retrieved from http://www.who.int/selection_medicines/list/en/

World Health Organization (WHO). (2010d). The international pharmacopoeia. Retrieved from http://www.who.int/medicines/publications/pharmacopoeia/overview/en/index.html

World Health Organization (WHO). (2010e). List of prequalified medicinal products available. Retrieved from http://apps.who.int/prequal/

World Health Organization (WHO). (2010f). Monitoring and evaluation: Core indicator package. Retrieved from http://www.who.int/medicines/areas/policy/monitoring/en/index.html

World Health Organization (WHO). (2010g). Rational use of medicines: Activities. Retrieved from http://www.who.int/medicines/areas/rational_use/rud_activities/en/index.html

World Health Organization (WHO). (2010h). Substandard medicines. Retrieved from http://www.who.int/medicines/services/counterfeit/faqs/06/en/

World Health Organization (WHO). (2010i). The WHO Prequalification Project. Retrieved from http://www.who.int/mediacentre/factsheets/fs278/en/

World Health Organization (WHO). (n.d.). *HA210 World Health Organization public assessment report*. Geneva, Switzerland: Author.

World Health Organization (WHO). (n.d.). *HA343 World Health Organization public assessment report*. Geneva, Switzerland: Author.

World Health Organization (WHO) & Health Action International (HAI). (2008). *Measuring medicine prices, availability, affordability and price components*. Geneva, Switzerland: WHO.

World Health Organization (WHO), UNAIDS, & UNICEF. (2008). *Towards universal access: scaling up priority HIV/AIDS interventions in the health sector: Progress report*. Geneva, Switzerland: WHO.

WorldMapper. (2008). Share of the world's pharmacists 2008. Retrieved from www.worldmapper.org

Wuliji, T. (2009). Current status of human resources and training in hospital pharmacy. *American Journal of Health-System Pharmacy*, 66(5), S56–S60.

Wuliji, T. (2010). *World medicines situation*. Geneva, Switzerland: World Health Organization.

CHAPTER

15

Health and the Economy

JENNIFER PRAH RUGER, DEAN T. JAMISON, DAVID E. BLOOM, AND DAVID CANNING

Health and healthcare systems interrelate with the economy in a number of ways, but the multiple causal mechanisms that define this relationship divide naturally into two categories. The first comprises the linkages between health and the growth rate and distribution of income. The second concerns the relationships among healthcare delivery institutions, health finance policies, and economic outcomes. The two major sections of this chapter follow this division of topics.

Figure 15-1 provides a summary of these linkages and a guide to the structure of the chapter. The first major section deals with relations between the health status of populations and income levels. Health and demography affect income (arrow F) through their effects on labor productivity, savings rates, investments in physical and human capital (education, for example), and age-structure effects. The current literature suggests that these effects may be more significant than previously thought, even as recently as

the early 1990s; these issues are addressed in the section titled "Economic Consequences of Ill Health."

The other direction of causality derives from income's impact on health and demography (arrow E). An important part of the literature on the health benefits of higher income assesses the extent to which income operates through improved capacity to purchase food and to have adequate sanitation, housing, and education, and through incentives for fertility limitation. The section titled "Economic Development's Consequences for Health" briefly discusses these points. Further, health systems as a whole play an important role in improving health and are themselves greatly influenced by health finance and related policies (arrows C and D). Other chapters in this volume deal with these issues.

Finally, wealthier countries tend to spend a larger percentage of their income per capita on health and to rely more substantially on public-sector finance than lower-income countries (arrow B). Conversely,

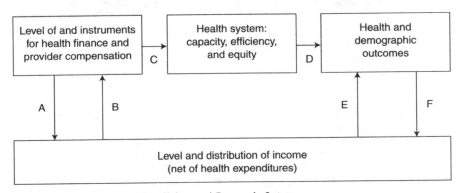

Figure 15-1 Health, Health Policies, and Economic Outcomes.

757

health finance and delivery mechanisms affect income level and distribution (arrow A) through their effects on incentives and institutional environments. Some health finance systems are, for example, more progressive than others, favorably affecting the distribution of income, whereas others have detrimental efficiency consequences through their effects on labor markets or on the adequacy with which financial risks are shared. The second major section of the chapter explores these linkages.

Whether the final objective of development policy is economic growth, poverty alleviation, or improved health, these domains are inextricably linked. Better information on the magnitude of the association between health and economic growth and of health systems and economic outcomes can aid academics and policy makers in understanding and devising health and development policies that will improve people's quality of life worldwide. This understanding allows the development of more balanced policy portfolios (Bloom & River Path Associates, 2000).

Health and Economic Development

The evidence presented here suggests that health is closely linked with economic growth and development. Figure 15-2 illustrates the multiple pathways through which illness can influence this outcome. The top half of the figure shows the age-structure effects of demographic transition as seen by a change in the dependency ratio, which has been a significant determinant of growth in East Asia, for example. High levels of fertility and child mortality (both in part a result of child illness), along with reductions in the labor force brought on by mortality and early retirement, can cause an increase in the dependency ratio that ultimately reduces income. Conversely, a reversal of these effects can decrease the dependency ratio, which increases per capita income. In addition, childhood health can affect adult health. Research points to a strong link between the health of adults and their level of health as children (Fogel, 2005; Kuh & Ben-Shlomo, 1997); an arrow in Figure 15-2 depicts that additional pathway between child health and eco-

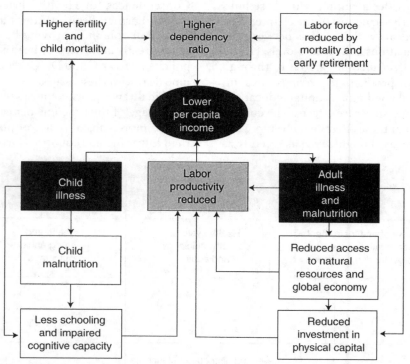

Figure 15-2 Channels Through Which Illness Reduces Income. *Source:* World Health Organization, *World Health Report 1999: Making a Difference* (Geneva, Switzerland: World Health Organization, 1999), p. 11. Adapted and reprinted with permission.

nomic outcomes. The lower half of Figure 15-2 illustrates the effects of illness and malnutrition, operating through other factors such as reduced investments in human and physical capital, in reducing labor productivity. Finally, reduced labor productivity has a direct impact on reducing per capita income. Economic conditions influence health as well. The relationship between health and economic development is causal in both directions.

Progress in health and other dimensions of development during the twentieth century constitutes one of humankind's greatest achievements. Rates of progress were so high that projecting them backward—or forward—in time suggests that never before and, probably, never again will so much be achieved in so short a period. Before turning to the more systematic discussion of health and economic development, it is worth touching on the broader context within which this relationship operates.

Table 15-1 provides examples of progress in five domains: health itself, fertility rates, physical growth (or nutritional status), cognitive growth, and income, linked in a web of mutual causation. Row 1 represents health using the life expectancy of Chilean females in the period 1910 to 1998 as an example. At the be-

ginning of this period, their life expectancy was 33 years; it then increased at an average rate of 1% per annum over 90 years to a level of 78 years in 1999 (World Health Organization [WHO], 1999). Had this rate been in effect for the preceding 70 years, life expectancy would have been 16 years in 1835, far lower than the actual level. If this rate were to continue, life expectancy would exceed 150 years by 2070—conceivable, but unlikely. For the other indicators, the twentieth century also stands out—in some cases more dramatically, in others less so.

The example of cognitive growth may be less familiar than the others. Evidence from an increasing number of studies around the world suggests major improvements in the average level of general, or "fluid," intelligence. The Dutch study cited in Table 15-1 is particularly suggestive. All Dutch males are screened (including an IQ test) for military service at approximately age 20. The study matched sons (1982 cohort) with fathers (1952 cohort) and found a 21-point gain. This gain is larger than that found in most studies, but is indicative of the general pattern. Flynn (1998) summarizes the Dutch and many similar studies (while placing caveats on how they should be interpreted).

Table 15-1	Human Progress in the Twentieth Century: Never Before, Never Again		
Welfare Indicator	**Example**	**Before and After**	**Rate**
Health (proxied by mortality)	Life expectancy, Chilean females (1910–1998)	33 years in 1910 78 years in 1998	1.0% per annum or 0.45 s.d.[a] per generation[b]
Total fertility rate[c]	TFR, Western Pacific Region (1950–1998)	5.9 in 1950 1.9 in 1998	−2.4% per annum or −0.53 s.d. per generation
Physical growth (height for age or BMI)	Height, 10-year-old Norwegian females (1920–1970)[d]	130.2 cm in 1920 139.6 cm in 1990	1.9 cm/decade or 0.84 s.d. per generation
Cognitive growth (general or "fluid" intelligence)	Dutch males' IQ (1982) relative to that of their own fathers (1952)	IQ = 100 in 1952 IQ = 121 in 1982	7 points per decade or 1.4 s.d. per generation
Income	Income per capita, Latin America (1913–1992), in 1990 dollars	$1,440 in 1913 $4,820 in 1992	1.5% per annum

[a]An estimate of the standard deviation (s.d.) of the variable's distribution at the initial time.

[b]A generation is defined to equal 30 years.

[c]The total fertility rate (TFR) is the expected number of children a woman would have if she gave birth at the then-current age-specific fertility rates.

[d]Source for 1970: G. H. Brundtland et al., 1975.

These examples illustrate the broad-based and substantial progress that forms the context of the following discussion of health and the economy.

Economic Consequences of Ill Health

Microeconomic analyses that study the link between health and economic outcomes focus on household-, family-, and individual-level data. Such studies typically look at the relationships between human resources, particularly education and health, and labor market outcomes (employment, wages and productivity, and age of retirement). It has become increasingly well established empirically that a person's health affects his or her labor performance (market and nonmarket). Work in this area demonstrates why the relationship between health and productivity is of special interest to low- and middle-income countries: Investments in health both contribute directly to individual productivity and complement investments in education and physical capital.

Macroeconomic studies provide evidence of a different sort by assessing the influence of health on national income in cross-country comparisons. This chapter focuses on such studies from low- and middle-income countries, although a number of examples from high-income countries are included. Currie and Madrian (1999) and Smith (1999) cover the research literature concerning health and labor market outcomes in the United States and other high-income countries and provide a careful discussion of problems of causality and statistical specification. More recently, Case, Fertig, and Paxson (2005) and Smith (2009) describe evidence of large effects of early childhood health on adult economic outcomes in Great Britain and the United States. This chapter notes those important issues but does not address them in a substantial way.

Households and Diseases

Health, Nutrition, and Productivity

The growing body of knowledge of the relationship between health and the earnings of individuals can be useful in designing policy interventions aimed at health improvement. These measures have the potential to enhance labor productivity, especially among populations in lower-income countries and among lower-income groups within countries.

Productivity as an adult depends on adult health. Nevertheless, an increasing body of evidence suggests that early childhood health and nutrition, particularly in utero and the first few years of life, have long-term benefits in the form of improved physical and cognitive development, better educational outcomes, and higher productivity and earnings as an adult. The Barker (1992) hypothesis argues that early childhood experiences have large effects on adult health.

Intervention studies have shown a link between investments in early childhood health and educational outcomes. Alderman, Hoddinott, and Kinsey (2006) examined the effect of early childhood nutrition on long-term child outcomes. Miguel and Kremer (2004) found that deworming in Kenya improved school attendance. Field, Robles, and Torero (2009) showed that iodine supplementation improved educational attainment in Tanzania. Clark and colleagues (2008) found that a malaria prevention intervention increased cognitive test scores in Kenya.

Hoddinott and colleagues (2008) found a very large effect of a childhood nutrition intervention for male children younger than three years of age on their productivity as adults in Guatemala, with wages in the treatment group being approximately 50% higher than those in the control group. In Sweden, Boman, Lindblad, and Hjern (2010) found that survivors of childhood central nervous system cancer attained lower educational levels, were less often employed, and had lower net incomes compared to other cancer survivors and the general population.

Such long-term studies linking an intervention in childhood to adult productivity and wages are rare. Rather, much of the work in this area is more indirect, with childhood health being linked to adult anthropometric measures such as height, weight, body mass index (BMI), and patterns of illness and disability (all measures or indicators of health), which are then linked to individuals' labor productivity as measured by wages or earnings.

Adult height is a marker for general health. Height and mortality have been found to be inversely related, implying that reductions in height can ultimately reduce an individual's number of productive working years (Schultz, 1997, 2002). Short height and low BMI have also been found to be associated with chronic morbidity in midlife (ages 20–50) and with male deaths in late life (Fogel, 1994). A number of other studies have assessed the effects of nutritional status on productivity in lower-income countries (Behrman, 1993; Deolalikar, 1988; Martorell, Melgar, Maluccio, Stein, & Rivera, 2010; Sahn & Alderman, 1988) and the cumulative impact of parental nutrition, childhood nourishment, and health over the course of the life cycle on adult height, which ultimately affects individuals' wage and earning potential.

| **Exhibit 15-1** | **Nutrient Intake and Time Allocation in Rwanda** |

Information on energy (calorie) intake and use can be difficult to obtain in all societies, but such data are especially difficult to gather in lower-income countries. Some people are self-sufficient, working primarily on their own land and in their own homes; because they do not receive monetary compensation in the marketplace, measuring the variables necessary to test implications for health is not easy. It can also be difficult to ascertain this relationship when health effects lag behind other changes; for example, simple measures, such as changes in dietary habits through protein intake and micronutrient supplementation for children, can prevent diseases later in the life cycle (Bhargava, 1994). Hence, some scholars analyze time allocation (from time allocation surveys, which document time spent on different activities, such as sleeping, resting or sitting quietly, work involving agriculture or heavy activities, or housework) and evaluate the relationship between time allocation and nutritional status to examine the energy intake, nutritional status, and health nexus.

In a 1982–1983 study of the time allocation patterns of adult men and women in approximately 110 Rwandan households surveyed four times, Bhargava (1997) found that low incomes and high food prices reduced households' energy intakes, resulting in more time spent resting and sleeping. The study also gathered statistics on age, consumption, production, protein intake, and weight and height (used to calculate body mass index). Subsequent analysis of these data revealed that the energy standard for active adult subsistence requires energy intakes of at least twice the basal metabolic rate.

The policy implications of this work are important. Interventions designed to improve nutrient intake and use through better health would enable individuals to carry out the activities necessary for active adult subsistence. Subsistence at higher activity levels would, in turn, enhance people's ability to purchase nutritious food in the marketplace, and dietary guidelines at a broad policy level should reflect the nutritional and energy needs for human activity.

In addition to the long-term effects of early childhood health and nutrition, adult health and nutrition have direct effects on productivity. Sahn and Alderman (1988) found that energy intake influenced wage offers for male and female labor in rural and urban areas of Sri Lanka, suggesting that better nutrition increases labor productivity. Martorell and colleagues' (2010) review of the long-term impact of a nutritional intervention found substantial improvements in future human capital and economic productivity from this program. Behrman (1993) also found, in a comprehensive literature review, that nutrition has direct effects on the labor productivity of poorer individuals in lower-income countries. Working in rural south India, Deolalikar (1988) found that although neither market wages nor farm output was affected by a worker's daily energy intake, both variables were influenced by weight-for-height ratios, indicating that chronic malnutrition has a significant effect on market wages and farm output. Evidence from Rwanda (described in Exhibit 15-1), however, shows direct effects of energy consumption operating through time allocation.

Thomas and Strauss (1997) have proposed two main reasons why household production studies should focus on health as an important determinant of productivity. First, they argue that the marginal productivity of good health is likely to be higher in lower-income countries than in higher-income societies because of lower absolute levels of health and different patterns of disease. In particular, the predominance of infectious diseases in lower-income countries causes higher rates of infant and child morbidity and mortality. The result can be ill-health consequences that are felt throughout the life cycle and not primarily at older ages, as is the case in higher-income countries.

Second, Thomas and Strauss argue that because physical strength and endurance affect employment opportunities in lower-income economies, the benefits of better health are likely to be larger in these contexts. For example, in one study, Indonesian men with anemia were found to have 20% lower productivity than men without it. In an experiment, men were randomly assigned to one of two groups, receiving either an iron supplement or a placebo. Anemic men who received the iron treatment increased their productivity to nearly the levels of nonanemic workers; these productivity gains were relatively large compared to the costs of treatment. Thus the most vulnerable—that is, the lowest-income individuals, the sickest persons, and those with the least education—are likely affected the most by improved health. Further, if there are thresholds of health status below which functioning and productivity are seriously impaired, policies that target those with the poorest health will yield the greatest increases in income. Bhargava and associates (2001) found strong evidence to support the plausible view that the effects of health on growth rates (using adult survival rates as the measure of health) are strongest at low levels of income.

In their earlier work in urban Brazil, Thomas and Strauss (Strauss & Thomas, 1995; Thomas & Strauss, 1997) analyzed the effects on wages of health indicators such as height and BMI, along with energy and protein intake, while controlling for educational variables that also contribute to earnings.[1] Including health variables in their analysis significantly reduced the effects of education on wages. These researchers found that height had a significant effect on wages (taller men and women earned more than shorter men and women), that higher BMI was associated with higher wages among males, and that this effect was most pronounced for less educated men. In addition, lower levels of energy and protein intake per person were associated with reduced wages for market workers, but not for self-employed individuals. A German study, however, demonstrated a nonlinear relationship between height and wages (Hübler, 2009), finding that women who were shorter than average and men who were taller than average had significant wage advantages over very short women or very tall men, respectively.

In Ghana, Schultz (1996) found that variations in adult height due to childhood health and nutrition inputs significantly affected wages; for example, a 1-cm height increase resulted in an 8% increase in male hourly wages and a 7% increase in female hourly wages. In Mexico, Knaul (1999) studied the productivity of investments in health and nutrition for women. The author analyzed the impact of age at menarche, or first menstruation (an indicator of cumulative health and nutritional status), on female labor market productivity, finding that investments in health and nutrition had significant effects on productivity. A 1-year decline in age of menarche was associated with a 25% increase in wages.[2] A report by Savedoff and Schultz (2000) cites a number of studies linking health to productivity and income in Latin America.

Human energy intake and nutritional deficiencies significantly affect people's ability to work. For example, a number of studies (Alderman & Linnemayr, 2009; Basta, Soekirman, Karyadi, & Scrimshaw, 1979; Gardner, Edgerton, Senewiratne, Barnard, & Ohira, 1975; Spurr, 1983) have demonstrated the influence of iron deficiency on oxygen consumption and the positive impact of iron supplementation on labor productivity. The effects of nutritional status on work performance are of interest to policy makers in designing food and economic programs to improve energy and nutrient intake.

In summary, the literature indicates a positive relationship exists among earnings, productivity, and energy intake. Higher earnings give people greater ability to purchase food, thereby improving their energy, nutrient intake, and health; improved health ultimately enhances productivity. Leibenstein (1957), Mirrlees (1975), and others have espoused the veracity of this set of relationships. Fogel (1994) also has done significant historical research in this area, suggesting that improvement in nutritional and health status contributed to the economic growth of England and France from approximately 1750 onward.

Disability and Income

In examining the productivity of household investments in health in Colombia, Ribero and Nunez (1999) found that an additional day of disability in a given month decreased male rural earnings hourly by 33% and female earnings by 13%. A disability in a given month was also detrimental to urban workers' wages, decreasing the hourly earnings of urban males by 28% and those of urban females by 14%. Height was also found to affect productivity significantly: A 1-cm height increase resulted in a 6.9% increase in urban female earnings and an 8% increase in urban male earnings.

Ribero and Nunez (1999) also evaluated the effects of public and private investments in health. They found that an increase in social security coverage in rural areas could result in a lower incidence and duration of illness, whereas increases in urban areas would result in a greater propensity to report illnesses. In addition, these researchers found that although basic service interventions, such as electricity and sewage or potable water, had very little effect on height and productivity, policies focused on providing adequate housing for those in need did have a positive impact on health and productivity.

---

[1] It is important to maintain a sharp distinction, as Strauss and Thomas have done, between nutrient intake and malnutrition. Nutrient intake is one determinant of nutritional status (as measured by anthropometric indicators such as height-for-age ratios, or biochemical indicators such as hematocrit for anemia). In many environments, infectious diseases will also be important determinants of malnutrition. For this reason, prevention or control of infection may often be more cost-effective for controlling malnutrition than attempts to improve diets through food transfers, food subsidies, or social marketing. (See Chapter 6 for more information on nutrition.)

[2] See also Knaul and Parker (1998) on the patterns over time and the determinants of early labor force participation and school dropout in Mexican children and youth.

Murrugarra and Valdivia (1999) studied the returns to health for Peruvian urban adults. Employing a two-stage process, these researchers first estimated the relationship between education and health; they then examined the effects of health on productivity (measured by wages), looking at different subsamples of the population (e.g., stratified by gender, age, location in the wage distribution, and type of employer, either public or private, small or large, or self-employed). The authors found that schooling's effects on health were positive, strong, and increased with age for urban males. They also found a positive effect of health on wages, controlling for education and income effects, which differed for different subgroups of the population. For example, among older, self-employed males, an additional sick day resulted in a 4.3% reduction in average hourly earnings. These males experienced greater effects due to illness than other groups: For instance, those at the lowest end of the earnings distribution experienced a reduction in average earnings due to an additional sick day of 3.8%, and those in the private sector experienced the weakest effect, with a 1.8% reduction in hourly earnings due to an additional sick day. The results for females were inconclusive.

More recently, a study by Sullivan and colleagues (2010) assessed the impact of rheumatoid arthritis on productivity in the United States. According to their analysis, even after adjusting for age, income, education, and chronic comorbidity, this autoimmune disease was associated with decreases in productivity, function, and employment.

Finally, disease and disability affect individuals' retirement decisions. For example, in Jamaica, Handa and Neitzert (1998) found that individuals with chronic illness faced an increased probability of retirement as compared with healthy individuals. In the United States, Dwyer and Mitchell (1999) studied the impact of mental and physical capacity for work on older men's retirement decisions. They found that health variables had more influence than economic factors on the decision to retire and estimated that men in poor health would retire, on average, one to two years earlier than those in good health.

In total, these studies suggest that health is related to productivity, both through the direct effects that adult height and chronic morbidity have on adult productivity and through the inverse relationship between height and mortality that can ultimately reduce an individual's number of productive working years. In addition, illness and disability have negative consequences on labor productivity, reducing hourly wages by as much as 33%. The studies summarized

in Exhibit 15-2 provide evidence that the link from health to productivity is causal in nature. These factors are particularly important in lower-income countries, where a significant proportion of the workforce is involved in agriculture and other forms of manual labor. Also, the negative effects of malnutrition during childhood can have lasting effects on human capacity, and the effects of improved health are probably greatest for those persons who are the most vulnerable: the lowest income, the sickest, and the least well educated.

Although the causal link between health and productivity levels can usually be determined only by applying statistical methods based on observation of populations, a more direct method is to use either actual or natural experiments to investigate the link. Almond (2006), for example, used the influenza pandemic of 1918 in the United States as a natural experiment. This pandemic caused health problems later in life for those with in utero exposure. By comparing the life courses of the members of this cohort with those cohorts immediately before and after it, Almond found that the 1918 influenza pandemic had a large negative impact on adult economic outcomes. More directly, Thomas and colleagues (2003) estimated the effects of a randomized controlled trial that provided iron supplementation and deworming medication to a population in Indonesia with high levels of iron-deficiency anemia, finding that the intervention had large effects on productivity levels and earnings for some workers.

Economic Costs of Particular Diseases

The economic effect of specific aspects of health status can be assessed by evaluating the economic burden created by particular diseases. The economic costs of particular diseases typically comprise two elements: (1) the direct costs of prevention and treatment, and (2) the indirect costs of labor time lost due to illness. Although empirical work in this area is limited, this section reviews economic analyses of three diseases—malaria, tuberculosis, and HIV/AIDS—with additional illustrative examples of the Onchocerciasis Control Program (OCP) and mental illness.

Malaria

Malaria, which remains one of the most significant public health problems in lower-income countries, claims approximately 1.1 million lives per year. In all WHO member states, the estimated total of disability-adjusted life years (DALYs) lost in 2004 due to malaria is calculated to be 34 million DALYs, or 2.2% of the total DALYs lost because of disease (WHO,

Exhibit 15-2	Do Health Changes Cause Income Changes?

When studying the relationships among different variables (e.g., health and wages), it is often difficult to disentangle the forces of mutual causation—that is, the strength of causation in each direction. In some studies, researchers attempt to go beyond standard statistical techniques, such as ordinary least-squares regression, in efforts to deal with both measurement error and the endogeneity of health. These studies require complicated multiple-staged statistical methods and produce results that are suggestive but seldom definitive. Three studies have used data allowing for a simpler, sharper assessment of causality and are illustrative of how data sets including non-income-related determinants of health can resolve the causality problem. Each study confirms a strong causal link from health to economic outcomes.

A British experiment (Moffett et al., 1999) evaluated the effectiveness of an exercise program for patients with lower back pain through a randomized controlled trial of the program compared with usual primary care management. The results indicated that at 1 year following initiation of the program, the intervention group showed significantly greater improvement compared to controls on a scale of back pain, and reported fewer (378) days off work compared with the control group, who took 607 days off work. Compared to controls, the intervention group used fewer healthcare resources.

Another study, conducted in the United States, traced the consequences for wealth status of a sudden health shock (Smith, 1999), evaluating the impact of the onset of chronic health problems (controlling for demographic factors, health risk behaviors, and preexisting conditions) and mild and severe new health conditions. In this study, it was found that even mild health problems may have lowered wealth accumulation by $3,620. The impact of new, severe health problems on savings was found to be a mean wealth reduction of approximately $17,000, or 7% of household wealth (per incident). Finally, among Americans aged 70 and older, a new health condition was found to lower wealth accumulation by approximately $10,000, half of which was found to take the form of a reduction in financial assets.

Finally, an experiment involving 6,000 households in Indonesia (Dow, Gertler, Schoeni, Strauss, & Thomas, 2003) examined the impact of price changes of publicly provided health services on labor force participation. By randomly selecting districts where fees were raised, and by holding fees in neighboring control districts constant, researchers found that compared to controls, test areas had declines in some health indicators and health care utilization. Higher prices were associated with more days spent in bed and greater limitations on daily activities, especially among the poor and among women who come from households with low economic and educational status. Finally, the study found that vulnerable groups in the test area had significant declines in labor force participation.

2008).[3] The high rates of morbidity and mortality caused by this disease suggest that it carries significant economic costs. (See Chapter 5.)

Chima, Goodman, and Mills (2003) and Malaney, Spielman, and Sachs (2004) have delineated the direct and indirect economic costs of malaria as follows:

- The direct costs of prevention (mosquito coils, aerosol sprays, bed nets, residual spraying, and mosquito repellents) and treatment (drugs, treatment fees, transport, and costs of subsistence at a health center)

- The indirect costs of labor time lost because of illness

Given these two components, household and public-sector expenditures are increased and labor inputs are decreased due to malaria. As a result of declines

in school attendance, lowered school performance, and increased cognitive impairment, human capital can also be reduced. For example, Bleakley (2010), by using the malaria eradication programs in the United States in the 1920s and in Brazil, Colombia, and Mexico in the 1950s as natural experiments, found that children in malarious areas in these countries born just after the eradication programs had significantly higher earnings than those born just before the programs were initiated.

Malaria has also been suggested to cause inefficiencies with respect to land use. Leighton and Foster (1993) estimated the total annual value of malaria-related production loss to be 2% to 6% of gross domestic product (GDP) in Kenya and 1% to 5% of GDP in Nigeria. Malaria-related costs as a percentage of total household costs for small farmers were 0.8% to 5.2% in Kenya and 7.2% to 13.2% in Nigeria.

Microeconomic studies of malaria tend to evaluate the costs of the disease in terms of its impact within a specific economic environment. Potentially more significant, however, is the effect of disease on economic opportunities. If a factory goes unbuilt in

---

[3] The World Bank (1993) introduced disease burden measurements based on DALYs, and the initial full publication of results appears in Murray, Lopez, and Jamison (1994).

a region because of malaria, for example, the consequences for income may be far more substantial than malaria's consequence for productivity in traditional agriculture. Gallup and Sachs (2001) advance this perspective, arguing for a macroeconomic approach that uses cross-country time-series data to capture effects that would go unobserved with collection of only household data. In particular, their work uncovered a significant negative relationship between malaria and GDP growth, with far greater estimated magnitude than reported in the household-level studies. Due to compounding, even small changes in the rate of economic growth can have large long-term effects. Gallup and Sachs suggest that the most important ways in which malaria affects long-run economic growth are through its effects on a country's ability to attract foreign direct investment and to create an environment suitable for modern economic growth. Thus allowing countries to undertake new enterprises, rather than just improving productivity in traditional enterprise, may be the most economically significant consequence of malaria control programs. Although the malaria data have some shortcomings, these findings have suggestive implications for policy makers, even if they are not entirely convincing.

Tuberculosis

Tuberculosis is a serious health threat across the globe. In 2004, deaths from tuberculosis in all WHO member states numbered approximately 1.5 million, representing 2.5% of all deaths (WHO, 2008). In 2007, 1.3 million new cases of tuberculosis occurred just in China (WHO, 2009). Tuberculosis is estimated to be four times more concentrated in lower-income populations than among the well-off (WHO, 1999). In addition, the considerable barriers to detecting this disease and to reducing its infectiousness exacerbate the impact of tuberculosis and increase the probability of transmitting it to others; indeed, only half of all tuberculosis cases are detected. If a patient does receive treatment, the risk of 5-year mortality is reduced to roughly 15%.

Tuberculosis is a disease that primarily affects adults, especially those in their most productive years. It is estimated that 77% of tuberculosis DALY cases and deaths occur among adults ranging in age from 15 to 59 years (Murray et al., 1994). (See Chapter 5.)

This section discusses two aspects of tuberculosis that have been addressed in the literature: (1) its economic burden, which necessarily compares different treatment options, and (2) the economic benefits and the cost-effectiveness of control, comparing the relative economic merits of different interventions. Exhibit 15-3 discusses the economic benefits of a tuberculosis control program in India.

The economic impact of tuberculosis, like malaria, comprises two components: (1) the direct costs of prevention and treatment, and (2) the indirect costs of earnings lost due to illness or mortality. Because tuberculosis largely affects adults in the most productive stage of their lives, its indirect costs can be quite high. Ahlburg (2000) provides a cost analysis for this disease in various lower-income settings.

In their study of patients presenting to a tuberculosis clinic in northwest Bangladesh, Croft, and Croft (1998) found a mean financial loss to the patient of $245, or 4 months' income (roughly 30% of annual family income based on an average annual income for a Bangladeshi family of $780). The breakdown of the $245 total loss of income was $115 of financial loss and roughly $130 of direct medical costs, consisting of $112 for medicine costs, $9 for doctor's fees, and $8.50 for laboratory costs. Of the 21 patients studied, 8 were forced to sell land or livestock to pay for their treatment. Geography was a significant factor in obtaining treatment: 6 of the 21 patients were able to walk to the clinic, but of the remaining 15 patients, 5 reported that transportation costs to and from the local clinic ($0.25–$1.25) placed a relatively significant burden on their family. In Tajikistan, Ayé and colleagues (2010) found that costs are highest in the early stages of tuberculosis treatment, imposing a significant economic barrier to commencing treatment and affecting treatment affordability.

Saunderson (1995) compared the costs and consequences of then-current treatment practices for tuberculosis in Uganda with a program based on treating ambulatory patients at their nearest health unit while they lived at home. He found that the total costs per patient for the current practice was £190 ($285) versus £115 ($172.50) for ambulatory care. The breakdown of costs for each program showed a total cost per patient to the health service of £55 ($82.50) for current practice and £65 ($97.50) for the ambulatory program. In addition, the total costs per patient were £134 ($201) for the current practice and £49 ($73.50) for the alternative program. Thus the largest difference between the two programs was patient costs: The ambulatory care program resulted in roughly half of the costs to the patient as compared with the costs of the current practice, primarily because of reduced costs before diagnosis (alternative program costs were cut in half due to greater access to the program), the elimination of a hospital stay, and the reduced costs due to work loss.

Exhibit 15-3 | **Economic Benefits of Tuberculosis Control in India**

Tuberculosis is one of the leading causes of ill health and death in India, with an estimated 4 million people in that country having tuberculosis in 1997. The health and economic consequences of tuberculosis infection are considerable: prolonged illness and premature mortality, medical costs, and indirect costs due to lost productivity. Although chemotherapy treatment options are available, these programs are often self-administered or are costly in terms of the direct medical costs of treatment in tertiary or hospital settings and in terms of the time necessary to receive care—sometimes as much as 12 months of treatment. Such self-administered and long-term treatment programs in tertiary facilities have limited effectiveness due to high relapse rates, low cure rates, high case fatality rates, and drug resistance.

WHO developed the DOTS (directly observed treatment, short course) regimen to alleviate some of the problems associated with the existing long-course and self-administered chemotherapy. Dholakia and Almeida (1997) attempted to estimate the potential health and economic benefits of successfully implementing the DOTS program in India, based on two primary assumptions: (1) DOTS will succeed in alleviating pulmonary tuberculosis in India, and (2) DOTS will reach 100% of tuberculosis patients with full and instantaneous coverage. The researchers found that, with a relatively high discount rate, a low percentage growth in labor productivity, and use of present value calculations for the future stream of benefits resulting from DOTS, the potential economic benefit to the Indian economy of this program amounted to approximately 4% of India's GDP in real terms, or $8.3 billion in 1993–1994.

Of course, the DOTS strategy will probably not be immediately 100% implementable, but rather will involve a phasing-in process in which personnel are trained, the drug supply system is reformed, and organizational and management changes are made. The longer the period of phase-in, the lower the present discounted value of economic benefits associated with DOTS. Dholakia and Almeida (1997) estimated that a phasing in of DOTS coverage in India over 10 years with a conservatively high discount rate of 16% would result in a present value of economic benefits of 2.1% of GDP (1993–1994), or $4.6 billion, with a 16% rate of return in real terms. This outcome translates into $750 million per year in tangible economic benefits from a successfully implemented DOTS program that costs $200 million per year.

In a cost-effectiveness analysis between the two programs at different levels of cure rate, the ambulatory program was found to be more cost-effective (at a total cost per cure of £230 [$345] for a 50% cure rate, £192 [$288] for a 60% cure rate, and £164 [$246] for a 70% cure rate) than the current practice (at a cost per cure of £380 [$570] for a 50% cure rate and £316 [$474] for a 60% cure rate).[4] In comparing the two programs, Saunderson (1995) concluded that savings from avoiding work loss had the greatest effect on cost per cure. Under the current program, the average time spent away from normal activities due to illness was 9.5 months (range: 1 week to 3 years). Interviews with patients revealed that many had spent this time visiting various clinics and hospitals in search of care. The shadow price for time away from work was assumed to be a nursing aide's salary (approximately £10 [$15] per month), for an average loss of £95 ($142.50). Also, 33 of 34 patients interviewed reported that illness had affected their work and income. Eight of 10 patients who had paid employment or business reported that they had stopped work or closed their business due to illness, and 23 of 24 farmers reported reduced work and lost production because of their illness. Five patients noted the need to remove their children from school because they could no longer pay school fees. The assumption was that ambulatory treatment could reduce time away from work by roughly 60%.

In northeastern KwaZulu-Natal (Hlabisa health district) in South Africa, Wilkinson, Floyd, and Gilks (1997) conducted an economic evaluation of the DOTS strategy and the conventionally delivered treatment for managing tuberculosis. They found that the total health system costs per patient in 1996 U.S. dollars were $649 for DOTS and $1,775 for conventional treatment. The total cost per case cured for DOTS was $740 and for conventional treatment $2,047, making DOTS 2.8 times less expensive overall than conventional treatment. In a scenario analysis of the best and worst cases, DOTS was found to be 2.4 to 4.2 times more cost-effective, with a cost of $890 per patient cured compared to the cost of con-

---

[4] For another cost-effectiveness analysis of alternative tuberculosis management strategies in South Africa, see Wilkinson, Floyd, and Gilks (1997).

ventional treatment, which ranged from $2,095 (best case) to $3,700 (worst case). Wilkinson, Floyd, and Gilks attributed the reduced expense of DOTS to reduced hospital stays.

In most of these studies, costs may be underestimated in the sense that they do not always include monetary equivalents of losses in the household's production due to illness (i.e., indirect costs); reduced efficiency of land use; transport, housing, and food costs during treatment; human capital loss (increased absenteeism and reduced performance at school for children of a household with an adult infected with tuberculosis); and the value of pain and suffering. What is clear, however, is that tuberculosis-related costs are substantial and that cost-effective means of control are available.

HIV/AIDS

Most studies find the economic effects of HIV/AIDS on the economy to be relatively small. For example, a study of the impact of HIV/AIDS on India's national economy (Anand, Pandav, & Nath, 1999) found that the estimated total annual costs of HIV/AIDS in India under low (1.5 million infected), medium (2.5 million), and high (4.5 million) prevalence scenarios were 7 billion, 20 billion, and 59 billion rupees ($200 million, $571 million, and $1.7 billion), respectively. AIDS treatment and productivity loss were the two major components of these costs. Anand and associates (1999) concluded that the estimated annual cost of HIV/AIDS (assuming a prevalence of 4.5 million persons) was roughly 1% of the GDP of India.

Conversely, in a study of 51 low- and middle-income and high-income countries that controlled for potentially confounding variables and corrected for simultaneity, Bloom and Mahal (1997) found that the AIDS epidemic—early in its course—had an insignificant effect on the growth of per capita income. Bloom, Rosenfield, and River Path Associates (2000), however, describe evidence of the economic effects of AIDS on individual businesses.

Over, Bertozzi, and Chin (1989) estimated direct and indirect costs attributable to a given HIV infection in the Democratic Republic of the Congo and Tanzania. Estimates of total costs per case of HIV infection ranged from $940 to $3,230 (1985 dollars) in the Democratic Republic of the Congo, and from $2,460 to $5,320 in Tanzania.

Cuddington (1993) and Cuddington and Hancock (1994) estimated that, assuming AIDS treatments are entirely financed from savings and that workers sick with AIDS are 50% as productive as they would be without AIDS, the growth rate of GDP would be reduced by 0.6 percentage point in Tanzania and by as much as 1.5 percentage points in Malawi owing to the HIV/AIDS pandemic. In 1992, Over estimated that (assuming 50% of AIDS treatment costs come from savings) GDP growth is slowed by 0.9 percentage point per year in the average country (among 34 sub-Saharan African countries), and per capita growth by 0.2 point. Ainsworth and Over (1994) obtained similar results in their analysis. The International Monetary Fund also commissioned assessments of the full range of macroeconomic consequences of the epidemic that document the diversity as well as the magnitude of the effects (Haacker, 2004).

One reason for the small financial effects found to be associated with the HIV/AIDS pandemic is that economic consequences are usually measured in terms of income per capita. A high death rate reduces both income and the number of people in the economy, causing a sharp reduction in total output but producing a more modest effect on income per capita. This relationship points to a weakness of using GDP per capita to measure economic burden of disease.

Jamison, Sachs, and Wang (2001) argue that the main burden of HIV/AIDS comprises the welfare loss to those with the disease who become ill and die. Thus using as a metric the income level of the survivors, as is done with income per capita, is inappropriate. When they valued decreases (or increases) in a country's mortality rates using now standard microeconomic estimates and added this factor to the change in per capita income, Jamison and colleagues (2001) found dramatic negative economic consequences of the epidemic in five countries of eastern Africa in the period after 1990. The importance of the direct welfare effects of good health is emphasized by Nordhaus (2003), who argues that the welfare gains from improved health and longevity in the United States in the twentieth century were greater than the welfare gains due to rising income levels over the period.

Although to date the economic effects of HIV/AIDS have been found to be relatively small, Bell, Devarajan, and Gersbach (2003) sound a warning note. They argue that the large number of orphans in countries with high AIDS mortality rates will lead to a lack of resources for education and the production of successive cohorts with lower levels of schooling and income. In particular, this trend may plunge sub-Saharan Africa into even greater poverty. Moreover, the economic impact of HIV/AIDS could take years to realize and may be much greater and more widespread than forecasts estimate (Veenstra & Whiteside, 2005).

Other Diseases

In a cost–benefit analysis of the Onchocerciasis Control Program (OCP) in West Africa, which seeks to prevent river blindness, Kim and Benton (1995) estimated OCP's net benefits in terms of net present value (NPV) and economic rate of return (ERR) over two project horizons: 1974 to 2002 and 1974 to 2012. Assuming 85% labor participation and land use, the NPV of labor and land-related benefits over a 39-year project horizon (1974–2012) ranged between $3.73 billion and $485 million, in 1987 constant dollars at discount rates of 3% and 10%, respectively. Under the same assumptions, the estimated ERR was approximately 20%. ERR was approximately 18% when using a project horizon of 29 years.

Smith and associates (2009) modeled the potential economic impact of pandemic influenza in the United Kingdom. They found that while effects could easily exceed 1% of GDP, appropriate response policies—including vaccination—could substantially attenuate this impact.

In their study of the impact of mental illness on annual income, Ettner, Frank, and Kessler (1997) found that psychiatric disorders resulted in noteworthy decreases in income for both women (18%) and men (13%). Robins and Regier (1991), in their analysis of the impact of mental health problems on income, found that 4.5% of women and 3% of men in the United States reported an inability to work or assume normal activities at some point in the past 3 months due to emotional stress. In reviewing a broad range of studies from high-income countries (mostly studies conducted in the United States), Currie and Madrian (1999) pointed out the particular significance of mental illness in terms of economic impact.

In contrast to the findings of many other condition-specific studies, Svedberg (2000), in a broad assessment of linkages between poverty and undernutrition, concluded that the links between malnutrition and poverty are probably relatively weak. In this finding, he differs from the reports in much of the literature cited earlier in this chapter.

Pandemics and Economic Outcomes

There is a growing concern about the potential economic impact of new infectious diseases. Several recent incidents include the outbreaks of severe acute respiratory syndrome (SARS) in 2003, H5N1 avian flu in 2006, and H1N1 swine flu in 2009. The outbreak of SARS, in particular, caused a large decline in international travel due to quarantines and fear of infection and worries of severe economic disruption (Wilder-Smith, 2006).

Brahmbhatt (2005) highlights two major types of economic costs that arise from such outbreaks: the costs of increased illness and death of affected people and animals, and the costs of control and coping strategies to mitigate effects of the pandemic. According to Brahmbhatt, the most immediate economic losses during the SARS outbreak were due to absenteeism, disruption of production, and severe decreases in tourism, mass transportation, retail sales, and hotel and restaurant use. Keogh-Brown and Smith (2008), however, found that in retrospect the effect of SARS on income levels was relatively short-lived and modest.

A study by Keogh-Brown, Smith, Edmunds, and Beutels (2009) examined the potential economic costs of a modern pandemic. While these researchers found that moderate GDP losses would ensue (ranging from 0.5% in mild pandemics to 2% in severe pandemics), behavioral changes to avoid infection could potentially double these costs. For example, the cost difference between closing schools for 4 weeks at a pandemic's peak and closing schools for all 13 weeks of a pandemic was estimated to be £27 billion ($44 billion) for the United Kingdom. An emphasis on preparedness, emergency procedures, risk assessment, and preventive actions at an outbreak's onset is potentially important to reduce the macroeconomic effects from such epidemics.

Smith (2006) argues that in the early stages of a new infectious disease, the key issue is risk, including the unknown dimensions of the threat. Thus, in the early stage of a pandemic, it is vital to obtain accurate assessments of the disease and the appropriate responses. In the absence of dissemination of such authoritative information, media speculation might potentially lead to inappropriate behavior. Kleinman and associates (2008) argue for a biosocial approach to new infectious diseases combining the speedy acquisition of a biological understanding of the disease with policies that get the relevant information, and policy prescriptions, into the public domain.

Health and Education

Health and nutritional problems can also have significant consequences for the educational success of many school-aged children. Such problems result not only in direct welfare losses, but also in losses of learning opportunities that are essential to the economic, social, and parental success of these individuals and, ultimately, to the larger society. The close link between health and school attendance and performance raises the question of how educational systems might intervene to improve conditions that undermine both health and educational success.

Figure 15-3 illustrates the different ways in which health, school participation, and learning outcomes are related, and depicts how health and school quality interventions can influence educational outcomes. The evidence supporting these relationships is discussed in this section. As demonstrated in Figure 15-3, school quality interventions can affect the learning rate, which, in conjunction with enrollment and attendance rates, can directly affect the distribution of learning in a given age cohort. The figure also illustrates that health-related interventions, through their influence on health and nutrition status, can enhance learning rates and participation, both of which contribute to learning outcomes. Likewise, school location policies have direct links to participation rates, which in turn influence learning.

Leslie and Jamison (1990) reviewed the links between health conditions and three important education problems in low- and middle-income countries:

- Children who are unprepared to begin school at the usual age
- The failure of many students to learn adequately in school
- The unequal participation of girls in schooling

Despite data limitations, their study found that several widespread health and nutritional problems clearly have negative consequences for school participation and performance. When children suffer from weakened or lower than expected physical capacity (and concomitant problems with cognitive ability, psychological well-being, and social competence), they may be incapable of attending school or may be developmentally limited. Lack of school readiness in the form of physical and cognitive abilities and social and communication skills can result in significantly lower than average school performance as compared to children's counterparts at national and international levels. When children are too sick to learn in school, they fail to obtain the minimal literacy and numeracy skills that are central not only to educational success but also to later economic and social achievements.

Leslie and Jamison (1990) suggest that seven categories of health conditions are likely to affect school participation or learning, and occur frequently in lower-income country contexts:

1. Nutritional deficiencies
2. Helminthic infections (including intestinal parasites and schistosomiasis)
3. Other infections
4. Disabilities
5. Reproductive and sexual problems (including premature fertility, sexual violence, and exposure to sexually transmitted infections)
6. Injury and poisoning
7. Substance abuse

Table 15-2 demonstrates that not all types of childhood illness and malnutrition are important for education, nor are these conditions all easily alleviated through school-based interventions. For example, in dealing with certain health conditions, such as early protein-energy malnutrition, school-based measures offer little help, whereas school is a potentially important venue for intervening against certain other

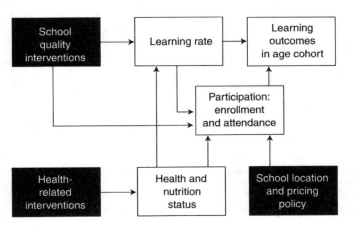

Figure 15-3 Health, School Participation, and Learning Outcomes. *Source:* D. T. Jamison and J. Leslie, "Health and Nutrition Considerations in Education Planning, 2. the cost and effectiveness of school-based interventions," 1990, Food and Nutrition Bulletin, 12(3). Adapted with permission of United Nations University.

conditions, such as tobacco use, that are important for health but not important for schooling.

In their summary of the relationships between the seven health conditions just mentioned and the three education problems (unpreparedness, failure to learn, and unequal participation by girls), Leslie and Jamison (1990) concluded that nutritional deficiencies have the most significant negative impact on education. Such deficiencies cause reduced cognitive function in both preschool and school-aged children and are directly reflected in poorer school attendance and achievement. These authors' review suggests that prenatal iodine deficiency can cause permanent mental retardation, and that chronic iodine deficiency can lead to less severe mental impairment among school-aged children and adults (see also Chapter 6). It also reveals that among infectious diseases, hookworm has a strong negative effect on cognitive function and Guinea worm negatively affects school attendance. Finally, although research on the links between education and reproductive health is limited, it is believed that the combined effects of early marriage, sexual vulnerability, and unwanted pregnancy at least partially influence the lower school participation rates of young females compared with those of males.

The question then arises as to what educational systems can do to improve the health and nutrition status of school-aged children. In a companion paper reviewing the costs and effectiveness of school-based interventions, Jamison and Leslie (1990) concluded that, given the current state of research on the health–education relationship, and the relatively low costs of well-designed and targeted programs, increased investment in child health and nutrition will benefit education. School-based interventions with the potential to improve learning, attendance and the participation of girls include improvements in school location and facilities; the presence of a school health worker or teacher who has been trained to screen for easily recognized health and nutrition problems and who has the ability to make referrals to local health facilities and administer first aid and basic medications; mobile health teams to deal with more extensive clinical problems such as vitamin A and iodine deficiencies and intestinal helminthic infections; school feeding to provide incentives for attendance and to address micronutrient deficiencies; and health, nutrition, and family planning education. A 2008 study by Clarke and colleagues, for example, found improved health and cognitive ability in semi-immune schoolchildren who received intermittent preventive treatment for malaria. School feeding is a frequently evaluated program and has been found to have a significantly positive effect on school attendance despite limited evidence of its effects on height or weight. School feeding also is by far the most costly of school-based programs, so its potential benefits need to be weighed carefully against the high costs. Using evidence of a very different sort on determinants of school attendance, Knaul and Parker (1998) found school

Table 15-2	Health Conditions and the Schools		
		Potential for Intervention[b]	
Condition	**Important for Education[a]**	**School-Based**	**Other**
Schistosomiasis (moderate to severe)	Yes	Yes	Yes
Iodine-deficiency disorders			
Anemia			
Short-term hunger			
Intestinal helminths (moderate to severe)			
Early protein-energy malnutrition	Yes	Low	Moderate
Diarrheal disease			
Acute respiratory illness			
Ill health of the parents of school-aged children			
Risk behaviors for chronic diseases (e.g., tobacco use)	No	Yes	Yes
Some immunizable diseases			
Mild schistosomiasis or intestinal helminthiasis			
Serious but infrequently occurring childhood diseases	No	No	Limited
Cataracts			
Most cancers			

[a]Conditions that are likely to affect school participation or learning and to occur relatively frequently in some environments.
[b]Conditions for which school-based interventions are likely to offer significant help.
Source: Leslie & Jamison, 1990. Adapted with permission of United Nations University.

participation in Mexico to be adversely affected by indicators of fertility in the child's household.

Health and nutrition from a child's earliest age, including influences in utero, can affect subsequent school performance. Glewwe and King (2001) have cited data from the Philippines to argue that nutritional status up to the age of two years can have significant effects on school outcomes. Miguel and Kremer (2004) noted significant effects on schooling outcomes from a randomized school-based deworming intervention. In their study, they found large-scale externalities to the program (due to the lower disease prevalence and transmission rates to those who did not receive the treatment) and an unwillingness to pay for the intervention despite its cost-effectiveness, indicating that public provision may be required for such programs.

In efforts to confront the health and nutrition problems that negatively affect girls' school participation rates, education planners can enhance sexual safety by paying attention to the location and gender basis of schools, by increasing the number of female teachers, and by improving school security. Other measures include the establishment of a sex, rape-prevention, and family-planning curriculum, and the dissemination of contraceptives and abortion referrals to reduce premature fertility and the onset of sexually transmitted infections. Evaluation of a school feeding program in India found greater positive effects on girls' enrollment as opposed to that of boys. In addition, experience from Bolivia suggests that programs that provide iodine and iron to micronutrient-deficient girls can enhance their cognitive function and school achievement. In particular, the Bolivia study found that a reduction in goiter was associated with improvements in IQ scores and that this relationship was stronger for school-aged girls than for boys. From the time of puberty, the incidence and severity of both anemia and iodine deficiency in girls substantially exceeds that in boys; hence, the greater intervention impact on girls is not surprising. Perhaps not coincidentally, female enrollment relative to male enrollment drops at puberty.

In addition to addressing cultural explanations for the education–health relationship, low-cost nutritional intervention will, in many cases, prove relevant and more amenable to policy making. On the question of causality between education and health, when Kawachi, Adler, and Dow (2010) and Schultz (1999) investigated links among schooling, income, and health, they found evidence suggesting schooling is causally related to improvements in health outcomes.

In an illustrative cost–benefit analysis, Jamison and Leslie (1990) suggested that "potential exists for benefits greatly to exceed costs for health and nutrition interventions in the schools" (p. 212).

Health and the Wealth of Nations

One of the main empirical tools used to understand variation in income levels and growth rates of countries is cross-country regression of economic growth (usually measured in terms of the growth rate of per capita GDP) on the variables believed to explain that growth.[5] Among the factors that are usually explored in such analyses are levels and patterns of educational attainment (schooling); health status (life expectancy, mortality rates, disease prevalence); population growth, density, and age structure; natural resource abundance; personal and government saving (investment rates); physical capital stock; trade policy, such as the degree of trade openness; quality of public institutions; and geography, such as the location and climate of a country (Bloom & Canning, 2000).

Research on the relationship between several specific variables and economic growth includes both directly linking economic performance and health variables, such as mortality rates and life expectancy, and indirectly linking health with economic growth, such as geography and demography indicators. Geography—especially tropical location—and disease burden are highly correlated, and have effects on economic performance. In contrast, demography, determined partly by health status, has age-structure effects that directly affect economic growth (WHO 2000). This section focuses on available empirical evidence estimating the influence of these various factors on a nation's overall level and rate of growth of income (see Figure 15-2).

Life Expectancy and Economic Outcomes

Life expectancy has been shown to be a powerful predictor of income levels and subsequent economic growth. Numerous studies have revealed that lower levels of mortality and higher levels of life expectancy have a statistically and quantitatively significant effect on income levels and growth rates (Barro & Lee, 1994; Bloom & Williamson, 1998; Jamison, Lau, &

---

[5] Conceptually quite distinct is an attempt by Cutler and Richardson (1998) to assess the value of health in the U.S. economy between 1970 and 1990. Assuming a value for a year in perfect health, one can estimate "health capital." This has increased over time in the United States, but more so for older adults than the young.

Wang, 2005; Radelet, Sachs, & Lee, 1997). In a study of determinants across countries of five-year economic growth rates, Bhargava and colleagues (2001) concluded that health's favorable impact on growth declined with a country's initial income level. The mechanisms through which this effect works are believed to be threefold: (1) the improvements in productivity that arise from a healthier workforce and less morbidity-related absenteeism, (2) the increased incentive that higher life expectancy gives individuals and firms to invest in physical and human capital, and (3) the increase in savings rates as working-age individuals save for their retirement years.

Jamison, Lau, and Wang (2005) combined their empirical estimates of the effects of adult survival rates on national income with country-specific estimates of improvements in survival rates to generate estimates of the contribution of health to economic growth. In the sample of 53 countries included in their study, their calculations suggest that, on average, 11% of total growth rate in per capita income was due to health improvements, although substantial variation across countries exists.

Bloom, Canning, and Sevilla (2004) provide a survey of the results of regression analyses that use life expectancy or other measures of mortality rates to explain economic growth. Their report indicates that findings in the literature of a large and significant impact of initial health status on subsequent economic growth rates are robust.

Historical studies reached similar conclusions using very different types of data. In a study of the determinants of the economic progress in Great Britain between 1780 and 1979, for example, Fogel (1997) estimated that 30% of the per capita growth rate can be explained by health and nutritional improvements.

Although the evidence of a large effect of health on economic growth is robust, the issue of how to interpret this result remains a thorny one. One possible explanation is that this result is the macroeconomic counterpart of the link between health and worker productivity. In their research, Shastry and Weil (2002) took the wage gains predicted by the microeconomic literature and calibrated how large an effect on output we would expect to see across countries due to health differences. They found that health differences, differences in physical capital, and differences in education were roughly equal in their importance in producing cross-country differences in income levels, supporting the view that health has a large macroeconomic effect. Weil (2007) found that eliminating health disparities among countries would reduce variance of log GDP per worker by 9.9%.

It is also possible that other mechanisms might underlie the link between population health and macroeconomic performance. Improvements in longevity are related to changes in age structure, so it might be the composition of the population, rather than the productivity of individual workers, that explains the health effect. This issue is discussed in the next section; the general finding is that the health effect of aggregate outcome persists even when age-structure effects are included in the model. For example, Bloom, Canning, and Sevilla (2004) find that higher life expectancies go hand in hand with an older, more experienced workforce, but it is the health effect—not the experience level of the workforce—that is important for economic growth.

An alternative explanation for the observation that life expectancy is important for economic growth is the hypothesis that increasing longevity increases the incentive to invest in education and to save for retirement (Kalemli-Ozcan, 2002). Bloom, Canning, and Graham (2003) have reported empirical evidence that life expectancy is linked to national savings rates. Alsan, Bloom, and Canning (2006) noted that health conditions have a significant impact on inward foreign direct investment, perhaps due to availability of a productive labor force or to attractive conditions for expatriate workers.

Another interpretation of the observed link between health and economic growth has been proposed by Acemoglu, Johnson, and Robinson (2003). They argue that health is linked to economic growth because the disease burden in low- and middle-income countries had an impact on the pattern of European settlement and the subsequent transference and development of institutions. This hypothesis proposes a historical link exists between health conditions and development but suggests that current improvements in health may have little effect on economic outcomes.

These findings indicate that for policy purposes, future macroeconomic research must go further than establishing the link between health and economic performance: It must show that improvements in health are linked to increases in income levels. One way of investigating such effects is through case studies of public health interventions that lead to dramatic health improvements. For example, Bleakley (2003) demonstrated that hookworm eradication in the southern states of the United States led to large increases in schooling levels in counties that previously had the highest infection rates, and that this trend had long-term consequences for earnings.

The weight of research evidence suggests, then, that improved health increases both individual income and national GDP per capita. Nevertheless, judging economic performance by GDP per capita fails to differentiate between situations in which health conditions differ: A country whose citizens have long lives clearly outperforms a country with the same GDP per person but lower life expectancy. Individual lifetime incomes are clearly higher in the first country, but numerous willingness-to-pay studies (Viscusi and Aldy [2003] summarize this literature) suggest that the economic value of reduced mortality exceeds by a factor of two or more the value of increased lifetime earnings. Usher's (1973) seminal paper first brought the value of mortality reduction into national income accounting. The previously mentioned paper by Jamison, Sachs, and Wang (2001) assessed the economic impact of the increased mortality rates from AIDS using Usher's methods. Bloom, Canning, and Jamison (2004) provide an introduction to this literature, suggesting that economic assessment of the intrinsic value of mortality change may substantially exceed its instrumental value in affecting GDP.

Demography and Growth

Health improvements also play a role in economic growth through their impact on demography. Acemoglu and Johnson (2007) argue that even if health improvements increase productivity of the individual, the reduced mortality rates will lead to a surge in population numbers that can depress income levels through a Malthusian effect of crowding on scarce resources such as land. This effect can be avoided, however, if fertility declines. Health advances in most high-income countries are associated with rapid declines in infant and child mortality rates. These declines, and increases in the proportion of surviving children, can substantially reduce desired fertility (Kalemli-Ozcan, 2002).

For example, in the 1940s, health improvements that led to changes in mortality and fertility rates in East Asia provided the impetus for a demographic transition. In the first phase of the demographic transition, an initial decline in infant and child mortality prompted a subsequent decline in fertility rates. These changes in mortality and fertility altered Asia's age distribution: The working-age population began growing much more rapidly than the youth dependent population. This resulted in a disproportionately high percentage of working-age adults, and led to increased rates of economic growth (Bloom, Canning, & Sevilla, 2002). Bloom and Williamson's (1998) work introducing demographic variables into an empirical model of economic growth suggest that changes in East Asia's

health and consequent changes in demography can explain one-third to one-half of the economic growth "miracle" experienced between 1965 and 1990.

Although this demographic dividend provides an opportunity for increasing wealth, it does not guarantee such results. East Asia's growth rates were achieved because both the government and private sectors were able to mobilize the growing workforce, successfully manage economic opportunities, adopt new industrial technologies, invest in education and human capital, and exploit global markets. These factors helped East Asia realize the economic growth potential created by the demographic transition.

The importance of demographic variables is supported by Jamison, Lau, and Wang (2005), who examined the role of total fertility rates in relation to economic levels using an aggregate-production function approach. These authors found a statistically significant negative relationship, similar to findings by Bloom and Freeman (1988), which showed that crude birth rates are negatively correlated with economic growth because they are associated with younger age distributions and lower labor force participation.[6] The link between mortality reduction and subsequent fertility reduction constitutes an important component of the total effect of health on development. The strength and causal nature of this link have been debated, but the direction of the evidence is now fairly clear. Schultz (1997), for example, concludes in a major review that "Whatever the cause of the mortality decline, the response of parents has been to reduce their births" (p. 418).

Bloom, Canning, and Malaney (2000) further developed this line of research by incorporating demography into a model of endogenous economic growth. They showed that, with the help of exogenous demographic influences and human and physical capital investments, countries can create a virtuous cycle of growth and thereby break free of a poverty trap (poor health affects low income, which in turn affects poor health).

Geography, Disease Burden, and Economic Growth

In their cross-country growth studies, Gallup, Sachs, and Mellinger (1999) focused on geographic factors as being among the empirical determinants of eco-

---

[6] In an early paper, Myrdal (1952) raised many of the issues dealt with in health economics in the years to come. Among other points, he noted the links between age distribution, fertility, health, and economic growth.

nomic growth. These researchers found that countries in tropical regions develop more slowly than those in temperate zones. The research suggests that, along with the effects of climate and geography on soil quality, this effect likely operates through an intermediate mechanism, the interaction of tropical climates and disease burdens: This interaction can have significant costs in terms of economic performance. Both high disease burdens and geographic isolation can separate countries from the global economy, denying them the benefits of trade, foreign direct investments, and technological interchange.

Economic Development's Consequences for Health

Previous sections in this chapter have discussed how health can lead to greater growth and reduced poverty. In fact, the causal relationship between health and development operates in both directions: Income influences health through a variety of intervening determinants. More distal determinants include housing, education, water, sanitation, nutrition, energy, health services, institutions, and industrial and agricultural policies. Industrial safety programs and environmental regulations, for example, have specific health objectives and are targeted at specific groups—namely, industrial workers and the general public. Housing policies aimed at subsidizing or providing housing for lower-income individuals have broader social and health objectives, but may also have concrete health impacts. Empowering women through better education, among other interventions, can enhance their capacity to improve their health and that of their families (Thompson, 2007). Marital status and family structure also play an important role in a family's economic status and health (Tipper, 2010). Education is strongly correlated with health in many studies in high-income countries as well, even after controlling for other factors, including income and medical care (Berger & Leigh, 1989; Farrell & Fuchs, 1982; Fuchs, 1993; Grossman, 1975; Kenkel, 1991). Quality of education, as measured by internationally standardized tests in mathematics, appears to be more important in this regard than years of schooling (Jamison, Jamison, & Hanushek, 2007).

The 1993 *World Development Report* (World Bank, 1993) provides an extensive overview of the determinants of health that are outside the health sector and their attractiveness from a policy perspective. For example, even if primary education offered no advantages for girls other than health benefits, education would still appear highly cost-effective.

Research has illuminated the various effects of income on health. Case (2004) demonstrated that pensions to the elderly in South Africa have a significant effect on the health status of household members. Pritchett and Summers (1996) found a link leading from income levels and education to health improvements in a macroeconomic study. Jamison, Sandbu, and Wang (2004), however, note that the Pritchett–Summers conclusion depends critically on these authors' (implicit) assumption that technical progress in health is the same in all countries. Even so, education's measured impact on health persists in their analysis.

There is also a growing body of information on health inequalities and the experience of relative deprivation as a cause of ill health. In the United Kingdom, for example, the Whitehall Study—a longitudinal study of behaviors and health status of more than 10,000 British civil servants—found that over a 10-year period males aged 40 to 64 in the lower grades (clerical and manual) of the civil service had an age-adjusted mortality rate that was 3.5 times higher than that for males in senior administrative grades (Marmot et al., 1991; Marmot & Theorell, 1988; Wilkinson, 1986). A gradient in mortality stretched across all levels of the civil service: Each status group had a higher mortality rate than the group immediately above it, which was not explainable by access to medical care or other primary goods, such as absolute levels of income, shelter, food, or education.

A Canadian study found that people in lower-income deciles had a lower health-adjusted life expectancy compared with people in higher-income deciles (McIntosh, Finès, Wilkins, & Wolfson, 2009). Likewise, a study in South Korea found that both men and women in lower socioeconomic positions as indicated by income and education and slightly less by occupation, had lower levels of self-reported health status and higher levels of morbidity, even after controlling for behavioral risk factories (Kim & Ruger, 2010). Moreover, these disparities were more pronounced for women than men.

Other research, aimed at confirming the Whitehall Study findings on a cross-national level, revealed a similar correlation between hierarchy and health. In a study of 11 countries belonging to the Organization for Economic Cooperation and Development (OECD), conducted from 1975 to 1985, Wilkinson (1990) used two measures of income inequality—the Gini coefficient and the ratio between the percentage of income flowing to the top and bottom 30% of a country's population. The analysis revealed an inverse relationship between income inequality in a country and the average national life expectancy. While nations with absolute levels of higher average income per capita had higher average life expectancy than those with a lower level of average national income (e.g., higher-income versus lower-income countries), the study suggested that greater income inequality within a country might also have a negative influence on life expectancy. Nations with a relatively flat income gradient, such as Japan and Sweden, had higher life expectancies than countries such as the United States and West Germany, which had steeper gradients. Moreover, in the United States, the sensitivity of mortality rates to socioeconomic status increased sharply between 1960 and the early 1980s (Preston & Elo, 1995). More recently, Liu and Hummer (2008) have noted widening gaps between educational level and self-rated health in middle-aged and older adults but a stable or narrowing gap in younger populations.

Other work has interpreted the apparent effect of income inequality on health as resulting from effects of ranking within a reference group that is much smaller than a country (Deaton, 2003; Deaton & Paxson, 2001; Karlsson, Nilsson, Lyttkens, & Lesson, 2010). If, for example, an academic had a low salary relative to other members within her discipline, this disparity might have a deleterious effect on health even if her absolute income was relatively high and she lived in a country where income was relatively evenly distributed. Even if individuals' reference groups are unobserved, individual income levels will provide partial information about the individuals' standing in their reference group (with the amount of information depending on the relative levels of within-group and across-group inequality). The mechanism of effect can generate the widely documented adverse effect of inequality on average health status even if there is no real effect of either within-group or between-group inequality on health. Deaton and Paxson's (2001) analyses using U.S. data support the conclusion of no effect. Zhang and Wang (2010), in contrast, found differences in development among children in eastern and western China that were related to regional economic status and living standards. More research is needed to extend the evidence base on how reference group rankings and socioeconomic inequalities influence health.[7]

An important question in assessing the historical determinants of health is how income, in relation to other factors, influences health improvements, especially during the twentieth century. Preston's (1980, 2007) work provides a broad framework for assessing income's impact, and his line of thought has influenced subsequent work. A WHO (1999) analysis, for example, examined these relationships. Figure 15-4 shows the results from this work and illustrates the relationship. From 1952 to 1992, mean income increased by approximately 66%, from roughly $1,500 to $2,500. The curves in Figure 15-4 indicate that the infant mortality rate (IMR) declined more than predicted (to 55 deaths per 1,000 births rather than to 116 deaths per 1,000 births) based on the 1952 relationship between income and IMR, suggesting that factors more important than income influence health. Historical analyses by Easterlin (1999) point to the same conclusion.

The WHO study and related World Bank analyses (Wang, Jamison, Bos, Preker, & Peabody, 1999) assessed the relative impact of three key areas on health improvements:

- Increases in average income levels
- Improvements in average education levels
- The generation and application of new knowledge

Researchers found that approximately 50% of health improvements were due to access to better technology, whereas the remaining gains resulted from income improvements and better education. Continued work along these lines (Jamison et al., 2004) has noted that country-specific differences in application of new knowledge are large indeed and, when properly accounted for, further reduce the apparent effect of income on health.[8]

Just as health conditions at any time improve with income level, so, too, might adverse income shocks have detrimental effects on health. Economic downturns—with their concomitant declines in employment and income, as well as rising uncertainty regarding employment and financial well-being—have been linked to increased morbidity and mortality, and to poor nutrition and mental health (Catalano, 2009; "The Economic Crisis and Suicide," 2009; "Protecting Health," 2008; Uutela, 2010).

---

[7] Note that the literature on inequalities in health is not, for the most part, about inequality in the univariate distribution of health, but rather generally about the strength of the effect of inequality in other variables (e.g., income) on health levels. Le Grand (1987) assessed univariate distribution of health or pure inequalities. Not surprisingly, these inequalities decline steadily with declines in overall mortality rates, even though the socioeconomic gradient may be getting steeper.

---

[8] Even though income differences may account for only a modest amount of cross-country variations in health outcomes over a period of several decades, the situation can be quite different within a given country at a given time.

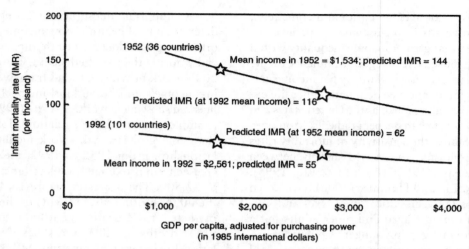

Figure 15-4 The Role of Improvements in Income in Reducing Infant Mortality Rates. *Note:* Results are based on a cross-sectional time-series regression that relates, at 5-year intervals, the natural logarithm of IMR to the natural logarithm of income, the square of the natural logarithm of income, and indicator variables for time.
Source: World Health Organization, *World Health Report 1999: Making a Difference* (Geneva, Switzerland: World Health Organization, 1999), p. 5. Reprinted with permission.

There are myriad channels through which an economic crisis may affect human health. First, loss of employment and reduction in wages can increase stress and lead to physical and mental health problems, including substance abuse, depression, and anxiety. For example, a recent review article reported relatively higher rates of psychological problems among unemployed adults as compared to their employed counterparts. The same review also noted that suicide rates in Asian and European countries increased as a result of past economic crises (Uutela, 2010). An important finding in this line of research is that the health effects of economic fluctuations and resulting unemployment can be ameliorated by social protection mechanisms that offset the loss of income (Stuckler, Basu, Suhrcke, Coutts, & McKee, 2009; Uutela, 2010).

Second, with less real income, individuals and households tend to spend less money on the promotion and preservation of health. This trend could mean reduced attention to primary care, inadequate adherence to medication regimens, and impaired access to high-quality food or adequate quantities of food. The Food and Agriculture Organization of the United Nations (FAO) reports that household attempts to cope with economic crises can put both child and adult nutrition and health status at risk. Such strategies include replacing more nutritious food with less nutritious and less expensive food options, reducing overall food consumption, and reducing the

frequency of healthcare visits (Brinkman, de Pee, Sanogo, Subran, & Bloem, 2009; FAO, 2009).

Third, fewer financial resources may be available for public health programs during and after times of economic crisis. During the recent economic crisis, high-income countries spent large sums of public money on "bailout" initiatives to generate higher levels of market liquidity. These policies may put global population health at risk, insofar as governments finance these macroeconomic policies through cuts in foreign assistance for health and cuts in their own future social spending ("Protecting Health," 2008).

Finally, individuals and households may spend down their savings and assets during economic crises, rendering them more vulnerable to future economic shocks.

The global economic crisis that began in 2008 has raised important and ongoing issues for population health. In discussing these issues, one must keep in mind the fact that the crisis came on the heels of the food and fuel crises of 2006–2008, which had already begun to erode people's health and the purchasing power of their income in a number of countries. In addition, the crisis began in high-income countries—unlike the financial crises of the 1980s and 1990s, which began in the low- and middle-income world. In low- and middle-income countries, the recent global recession has meant declines in exports, foreign direct investment, remittances, and donor aid, as well as rising rates of unemployment. Government budgets have also been negatively affected, which in turn has had detrimental effects on health-sector funding.

The true magnitude of the health effects of the recent economic crisis is largely unknown, and the lack of systematized monitoring of the situation has been noted (Richards, 2009). In addition, little is known about the distribution of impacts across the income spectrum. For some parts of the population, reductions in income might potentially lead to improved health behavior and reductions in risky behavior, such as increased walking or biking in place of driving (Catalano, 2009). For the most part, however, available data indicate an overall negative impact on population health from such economic downturns. FAO (2009), for example, has reported on problematic consequences of the recent economic crisis in Armenia, Bangladesh, Ghana, Nicaragua, and Zambia. In Nicaragua, the crisis has led to a decline in the consumption of meat and dairy products, which provide macronutrients and micronutrients that are particularly vital for young children and women who are pregnant or lactating. The FAO's Zambia case documents severe impacts of the crisis on healthcare access and utilization: Workforce reductions in the mining sector resulted in the loss of both income and benefits provided by mining companies. This, in turn, has translated into a loss of access to the hospitals and clinics established by the companies, which provided not only antiretroviral treatment to HIV-positive individuals, but also nutritious diets (FAO, 2009).

Implications of the economic downturn for the health system have also been explicated. For example, U.S. hospitals have reported increases in uncompensated care and reductions in revenues as a result of the crisis. In response, many hospitals have postponed capital investments, such as infrastructure renovations, purchasing of equipment, or upgrades to information technology systems (American Hospital Association [AHA], 2008).

Some evidence also indicates that public health programs have experienced negative effects as a result of the recent economic crisis. The Joint United Nations Program on HIV/AIDS (UNAIDS) reports that funding by donor governments was flat in 2009, following major increases in every year since 2002 (Kates, Boortz, Lief, Avila, & Gobet, 2010; Roehr, 2010). Survey data collected in 71 countries in 2009 indicate that scale-up of antiretroviral treatment programs was at risk of being stalled in many of these countries (UNAIDS, 2009). Interruptions in such treatment can have serious impacts on HIV transmission rates, as HIV-positive individuals off treatment become more infectious and HIV-positive pregnant women without adequate treatment are at increased risk of delivering babies infected with HIV. Without proper treatment, it is expected that the incidence of other life-threatening illness will increase (e.g., tuberculosis and other AIDS-related conditions). Drug resistance is another serious risk of interrupted treatment of HIV/AIDS and related conditions: It pushes more people on to more expensive second-line therapies, thereby burdening both individuals and health systems (UNAIDS, 2009) and putting the general population at risk of developing drug-resistant infection.

Although a full picture of the recent crisis's impact on health is lacking, we can look to past crises to shed some light on this issue. For example, Frankenberg, Thomas, and Beegle (1999) examined data contained in the Indonesia Family Life Surveys to study the impact of the 1998 economic crisis on household expenditure, employment, education, utilization of healthcare and family planning services, and health outcomes. Although their study found little evidence of a negative impact of the crisis on health outcomes, perhaps because of the narrow time frame, it revealed that the economic stress had negative impacts on health-seeking behavior and health system operations. In particular, the study noted decreased use of public health services by both adults and children, declines in vitamin A supplementation for children, medication and supply stockouts at public facilities, and price increases in both public and private health facilities.

Similarly, an AusAid (1999) report explored the magnitude of the health impacts of the 1997–1998 Asian economic crisis. The report cited a sharp increase in the price of pharmaceuticals, declines in vitamin A intake, and declines in the frequency of child healthcare visits during this period.

In another study of the link between macroeconomic crises and health, Brainerd (1998) examined the effects of market reform on mortality in Russia and other transition economies in the late 1980s and early 1990s. Standardized death rates in these countries increased in the period from 1989 to 1994, with Russia and Latvia experiencing the greatest increases—more than 50%. Brainerd provided strong evidence of a significant positive association between unemployment and the standardized death rate for adult males across 15 countries in the former Soviet Union.

Past experience has also demonstrated that the health of the poor is especially vulnerable to economic downturns. FAO (2009) reviewed the impact of past crises on nutrition and health among the poor. For example, Cameroon's crisis of the 1990s was associated with an increase in the prevalence of underweight children, especially among the poorest half of the population. As another example, Zimbabwe's drought of the mid-1990s caused losses in real income, leading to stunting among young children in the poorest households—a phenomenon that has been linked to cognitive impairments and reduced earnings during adulthood (FAO, 2009).

If past crises are any indication of what can be expected from the recent global economic crisis, the full effects are likely to be serious, widespread, and long-lasting, with significant implications for other realms of well-being. In a special April 2009 issue of *Global Social Policy*, scholars tackled the subject of economic crisis and children in East Asia. Using data from the 1997 Asian economic crisis, Bhutta and colleagues (2009) estimated the potential impacts of the recent global economic downturn on child health in East Asia and the Pacific. Their projections suggest that the crisis could have severe health impacts, including a 10% to 20% increase in maternal anemia, a 5% to 10% increase in low birth weight, a 3% to 7% increase in childhood stunting, an 8% to 16% increase in childhood wasting, and a 3% to 11% increase in overall under-five morality (Bhutta et al., 2009).

Health and Economic Development Policy

There is increasing recognition that health plays a vital role in human development. It is valuable both directly, as a source of welfare in itself, and indirectly, as a form of human capital that promotes economic development. Becker, Philipson, and Soares (2005) have estimated that welfare gains from health improvements over the last 50 years in low- and middle-income countries were approximately equal to the welfare gains from income improvements, highlighting the direct importance of health. The idea that health is an important input into macroeconomic growth was also recognized by WHO's Commission on Macroeconomics and Health (2001).

More recently, a panel of experts taking part in the Copenhagen Consensus (CC) 2008 sought to rank a wide range of potential interventions in terms of their ability to advance global welfare, and particularly the welfare of low- and middle-income countries. Given that there is a limited budget for such interventions, the CC participants examined the evidence base to determine the most cost-effective manner in which to spend development money to promote global welfare. Their top-ranked intervention was micronutrient supplements for children. In total, 6 of the top 10 interventions involved disease control or nutrition, including deworming and vaccination programs.

In a challenge paper on communicable diseases for the 2004 CC, Mills and Shillcutt (2004) reviewed the economic benefits of reducing the burden of communicable disease relative to controlling malaria and HIV/AIDS and strengthening basic health services. Their analysis revealed that many health interventions and programs had a favorable benefit–cost ratio. Data suggest that investment in areas of communicable disease control such as malaria and HIV/AIDS will yield high investment returns, especially in the poorest populations.

For the 2008 CC, Jamison, Jha, and Bloom (2007) wrote a challenge paper identifying priorities for disease control. The authors identified seven highly cost effective key priority interventions that address major disease burdens. These seven priorities (along with their benefit–cost ratios) are as follows:

- The appropriate case finding and treatment of tuberculosis (30:1)
- Managing heart attacks with low-cost drugs (25:1)
- Prevention and treatment package for malaria control (20:1)
- Expanding childhood immunization coverage (20:1)
- Tobacco taxation (20:1)
- Combination prevention of HIV/AIDS (12:1)
- Expanding surgical capacity at the district hospital level (10:1)

Even if costs increased threefold, these seven priority areas would still be cost-effective solutions for major disease burdens worldwide. Lomborg (2009) sets out the evidence base for the proposed interventions and the decisions made by the panel of experts.

Health Systems and Economic Outcomes

An important aspect of the link between health and economic development is how the characteristics of a particular healthcare system, especially health financing policies, affect economic performance.[9] Health care is one of the largest sectors of the world economy, accounting for 9.7% of the total global

---

[9] Chapter 12 provides a description of the main financing mechanisms of health systems; this section has a more detailed presentation of specific aspects of these arrangements in terms of their economic and equity impacts.

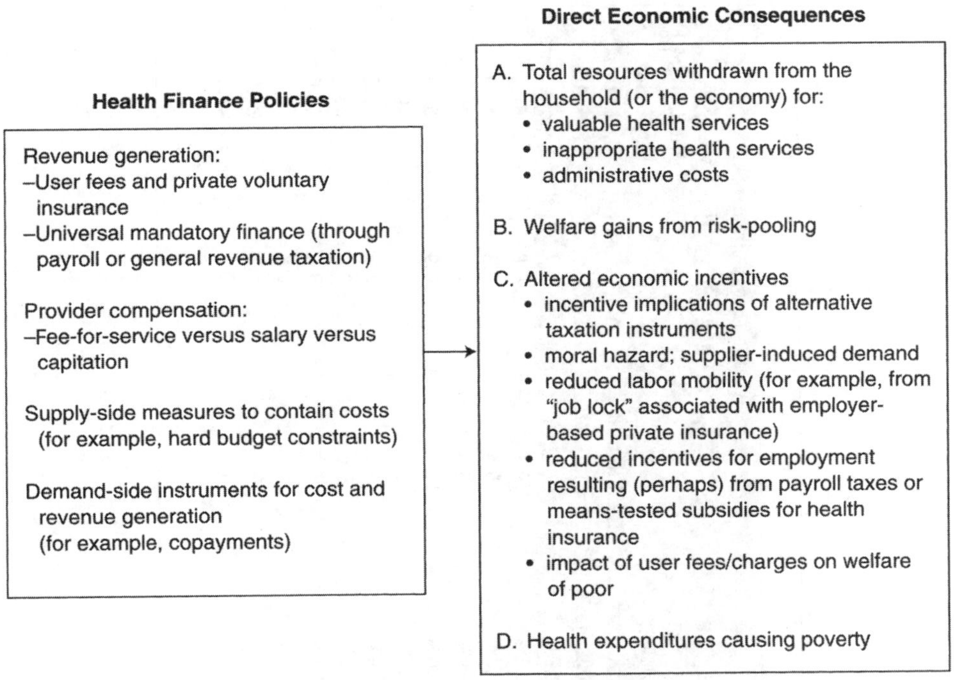

Direct Economic Consequences

Health Finance Policies

Revenue generation:
−User fees and private voluntary insurance
−Universal mandatory finance (through payroll or general revenue taxation)

Provider compensation:
−Fee-for-service versus salary versus capitation

Supply-side measures to contain costs (for example, hard budget constraints)

Demand-side instruments for cost and revenue generation (for example, copayments)

A. Total resources withdrawn from the household (or the economy) for:
  • valuable health services
  • inappropriate health services
  • administrative costs

B. Welfare gains from risk-pooling

C. Altered economic incentives
  • incentive implications of alternative taxation instruments
  • moral hazard; supplier-induced demand
  • reduced labor mobility (for example, from "job lock" associated with employer-based private insurance)
  • reduced incentives for employment resulting (perhaps) from payroll taxes or means-tested subsidies for health insurance
  • impact of user fees/charges on welfare of poor

D. Health expenditures causing poverty

Figure 15-5 Economic Consequences of Health Finance Policies.

product in 2007 (World Bank, 2010), and healthcare funding has significant potential to affect economic development and growth. This influence can operate at both a macroeconomic and a microeconomic level.

As Figure 15-5 illustrates, health finance policies can have direct economic consequences in one of four ways:

- The total resources withdrawn by healthcare systems from the economy (e.g., in terms of health expenditure in relation to GDP)
- The extent to which these systems provide welfare gains that can be achieved from risk pooling
- The incentives that health finance policies can create in terms of the labor market and consumer and provider behavior
- The extent to which health expenditures generate or perpetuate poverty

As introduced in Chapter 12 and as shown in Figure 15-5, financing policies can take a number of different forms (e.g., user fees, private voluntary insurance, universal mandatory finance, public health and social insurance, and supply- and demand-side measures

for cost control and revenue generation), depending on the type of healthcare system. This section reviews the relationship between healthcare systems and the economy and discusses particular issues within this arena that need to be addressed. Hsiao (2000) addresses many of the same issues from a rather different perspective.

Total Resources Withdrawn from the Economy

Countries tend to devote more resources and increasing shares of their national income to health care as their income increases. Lower-income countries, on average, spend less than wealthier countries on health on a per capita basis, in terms of percentage of GDP and in terms of public spending on health. This leads to a lower level and a less equitable distribution of health care and public health services—and ultimately of health—in these societies. However, although health care affects health, it is not the only determinant of health. As Table 15-3 illustrates, in 2007, low-income countries spent an average of $27 per capita on health as compared with $164 for middle-income countries and $4,405 for high-income countries. South Asia ($36), East Asia and the Pacific ($96),

Table 15-3   Health Expenditures by Income Group and Region, 2007

Region or Income Group	Total Population (millions, 2007)	GNI Per Capita (2007 US$)	Health Expenditures			Average Across Countries Spent on Health	
			Total Health Expenditure Per Capita (2007 US$)	Total Health Expenditure as a Percentage of GNI	Total Health Expenditure (% of GDP)	Public-Health Expenditure (% of GDP)	Public-Health Expenditure (% of total) Health Expenditure
World	6,620	8,046	809	10.1%	9.7	5.8	59.6
Low income	956	461	27	5.8%	5.4	2.3	41.9
Middle income	4,602	2,765	164	5.9%	5.4	2.7	50.2
High income	1,061	37,833	4,406	11.6%	11.2	6.9	61.3
Low & middle income	5,559	2,371	141	5.9%	5.4	2.7	49.9
East Asia & Pacific	1,916	2,190	96	4.4%	4.1	1.9	46.2
Europe & Central Asia	442	6,013	396	6.6%	5.6	3.7	65.7
Latin America & the Caribbean	560	5,888	475	8.1%	7.1	3.4	48.6
Middle East & North Africa	319	2,795	151	5.4%	5.5	2.8	50.8
South Asia	1,523	879	36	4.1%	4	1.1	27.5
Sub-Saharan Africa	799	966	69	7.1%	6.4	2.6	41.1

GNI = gross national income.

and sub-Saharan Africa ($67) spent the least of the low- and middle-income regions, whereas Europe and Central Asia ($396) and Latin America and the Caribbean ($475) spent the most for that group of regions. In the very lowest-income countries, annual health spending can be as low as $2 or $3 per capita, and most of that spending comes from private sources (World Bank, 2010).

In terms of percentage of GDP, as shown in Table 15-3, in 2007, low- and middle-income countries, on average, spent 5.4% of GDP on health, whereas high-income countries spent 11.2% of GDP on health. Among low- and middle-income regions, South Asia (4.0% of GDP) spent the least on health, whereas Latin America and the Caribbean spent the most, at approximately 8.1% of GDP (World Bank, 2010).

Both health spending generally and the public share of health spending increase with increases in national and per capita income. As shown in Table 15-3, the public share of health expenditures (as a percentage of total health spending) was 42% in low-income countries, 50% in middle-income countries, and 61% in high-income countries in 2007. Among low- and middle-income countries, regions such as Europe and Central Asia have the largest public share (66%) of health spending, and South Asia has the smallest (28%) (World Bank, 2010).

According to Schieber and Maeda (1997), the income elasticity of demand for health services—defined as the percentage change in health expenditures

as a result of a 1% change in income—in 1994 was roughly 1.13 worldwide, and in a range of 1.47 for high-income countries, 1.19 for middle-income countries, and 1.00 for low-income countries. Thus, for every 1% increase in per capita income, public health expenditures will increase by 1.47% in middle- and high-income countries, by 1.19% in middle-income countries, and by 1.00% in lower-income countries. As these data indicate, the increase in health expenditures in low-income countries is less responsive to increases in income than it is in middle- and high-income countries. Figures 15-6 and 15-7 show the relationships between income and health spending and between income and public health spending, respectively. In addition, Schieber and Maeda (1997) found that private health spending (income elasticity of 1.02) is less responsive to increases in per capita income than public health spending (income elasticity of 1.21).

A recent study by Lu and colleagues (2010) analyzed government spending on health in low- and middle-income countries. These researchers found that development assistance for health (DAH) to low-income governments had negatively affected domestic government spending on health, but that DAH to nongovernmental sectors positively affected domestic government health spending. Some of the implications of lower levels of spending in lower-income countries include lower levels of capital stock, such as clinics, hospitals, and inpatient beds; lower levels of human resources, such as physicians and providers;

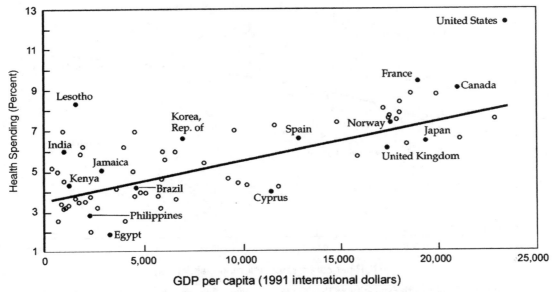

Figure 15-6 Percentage of GDP Spent on Health. *Source:* International Bank for Reconstruction and Development, World Bank, World Development Report (Washington, DC: World Bank, 1993), p.110. Reprinted with permission.

and lower levels of service use, such as outpatient and inpatient visits. Comprehensive data are very scarce for low-income countries, but the number of hospital beds per 1,000 population appears to be much higher in high-income countries (6.2 in 2006) as compared with middle-income countries (2.2 in 2003) and low-income countries (e.g., 0.8 in the Democratic Republic of Congo and 1.4 in Kenya in 2004) (World Bank, 2010). Among the regions worldwide, Eastern Europe and Central Asia had the greatest number of hospital beds per 1,000 population (7.1 in 2006), and South Asia (0.9 in 2003) had one of the lowest.

This pattern persists when analyzing physicians per 1,000 population: High-income countries (2.6 in 2002) fared better than middle-income countries (1.3 in 2005) and low-income countries (e.g., 0.1 in the Democratic Republic of the Congo, 0.3 in Madagascar, and 0.1 in Kenya in 2004) on this indicator of health system infrastructure. Comparing different regions of the world, the number of physicians per 1,000 population was highest in Eastern Europe and Central Asia (3.1 in 2006), whereas South Asia (0.5 in 2005) had one of the lowest ratios.

Many economists view the evidence regarding the income elasticity of expenditures on health as indicative of the nature of health as a normal consumption good. In the last decade, there has been an upsurge of interest in the nature of health care as an investment good. Expenditures on health care can lead to improvements in health status that, in turn, promote income growth, and the efficiency and equity of health systems are important in both improving health and affecting income, productivity, and the overall economy. Lower-income countries, in particular, tend to under-invest in health, leaving their populations vulnerable to disease and disability and ultimately affecting the countries' labor productivity and growth. They also have health systems that are often highly inefficient at both macroeconomic and microeconomic levels, and are highly inegalitarian in both financing and delivery.

Health System Efficiency and Equity
Macroeconomic Efficiency

Health system efficiency at the macroeconomic level describes the relationship between aggregate healthcare expenditures and health outcomes. There is considerable variation in both health expenditures and health outcomes by country. For example, in 2008, life expectancy at birth ranged from 44 years in Afghanistan and Zimbabwe, 45 years in Lesotho and Zambia, and 46 years in Swaziland to 82 years in France, Hong Kong, Iceland, Italy and Switzerland, and 83 years in Japan and Liechtenstein (World Bank, 2010). Under-five mortality rates per 1,000 live births in 2008 ranged from 257 deaths in Afghanistan and 220 deaths in Angola to 2 deaths in San Marino and Liechtenstain and 3 deaths in Luxembourg, Singapore, Iceland,

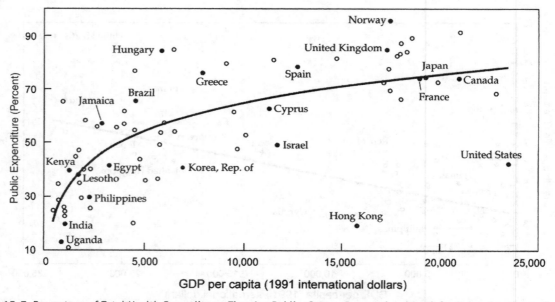

Figure 15-7 Percentage of Total Health Expenditures That Are Public. *Source:* International Bank for Reconstruction and Development, World Bank, World Development Report (Washington, DC: World Bank, 1993), p.110. Reprinted with permission.

Sweden, and Finland (World Bank, 2010). Many factors influence health outcomes, but some countries certainly appear to be more efficient in the use of healthcare resources than others.

Expenditures on health systems, however, often correlate poorly with outcomes. For example, in 2007 India spent 4.1% of its GDP (26% in the form of public spending) to achieve a 2007 IMR of 54 per 1,000 and an average life expectancy at birth in 2007 of 63 years. By comparison, in the same year China spent 4.3% of its GDP (45% in the form of public spending) to achieve a 2007 IMR of 19 per 1,000 and an average life expectancy at birth in 2007 of 73 years (World Bank, 2010). In the same year, Mauritius spent 4.2% of its GDP (49% in the form of public spending) to achieve a 2007 IMR of 15 per 1,000 and an average life expectancy at birth in 2007 of 73 years. Among higher-income countries, the patterns are similar. For example, in 2007 the United States spent 16% of its GDP (46% in the form of public expenditures) to achieve a 2007 IMR of 7 per 1,000 and an average life expectancy in 2007 of 78 years. The United Kingdom spent 8.4% of its GDP (82% in the form of public expenditure) and Japan spent 8.0% of its GDP (81% in the form of public expenditure) to achieve 2007 IMRs of 5 per 1,000 and 3 per 1,000, respectively, and average life expectancy at birth in 2007 of 80 and 83 years, respectively. Finally, in the same time period, France spent 11.0% of its GDP (79% in the form of public expenditure) and Germany spent 10.4% of its GDP (77% in the form of public expenditure) to achieve 2007 IMRs of 3 and 4 per 1,000, respectively, and an average life expectancy at birth of 81 and 80 years, respectively (World Bank, 2010).

Wang and colleagues (1999) present systematic data on 115 countries for the period 1960 to 1991 on country performance relative to income (or income and education) on several health indicators. These performance measures are intended to catalyze discussion of the role of health system characteristics as partial explanations. Wang and colleagues' evidence suggests that health systems vary in the efficiency with which they produce health. Of course, healthcare services are merely one of multiple determinants of health. Some countries obtain better health for less money; others obtain good health by spending more; and some seem to be in a situation of diminishing marginal returns to increases in healthcare expenditures.

In lower-income countries, it is often the case that very little health is obtained for the money spent. When total health spending is as low as it is in some lower-income countries (e.g., 2% to 3% of GDP), the resources allocated are insufficient to cover even the minimum necessary care. Thus even the most basic package of preventive and clinical services is not available to the whole population. Inadequate allocations of public and private resources to health can lead to continued poverty and stifled development. These countries require increases in money spent (especially equally distributed public resources) on the most basic and cost-effective services. At the other end of the spectrum, countries such as the United States, France, Germany, and Switzerland, which spend more than 9% of GDP on health, have a tripartite health policy focus of increasing access and improving quality with a central emphasis on controlling and decreasing healthcare costs.

Although scant evidence of the economic impact of greater spending on health has been published, some economists suggest that higher health expenditures might reduce a country's relative productivity in the global economy due to the large costs of health benefits for the labor force, and due to resultant reduced investments in other sectors of the economy. The labor market effects of certain health policies are addressed later in this section, but it is not clear that overall productivity and growth are severely hindered by very high health expenditures. It is not possible to determine the most efficient level or percentage of health spending for any given economy. Given the wide range of spending on health care, the challenge is to increase spending among lower-income countries and to analyze spending in both higher- and lower-income countries. The aim is to develop methods to enhance the efficient production of health within health systems.

Microeconomic Efficiency

Microeconomic efficiency focuses on getting the best return on existing resources and reducing the waste and inefficiency that some systems generate. Allocative inefficiency occurs when resources are allocated not to activities that are highly cost-effective, but rather to those that are costly and offer a low return in terms of effectiveness. Efficiency entails allocating resources to the most cost-effective way of achieving given health objectives (e.g., investing in cost-effective preventive measures, such as immunizations for certain diseases or behavioral modification, rather than spending extensively at later stages of the health cycle through high-cost tertiary services). A health system is allocatively inefficient when greater gains could be achieved with a different pattern of resource use. The 1993 *World Development Report* (World Bank, 1993) concluded that improvements in allocative efficiency of health systems in lower-income countries could be achieved through the introduction of basic cost-effective intervention packages for the most common conditions in a given country.

Technical inefficiencies occur when the pattern and level of resources (human, financial, and physical) do not adequately meet the level of health (or access) outcomes possible with that degree of resource commitment. In lower-income countries, scarcity of providers and basic clinic and hospital resources, in addition to poor quality and accessibility of facilities (ill-equipped and run-down infrastructure) and providers (poorly trained and unqualified), contribute to a failure to meet the health needs of populations.

In higher-income countries, the focus has been on assessing and improving the efficiency of particular aspects of health systems, including cost and use-control measures on the supply and demand sides of the healthcare market, medical care appropriateness, and healthcare administration. These topics are ad-

dressed in Exhibits 15-4 and 15-5. In addition, some health systems in higher-income countries have begun explicitly to prioritize or ration health services in an effort to improve the allocative efficiency and public acceptability of their health systems.

Equity

Equity in health policy should focus on the financing, delivery, and allocation of healthcare services (Ruger, 1998, 2003b, 2004a). Two important dimensions of equity include vertical and horizontal equity.

In terms of financing, vertical equity refers to the requirement that health care be financed by ability to pay—that is, contributions to the cost of health care must be determined by income status. Some mechanisms for raising revenues for healthcare expenditures are more progressive than others (Van Doorslaer, Wagstaff, & Rutten, 1993). Horizontal financial equity means that individuals with the same ability to pay

Exhibit 15-4	Costs of Healthcare Administration?

One aspect of health system inefficiency is the perception of some administrative expenditures as wasteful. Comparisons of different health systems suggest that administrative costs can be an important factor in the level and rate of change in healthcare spending.

Single-payer plans are claimed to be advantageous because they tend to centralize and, therefore, reduce the costs of healthcare administration—a significant issue around the world. International comparisons of international health systems show that administrative costs as a percentage of total costs vary by country and financing mechanism. These large differences suggest, at first glance, wasteful and inefficient use of resources in some countries. Several national (United States) and cross-national (OECD countries) studies have attempted to estimate such costs (Bovbjerg, 1995; Gauthier, Rogal, Barrand, & Cohen, 1992; Poullier, 1992; U.S. Congress, 1994; Woolhandler & Himmelstein, 1991, 1997; Woolhandler, Himmelstein, & Lewontin, 1993). One study found that in 1987, U.S. healthcare administration cost between $96.8 billion and $120.4 billion ($400 to $497 per capita), equivalent to 19.3% to 24.1% of total healthcare spending (Woolhandler & Himmelstein, 1991). The same study found that administrative costs in the United States were 60% higher than in Canada and 97% higher than in the United Kingdom.

Another study, employing OECD data from 1991 and 1992, compared costs of healthcare administration across 20 high-income countries. With respect to administrative costs, the United States had the highest (and Germany the second highest) per capita spending for health administration. The authors concluded that administrative costs were higher in insurance-based systems than in direct-delivery systems. Insurance-based systems are more complex and involve multiple, decentralized payers, all of which contribute to higher administrative costs (Poullier, 1992).

Illustrating the unusual character of the health sector among sectors of the economy, the available research suggests that single-payer systems (in which a single authority processes claims and pays providers directly for services) have lower administrative costs compared to multiple-payer systems. Single-payer systems accrue benefits by standardizing, consolidating, and integrating functions. Such systems are well situated to take advantage of efficiency gains from standardization and of technological advances in information systems, especially electronic claims transmission and magnetic card technology. Even without a single-payer system, standardization and reform could reduce costs for multiple payers. For instance, introducing a common electronic administrative system (common formats and standards) that connects multiple systems of insurance and medical information through the use of "smart cards" could improve health system performance. These technologies could bring a number of health administrative functions under common guidelines, thereby improving communication, claims processing, and use review.

continued

Exhibit 15-4   continued

Ultimately, the costs and benefits of health administrative reforms must be assessed to determine any health system's cost-effectiveness. Although certain administrative costs might be reduced without the loss of benefits to individuals or to society, others might not. The extent to which the results of administrative reforms are categorized as benefits or costs will also depend on the value that is placed on any given economic or health-related outcome. Such values might vary from one community to another. In general, administrative activities that clearly deliver benefits to patients and the health system should be prioritized, and in some cases beneficial administrative activities can be provided more efficiently. For example, benefit management costs—including data collection, clinical evaluation, and statistical analysis—confer consumer benefits by improving healthcare quality, enhancing patients' decision-making autonomy, and reducing inappropriate care. These activities will become an increasingly valuable tool as additional information on effective and cost-effective health service delivery becomes available.

Exhibit 15-5   **Medical Care Appropriateness and Resource Allocation**

While achieving a broad spread of risk, health insurance can, in principle, lead to incentives for too much medical care. When people are insured, they do not individually bear the costs of the medical services they consume, so some individuals may perceive that they have an incentive to overconsume healthcare resources. (Countering these financial incentives are other costs of seeking care, such as time, pain, and inconvenience.) This central problem of any insurance plan, which is called the moral hazard problem, has spawned a number of efforts to ensure medical care appropriateness and efficient resource allocation within insurance plans, both public and private. The private insurance markets have developed a number of techniques for assessing and enforcing medical care appropriateness.

The first approach is economic. Health economists endeavor to reduce overuse of health care through the use of various economic incentives on both the supply and demand sides of the healthcare market. On the demand side, copayment plans and health insurance deductibles, which require patients to pay a portion of the price of a given medical procedure, reduce use rates. On the supply side of the healthcare market, price, budgetary, and salary incentives, such as prospective and capitated payment plans and global budgets, deter physicians and hospitals from providing excess care. These incentives force physicians and hospitals to internalize costs in the process of health service delivery and, therefore, encourage them to provide the most cost-effective services. The rise of healthcare financing and delivery institutions, such as managed care organizations, is a result of these efforts.

Studies have shown that these economic devices are effective in reducing healthcare use. For instance, in a randomized controlled health insurance experiment, researchers found that increasing patient copayments as part of health insurance reduced demand for healthcare services, in some cases by as much as 40% (RAND Health Insurance Experiment; see Newhouse, 1993). In practice, however, copayments are eliminated for expensive procedures, thereby attenuating the usefulness of copayments in cost containment.

In addition, cross-cultural comparisons of national health systems provide evidence for the effectiveness of capitation and global budgeting in reducing health care use (e.g., Aaron & Schwartz, 1984). However, because these economic approaches are devoid of clinical input, they act as blunt instruments in achieving their objective: In most cases, they reduce medically appropriate as well as inappropriate care. Without the ability to discriminate between productive and unproductive care, these tools can have deleterious health consequences and can be highly inegalitarian.

Distinguishing between types of care requires clinical input to create a system of assessing and ranking which treatments are medically appropriate for a given health condition. At least one existing model attempts to do just that: the RAND/UCLA appropriateness method. This method encompasses multiple stages of collecting and interpreting data about specific procedures from literature and clinicians, with the goal of developing guidelines for appropriate care. Since 1986, more than 30 studies using this method have been conducted to examine the appropriateness of procedures (see accompanying table). The resulting literature suggests that the percentage of inappropriate use across procedures ranges from 2.4% to 75%, whereas the percentage of appropriate care ranges from 35% to 91%, and the percentage of equivocal use ranges from 7% to 32%.*

continued

Exhibit 15-5	continued

Ultimately, attempts to achieve the optimal level of health status from any given amount of resources will require a joint economic and clinical solution. Social scientists and clinicians should continue to study the magnitude and determinants of inappropriate care and to harness technological advances to create effective information systems and accessible guidelines for medical care. Economic incentives should follow and complement clinical progress, albeit not to the exclusion of professional incentives. As the evidence on the magnitude and determinants of inappropriate care accumulates and becomes more widely understood, economists and health policy analysts should be able to create policy instruments that give an incentive for physicians, patients, and planners to provide productive care. Particular attention should be paid to encouraging and training physicians by rewarding the provision of appropriate care and correcting for the provision of inappropriate care.

*See also Bernstein et al. (1993); Brook (1992, 1994, 1995, 1997); Brook, Kamberg, Mayer-Oakes, Beers, Raube, & Steiner (1990); Brook & Lohr (1985, 1986, 1987); Brook, Park, Chassin, Solomon, Keesey, & Kosecoff (1990); Carlisle et al. (1992); Chassin, Kosecoff, Solomon, & Brook (1987); Hilborne et al. (1993); Kleinman, Kosecoff, Dubois, & Brook (1994); Leape, Hilborne, et al., (1993); Leape, Park, Solomon, Chassin, Kosecoff, & Brook (1990); Winslow, Kosecoff, Chassin, Kanouse, & Brook (1988); and Winslow, Solomon, Chassin, Kosecoff, Merrick, & Brook (1988).

Medical Appropriateness and Healthcare Use		
Author(s)	**Sample/Procedure**	**Magnitude of Appropriateness**
Winslow, Solomon, Chassin, Kosecoff, Merrick, & Brook (1988)	Random sample of 1,302 Medicare patients in three geographic areas who had a carotid endarterectomy in 1981.	Estimated the appropriateness of carotid endarterectomy. Found 35% appropriate, 32% equivocal, and 32% inappropriate. Concluded that carotid endarterectomy was substantially overused in three geographic areas studied.
Bernstein et al. (1993)	Retrospective cohort study. Random sample of all non-emergency, non-oncological hysterectomies performed in seven managed care organizations, over a 1-year period.	Roughly 16% inappropriate, and only one plan had significantly more hysterectomies rated inappropriate compared with the group mean (27%, unadjusted). Age and race adjustments did not affect percentage appropriate.
Leape, Hilborne, et al. (1993)	Random sample of 1,338 patients from 15 different hospitals undergoing isolated coronary artery bypass graft surgery in New York state in 1990.	Nearly 91% appropriate, 7% equivocal, and 2.4% inappropriate. Low inappropriateness rate differs significantly from the 14% rate found in 1979, 1980, and 1982 studies. Rates did not vary by hospital, hospital location, volume, or teaching status.
Winslow, Kosecoff, Chassin, Kanouse, & Brook (1988)	Appropriateness of coronary artery bypass surgeries performed in three randomly selected hospitals in a western state. Data obtained from medical records with 488 indications; 386 cases from years 1979, 1980, and 1982.	Found 56% appropriate, 30% equivocal, and 14% inappropriate. The percentage of appropriate procedures varied by hospital, from 37% to 78%, but did not vary by patient age.
Kleinman, Kosecoff, Dubois, & Brook (1994)	Appropriateness of tympanostomy tube surgery for recurrent acute otitis media and/or otitis media with effusion. Random selection of subsample (6,611) of cases deemed appropriate by use review firm methodology. Represented otolaryngologists, in practices from 49 states and the District of Columbia.	Found 41% of proposals appropriate, 32% equivocal, and 27% inappropriate. Concluded that roughly 25% of tympanostomy tube insertion procedures for children were proposed for inappropriate indications and 30% for equivocal ones.

Note: All studies cited employed the RAND/UCLA appropriateness method.

should contribute the same amount to financing health expenditures regardless of medical need, gender, marital status, geography, age, or employment status.

In terms of delivery, vertical equity refers to the requirement that individuals with different needs should receive different amounts and levels of health services. Horizontal equity means that individuals with equal needs should receive equal medical treatment (Van Doorslaer et al., 1993).

One aspect of health equity involves a concern for the status—both health and financial—of the most disadvantaged segments of society (Anand, Diderichsen, Evans, Shkolnikov, & Wirth, 2001; Ruger, 1998, 2006a). Improving equity and improving the conditions of the very poor or worse-off may often go together, but sometimes they do not, in which case tradeoffs are required (Anand et al., 2001; Ruger, 1998, 2004a) as well as a comprehensive analysis of health equity (Ruger, 2006b).

In the 1990s, many OECD countries initiated reforms designed to improve the efficiency and responsiveness of their health systems. Hurst (2000) provides an overview of the achievements of these systems, and of their reforms, while pointing to an essential tension that increasingly confronts public policy in these countries. This tension results from upward pressures on costs (for technological and demographic reasons), core commitments to universal public (or publicly mandated) funding for reasons of efficiency as well as equity, and general reluctance to raise taxes. Feachem (2000) suggests that in the United Kingdom, both radical reform of delivery institutions and increased resources will be required; Enthoven (2000) reviews the history and lessons from the (incomplete) reforms of the U.K. National Health Services in the past decade.

Preker, Harding, and Travis (2000) analyze these experiences from the perspective of "new institutional economics" to reach a number of important conclusions about the evolving roles of the public and private sectors in the health sector. To quote their main findings concerning the public-sector role, "Consequently, in parallel with moving out of the area of production of goods and services, in many low-income and middle-income countries it may be desirable to have . . . greater public sector involvement in health care financing, knowledge generation, and the provision of human resources" (p. 788).

Welfare Gains from Risk Pooling

Insurance involves collective risk reduction, reduced financial risks, and increased human welfare. Insurance reduces risks in the aggregate by pooling a large number of people with similar, small, individual risks. This practice enables insurers to increase aggregate predictability even when given health episodes remain unpredictable. Insurers are able to predict the probability of financial loss occurrence with greater precision when the risk pool is large.

While collective risk reduction in the form of risk pooling through insurance can lead to economic and welfare benefits, many health systems in low- and middle-income countries fail to take advantage of it (Ruger, 2003b). Analyzing health insurance from an even broader conceptual framework, one might argue that universal health insurance is necessary to achieve human flourishing and that, by protecting people from both ill health and its economic consequences, universal health insurance coverage's central ethical aim is keeping people healthy and enhancing their security (Ruger, 2007).

Risk Pooling Mechanisms

Several aspects of health insurance are rooted in the risk-averse nature of human beings. Without insurance, if a person suffers a medical catastrophe, he or she may not have the financial resources to pay the large sums required for treatment. Instead, a person would prefer, and could better afford, to pay a relatively small amount of money on a regular basis to avoid a large financial loss at one time. This provides for "smoothing" or "evening out" financial payments for adverse health events as well as for pooling of risks. Public finance of specific health interventions has quantifiable economic benefits (Jamison, 2009) for risk reduction that can be considered alongside those interventions' impact on health outcomes.

By pooling a large number of people and, therefore, a large number of adverse health events, insurance companies are better able to predict the occurrence of these events and to spread the financial risk. Pooling risks across people is more efficient than pooling risks within individuals but across time. For example, if the risk of an adverse health event that costs $2,000 is 1 in 1,000, and 1,000 people paid $2 each into an insurance pool, then the cost of the health event would be covered should it occur. In this case, each individual would have paid $2, rather than being exposed to the risk of paying $2,000.

Pooling risks within individuals across time (i.e., a medical savings account) can generate potential inefficiency, even though some effectively implemented examples exist (e.g., Singapore). Continuing the preceding example, if an individual saved $2 per year to cover a potential cost of $2,000, it would take that person 1,000 years to cover the cost; saving $20 per year would require 100 years; and saving $50 per year would take 40 years. Pooling across individuals is more efficient than pooling within individuals over time, because the same protection against the potential financial loss of $2,000 is achieved through a yearly payment of $2 versus a payment of $2 per year for 1,000 years or perhaps saving $50 per year for 40 years.

Because people are risk averse, risk pooling provides welfare benefits in protecting people from large financial losses that result from catastrophic health events.

Insurance Versus Direct Purchase

Given its benefits, insurance is a preferred mechanism for financing personal health care services for high-cost, low-probability health events.[10] However, it may not necessarily be the preferred method of payment for low-cost, high-probability health events, because individuals have the ability to plan and save for such occurrences, depending on the relative expense of the event. If the service is relatively inexpensive and highly probable, risk pooling may be less beneficial, especially given that administrative costs and expected profits associated with insurance can be high. Attempting to divide services between those who are covered and those who are not covered entails its own set of problems: Should individuals with different incomes have different cutoffs? Is the incentive for early (usually less costly) care reduced? Will individuals attempt to move to venues (usually hospitals) where care is free but may be less efficiently provided? For all these reasons, most national health services cover routine care, and appear to do so at modest administrative costs.

The financial burden of a direct-purchase system falls disproportionately on the poor, who are more price sensitive than the rich, and who typically have more health problems and higher health costs. As a result, the poor underutilize services (many of which are medically necessary) in such a system. WHO's *World Health Reports* for 1999 and 2000 provide valuable discussions of these issues (WHO, 1999, 2000).

Degrees of Risk Sharing

Figure 15-8 (drawn from *World Health Report 1999*) demonstrates the different ways financing and provider mechanisms distribute risks among patients, providers, and third-party insurers. Government finance works as a form of insurance in this context, by shifting risk away from the individual. When patients carry the full financial risk of healthcare costs, they pay for all services on an out-of-pocket basis. This makes patients susceptible to significant financial loss when expensive adverse health events occur. The majority of health financing plans in low- and middle-income countries use this type of arrangement, which tends to be the least equitable, efficient, and organized form of payment.

While private for-profit insurers pool risks to a certain extent, their main strategy is risk segmentation—insuring only the lowest-risk individuals—to maximize profits. This practice—known as cream skimming or cherry picking—is not an efficient or equitable way to spread risk from the perspective of society as a whole. In addition, the existence of private insurance can create a two-tiered system (one in which different groups obtain different sets of benefits) and can exacerbate inequities of access without efforts to enhance the quality and equity of services (typically public) for those in lower-income groups. It is also possible to have a system in which providers, such as hospitals, clinics, or practitioners, assume the financial risks of healthcare costs—a practice that is becoming increasingly common in the United States.

Informal Community Financing and Risk Pooling

Informal community financing can be a useful solution to the risk pooling and health insurance constraints seen in low- and middle-income countries where neither government risk sharing (which often redistributes wealth through subsidies) nor private or social health insurance exists on a large scale. Such plans are typically rural, informal, and nongovernmental in nature, and involve either voluntary or compulsory risk pooling through a community fund to which individuals contribute prepayment of premiums that entitle them to postservice payments of

---

[10] Public insurance pools health risks through public financing from general taxes or other public revenue sources that are collected through a government mandate (e.g., through a social security program, earmarked taxes, or an employer mandate). Social insurance is also a form of compulsory universal health insurance coverage that is typically implemented under the auspices of a social security–type program and is usually financed by employer and employee contributions to government or nonprofit insurance funds. Social insurance funds usually pool risks through social insurance financed from mandatory earmarked payroll taxes set aside specifically for social programs. Public and social health insurance provision can help alleviate many of the insurance market failures that occur with private insurance markets, and the dominant provision of public insurance obviates the need for health insurance regulation.

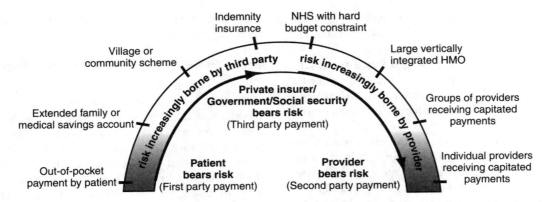

Figure 15-8 Risk-Sharing Arrangements: The Impact of Different Financing Schemes and Provider Payment *Source:* World Health Organization, *World Health Report 1999: Making a Difference* (Geneva, Switzerland: World Health Organization, 1999), p. 39. Reprinted with permission.

certain health services defined by the community. As Figure 15-8 suggests, these plans can shift risk substantially toward the collective. Some plans obtain contributions from employers and governments. Often, the community fund also manages the organization and provision of care (including immunizations and pharmaceuticals), creating a structure similar to an integrated health maintenance organization.

In their analysis of 82 health insurance plans for people outside formal-sector employment, Bennett, Creese, and Monasch (1998) found that, with the exception of China's rural medical plan, few plans covered very large populations or even high proportions of the eligible population, and many plans faced significant problems of adverse selection. In addition, nearly all of the plans depended on external subsidies. Very few plans served the poorest households, but instead were targeted toward the rural middle class. In terms of delivery, plan managers failed to focus sufficiently on efficiently delivering high-quality health care.

The administrative structure and practice of plans also varied widely, with some focusing on insuring against primary care risks and others against tertiary or hospital care risks. Administrative costs for plans ranged from 5% to 17% of total costs, which is low compared with pluralistic systems with multiple insurers (e.g., the U.S. system, which has administrative costs in the range of 19% to 24%) and compared with Western national health insurance systems (e.g., the Canadian system, which has administrative costs in the range of 8% to 11%). Many of the plans that were primarily based on tertiary care (e.g., in Nkoranza in Ghana, Masisi in the Democratic Republic of the Congo, Korea, and Taiwan) had problems with over-

use of services and cost escalation, whereas plans that were primary care oriented employed primary care physicians as gatekeepers to control use and costs. Plan managers were found to be highly inefficient in financial planning.

In terms of equity, Bennett, Creese, and Monasch (1998) found that although nearly all of the insurance plans they studied had community-rated insurance premiums (whereby everyone pays the same amount), the premiums were flat rated and, therefore, regressive in nature. Other taxation or payment measures that associate tax rates with income level (e.g., direct taxes and higher tax rates for higher incomes on a gradient basis) are more progressive than such plans. With the exception of a few plans, no exemptions or subsidies were provided for those individuals who had difficulty affording membership in the plan—premiums amounted to 5% to 10% of an annual household budget in some plans, such as that in Nkoranza district, Ghana. Because the low-income population often could not afford to begin or maintain payments in a plan, they were forced to pay user fees for health services.

The same authors also assessed use patterns of different plans and concluded that households located closer to a health facility were more likely to enroll in insurance plans and had higher use rates than those living farther away. Thus geography played an important role in use patterns. This geographic effect could create adverse selection problems, whereby those living farther from a health facility drop out of the plan, increasing premiums for the remaining members and leading to further withdrawals. In addition, the authors noted a number of structural features that contributed to poor financial sustainability: small scale, adverse selection leading to smaller risk pools and higher costs, significant administrative structures, and costs.

Although risk pooling and insurance are generally preferred to direct purchase of health care due to their efficiency and welfare gains, they also have significant incentive-altering effects that reduce efficiency and equity in other areas of the health system. For this reason, public and private policy is increasingly shifting risk from government (or third-party private insurers) to providers, by moving clockwise around the circle depicted in Figure 15-8. In addition, the mechanisms through which funds are obtained to finance health insurance affect patients' behavior. Exhibit 15-6 explains two types of health insurance market failures that result from the altered incentives of health insurance, and the next section addresses many of the incentive effects of various health financing policies.

Health Financing Policies and Their Incentives

The evidence presented earlier in this chapter suggests that lower-income countries underinvest in health, and their use of already low health investments is often inefficient and inequitable. These factors contribute to lower economic growth and lead to poor health and economic outcomes. To improve these outcomes, lower-income countries face the challenge of raising political support and revenues to sustain greater public investments in health and to improve efficiency in use of both public and private resources (McIntyre, Thiede, Dahlgren, & Whitehead, 2006). In addition, many health systems in lower-income countries fail to take advantage of the eco-

---

Exhibit 15-6   Insurance Market Failures: Adverse Selection and Moral Hazard

Insurance market failures, credit shortages, and information asymmetries and insufficiencies can inhibit individuals from realizing the economic benefits of collective risk reduction through risk pooling and efficient insurance systems. Thus a rationale exists for public financing of healthcare services or for strong regulation of private health insurance markets. Two commonly noted forms of health insurance market failure are adverse selection and moral hazard.

Adverse Selection

Adverse selection occurs when individuals who are sicker than average self-select into plans that offer better benefits than other plans. This selection increases premiums, making it more likely that average or healthier than average individuals will opt out of these plans. If healthier individuals opt out, then spreading risk across the population is no longer possible, because only the sickest persons are left in the plan. The result is a spiraling effect in which premiums increase and risk pooling disintegrates. In just 3 years in the late 1990s, for example, the indemnity insurance option in the UCLA staff health plan rose from $200 per month to more than $1,000 per month, as all but those at highest risk opted for managed care (available at a premium of less than $50 per month).

Insurance companies attempt to combat adverse selection by screening high-risk individuals through mechanisms such as excluding preexisting conditions from coverage, refusing coverage, requiring medical exams, and having waiting periods. These costly insurance company strategies further add to the instabilities in health insurance markets. Regulating insurers, offering insurance through groups (e.g., employers), and requiring mandatory public insurance can help alleviate these problems in the private health insurance market.

Moral Hazard

Moral hazard occurs when people are insured and, therefore, do not have to pay the full costs of health care. As a consequence, they have a reduced incentive to avoid certain healthcare costs, which results in behavior that may actually increase the probability that an event that has been insured against occurs. This feature can be present in either public or private insurance systems. To mitigate moral hazard, insurers incorporate cost sharing, benefit limitation, frequent renewability, and management features into the health insurance system.

Equity

Ill health and financial ruin resulting from catastrophic illness may lead to poverty and income inequality, thereby bolstering efficiency arguments for government financing of healthcare services for the low-income population and other vulnerable groups. Equitably financed health systems raise revenues based on people's ability to pay, and equitable delivery systems allocate resources based on people's medical care needs (Ruger, 1998, 2004a). Although often goals can be achieved only at some cost in efficiency, this tradeoff is far less acute in health finance precisely because of the insurance market failures just discussed. Private health insurance markets will not ensure equitable revenue generation for healthcare financing, the equitable distribution of health insurance, or the equitable allocation of health resources. Regulation and public financing are required to achieve equitable as well as efficient outcomes in health finance and delivery.

nomic and welfare benefits that accrue from collective risk reduction in the form of risk pooling, and from analytical efforts to set priorities through improvements in allocative and technical efficiencies. Constraints that are particular to lower-income countries include low personal income, a large informal or subsistence sector that is exempt from income taxation, and low administrative and tax collection capacity—all of which result in low levels of insurance and risk pooling; health-related capital stock, such as facilities, equipment, beds, and pharmaceutical products; and human resources, such as physicians and nurses. In general, lower-income countries are characterized by greater inequality in income distribution compared to higher-income economies because they employ less targeted approaches and have lower levels of public expenditure.

Increasing lower-income countries' overall and public investments in health—and ensuring equitable and efficient use of those resources—is essential to improving health and economic growth and to reducing poverty. However, revenue generation policies have their own economic and equity implications that must be analyzed to ensure that efforts to finance health investments do more good than harm. This section assesses the economic and equity consequences of various financing mechanisms—namely, taxation; insurance funding, especially as it affects employment; and user fees or user charges and their effect on the welfare of the low-income population. Certain choices among financing and provider compensation options can create conditions for excessive spending on health, which appears to be an emerging problem in middle-income countries.

Taxation

In terms of economic efficiency and revenue generation, most forms of taxation (with the exception of lump-sum or poll taxes) distort the consumption and production decisions made by individuals, households, and firms, resulting in a cost (a deadweight loss) that must be considered when devising health financing plans involving public taxation. Lump-sum and poll taxes, which avoid these burdens, are less desirable on equity grounds and are typically infeasible politically (Schieber & Maeda, 1997).

Although taxation can be inefficient due to the deadweight loss created by distorting production and consumption decisions, it can also be effective in generating revenue. In addition, it serves as a primary mechanism for some types of investment in the economy. Moreover, it can be a means for enhancing equity through subsidies and transfers if progressive

taxation is employed. A difficulty with general tax revenues in all countries, and especially in lower-income nations, is that budget allocations by sector depend on the political support that a given sector generates. In such intersectoral budgetary decisions, health care often loses out to other, more popular sectors. This situation is especially likely to occur when budget projections are overestimated, leaving a shortfall to be made up through budget cuts, as is the case in many lower-income countries. Finally, taxation capacity can be limited in lower-income countries because of underdeveloped and inefficient administrations.

Medical Care Demand Effects of Expanding Private Insurance

The economic impact of expanding private insurance is believed to consist of increased demand for private insurance, and reduced demand for public insurance, among those with the ability to pay the increased insurance rates (i.e., higher-income groups). Jamaica, for example, has experienced such a transition. Gertler and Sturm (1997) studied the demand for public and private medical care with the expansion of private-sector insurance in Jamaica. Jamaica has a universal public healthcare system in which anyone can use public facilities free of charge, and access to facilities by all groups has been found to be quite good. Jamaica also has a significant private-sector healthcare market in which higher-quality services are offered at higher prices. Gertler and Sturm (1997) found that private insurance coverage was concentrated primarily among the higher-income groups, a factor that then freed up public resources for lower-income individuals (see Table 15-4 for results). This stratification also creates a two-tiered system of health care, in which higher-income groups obtain private care through private insurance companies, and lower-income groups obtain publicly financed, and often publicly provided, care.

The work of Gertler and Sturm is especially relevant in the context of low- and middle-income countries, because health care financed by governments in these settings often subsidizes the wealthier groups in society. For example, in Indonesia the lowest income quintile consumes less than 14% of public-sector healthcare expenditures, while the highest income quintile consumes more than 30% (Van de Walle, 1994).

Gertler and Sturm (1997) found that introducing mandated private insurance induced covered individuals to favor perceived higher-quality services in the private sector over public sector insurance, and that this shift reduced the total public health expenditure on health care. These authors also suggested that

Table 15-4	The Estimated Effect of Health Insurance on the Demand for Medical Care					
	Preventive Care Visits per Month			Curative Care Visits per Month		
	Public	Private	Total	Public	Private	Total
Insurance	0.138	0.473	0.611	0.022	0.089	0.111
No insurance	0.191	0.221	0.412	0.040	0.065	0.105
Difference	−0.053	0.252	0.199	−0.018	0.024	0.006

Source: Gertler & Sturm, 1997. Reprinted with permission from Elsevier Science.

this policy shift improved the targeting of public healthcare services toward the low-income population. Their simulations suggest that "a reduction in total public sector visits from expanding health insurance to the top half of the income distribution implies: (1) a reduction in public expenditures of about 33 percent, (2) an increase in the share of public expenditures captured by the poor by about 25 percent, and (3) a shift in the mix of subsidies away from curative in favor of preventive care" (p. 255). This shift could result in significant cost savings for the public-sector and improve targeting of subsidies to the low-income population and toward preventive services.

Employer-Related Health Insurance

Some aspects of employer-related health insurance (ERHI) have economic consequences that are worthy of consideration. Securing health insurance through formal employment is typical where the formal employment sector is substantial (higher-income as opposed to lower-income settings) because an individual's income is higher, identifiable, taxed, and subsidized, and because organization of such a system is more feasible through formal employment. The extent to which national insurance plans are successful can depend on the size and nature of the formal employment and private insurance sectors and government administrative capacity.

Employer-related (or employment-based) health insurance is primarily an U.S. phenomenon, although recent reforms in countries such as Morocco underscore the interest in employing payroll-based health insurance plans to extend coverage to the population of formal public- and private-sector employees (Ruger & Kress, 2007). In the United States, approximately 90% of Americans who are covered by private health insurance obtain this coverage through their employer. Of the total compensation package for U.S. civilian workers in 2009, health benefits coverage accounted for approximately 27% of benefits expenditures and

8.2% of the total compensation package (U.S. Bureau of Labor Statistics, 2010).

The link between employment and health insurance in the United States has historical roots in mid-twentieth-century legislation and policies devised to deal with the excess demand for labor in the aftermath of World War II. In particular, two policy efforts confirmed the employment–health insurance link: (1) congressional efforts to restrict wage increases after World War II, which resulted in employer competition for employees on the basis of nonwage benefits such as pensions and health insurance, and (2) tax laws that exempted benefits from taxation, making them a tax-deductible expenditure of business for employers. Both measures created an incentive for employers to offer health insurance as a benefit of employment (Federal Reserve Bank of San Francisco, 1998).

In reality, although employers advertise health insurance as an employer-subsidized benefit, it is the employees who pay for the cost of these services through reduced real wages (except in cases where, as in the United States after World War II, core wages have been artificially capped). Given the established employment–health insurance link in the United States, the market for employer-related health insurance has a number of implications for employee decisions regarding job mobility, retirement, and labor supply.

Job Mobility

Job-lock is a relatively new term used to describe the situation in which employees are reluctant to change jobs because they fear losing their health insurance coverage. It might occur, for example, when an individual does not take a better job at a new company because of differences in health insurance coverage between the old job and the new one. Such health insurance differences for this individual might involve the requirement of a waiting period of several months before health insurance can be obtained, or it might mean that the new employer's coverage excludes healthcare services that treat one of his or her family's preexisting conditions. Because of the disparities between jobs in the availability and scope of health insurance, and despite potential gains in productivity and income, employees facing these circumstances are reluctant to change jobs.

Reduction of job mobility not only limits workers' freedom, choice, and income, but also has implications for the productivity of the national economy if employees are reluctant to take new jobs that will enhance their individual productivity. Although it has long been surmised that job-lock exists, over the last decade and a half empirical evidence has accumulated to document the magnitude of this phenomenon in the labor market.

Magnitude of Job-lock

From 1994 to 1996, at least five studies examined the effects of ERHI on job mobility, productivity, and welfare (e.g., welfare loss from job-lock is the productivity losses associated with decreased worker mobility). A review of this literature (Table 15-5) demonstrates that ERHI does deter worker mobility: These studies typically reported a 20% to 40% reduction in mobility rates due to ERHI, depending on

workers' marital status, gender, and family size (Buchmueller & Valletta, 1996; Cooper & Monheit, 1993; Holtz-Eakin, 1994; Madrian, 1994; Monheit & Cooper, 1994). One study found that after controlling for pension receipt, job tenure, and spouse job change, strong evidence existed for the presence of job-lock among women, but not among men (Buchmueller & Valletta, 1996). Another study found that reductions in job mobility due to ERHI were highest for two specific groups: (1) married men with large families and (2) married men with pregnant wives (Madrian, 1994).

Fewer studies have been done on the effects of ERHI on worker productivity and macroeconomic efficiencies. However, one such study concluded that in 1987 the economic productivity loss due to job-lock accounted for approximately 0.5% of the total U.S. wage bill—$3.7 billion in annual wages out of $1.262 trillion total, assuming full-time and full-year employment (Monheit & Cooper, 1994). The authors suggest that this figure can be explained by the fact that these effects are relatively short-lived and affect a relatively small number (1 million of 61 million) of workers. To obtain an estimate of the net effect of ERHI on economic efficiency, these efficiency losses

Table 15-5	Employment-Related Health Insurance (ERHI) and Job Motility: Estimates of Job-Lock in the United States	
Author(s)	**Sample/Method**	**Magnitude of Job-Lock**
Madrian (1994)	1987 National Medical Expenditure Survey (NMES). Sample of married men aged 20–55. Estimated probit equation of likelihood of job change and examined three experimental groups using a difference-in-difference approach.	Estimated that mobility rates decreased by 30% to 31% for those with employment-provided health insurance coverage compared with those without such coverage. Mobility rates were reduced by 33% to 37% for those married men with employment-related coverage and large families. Mobility rates decreased by 67% for those with employment-related coverage and pregnant wives.
Holtz-Eakin (1994)	1984 Panel Study of Income Dynamics (PSID). Full-time workers aged 25–55. Used a difference-in-difference approach.	Found no statistically significant results. For job changes during 1984–1985, mobility rates for married men declined by 1.59 percentage points, and rates for single women declined by 1.06 percentage points.
Gruber and Madrian (1994)	Survey of Income and Program Participation (1985, 1986, 1987).	Found that state and federal policy to mandate continuation of coverage increased the job mobility of prime-age male workers. Suggested that job-lock may result from short-run (as opposed to long-run) employee concerns over portability.

continued

Table 15-5	continued	
Author(s)	**Sample/Method**	**Magnitude of Job-Lock**
Monheit and Cooper (1994)	1987 National Medical Expenditure Survey (NMES). Reviewed literature and studied the nature of welfare loss associated with job-lock.	The authors reviewed the literature on job-lock and found that studies typically reported a 20% to 40% reduction in mobility rates due to ERHI, depending on worker marital status, gender, and family size. Examined welfare loss due to job-lock and found that the magnitude of welfare loss was $4.8 billion, less than 1% of the wage bill of those affected.
Buchmueller and Valletta (1996)	1984 Survey of Income and Program Participation (SIPP). Included pension receipt, job tenure, and spouse job change to estimate ERHI effects on job mobility.	Found for dual-earner married men and women, strong evidence of job-lock among women, but weak evidence of job-lock among men.

ultimately must be weighed against potential efficiency gains (currently not estimated) that may result from ERHI.

Alleviating or Eliminating Job-Lock

At least three strategies can be employed to mitigate the effects of ERHI on job mobility:

- Maintain ERHI, but ensure health insurance coverage is fully portable across jobs
- Maintain ERHI, but disallow insurers from excluding coverage of preexisting medical conditions
- Disassociate health insurance from employment altogether

There is limited empirical evidence concerning the effectiveness of these policy options, but one study did find that short-term (3 to 20 months) "continuation of coverage" mandates (i.e., policies that give individuals a specific period of time to purchase health insurance through their former employers) had a positive effect on worker mobility (Gruber & Madrian, 1994). These results suggest that job-lock may result from short-term (as opposed to long-term) employee concerns over health insurance portability.

Retirement

The decision to retire or continue working is also heavily influenced by ERHI status. This relationship is especially strong because the quantity and frequency of medical expenses increase with age, as does the difference between the costs of employer-related health insurance and the insurance policies that can be purchased individually on the open market (Gruber & Madrian, 1995). In some circumstances, older individuals cannot even purchase individual market-based policies.

In their analysis of the impact of continuation-of-coverage laws on retirement decisions, Gruber and Madrian (1995) found that the ability to purchase an employment-based plan from a former employer at the same price as if one were employed increases the odds of early retirement (because the individual is no longer working, employees still working will be forced to pay for the subsidy provided to retired workers). According to these authors, the degree to which the likelihood of early retirement increases depends on the duration of the ability to purchase post-retirement insurance and the quality of the employer-based post-retirement and publicly offered health insurance options. More specifically, Gruber and Madrian found that among men aged 55 to 64 who are too young for Medicare (which commences at age 65), each additional year of continued coverage increases the likelihood of retiring by 30%.

In a different study, Manski and associates (2010) assessed dental care coverage and retirement. They found that people in the labor force were much more likely to have dental insurance than those who were not working.

Labor Supply

Most employers do not offer health benefits to part-time employees. In addition, many low-wage earners in service-sector positions (e.g., fast-food service employees) do not receive health insurance as a benefit of employment; low-wage earners typically do not receive benefits because their earnings are too low to pass on the premium costs. These factors provide an incentive for those who need or value health insurance to choose full-time over part-time employment.

In their analysis of married women's decisions to work on a full- or part-time basis, Buchmueller and Valletta (1999) found that wives frequently switched from nonparticipation to work so as to obtain health insurance. Their estimates demonstrate a 15% to 36% increase in married women's labor supply associated with a lack of their husbands' health insurance coverage.

Labor Market Effects of Introducing National Health Insurance in Canada

One of the negative economic impacts of introducing national health insurance in a given country is believed to be the deadweight loss and increased unemployment resulting from altered production and consumption decisions due to the necessary increases in payroll taxes.[11] Economic theory predicts that increases in payroll taxes will result in economic activity and deadweight losses as a result of altered production and consumption decisions in the economy. At the same time, theory points to efficiency gains from effectively implemented risk-pooling arrangements.

From the early 1960s to the early 1970s, Canada moved from a primarily private insurance–based healthcare system to a national health insurance system financed primarily through lump-sum premiums or general revenue financing, with management decentralized to the provincial level. National health insurance in Canada provides coverage to all citizens.

Gruber and Hanratty (1993) studied the effects of Canada's "natural experiment" of transitioning from ERHI (roughly 70% of the population was covered by private health insurance in the mid-1960s) to national health insurance. In examining employment, wages, and hours across eight industries and 10 provinces from 1961 to 1975, they found that, after national health insurance was introduced, average hours were unchanged despite that fact that both employment and wages increased. These results were robust to a number of model specifications (different analyses) that controlled for the potential endogeneity of national health insurance and provincial and industry effects.

The authors suggest that these results might be explained by the notion that the introduction of national health insurance systematically increases labor demand across all sectors of the economy due, at least

in part, to the increases in labor productivity that result from increases in job mobility or health improvements in the labor force. Despite some noted differences in the costs of medical and hospital care, the authors believe that the pre–national health insurance system in Canada is sufficiently similar to that in the United States for this Canadian experiment to offer useful evidence of the effects of a similar transition in the United States following recent national health reform legislation.

The Impact of Private User Fees or Public User Charges on the Welfare of the Poor

Private user fees are part of a system in which patients pay directly, on an out-of-pocket basis, for healthcare services. These fees can take the form of payment for the whole charge, partial payment for a service, a copayment (a flat amount per visit), or coinsurance (a percentage of the cost of the service). User charges are fees paid by patients for publicly provided services and constitute public revenues. User fee/user charge financing is designed as a demand-side and revenue-generation measure with the goal of improving allocative efficiency in the healthcare system by making patients more cost conscious in healthcare decision making. In addition to controlling use, user charges have been designed to raise revenues and to decrease the government's financial burden in the health sector, to increase coverage and the quality of care by increasing resources for the health sector, and to increase efficiency in health service delivery.

Higher-income countries promote these types of payments to reduce healthcare use by making consumers more conscious of healthcare costs. Cost sharing, in particular, shifts the financial risk of healthcare costs toward patients. A recent review by Remler and Greene (2009) found that cost sharing can reduce utilization of inappropriate healthcare services, thereby reducing costs. However, in some cases, such as with maintenance drug use among chronically ill patients, cost sharing reduces utilization of critical healthcare goods and services and, therefore, may have negative effects on a patient's health—and on future healthcare costs. Thus Remler and Greene dub cost-sharing a "blunt instrument." Evidence suggests that these mechanisms have been successful in reducing use of healthcare goods and services, regardless of whether reduced health care is medically appropriate (Newhouse, 1993). User fees have a greater health and income impact on the poor and medically indigent because these groups decrease their use of both necessary and unnecessary health care in response to such fees.

---

[11] Currie and Madrian (1999) provide an excellent overview and additional references concerning the labor market effects of health insurance, with an emphasis on the situation in the United States. See also Gruber and Hanratty (1993) and Hanratty (1996).

Rather than employ user fees or user charges, an alternative system of promoting allocative efficiency, or medical care appropriateness, has emerged to reduce inappropriate care while ensuring that appropriate and necessary care reaches those in need. This system has been tested in the United States and is discussed in Exhibit 15-5.

The evidence from a number of in-country experiences with user fees or user charges demonstrates that, for the most part, such fees have not proved overwhelmingly successful in enhancing efficiency, raising revenue, or improving equity. With respect to revenue generation, user charges have failed to provide more than 5% of ministry of health recurrent costs in sub-Saharan Africa (Wang'ombe, 1997). Programs in China have been much more successful in cost recovery (24% to 36% of the ministry of health's recurrent expenditures recovered) than have programs in sub-Saharan Africa, where an average of 5% of operating costs are recouped through user charges. This figure is probably an underestimate of the net yield because the administrative costs of collecting fees must also be considered. In many cases, it is likely that the net yield is near zero or negative for cost recovery. Moreover, because systems are not raising enough revenues from user fees or user charges, little additional money is available to channel into improved quality and system reform, especially for public health services targeted at low-income populations, which are especially hard hit by the lack of additional money. Funding for these efforts still must stem from the ministry of health's budget.

A review of the literature on user financing of basic social services by Reddy and Vandemoortele (1996) further supports the contention that user fees and user charges generally have had negative effects on health system use and very little success in raising revenue to cover governmental recurrent costs. As shown in Table 15-6, recent estimates of price elasticity of demand for health care in a number of countries provide compelling evidence that user fees are associated with significant reductions in use rates, especially among low-income segments and children. The magnitude of revenues raised through health cost recovery in Africa ranges from roughly 0.5% to 20% of the recurrent budget of the ministry of health.

Additional evidence indicates that user fees or user charges reduce use, but the overall efficiency effects are unclear given that these reductions occur with both necessary and unnecessary care. In his review of the literature on user charges, Creese (1991) found that user fees decrease use of the health system, especially among the patients at greatest risk and for

whom the most cost-effective preventive and treatment options are appropriate. In the Democratic Republic of the Congo, for instance, relative increases in the cost of health care (as compared with the cost of other consumer products) led to significant decreases in the demand for treatment measures, especially for prenatal care and interventions for children younger than age 5. The magnitude of the reduction was significant: The overall use rate fell from 37% to 31%, and the coverage rate for prenatal visits fell from 95% to 84% (De Bethune, Alfani, & Lahaye, 1989). As Creese (1991) notes, these study results indicate that the demand for health care is more price elastic among lower-income individuals than among higher-income groups. The cost-recovery rate through user charges was insignificant.

Efficiency gains from these mechanisms have also been modest. Some evidence suggests that the use of graduated user charges (higher fees for hospitals and lower fees for health centers) aimed at improving technical efficiency (delivering primary care at low-level health centers and tertiary care at high-level hospitals) has been successful (Collins, Quick, Musau, Kraushaar, & Hussein, 1996). Some countries— namely, Côte d'Ivoire, Mali, Namibia, Zambia, and Zimbabwe—have implemented graduated user charges with some successes in technical efficiency (e.g., better use of referrals, and better patterns of use for both primary care received at lower-level facilities such as health centers and tertiary care received at higher-level facilities such as hospitals) (Barnum & Kutzin, 1993; Bennett & Ngalande-Banda, 1994).

In Ghana, Creese (1991) notes a sharp reduction in the use of the health system as a result of large increases in healthcare fees. Reduced use was sustained over a 2-year period (Waddington & Enyimayew, 1990). Although the cost-recovery rate of this policy (15%) was fairly high compared with some other projects, the demand likely shifted from health care sought in government facilities to rural, unlicensed sellers of drugs, which had potentially significant ramifications for health. Finally, Creese (1991) noted a sharp decrease in demand following a policy decision in Swaziland to raise charges at government health units by 300% to 400% (to the same fee levels as mission providers), without raising quality. The resultant decrease in use of government healthcare facilities was 32%, but this decrease was coupled with a 10% increase in use of mission facilities; the overall drop in use was 17%. Use continued to decrease over the course of the year following the policy change, and a disproportionate drop in use

Table 15-6	Estimates of Price Elasticity of Demand for Health Care			
Study	**Location and Year of Data**		**Results**	
Jimenez (1987)	Ethiopia (1985)	Overall	−0.05 to −0.50	
Jimenez (1987)	Sudan (1986)	Overall	−0.37	
Yoder (1989)	Swaziland (1985)	Overall	−0.32	
Gertler and van der Gaag (1988)	Côte d'Ivoire (1985)		**Rural Hospitals**	
		Income Quartile	**Adults**	**Children**
		Lowest	−0.47 to −1.34	−0.65 to −2.32
		Second	−0.44 to −1.27	−0.58 to −1.98
		Third	−0.41 to −1.18	−0.49 to −1.60
		Highest	−0.29 to −0.71	−0.12 to −0.48
Gertler and van der Gaag (1988)	Peru (1985)		**Rural Hospitals**	
		Income Quartile	**Adults**	**Children**
		Lowest	−0.57 to −1.36	−0.67 to −1.72
		Second	−0.38 to −0.91	−0.48 to −1.20
		Third	−0.16 to −0.37	−0.22 to −0.54
		Highest	−0.01 to −0.04	−0.03 to −0.09
Sauerborn, Naugtara, and Latimer (1994)	Burkina Faso (1985)	Overall	−0.79	
		Age Groups		
		<1	−3.64	
		1–14	−1.73	
		15+	−0.27	
		Income Quartile		
		Lowest	−1.44	
		Second	−1.21	
		Third	−1.39	
		Highest	−0.12	

Source: Reddy & Vandemoortele, 1996. Reprinted with permission.

(especially for use of government services for sexually transmitted and respiratory infections) occurred among the lower-income groups (Yoder, 1989).

The equity effects of user fees and user charges are not favorable. Although some healthcare economists initially argued that equity can be improved through the use of user fees or user charges due to increased service availability and quality (from increased revenues) and better use (from price effects on demand) (De Ferranti, 1985), the subsequent evidence does not necessarily support this argument. For these factors to be equity enhancing, the government would need to ensure that increased revenues are reinvested and targeted toward services that directly affect the low-income segments, and to ensure that low-income and vulnerable groups are exempted from many user fees and charges and offered public subsidies instead.

Evidence from sub-Saharan Africa suggests that patients are highly sensitive to user charges and fees (Bennett & Ngalande-Banda, 1994; Gertler & van der Gaag, 1990; Mwabu & Wang'ombe, 1995; Waddington & Enyimayew, 1990). Although nearly all sub-Saharan African user fee and user charge programs offer exemptions for the poor through means testing, this method is difficult to implement in many countries and can be exploited by higher-income groups.

Health Expenditures and Poverty

For those persons without insurance coverage, high health expenditures relative to income either can preclude treatment because of income insufficiencies or, if medical treatment options are pursued, can pose a major financial burden. Although the evidence on this subject is scant, a few studies have elucidated the implications both of falling ill and of facing catastrophic health expenditure.

For example, in their analysis of the post–Cooperative Medical System era in China, Liu and associates (1996) found that high health expenditures were a major cause of poverty in rural areas. Healthcare costs were found to be high relative to a rural farmer's income: To pay for an episode of hospitalization at a county hospital, low-income farmers often had to spend roughly 1.2 years of disposable income. As Table 15-7 demonstrates, the cost of an outpatient visit as a percentage of weekly income for the lowest-income households varied from 38% in a village facility to 151% at a township provider and 170% in a county facility. In addition, 18% of households using health services had health expenditures that exceeded their total household income in 1 year (1993). In addition, 24.5% of the 11,044 rural households surveyed borrowed or became indebted, and 5.5% sold or mortgaged properties to pay for health care. In their survey of 30 counties, the authors found that as a result of these burdensome payments, 47% of medically indebted households suffered from hunger.

In Vietnam, Nguyen et al. (under review) found decreased consumption of food, education, and production means for households in the lowest income quartile who had inpatient treatment and high levels of outpatient treatment over the past 12 months. These authors' findings suggest that financial strain from health expenses can create or exacerbate poverty and poor health, particularly for persons living in low-income households. Nguyen and colleagues recommend health policy reforms to reduce the out-of-pocket payments in Vietnam that result in this economic and social burden.

In a preliminary study of people's ability to cope with catastrophic health shocks in Indonesia, Prescott and Pradhan (1999) found that out-of-pocket health expenditures were highly skewed, suggesting that, relative to their income, a proportion of the population faced catastrophic levels of health expenditures. In South Korea, Ruger and Kim (2007) found that out-of-pocket spending was regressive: Lower-income groups paid disproportionately greater percentages of their income compared with higher-income groups. Individuals who had both multiple chronic conditions and relatively low incomes were especially vulnerable. Social risk management mechanisms, in the form of insurance for civil servants and budget subsidies for publicly provided services, generally benefited the better-off, whereas lower-income households were forced to reduce demand (especially for inpatient services) and spend less on medical care. With respect to policy measures employed to alleviate the burden on poorer households, Ruger and Kim suggest that efforts to ensure universal coverage through budget subsidies targeting the poor and through insurance options can significantly reduce, but will not eliminate, the catastrophic shocks experienced by lower-income households.

Finally, Fabricant, Kamara, and Mills (1999) showed that in Sierra Leone, rural low-income populations were disproportionately disadvantaged by user charges for health care, in that they paid a higher percentage of their incomes for health care compared to wealthier households. The authors concluded that greater accessibility to basic health facilities and greater reliance on additional resources generated through improved efficiency and cross-subsidization would relieve much of the financial burden placed on these lower-income households. Insurance and prepayment plans also would help reduce the financial burden of health expenditure.

Table 15-7	The Financial Burden of Healthcare Costs for Households with Different Income Levels in China's Poverty Regions	
Level of Facilities	**Households with per Capita Income of 200 Yuan**	**Households with per Capita Income of 400 Yuan**
	Cost of an Outpatient visit as a Percentage of Weekly Income	
Village	38%	36%
Township	151%	71%
County	170%	84%
	Cost of an Inpatient Episode as a Percentage of Annual Income	
Township	28%	22%
County	116%	138%

Source: Liu, Hu, Fu, & Hsiao, 1996. Reprinted with permission from Elsevier.

Conclusion

The World Bank's 1980 *World Development Report* on human resources and poverty examined the interrelations between poverty (in terms of low income) and health, education, nutrition, and fertility levels. Table 15-1 points to the enormous progress in the twentieth century in several of these domains—albeit progress substantially denied to the world's lowest-income billion persons. The upper panel of Figure 15-9, reproduced (and modified) from the 1980 report, illustrates both the possible relationships among these variables and the entry points for policy operating through them. Although the World Bank report in-

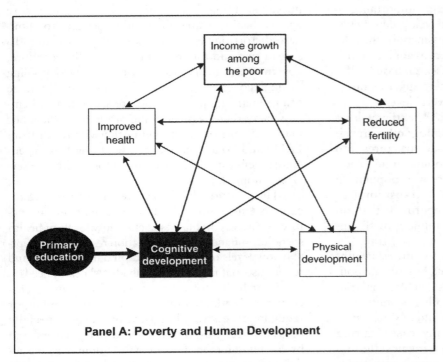

Panel A: Poverty and Human Development

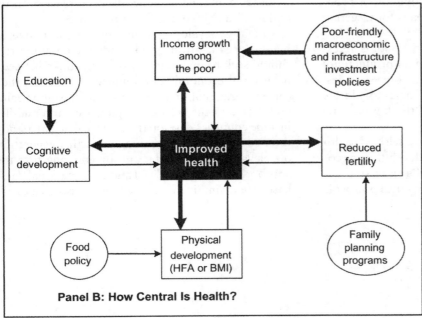

Panel B: How Central Is Health?

Figure 15-9 Health and Development. *Note:* HFA = height for age; BMI = body mass index. *Source:* International Bank for Reconstruction and Development, World Bank, World Development Report (Washington, DC: World Bank, 1980). Adapted with permission.

dicates the importance of public action in each domain, it concludes that expansion and improvement in primary education, particularly for girls, is the critical priority in most countries. The information presented in this chapter suggests a more central role for health, at least for low-income regions with current high levels of illness. The lower panel of Figure 15-9 places health in this central role.

The consequences of health and health policy for economic development are of major importance to policy makers in the health and development fields. This chapter has provided an assessment of the relevant conclusions from the literature available on this subject, but recognizes that the research base itself is limited. The analysis presented here suggests directions for government policy at several levels.

First, it is useful to encourage policies that will accelerate the speed of favorable demographic transitions and incorporate changing age structures into government policies aimed at schooling and job creation. The changing age structure of a population that results from the demographic transition (see Chapter 1) provides a window of opportunity that can lead to a transitory boost in economic growth, enabling a country to break free of a poverty trap.

Second, a central goal of many countries' health-sector development strategies should be to create policies to control infectious diseases, such as malaria, tuberculosis, HIV/AIDS, and sexually transmitted infections, by providing information and resources necessary for avoiding, and in many cases, curing infection. Categorical control policies against the major diseases affecting low-income populations probably represent the most efficient means for targeting public expenditures to them.

Third, improving the health of the poor is necessary to alleviate poverty. The marginal productivity of health is probably higher in low-income societies, and governments should develop policies to address the health and economic needs of the low-income population.

Efforts also must be made to assess selected health policies based on their effects on both health and economic outcomes (Ruger, 2003a, 2004b). First, practitioners should promote the use of clinical protocols to improve health outcomes and enhance efficient healthcare spending. Economic incentives to decrease healthcare use (e.g., copayments, deductibles, capitated payments, and global budgets) do not necessarily distinguish between types of care (appropriate versus inappropriate) and the needs of patients, and they can have a disproportionate impact on the poor and medically indigent.

Second, governments and policy makers should pursue sustainable healthcare financing to insure against health-related financial losses and to eliminate distortions in the market for health care. To spread risk and minimize insurance market failure, governments can (1) encourage universal risk pooling through government mandates and taxes; (2) pursue health financing policies that are separate from employment, thereby preempting or reducing the labor market distortions that might otherwise result from ERHI; and (3) discourage the use of user fees to generate revenue and reduce demand for healthcare services among the poor.

Third, efforts should be taken to improve healthcare systems characterized by inadequate infrastructure and access. In many societies, low levels of health spending and inequitable allocation result in unacceptably low levels of capital stock, human resources, and service use that fail to meet individuals' health needs.

Fourth, health planners should promote efficient health administration policies by avoiding or reducing excessive administrative costs, especially those between hospitals and third-party payers, and by encouraging the efficient use of administrative activities to monitor and reduce the occurrence of costly and medically inappropriate procedures.

Finally, development institutions, nongovernmental organizations, and academic communities should seek to investigate further the links between health and economic development. Primarily, they can encourage continued efforts to understand health and development links by helping low- and middle-income countries develop their own capacity to study these connections; by encouraging further generation of relevant primary data; and by ensuring that the appropriate household-level and cross-national databases are maintained, updated, and accessible to all.

Acknowledgments

The original version of this chapter was prepared for the 1998 transition team of the then-incoming World Health Organization Director-General Dr. G. H. Brundtland. Preparation of that version was supported by grants from the Royal Norwegian Ministry of Foreign Affairs to WHO and the World Bank. The WHO Commission on Macroeconomics and Health supported extension and revision, and discussions with the commission's chair, Jeffrey Sachs, provided valuable ideas and feedback during preparation of this chapter. Earlier versions of this chapter have been published in 2001 and 2006. Conclusions and opinions are those of the authors and not necessarily those of any of the sponsoring agencies. Felicia Knaul, Lawrence Lau, Michael Merson, Pia Malaney, and Anne Mills also made valuable suggestions and comments on earlier drafts. Leslie Evans prepared the tables and graphics, Christina Lazar provided research assistance, and Elizabeth Cafiero and Marija Ozolins provided research and editorial assistance.

• • • Discussion Questions

1. In what ways, and to what extent, do major diseases such as tuberculosis, malaria, and HIV/AIDS affect the income and well-being of people living in low- and middle-income countries?

2. What can policy makers and practitioners do in non-health-service-related settings, such as schools, to improve the health and well-being of girls and boys in low- and middle-income countries?

3. How do changes in fertility and mortality patterns work to influence the level and capacity of those persons contributing to economic production in a given society?

4. Why is the concept of risk pooling in financing healthcare services so important?

5. What are the health, healthcare service use, and economic effects of making people pay part of the costs of medical services?

6. How have recent pandemics directly and indirectly affected national and global economies?

7. Which cost-effective solutions have been identified to address major international disease burdens and improve global welfare?

• • • References

Aaron, H., & Schwartz, W. (1984). *The painful prescription: Rationing hospital care*. Washington, DC: Brookings Institution.

Acemoglu, D., & Johnson, S. (2007). Disease and development: The effect of life expectancy on economic growth. *Journal of Political Economy, 115*(6), 925–985.

Acemoglu, D., Johnson, S., & Robinson, J. A. (2003). Disease and development in historical perspective. *Journal of the European Economic Association, 1*(2–3), 397–405.

Ahlburg, D. A. (2000). *The economic impacts of tuberculosis* (WHO/CDS/STB/2000.5). Geneva, Switzerland: World Health Organization.

Ainsworth, M., & Over, M. (1994). Aids and African development. *World Bank Research Observer, 9*, 203–240.

Alderman, H., Hoddinott, J., & Kinsey, B. (2006). Long term consequences of early childhood malnutrition. *Oxford Economic Papers, 58*(3), 450–474.

Alderman, H., & Linnemayr, S. (2009). Anemia in low-income countries is unlikely to be addressed by economic development without additional programs. *Food Nutrition Bulletin, 30*(3), 265–269.

Almond, D. (2006). Is the 1918 influenza pandemic over? Long-term effects of in utero influenza exposure in the post-1940 U.S. population. *Journal of Political Economy, 114*(4), 672–712.

Alsan, M., Bloom, D. E., & Canning, D. (2006). The effect of population health on foreign direct investment inflows to low- and middle-income countries. *World Development, 34*(4), 613–630.

American Hospital Association (AHA). (2008). *Report on the economic crisis: Initial impact on hospitals*. Retrieved from http://www.aha.org/aha/content/2008/pdf/081119econcrisisreport.pdf

Anand, K., Pandav, C. S., & Nath, L. M. (1999). Impact of HIV/AIDS on the national economy of India. *Health Policy, 47*, 195–205.

Anand, S., Diderichsen, F., Evans, T., Shkolnikov, V. M., & Wirth, M. (2001). Measuring disparities in health: Methods and indicators. In T. Evans, M. Whitehead, F. Diderichsen, A. Bhuiya, & M. Wirth (Eds.), *Challenging inequities in health: From ethics to action* (pp. 49–67). London: Oxford University Press.

Australian Agency for International Development (AusAID). (1999). *Impact of the Asia crisis on children: Issues for social safety nets*. Retrieved from http://www.ausaid.gov.au/publications/pdf/impact-asiacrisis-children1999.pdf

Ayé, R., Wyss, K., Abdualimova, H., & Saidaliev, S. (2010). Household costs of illness during different phases of tuberculosis treatment in Central Asia: A patient survey in Tajikistan. *BioMed Central Public Health, 10*(18).

Barker, D. J. P. (1992). *The fetal and infant origins of adult disease*. London: BMJ Books.

Barnum, H., & Kutzin, J. (1993). *Public hospitals in developing countries: Resource use, cost, financing*. Baltimore, MD: Johns Hopkins University Press for the World Bank.

Barro, R., & Lee, J. W. (1994). Sources of economic growth. *Carnegie–Rochester Conference Series on Public Policy, 40*, 1–46.

Basta, S. S., Soekirman, M. S., Karyadi, D., & Scrimshaw, N. S. (1979). Iron deficiency anemia and the productivity of adult males in Indonesia. *American Journal of Clinical Nutrition, 32*, 916–925.

Becker, G. S., Philipson, T. J., & Soares, R. R. (2005). The quantity and quality of life and the evolution of world inequality. *American Economic Review, 95*, 277–291.

Behrman, J. (1993). The economic rationale for investing in nutrition in developing countries. *World Development, 21*(11), 1749–1771.

Bell, C., Devarajan, S., & Gersbach, H. (2003). *The long-run economic costs of AIDS: Theory and an application to South Africa* (Policy Research Working Paper No. WPS 3152). Washington, DC: World Bank.

Bennett, S., Creese, A., & Monasch, R. (1998). *Health insurance schemes for people outside formal sector employment* (Division of Analysis, Research and Assessment Paper No. 16). Geneva, Switzerland: World Health Organization.

Bennett, S., & Ngalande-Banda, E. (1994). *Public and private roles in health: A review and analysis of experience in sub-Saharan Africa* (Strengthening Health Services Paper 6). Geneva, Switzerland: World Health Organization.

Berger, M. C., & Leigh, J. P. (1989). Schooling, self-selection and health. *Journal of Human Resources, 24,* 435–455.

Bernstein, S. J., McGlynn, E. A., Siu, A. L., Roth, C. P., Sherwood, M. J., Keesey, J. W., et al. (1993). The appropriateness of hysterectomy: A comparison of care in seven health plans. *Journal of the American Medical Association, 269,* 2398–2402.

Bhargava, A. (1994). Modeling the health of Filipino children. *Journal of the Royal Statistical Society, Series A, 157,* 417–432.

Bhargava, A. (1997). Nutritional status and the allocation of time in Rwandese households. *Journal of Econometrics, 77,* 277–295.

Bhargava, A., Jamison, D., Lau, L., & Murray, C. (2001). Modeling the effects of health on economic growth. *Journal of Health Economics, 20*(3), 423–440.

Bhutta, Z. A., Bawany, F. A., Feroze, A., Rizvi, A., Thapa, S. J., & Patel, M. (2009). Effects of the crises on child nutrition and health in East Asia and the Pacific. *Global Social Policy, 9,* 119–143.

Bleakley, H. (2003). Disease and development: Evidence from the American South. *Journal of the European Economic Association, 1*(2), 376–386.

Bleakley, H. (2010). Malaria eradication in the Americas: A retrospective analysis of childhood exposure. *American Economic Journal: Applied Economics, 2*(2), 1–4.

Bloom, D. E., & Canning, D. (2000). The health and wealth of nations. *Science, 287,* 1207–1209.

Bloom, D. E., Canning, D., & Graham, B. (2003). Longevity and life cycle savings. *Scandinavian Journal of Economics, 105,* 319–338.

Bloom, D. E., Canning, D., & Jamison, D. T. (2004). Health, wealth and welfare. *Finance and Development, 41,* 10–15.

Bloom, D. E., Canning, D., & Malaney, P. (2000). Population dynamics and economic growth in Asia. *Population and Development Review, 26*(suppl), 257–290.

Bloom, D. E., Canning, D., & Sevilla, J. (2002). *The demographic dividend: A new perspective on the economic consequences of population change* (MR-1274). Santa Monica, CA: RAND.

Bloom, D. E., Canning, D., & Sevilla, J. (2004). The effect of health on economic growth: A production function approach. *World Development, 32*(1), 1–13.

Bloom, D. E., & Freeman, R. B. (1988). Economic development and the timing and components of population growth. *Journal of Policy Modeling, 10*(1), 57–82.

Bloom, D. E., & Mahal, A. S. (1997). Does the AIDS epidemic threaten economic growth? *Journal of Econometrics, 77,* 105–124.

Bloom, D. E., & River Path Associates. (2000). Social capitalism and human diversity. In Organization of Economic Cooperation and Development, *The creative society of the 21st century* (pp. 25–78). Paris: Author.

Bloom, D. E., Rosenfield, A., & River Path Associates. (2000). A moment in time: AIDS and business. *AIDS Patient Care and STDs, 14*(9), 509–517.

Bloom, D. E., & Williamson, J. G. (1998). Demographic transitions and economic miracles in emerging Asia. *World Bank Economic Review, 12*(3), 419–455.

Boman, K. K., Lindblad, F., & Hjern, A. (2010). Long-term outcomes of childhood cancer survivors in Sweden: A population-based study of education, employment, and income. *Cancer, 116*(5), 1385–1391.

Bovbjerg, R. R. (1995). The high cost of administration in health care: Part of the problem or part of the solution? *Journal of Law, Medicine & Ethics, 23,* 186–194.

Brahmbhatt, M. (2005, September 23). *Avian influenza: Economic and social impacts.* Washington, DC: World Bank.

Brainerd, E. (1998). Market reform and mortality in transition economies. *World Development, 16*(11), 2013–2027.

Brinkman, H. J., de Pee, S., Sanogo, I., Subran, L., & Bloem, M. W. (2009). High food prices and the global financial crisis have reduced access to nutrition food and worsened nutritional status and health. *Journal of Nutrition, Supplement: The Impact of Climate Change, the Economic Crisis, and the Increase in Food Prices on Malnutrition,* 153S–161S.

Brook, R. H. (1992). Improving practice: The clinician's role. *British Journal of Surgery, 79,* 606–607.

Brook, R. H. (1994). The RAND/UCLA appropriateness method. In K. A. McCormick, S. R. Moore, & R. A. Siegel, *Clinical practice guideline development: Methodology perspectives* (AHCPR Publication No. 95-0009) (pp. 59–70). Rockville, MD: Public Health Service.

Brook, R. H. (1995). Medicare quality and getting older: A personal essay. *Health Affairs, 14*(4), 73–81.

Brook, R. H. (1997). Managed care is not the problem: Quality is. *Journal of the American Medical Association, 278,* 1612–1614.

Brook, R. H., Kamberg, C. J., Mayer-Oakes, A., Beers, M. H., Raube, K., & Steiner, A. (1990). Appropriateness of acute medical care for the elderly: An analysis of the literature. *Health Policy, 14,* 225–242.

Brook, R. H., & Lohr, K. N. (1985). Efficacy, effectiveness, variations, and quality: Boundary-crossing research. *Medical Care, 23*(5), 710–722.

Brook, R. H., & Lohr, K. N. (1986). Will we need to ration effective health care? *Issues in Science and Technology, 3,* 68–77.

Brook, R. H., & Lohr, K. N. (1987). Monitoring quality of care in the Medicare program: Two proposed systems. *Journal of the American Medical Association, 258,* 3138–3141.

Brook, R. H., Park, R. E., Chassin, M. R., Solomon, D. H., Keesey, J., & Kosecoff, J. (1990). Predicting the appropriate use of carotid endarterectomy, upper gastrointestinal endoscopy, and coronary angiography. *New England Journal of Medicine, 323,* 1173–1177.

Brundtland, G. H., Liestol, K., & Walloe, L. (1975). Height and weight of school children and adolescent girls and boys in Oslo 1970. *Acta Paediatrica Scandinavica, 64,* 565–573.

Buchmueller, T. C., & Valletta, R. G. (1996). The effects of employer-provided health insurance on worker mobility. *Industrial and Labor Relations Review, 49*(3), 439–455.

Buchmueller, T. C., & Valletta, R. G. (1999). The effect of health insurance on married female labor supply. *Journal of Human Resources, 34*(1), 42–70.

Carlisle, D. M., Siu, A. L., Keeler, E. B., McGlynn, E. A., Kahn, K., Rubenstein, L. V., & Brook, R. H. (1992). HMO vs. fee-for-service care of older persons with acute myocardial infarction. *American Journal of Public Health, 82,* 1626–1630.

Case, A. (2004). Does money protect health status? Evidence from South African pensions. In D. Wise (Ed.), *Perspectives on the economics of aging* (pp. 287–312). Chicago: University of Chicago Press.

Case, A., Fertig, A., & Paxson, C. (2005). The lasting impact of childhood health and circumstance. *Journal of Health Economics, 24,* 365–389.

Catalano, R. (2009). Health, medical care, and economic crisis. *New England Journal of Medicine, 360*(8), 749–751.

Chassin, M. R., Kosecoff, J., Solomon, D. H., & Brook, R. H. (1987). How coronary angiography is used: Clinical determinants of appropriateness. *Journal of the American Medical Association, 258,* 2543–2547.

Chima, R., Goodman, C., & Mills, A. (2003). The economic impact of malaria in Africa: A critical review of the evidence. *Health Policy, 63,* 17–36.

Clarke, S. E., Jukes, M. S., Njagi, J. K., Khasakhala, L., Cundill, B., Otido, J., et al. (2008). Effect of intermittent preventive treatment of malaria on health and education in schoolchildren: A cluster-randomised, double-blind, placebo-controlled trial. *Lancet, 372,* 127–138.

Collins, D., Quick, J. D., Musau, S. N., Kraushaar, D. L., & Hussein, M. (1996). The fall and rise of cost-sharing in Kenya: The impact of phased implementation. *Health Policy and Planning, 1*(61), 52–63.

Commission on Macroeconomics and Health. (2001). *Macroeconomics and health: Investing in health for economic development.* Geneva, Switzerland: World Health Organization.

Cooper, P. F., & Monheit, A. C. (1993). Does employment-related health insurance inhibit job mobility? *Inquiry, 30*(4), 400–416.

Creese, A. L. (1991). User charges for health care: A review of recent experience. *Health Policy and Planning, 6*(4), 309–319.

Croft, R. A., & Croft, R. P. (1998). Expenditure and loss of income incurred by tuberculosis patients before reaching effective treatment in Bangladesh. *International Journal of Tuberculosis and Lung Disease, 2*(3), 252–254.

Cuddington, J. T. (1993). Modelling the macroeconomic effects of AIDS with an application to Tanzania. *World Bank Economic Review, 7*(2), 173–189.

Cuddington, J. T., & Hancock, J. D. (1994). Assessing the impact of AIDS on the growth path of the Malawian economy *Journal of Economic Development, 43,* 363–368.

Currie, J., & Madrian, B. C. (1999). Health, health insurance and the labor market. In O. Ashenfelter & D. Card (Eds.), *Handbook of labor economics* (Vol. 3, pp. 3309–3416). New York: Elsevier Science.

Cutler, D. M., & Richardson, E. (1998). The value of health: 1970–1990. *American Economic Review, 88,* 97–100.

Deaton, A. (2003). Health, inequality, and economic development. *Journal of Economic Literature, 41*(1), 113–158.

Deaton, A., & Paxson, C. (2001). Mortality, education, income and inequality among American cohorts. In D. Wise (Ed.), *Themes in the economics of aging* (pp. 129–170). Chicago: University of Chicago Press.

De Bethune, X., Alfani, S., & Lahaye, J. P. (1989). The influence of an abrupt price increase on health service utilization: Evidence from Zaire. *Health Policy and Planning, 4,* 76–81.

De Ferranti, D. (1985). *Paying for health services in developing countries: An overview* (Staff Working Paper 721). Washington, DC: World Bank.

Deolalikar, A. B. (1988). Nutrition and labor productivity in agriculture: Estimates for rural South India. *Review of Economics and Statistics, 70*(3), 406–413.

Dholakia, R. H., & Almeida, J. (1997). *The potential economic benefits of the DOTS strategy against TB in India.* Geneva, Switzerland: Global TB Program of the World Health Organization, Research and Surveillance Unit.

Dow, W. H., Gertler, P., Schoeni, R. F., Strauss, J., & Thomas, D. (2003). *Health care prices, health, and labor outcomes: Experimental evidence* (Population Studies Center Report No. 03-542). Ann Arbor, MI: University of Michigan.

Dwyer, D. S., & Mitchell, O. S. (1999). Health problems as determinants of retirement: Are self-rated measures endogenous? *Journal of Health Economics, 18,* 173–193.

Easterlin, R. A. (1999). How beneficent is the market? A look at the modern history of mortality. *European Review of Economic History, 3*(3), 257–294.

The economic crisis and suicide. (2009). *British Medical Journal, 338,* b1891.

Enthoven, A. (2000). In pursuit of an improving National Health Service. *Health Affairs, 19,* 102–119.

Ettner, S., Frank, R., & Kessler, R. (1997). The impact of psychiatric disorders on labor market outcomes. *Industrial and Labor Relations Review, 51*(1), 64–81.

Fabricant, S. J., Kamara, C. W., & Mills, A. (1999). Why the poor pay more: Household curative expenditures in rural Sierra Leone. *International Journal of Health Planning and Management, 14*(3), 179–199.

Farrell, P., & Fuchs, V. (1982). Schooling and health: The cigarette connection. *Journal of Health Economics, 1,* 217–230.

Feachem, R. G. A. (2000). The future of the NHS: Confronting the big questions. *Health Affairs, 19,* 128–129.

Federal Reserve Bank of San Francisco. (1998). *Economic letter* (No. 98-12). San Francisco: Author.

Field, E., Robles, O., & Torero, M. (2009). Iodine deficiency and schooling attainment in Tanzania. *American Economic Journal: Applied Economics, 1*(4), 140–169.

Flynn, J. R. (1998). IQ gains over time: Toward finding the causes. In U. Neisser (Ed.), *The rising curve: Long-term gains in IQ and related measures* (pp. 25–66). Washington, DC: American Psychological Association.

Fogel, R. W. (1994). Economic growth, population theory, and physiology: The bearing of long-term processes on the making of economic policy. *American Economic Review, 84*(3), 369–395.

Fogel, R. W. (1997). New findings on secular trends in nutrition and mortality: Some implications for population theory. In M. R. Rosenzweig & O. Stark (Eds.), *Handbook of population and family economics* (Vol. 1A, pp. 433–481). Amsterdam: Elsevier Science.

Fogel, R. W. (2005). Changes in the disparities in chronic diseases during the course of the 20th century. *Perspectives in Biology and Medicine, 48* (1 suppl), S150–S165.

Food and Agriculture Organization (FAO). (2009). *The state of food insecurity in the world 2009: Economic crises impacts and lessons learned.* Rome: Author.

Frankenberg, E., Thomas, D., & Beegle, K. (1999). *The real costs of Indonesia's economic crisis: Preliminary findings from the Indonesia Family Life Surveys.* RAND Labor and Population Program Working Paper Series 99-04. Los Angeles: RAND and UCLA.

Fuchs, V. R. (1993). *The future of health policy.* Cambridge, MA: Harvard University Press.

Gallup, J. L., & Sachs, J. (2001). The economic burden of malaria. *American Journal of Tropical Medicine and Hygiene, 64*(1–2 suppl), 85–96.

Gallup, J. L., Sachs, J., & Mellinger, A. D. (1999). Geography and economic development. *International Regional Science Review, 22,* 179–232.

Gardner, G. W., Edgerton, V. R., Senewiratne, B., Barnard, R. J., & Ohira, Y. (1975). Physical work capacity and metabolic stress in subjects with iron deficiency anemia. *American Journal of Clinical Nutrition, 30,* 910–917.

Gauthier, A. K., Rogal, D. L., Barrand, N. L., & Cohen, A. B. (1992). Administrative costs in the U.S. health care system: The problem or the solution? *Inquiry, 29,* 308–320.

Gertler, P., & Sturm, R. (1997). Private health insurance and public expenditures in Jamaica. *Journal of Econometrics, 77,* 237–257.

Gertler, P., & van der Gaag, J. (1988). *Measuring the willingness to pay for social service in developing countries.* Washington, DC: World Bank.

Gertler, P., & van der Gaag, J. (1990). The willingness to pay for medical care. Baltimore: Evidence from two developing countries. Baltimore, MD: Johns Hopkins University Press.

Glewwe, P., & King, E. M. (2001). The impact of early childhood nutritional status on cognitive development: Does the timing of malnutrition matter? *World Bank Economic Review, 15*(1), 81–113.

Grossman, M. (1975). The correlation between health and schooling. In N. E. Terleckyj (Ed.), *Household production and consumption* (pp. 147–224). New York: National Bureau of Economic Research, Columbia University Press.

Gruber, J., & Hanratty, M. (1993). *The labor market effects of introducing national health insurance: Evidence from Canada* (Working Paper No. 4589). Cambridge, MA: National Bureau of Economic Research.

Gruber, J., & Madrian, B. C. (1994). Health insurance and job mobility: The effects of public policy on job-lock. *Industrial and Labor Relations Review, 48*(1), 86–102.

Gruber, J., & Madrian, B. C. (1995). Health insurance availability and the retirement decision. *American Economic Review, 85*(4), 938–948.

Haacker, M. (2004). *The macroeconomics of HIV/AIDS.* Washington, DC: International Monetary Fund.

Handa, S., & Neitzert, M. (1998). *Chronic illness and retirement in Jamaica* (Living Standards Measurement Study Working Paper No. 131). Washington, DC: World Bank.

Hanratty, M. (1996). Canadian national health insurance and infant health. *American Economic Review, 86*(91), 276–284.

Hilborne, L. H., Leape, L. L., Bernstein, S. J., Park, R. E., Fiske, M. E., Kamberg, C. J., et al. (1993). The appropriateness of use of percutaneous transluminal coronary angioplasty in New York state. *Journal of the American Medical Association, 269,* 761–765.

Holtz-Eakin, D. (1994). Health insurance provision and labor market efficiency in the United States and Germany. In R. M. Blank (Ed.), *Social protection versus economic flexibility* (pp. 157–188). Chicago: University of Chicago Press.

Hoddinott, J., Maluccio, J., Behrman, J., Flores, R., & Martorell, R. (2008). Effect of a nutrition intervention during early childhood on economic productivity in Guatemalan adults. *Lancet, 371*(9610), 411–416.

Hsiao, W. (2000). *What should macroeconomists know about health care policy? A primer.* Washington, DC: International Monetary Fund.

Hübler, O. (2009). The nonlinear link between height and wages in Germany, 1985–2004. *Economics and Human Biology, 7*(2), 191–199.

Hurst, J. (2000). Challenges for health systems in member countries of the Organisation for Economic Co-operation and Development. *Bulletin of the World Health Organization, 78,* 751–760.

Jamison, D. T. (2009, October). *Financial protection and cost-effectiveness analysis in health.* Paper presented at the McArthur Foundation Forum on Benefit–Cost Analysis in Social Policy, Washington, DC.

Jamison, D. T., Jha, P., & Bloom, D. E. (2007). *Disease control.* Paper prepared for the Copenhagen Consensus, 2008.

Jamison, D. T., Lau, L. J., & Wang, J. (2005). Health's contribution to economic growth in an environment of partially endogenous technical progress. In G. Lopez-Casasnovas, B. Rivera, & L. Currais (Eds.), *Health and economic growth* (pp. 67–91). Cambridge, MA: MIT Press.

Jamison, D. T., & Leslie, J. (1990). Health and nutrition considerations in education planning. 2. The cost and effectiveness of school-based interventions. *Food and Nutrition Bulletin, 12*(3), 204–214.

Jamison, D. T, Sachs, J., & Wang, J. (2001). *The effect of the AIDS epidemic on economic welfare in sub-Saharan Africa* (Working Paper WG 1). Geneva, Switzerland: World Health Organization Commission on Macroeconomics and Health.

Jamison, D. T., Sandbu, M., & Wang, J. (2004). *Why has infant mortality declined at such different rates in different countries?* (Working Paper No. 21). Bethesda, MD: Disease Control Priorities Project.

Jamison, E. A., Jamison, D. T., & Hanushek, E. A. (2007). The effect of education quality on income growth and mortality decline. *Economics of Education Review, 26,* 771–788.

Jimenez, E. (1987). *Pricing policy in the social sectors: cost recovery for education and health in developing countries.* Baltimore, MD: Johns Hopkins University Press.

Kalemli-Ozcan, S. (2002). Does the mortality decline promote economic growth? *Journal of Economic Growth, 7,* 411–439.

Karlsson, M., Nilsson, T., Lyttkens, C. H., & Lesson, G. (2010). Income inequality and health: Importance of a cross-country perspective. *Social Science and Medicine, 70,* 875–885.

Kates, J., Boortz, K., Lief, E., Avila, C., & Gobet, B. (2010). *Financing the response to AIDS in low-and middle-income countries: International assistance from the G8, European Commission and other donor governments in 2009.* The Henry J. Kaiser Family Foundation & UNAIDS. Retrieved from http://www.stimson.org/images/uploads/research-pdfs/2009_Report.pdf

Kawachi, I., Adler, N. E., & Dow, W. H. (2010). Money, schooling, and health: Mechanisms and causal evidence. *Annals of the New York Academy of Sciences, 1186,* 56–68.

Kenkel, D. S. (1991). Health behavior, health knowledge, and schooling. *Journal of Political Economy, 99,* 287–305.

Keogh-Brown, M., & Smith, R. (2008). The economic impact of SARS: How does the reality match the predictions? *Health Policy, 88*(1), 110–120.

Keogh-Brown, M. R., Smith, R. D., Edmunds, J. W., Beutels, P. (2009). The macroeconomic impact of pandemic influenza: Estimates from models of the United Kingdom, France, Belgium and the Netherlands. *European Journal of Health Economics.* doi: 10.1007/s10198-009-0210.1

Kim, A., & Benton, B. (1995). *Cost–benefit analysis of the Onchocerciasis Control Program (OCP)* (World Bank Technical Paper No. 282). Washington, DC: World Bank.

Kim, H.-J., & Ruger, J. (2010). Socioeconomic disparities in behavioral risk factors and health outcomes by gender in the Republic of Korea. *BMC Public Health,* 10(1):195

Kleinman, A. M., Bloom, B. R., Saich, A., Mason, K. A., & Aulino, F. (2008). Introduction: Avian and pandemic influenza: A biosocial approach. *Journal of Infectious Diseases, 197,* S1–S3.

Kleinman, L. C., Kosecoff, J., Dubois, R. W., & Brook, R. H. (1994). The medical appropriateness of tympanostomy tubes proposed for children younger than 16 years in the United States. *Journal of the American Medical Association, 271,* 1250–1255.

Knaul, F. M. (1999). *Linking health, nutrition and wages: The evolution of age at menarche and labor earnings among adult Mexican women* (Working Paper Series R-355). Washington, DC: Inter-American Development Bank.

Knaul, F. M., & Parker, S. M. (1998). *Patterns over time and determinants of early labor force participation and school dropout: Evidence from longitudinal and retrospective data on Mexican children and youth.* Paper presented at the 1998 meeting of the Population Association of America.

Kuh, D., & Ben-Shlomo, Y. (Eds.). (1997). *A life course approach to chronic disease epidemiology.* Oxford, UK: Oxford University Press.

Leape, L. L., Hilborne, L. H., Park, R. E., Bernstein, S. J., Kamberg, C. J., Sherwood, M., & Brook, R. H. (1993). The appropriateness of use of coronary artery bypass graft surgery in New York state. *Journal of the American Medical Association, 269,* 753–760.

Leape, L. L., Park, R. E., Solomon, D. H., Chassin, M. R., Kosecoff, J., & Brook, R. H. (1990). Does inappropriate use explain small-area variations in the use of health care services? *Journal of the American Medical Association, 263,* 669–672.

Le Grand, J. (1987). Inequalities in health: Some international comparisons. *European Economic Review, 31,* 182–191.

Leibenstein, H. (1957). *Economic backwardness and economic growth.* New York: John Wiley & Sons.

Leighton, C., & Foster, R. (1993). *Economic impacts of malaria in Kenya and Nigeria* (Major Applied Research Paper No. 6). Bethesda, MD: Abt Associates.

Leslie, J., & Jamison, D. T. (1990). Health and nutrition considerations in education planning. 1: Educational consequences of health problems among school-age children. *Food and Nutrition Bulletin, 12,* 204–214.

Liu, Y., Hu, S., Fu, W., & Hsiao, W. C. (1996). Is community financing necessary and feasible for rural China? *Health Policy, 38*(3), 155–171.

Liu, H., & Hummer, R. A. (2008). Are educational differences in U.S. self-rated health increasing? An examination by gender and race. *Social Science and Medicine, 67,* 1898–1906.

Lomborg, B. (2009). *Global crises, global solutions.* Cambridge, UK: Cambridge University Press.

Lu, C., Schneider, M. T., Gubbins, P., Leach-Kemon, K., Jamison, D., & Murray, C. J. L. (2010). Public financing of health in developing countries: A cross-national systematic analysis. *Lancet, 375,* 1375–1387.

Madrian, B. C. (1994). Employment-based health insurance and job mobility: Is there evidence of job-lock? *Quarterly Review of Economics, 109*(1), 27–54.

Malaney, P., Spielman, A., & Sachs, J. (2004). The malaria gap. *American Journal of Tropical Medicine and Hygiene, 71*(suppl 2), 141–146.

Manski, R. J., Moeller, J., Schimmel, J., St Clair, P. A., Chen, H., Magder, L., & Pepper, J. V. (2010). Dental care coverage and retirement. *Journal of Public Health Dentistry, 70*(1), 1–12.

Marmot, M. G., Smith, G. D., Stansfeld, S., Patel, C., North, F., Head, J., et al. (1991). Health inequalities among British civil servants: The Whitehall II study. *Lancet, 337,* 1387–1393.

Marmot, M. G., & Theorell, T. (1988). Social class and cardiovascular disease: The contribution of work. *International Journal of Health Services, 18,* 659–674.

Martorell, R., Melgar, P., Maluccio, J. A., Stein, A. D., & Rivera, J. A. (2010). The nutrition intervention improved adult human capital and economic productivity. *Journal of Nutrition, 140,* 411–414.

McIntosh, C. N., Finès, P., Wilkins, R., & Wolfson, M. C. (2009). Income disparities in health-adjusted life expectancy for Canadian adults, 1991 to 2001. *Health Reports, 20,* 55–64.

McIntyre, D., Thiede, M., Dahlgren, G., & Whitehead, M. (2006). What are the economic consequences for households of illness and of paying for health care in low- and middle-income country contexts? *Social Science and Medicine, 62*(4), 858–865.

Miguel, E., & Kremer, M. (2004). Worms: Identifying impacts on education and health in the presence of treatment externalities. *Econometrica, 72*(1), 159–217.

Mills, A., & Shillcutt, S. (2004). Communicable diseases. In B. Lomborg (Ed.), *Global crises, global solutions* (pp. 62–128). Cambridge, UK: Cambridge University Press.

Mirrlees, J. (1975). A pure theory of underdeveloped economies. In L. G. Reynolds (Ed.), *Agriculture in development theory.* New Haven, CT: Yale University Press.

Moffett, J. K., Torgerson, D., Bell-Syer, S., Jackson, D., Llewlyn-Phillips, H., Farrin, A., & Barber, J. (1999). Randomized controlled trial of exercise for low back pain: Clinical outcomes, costs, and preferences. *British Medical Journal, 319,* 279–283.

Monheit, A. C., & Cooper, P. F. (1994). Health insurance and job mobility: Theory and evidence. *Industrial and Labor Relations Review, 48*(1), 68–85.

Murray, C. J. L., Lopez, A. D., & Jamison, D. T. (1994). The global burden of disease in 1990: Summary results, sensitivity analysis, and future directions. In C. J. L. Murray & A. Lopez (Eds.), *Global comparative assessments in the health sector: Disease burden, expenditures, and intervention packages* (pp. 97–138). Geneva, Switzerland: World Health Organization.

Murrugarra, E., & Valdivia, M. (1999). *The returns to health for Peruvian urban adults: Differentials across genders, the life-cycle and the wage distribution* (Documento de Trabajo R-352). Washington, DC: Inter-American Development Bank.

Mwabu, G., & Wang'ombe, J. (1995). *User charges in Kenya: Health service pricing reforms in Kenya, 1989–1993: A report on work in progress with support from the International Health Policy Program.* Washington, DC: International Health Policy Program.

Myrdal, G. (1952). Economic aspects of health. *Chronicle of the World Health Organization, 6,* 203–218.

Newhouse, J. P. (1993). *Free for all? Lessons from the RAND health insurance experiment.* Cambridge, MA: Harvard University Press.

Nguyen, K. T., Khuat, O. T. H., Ma, S., Pham, D. D., Khuat, G. T. H, & Ruger, J. P. (Under review). Impact of health expenses on household capabilities and resource allocation in Hanoi, Vietnam.

Nordhaus, W. (2003). The health of nations: The contribution of improved health to living standards. In K. H. Murphy & R. H. Topel (Eds.), *Measuring the gains from medical research: An economic approach* (pp. 9–40). Chicago: University of Chicago Press.

Over, M. (1992). *The macroeconomic impact of AIDS in sub-Saharan Africa* (Population and Nutrition Technical Working Paper No. 3.). Washington, DC: World Bank.

Over, M., Bertozzi, S., & Chin, J. (1989). Guidelines for rapid estimation of the direct and indirect costs of HIV infection in a developing country. *Health Policy, 11,* 169–186.

Poullier, J.-P. (1992). Administrative costs in selected industrialized countries. *Health Care Financing Review, 13*(4), 167–172.

Preker, A. S., Harding, A., & Travis, P. (2000). "Make or buy" decisions in the production of health care goods and services: New insights from institutional economics and organizational theory.

Bulletin of the World Health Organization, 78, 779–790.

Prescott, N., & Pradhan, M. (1999, February). *Coping with catastrophic health shocks.* Revised draft prepared for the Conference on Poverty and Social Protection, Inter-American Development Bank, Washington, DC.

Preston, S. H. (1980). Causes and consequences of mortality decline in less developed countries during the twentieth century. In R. A. Easterlin (Ed.), *Population and economic change in developing countries* (pp. 289–360). Chicago: University of Chicago Press.

Preston, S. H. (2007). The changing relation between mortality and level of economic development. *International Journal of Epidemiology, 36,* 484–490.

Preston, S. H., & Elo, I. T. (1995). Are educational differentials in adult mortality increasing in the United States? *Journal of Aging and Health, 7,* 476–496.

Pritchett, L., & Summers, L. (1996). Wealthier is healthier. *Journal of Human Resources, 31*(4), 841–868.

Protecting health during the economic crisis. (2008). *Lancet, 372,* 1520.

Radelet, S., Sachs, J. D., & Lee, J.-W. (1997). *Economic growth and transformation* (Development Discussion Paper No. 609). Cambridge, MA: Harvard Institute for International Development.

Reddy, S., & Vandemoortele, J. (1996). *User financing of basic social services: A review of theoretical arguments and empirical evidence.* New York: Office of Evaluation, Policy and Planning, UNICEF.

Remler, D. K., & Greene, J. (2009). Cost-sharing: A blunt instrument. *Annual Review of Public Health, 30,* 293–311.

Ribero, R., & Nunez, J. (1999). *Productivity of household investment in health: The case of Colombia* (Working Paper R-354). Washington, DC: Inter-American Development Bank.

Richards, T. (2009). Governments must act now to prevent slide into poverty and ill health after recession. *British Medical Journal, 339,* b4087.

Robins, L. N., & Regier, D. A. (1991). *Psychiatric disorders in America: The epidemiologic catchment area study.* New York: Free Press.

Roehr, B. (2010). International AIDS relief stagnated in 2009. *British Medical Journal, 341,* c3942.

Ruger, J. P. (1998). *Aristotelian justice and health policy: Capability and incompletely theorized agreements.* Unpublished doctoral dissertation, Harvard University, Cambridge, MA.

Ruger, J. P. (2003a). Health and development. *Lancet, 362,* 678.

Ruger, J. P. (2003b). Catastrophic health expenditure. *Lancet, 362,* 996–997.

Ruger, J. P. (2004a). Health and social justice. *Lancet, 364*(9439), 1075–1080.

Ruger, J. P. (2004b). Ethics of the social determinants of health. *Lancet, 364*(9439), 1092–1097.

Ruger, J. P. (2006a). Health, capability, and justice: Toward a new paradigm of health ethics, policy, and law. *Cornell Journal of Law and Public Policy, 15*(2), 101–187.

Ruger, J. P. (2006b). Toward a theory of a right to health: Capability and incompletely theorized agreements. *Yale Journal of Law and the Humanities, 18,* 273–326.

Ruger, J. P. (2007). The moral foundations of health insurance. *Quarterly Journal of Medicine, 100*(1), 53–57.

Ruger, J. P., & Kim, H.-J. (2007). Out-of-pocket healthcare spending by the poor and chronically ill in the Republic of Korea. *American Journal of Public Health, 97*(5), 804–811.

Ruger, J. P., & Kress, D. (2007). Health financing and insurance reform in Morocco. *Health Affairs, 26*(4), 1009–1016.

Ruger, J. P., Malaney, P., Jamison, D., & Bloom, D. (1998). *Health, Health Policy, and Economic Out-comes.* Final Report for Health and Development Satellite, World Health Organization Director-General Transition Team, World Health Organization, 12 August.

Sahn, D. E., & Alderman, H. (1988). The effect of human capital on wages, and the determinants of labor supply in a developing country. *Journal of Development Economics, 29*(2), 157–183.

Sauerborn, R., Nougtara, A., & Latimer, E. (1994). The elasticity of demand for health care in Burkina Faso: Differences across age and income groups. *Health Policy & Planning, 9*(2), 185–192.

Saunderson, P. R. (1995). An economic evaluation of alternative programme designs for tuberculosis control in rural Uganda. *Social Science Medicine, 40*(9), 1203–1212.

Savedoff, W. D., & Schultz, T. P. (2000). *Wealth from health: Linking social investments to earnings in Latin America.* Washington, DC: Inter-American Development Bank.

Schieber, G., & Maeda, A. (1997). A curmudgeon's guide to financing health care in developing countries. In G. J. Schieber (Ed.), *Innovations in health care financing: Proceedings of a World Bank conference, March 10–11, 1997* (World Bank Discussion Paper No. 365) (pp. 1–38). Washington, DC: World Bank.

Schultz, T. P. (1996). *Wage rentals for reproducible human capital: Evidence from two West African countries.* New Haven, CT: Yale University, Economic Growth Center.

Schultz, T. P. (1997). Assessing the productive benefits of nutrition and health: An integrated human capital approach. *Journal of Econometrics, 77,* 141–158.

Schultz, T. P. (1999). Health and schooling investments in Africa. *Journal of Economic Perspectives, 13*(3), 67–88.

Schultz, T. P. (2002). Wage gains associated with height as a form of health human capital. *American Economic Review, 92,* 349–353.

Shastry, G. K., & Weil, D. N. (2002). How much of cross-country income variation is explained by health? *Journal of the European Economic Association, 1,* 387–396.

Smith, J. P. (1999). Healthy bodies and thick wallets: The dual relation between health and economic status. *Journal of Economic Perspectives, 13*(2), 145–166.

Smith, J. P. (2009). The impact of childhood health on adult labor market outcomes. *Review of Economics and Statistics, 91*(3), 478–489.

Smith, R. D. (2006). Responding to global infectious disease outbreaks: Lessons from SARS on the role of risk perception, communication and management. *Social Science & Medicine, 63*(12), 3113–3123.

Smith, R. D., Keogh-Brown, M. R., Barnett, T., & Tait, J. (2009). The economy-wide impact of epidemic influenza on the UK: A computable general equilibrium modeling experiment. *British Medical Journal, 339.*

Spurr, G. B. (1983). Nutritional status and physical work capacity. *Yearbook of Physical Anthropology, 26,* 1–35.

Strauss, J., & Thomas, D. (1995). Human resources: Empirical modeling of household and family decisions. In J. Behrman & T. N. Srinivasan (Eds.), *Handbook in development economics* (Vol. 3A) (pp. 1883–2023). Amsterdam: Elsevier Science.

Stuckler, D., Basu, S., Suhrcke, M., Coutts, A., & McKee, M. (2009). The public health effect of economic crises and alternative policy responses in Europe: An empirical analysis. *Lancet, 374,* 315–323.

Sullivan, P. W., Ghushchyan, V., Huang, X. Y., & Globe, D. R. (2010). Influence of rheumatoid arthritis on employment, function, and productivity in a nationally representative sample in the United States. *Journal of Rheumatology, 37*(3), 544–549.

Svedberg, P. (2000). *Poverty and undernutrition: Theory, measurement and poverty.* Oxford, UK: Oxford University Press.

Thomas, D., & Strauss, J. (1997). Health and wages: Evidence on men and women in urban Brazil. *Journal of Econometrics, 77,* 159–185.

Thomas, D., Frankenberg, E., Friedman, J., Habicht, J.-P., Hakimi, M., Jaswadi, et al. (2003). *Iron deficiency and the well-being of older adults: Early results from a randomized nutrition intervention.* Unpublished manuscript, University of California–Los Angeles.

Thompson, J. E. (2007). Poverty, development, and women: Why should we care? *Journal of Obstetric, Gynecologic and Neonatal Nursing, 36*(6), 523–530.

Tipper, A. (2010). Economic models of the family and the relationship between economic status and health. *Social Science and Medicine.* [Epub ahead of print].

UNAIDS. (2009). *The global economic crisis and HIV prevention and treatment programmes: Vulnerabilities and impact.* Geneva, Switzerland: Author.

U.S. Bureau of Labor Statistics. (2010). *Economic news release: Employer costs for employee compensation news release text.* Washington, DC: Author.

U.S. Congress. (1994). *International comparisons of administrative costs in health care* (Office of Technology Assessment Publication No. BP-H-135). Washington, DC: U.S. Government Printing Office.

Usher, D. (1973). An imputation to the measure of economic growth for changes in life expectancy. In M. Moss (Ed.), *The measurement of economic and social performance* (pp. 193–226). Chicago: University of Chicago Press for National Bureau of Economic Research.

Uutela, A. (2010). Economic crisis and mental health. *Current Opinion in Psychiatry, 23,* 127–130.

Van de Walle, D. (1994). The benefit-incidence of social sector public expenditures in Indonesia. *World Bank Economic Review, 8,* 115–134.

Van Doorslaer, E., Wagstaff, A., & Rutten, F. (1993). *Equity in the finance and delivery of health care: An international perspective.* Oxford, UK: Oxford University Press.

Veenstra, N., & Whiteside, A. (2005). Economic impact of HIV. *Best Practice and Research Clinical Obstetrics and Gynaecology, 19*(2), 197–210.

Viscusi, W. K., & Aldy, J. E. (2003). The value of a statistical life: A critical review of market estimates from around the world. *Journal of Risk and Uncertainty, 27*, 5–76.

Waddington, C., & Enyimayew, K. (1990). A price to pay, part 2: The impact of user charges in the Volta region of Ghana. *International Journal of Health Planning and Management, 5*(4), 287–312.

Wang, J., Jamison, D. T., Bos, E., Preker, A., & Peabody, J. (1999). *Measuring country performance on health: Selected indicators for 115 countries.* Washington, DC: World Bank.

Wang'ombe, J. (1997). Cost recovery strategies in sub-Saharan Africa. In G. J. Schieber (Ed.), *Innovations in health care financing: Proceedings of a World Bank conference, March 10–11, 1997* (World Bank Discussion Paper No. 365, pp. 155–161). Washington, DC: World Bank.

Weil, D. N. (2007). Accounting for the effect of health on economic growth. *Quarterly Journal of Economics, 122*, 1265–1306.

Wilder-Smith, A. (2006). The severe acute respiratory syndrome: Impact on travel and tourism. *Travel Medicine and Infectious Disease, 4*(2), 53–60.

Wilkinson, D., Floyd, K., & Gilks, C. F. (1997). Costs and cost-effectiveness of alternative tuberculosis management strategies in South Africa: Implications for policy. *South African Medical Journal, 87*(4), 451–455.

Wilkinson, R. G. (Ed.). (1986). *Class and health: Research and longitudinal data.* New York: Tavistock.

Wilkinson, R. G. (1990). Income distribution and mortality: A natural experiment. *Health and Illness, 12*, 391–412.

Winslow, C. M., Kosecoff, J. B., Chassin, M., Kanouse, D. E., & Brook, R. H. (1988). The appropriateness of performing coronary artery bypass surgery. *Journal of the American Medical Association, 260*, 505–509.

Winslow, C. M., Solomon, D. H., Chassin, M. R., Kosecoff, J., Merrick, N. J., & Brook, R. H. (1988). The appropriateness of carotid endarterectomy. *New England Journal of Medicine, 318*, 721–727.

Woolhandler, S., & Himmelstein, D. U. (1991). The deteriorating administrative efficiency of the U.S. health care system. *New England Journal of Medicine, 324*(18), 1253–1258.

Woolhandler, S., & Himmelstein, D. U. (1997). Costs of care and administration at for-profit and other hospitals in the United States. *New England Journal of Medicine, 336*(11), 769–774.

Woolhandler, S., Himmelstein, D. U., & Lewontin, J. P. (1993). Administrative costs in U.S. hospitals. *New England Journal of Medicine, 329*(6), 400–403.

World Bank. (1980). *World Bank development report.* Washington, DC: Author.

World Bank. (1993). *World development report 1993: Investing in health.* New York: Oxford University Press.

World Bank. (2010). *World development indicators.* Washington, DC: Author.

World Health Organization (WHO). (1999). *World health report 1999: Making a difference.* Geneva, Switzerland: Author.

World Health Organization (WHO). (2000). *World health report 2000. Health systems: Improving performance.* Geneva, Switzerland: Author.

World Health Organization (WHO). (2008). *The global burden of disease: 2004 update.* Geneva, Switzerland: Author.

World Health Organization (WHO). (2009). *Tuberculosis control in the Western Pacific Region: 2009 report.* Geneva, Switzerland: Author.

Yoder, R. A. (1989). Are people willing and able to pay for health services? *Social Science and Medicine, 29*, 35–42.

Zhang, Y. X., & Wang, S. R. (2010). Differences in development among children and adolescents in eastern and western China. *Annals of Human Biology.* [Epub ahead of print].

Evaluations of Large-Scale Health Programs

CESAR G. VICTORA, DAMIAN WALKER, BENJAMIN JOHNS, AND JENNIFER BRYCE

Why We Need Large-Scale Impact Evaluations

In spite of large investments aimed at improving health outcomes in low- and middle-income countries, there is a growing realization that few such programs and initiatives have been properly evaluated ("Evaluation," 2011; Evaluation Gap Working Group, 2006; Oxman et al., 2010). In addition, current interest in results-based financing (World Bank, 2010) is increasing the pressure on funders and implementers to carry out impact evaluations.

The Evaluation Gap Working Group (2006) has summarized the issue well:

Each year billions of dollars are spent on thousands of programs to improve health, education and other social sector outcomes in the developing world. But very few programs benefit from studies that could determine whether or not they actually made a difference. This absence of evidence is an urgent problem: it not only wastes money but denies poor people crucial support to improve their lives.

This chapter covers a specific area of evaluation science: the rationale for and design and implementation of summative evaluations of programs being scaled up—that is, being delivered to large populations (Mangham & Hanson, 2010). The chapter does not cover formative evaluations, which are aimed at improving program design prior to large-scale implementation, nor does it address program evaluations using qualitative methods.

The focus here is on evaluating the implementation of programs at scale that are aimed at delivering

several biological and/or behavioral interventions simultaneously. Most, if not all, interventions packaged in these programs have been submitted to randomized trials that established their efficacy—for example, vaccines, antibiotic or antiviral drugs, micronutrients, and insecticide-treated nets. Thus little doubt exists that these interventions would reduce mortality and improve health status, if delivered with appropriate quality to those who need them.

International and bilateral organizations often pay lip service to the need for evaluations of their large-scale initiatives. Some even pledge a given proportion of their program budgets for evaluation. Despite these lofty statements, very few comprehensive evaluations of large health programs have been carried out, perhaps because independent evaluations can be threatening, given their potential for revealing shortcomings or lack of impact of a program.

Such evaluations often include several players with different—and sometimes conflicting—interests: the funders of a program or initiative (e.g., foundations or bilateral organizations); program implementers (e.g., international organizations such as the World Health Organization [WHO] or UNICEF, their country missions, and national government counterparts); and the external evaluation team. In this chapter, we provide our perspective as independent evaluators. Although we focus on the technical aspects of design, implementation, and analyses, we also use our experience in a number of multicountry studies to highlight the political tensions that inevitably underlie evaluation science.

Throughout this chapter, three evaluations are consistently used as examples: the Multi-Country Evaluation of the Integrated Management of Childhood

Illness (Exhibit 16-1), a retrospective evaluation of the Accelerated Child Survival and Development Initiative (Exhibit 16-2), and an evaluation of the Tanzanian national voucher scheme for insecticide-treated nets (Exhibit 16-3).

Planning the Evaluation

Who Will Carry Out the Evaluation?

Internal evaluations are carried out by the implementing institutions themselves, sometimes with the help of external consultants for specific tasks. Such evaluations often address levels of inputs and utilization (e.g., whether expected quantities of drugs or mosquito nets were procured and distributed) and issues related to process (e.g., surveys of the quality of care being provided or the frequency of supervision). Less frequently, internal evaluations include population-based coverage surveys, which may be subcontracted to consultants. Internal evaluations are classified into two main categories: Either they are formative—that is, aimed at improving the program in its early implementation stage—or they are summative—that is, attempting to document an effect of the program on coverage levels or on health indicators. They may or may not include a comparison with other areas without the program. The main characteristic of internal evaluations is the lack of independence between implementers and evaluators, which creates an obvious conflict of interest because the continuity of funding for the program is affected by evaluation results. Nevertheless, internal evaluations are essential for fine-tuning a program.

External, or independent evaluations, are carried out by researchers who are not involved in implementation. As a rule, the evaluation is funded by a third party—either the institution that provided funds for the implementation agency or an outside agency, such as the International Initiative for Impact Evaluation (3ie; http://www.3ieimpact.org/). Although external evaluators must collaborate closely with the implementation team—as will be discussed later in this chapter—they

---

Exhibit 16-1 **The Multi-Country IMCI Evaluation**

Integrated Management of Childhood Illness (IMCI) is a strategy for reducing mortality among children younger than five years of age, and is supported by WHO, UNICEF, and their technical partners (Tulloch, 1999). IMCI began with a set of case management guidelines for the integrated management of sick children in a first-level health facility designed to address the major causes of child mortality and undernutrition. It was soon extended beyond improving health worker skills to the improvement of health systems support (including supervision, drug supply, and health information systems) and promotion of 12 key family and community practices related to child health—such as appropriate care seeking and home management of illnesses—that would act synergistically with improving health worker skills at the facility level. IMCI was first introduced at country level in 1996 by Tanzania and Uganda. Within a decade, however, this strategy had been adopted at national level by ministries of health in more than 100 countries. Further information on IMCI is available at http://www.who.int/child_adolescent_health/topics/prevention_care/child/imci/en/index.html.

The Multi-Country Evaluation of IMCI Effectiveness, Cost and Impact, more simply known as MCE, provided information to ministries of health and technical assistance partners about the barriers to IMCI implementation at the ground level, the effects of the strategy on health services and communities, the cost of the program, and the number of lives it can save. A special focus was to provide the information needed to help countries adapt and improve on the strategy so that it could be fully implemented and delivered equitably and on a large scale. Although the evaluation was coordinated by WHO, all technical and scientific decisions were made by a technical advisory group of independent evaluators; in all countries, there were national academic counterparts who participated in designing the studies and carried out the fieldwork and data analyses.

Twelve countries participated in the initial round of MCE assessments and data collection about IMCI implementation. More in-depth studies were conducted in five countries: Bangladesh, Brazil, Peru, Tanzania, and Uganda. The study design varied according to the geographical spread of implementation. In Tanzania, two districts where IMCI was already being implemented were compared with two matched neighboring districts, taking advantage of the fact that all four districts had demographic surveillance efforts already under way. In Brazil, municipalities with strong, weak, or no IMCI implementation were compared. In Peru, the association between implementation strength and coverage and impact was investigated in all 24 departments in the country, whereas in Uganda a similar approach was used in 10 districts. Finally, in Bangladesh, it was possible to randomize 10 health facility catchment areas to IMCI and 10 areas to routine child health services.

Detailed descriptions of the MCE methods and results are available in various publications (Bryce, Victora, Habicht, Black, & Scherpbier, 2005; Bryce, Victora, Habicht, Vaughan, & Black, 2004) and on the study website: http://www.who.int/imci-mce/overview.htm.

Exhibit 16-2 | **The Retrospective Evaluation of the Accelerated Child Survival and Development Program**

The Accelerated Child Survival and Development program (ACSD) was implemented by UNICEF in 11 West African countries between 2001 and 2005 with support from the Canada International Development Agency. The aim of ACSD was to increase coverage for proven interventions grouped in three broad packages, labeled as EPI+ (immunizations, vitamin A supplementation, insecticide-treated nets), IMCI+ (case management of malaria, diarrhea, and pneumonia; breastfeeding promotion) and ANC+ (antenatal and delivery care, postnatal vitamin A supplementation, intermittent presumptive treatment of malaria). The ultimate aim of the program was to reduce under-five mortality by 20%.

In each participating country, ACSD high-impact districts were selected to scale up these interventions rapidly to full coverage. At the same time, a smaller set of interventions were supported, to a greater or lesser extent, in additional districts in each country—the so-called ACSD expansion areas. The countries that first moved ahead with rapid implementation were Benin, Ghana, Mali, and Senegal. More information on ACSD is available at the following website: www.unicef.org/health/index_childsurvival.html.

UNICEF commissioned the Bloomberg School of Public Health at Johns Hopkins University to conduct an independent retrospective evaluation of the ACSD project. The objective was to provide valid and timely evidence to child health planners and policy makers about the effectiveness of the ACSD project in reducing child mortality and improving child nutritional status, as a basis for strengthening child health programming in the future. From 2006 to 2008, the evaluation team reviewed documentation on ACSD implementation, evaluated intervention coverage using standard international indicators, and measured the program's impact, focusing on under-five mortality in Benin, Ghana, and Mali. An evaluation in Senegal was also started but could not be completed due to a lack of information on comparison areas. Because the evaluation was retrospective, information on coverage and mortality was obtained through reanalyses of national surveys, comparing the ACSD high-impact districts with the remaining rural districts in the country.

The evaluation results are available in a publication (Bryce et al., 2010) and at the following website: http://www.jhsph.edu/dept/ih/IIP/projects/acsd.html.

Exhibit 16-3 | **Evaluation of the Tanzanian National Voucher Scheme for Insecticide-Treated Nets**

Insecticide-treated nets (ITNs) are a cost-effective means of preventing malaria, which remains one of the major killers of children younger than the age of five in Africa. The Tanzania National Voucher Scheme is a targeted subsidy program that relies on the commercial sector to distribute ITNs throughout the country. Every pregnant woman who attends antenatal care in a government or nongovernmental organization (NGO) facility is eligible to receive a voucher that can be used as part payment for an ITN.

The Tanzania National Voucher Scheme was rolled out gradually, starting in late 2004 in districts near Dar es Salaam and ending with some of the most remote districts in the country 18 months later. Program managers decided that a phased roll-out was necessary on programmatic grounds because of the size of the country. It was not feasible or acceptable to randomize districts by roll-out phase. Nevertheless, the gradual scale-up allowed the evaluation team to compare areas with and without the voucher scheme at three points in time using cross-sectional household and facility surveys. Within-district changes were compared in the analysis with the length of time that the program had been operating in each district to determine whether program duration was associated with increases in net coverage.

The objectives of this study were to assess the changes in the level and socioeconomic distribution of ITN coverage over the period 2005–2007, during which the voucher scheme was initiated and expanded to a national scale, and to examine the link between program duration and change in household net ownership as a measure of program impact.

The evaluation was carried out by a team of U.K.- and Tanzania-based investigators (Hanson, Marchant, et al., 2009; Hanson, Nathan, et al., 2008; Mulligan, Yukich, & Hanson, 2008). Particular emphasis was given to describing the intermediate steps in the process leading to high ITN coverage, as well as to the assessment of costs and of impact of the program on reducing socioeconomic inequalities in net ownership.

---

retain a level of independence that is essential for ensuring the credibility of the evaluation findings and can contribute to both formative and summative evaluations. In both the IMCI (Lambrechts, Bryce, & Orinda, 1999) and ACSD evaluations (UNICEF, 2005), the results of internal evaluations proved to be more optimistic than later results from the independent team's external evaluation. This chapter focuses on external evaluations.

In-country research institutions that are independent of program evaluation can and should play an important role in these evaluations, bringing context-relevant experience and expertise to the team, serving as a first point of contact with program implementers, and providing continuity in the dissemination and eventual uptake of evaluation findings. The selection of the in-country research partners should be based on objective criteria that include research capacity relevant to the evaluation design and credibility with the ministry of health. Partnerships between in-country and external research institutions can result in expanded capacity and objectivity that will contribute to the success of the evaluation.

What Are the Evaluation Objectives?

The first task of the evaluation team is to review the available documentation on program objectives and goals, and to turn these items into evaluation objectives. This transformation is best achieved by involving implementers and funders at the very beginning of the evaluation design process.

An early decision is to agree upon what is being evaluated. For example, the MCE external evaluation team found it particularly difficult to define IMCI for the purpose of the evaluation, because the strategy required local adaptation and was implemented at different speeds in each setting. Thus an early challenge for the team was to decide whether the evaluation would be designed to assess the strategy as a whole or to assess each of the three component parts (community, health facilities, health systems) individually. Similarly, the ACSD strategy (Exhibit 16-2) included three packages—EPI+, IMCI+, and ANC+— that were implemented with variable intensities in different countries. Although it may be tempting to try to design the evaluation in ways that disentangle the effects of different components, in practice this parsing is often impossible, because one cannot predict which components will end up being more strongly implemented, and in which part of the country. Also, many strategies are designed to take advantage of the potential synergies among its components—for example, IMCI—so that trying to break down their effects contradicts the entire concept underlying the program. A related issue is the challenge of trying to attribute program impact to a single donor when a program is funded by several sources, each of which supports one or more components. The definition of what is being evaluated must be agreed upon with evaluation funders and program implementers early in the process of evaluation design.

Large-scale programs and initiatives often establish quantitative goals in terms of what they expect to achieve. These aims are frequently expressed in terms of coverage (e.g., 70% of all pregnant women

receiving a long-lasting mosquito net) or impact (e.g., a 25% reduction in under-five mortality). Program goals are often expressed in ways that allow different interpretations. For example, the target coverage of a program based in health facilities could be calculated for the whole population or only for those living within a given distance (catchment area) of the facility.

A more complex example is how to interpret a "25% reduction in mortality." In this case, four interpretations are possible:

- Endline mortality being 25% lower in program areas than baseline levels in the same areas

- Endline mortality being 25% lower in program areas than in comparison areas (regardless of baseline differences)

- The reduction in mortality from baseline to endline in program areas being 25% greater than the corresponding reduction in comparison areas

- The rate of decline over time in the program areas being 25% faster than the rate of decline in comparison areas (e.g., 5% annual decline in program and 4% annual decline in comparison areas)

These four options have very different implications for study design and sample size calculations, and it is essential to reach agreement on a common interpretation at the very beginning of the evaluation.

Once the overall evaluation objectives are defined, they must be broken down into specific evaluation questions that the study will try to answer. These questions are detailed later in this chapter.

The ultimate objective of an evaluation is to influence decisions. Evaluation objectives and design depend on who the decision maker is and which types of decisions will be taken as a consequence of the findings. Program funders—for example, high-income-country organizations providing aid to health programs in low-income countries—are typically interested in providing evidence to their governments and taxpayers that their funds led to a measurable impact on health outcomes, such as mortality. The decisions to be made in such cases include whether to continue funding the program and at what level, and whether the program strategy needs to be reformulated. Funders often work on a short timeline: They need results soon, in accordance with funding and electoral cycles. They also tend to be more interested in impact measurement than in intermediate results such as inputs, processes, outputs, or outcomes (these terms are defined later in this chapter).

In contrast, local implementers—for example, senior officials at the ministry of health—may seek reassurance that the program is moving in the right direction, that the quality of services is adequate, and that high population coverage is being or will be achieved. Their decisions are primarily related to improving the program through specific actions. Evaluation results may also have an important role in advocacy and provide political gains at country level.

Later in this chapter, we describe how important it is to build a conceptual model that takes into account the different needs of different partners and the decisions they must make as a result of the evaluation findings. Obtaining information on health impact measures such as mortality is important, but just as important is to understand why the program had—or failed to have—a measurable impact.

When to Plan the Evaluation?

Many advantages accrue from planning the evaluation at the time the program is being designed. Early-onset, prospective evaluations allow collection of baseline data before implementation starts. They also allow thorough, continuing documentation of program inputs and the contextual variables that may affect the program's impact. Under some circumstances, early planning may enable the evaluation team to influence how the program is rolled out, thereby improving the validity of future comparisons. A disadvantage of prospective evaluations including a program and a comparison group is that program implementation may change over time for reasons that are outside the control of the evaluation team—for example, similar activities may be implemented in the comparison districts, or some of the program districts may have insufficient implementation.

In reality, evaluation is often an afterthought. Studies are frequently launched when implementation is already under way—and in some cases after the program cycle is completed. Such retrospective evaluations have important limitations. Documentation requires the reconstruction of project assumptions and activities by requesting the assistance of project implementers to produce records of activities and inputs. In such cases, the resulting information is often incomplete, inconsistent, and difficult to verify. Baseline data are often unavailable, and even where they exist, they may be of poor quality, be based on sample sizes that are too small to address the evaluation questions, or lack information on all needed indicators. The importance of carrying out evaluations prospectively cannot be over-emphasized.

How Long Will the Evaluation Take?

The answer to this question depends on whether the evaluation is retrospective, prospective, or a mixture of both techniques (ambispective) (Kleinbaum, Kupper, & Morgenstern, 1982). Fully prospective evaluations include several sequential steps:

1. Collect baseline information
2. Wait until the large-scale program is fully implemented and reaches high population coverage
3. Allow time for a biological effect to take place in participating individuals
4. Wait until such effect can be measured in an endline survey
5. Clean the data and conduct the analysis

Each step can easily take one year, often longer. In our experience, Step 2 usually takes longer than initially anticipated, due to delays in staff deployment, training, and commodity procurement. Step 3 can be fairly short for interventions with a rapid effect on outcomes—for example, case management of disease episodes or interventions that prevent disease transmission such as insecticide-treated nets or indoor residual spraying for the prevention of malaria can reduce mortality rapidly. The time needed for an intervention to achieve its biological effect can be much longer for interventions that require changes in behavior, such as changing breastfeeding practices to improve nutrition. Step 4 can also slow down the production of final results. For example, assessment of child mortality is retrospective, and often the calendar midpoint of the mortality estimate is one to two years prior to the date of the endline survey. Cleaning the data and conducting a full analysis (Step 5) is often overlooked when planning an evaluation, but requires considerable time and effort to do well.

Donors, policy makers, and evaluation funders frequently organize their work in periodic cycles of five years or less. Prospective impact evaluations of complex programs under real-life conditions, however, often require longer time frames. Because few policy makers are willing to wait so long for study results, it is important that data on intermediate outcomes, such as quality of care or achieved coverage, become available in the first year or two of the evaluation. This issue is discussed in further detail in the section on implementation.

Where Will the Evaluation Be Carried Out?

Many large-scale programs are implemented simultaneously in more than one country. An early decision for the evaluation team is to select those countries that will participate in the study. This decision is usually taken in agreement with the implementation agencies, and will depend on factors such as the likely strength of the implementation (or, for retrospective or ambispective evaluations, the strength of implementation to date), the availability of local research partners, and the need for the group of countries to be reasonably representative of geographic areas or epidemiologic patterns (e.g., the presence or absence of high levels of HIV/AIDS or malaria). For example, when evaluating a program being rolled out in many low- and middle-income countries, selection criteria should include both characteristics that are desirable in all participating countries (e.g., political stability, availability of local research partners, likelihood of strong implementation of the program) and characteristics that are desirable in the set of countries as a whole (e.g., representation of countries that reflect the diversity of all implementing countries in terms of geography, health system strength, and epidemiological profiles).

It is important to keep track of the rationale for selecting some countries and not others, because these criteria will affect the external validity—or generalizability—of the evaluation findings (Bryce, Victora, et al., 2004). For example, if the evaluation is conducted only in countries that have performed well in implementing the program, then it is more likely that an impact of the program may be detected, but extrapolating to all implementing countries may not be justified.

The IMCI evaluation was largely prospective. Thus, although the 5 countries selected for in-depth evaluation were judged to best meet the selection criteria among the 12 originally assessed, there were wide variations in the strength of implementation and, therefore, reasonable external validity to support generalization of the findings (Bryce, et al., 2005). The ACSD evaluation in West Africa was retrospective, and UNICEF preselected 4 countries among the 11 participating in the program based on the fact that they were judged to have the strongest implementation of all program components. This decision likely introduced a positive bias into the design and limited the extent to which the results could be generalized to the remaining countries (Bryce et al., 2010).

Once the country or countries for the evaluation are defined, there is a need to select which districts will be included in the study or, less commonly, to design an evaluation that covers all districts in the country; these options are discussed later in this chapter. As discussed in the context of country selection, the criteria by which districts are chosen may strongly influence the external validity of the evaluation results.

Developing an Impact Model

The development of an impact model—also known as an operational model, a model of change, or a conceptual framework—for the program's assumed effects is an essential step in designing an evaluation of a large-scale program. The model should lay out how it is expected that the program inputs will lead to an effect on health.

A commonly used framework includes the following sequence: inputs → process → outputs → outcomes → impact. Inputs can include such diverse items as staff, drugs, and equipment or teaching materials. Process can include training, logistics, and management. Examples of outputs are the number of contacts with the population—for example, health services attendance rates or mosquito nets distributed. Outcomes are often expressed in terms of coverage with a given intervention—for example, the percentage of women giving birth at a healthcare facility or the proportion of children sleeping under an insecticide-treated mosquito net. Finally, impact refers to a change in health status—for example, reduced mortality or improved nutrition. This generic framework has to be adapted to each particular program. Exhibit 16-4 describes the IMCI strategy and its impact model (Bryce, Victora, Habicht, Black, & Scherpbier, 2005; Bryce, Victora, Habicht, Vaughan, & Black, 2004).

In the Tanzania ITN evaluation (Exhibit 16-3), a detailed model was designed that included several necessary steps for the voucher scheme processes to translate into effective coverage: Vouchers needed to be in stock; women needed to attend antenatal services; women had to receive and redeem their voucher; and women needed to sleep under the voucher net. Evidence from three sequential surveys was used to assess intermediate steps in the program pathway so as to inform judgments about its effect (Hanson et al., 2009).

Impact models are essential for several reasons. For instance, they help clarify the expectations of program planners and implementers, by laying them out clearly. They help estimate sample sizes, by defining what needs to be measured and what the magnitude of effects is likely to be. Most importantly, models contribute to the development of the evaluation proposal. For example, each box in Figure 16-1 generated relevant evaluation questions, indicators, and data collection strategies. The need to measure

Exhibit 16-4	**The IMCI Impact Model**

Figure 16-1 shows a simplified model of the pathways through which the developers of the strategy believed that IMCI would improve child health and nutrition. This model was originally developed by the evaluation team and refined through consultations with IMCI developers. For each box in the model, the evaluation team developed appropriate indicators and data collection procedures. The evaluation questions addressed the assumptions underlying this model, shown by the arrows in the figure. The impact model formed the backbone of the evaluation, serving as a common frame of reference for the evaluation team and program implementers, supporting estimates of needed sample sizes for various evaluation components, and providing a map for the data analysis that showed clearly the expected associations to be tested.

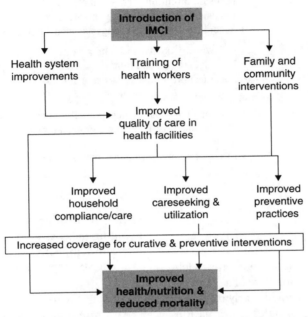

Figure 16-1 Example of an Impact Model: The Multi-Country Evaluation of IMCI (Integrated Management of Childhood Illness. *Source:* Bryce, Jennifer, Cesar G Victora, Jean-Pierre Habicht, Robert E Black, Robert W Scherpbier and on behalf of the MCE-IMCI Technical Advisors. *Health Policy and Planning.* 2005 (20supp1) "Programmatic pathways to child survival: results of a multi-country evaluation of Integrated Management of Childhood Illness" Figure 2. Page 4.

improved health worker performance, for instance, led to the development of health facility surveys based on the IMCI clinical guidelines, which were then implemented in several countries participating in the evaluation. Also, impact models help guide the analyses and attribution of the results—for example, if the evaluation finds a reduction in mortality in the absence of changes in the intermediate outcomes laid out in the model, it is unlikely that the observed impact can be attributed to the program.

Two other reasons for building impact models upfront can be cited. In a dynamic evaluation setting with feedback to implementers (described later in this chapter), models can help track changes in assumptions as these evolve in response to early evaluation findings. Models help implementers and evaluators stay honest about what was expected—unfortunately, program managers may be tempted to reinvent history by changing expectations as programs are rolled out and initial expectations are shown to be unrealistic.

The steps involved in developing and checking an impact model are summarized in Table 16-1. Impact models describe how a given program is expected to affect health. A later section of this chapter discusses how such models fit into a broader conceptual framework of factors influencing health status, which go beyond any given program and attempt to capture other determinants of health.

Table 16-1	Steps in the Development of an Impact Model
Step	**Details**

Learn about the program	▸ Read documents
	▸ Interview planners and implementers
	▸ Carry out field visits to future implementation areas
	▸ Use special techniques as needed
	  –Card-sorting exercise
	  –Challenges

Develop drafts of the model	▸ Focus on intentions and assumptions ▸ Document responses from implementers ▸ Record iterations and changes as model develops

Quantify and check assumptions	▸ Review existing evidence and literature
	▸ Identify early results from the evaluation
	  –Documentation: What was actually done?
	  –Outcomes: Are assumptions confirmed?

Use and evaluate the model	▸ Develop an evaluation design, testing each assumption if possible ▸ Plan for analysis, including contextual factors ▸ Analyze ▸ Interpret results with participation by implementers

A Stepwise Approach to Impact Evaluations

Figure 16-2 summarizes the basic stepwise approach to conducting an impact evaluation. Use of a stepwise approach allows evaluators to provide early feedback to program implementers and to halt the evaluation at midcourse if the implementation is not sufficiently strong to produce a measurable impact, thereby avoiding the costly surveys needed for assessing coverage and impact.

The six steps are as follows:

1. *Assess the technical soundness of implementation plans in light of local epidemiological and health services characteristics.* It is not un-

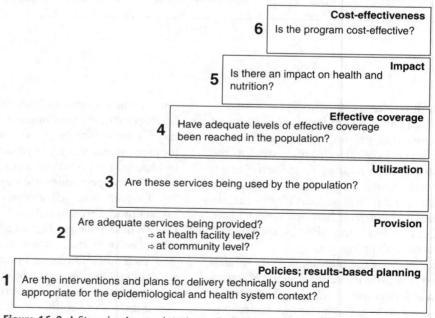

Figure 16-2 A Stepwise Approach to Large-Scale Impact Evaluations.

usual for programs to be imported into a country without a proper assessment of whether they address the leading causes of morbidity and mortality, or without a realistic evaluation of the health systems characteristics required for making the program work. In recent years, a variety of tools for estimating the impact of interventions in different epidemiological contexts have been developed. When considering the evaluation of a health facility–based program in Niger in the late 1990s, for example, the study was dismissed when a desk review showed an average of 0.5 annual visit per under-five child in the country, suggesting that the health systems were not strong enough to deliver the program in a short time frame. The Lives Saved Tool (LiST), which is described in detail later in this chapter, can contribute to this initial assessment (Johns Hopkins Bloomberg School of Public Health, n.d.).

2. *Investigate whether the quantity and quality of the program being provided are compatible with a potential impact.* The evaluation team makes this judgment using the documentation of program activities, combined—if applicable—with surveys assessing the quality of care being provided. For example, in the IMCI evaluation in Uganda, a health facility survey showed that quality of care was much lower than expected even after training large numbers of health workers in IMCI, and the evaluation was interrupted at this stage (Pariyo, Gouws, Bryce, & Burnham, 2005).

3. *Assess whether data on outputs or utilization suggest that an impact is likely.* Even if the program inputs seem sufficient in terms of quantity and quality, uptake by the population may be limited. For example, if the number of insecticide-treated nets (ITNs) effectively distributed in a country is much smaller than the number necessary to achieve adequate coverage in the target population, continuing the study to measure health impact would be unwarranted. This step is usually assessed through documentation of program outputs; it does not require household surveys.

4. *Check whether adequate coverage has been reached.* Even if outputs appear to be adequate, it is necessary to check whether they have effectively reached the population and are being used by the target groups. Making this determination usually requires a population survey, which will cost much more than assessing the preceding steps on the basis of documentation. Continuing with the ITN example, the nets that were distributed may have been sold to those not in the intervention area, or they may have been used by the heads of households instead of by the pregnant women and young children who constitute the primary targets of the program. Assessment of coverage applies not only to interventions based on commodities such as ITNs or vaccines, but also to health-related behaviors—for example, condom use, breastfeeding, or care seeking.

5. *Assess the impact on health.* Measuring health impact often requires costly surveys, and the stepwise approach may reveal shortcomings in the preceding steps that suggest an impact is unlikely. Impact attribution requires ruling out alternative explanations for the observed findings. This may prove to be difficult—and sometimes impossible, no matter how hard funders and implementers would like to produce an unequivocal statement. These issues are discussed in greater detail later in this chapter.

6. *Measure cost-effectiveness.* If there is evidence of an impact, the next question relates to cost-effectiveness. Measurement of program costs is discussed in subsequent sections of this chapter.

Types of Inference and Choice of Design

There is no single "best" design for evaluations of large-scale programs. Different types of decisions require different degrees of certainty to support their decisions. Whereas some decisions require randomized trials, other decisions may be adequately taken with observational studies. Also, the manner in which programs are rolled out often limits the scope of possible approaches to evaluation.

In real-world evaluations, the program of interest often accounts for a small part of the variability in the outcomes. Figure 16-3 presents a simplified framework showing that health outcomes may be also influenced by socioeconomic factors, by changes in existing health services in the public and private sectors (that are outside the scope of the program of interest), and by other programs in the health and other sectors present in the same geographical areas. We

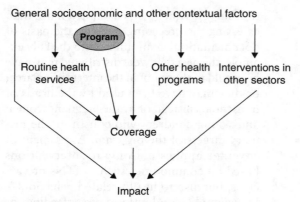

Figure 16-3 Simplified Conceptual Framework of Factors Affecting Health, from the Standpoint of Evaluation Design.

will refer to this framework when describing different evaluation designs.

Habicht et al. (1999) proposed that evaluations can be classified as one of three types in terms of strength of inference, according to the ways in which the factors described in Figure 16-3 are handled. The types of inference are discussed below in relation to possible evaluation designs.

Adequacy Evaluations

Adequacy evaluations assess whether initial targets were met in the program areas or, at the very least, whether trends moved in the expected direction in terms of coverage or impact measures. For example, for a health manager it may be sufficient to establish that 80% coverage with an intervention (e.g., a vaccine) has been reached in the district; this evidence is sufficient to support the continuation of the strategy for delivering this intervention. The manager does not require direct measurement of health impact, because the vaccine is already known to save lives in similar populations. Nevertheless, if appropriate, modeling tools (such as LiST, which is described later in the chapter) may be used to estimate the intervention's health impact.

Adequacy evaluations are often based on before-and-after studies in the program areas only, aimed at measuring progress in coverage or impact indicators. If the intervention included in the program is new to the geographical area, adequacy evaluations may be limited to an endline survey. Such a design is particularly suited to studies of coverage, in which a direct link exists between the program and the frequency of the intervention's use in the population.

Use of adequacy evaluations for impact assessments is more complex. Because adequacy evalua-

tions do not include a comparison group, important underlying assumptions are made—in particular, that none of the factors shown in Figure 16-3 except for the program of interest has changed over time.

Nevertheless, adequacy evaluations are often the only alternative for programs that are scaled up rapidly and reach whole populations. For example, introduction of the *Haemophilus influenzae* type b (Hib) vaccine in Uruguay was associated with virtual disappearance of Hib disease (Pan American Health Organization [PAHO], 1996). Also, adequacy evaluations are often the only approach to estimate the impact on health of policy changes effected through legislation—for example, salt iodization or changes in antimalarial drug regimens.

Even if more complex analyses are being planned, adequacy of program coverage should always be reported. For example, in the Tanzania voucher evaluation (Exhibit 16-3), steady increases in national coverage of any net and ITNs were observed over the study period. ITN use among infants increased from 16% in the baseline survey to 34% in the endline survey (Hanson et al., 2009), showing important progress in this area but also revealing considerable room for improvement. Subsequent analyses determined that increases were significantly stronger in early-implementation districts.

Adequacy evaluations may produce valid results if (1) the causal pathway is relatively short and simple, (2) the expected effect is large, and (3) confounding is unlikely—that is, other factors in Figure 16-3 are either unchanged or are unrelated to the impact measure. These three conditions held, for example, in the Uruguay Hib example. For most health programs and interventions, however, these conditions do not hold, and more complex evaluation designs are needed.

In summary, adequacy evaluations are very useful for assessing coverage outcomes, but more often than not they are insufficient for establishing the health impact of a specific intervention.

Plausibility Evaluations

Plausibility evaluation designs aim to document the health impact of an intervention and to rule out alternative explanations by including a comparison group and addressing confounding variables. Such evaluations are particularly useful when randomized allocation of the program is not possible due to ethical, practical, or political reasons—situations that in real life evaluations constitute the norm rather than the exception. Plausibility evaluations are also useful to demonstrate the large-scale effectiveness of programs or interventions whose efficacy has already been demonstrated in smaller-scale studies. These evaluations may avoid some of the artificiality of randomized controlled trials (RCTs), which often address efficacy, by studying health impact under real-life, less-than-perfect implementation conditions. For this reason, the external validity of plausibility evaluations is likely greater than for tightly controlled trials (Victora, Habicht, & Bryce, 2004).

Several types of design may be used in a plausibility evaluation, some of which are described next.

Before-and-After Study in Program and Comparison Areas

A very commonly used type of study design is the before-and-after program-comparison design. In this design, one or more areas—say, districts—with the program being evaluated are compared with districts without the program (Figure 16-4). Because health impact indicators may be affected by several factors other than the program, it is essential to document changes on the nonprogram factors depicted in Figure 16-4, in both program and comparison districts. If these factors differ at baseline from one set of districts to the other, or if they evolve over time in different ways, they may bias the results of the evaluation.

A detailed discussion of design issues with this type of evaluation is outside the scope of this chapter, but some common recommendations are as follows:

- Select as many districts as possible with and without the programs. Detailed sample size calculations are needed, but ideally aim at 10 or more districts in each group.

- In the data analyses, treat the districts as the units, not the individuals living in the districts. This means that the sample size will be, for example, 10 districts in the program group, rather than the number of individuals surveyed.

- When the number of districts with the program is small, select comparison districts from the larger pool of districts without the program by matching them to the program districts according to key characteristics—the most important of which are baseline levels of the main impact indicator.

- Collect detailed information on all nonprogram factors listed in Figures 16-3 and 16-4.

- Take nonprogram factors into account in the data analyses by treating them as potential confounding factors and considering them in the interpretation of results (Cousens et al., 2009).

The before-and-after program-comparison design is well suited to evaluate the introduction of large-scale programs delivering interventions whose efficacy has already been demonstrated under experimental conditions, but that have yet to be scaled up. In this case, the comparison areas are completely devoid of the program's interventions—hence evaluators often refer to them as "virgin" or "untouched" comparison areas.

Many large-scale evaluations, however, address new strategies for accelerating the delivery of biological or behavioral interventions that are already being implemented, to a greater or lesser extent, in other

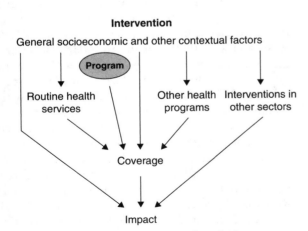
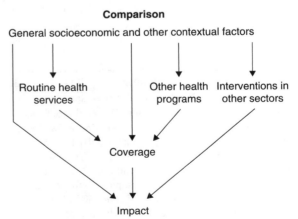

Figure 16-4 Schematic Program-Comparison Design.

districts in the same country. An example is the ACSD initiative in West Africa (Exhibit 16-2). This program represented a renewed effort to intensify the delivery of vaccines, ITNs, vitamin A, antenatal care, breast-feeding promotion, and case management of pneumonia, diarrhea, and malaria. An evaluation of ACSD showed that, paradoxically, some of these interventions had higher coverage in districts without ACSD than in districts with ACSD (Bryce et al., 2010). In such cases, the program-comparison design does not make much sense and other alternatives are required.

The Ecological Dose-Response Design

When a program includes biological or behavioral interventions that are being promoted throughout a country, a dose-response design may be the most appropriate evaluation approach. For example, health worker training in IMCI was disseminated throughout Peru in the late 1990s, but training coverage varied markedly by district (Huicho, Davila, Gonzales, Drasbek, Bryce, & Victora, 2005). Figure 16-5 shows the percentage reduction in under-five mortality in the period 1996–2000 for the 24 departments in the country, by levels of IMCI training coverage for health facility workers. Rapid reductions in mortality occurred, ranging from 20% to 50% in all departments, but no clear association with IMCI training was established.

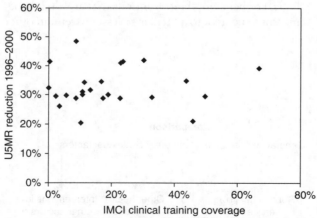

Figure 16-5 Scatter Diagram of Under-Five Mortality Reduction from 1996 to 2000 According to IMCI Clinical Training Coverage in Peru (each point represents one department). *Source:* Huicho, Luis, Miguel Dávila, Fernando Gonzales, Christopher Drasbek, Jennifer Bryce and Cesar G Victora. *Health Policy and Planning.* 2005 (20supp1) "Implementation of the Integrated Management of Childhood Illness strategy in Peru and its association with health indicators: an ecological analysis."

In light of widespread scaling up of health interventions in many countries, dose-response designs may become increasingly useful in the future. Exhibit 16-5 proposes an approach to such studies.

Randomized (Probability) Evaluation Designs

Randomized designs are the gold standard for achieving internal validity. Because health programs are delivered to groups rather than individuals, cluster-randomized trials are appropriate for their evaluation (Donner & Klar, 2000). Random allocation of clusters of individuals—for example, districts—to receive or not to receive the program or intervention increases the likelihood that the two study arms will be highly comparable in terms of confounding variables, including those that cannot be measured directly.

This situation is particularly likely to hold when the number of clusters available for randomization is large. If the number is small—as is often the case for large-scale programs delivered at the district level—the program and comparison groups may still differ substantially in terms of baseline confounding factors, in spite of randomization. In these cases, constrained randomization may be used to improve comparability of the two study arms (Moulton, 2004).

Even programs that consist of packages of proven interventions may be evaluated through randomized trials. All districts in a country would be listed, possibly stratified in categories of risk (e.g., high, medium, or low frequency of the main study outcome), and then allocated randomly within each stratum either to receive the program under routine conditions of implementation or to not receive it. Politicians and managers—as well as members of the population—need to agree with the process of randomization, as do all involved district authorities and implementation partners.

In practice, a variety of ethical, political, and practical barriers to randomizing districts to receive or not to receive a program may exist (Black, 1996; Victora et al., 2004). For instance, large-scale programs usually encompass biological and behavioral interventions whose efficacy has already been established in RCTs in smaller populations, so that withholding them from population groups for the purpose of evaluation is difficult to justify. Political barriers arise from a similar source: Policy makers are understandably reluctant to withhold proven interventions from the population for the purpose of research. Practical barriers include the assumptions within an RCT that the researcher controls the pace and quality of intervention delivery and that the intervention does not change over time—criteria that cannot be

| Exhibit 16-5 | **The Evaluation Platform Design** |

The prevailing evaluation paradigm assumes that programs are implemented in a few districts and not in the rest of the country. Changes in service provision, utilization, coverage, and sometimes health impact are documented over time, and gains in the intervention districts relative to comparison areas are attributed to the program, reflecting the assumption that any improvement is a direct result of program inputs. The counterfactual supposition is that in the absence of the program, outcomes in the target districts would have shown trends similar to those in the comparison areas. Several types of bias may compromise this comparison, including selection biases (e.g., districts chosen for the program may have special characteristics that favor implementation) and confounding factors. This traditional evaluation design remains popular despite its limitations because no feasible alternatives may exist to it; if properly conducted and analyzed, such evaluations often provide valuable information.

Recent experience in evaluating large-scale programs and initiatives suggests that this traditional design has important limitations in the current development context. "Untouched" comparison areas are seldom available because similar biological or behavioral interventions are often being scaled up by other programs or initiatives—with greater or lesser success—in different geographical areas. As a consequence, populations in the comparison area are often exposed to interventions that are similar to those promoted in the program area. For example, in the ACSD evaluation (Exhibit 16-2) in Mali, several of the comparison districts were receiving virtually the same interventions as the program districts, with support from other donors. Even in situations where a program is planned to be scaled up in several districts, the reality is that implementation speed tends to vary from district to district, as was the case in the Tanzania ITN voucher study. Therefore, in many circumstances dose-response analyses relating implementation strength to coverage and health impact make more sense than comparisons of program and nonprogram districts.

To further complicate the issue of attribution, health status is influenced by a myriad of factors other than an individual program. At least four categories of contextual factors must be considered (Victora, Schellenberg, et al., 2005), as suggested in Figure 16-3: (1) preexisting health services, whether public or private; (2) the presence of new health programs other than the one being evaluated; (3) the presence of interventions in other sectors that may affect health (e.g., water, sanitation, or education); and (4) overall socioeconomic and environmental conditions. This broad framework of determinants of health requires that evaluations go well beyond the health sector. For this reason, evaluations of all health programs require careful documentation of contextual factors and their incorporation in data analyses and interpretation.

As a consequence, instead of the current practice of evaluating one program at a time, it makes much more sense to develop a broad evaluation platform to assess all of the multiple programs that are in place within a country. For example, partners can work with national and local governments to support nationwide assessments of programs in different areas: maternal and child health; reproductive health; disease-specific control programs, including those for malaria and HIV/AIDS; and efforts aimed at strengthening health systems (Global Initiative to Strengthen Country Health Systems Surveillance [CHeSS], 2008).

A strong rationale supports the practice of looking beyond a single program at a time. Although the specific indicators and some of the data collection needs will vary depending on the program, many of the contextual factors will be the same across several programs. Also, the presence of a given program may confound the effect of another program. This type of entanglement was noted in the ACSD evaluation, where similar programs were present in the comparison districts. It also affected the Tanzania ITN evaluation because some of the districts had free distribution of ITNs side by side with the voucher scheme. Lastly, one program may have detrimental side effects on other programs (e.g., the heated debate about whether HIV/AIDS programs are weakening health systems), and these will be detected using the platform approach (Yu, Souteyrand, Banda, Kaufman, & Perriens, 2008).

This proposed approach has been described as the *evaluation platform* (Victora et al., 2009), which would include the following steps:

1. Develop and regularly update a district database that includes existing demographic, epidemiological, socioeconomic, and health infrastructure variables, derived from sources such as censuses, economic surveys, poverty maps, and service availability censuses. All districts in a country—or in a subnational region—would be included.
2. Conduct an initial survey (or build on existing and future household surveys), to be repeated every three years or so, to measure coverage levels for proven interventions and health status. Ideally this survey would also allow estimation of mortality and prevalence of biomarkers.
3. Establish a continuous monitoring system for documenting provision, utilization, and ideally quality of interventions at the district level, with mechanisms for prompt reporting to local, national, and international audiences.

This platform would allow multiple analyses based on ecological designs, with the unit of intervention being the district. It would support the comparison of various combinations of interventions and delivery strategies—including the assessment of a range of intervention intensities—in regard to changes in health impact measures, while considering confounding factors. Such an approach is likely to cost less than the aggregate costs of conducting multiple separate evaluations, and to generate more and better information about the effects of specific programs, both alone and in combination.

Exhibit 16-6	Large-Scale RCTs: The Progresa and Seguro Popular Evaluations in Mexico

Mexican policy makers and researchers have pioneered the use of RCTs for large-scale program evaluation in low- and middle-income countries. Two large studies have attracted special attention: the evaluations of Progresa, a program that included conditional cash transfers (Rivera, Sotres-Alvarez, Habicht, Shamah, & Villalpando, 2004), and of Seguro Popular, a health insurance initiative (King et al., 2009).

Progresa was a large-scale, incentive-based development program with a built-in nutritional intervention. Taking advantage of the lack of resources for covering all eligible families in the country at the same time, the evaluators designed a two-wave stepped wedge trial. Of 347 poor rural communities in 6 central Mexican states, 205 were randomly assigned to immediate launch of the program in 1998 and another 142 to initiate the program 2 years later (Rivera et al., 2004). Random samples of children in those communities were surveyed at baseline, and again at 1 and 2 years afterward. Participants, all of whom came from low-income households within each community, were selected on the basis of an index of household assets.

Progresa provided micronutrient-fortified foods for women and children and health services and cash transfers for the family. The original design sought to provide a 2-year window during which Progresa would be implemented in the intervention but not in the comparison communities, but political pressure to accelerate the program led the comparison communities to start receiving the program more than 1 year earlier than originally planned, in late 1999 rather than in early 2001. In addition, nearly half of all young children (younger than age 6 months) were lost to follow-up by the time of the 2-year follow-up. Progresa was associated with better growth in height among the poorest and younger infants, but not in the sample as a whole. After 1 year, mean hemoglobin values were higher in the intervention group than in the comparison group, but there were no differences in hemoglobin levels between the two groups at year 2, after both groups were receiving the intervention.

The second evaluation involved an innovative cluster trial of health insurance—Seguro Popular—in Mexico, one of the largest randomized health policy experiments ever carried out. Policy makers in 13 of the 32 Mexican states agreed to join the study. From more than 7,000 clusters (health facility catchment areas) in these 13 states, the evaluators "negotiated access to 74 cluster pairs in seven states, with inclusion based on necessary administrative, political, and other criteria" and then randomly assigned one health cluster from each pair to receive the Seguro Popular program. The main finding was a reduction in catastrophic expenditures in health of 1.9 percentage points. Although program resources reached the poor, contrary to expectations, they did not have any effects on medication spending, utilization of health services, or health outcomes after 10 months of follow-up. The authors (King et al., 2009) recognize that the short implementation period may have precluded documenting an impact on outcomes that are unlikely to change rapidly. They also note that the program varied considerably across areas.

These two Mexican trials make an important contribution to the literature on the evaluation of large-scale programs, but they also reveal that RCTs are not a panacea for all evaluation ills. First, obtaining agreement of policy makers at all levels—from national to local—is not a trivial matter, and external validity may be affected because of low compliance with randomization at local level. That may have been the case in the Seguro Popular trial, in which 74 cluster pairs were non-randomly selected from over 7,000 clusters.

Second, both trials show that getting policy makers and managers to accept randomization is a major achievement, but ensuring their continued support during the trials is also essential. In both studies, the patience of decision makers was shorter than what would be required for a full assessment of the intervention's impact. Both trials demonstrated that, when taken out of their traditional context—that is, efficacy studies that are completely under the control of researchers—RCTs do not perform well for the evaluation of large-scale, real-life programs.

met when evaluating strategies or programs that are being scaled up by governments and their partners and often refined in response to early experience or intermediate results from the evaluation.

These barriers to RCTs tend to counterbalance the increased internal validity associated with their use, so it is not surprising that randomized designs are rare in large-scale effectiveness evaluations. In addition, evaluators are often called in when it has already been decided which areas will receive—or are already receiving—the program and, therefore, cannot influence its deployment.

Among the few examples of RCTs used for evaluation programs affecting health outcomes are two Mexican studies, which are summarized in Exhibit 16-6.

Stepped Wedge Design

An attractive alternative to the RCT is the stepped wedge design, a variation of randomized cluster trials

(Brown & Lilford, 2006). This strategy should not be confused with the stepwise approach to evaluation described in Figure 16-2. A stepped wedge design makes use of implementation timetables that specify introduction of the program or strategy earlier in some geographical areas than in others. This phased roll-out allows evaluators to use the later-implementation areas as comparison groups for the earlier-implementation areas.

A hypothetical example of a randomized stepped wedge design follows. The capacity to train health workers or to procure a commodity is limited, so that only a few districts can be covered in the first year of the program. These areas are selected randomly from all districts in the country, and start to receive the program. In the following year, another wave of districts is selected from those without the program, and so forth, until all districts are covered. At any given time until the last implementation wave is complete, there will be districts with the program and districts without the program; the latter provide a randomized comparison group.

This design has advantages from an ethical standpoint, because it would not have been possible to implement the program in all districts at the same time, and selection of program districts is random. Nevertheless, fewer than 20 such trials have been published in the literature (Brown & Lilford, 2006), and none of these reports have dealt with large study units such as districts. Instead, the study units in most cases were health facilities, vaccination teams, or small communities.

As with standard RCTs, practical constraints to implementing stepped wedge trials at the district level in low- and middle-income countries exist:

- It may be difficult to explain the randomization process to district authorities and convince them that there are no hidden allocation biases.

- National governments are often reluctant to leave any district completely devoid of a program. Instead, they may attempt to be "equitable" by allocating some amount of resources to all districts.

- Other bilateral or international organizations delivering health programs in the country already have their favorite districts, and may continue to implement activities that are similar to the program.

- Many infectious diseases demonstrate marked seasonal or cyclical patterns, and it may be difficult to distribute implementation waves of

districts over time so that temporal patterns do not affect the interpretation of results.

- Implementation timetables are subject to many influences, and often change over time, which may weaken the design.

- This design can be used only for programs or strategies that are unlikely to have effects beyond the border of a district. It would not be appropriate, for example, in evaluations of mass-media campaigns.

These reasons may explain why stepped wedge designs, although available since the 1980s, have never enjoyed great popularity despite their theoretical advantages (Brown & Lilford, 2006).

Even if a randomized stepped wedge design is not possible, evaluators may take advantage of the fact that some programs are implemented gradually, in one group of districts at a time, and analyze the data as a stepped wedge trial. For example, the Reach Every District approach to scale up immunizations and other child survival interventions in Mozambique started in 33 of the country's 148 districts in 2008, and new waves of coverage for 33 districts were expected to be initiated every year until the whole country is covered. In this example, the order in which districts start implementation is not random, so the design falls into the "plausibility evaluation" category, with its corresponding caveats.

Defining the Indicators and Obtaining the Data

Documentation of Program Implementation

Obtaining detailed data on program implementation is essential because—unlike what happens in tightly controlled, small-scale trials—large-scale programs often fail to deliver what was originally proposed. The ACSD evaluation showed, for example, that whereas vaccines and vitamin A supplements reached high coverage in the target districts, other equally important parts of the ACSD package—such as insecticide-treated nets—were affected by unforeseen stock-outs that resulted in insufficient distribution of these items to the population.

It is often assumed that data on program implementation are readily available from those involved in delivering the program. Our experience, however, shows that this is rarely the case. In the IMCI evaluation, even relatively simple data on how many trained health workers were active in a district proved very difficult to obtain. In the retrospective ACSD evaluation, obtaining data on the early stages of the program was difficult because records were often incomplete, and some key staff involved in setting up the program were no longer available to be interviewed.

Documentation efforts should strive to cover the following topics, drawn from the conceptual framework for the program (Figure 16-1) and reflecting the stepwise approach (Figure 16-2):

- Describe the original program proposal: development, adaptation, program strategies and activities, associated policies, and delivery strategies.

- Describe how the original proposal changed over time, and why—for example, whether a result of internal decisions or due to feedback by the evaluation team.

- Quantify the program inputs, processes, and outputs—for example, the number of health workers that were trained, the types of commodities that were procured and distributed, the type and frequency of supervision activities, utilization by the target population of the services being provided, and the frequency and nature of community-level activities.

- Describe contextual factors (e.g., epidemiological, health systems, demographic or sociocultural characteristics) that may affect the program's impact.

Methods for documentation include desk reviews of program and policy documents, training materials, workshop and supervision reports, and administrative records related to program inputs and outputs. This step may also require talking to implementers, conducting in-depth interviews, and conducting focus group discussions.

The ultimate objective of documentation is to go beyond program objectives and goals to understand what actually took place at the population level. Systematic documentation is essential for understanding why a program achieved—or failed to achieve—its intended effect. Qualitative studies are often a useful adjunct to documentation.

In terms of the stepwise design described in Figure 16-2, documentation is essential for assessing the first question: Are the interventions and plans for delivery technically sound and appropriate for the epidemiological and health system context? Such documentation will also contribute to addressing the second question—Are adequate services being provided at facility and community level?—by providing quantitative information on implementation activities.

Measurement of Intervention Quality

Health programs include interactions between health workers and the target population, with or without the provision of commodities. A behavioral change and communications intervention may include individual or group sessions; a vaccination program will include delivery of the vaccine to the target population; and case management interventions will include interaction between a community or facility-based provider and a patient, often followed by provision of drugs. While documentation will provide quantitative information on these interactions, it is also important to assess their quality.

Survey methods are available for this purpose. Typically, a multistage sampling scheme is used to select units within the program areas—for example, health facilities or communities; within these units, health workers involved in service delivery are then sampled. Next, the interaction between these workers and members of the population is observed. Many survey tools also include a description of the facilities where health workers operate (e.g., the physical space, drug supply, equipment) and incorporate exit interviews to check user satisfaction. For case management surveys, a second examination of the same patient by a gold-standard examiner is often included, which is then compared with the original conduct of the health worker. The quality of case management for rarely occurring events is sometimes assessed through the use of written or oral scenarios. Further details of how to conduct these surveys, and standard indicators to be used, are available elsewhere (Gouws, Bryce, Pariyo, Armstrong Schellenberg, Amaral, & Habicht, 2005).

Measuring Coverage

Although population coverage can sometimes be estimated from utilization statistics (e.g., dividing the number of births reported by skilled attendants by the estimated number of births in the population), in most instances coverage measurement requires household surveys. This technique is necessary because there may be population movements—for example, mothers from a neighboring district coming to the focus district to give birth—and because the availability of simple data on commodities disbursed (e.g., antibiotics, oral rehydration solution [ORS] packets, or ITNs) does not guarantee that those items reached, and were used by, those in need.

Many low- and middle-income countries now have regular surveys on maternal and child health, such as Demographic and Health Surveys (DHS; Measure DHS, n.d.) or UNICEF's (n.d.) Multiple Indicator

Cluster Surveys (MICS) that are carried out every three to five years in a given country. In addition, surveys may assess coverage of disease-specific programs, such as malaria indicator surveys (MIS; Measure DHS, "Malaria Indicator Surveys," n.d.) and HIV/AIDS indicators surveys (Measure DHS, "AIDS Indicators Surveys," n.d.). The frequency of such surveys is likely to increase as the Millennium Development Goals (MDG) 2015 deadline approaches.

These types of surveys include standard indicators, usually defined by multi-institutional or inter-agency working groups. It is essential that program evaluations comply with agreed-upon indicators, to allow comparability of the results with those from other evaluations and studies.

There are several scenarios in which surveys may be used as part of evaluations:

- A national survey (e.g., DHS or MIS) is carried out at a suitable time for the evaluation, and the number of households sampled in the program and comparison areas is sufficiently large to yield precise estimates. This was the case in the Peru IMCI evaluation, which was largely based on DHS data (Huicho et al., 2005).

- A national survey as described above is planned, but needs to be oversampled in program and/or comparison areas. This was done in the ACSD evaluation in West Africa (Bryce et al., 2010).

- No suitable surveys are planned, and the evaluation team has to carry out its own survey in program and comparison areas. This was the case in the Tanzania IMCI evaluation (Schellenberg, 2004).

Survey samples are usually insufficient for providing precise coverage estimates at the district level. There are a few exceptions, however, such as the Malawi 2010 DHS, which sampled 1,000 households per district, and the India Reproductive and Child Health Surveys, which had a total sample of more than 600,000 households (India Ministry of Health and Family Welfare, 2006).

Even if the number of sampled households per district is small and few programs are implemented in a single district, pooling across several districts may result in sufficient numbers of individuals to assess coverage. It is often argued that survey results should not be pooled, because few national surveys are designed to provide probability samples at the district level. Nevertheless, these surveys systematically present tables stratified by age, socioeconomic, and ethnic categories, even though the sample was not designed to be strictly representative of such subgroups. In practice, most nationally representative surveys employ implicit stratification within each district by listing enumeration areas in a geographical sequence and systematically sampling these areas; as a result, households included in the sample tend to be spread throughout the districts. By giving due attention to sampling weights, groups of districts where a program was implemented may be separated from a national survey for the purposes of assessing coverage (Rao, 2003; West, Berglund, & Heeringa, 2008).

A prerequisite for disaggregating survey data by district is the presence of a geographical stratifier variable in the database. For example, some surveys that include serological testing for HIV/AIDS are "scrambled"—that is, information on location of the study clusters is obliterated to make it impossible to identify HIV-positive subjects using information on cluster, age, number of children, and so on. Although the ethical concern behind this practice is laudable, in practice it may preclude the use of surveys for evaluation of other programs. It would make much more sense to use stand-alone surveys when collecting such samples, so as to avoid the concern that a single disease might eliminate the possibility of evaluating several other programs.

Due to the high cost of surveys, other alternatives are worth exploring, such as using National Immunization Days (NID) to collect information on coverage or health outcomes related to other programs than those delivered at the NID—for example, breastfeeding promotion or nutritional status (Santos, Paes-Sousa, Silva, & Victora, 2008). As long as coverage of NID attendance is high (say, 90% or so), coverage of other programs can be estimated with little bias.

Measuring or Modeling Impact

Some programs express their main goals in terms of coverage indicators, and as a consequence impact measurement is not necessary. This is the case, for example, with a vaccination program that seeks to reach high coverage with a vaccine (e.g., rotavirus vaccine) whose efficacy is well established. For such an evaluation, if high coverage is documented, there is no need for expensive and complex assessments of the incidence of diarrhea due to rotavirus.

Many funders, however, wish to go back to their constituencies armed with hard data on the health impact of the intervention—for example, the number of lives saved by their actions. Some initiatives, such as the Catalytic Initiative to Save a Million Lives (http://www.acdi-cida.gc.ca/acdi-cida/acdi-cida

.nsf/eng/NAD-1249841-JLG), have actually incorporated their quantitative goals into their program title.

Impact measurement is often included in surveys that also measure coverage. Nevertheless, assessing impact indicators usually makes coverage surveys much more complex. Issues that influence the measurement of impact in program evaluations include the following:

- *How difficult is the measurement?* For example, will impact be assessed through interviews (e.g., full birth histories of women of reproductive age, aimed at assessing child mortality; infant feeding practices), or is there a need for measurements or collection of biological specimens? Measuring child underweight with a weighing scale is easier than measuring stunting, which requires substantial training of interviewers and more sophisticated equipment. Drawing blood samples adds another level of logistical complications, including equipment, interviewer safety concerns, and issues related to processing, transportation, storage, and analysis of samples. If data on causes of death are needed—often an important consideration for attributing success to a program—there will be additional requirements in terms of interviewer training and sample size.

- *How rare is the event being measured?* The frequency of the impact measure in the population is key for determining sample sizes. Rare events (e.g., mortality or, even worse, cause-specific mortality) require larger sample sizes than more frequent events (e.g., stunting or malaria parasitemia in an endemic area). Some events (e.g., maternal mortality) are so infrequent that the samples required are prohibitively large, leading evaluators to rely on proxy measures such as coverage of interventions known to reduce mortality. In the case of cluster surveys, evaluators also need to take into account the "design effect" (Cochran, 1977): Events that are evenly spread throughout the population require samples that are smaller than events that are highly clustered, as is the case for some transmissible diseases. For impact measures such as mortality rates, sample sizes may be reduced by using deaths in the last two or three years before the survey, rather than deaths in the last year. This approach requires full implementation of the program throughout the mortality measurement period, as otherwise its full effect will not be picked up.

- *How large is the effect to be detected?* Picking up large effects requires smaller samples than detecting small effects. For example, detecting a 25% reduction in under-five mortality over a certain period, relative to baseline levels, will require much smaller samples than detecting a 15% decline. Even larger sample sizes are needed to detect a 25% difference between the annual rates of mortality decline in program and comparison areas—for example, 10% and 8% per year, respectively.

Recent advances have led to the development of modeling tools that allow the estimation of under-five mortality trends based on measured changes in coverage. Exhibit 16-7 describes the Lives Saved Tool (LiST), which is becoming widely used for this purpose (Bryce, Friberg, et al., 2010).

Exhibit 16-7 | **LiST: An Example of Mortality Modeling Software**

Software for modeling changes in mortality on the basis of coverage data is a useful tool for impact assessments. In the maternal, newborn, and child health (MNCH) field, the Lives Saved Tool (LiST) allows users to estimate the impact of scaling up proven interventions by defining and running multiple country-, state-, or district-specific scenarios. LiST was designed to enable ministry of health personnel, program managers, and academics to combine the best scientific evidence about the effectiveness of interventions with information about cause of death and current coverage of interventions to inform their planning and decision making, help prioritize investments, and evaluate existing programs (Boschi-Pinto, Young, & Black, 2010).

LiST uses data on baseline mortality rates and causes of death to estimate the number of maternal, under-five, infant, and neonatal deaths that can be averted both by cause and by intervention, as intervention coverage increases. It is programmed into a demographic software package called Spectrum, which has been widely used for 20 years and is designed to predict population changes over time by age and sex (Stover, McKinnon, & Winfrey, 2010). The data in this module are based on the 2008 United States population projections, which facilitate estimates of population growth through 2050. In using

(continued)

Exhibit 16-7	Continued

this platform, LiST also links with other modules within Spectrum such as AIM, which models UNAIDS data for each country, and FamPlan, which estimates the impact of family planning on the number of births.

LiST and other modeling software are used in two ways in evaluations of large-scale programs. First, they can help assess whether the interventions being promoted by the program are appropriate to the cause of death profile of the program area and suggest what the likely impact mortality will be if scaling up is successful. This information can help evaluators complete the first step in the stepwise model described in Figure 16-2: Are the interventions relevant to the epidemiological context? The second and most important use of LiST and similar software is to translate changes in coverage measured through surveys into expected mortality impact. When direct impact measurement is not feasible or too expensive, LiST can provide a reasonable estimate of how much mortality decline can be obtained from the measured coverage gains.

The LiST website (www.jhsph.edu/IIP/list) is the gateway for downloading the tool. It provides instructions on this software's use, as well as the latest results of intervention reviews and validation studies.

Describing Contextual Factors

In impact evaluations, contextual factors are variables external to the program that can confound or modify its observed effect (Victora et al., 2005). Confounding occurs when changes in these external variables differ in program and comparison areas. For example, crop failures, natural disasters, or establishment of new health facilities (or presence of other programs) may occur in one area, but not in others. The ACSD evaluation showed an apparent impact of the intervention on undernutrition prevalence, but documentation of contextual factors identified a famine in some of the comparison districts; once these effects were excluded from the comparison group, there was no longer any evidence of a positive impact of the program (Bryce et al., 2010). Control of confounding factors is essential for improving the internal validity of the evaluation.

Effect modification occurs when certain baseline conditions—for example, the level and causes of mortality, or the strength of health systems—either contribute to or detract from the observed impact of the program. Effect modification is particularly relevant to external validity, or the ability to generalize from the evaluation findings. In the IMCI evaluation in Tanzania, for example, the success of this facility-based intervention may have been largely dependent on the high utilization of health services by sick children, even before IMCI was implemented (Schellenberg et al., 2004). Given this dependency, expecting a similar impact in low-utilization settings such as most other sub-Saharan African countries may not be realistic.

Data on contextual factors come from a variety of sources. Most low- and middle-income countries already have a number of databases maintained by governmental, international, or partner institutions, with information disaggregated at the provincial or district level. Table 16-2 identifies sources of information on a variety of contextual factors; this listing was prepared for an evaluation of the Catalytic Initiative to Save One Million Lives in Mozambique.

If quantitative information is available for all geographical areas included in the evaluation, contextual factors may be formally included in the statistical analyses models as covariates. Even if information is incomplete or unquantifiable, contextual factors may help interpret the evaluation findings.

The process of obtaining information on contextual factors is part of the documentation exercise described previously. It can be often done by the same team collecting data on program implementation.

Measuring Costs

Cost data can be used in many different ways to inform decisions about public health programming, and are a key component of large-scale program evaluations. They contribute to understanding the budgetary implications of health programs and are needed to perform economic analyses such as those assessing cost-effectiveness. Cost data can help answer questions not only about how much money programs cost, but also about where the costs are incurred (e.g., by patients, at a particular service level, at higher levels), how programs operate, and which factors are hindering program scale-up. Moreover, such data can help to answer questions about the relationship between costs and other aspects of health care, such as the quality of services, which are public health goals in their own right (Bishai et al., 2008). Finally, cost data can be used in conjunction with data on utilization and household assets to understand the equity implications of a program.

Table 16-2	Examples of Data Available from Existing Databases at the District and Provincial Level in Mozambique and Sources and Information	
Category	**Examples**	**Source**
Socioeconomic factors	Household assets Family income and poverty Parental education and occupation Unemployment Land tenure Economic crises (inflation rates, crop failures, floods)	2007 census Economic censuses and surveys National Institute of Statistics
Demographic factors	Population density Fertility patterns Family size Ethnic groups	2007 census
Environmental characteristics	Water supply Sanitation Urbanization Housing Rainfall Altitude	2007 census National Meteorological Institute
Baseline health conditions	Under-five mortality Prevalence of malnutrition HIV prevalence Malaria transmission patterns	2007 census 2008 MICS Malaria and HIV surveys
Health services characteristics	Availability of health services (e.g., hospitals, clinics) in public and private sectors Population/facility ratio Health worker staffing patterns Health worker pay Drug supply Baseline utilization rates Availability of referral services Strength of district health management team District health budget (overall and for child health)	Health Metrics Network Ministry of Health Information Systems UNFPA Needs Assessment Survey WHO Service Availability Mapping
Presence of other projects and programs that may affect health status	Micronutrients Indoor residual spraying Immunizations HIV programs Others	UNICEF World Health Organization Network of Organizations Working in Health and HIV/AIDS (NAIMA) Official Development Assistance to Mozambique Database (ODAMOZ)

Figure 16-6 presents a conceptual diagram of the total costs involved in the scale-up of health programs. The x-axis represents the time from before the start of the scale-up program until the target levels of coverage (or mortality reduction) have been achieved, or until the end of the evaluation. The y-axis represents the annualized, total costs of health services, where higher levels of coverage are associated with higher levels of total costs.

Five cost categories are incorporated in the framework depicted in Figure 16-6. *Area A*, the rectangular region above the x-axis, represents the total amount of resources used for health services at the beginning of the observation period.

Area B represents the change in total costs normally associated with secular trends in most health systems. It could also be thought of as the change in area A over time due to changing population, infla-

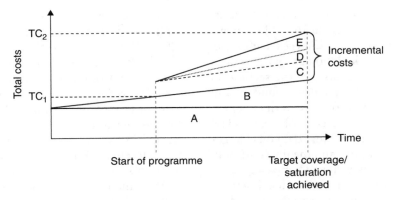

Figure 16-6 Conceptual Framework for Assessing the Cost of Rapid Scale-Up.
Source: Assessing the costs and cost-effectiveness of rapid- scale up for . . .
p. 10 Figure 2 http://www.jhsph.edu/bin/c/g/CI_costeffectiveness.pdf

tionary pressures, and the introduction of new technologies, among other factors. In Figure 16-6, secular trends are seen as increasing total costs, which is normally—albeit not universally—the case. This does not conceptually imply that average or marginal costs are necessarily increasing, nor is there any particular reason to believe that secular trends will affect total costs in a linear way as depicted in the diagram; this depiction is provided here for simplicity's sake. Note that secular trends will affect the total costs of a health program both before and after its implementation.

Area C represents the start-up costs associated with the scale-up; these costs are specific to the scale-up program and, therefore, are added to the costs represented in areas A and B. In economic terms, the start-up costs will be annualized over the lifetime of the program; thus they are shown in Figure 16-6 as remaining constant over time, although this again may not necessarily be the case. The size of area C to some extent depends on the time frame of the evaluation.

Area D represents the operational program-level costs associated with the scale-up; these costs are specific to the scale-up program and, therefore, are added to the costs represented in areas A and B. Again, there is no predetermined pattern for how these costs will change over time; for convenience, they are depicted here as increasing with the expansion of scale-up activities.

Area E represents the additional costs due to the increased service utilization under the scale-up program. Again, if scale-up increases coverage, total costs should increase, but there is no a priori reason to believe that unit costs will remain constant, increase, or decrease. Area E must be assessed as part of the economic component of the impact evaluation. Note

that any changes in unit costs due to program scale-up are also likely to affect the unit costs associated with areas A and B.

The costs associated with areas C and D may be estimated using four different methods:

1. *Documentation approach*: Costs are estimated by documenting the costs of activities and then identifying which costs are unique to the scale-up. This process was discussed earlier in the section on documentation.

2. *First difference approach*: The costs for areas C and D are estimated by calculating program costs at baseline and subtracting these baseline costs from the total program costs observed after implementation. This initial approach ignores secular trends.

3. *Aggregate difference approach*: Costs are estimated by subtracting the program costs in control districts from the program costs in the scale-up districts after scale-up has occurred (Johns Hopkins Bloomberg School of Public Health, n.d.). This approach assumes that the baseline costs in control and rapid-scale up areas are the same.

4. *Difference-in-difference approach*: Methods 2 and 3 can be combined to control for secular trends. With this approach, program costs are collected before and after rapid scale-up in both control and implementation districts, and the difference in costs in the control districts is interpreted as the secular trend in program costs, and taken out of the difference in costs between the two time points in the scale-up districts (Adam et al., 2004).

Similar methods are used to estimate the costs that make up area E, although further adjustments may be necessary. Tracking time-series cost data by activity may allow for the calculation of total, average, and marginal/incremental costs (see the section on analyzing costs and cost-effectiveness, found later in this chapter, for a definition of these terms) per recipient in both the scale-up and control areas and by different levels of coverage, because data on changes in the utilization, population, and the unit costs will be available. Using the full change (comparing baseline to full implementation—that is, the first difference approach) in unit costs in the scale-up areas would assume that all changes in the unit costs of service delivery and the utilization rate are attributable to the scale-up, which ignores the influence of secular trends. Secular trends may be controlled for using comparison areas (i.e., via the aggregate or difference-in-difference approaches described earlier).

Given the concerns related to estimating area E, it is important to clarify which factors may influence costs apart from the program of interest. Three kinds of variables may potentially influence costs: patient-level variables, facility-level variables, and contextual variables (Hussey et al., 2009). Each of these is discussed in turn.

Patient-Level Costs

A great deal of the existing cost-effectiveness literature has been devoted to controlling for differences in costs due to variation in patient-level characteristics; most of this work has been conducted in high-income countries. Variables that have been found to be important include case mix or severity of illness (Hofer et al., 1999; Powell et al., 2003; Tucker et al., 1996), sex, age, living conditions, race/ethnicity, and other socioeconomic variables (Grieve et al., 2005; Hussey et al., 2009).

Facility-Level Characteristics

Facility-level variables encompass factors that affect costs at the provider level. Quality is one frequently cited example (Amorin et al., 2008; Bishai et al., 2008), although one recent review found that many authors fail to control for it for when examining efficiency measurement (Hussey et al., 2009). The scale of services (e.g., the number of patients seen) and the number and types of outputs for a particular health service provider (i.e., the scope of service provision) may influence the unit costs and total costs of delivering service (Jacobs et al., 2006). Technical efficiency—the ability to maximize outputs for a given set of inputs or to minimize inputs for a given set of outputs—may also influence unit costs at the facility level (Adam et al., 2005, 2008; Baltussen et al., 2003; Bryce et al., 2005; Jacobs et al., 2006). Other variables that have been used to control for costs include the way in which a health provider is reimbursed (Grieve et al., 2005) and the type of ownership (Hollingsworth, 2003), although the latter consideration really reflects technical efficiency.

The effect of economies of scale on unit costs has been shown to be important for primary health care in low- and middle-income countries (Berman et al., 1989). It has also been increasingly studied in disease-specific contexts, where it has been shown to influence costs (Guinness et al., 2005; Kumaranayake, 2008; Marseille et al., 2004; Valdmanis et al., 2003). Technical efficiency has been less frequently studied, although at least one study from a low- and middle-income country indicates that health centers may have different costs due to different levels of technical efficiency (Masiye et al., 2006). Quality may either increase costs or lower costs. All three of these factors may have an influence on the costs of health services.

Contextual Variables

Variables that are outside the control of the health provider, yet reflect the environment in which the provider operates, may also have an influence on the costs of services. The IMCI cost study from Brazil mentioned that average income in a municipality may have an influence on utilization rates and, therefore, on the scale of services (Adam et al., 2009). Geographic features of an area may influence the cost of transport, supervision, and training as well as patients' ability to access care due to the need to travel for greater distances and over difficult terrain (Johns & Torres, 2005; Over, 1986). The reimbursement of human resources may change in different areas, either due to differences in costs of living (Jacobs et al., 2006) or due to the need for incentives to entice personnel to work in remote areas (Barnighausen et al., 2009). The degree of competition between providers within an area may also influence efficiency and therefore costs, but be outside the control of an individual provider (Jacobs et al., 2006).

Previous studies of the costs of large-scale child health interventions in low- and middle-income countries have, by and large, relied on cross-sectional data collection after the program was implemented, as was the case in three of the four countries participating in the IMCI evaluation (see Exhibit 16-8). Although these studies plausibly established that IMCI did not increase the cost of child health programs by a great

Exhibit 16-8	The Cost of Child Health Services: The Multi-Country IMCI Evaluation

The cost of child health services delivery has been most recently and notably studied in conjunction with the evaluation of the IMCI program in Bangladesh, Brazil, Tanzania, and Uganda that was described in Exhibit 16-1 (Adam et al., 2005, 2009; Amorim et al., 2008; Bishai et al., 2008). In this assessment, costs were estimated from the societal perspective (providers and households).

Standard MCE cost questionnaires were developed and adapted for use in each country. They consisted of four questionnaires to collect data at the national, district, facility, and community levels, respectively. At national level, data on the following IMCI-related activities were collected: planning and orientation meetings, preparation of IMCI training materials (including translation, adaptation, and printing of guidelines and training materials) and training of national trainers, and administration. Data collection at the district level included training of trainers related to IMCI, supervision for IMCI activities related to under-five children, and administrative costs of under-five care. The cost questionnaire at the first-level health facility collected data on personnel (including volunteer labor, if any), drugs, capital items, number of patient visits by type, and staff time allocation based on a time-and-motion study. Data collection of household costs was based on a two-week morbidity module in a household survey. Information on costs incurred during under-five illness episodes in the two weeks prior to the survey were collected for each child in the household.

In Brazil, Tanzania, and Uganda, no baseline cost data were collected because the evaluations were commissioned after implementation of the program was already under way, when it was no longer possible to collect baseline costs. Therefore, costs were collected after the implementation of IMCI had occurred in the intervention districts, and other matched districts without IMCI were used as comparison districts (Adam et al., 2005, 2009; Amorim et al., 2008; Bishai et al., 2008). Only in Bangladesh, where a fully prospective IMCI evaluation was carried out, were baseline costs collected (S. Arifeen, personal communication). The need to collect baseline costs is another strong reason for undertaking prospective assessment, rather than ambispective or retrospective evaluations.

Given the fact that the evaluations from Brazil, Tanzania, and Uganda were not prospective and, therefore, lacked baseline data, the results proved somewhat difficult to interpret. For example, the study from Tanzania found that the costs at the household and health center (primary healthcare level) were almost the same between the IMCI and comparison areas, while costs at the hospital level and at the district level were higher in the comparison areas than in the IMCI districts. Given the nature of the data collection, the reasons for this difference could not be explained; the authors concluded it could be due to decreased referrals after IMCI training, or to factors not related to IMCI (Adam et al., 2005). Without baseline data, it is difficult to know, from this study, what the costs of IMCI were, and to what extent they increased (or decreased) the costs of providing child health care.

A similar analysis done in Brazil found that costs were higher at hospital and municipal levels in IMCI areas than in comparison areas, but lower at primary healthcare levels, although the authors did not find a statistically significant ($p < 0.05$) difference between the two areas for the total costs (Adam et al., 2009). The study in Brazil tried to control for other differences between IMCI and control areas by including variables for facility location and population in the catchment areas of the health centers. This construction suggested that IMCI is endogenously related to total costs via the number of visits per child. That is, IMCI may improve quality, so that people become more likely to attend the clinic; this greater volume of patients then increases total costs but also alters the unit costs of delivering services (Adam et al., 2009).

deal in comparison with areas that did not implement IMCI, they did not ascertain the costs of the IMCI program. As when measuring the effects of a program, to establish a causal link between an intervention and the costs of that intervention, it is not sufficient to establish that areas with a program have different (or similar) costs compared to areas that did not have the program. Rather, it is also necessary to establish that the differences (or similarities) are not due to differences at baseline. Thus data on factors that may influence costs, as well as data on the costs themselves, need to be collected and analyzed at baseline to establish the extent to which they influence

costs, or may result in differences in costs after the program has been implemented.

Data Collection Methods

There are three principal methods of estimating costs: modeled costing, top-down costing, and bottom-up costing. Within each of these methods, multiple sources or ways of collecting data may be employed. These techniques are complementary methods that can be used simultaneously to obtain a comprehensive collection of cost data, and for cross-checking the results from each strategy. Modeled cost analysis should be done only before or at the very start of the scale-up program, whereas top-down costing is usually done retrospectively, although it could be carried out on a repeated basis. Bottom-up costing is usually cross-sectional, so it could also be performed on a repeated basis.

Model-Based Cost Estimates Using Existing Data

Models such as the Lives Saved Tool (LiST) can be used to derive an ex ante cost-effectiveness ratio to inform policy makers of an expected level of cost-effectiveness for their planned activities. Both the unit costs of delivering services and the program-level costs of operating the scale-up effort need to be estimated to carry out model-based cost or cost-effectiveness analyses. Full provider- and patient-perspective analyses may not be feasible given the available data. Any comparison with later results should be adjusted to account for the perspective used in the initial analysis. Modeled unit costs can be estimated based on any of the following methods. The preferred methods, which reflect the most context-specific data, are listed first. Nevertheless, different methods can be used to derive unit costs to the extent possible to perform sensitivity analysis.

1. Unit costs can be collected during a baseline survey of health service providers (e.g. health centers, hospitals, and minimally trained health workers in the community). If such data are collected during the evaluation or are available from another study recently undertaken in the country, they can be used either directly or with adjustments due to anticipated changes in utilization.

2. Unit costs can be based on estimates made in previously undertaken econometric studies. It is recommended that WHO-CHOICE (http://www.who.int/choice/costs/en/) unit costs be used because they are available on a country-by-country basis. WHO-CHOICE unit costs include human resources but exclude drug items; thus excluded costs must be estimated using method 3.

3. Unit costs can be estimated based on treatment protocols (and estimated staff time if options 1 and 2 are not used). Although this method suffers from the bias that medical personnel rarely follow treatment protocols, it does allow for a relatively quick assessment of the potential costs of delivery of the program. An alternative, and more desirable, approach is to elicit resource usage from providers using vignettes; this approach requires additional time and resources, however.

Two principal methods of measuring costs are used: top-down costing and bottom-up costing. These methods are seen as complementary methods that can be used to obtain a complete collection of cost data and for cross-checking each other.

Bottom-Up Cost Analysis

Bottom-up costing involves three aspects:

1. An ingredients approach, in which the total quantities of goods and services employed in delivering health care are measured, and multiplied by their respective input prices (or unit costs).

2. Surveys of patients and/or caregivers to collect information on the costs associated with accessing and receiving care. Costs at this level reflect both out-of-pocket payments made to access and receive care and the opportunity costs of patients' and caregivers' time.

3. Detailed review of program accounting and expenditure reports to estimate program-level costs.

Bottom-up costing was used in all sites in the IMCI evaluation where costs were assessed.

Top-Down Cost Analysis

Some evidence indicates that increased funding, by itself, does not always result in more or better services. Various barriers to the effective usage of funds—such as leakage, corruption, and poor incentive structures—can have a detrimental impact on the effective use of funds (India Ministry of Health and Family Welfare, 2006). Thus the costs collected using the bottom-up approach may "miss" some financial expenditures and provide an unrealistic estimate of the true costs of services. The top-down and bottom-up approaches provide different bases from which to estimate total costs; thus they represent complementary means of assessing the accuracy of the data collected.

The top-down approach focuses on financial expenditure data, linking these data to other resources such as staff and services and population data. Data are collected by reviewing records and conducting interviews at pertinent governmental levels about the financial flows and costs of health services.

Allocation Methods

Some resources (e.g., staff, facility space, transportation) may be fully dedicated to the program being evaluated, in which case their full costs should be included in the estimation. In contrast, overhead (capital and administrative) costs may need to be allocated between the program being evaluated and other health or development activities. For example, structural overhead costs, such as for staff not involved in direct patient contact, may be allocated according to utilization variables (e.g., the percentage of visits that involve children). However, equipment, facility costs, and staff costs that are shared between different types of patients are usually allocated according to the amount of staff time spent on particular activities.

The gold-standard methodology for determining the proportion of time staff spent on particular activities comprises time-motion studies (Bratt et al., 1999). While provider interviews tend to underestimate nonproductive time (Bratt et al., 1999), this bias may not be as important when assessing relative time spent between activities. Time-motion studies were part of the IMCI evaluations in Tanzania, Brazil, and Bangladesh.

Incorporating Equity in the Evaluation

There is growing concern that programs and interventions may fail to reach those who need them most, and that overall progress in health indicators can hide important gender, socioeconomic, or ethnic group differences. Assessing the impact of a program on equity, therefore, is becoming increasingly more important.

The focus on equity can start at an early stage in the evaluation, by assessing whether programs are being deployed in those districts where they are most needed (i.e., in those with highest mortality and lowest standard of living). These analyses require combining data on baseline contextual factors with implementation strength—an approach that is further discussed in the later section on data analysis.

Another step to address equity concerns is to ensure that—within program areas—the evaluation team can document the degree to which different population subgroups (stratified by gender, socioeconomic position, urban versus rural residence, and ethnic group, for example) are benefiting from the interventions being promoted. Similar information should be collected for nonprogram areas. This effort requires ensuring that the data collection tools used for the evaluation incorporate the information required to classify families or individuals according to the stratification variables to be used in the analyses. Simple and reasonably accurate measurement of socioeconomic position is now possible in household surveys, using principal component analyses of household assets to classify families into five equal groups, or wealth quintiles (O'Donnell, Van Doorslaer,

Wagstaff, & Lindelow, 2007). Because it is possible to calculate aggregate indicators of inequality that use information from the whole population rather than a single subgroup (see the later section on data analysis), in most cases there is no need to expand the original sample sizes to perform such analyses. The three evaluations described in Exhibits 16-1, 16-2, and 16-3 incorporated equity analyses using these tools (Bryce et al., 2010; Hanson et al., 2009).

Incorporation of the equity dimension in program evaluations is no longer an option, given its importance and the wide availability and simplicity of existing tools. Rather, it is a requirement for public health interventions.

Carrying Out the Evaluation

In prospective evaluations, there is a need for continued interaction between the evaluation and implementation teams.

Starting the Evaluation Clock

In a prospective evaluation, documentation of program implementation will help assess how rapidly the interventions are being rolled out. This information should be used to plan the timing of post-baseline data collection on coverage and impact indicators. If outcomes are measured too early, there is a risk that the full effect of the program may not be captured. This was the case, for example, in a randomized evaluation of the Mexican Seguro Popular program, in which—for reasons beyond the control of the investigators—the endline survey took place only 10 months after the program was launched (King et al., 2009).

In the IMCI evaluation in Tanzania, formal meetings between the evaluation and implementation teams were held to decide whether the "evaluation clock" should be started—that is, whether data collection for assessing outcomes could be carried out. In the retrospective ACSD evaluation, similar discussions led to the identification of three periods: baseline (pre-program), phase-in, and endline (program fully implemented); each period lasted 18 to 24 months. The main analyses of program impact included comparisons between the endline and baseline phases.

Feedback to Implementers and Midstream Corrections

In classical efficacy trials, the interventions are defined a priori and remain unchanged during the study. This is not the case for large-scale programs including proven interventions, where midstream corrections are commonly undertaken to increase coverage and improve quality. Such corrections may result from the implementation team's own assessment of how the program is performing, based on internal monitoring. Changes may also arise in response to feedback from the evaluation team, as indicated in the earlier discussion of documentation. In prospective program evaluations, it would be unethical for the evaluators not to provide feedback on obvious implementation shortcomings.

Feedback from evaluators may also improve the program. This type of change may affect the external validity of the study findings, but in light of the ethical imperative this difficulty is unavoidable. To minimize this problem, it is essential that feedback should be provided in a structured manner—for example, in one session conducted every three to six months. All feedback and any resulting actions should be carefully documented and reported as part of the final evaluation results. Plans for feedback should be developed and agreed upon with program implementers in advance. In the IMCI evaluations, for example, an agreement was made that feedback would be provided at the national level first, so that further dissemination of the feedback to the district level and below could be conducted under the leadership of the ministry of health.

Ongoing feedback is not relevant to retrospective evaluations. Nevertheless, whatever the design of the evaluation, it is important to provide feedback to implementers and policy makers at the end of the study. This point is discussed later in the section on dissemination of evaluation results.

Linking the Independent Evaluation to Routine Monitoring and Evaluation

All programs must include internal monitoring and evaluation systems. Monitoring typically includes documenting program inputs and outputs—for example, the number of health workers trained, the number of ITN vouchers distributed, or the number of mothers attending breastfeeding promotion activities.

As far as possible, the independent evaluation data collection activities should be integrated with routine monitoring, such as by including the same data sources and indicator definitions. Because the data quality needs for a rigorous evaluation often exceed those required for routine monitoring, however, it may be necessary to set in place a parallel data collection or data quality checks system. This structure should not be viewed as a replacement for routine monitoring activities, which must continue during and after the independent evaluation. It is also important

to provide feedback to implementers when shortcomings are identified through routine monitoring.

Similarly, the presence of an independent evaluation does not replace the need for focused internal evaluations aimed at fine-tuning the program. As far as possible, these two exercises should be coordinated so that they complement each other.

Data Analyses

Data analyses should be driven by the evaluation questions, and should make full use of the data collected on implementation strength, quality, and outcomes—complemented by data on costs and contextual factors. Integrating data from different sources in a comprehensive and logical plan of analysis is not an easy task, and its success requires careful forward planning from the time the evaluation is being designed.

Issues in the analyses of nonrandomized evaluations are reviewed elsewhere (Cousens et al., 2009), but the following basic concepts should certainly drive the plan of analyses:

- The units of analysis should be the same as the geographical units where the program is being implemented (e.g., districts).
- The sample size is the number of districts, not the total number of individuals surveyed in all study districts.
- Detailed analyses of baseline comparability are essential.
- Standard stratification and regression techniques will often be appropriate, but attention must be given to the number of degrees of freedom, which will often be small as a result of the number of districts available for analyses.
- Propensity scores may be useful for summarizing several confounders (Sturmer, Joshi, Glynn, Avorn, Rothman, & Schneeweiss, 2006), particularly when the number of degrees of freedom is small.
- Comparisons between program and nonprogram areas, when baseline data exist, may rely on the difference-in-differences approach. This method focuses on the net change in each set of districts.
- Multilevel analyses may be appropriate if the data structure is hierarchical—for example, districts within the program area, health facilities within each district, providers within each facility, and patients seen by each provider.
- The plan of analysis should ideally examine all assumptions included in the conceptual

Table 16-3	Proposed Approaches for Data Analyses, According to Each Objective of a Hypothetical Evaluation of a Maternal, Newborn, and Child Health Program
Research Question/Objective	**Analytical Approach**

Primary Objectives

Research Question/Objective	Analytical Approach
1. Will the program-focus districts implement maternal, newborn, and child health (MNCH) interventions more strongly and at higher levels of quality than other districts in the country?	Comparison of implementation strength in program and nonprogram districts
2. Will the program-focus districts achieve greater increases in coverage of MNCH interventions than other districts in the country?	Comparison of changes in coverage over time in program and nonprogram districts
3. Will the program-focus districts achieve greater health impact (reductions in mortality and undernutrition) than other districts in the country?	Comparison of changes in impact indicators over time in program and nonprogram districts
4. How much did the program cost compared to other approaches, and how does their cost-effectiveness compare?	Comparison of costs and cost-effectiveness in program and nonprogram districts
5. Among all districts in the country, will those with stronger implementation of MNCH interventions achieve higher coverage levels than those with weaker implementation?	Dose-response analyses: regression of changes in coverage over time on implementation score
6. Among all districts in the country, will those with stronger implementation of MNCH interventions achieve greater health impact (reductions in mortality and undernutrition) than those with weaker implementation?	Dose-response analyses: regression of changes in impact indicators over time on implementation score
7. How much did the implementation cost, and is it cost-effective?	Dose-response analyses relating implementation costs to impact
8. If there is evidence of an impact, can external explanations for these associations be ruled out?	Incorporation of relevant confounding factors in the preceding analyses

Secondary Objectives

Research Question/Objective	Analytical Approach
9. Was the program focused on the districts where it was most needed, in terms of baseline health and socioeconomic characteristics?	Stratification of all districts according to baseline characteristics, and comparison of strata in terms of implementation strength
10. Did implementation of the program contribute to reducing socioeconomic and other inequities in MNCH indicators?	Analyses of time trends in inequalities in coverage and impact indicators, according to strength of implementation of program
11. Are there positive or negative effects of the program in terms of health systems, other health programs, or related indicators?	Comparison of health systems indicators and coverage of other interventions, according to strength of implementation of the program
12. Are changes in program implementation and in intervention coverage compatible with the observed impact on mortality and nutrition?	Comparison of actual changes in impact indicators with those predicted by modeling changes in intervention coverage (LiST)

model (i.e., all the arrows in the model). An example is provided in Table 16-3.

- The plan of analyses should be flexible, as real-world implementation may occur in ways that are not planned ahead of time.

Table 16-3 shows possible research questions for evaluating a hypothetical maternal, newborn, and child health program (MNCH) in a country in sub-Saharan Africa. The program includes several MNCH interventions, and will be initially rolled out in a limited number of districts. A stated objective of the program is to eventually scale up the program to all districts in the country, but this step will depend on further partner and governmental buy-in and additional funding. This somewhat vague implementation plan is typical of many health programs in low- and middle-income countries. A good example is the ACSD program (Exhibit 16-2), in which the full package was implemented in selected high-impact districts but a smaller set of interventions were scaled up nationally.

The analytical approaches suggested in Table 16-3 encompass the traditional program-versus-nonprogram districts comparison as well as dose-response analyses, such as those carried out in the context of an evaluation platform (Exhibit 16-5). Of the primary objectives, questions 1–4 may be addressed through a traditional comparison of two groups of districts (with or without the program). As pointed out earlier, such comparisons are often favored by funders, but may make little sense if the same or similar interventions are also present in the comparison areas. Answering questions 5–7 requires dose-response analyses, and goes beyond the simple stratification of districts in two groups. If a stepped wedge design is used for the evaluation, these questions can be tailored to this type of analytical approach (Hussey & Hughes, 2007).

Question 8 is fundamental for both approaches: It requires control of confounding factors to address the issue of attribution of an observed impact to a given program. In a context in which multiple programs are being studied simultaneously through an evaluation platform approach, the presence of other programs may also be included as a confounding factor. For example, the Tanzania ITN voucher evaluation showed that the program's effect persisted even after taking into account the large number of free ITNs that were distributed in some districts in 2005 (Hanson et al., 2009).

Questions 9–12 represent secondary objectives of the hypothetical program evaluation. Question 9 assesses whether programs are being deployed where they are most needed. Implementers often state that they are prioritizing the poorest or highest-mortality districts, but studies have shown that this is not always true (Victora et al., 2006). Identification of indicators of baseline mortality, poverty levels, or health systems strength available in the district database (Exhibit 16-5) will help answer this question.

A related question is number 10, which assesses changes in health inequalities between population subgroups. Earlier in this chapter, we described the importance of collecting information on gender, socioeconomic position, urban versus rural residence and ethnic group during surveys commissioned by the evaluation. Several approaches may be used to express the magnitude of inequality, and how this level evolves over time in program and nonprogram areas. In particular, use of concentration indices and

of slope indices of inequality has become increasingly popular (O'Donnell et al., 2007; PAHO, 1999; Pamuk, 1985; Wagstaff, Paci, & van Doorslaer, 1991).

Question 11 relates to side effects of the program, which are often unintended and overlooked. Evaluators can address this question by collecting relevant information on the implementation and coverage of other health programs, such as through an evaluation platform approach.

Finally, question 12 relies on statistical modeling to check whether the observed impact on health status is compatible with the magnitude of changes in coverage of the interventions being promoted. In the case of maternal, newborn, and child mortality, the LiST software (Exhibit 16-7; Johns Hopkins Bloomberg School of Public Health, n.d.) may be used to conduct these simulation exercises. Demonstration that the degree of mortality decline can be explained by changes in coverage is a strong argument that reinforces the impact model and increases the ability to attribute the health impact to the program interventions.

For evaluations that do not go as far as measuring mortality impact—for example, most evaluations in the field of maternal health and of HIV/AIDS programs—use of LiST or similar simulation tools can provide evidence to funders and national policy makers that observed improvements in coverage are most likely contributing to reducing mortality rates.

Analyzing Costs and Cost-Effectiveness

A number of process, intermediate, and outcome indicators are available to be compared with cost; these indicators are summarized in Table 16-4. To the extent possible, all of these indicators should be used, because each provides useful information. However, the minimum set of recommended indicators includes the following items:

- Cost per beneficiary
- For curative services, the cost per person treated
- For preventive services, the cost per preventive item delivered
- Cost per death averted

Costs should be presented in the currency most relevant for the target audience. In most cases, this means that results should be presented in local currency units (for national policy makers), in U.S. dollars (for donors and program managers in other countries), and in purchasing power parity adjusted dollars (for comparison with other studies and for international policy makers). The website found at

Table 16-4	Types of Process, Intermediate, and Outcome Indicators and Data Needed		
Type of Indicator	**Indicator**	**What the Indicator Measures**	**Additional Data Needed for the Indicator**
Process	Ex ante cost-effectiveness	Expected costs and value for money	Budget projections, work plans, coverage targets
Process	Incremental/total cost per person treated	Services provided	Utilization rates
Process	Incremental/total cost per preventive item delivered (e.g., bed net or vitamin A capsule)	Services provided	Utilization rates
Process	Cost per capita	Services provided, program effort, and sustainability	Population
Intermediate	Incremental/total cost per patient correctly treated	Treatment leading to health gains	Utilization rates adjusted by quality
Intermediate/outcome	[Marginal] cost of quality improvement	Improvements in services due to program	Quantitative measure of quality improvements
Outcome	Incremental cost per death averted	Mortality reduction	Mortality rates
Outcome	Incremental cost per life year gained	Mortality reduction	Mortality rates and age of death (and life expectancy)
Outcome	Incremental cost per DALY averted	Mortality and morbidity reduction	Mortality rates, age of death (and life expectancy), average morbidity associated with diseases, correct treatment by disease

Source: Evaluation Gap Working Group, 2006.

http://www.who.int/choice/costs/ppp/en/index.html offers more details about purchasing power parity adjusted dollars.

Total costs are defined as the sum of all costs associated with a particular scale of activity and are derived by summing all the costs incurred during production (e.g., the costs of providing a vaccination service). For example, costs at facilities can be estimated using the bottom-up approach by multiplying unit costs by the number of patients visiting health facilities; the unit costs may be weighted if the sampling scheme was stratified by type of facility.

Average costs are measures of the total costs of production associated with each unit of output. They indicate the resource requirements for each unit of output and are calculated by dividing total costs by the number of units of output (e.g., cost per vaccination provided).

Marginal costs are measures of the resources associated with a small change in the output of health care. Most economic decisions do not focus on whether to produce all or nothing, but rather concern small changes in the existing scale of an activity. The concept of marginal cost addresses the change in costs associated with increasing or decreasing output by one unit; it is derived by calculating the change in total costs for that one unit. In practice, it is rare for output to change by one unit, so the marginal cost of a particular program is often approximated by dividing the change in total costs associated with a larger change in production by the change in production (e.g., change in total costs ÷ change in number of vaccinations). For example, an evaluator might identify the cost of extending the same vaccination service to another village and divide this value by the additional number of vaccinations to obtain the marginal costs.

Incremental costs are defined as the difference in cost between two alternatives—for example, the difference in costs between a district without scale-up activities and a district with scale-up activities.

Once the incremental cost has been established, it can be compared with the incremental benefits to determine the *incremental cost-effectiveness ratio*

(ICER). At the very least, cost-effectiveness should be calculated using deaths averted as the denominator. Other metrics (e.g., life-years saved, DALYs averted) can be applied if relevant for a particular country, although these metrics also imply different analytic horizons or time frames.

The *ceiling ratio* is the relative cost-effectiveness value against which the acceptability of ICERs is judged. If the value of an ICER is below the ceiling ratio, an intervention is deemed acceptable on grounds of cost-effectiveness. Based on the recommendation of the Commission on Macroeconomics and Health (CMH, 2001), WHO classifies interventions as "highly cost-effective" for a given country if results show that they avert a DALY for less than the per capita national GNI or GDP, and as "cost-effective" if this value is less than three times the per capita national GNI. The choice of ceiling ratios is affected by the decision maker's valuation of a unit of health gain and is a particularly crucial and politically sensitive element of economic evaluation.

We suggest placing findings in a broader context by comparing them to other economic evaluations that have been undertaken in the same or neighboring countries after adjustments have been made for inflation. Placing results in the context of a ceiling ratio provides a general picture of the program's value for money, but does not address the issue of whether the intervention represents the best use of additional resources. Comparing the results to other studies will partly alleviate this problem. It also informs the decision maker about other options to the program besides "doing nothing," "the status quo," or what is happening in the comparison areas. Note, however, that the methods and assumptions in other studies may be different from those employed here or in comparison with each other, which makes these comparisons problematic. Results need to be interpreted with these shortcomings made clear.

Interpretation and Attribution

Adequacy evaluations were discussed earlier in this chapter, in the design section. These assessments typically include a before and after comparison of outcomes within the program areas, without an external comparison. The conclusion may be that outcome indicators improved, remained unchanged, or worsened. Such evaluations may be useful for assessing changes in coverage and attributing them to a given program, but are rarely sufficient for attributing impact. Therefore, adequacy evaluations per se have a limited role in attribution.

Nevertheless, assessment of the adequacy of impact indicators—whether or not they improved over time—is essential, even in more complex plausibility evaluations that also include a comparison group. Because every plausibility evaluation provides the opportunity to assess adequacy, it is possible to interpret these findings jointly. Table 16-5 shows how combining adequacy and plausibility may help interpret results and attribute them to a given program. (Table 16-5 is based on a program-versus-nonprogram areas design, but it can be adapted to dose-response and stepped wedge designs as well.) The plausibility find-

Table 16-5	Joint Interpretation of Findings from Adequacy and Plausibility Analyses		
How Did Program Areas Fare Relative to Nonprogram Areas? (Plausibility Assessment)	**How Did Impact Indicators Change Over Time in the Program Areas (Adequacy Assessment)**		
	Improved	**No Change**	**Worsened**
Better	Both areas improved, but the program led to faster improvement	Program provided a safety net	Program provided a partial safety net
Same	Both areas improved to a similar extent; no evidence of an additional program impact	No change in either area; no evidence of program impact	Indicators worsened in both areas; no evidence of a safety net
Worse	Both areas improved, particularly nonprogram areas; presence of the program may have precluded the deployment of more effective strategies	Program precluded progress; presence of the program may have hindered the deployment of more effective strategies	Program was detrimental; presence of the program may have hindered the deployment of more effective strategies

ings are assumed to be not confounded—that is, unaffected by changes in contextual factors.

Our experience with large-scale evaluations is that implementers often concentrate on adequacy findings (e.g., did mortality rates fall?). Although this understanding is important, the result does not necessarily mean that the program can be held responsible for the observed success, as in some cases the comparison areas did just as well. An example is the Bangladesh IMCI evaluation (Arifeen et al., 2009).

Table 16-5 also shows situations in which no improvement occurred in the program areas but nonprogram areas fared worse. This outcome would support a safety net effect in which the program helped offset the deterioration in external factors.

Finally, there is the possibility that the program displaced a more efficient program or strategy. This outcome may have occurred in the ACSD evaluation in Mali (Bryce et al., 2010), where documentation of program implementation and contextual factors showed that other funding agencies were supporting the scale-up of similar MNCH interventions as ACSD in most districts from the comparison area.

Ensuring the internal validity of an evaluation requires several measures that were described earlier in this chapter. These steps include taking into account baseline comparability, documenting and adjusting for important confounding factors, ensuring valid measurement of implementation and outcomes, and using appropriate analytical strategies. An equally important consideration is to document changes in the intermediate steps laid out in the impact model, and to show that these outcomes are consistent with the impact findings.

Plausibility that the impact findings can be attributed to the intervention does not depend on a single finding or analysis, but rather on the progressive accumulation of evidence supporting the hypothesis that the observed impact is due to a program. This type of buildup was noted in the Tanzania ITN voucher evaluation (Hanson et al., 2009).

Attribution is a central issue in evaluation and should be considered prior to deciding on an evaluation design. When multiple agencies or programs are active in the same country promoting similar interventions, it is difficult, if not impossible, to attribute any observed improvements to a single partner. A more sensible approach in such situations is to adopt a "contributorship" model of attribution, in which all those who contribute to a program are acknowledged and successes or failures are shared among them. Doing a good job on the documentation component of the evaluation should make this type of joint attribution possible.

Evaluators are sometimes requested not only to provide evidence that overall impact can be attributed to a program, but also to assess which of several program components or interventions played the most important role. As mentioned in the description of the IMCI and ACSD programs, it is usually impossible to disentangle these different components, unless there are few interventions, the various interventions address different causes of morbidity and mortality, and little comorbidity exists between these causes. A similar issue arises when different funders support separate interventions that are packaged in the same program, in which case separate attribution of results is seldom possible. Funders and implementers must become aware early on that these types of attribution are not feasible.

Disseminating Evaluation Findings and Promoting Their Uptake

Evaluators have an ethical responsibility to make their findings available so that they can be used to guide program implementation and future evaluations. The provision of feedback to program implementers was addressed earlier in this chapter; the same principles apply to the final results addressing the evaluation questions. Dissemination activities should be planned and carried out with several audiences in mind:

- *Policy makers and program implementers at country level.* These audiences should be carefully defined, and are likely to include district managers and even communities as well as national-level decision makers. Dissemination channels can take various forms, including face-to-face presentations and print materials. For example, in the IMCI evaluation, meetings with policy makers were held to define the need for specially designed policy briefs, which were then developed by the evaluation team using a format and style that was accessible to national decision makers.

- *Global scientific public health communities.* Evaluators have a responsibility to publish their findings in peer-reviewed scientific journals, and especially those likely to reach readers who can make use of the findings. Presentations at professional conferences usually reach a smaller audience but can also be useful. The latter forums offer an opportunity for younger members of the evaluation team to gain visibility and experience in presenting to colleagues.

Our experience indicates that generating interest in and uptake of the results of large-scale program evaluations is an ongoing process, and often requires several attempts using multiple channels. One strategy that can help in this regard is to ensure that those who can make use of the findings are involved from the start in defining the evaluation questions and are kept informed of the progress of the evaluation and its intermediate results.

Working in Large-Scale Evaluations

Conducting large-scale evaluations is not for the faint-hearted. This chapter has focused on the technical aspects of designing and conducting an evaluation, mentioning only in passing some of the political and personal challenges involved. We close the presentation here by highlighting a selection of these issues, all of which are crucial for designing an evaluation that can produce sound evidence that is widely used to improve public health practice and programs.

First, good evaluations require effective communication. Exhibit 16-9 lists some common misperceptions about evaluation and evaluators from the perspective of those implementing or funding programs, and vice versa.

Second, good evaluations require a broad range of skills and techniques, as well as an interdisciplinary approach. Evaluators should have sufficient experience and a multifaceted "toolbox" to respond to the specific questions posed by stakeholders, rather than just those questions they have been trained to answer. This goal is often best accomplished by establishing an evaluation team, as was done in all of the large-scale evaluations used as examples in this chapter.

Third, good evaluations require patience and flexibility. Large-scale evaluations can move only as fast as implementation, and real-world programs are vulnerable to frequent delays, setbacks, and false starts. Timetables for program implementation often slip or are changed for reasons outside the control of the evaluation team. In-country research partners have many demands on their time, and capacity-building exercises are often needed as a precursor to full analysis of the data. Evaluation results may sit on a shelf until political circumstances or changes in leadership provide an opportunity for them to be incorporated

---

Exhibit 16-9 | **Building Stronger Bridges Between Implementers and Evaluators**

Table 16-6 lists some of the things implementers say about evaluators, and evaluators say about implementers. In a perfect world, these perceptions would be brought into alignment and both groups would recognize the value of sound evaluation as a contribution to strong programs. Making this synchrony happen is a challenge that must be faced every day, in every evaluation.

Table 16-6 | **What Are They Saying?**

Implementers About Evaluators and Evaluations	Evaluators About Program Implementers and Implementation
• Not tied to the realities of the field; too academic	• Don't understand the importance of external, independent evaluations
• Too slow in producing results	• Underestimate the need for data checking and time for analysis before sharing results
• Cost too much; resources would be better spent in doing more implementation	• Need to recognize and act on intermediate results more rapidly
• Can bring only bad news	• Want to "cherry pick" the findings to support their own program
• Too focused on impact rather than process (black box)	• Don't understand that evaluation is a technical discipline and requires special training to be done well
• Insensitive to the policy process—produce results that are too late, too negative, insufficiently action oriented	• Need to do more internal monitoring and documentation of their own programs and to cover such costs from their budgets, rather than expect evaluators to do these tasks
• We could do a better job ourselves, from within the program	

into program plans. Ideal designs (based on textbooks like this one) must often be modified to reflect what is possible and affordable in specific country contexts.

This chapter extends an invitation to readers to become engaged in the science of large-scale evaluations, either as evaluators themselves or as informed consumers and supporters. Few formal training programs for public health evaluators exist, although the number has increased in recent years. Making a commitment to evaluation often requires seeking out and using resources from a variety of disciplines, and bringing them together into an effective mix of skills. Recent efforts to establish a community of practice—for example, the 3ie initiative—should be continued and expanded to support this emerging culture and to ensure that more and better evaluations of large-scale programs are supported in the future.

● ● ● References

Adam, T., Edwards, S. J., Amorim, D. G., Amaral, J., Victora, C. G., & Evans D. B. (2009). Cost implications of improving the quality of child care using integrated clinical algorithms: Evidence from Northeast Brazil. *Health Policy 89*, 97–106.

Adam, T., Ebener, S., Johns, B., & Evans, D. B. (2008). Capacity utilization and the cost of primary care visits: Implications for the costs of scaling up health interventions. *Cost Effectiveness and Resource Allocation, 6*, 22.

Adam, T., Manzi, F., Schellenberg, J. A., Mgalula, L., de Savigny, D., & Evans, D. B. (2005). Does the integrated management of childhood illness cost more than routine care? Results from the United Republic of Tanzania. *Bulletin of the World Health Organization, 83*, 369–377.

Adam, T., Bishai, D., Kahn, M., & Evans, D. (2004). Methods for the costing component of the multi-country evaluation of IMCI. Geneva, Switzerland: World Health Organization.

Amorim, D. G., Adam, T., Amaral, J. J., Gouws, E., Bryce, J., & Victora, C. G. (2008). Integrated management of childhood illness: Efficiency of primary health in Northeast Brazil. *Revista de saude publica 42*, 183–190.

Arifeen, S. E., Hoque, D. M., Akter, T., Rahman, M., Hoque, M. E., Begum, K., et al. (2009). Effect of the Integrated Management of Childhood Illness strategy on childhood mortality and nutrition in a rural area in Bangladesh: A cluster randomised trial. *Lancet, 374*(9687), 393–403.

Baltussen, R., Adam, T., Tan-Torres, E. T., Hutubessy, R., Acharya, A., Evans, D. B., et al. (2003). Methods for generalized cost-effectiveness analysis. (Eds.) In *WHO Guide to Cost-Effectiveness Analysis, 2*, 106. Geneva, Switzerland: World Health Organization.

Barnighausen, T., & Bloom, D. E. (2009). Financial incentives for return of service in underserved areas: A systematic review. *BMC Health Services Research, 9*, 86.

Berman, P., Brotowasisto, Nadjib, M., Sakai, S., & Gani, A. (1989). The costs of public primary health care services in rural Indonesia. *Bulletin of the World Health Organization, 67*, 685–694.

Bishai, D., Mirchandani, G., Pariyo, G., Burnham, G., & Black, R. (2008). The cost of quality improvements due to integrated management of childhood illness (IMCI) in Uganda. *Health Economics, 17*, 5–19.

Black, N. (1996). Why we need observational studies to evaluate the effectiveness of health care. *British Medical Journal, 312*(7040), 1215–1218.

Boschi-Pinto, C., Young, M., & Black, R. (2010). The child health epidemiology reference group reviews of the effectiveness of interventions to reduce maternal, neonatal and child mortality. *International Journal of Epidemiology, 39*(1 suppl), i3–i6.

Bratt, J. H., Foreit, J., Chen, P. L., West, C., Janowitz, B., De Vargas, T. (1999). A comparison of four approaches for measuring clinician time use. *Health Policy and Planning, 14*, 374–381.

Brown, C. A., & Lilford, R. J. (2006). The stepped wedge trial design: A systematic review. *BMC Medical Research Methodology, 6*, 54.

Bryce, J., Friberg, K., Kraushaar, D., Nsona, H., Afenyadu, G., Nare, N., et al. (2010). LiST as a catalyst in program planning: Experiences from Burkina Faso, Ghana and Malawi. *International Journal of Epidemiology, 39*(1 suppl), i40–i47.

Bryce, J., Gilroy, K., Jones, G., Hazel, E., Black, R. E., & Victora, C. G. (2010). The accelerated child survival and development programme in west Africa: A retrospective evaluation. *Lancet, 375*(9714), 572–582.

Bryce, J., Victora, C. G., Habicht, J. P., Black, R. E., & Scherpbier, R. W. (2005). Programmatic pathways to child survival: Results of a multi-country evaluation of Integrated Management of Childhood Illness. *Health Policy and Planning, 20*(suppl 1), i5–i17.

Bryce, J., Victora, C. G., Habicht, J. P., Vaughan, J. P., & Black, R. E. (2004). The multi-country evaluation of the Integrated Management of Childhood Illness strategy: Lessons for the evaluation of public health interventions. *American Journal of Public Health*, 94(3), 406–415.

Cochran, W. G. (1977). *Sampling techniques*. 3rd ed. New York: John Wiley & Sons.

Commission on Macroeconomics and Health. (2001). Macroeconomics and health: Investing in health for economic development. Geneva, Switzerland: World Health Organization.

Cousens, S., Hargreaves, J., Bonell, C., Armstrong, B., Thomas, J., Kirkwood, B. R., et al. (2009). Alternatives to randomisation in the evaluation of public-health interventions: Statistical analysis and causal inference. *Journal of Epidemiology and Community Health*, 6, 6.

Donner, A., & Klar, N. (2000). *Design and analysis of cluster randomization trials in health research*. London: Arnold.

Evaluation: The top priority for global health. (2011). *Lancet*, 377, 85–95.

Evaluation Gap Working Group. (2006). *When will we ever learn? Improving lives through impact evaluation*. Washington, DC: Center for Global Development. Retrieved from http://www.cgdev .org/content/publications/detail/7973.

Global Initiative to Strengthen Country Health Systems Surveillance (CHeSS). (2008). *Summary report of a technical meeting and action plan*. Bellagio, Italy: Bellagio Rockefeller Center.

Gouws, E., Bryce, J., Pariyo, G., Armstrong Schellenberg, J., Amaral, J., & Habicht, J. P. (2005). Measuring the quality of child health care at first-level facilities. *Social Science & Medicine*, 61(3), 613–625.

Grieve, R., Nixon, R., Thompson, S.G., & Normand, C. (2005). Using multilevel models for assessing the variability of multinational resource use and cost data. *Health Economics*, 14, 185–196.

Guinness, L., Kumaranayake, L., Rajaraman, B., Sankaranarayanan, G., Vannela, G., Raghupathi, P., et al. (2005). Does scale matter? The costs of HIV-prevention interventions for commercial sex workers in India. *Bulletin of the World Health Organization*, 83, 747–755.

Habicht, J. P., Victora, C. G., & Vaughan, J. P. (1999). Evaluation designs for adequacy, plausibility and probability of public health programme performance and impact. *International Journal of Epidemiology*, 28(1), 10–18.

Hanson, K., Marchant, T., Nathan, R., Mponda, H., Jones, C., Bruce, J., et al. (2009). Household ownership and use of insecticide treated nets among target groups after implementation of a national voucher programme in the United Republic of Tanzania: Plausibility study using three annual cross sectional household surveys. *British Medical Journal*, 2, 239.

Hanson, K., Nathan, R., Marchant, T., Mponda, H., Jones, C., Bruce, J., et al. (2008). Vouchers for scaling up insecticide-treated nets in Tanzania: Methods for monitoring and evaluation of a national health system intervention. *BMC Public Health*, 8, 205.

Hofer, T. P., Hayward, R. A., Greenfield, S., Wagner, E. H., Kaplan, S. H., Manning, W. G. (1999). The unreliability of individual physician "report cards" for assessing the costs and quality of care of a chronic disease. *Journal of the American Medical Association*, 281, 2098–2105.

Hollingsworth, B. (2003). Non-parametric and parametric applications measuring efficiency in health care. *Health Care Management Science*, 6, 203–218.

Huicho, L., Davila, M., Gonzales, F., Drasbek, C., Bryce, J., & Victora, C. G. (2005). Implementation of the Integrated Management of Childhood Illness strategy in Peru and its association with health indicators: An ecological analysis. *Health Policy Plan*, 20(suppl 1), i32–i41.

Hussey, P. S., de Vries, H., Romley, J., Wang, M. C., Chen, S. S., Shekelle, P. G., et al. (2009). A systematic review of health care efficiency measures. *Health Services Research*, 44, 784–805.

Hussey, M. A., & Hughes, J. P. (2007). Design and analysis of stepped wedge cluster randomized trials. *Contemporary Clinical Trials*, 28(2), 182–191.

India Ministry of Health and Family Welfare. (2006). *Reproductive and child health survey*.

Jacobs, R., Smith, P., & Street, A. (2006). Measuring efficiency in health care: Analytic techniques and health policy. Cambridge, UK: Cambridge University Press.

Johns, B., & Torres, T. T. (2005). Costs of scaling up health interventions: A Systematic review. *Health Policy and Planning*, 20, 1–13.

Johns Hopkins Bloomberg School of Public Health, Department of International Health. (n.d.). LiST: An evidence-based decision-making tool for estimating intervention impact. Retrieved from http://www.jhsph.edu/dept/ih/IIP/list/index.html

King, G., Gakidou, E., Imai, K., Lakin, J., Moore, R. T., Nall, C., et al. (2009). Public policy for the poor? A randomised assessment of the Mexican universal health insurance programme. *Lancet*, 373(9673), 1447–1454.

Kleinbaum, D. G., Kupper, L. L., & Morgenstern, H. (1982). *Epidemiologic research: Principles and quantitative methods*. Hoboken, NJ: John Wiley & Sons.

Kumaranayake, L. (2008). The economics of scaling up: Cost estimation for HIV/AIDS interventions. *AIDS*, 22 (1 Suppl), S23–S33.

Lambrechts, T., Bryce, J., & Orinda, V. (1999). Integrated management of childhood illness: A summary of first experiences. *Bulletin of the World Health Organization*, 77(7), 582–594.

Mangham, L. J. & Hanson, K. (2010). Scaling up in international health: What are the key issues? *Health Policy and Planning*, 25(2), 85–96.

Marseille, E., Dandona, L., Saba, J., McConnel, C., Rollins, B., Gaist, P., et al. (2004). Assessing the efficiency of HIV prevention around the world: Methods of the PANCEA project. *Health Services Research*, 39, 1993–2012.

Masiye, F., Kirigia, J. M., Emrouznejad, A., Sambo, L. G., Mounkaila, A., Chimfwembe, D., et al. (2006). Efficient management of health centres human resources in Zambia. *Journal of Medical Systems*, 30, 473–481.

Measure DHS. (n.d.). AIDS indicators surveys: AIS overview. Retrieved from http://www.measuredhs.com/aboutsurveys/ais/start.cfm

Measure DHS. (n.d.). Demographic and health surveys: DHS overview. Retrieved from http://www.measuredhs.com/aboutsurveys/dhs/start.cfm

Measure DHS. (n.d.). Malaria indicator surveys. Retrieved from http://www.measuredhs.com/aboutsurveys/mis/start.cfm

Measure DHS. (2010). Malawi: Standard DHS, 2009. Retrieved from http://www.measuredhs.com/aboutsurveys/search/metadata.cfm?surv_id=333&ctry_id=24&SrvyTp

Moulton, L. H. (2004). Covariate-based constrained randomization of group-randomized trials. *Clinical Trials*, 1(3), 297–305.

Mulligan, J. A., Yukich, J., & Hanson, K. (2008). Costs and effects of the Tanzanian national voucher scheme for insecticide-treated nets. *Malaria Journal*, 7, 32.

O'Donnell, O., Van Doorslaer, E., Wagstaff, A., & Lindelow, M. (2007). *Analyzing health equity using household survey data: A guide to techniques and their implementation*. Washington, DC: World Bank Publications.

Oxman, A. D., Bjorndal, A., Becerra-Posada, F., Gibson, M., Block, M. A., Haines, A., et al. (2010). A framework for mandatory impact evaluation to ensure well informed public policy decisions. *Lancet*, 375(9712), 427–431.

Pamuk, E. R. (1985). Social class inequalities in mortality from 1921 to 1972 in England and Wales. *Population Studies*, 39, 17–31.

Pan American Health Organization (PAHO). (1996). Impact of Uruguay's introduction of the *Haemophilus influenzae* type b (Hib) vaccine. *EPI Newsletter*, 18, 6.

Pan American Health Organization (PAHO). (1999). Health analysis: Risks of dying and income inequalities. *Epidemiology Bulletin*, 20(4), 7–10.

Pariyo, G. W., Gouws, E., Bryce, J., & Burnham, G. (2005). Improving facility-based care for sick children in Uganda: Training is not enough. *Health Policy and Planning*, 20(suppl 1), i58–i68.

Rao, J. K. N. (2003). *Small area estimation*. Hoboken, NJ: Wiley Interscience.

Rivera, J. A., Sotres-Alvarez, D., Habicht, J. P., Shamah, T., & Villalpando, S. (2004). Impact of the Mexican program for education, health, and nutrition (Progresa) on rates of growth and anemia in infants and young children: A randomized effectiveness study. *Journal of the American Medical Association, 291*(21), 2563–2570.

Santos, L. M., Paes-Sousa, R., Silva, J. B. Jr., & Victora, C. G. (2008). National Immunization Day: A strategy to monitor health and nutrition indicators. *Bulletin of the World Health Organization, 86*(6), 474–479.

Schellenberg, J. R. A., Adam, T., Mshinda, H., Masanja, H., Kabadi, G., Mukasa, O., et al. (2004). Effectiveness and cost of facility-based Integrated Management of Childhood Illness (IMCI) in Tanzania. *Lancet, 364*(9445), 1583–1594.

Stover, J., McKinnon, R., & Winfrey, B. (2010). Spectrum: A model platform for linking maternal and child survival interventions with AIDS, family planning and demographic projections. *International Journal of Epidemiology, 39*(1 suppl), i7–i10.

Sturmer, T., Joshi, M., Glynn, R. J., Avorn, J., Rothman, K. J., & Schneeweiss, S. (2006). A review of the application of propensity score methods yielded increasing use, advantages in specific settings, but not substantially different estimates compared with conventional multivariable methods. *Journal of Clinical Epidemiology, 59*(5), 437–447.

Tucker, A. M., Weiner, J. P., Honigfeld, S., Parton, R. A. (1996). Profiling primary care physician resource use: Examining the application of case mix adjustment. *Journal of Ambulatory Care Management, 19*, 60–80.

Tulloch, J. (1999). Integrated approach to child health in developing countries. *Lancet, 354*(suppl 2), SII16–SII20.

UNICEF. (2005). Accelerating child survival and development: A results-based approach in high under-five mortality areas: Final report to CIDA. New York: Author.

UNICEF. (n.d.). Childinfo: Multiple indicator cluster surveys (MICS). Retrieved from http://www.childinfo.org/mics.html

Valdmanis, V., Walker, D., & Fox-Rushby, J. (2003). Are vaccination sites in Bangladesh scale efficient? *International Journal of Technology Assessment in Health Care, 19*, 692–697.

Victora, C. G., Black, R. E., & Bryce, J. (2009). Evaluating child survival programmes. *Bulletin of the World Health Organization, 87*(2), 83.

Victora, C. G., Habicht, J. P., & Bryce, J. (2004). Evidence-based public health: Moving beyond randomized trials. *American Journal of Public Health, 94*(3), 400–405.

Victora, C. G., Huicho, L., Amaral, J. J., Armstrong-Schellenberg, J., Manzi, F., Mason, E., et al. (2006). Are health interventions implemented where they are most needed? District uptake of the integrated management of childhood illness strategy in Brazil, Peru and the United Republic of Tanzania. *Bulletin of the World Health Organization, 84*(10), 792–801.

Victora, C. G., Schellenberg, J. A., Huicho, L., Amaral, J., El Arifeen, S., Pariyo, G., et al. Context matters: Interpreting impact findings in child survival evaluations. *Health Policy Plan 2005, 20*: i18–31.

Wagstaff, A., Paci, P., & van Doorslaer, E. (1991). On the measurement of inequalities in health. *Social Science & Medicine, 33*(5), 545–557.

West, B. T., Berglund, P., & Heeringa, S. G. (2008). A closer examination of subpopulation analysis of complex-sample survey data. *Stata Journal, 8*(4), 520–531.

World Bank. (2010). Results-based financing. Retrieved from http://web.worldbank.org/WBSITE/EXTERNAL/TOPICS/EXTHEALTHNUTRITIONANDPOPULATION/EXTHSD/0,,menuPK:376799~pagePK:149018~piPK:149093~theSitePK:376793,00.html

Yu, D., Souteyrand, Y., Banda, M. A., Kaufman, J., & Perriens, J. H. (2008). Investment in HIV/AIDS programs: Does it help strengthen health systems in developing countries? *Global Health, 4*, 8.

17

Cooperation in Global Health

GILL WALT, KENT BUSE, AND ANDREW HARMER

Why do countries cooperate in global health? This chapter explores this question, focusing on the cooperation process, the institutions and actors involved in global health cooperation, the ways in which they have changed over the past 50 years, and the implications that these factors may have for future health policies around the world. A policy approach provides the theoretical framework, drawing on a number of disciplines and focusing on the interaction among context, actors, and processes (Walt & Gilson, 1994).

As suggested in this chapter, there has been a shift from international to global cooperation and from vertical representation to horizontal participation in global health in recent times. Vertical representation describes the relationship between the state and international organizations that make up the United Nations (UN) system, which was established in the mid-1940s to represent the interests of all states and promote cooperation between them. By 2000, global cooperation was determined less by formal vertical representation between the state and international organizations than by horizontal partnerships and alliances among many different bodies, including the state, UN agencies, industry, and nongovernmental organizations (NGOs). It is this shift to more diverse actors and inclusive decision-making processes that characterizes the notion of "global" as compared to "international" health (Koplan et al., 2009).

The chapter starts by describing the analytical framework of global health cooperation. It goes on to identify the actors (including the state) in global health, and to ask why states cooperate, and through which mechanisms. The second half of the chapter analyzes the shifts in global cooperation, demonstrating how vertical representation has been replaced by hor-

izontal participation, and describing the implications of these shifts for global health policy.

The Policy Framework

Many of the earlier chapters in this book have focused on the content of policy: current problems in communicable diseases (e.g., increasing rates of sexually transmitted diseases) or nutrition (e.g., lack of vitamin A leading to blindness), and the sorts of policies employed to address these problems (e.g., training primary health workers to recognize the signs and symptoms of sexually transmitted infections, or introducing vitamin A into routine immunization programs). Some of the chapters have also explored how health systems have been designed and managed to put these policies into practice by emphasizing primary healthcare (PHC) systems or decentralization of management. This chapter provides an understanding of global health policy by focusing on the roles of actors and the ways in which they are affected by, and influence, the context and processes within which policies are made and implemented.

Actors may be individuals (e.g., a minister of health), or groups (e.g., the National Association of Nurses), but institutions (e.g., a university or the World Bank) and even states (e.g., the United States) also are considered actors. Although actors may be involved in national or global policy, it should not be assumed that all groups, institutions, or states act with one voice, or that there are not quite different, and sometimes contending, groups of actors within institutions. The World Bank, for example, acts according to a particular mission but is made up of individuals who do not necessarily agree with one another or with the World Bank's policy on a particular issue.

Because actors are the center of analysis in this chapter, it is helpful to differentiate ways of referring to them. Individuals can be all-important, but alone are not likely to be very effective. Their influence arises because they lead social movements (i.e., bring people together, usually in protest or to promote a particular cause) or are key members of organizations. For example, it was the combination of a charismatic leader, Zachie Achmat, and the dynamic South African NGO, the Treatment Action Campaign, that gave this organization its high profile and successful reputation in the 2000s (Fassin & Schneider, 2003).

Understanding organizations and their roles within global health is central to understanding how change comes about. Organizations differ in their reputations, of course. Some are strong, with high levels of influence because of their wealth, knowledge, research, professional expertise, and contribution to the economy. Such organizations (and individuals within them) are likely to have considerable access to other influential individuals in key government departments, corporations, academic institutions, and so on, and be able to influence ideas and policies. However, reputations are not set in stone, and organizations have to adapt and change with time. The World Health Organization (WHO), for example, was held in high regard until the 1980s, after which it struggled to retain its earlier authority.

In this chapter, actors refers to individuals and institutions such as UNICEF, WHO, or public–private partnerships at the global level. Ministries of health (MOHs) at the national level and, more broadly, governments or states are also actors. The state is an abstract notion, but generally refers to all the authoritative decision-making bodies within a specific geographic border. It is legally supreme, and can use force to achieve its ends. The state's lawmaking occurs through government—a narrower concept that includes the public institutions, such as the legislative body, the executive, the bureaucracy, and ministries or departments of state. The judiciary, which is part of government, is responsible for interpreting and applying the law. All governments are organized into different levels, and subnational bodies or local authorities may also be referred to as policy actors. A lively contemporary debate addresses the role of the state, including how trends in globalization are affecting it and reducing its role (Stiglitz, 2002). In this chapter, however, the state is assumed to be a central player in global health cooperation, although, as will be shown, its role has changed.

Context refers to a myriad of external factors that affect the way policy is formulated and implemented. Political and economic instability in a country or region may mean that domestic policy makers are prepared to support only short-term, or incremental, changes to policy for fear of losing power; it may mean that internationally agreed-upon policies on immunization campaigns, for example, cannot be executed. A newly elected government may have the legitimacy to introduce major change, as happened in South Africa in 1994 when free health services were introduced for all children younger than the age of 6 years. Political transformation in Eastern Europe in the wake of the fall of the Soviet bloc led to a host of health reforms being introduced in the countries of the former Soviet Union. Similarly, a new leader in a UN agency may have added legitimacy to initiate new policies; for example, in 1998, after years of taking a very cautious approach on tobacco and its harmful effects on health, a high-level campaign advocating tobacco control was initiated by a new director-general in WHO (Exhibit 17-1). Multiethnicity, linguistic plurality, and the position of women all influence policy at both national and international levels. For example, people may not have the same trust or confidence in a health professional, a scientist, or a consultant who is a member of another ethnic or national group or who does not speak their language. Contextual factors may be specific to particular countries or common globally (as with world economic recessions, for example, which affect the availability of domestic and international resources to implement health policies).

The *process of policy making* is influenced by the history and role of the different institutions of government. Policy processes can be described as occurring in different phases:

- How issues get onto the policy agenda (Is there a role for the media?)

- Who is consulted in the formulation and design of policy (Are policies made by a handful of bureaucrats or politicians, or are they discussed with managers and interest groups, such as patient groups or consumers?)

- How policies are communicated, executed, regulated, and assessed (Is policy making a top-down process? Are policies monitored?)

Similar questions affect policy processes at the global level: Do industrialized countries dominate international organizations and decide how and where resources should be allocated?

| Exhibit 17-1 | The Framework Convention on Tobacco Control |

Tobacco kills almost 5 million people each year. If current trends continue, it is projected to kill 10 million people per year by 2020, with 70% of those deaths occurring in low- and middle-income countries. Tobacco also takes an enormous toll in healthcare costs, lost productivity, and, of course, the intangible costs of the pain and suffering inflicted upon smokers, passive smokers, and their families. In 2003, after 4 years of negotiations, the World Health Assembly unanimously endorsed the Framework Convention on Tobacco Control. This occasion marked the first time WHO had used its constitutional authority in global health to develop an international treaty.

The convention was launched because many perceived that "the tobacco industry's use of international trade agreements, cigarette smuggling, and global marketing techniques" had undermined national control measures and rendered them insufficient to control the tobacco epidemic (Gilmore & Collin, 2002, p. 846). The WHO-sponsored agreement included provisions for the enactment of comprehensive bans on tobacco advertising, promotion, and sponsorship; large, rotating health warnings on packaging; and the prohibition of misleading descriptors such as light or mild.

A large majority of countries backed the convention, and in 2010 there were 168 signatories or parties to the convention. However, according to the 2009 summary report on global progress, implementation levels vary among countries. There is higher implementation of measures on packaging and labeling and sales to, or by, minors than of provisions dealing with more contentious issues such as disclosure of marketing expenditure by the tobacco industry (WHO, 2009).

Who Are the Actors in Global Health?

There has been a huge increase in the number and diversity of actors involved in global health since the establishment of the UN system at the end of World War II. The UN was conceived as a system to maintain peace and security in a world that had been torn by strife—"to save succeeding generations from the scourge of war" (Childers & Urquhart, 1994, p. 11). At its center was the sovereign nation-state (able to exercise rule that is supreme, exclusive, and comprehensive over a given territory), which could become a member of the different organs and agencies of the UN. The largest specialized agencies of the UN are the Food and Agriculture Organization (FAO), the International Labor Organization (ILO), the UN Educational, Scientific and Cultural Organization (UNESCO), and WHO. In addition to the specialized agencies, a number of other funds and programs exist, such as UNICEF and UNAIDS. The latter, which was established in 1996 to coordinate the HIV-related work of the UN, was the first UN body to have civil society representatives on its governing body.

The international organizations that made up the UN were established to facilitate exchange and contact between all member states and to coordinate overseas development assistance provided collectively by some nation-states to others, which were then expected to use this aid in their exercise of national sovereignty. In this system of formal, vertical representation, member states decided the policies and activities of the international organizations. Only limited interaction occurred between these representative bodies and civil society organizations.

Actors in Health at the Global and Regional Levels

Founded in 1948, WHO is the UN's designated specialized agency in health, expected to play a leading role in coordinating international health activities. With headquarters in Geneva, Switzerland, WHO boasts an unusually decentralized structure of 6 regional offices plus offices in 145 countries. The Pan American Health Organization (PAHO), representing the Americas, and the South-East Asia Regional Office (SEARO), representing countries in the South East Asia region, are 2 of the 6 WHO regional offices.

Other organizations within the UN system also have some responsibilities in health. The more active of these are the first five listed in Table 17-1, although some of the others, such as the World Trade Organization (WTO), are important for particular issues such as intellectual property rights, which indirectly govern the costs of pharmaceuticals as well as trade in health services.

Cooperation in health, however, has not been limited to collaboration through the UN and its agencies involved in health. Bilateral organizations, such as the United Kingdom's Department for International Development (DFID), the Swedish International Development Agency (SIDA), and the U.S. Agency for International Development (USAID), among many others, have played important roles at international and regional levels and in many countries. These agencies are often the main contributors to international health programs through UN organizations, but they also provide assistance to lower-income countries through government-to-government agreements known as bilateral aid. In the 2000s, the number of governments providing bilateral aid increased,

Table 17-1	United Nations Health-Related Organizations

World Health Organization (WHO)

World Bank

UN Children's Fund (UNICEF)

UN Population Fund (UNFPA)

Joint United Nations Programme on HIV/AIDS (UNAIDS)

UN Development Program (UNDP)

UN Educational, Scientific and Cultural Organization (UNESCO)

Food and Agriculture Organization (FAO)

World Food Program (WFP)

UN High Commissioner for Refugees (UNHCR)

International Labor Organization (ILO)

UN Environment Program (UNEP)

UN Office on Drugs and Crime (UNODC)

World Trade Organization (WTO)

expanding to include China and the Persian Gulf states, among others.

International NGOs—increasingly referred to as civil society organizations (CSOs)—have also made critical contributions to health development at both the global and domestic levels (see Exhibit 17-2).

Although no definitive definition of CSOs exists, there is general agreement that these groups are typically voluntary, nonformal, and noncommercial associations of individuals who share some common cause or goal. NGOs or CSOs make up a broad group of agencies of considerable complexity. They include church missions providing health care to isolated rural communities; agencies such as Oxfam, which may be involved in advocacy on behalf of lower-income countries (e.g., on debt relief) or may be working with local groups (AIDS support groups, for example); and private foundations, such as the Rockefeller, Ford, and the Bill and Melinda Gates Foundations.

The corporate sector has also become more involved in health activities over the last decades, at both the global level (e.g., more than 1,000 companies are members of the Global Health Initiative of the World Economic Forum, established to increase the quantity and quality of business programs fighting HIV/AIDS, tuberculosis, and malaria) and the local level. For example, companies such as Heineken, Anglo-America, and Coca-Cola have introduced antiretroviral treatment programs for their workers in Africa (Exhibit 17-3).

When the UN was established in the middle of the twentieth century, there were few actors in health, the role of the private sector and CSOs was small, and WHO played the dominant role. By the end of the century, many more actors were interested in health activities, and they were increasingly forming alliances, networks, and partnerships across public and private sectors to tackle health issues.

Exhibit 17-2	An Expanding Global Role for Civil Society Organizations

One of the most successful global civil society actions in the new millennium has been improving access to medicines, a movement spearheaded by Médicins Sans Frontières (MSF) in the late 1990s. Working in tandem with groups such as Oxfam and Ralph Nader's Consumer Project on Technology, among others, MSF sought to prevent the multinational pharmaceutical industry from exploiting emerging agreements through the World Trade Organization that attempted to block the production of generic medicines in middle-income countries such as Brazil, India, South Africa, and Thailand. Many national NGOs joined the global campaign and lobbied together on these issues. Schneider (2002) reports that in one week in 2001, when a number of pharmaceutical manufacturers took the South African government to court (withdrawing from the court hearing only at the last minute) to prevent regulatory measures to reduce the cost of AIDS drugs, 27 protest activities were reported on the website of the South African NGO Treatment Action Campaign (TAC), involving 12 countries, including the United States, Canada, the United Kingdom, Brazil, and the Philippines.

Lobbying for the Framework Convention on Tobacco Control also took off when the actions of the groups supporting the convention were enhanced by the formation and development of the Framework Convention Alliance (FCA). Initially, civil society groups involved in discussions regarding tobacco control were largely confined to high-income-country NGOs and international health–based NGOs. FCA was formed as a loose international alliance to support the development and ratification of an effective convention and to engage a larger group of CSOs in the process of drawing up the convention. By 2003, FCA encompassed more than 180 NGOs from over 70 countries and had established itself as an important lobbying alliance (Collin, 2004).

Exhibit 17-3	**Coca-Cola, AIDS, and Nongovernmental Organizations**

The Business section of London's *Guardian* newspaper reported in April 2004 on "sisters who stirred the conscience of Coca-Cola" as an illustration of the way in which faith-based organizations have lobbied for greater corporate responsibility among a number of different industries over a number of decades (Pratley, 2004). The Interfaith Center on Corporate Responsibility, which is an organization of 275 faith-based groups, claims an investment portfolio of $110 billion. Its financial heft strengthens the organization's position in negotiations with industry and enables it to put forth resolutions to company shareholder and annual meetings. As a result, the Interfaith Center on Corporate Responsibility has been able to influence a number of companies to at least pass resolutions calling on Coca-Cola to review the economic impact of its operations on the HIV/AIDS pandemic in Africa. Although "not a revolutionary step," the significance of Coca-Cola's resolution lies in the commitments the company has already made to provide antiretroviral drugs to employees. Although ultimately it is in Coca-Cola's self-interest to treat its employees, knowing that the epidemic is also killing its customers and potential customers, other companies have been slow to act or to think more broadly about HIV-preventive measures (Pratley, 2004, p. 26).

Linking Global and Regional Actors with Local Actors

All states take some responsibility for their own health and health services, although the resources they have available differ markedly. As explained in Chapter 12 on the design of health systems, most resources for health are generated domestically, although governments may also receive significant aid from multilateral, bilateral, or NGO sources. In some low-income countries the health budget is heavily subsidized from external sources such as the Global Fund to Fight AIDS, Tuberculosis, and Malaria (the Global Fund).

While states are responsible for health policy within their own borders, they also send representatives to participate in global policy discussions about health at the international level. For example, most states are members of WHO. Every year they send a delegation—usually the minister of health and some officials from the health ministry—to attend the World Health Assembly (WHA) held at WHO's headquarters in Geneva. It is at the WHA that international policies on health are discussed, and ministers of health commit to programs and measures they will introduce or support when they return home. Membership in WHO entitles each state to vote on an equal basis, although membership contributions are based on population size and wealth.

Even though there may be considerable consensus on policies decided at the WHA, all states are sovereign entities; if they do not adhere to, or implement, recommendations agreed to at the international level, there is little that WHO can do. Its only sanctions are based on its authority and reputation. Exhibit 17-1, which describes the Framework Convention on Tobacco Control, illustrates how states may sign up to a particular policy, yet prove slow to enact it within their own borders.

States may also serve on a rotational basis on the boards of governors of other UN agencies, such as UNICEF or the United Nations Population Fund (UNFPA). Moreover, they may apply for membership in the international financial institutions (IFIs), such as the World Bank and International Monetary Fund, where membership is subject to financial subscription and other economic criteria, and voting is weighted according to the number of shares held by each member.

States also engage with regional bodies such as the six offices of the WHO, participating as members in their decision making. For example, the Eastern Mediterranean Regional Office (EMRO) and the Western Pacific Regional Office (WPRO) hold many meetings for countries in their respective regions, and have considerable power and autonomy to establish regional policies. States may also be involved in other regional bodies that have a strong economic or political focus (or both) and may or may not include health in their jurisdictions. Examples include the European Union (EU); the Organization for Economic Cooperation and Development (OECD), which includes not only all the industrialized nations but also Turkey and Thailand, among others; and the Association of Southeast Asian Nations (ASEAN). All of these organizations provide a forum in which to discuss health-related issues of concern to the region and may issue guidance, which may be binding on member states, although adherence to policies will depend on the authority and consensus on which they are based.

The links described so far are vertical and representational—that is, between states (national governments) and multilateral agencies at the global and regional levels. States are represented on those bodies and have a say in decision making, although their power to influence those decision-making processes will differ. States also retain considerable autonomy in their decision to reject, adopt, and adapt policies proposed by international and regional organizations.

At the national level, however, the state links with a variety of different agencies in expanding horizontal relationships, based more on participation than on representation. Not only will the state have dealings with a myriad of national NGOs or CSOs, but it may also engage with multilateral agencies such as WHO or UNICEF; bilateral agencies such as USAID and SIDA; international NGOs such as MSF or Oxfam; and, increasingly, global health initiatives that do not necessarily have a continuing presence in the country but that offer large amounts of aid for specific health interventions. Just in the area of HIV/AIDS, several such initiatives have been launched. For example, the Clinton Foundation has brokered deals between donors and poor countries such as Mozambique, Rwanda, and Tanzania for AIDS drugs and with pharmaceutical companies to lower the price of antiretroviral drugs; between 2003 and 2008, U.S. President George W. Bush's Emergency Plan for AIDS Relief (PEPFAR) provided $15 billion to countries in Africa and the Caribbean. The Global Fund had by March 2010 disbursed approximately $10 billion to 144 countries (Exhibit 17-4).

Although all of these relationships bring much-needed resources to poor countries and are generally welcomed, they also have some costs. For instance, they target particular diseases and conditions and ignore others, are costly to establish and monitor, and may lead to potential neglect of other parts of the health system. Moreover, their effects are difficult to assess. One analysis of evidence on the effect of global health initiatives on countries' health systems concluded that such initiatives had both negative and positive effects (WHO Maximizing Positive Synergies Collaborative Group, 2009) (Exhibit 17-5).

Why Do States Cooperate?

Cooperation in health has a long history. Between 1851 and 1909, 10 international meetings were held to discuss quarantine and other measures to deal with epidemics of plague and cholera. Although most of these early meetings were conducted on an ad hoc basis and largely limited to epidemic intelligence gathering between scientists or professionals, they led to international agreements on common approaches for the control and treatment of infectious diseases. After the two world wars in the first half of the twentieth

---

Exhibit 17-4	The Global Fund to Fight AIDS, Tuberculosis, and Malaria

The Global Fund to Fight AIDS, Tuberculosis, and Malaria (the Global Fund) was established in January 2002 to attract, manage, and disburse additional resources to countries to control three diseases having a devastating impact in poor countries, especially in sub-Saharan Africa. The Global Fund is a public–private partnership that is governed by a board (18 voting and 5 nonvoting members) and supported by a secretariat of approximately 650 staff in Geneva, Switzerland. It describes itself as a financing mechanism, with a mandate to "Raise it, spend it, prove it."

By 2010, the Global Fund had supported programs that had saved 4.9 million lives, allocated more than $19 billion, and disbursed $10 billion to 144 countries (Global Fund, 2010).

Countries apply for Global Fund support by submitting proposals via the Country Coordinating Mechanism (CCM). These suggestions are then assessed by a technical review panel of independent experts and considered for approval by the board. The CCM is a partnership tasked with preparing proposals for Global Fund support, selecting principal recipient(s), and overseeing and monitoring implementation of successful applications. The Global Fund requires CCMs to include "broad representation from governments, NGOs, civil society, multilateral and bilateral agencies and the private sector."

The Global Fund has a reputation for being open and flexible, but also tough. It uses a performance-based funding system that allows it to suspend grants if it finds accounting inconsistencies or if fraud is reported to its Office of the Inspector General, an independent unit directly responsible to the board. In 2005, the Global Fund terminated a grant to Myanmar (Burma), and it suspended grants to a number of countries including Nigeria, Pakistan, Uganda, South Africa, and Senegal at various times in the mid-2000s (Salaam-Blyther, 2008).

Given the success of the Global Fund in raising and disbursing funds, a debate resurfaced in the late 2000s about extending its mandate, either informally or formally, to include funding for other health problems in low- and middle-income countries. For example, in 2009 Cometto and colleagues proposed a global fund for meeting the health Millennium Development Goals (MDGs). Proponents contend that this expansion would improve coherence in global health, although others are concerned that the urgency and focus on three original diseases would be lost (Cometto et al., 2009).

Exhibit 17-5 | **How Do Global Health Initiatives Affect Health Systems?**

Global health initiatives (GHIs) are defined in different ways (Biesma, Brugha, Harmer, Walsh, Spicer, & Walt, 2009) but they share some common characteristics: a focus on specific diseases or selected interventions, commodities, or services; significant financial resources; and inputs linked to performance.

Among the largest GHIs are those concerned with HIV/AIDS: the Global Fund, the World Bank (through its HIV/AIDS programs), and the President's Emergency Plan for AIDS Relief (PEPFAR). By 2007, these three GHIs accounted for more than two-thirds of external funding for HIV/AIDS and malaria in highly affected countries; and the disease control budgets of these countries have become highly dependent on these funds. As antiretroviral drugs (ARVs) became more accessible through the GHIs, and were rolled out by what were recognized to be weak health systems, the spotlight focused on GHI funding for HIV/AIDS. Was it undermining other parts of the health service, by focusing so much attention and such high levels of resources on just one disease, or was the influx of funds helping to strengthen other parts of health care (Shiffman, 2008)?

To answer this question, a WHO-convened group of collaborating bodies explored the synergies between GHIs and health systems by reviewing the existing evidence to assess both positive and negative effects for health systems of large injections of funds for specific diseases (WHO Maximizing Positive Synergies Collaborative Group, 2009). The picture that emerged was mixed and highly contextualized, and, given a weak evidence base, demonstrated both positive and negative effects.

Clear evidence was found that GHI funding had increased access and uptake of HIV/AIDS services, and many countries reported rapid ARV roll-out. On average, coverage of ARVs for prevention of mother-to-child transmission in HIV in Africa increased from 9% to 33% between 2004 and 2007. A few countries reported that HIV-specific resources were used more broadly to invest in construction of health facilities, improvements in laboratories, or training health workers, all of which had a positive effect on primary health services. In Haiti, implementation of an integrated package of HIV prevention, treatment, and care services led to dramatic improvements in the quality of primary health care in general—correlating with a fivefold increase in prenatal visits and vaccinations. In Rwanda, one study found that after basic HIV services were introduced in primary healthcare facilities, the average number of people screened for syphilis at these facilities increased from 1 to 79 per month, and growth monitoring occurring at the facilities increased by nearly 30%.

However, as access to AIDS services increased, so did the burden on health workers, potentially demotivating a poorly paid workforce. Some health workers were attracted away from the public sector to work in GHI-funded AIDS programs. On the whole, GHIs have not sufficiently and systematically identified and leveraged investments in disease-specific programs to support countries' overall health systems.

---

century, such cooperation expanded. The Marshall European Recovery Program of 1948 to 1952, in which the United States gave $13 billion to rebuild the economies of Western Europe (Basch, 1999), introduced an era of extensive global aid for many development activities, including support for health services in low-income countries.

The latter half of the twentieth century witnessed an increase in trade, travel, and improved communication—some of the factors commonly assumed to have led to globalization of the world economy. These factors have highlighted risks that states by themselves cannot address adequately within their national borders. Such risks include new and emerging infectious diseases, resulting in part from the increased prevalence of drug-resistant pathogens; exposure to dangerous substances, such as contaminated foodstuffs or banned and toxic substances; environmental exploitation, leading to pollution and such conditions as respiratory disorders; and violence, resulting from the huge production and sales of arms as well as chemical and biological weapons.

Although most of the direct health problems are addressed by domestic health policies decided at the national level, some depend on international collaboration. No one state can, by itself, resolve the risks and problems just detailed. Recognizing this concern, many scholars have attempted to identify global public goods, defined as activities that countries introduce in collaboration with others, for which national action on its own is ineffective or impossible to organize or encourage. By definition, benefits from a global public good accrue widely, and not just to the entity that pays for them (public goods are defined by their attributes of being non-excludable and nonrival in consumption). Many international meetings are held to try to reach agreement among countries on norms and standards regarding pollution levels, the trafficking of illegal drugs, nuclear tests, and other policies from which all will benefit.

Although states may recognize the benefits of promoting international public goods, cooperation is not always easy to achieve because of conflicting interests. Bad behavior in one country that affects its innocent neighbors may demand interventions that are difficult to implement. For example, excessive and indiscriminate use of antibiotics in both high-income and low-income countries has created drug resis-tance, making it more difficult to treat some diseases. Concerted action is needed to combat resistance, but is complex, given that it means changing the behavior of patients who do not complete their antibiotic prescriptions, or of physicians who overprescribe antibiotics, or controlling and regulating the production or importation of high-quality antibiotics. Similarly, gaining cooperation on issues such as controlling pollution or activities that may lead to global warming is also highly problematic, as was demonstrated at the Copenhagen climate change meeting in Denmark in 2009, when delegates were unable to agree on a program of action.

Even where consensus exists regarding the value of international public goods produced through international cooperation (cooperation on research to find an AIDS vaccine, for example, or campaigning to eradicate smallpox from the world), achieving international goals can be difficult, and gains may be visible only in the long run (Smith & MacKeller, 2007). One example relates to virus sharing, which is a rec-

ognized global goal to help address future influenza pandemics, but one in which global collaboration broke down in the late 2000s because of lack of trust between countries (Exhibit 17-6).

States may also decide to act collectively at the international level because of shortcomings or lack of resources in particular national health systems. Development aid, for example, aims to build and strengthen capacity in low-income countries through technical assistance, grants, or loans. As Howson, Fineberg, and Bloom (1998, p. 586) point out, such engagement has as much significance for high-income countries as for low-income countries:

All developed countries have a vital and direct stake in the health of people around the world; this stake derives both from enduring traditions of humanitarian concern and from compelling reasons of enlightened self-interest. Considered involvement can serve to protect citizens, improve indigenous economies, and advance national and regional interests on the world stage.

At the extreme, states may cooperate with others because of the threat of force. This scenario is un-

---

Exhibit 17-6	**Global Cooperation Falters over Avian Flu**

Since 1952, WHO's member countries have voluntarily participated in the Global Influenza Surveillance Network (GISN) by donating influenza virus samples for analysis to one of five WHO Collaborating Centers. In 2006, for example, Indonesia contributed specimens from 56 positive cases of H5N1 virus. Data from these Centers is then shared globally through WHO's online program, FluNet. In 2007, a "geopolitical storm" broke out when Indonesia's minister of health (IMOH) announced that the country would no longer share its H5N1 (avian flu) virus samples with the "imperialist" WHO (Forster, 2009, p. 46).

Indonesia was incensed to discover that, in 2006, results of tests on its virus samples conducted by WHO-affiliated laboratories were presented at international conferences without Indonesia's prior permission. Further, it transpired that WHO laboratories had been distributing samples of donated viruses to Western pharmaceutical companies—in violation of WHO's own guidelines on virus sharing—and that an Australian vaccine company planned to develop a vaccine against H5N1 using one of Indonesia's donated virus samples (Sedyaningsih, Isfandiri, Soendoro, & Supari, 2008).

Indonesia withdrew its support for GISN, refused drug and vaccine supplies from WHO, and insisted on national ownership rights over its samples as well as control over where and to whom they were distributed (Forster, 2009). The IMOH argued that the practice of distributing donated virus samples to Western pharmaceutical companies was inequitable, as it allowed these corporate entities to develop a vaccine from the samples and sell them back to low- and middle-income countries—often at an unaffordable cost (Sedyaningsih et al., 2008). Despite a number of high-level meetings and a World Health Assembly (WHA) resolution to promote "transparent, fair and equitable sharing of the benefits" of virus sharing, Indonesia continued to argue that the system impeded access to vaccines and was not transparent.

In May 2008, the IMOH announced that Indonesia would no longer report human cases and deaths of H5N1 on a case-by-case basis, saying, "The conspiracy between superpower nations and global organizations is a reality. It isn't a theory, isn't rhetoric, but it's something I've experienced myself" (quoted in Forster, 2009, p. 47). In February 2010, the Indonesian Health Ministry's director-general of disease control and environmental health told the *Jakarta Post* that "our [Indonesia's] position [on virus sharing] remains the same" and that the new health minister would be attending the 63rd WHA in May 2010 to negotiate a fairer global system of virus sharing (Budlanto, 2010). After lengthy deliberations, a working group at WHO reached agreement on a framework for sharing vaccine strains among other things, to be presented to the World Health Assembly in May 2011.

likely in international health, but coercion may occur at the domestic level. Greenough (1995) argues, for example, that at the end of the smallpox campaign in India and Bangladesh, some force was exerted on families who were reluctant (for religious reasons, for example) to have their children vaccinated. Coercion has also sometimes been used in tuberculosis (and AIDS) programs. In 1993, for example, a New York City health code was amended to authorize the city's commissioner of health to detain any noninfectious individual "where there is substantial likelihood . . . that he or she cannot be relied upon to participate in and/or to complete an appropriate prescribed course of medication for tuberculosis." Between 1993 and 1998, more than 200 noninfectious patients were detained in New York under this rationale—many for long periods, including some for more than two years (Coker, 1999). As of early 2010, 57 countries had in place restrictions on entry or stay for people living with HIV.

Most relations in health are not directly coercive, although states may have little room to maneuver because of pressure from international organizations, the media, or neighboring states. In investigating the use of World Bank policy conditions in structural adjustment programs, for example, Killick, Gunatillaka, and Marr (1998, p. 11) distinguish between "pro forma" and "hard core" conditionality. They argue that the former may well be voluntary, based on consensus, because the recipient essentially agrees with the range of measures suggested by the lender; alternatively, the agreement may be based on the perceived authority of the international organization. Similarly, in conflict situations, where displaced persons have crossed borders, neighboring states may believe they have to make some response in spite of their own lack of resources or potential conflict with their own populations. Hard-core conditionality, by contrast, consists of "measures that would not otherwise be undertaken or taken within the time frame desired by the lender" (Killick et al., 1998, p. 11) but that are accepted by recipients because they need the funds.

Another reason for states to cooperate is perceived threats to their security. Several countries, led by the United States, consider global health problems, including HIV/AIDS and other infectious disease epidemics, to be security threats. Feldbaum and associates (2004) compared two security documents before and after the terrorist attacks in the United States on September 11, 2001. One document, published in 1998, discussed public health only as a secondary issue to bioterrorism and environmental degradation, mentioning HIV/AIDS only once. The

2002 document, by comparison, discussed public health issues in six of the nine chapters, with HIV/AIDS being referred to seven times. This change in perception has led to increased support for global health activities by the security and foreign policy communities, and more collaboration on issues such as bioterrorism. In 2007, WHO selected health security as the theme of its annual report: *A Safer Future: Global Public Health Security in the 21st Century*.

How Do States Cooperate?

States come together in many formal and informal ways that result in levels of cooperation. For example, the UN may arrange large international meetings, attended by delegations or representatives from states, international organizations, NGOs, private-sector companies, and others. Specialized meetings may be held, such as the WHA, to which member states send representatives from MOHs, or World Bank annual meetings, attended by ministers of finance and national and international bankers. Alternatively, experts in a particular field may convene in small meetings. WHO, for example, uses expert committees of academics, professionals, and scientists to establish norms and standards, such as which drugs should be included in an essential drugs list or whether hepatitis B vaccine should be included in routine infant immunization schedules. Activities in international health cooperation occur in three areas (Lucas et al., 1997):

- Consensus building and advocacy
- Cross-learning and transfer of knowledge
- Production and sharing of global public goods

Consensus Building and Advocacy

Many of the high-profile UN meetings that take place all over the world are exercises in building consensus on particular themes, with follow-up advocacy. UN conferences are usually agreed to by the General Assembly, and arranged outside the regular framework of the UN and its agencies, although they frequently involve inputs in the form of proposals and secretarial provision from those bodies (Taylor, 1993). These gatherings are highly formalized and orchestrated, with many groups holding preconference meetings to prepare background papers and recommendations. Originally, UN conferences were attended only by formal delegations representing governments, but over time they have opened to allow the participation of independent groups of NGOs, the media, and others.

In the 1990s, for example, meetings receiving a great deal of media attention were held in Rio de Janeiro, Brazil, and Kobe, Japan (on the environment); in Copenhagen, Denmark (on social-sector support); in Beijing, China (on women); and in Cairo, Egypt (on reproductive health). The 1994 meeting in Cairo, titled the International Conference on Population and Development, followed two earlier meetings, in 1974 in Bucharest and 1984 in Mexico, and is an example of how consensus building, plus other activities, changed attitudes and approaches to population issues over two decades. In the 40 years of discussions on population growth, ideas evolved to a considerable extent. In the 1950s and 1960s, discussion largely focused on regulating population growth through family planning programs and was highly contested, partly for religious reasons and partly because of disagreement on the relationship between population growth and development. By the 1990s, family planning programs were universally accepted (with dispute only over the role of abortion), but the increased participation of women's groups in international discussions had broadened the emphasis from contraception to reproductive health and rights. Over four decades, considerable energy was expended on advocacy to change public opinion and the views of key policy makers, with Western donors exercising significant influence on initially reluctant low- and middle-income countries through policies such as generous funding of family planning programs.

Cross-Learning and Transfer of Knowledge

Cooperation in health also occurs through exchange of experience and transfer of knowledge. One of the great strengths of international organizations is that they can overlook political, geographical, or cultural barriers and draw on "epistemic communities"—that is, networks of professionals with recognized expertise and competence in a particular domain and an authoritative claim to policy-relevant knowledge within that domain or issue area (Haas, 1992). WHO, for example, can call on a worldwide network of scientist groups, academics, technicians, and practitioners to provide up-to-date assessments and evidence on a range of health matters, from new technologies to emerging problems. From such meetings emerge consensus statements (e.g., which measures health professionals can use to protect themselves when working with infectious diseases), guidelines and manuals (e.g.,

how to treat childhood diarrheas, appropriate vaccine schedules, how to train community health workers), and various measures of best practice.

Cross-learning may also occur at the regional level, with regional bodies bringing states together to transfer information and experience. In the 1980s, PAHO set up interregional coordinating committees to assist in polio eradication in the Americas, establishing monitoring systems of immunizable diseases and training nationals in their use. Cooperation was also promoted among these countries by PAHO's establishment of a revolving fund for the purchase of vaccines and related supplies for national immunization programs.

Scholarships, study visits, and training are all mechanisms used by international, regional, and national bodies to stimulate cross-learning.

Producing and Sharing International Public Goods

By producing agreements on international public goods, countries all over the world agree to adopt and use technical standards, norms, and ways of tackling particular issues. Achieving global consensus occurs through the sorts of mechanisms already discussed: meetings of experts and, often, ratification by international, regional, or national bodies. The sorts of activities covered by such international cooperation in health include agreements on technical standards (of vaccines and drugs), the establishment of norms (for the classification and control of diseases), research on questions considered to be high priority (e.g., on HIV), and the setting up of global surveillance systems (e.g., the Global Outbreak and Alert Response Network [GOARN], which played a critical role in the containment of SARS in 2003). For example, WHO and the FAO together make up the Codex Alimentarius Commission, which sets food safety standards in relation to, among other things, food additives, veterinary drug and pesticide residues, contaminants, and standards of hygienic practice.

When there is a failure to produce what would be an international public good, either because it is too costly (e.g., new medicines for malaria) or because industry anticipates negligible returns on its investment (e.g., vaccines against diseases that affect few people), partnerships may be formed between different organizations to overcome market failure. For example, to help in the development of a vaccine against HIV, a number of donors established the International AIDS Vaccine Initiative (IAVI) in 1996 to ensure the development of safe, effective, accessible, preventive HIV vaccines for use throughout the world. Funded by a number of large foundations, private-sector companies, UNAIDS, the World Bank, and government development agencies, IAVI has established a network of clinical trial research centers in southern and eastern Africa, set up an immunology laboratory in London to coordinate clinical trials, and established a vaccine laboratory in New York to convert the research done within IAVI's consortia into viable vaccine candidates.

The Changing Nature of Global Cooperation

Vertical Tiers of Representation: 1950s–1990s

The high ideals of the UN system, which would bring peace, law, reason, and security to a war-torn world, were short-lived. As domination of membership of the UN by a few high-income countries was challenged by newly independent nations in the late 1960s and early 1970s, the UN agenda became broader and its decisions less predictable. Growth in nation-state membership of the UN was accompanied by a considerable shift in autonomy between its component parts, and, in contradiction to original hopes, it appeared increasingly competitive and difficult to coordinate.

Financing of the UN also became less predictable. By the 1970s, member states began to renege on their membership contributions. In 1993, the UN Secretary-General pointed out that halfway through the year arrears stood at $572 million, or half the year's needed resources. Only 47 (of 186) states had fully paid their regular budget assessments—19 high-income and 28 low- and middle-income countries. These tensions within the UN in general were reflected in its specialized agencies.

Because WHO was designated by the UN as the lead international organization in health, "directing and coordinating international health work," and for many years was so recognized, it is worth understanding how this organization changed between the 1950s and 2000.

WHO: Membership Becomes More Inclusive

From the outset, WHO was essentially autonomous, accountable only to its member states and financing and governing bodies. As its membership expanded, however, its policies became less consensual and its funding suffered.

Most nations were eager to join WHO when it was established in 1948, and the 55 original members rapidly expanded to 189 in 1998 (Lee, 1998), with most managing to find the resources to make the requisite financial contribution. The real growth of membership occurred in the 1960s, and by the 1970s heterogeneity was evident in the different goals and strategies of different member states. What had been a largely colonized world, dominated by a few industrialized powers, was transformed into a polity of sovereign states, in which members of what was then referred to as the "Third World" formed important groupings such as the Non-Aligned Movement, or the Group of 77. After the breakup of the Soviet Union, 25 more states joined the organization, largely from the newly independent states of central and eastern Europe.

As newly independent states joined the organization, new delegations rapidly became more familiar with its workings and more confident about drawing attention to problems in the low-income member states, and they called for greater levels of technical cooperation. By 1966, more than half of WHO's budget was devoted to operational activities in low- and middle-income countries, in contrast to, say, the ILO's 8%. As technical cooperation grew from the 1960s, differentiation between member states also sharpened: By the 1970s, the high-income member states were increasingly seen as "donors," supporting middle- and low-income member states. Although all member states had an equal vote at the policy-determining, annual World Health Assembly held in Geneva, Switzerland, many believed that the countries that contributed more financially had more influence in decision making.

WHO: Policies Become Less Consensual

The consensual policy environment enjoyed by WHO in its early days (albeit one punctuated by debates over issues such as population growth in the early 1950s) was challenged by the growth in membership. Health policies shifted from a technological, disease orientation to a more developmental, multisectoral primary healthcare (PHC) approach in the late 1970s.

With the change in emphasis, interests and ideas about health diversified, and consensus began to break down. For example, one of the main PHC policies was to introduce the concept of an essential drugs list—a restricted list of only the most common and useful drugs to be used in the public sector, especially at primary health facility levels. Although essential drugs lists represented significant savings for countries that were importing large numbers of nonessential, and sometimes even harmful, drugs, the medical profession and pharmaceutical industry generally were not in favor of this policy, which WHO promoted strongly. At one point the United States was accused of bending to pressure from its own pharmaceutical industry to withhold its contribution to WHO (Kanji, Hardon, Harnmeijer, Mamdani, & Walt, 1992).

Conflict also occurred over the interpretation of PHC policies between UNICEF and WHO, the two agencies that had sponsored the international meeting on PHC at Alma Ata in 1978. During the early 1980s, WHO's Director-General publicly expressed irritation with what he saw as UNICEF's selective, top-down approach to primary health care —specifically the perceived "vertical" nature of its GOBI interventions (interventions directed at growth monitoring, oral rehydration, breastfeeding, and immunization) (Mahler, 1983).

WHO: Funding Becomes More Exclusive

Alongside the expansion of WHO's membership, its funding base changed. In 1948, the organization relied largely on a regular budget ($6 million in 1950) made up of member states' contributions based on a formula taking into account population size and gross national product (GNP). Beginning in 1960, this regular budget was supplemented by modest voluntary donations (known as extrabudgetary funds) that came from other multilateral agencies or donors. For example, by 1971 the regular budget had grown to $75 million, to which $25 million was donated as extrabudgetary funds from the United Nations Development Program (UNDP) and UNFPA. Such extrabudgetary funds grew as particular donors (often the higher-income member states, such as the European countries and the United States) gave additional funds to WHO for particular programs—an unprecedented $100 million toward AIDS in the period from 1989 to 1991, for example. By 2004, approximately 66% of WHO's budget came from extrabudgetary sources, as opposed to 25% in 1971.

Extrabudgetary funds played an important supplementary role because WHO's regular budget was under significant pressure, largely because of member states' decision to adopt a policy of zero growth in real terms of the budgets allocated to all of the specialized agencies, but partly because of the nonpayment of contributions. In 2004, the Director-General of WHO noted, "I am concerned that US$50 million, or 6% of assessed contributions, were not paid. Total unpaid assessed contributions, including amounts due for previous financial periods, is US$138 million. Within this figure, long-term arrears stand at US$88 million, having increased from US$82 million at the end of the biennium 2000–2001" (WHO, 2004).

Although extrabudgetary funds supplemented WHO's budget in the short term, they increased the difficulty in ensuring coordination and continuity because of changing donor interests and short-term financial commitments, and they led to dependence on a small number of donors. In the 1990s, 10 countries provided 90% of all extrabudgetary funds, and the same countries provided more than half of the regular budget through assessed contributions. "In effect, voluntary contributions increase the risk of placing institutions in the thrall of those who give them the money" (Taylor, 1993, p. 378). In the 1990s, investigators into the role of such funds agreed cautiously that there was some truth in the assertion that a small number of donors to WHO were "driving health policy," but concluded that donor involvement had brought many advantages to the organization as a whole (Vaughan, Mogedal, Walt, Kruse, Lee, & de Wilde, 1996).

Changes in membership and financing led to more friction over health policies, and resulted in two contradictory trajectories. On the one hand, WHO was perceived as a universalist, inclusive membership organization, with a reputation for being neutral in dealing with its member states (in contrast to bilateral organizations, which were seen to be partial for geopolitical or historical reasons). Until the 1980s, its reputation was unassailable. On the other hand, by the 1990s, WHO was seen as increasingly dependent on a few donor member states whose interests dominated the activities of the organization, and dissatisfaction with the organization was apparent. Critics suggested it was inward-looking and bunkered against external criticism.

Attempts to reform the organization were initiated in the early 1990s, but the scope, nature and pace of change were limited and deemed to be slow. Questions were raised openly about WHO's effectiveness as an international organization, as well as its capacity to fulfill its leadership role (Godlee, 1994, 1995). For example, some critics argued that WHO was slow in establishing a response to AIDS; that it was UNICEF and other agencies that led the way on polio eradication and universal child immunizations; and that the organization did not identify the serious deficit in health financing during the 1980s, thereby allowing the World Bank to define health reform policies for the 1990s. Many viewed WHO's loss of leadership as due to its organizational mold, which favored vertical representation between ministries of health, WHO regional offices, and the Geneva headquarters, and which had not adapted to the political and economic changes that favored greater and more diverse participation in health.

Moving Toward Horizontal Participation: 1990s–2000s

The last decades of the twentieth century were dominated by neoliberal political and economic thinking, which changed the health policy environment. Among international organizations, the World Bank played a major part in this change, increasingly turning its attention to the social sectors, including health. In 1980, the World Bank published its Health Sector Policy Paper and began direct lending for health services for the first time. At the same time, Western governments, concerned with rising costs of health care, began to review their own health systems, and the era of health reforms was introduced, looking toward increased competition in delivery of health services and different forms of financing health systems, among other changes. Health reforms came at a time of considerable financial constraint—world economic recession, indebtedness among many low-income countries, disillusionment with the overextended role of the state—and rapidly became part of a wider program of economic and structural reforms sought by the World Bank and other donors in many low- and middle-income countries.

As the focus on health policies shifted from the delivery of PHC to concerns about financing health systems, WHO lost ground to the World Bank. One commentator suggested the World Bank had become "the new 800 lb gorilla in world health care" (Abbasi, 1999, p. 866) as it led discussions on health reforms. These proposals were articulated in the World Bank's 2003 report entitled *Investing in Health,* which recommended (among other things) that government introduce private or social insurance plans and foster competition in the delivery of health services. Other actors from civil society and the private, for-profit sector were also taking a close interest in the health sector, and changes in the role of the state paved the way for other actors to become involved in global health.

The Changing Role of the State

Although the extent of the state's role in the provision of services—whether health, education, or social security—has differed from country to country, there is no doubt that its size and scope expanded hugely during the twentieth century, especially in high-income countries.

Until the late 1970s, there was little challenge to the role of the state in its provision of health services, although differences among roles were apparent in different parts of the world. Most Latin American health systems were segmented between MOHs, which provided health services for the low-income population, and better-endowed institutes of social security, which provided services for workers and their families. In Asia, MOHs functioned within very pluralistic health systems, with a flourishing private sector. In Africa, MOHs were often the main providers of health services for urban populations, and with the extension of primary health services in the 1970s and 1980s, for rural populations; however, NGOs such as missions were also important providers in rural areas, and the informal private sector (e.g., drug sellers, traditional midwives) provided much first-contact care.

By the final decades of the twentieth century, however, the political and economic landscape looked different. Fueled partly by the rise of neoliberal economic policies and partly by disillusionment with what were perceived as overextended, corrupt, inefficient, and nondemocratic states in many low- and middle-income countries, donors (and the World Bank) began to look beyond the state and MOHs to the private sector. Notably, they began to promote reforms to health systems that would divest ministries of some of their service roles and extend them to the private sector (see Chapter 12). To achieve such reforms, donors began to attach conditions to their loans and grants to low- and middle-income countries. For example, a donor might agree to provide a grant (or a loan, in the case of the World Bank) to support the health system, but only on the condition that the MOH decentralize its authority, introduce user fees for publicly provided services, or pass legislation facilitating private practice.

The Rise of Civil Society

Although the notion of "civil society" has a long genesis, it has become common parlance in the development literature only in the past two decades. This phrase usually refers to all those organizations that exist in the space between the state and the household. Some definitions include the private, for-profit sector as part of civil society; others prefer to differentiate between those organizations that form part of the private, corporate sector and those organizations that are essentially nonprofit—most NGOs would fit into the latter category.

Donors to global health initiatives have supported the notion of civil society for a number of reasons. By the 1990s, the health sector provided many examples of NGOs that had demonstrated an impact on development, as measured by mortality and morbidity in small communities, through a variety of different interventions. They were perceived to be effective, innovative, and able to reach the grassroots level in a way that governments and multilateral or bilateral donors could not.

In the 1990s, donors began funding a wider range of CSOs, whose members often participated in lobbying and other political activities. Support for such groups was seen as a way to build up democracy—by providing outlets for citizens to voice their demands—and to promote social capital, which would lead to improved economic performance. The idea of social capital came from Robert Putnam, who suggested that the difference between the prosperous Italian north and the low-income south was explained by trust, family and civic responsibilities, and sharing a public spirit—all of which represent the cement that holds society together, and which were apparent in the north of Italy but not in the south (Putnam & Nanetti, 1995). Donors saw NGOs and CSOs as ways to build up social capital, as well as to provide antidotes to the supposedly bloated, autocratic, and inefficient state.

Civil society organizations also became far more active in the last decades of the twentieth century, moving from largely service-delivery roles to much more active advocacy and lobbying, and forming networks across national boundaries. The People's Health Movement, for example, was set up following the 1st People's Health Assembly held in Savar, Bangladesh, in January 2001. It represented a response to dissatisfaction with international health organizations and frustration at the failure of governments to achieve the "health for all" goals enshrined in the 1978 Alma Ata Declaration (Chowdury & Rowson, 2000). The Movement continues to champion a radical, people-centered approach to public health (People's Health Movement, 2009).

Other transnational groups have been successful in a variety of ways. For example, they have reframed global debates on debt and trade, argued for changes in policy on the use of DDT in malaria, and drawn attention to neglected areas—for example, access to essential drugs.

The Rise of the Private, Commercial Sector

In this chapter, private, for-profit organizations are considered sufficiently distinct from CSOs to warrant separate discussion. Commercial activity in health has grown, and, with trade liberalization in global markets, is likely to expand further (Pollock & Price, 2003). In many countries, foreign investment in the health sector, which was once forbidden or heavily restricted, has opened up. For example, states are

increasingly allowing foreign hospital management companies to invest in local hospitals and in health insurance, often as joint ventures with local, domestic partners. Although some of these moves may be beneficial—for example, the entry of new insurance companies in Brazil is said to have increased coverage of the population by offering improved insurance packages and to have brought down administrative costs—foreign investors may also increase inequities within and between countries because it is in their financial best interests to invest in those areas where there is relatively high per capita income. This strategy may improve access and services for those who can pay, but also attracts workers from the public sector into the private sector (Zarrilli & Kinnon, 1998).

Although some private companies are very powerful, with annual turnovers several times larger than the GNP of many lower-income countries, some observers suggest they are taking a broader view of their social responsibilities—if only out of enlightened self-interest—partly because of the actions of CSOs pressuring for particular changes in policies. A number of examples can be cited in which international environmental, human rights, and faith-based groups managed to change companies' policies. In the United States, Coca-Cola bowed to the lobbying of the Interfaith Center on Corporate Responsibility, among other groups, and agreed in 2004 that all of the company's HIV-positive employees in Africa would receive free antiretroviral drugs (as discussed in Exhibit 17-3). There is little doubt that the prices of the antiretroviral drugs of several pharmaceutical transnational companies were lowered considerably after 2000 largely as a result of pressure and lobbying from CSOs.

In addition, pharmaceutical companies have sometimes offered large donations of drugs to help control or eradicate diseases in low-income countries. For instance, in 1998 the pharmaceutical company Pfizer announced the establishment of the International Trachoma Initiative, in partnership with the United States' Edna McConnell Clark Foundation and others, to eliminate blinding trachoma. The pharmaceutical company provides the antibiotic Zithromax free of charge in 18 out of 56 countries in which this infection is endemic, and it supports national trachoma control programs.

Other pharmaceutical companies have lowered their prices on some antiretroviral drugs so as to increase access to these agents to persons with HIV/AIDS in very poor countries, where the great majority of people cannot afford their high cost. This reduction was achieved over a long decade of painful negotiation (UNAIDS, for example, initiated a dialogue about lowering prices with some pharmaceuti-

Exhibit 17-7	How Civil Society Groups Affected Access to Medicines in Thailand

In Thailand, civil society groups have been key to challenging the practices of the multinational pharmaceutical industry and governments of high-income countries in their quest for improved access to medicines. Such groups include the Thai Foundation for Consumers, the Thai NGO Coalition on AIDS, the Thai Network for People Living with HIV/AIDS, and the international NGO Médicins Sans Frontières, working with national academics and the Law Society of Thailand. Besides lobbying on issues related to patent protection, providing information, and supporting activities for people living with AIDS, these CSOs have been involved in legal proceedings. For example, in 2001 they filed a lawsuit to try to revoke the patent of a Bristol-Myers Squibb antiretroviral drug, didanosine. The action began with the CSOs' attempts to persuade the Thai Ministry of Health to issue a compulsory license for this drug. Compulsory licensing allows governments to overturn patents and produce and sell generic medicines at prices far lower than those charged for branded products. Although the final court ruling was complex, the lawsuit set an important precedent, establishing that essential drugs are not just another consumer product but a human right, and that patients are injured by patents.

One of the intriguing aspects of the Thai civil society groups' activities was the link forged with like-minded groups across borders. Thai groups were supported by U.S. AIDS activists who demonstrated in Washington, D.C. against Bristol-Myers Squibb and the U.S. government regarding their repressive trade policies with respect to drugs for HIV/AIDS (Ford, Wilson, Bunjumnong, & Van Schoen Angerer, 2004).

cal companies in the late 1990s), but it was not until a network of active and vocal CSOs began lobbying that the pharmaceutical industry began to respond to demands for increased access (Nattrass, 2008).

Although strides have been made toward improving access to certain drugs—antiretroviral agents being the most prominent example—such moves have been complex, slow, and controversial. As Exhibit 17-7 demonstrates, CSOs have had to go to court to win concessions in Thailand, and Brazil and South Africa have had to fight battles at the global and local level to improve access to drugs. Difficult questions about the potential for antiretroviral resistance if drugs are not carefully handled have also arisen, and concern remains that prevention has not received as much attention as treatment—although in reality the two are linked.

During the 1990s, a series of meetings between organizations in the private and public sectors was held to address concerns about the lack of research and development in vaccines, and the apparent slowness of many countries to include new vaccines in their immunization programs. Such meetings resulted in discussions of a number of new policies, including removal of price controls and establishment of a global fund for vaccines to encourage pharmaceutical companies to invest in research and development of vaccines for low-income countries that might have difficulties in buying such vaccines. One result of these discussions was the International AIDS Vaccine Initiative. Another was the establishment of the Global Alliance for Vaccines and Immunization (GAVI Alliance) in 1999 to "fulfill the right of every child to be protected against vaccine-preventable diseases of public health concern." These public–private

vaccine initiatives have been followed by a host of others, including the Pediatric Dengue Vaccine Initiative, the Malaria Vaccine Initiative, the European Malaria Vaccine Initiative, the Human Hookworm Vaccine Initiative, the Meningitis Vaccine Project, and the Pneumococcal Vaccines Accelerated Development and Introduction Plan. The biggest funder of vaccine research and development is the Bill and Melinda Gates Foundation, which in 2010 announced a plan to spend $10 billion on vaccine programs over the next decade.

From 2000: Boarding the Millennium Train

The new millennium provided an impetus for change in the way that global health was addressed. Indeed, the first decade of the twenty-first century looked very different from 1950. In September 2000, world leaders came together at the United Nations headquarters in New York to adopt the United Nations Millennium Declaration. Three particular actions stemmed from this UN Millennium Summit.

First, world leaders committed to an agreed set of eight time-bound and measurable goals—the Millennium Development Goals (MDGs)—and targets for combating poverty, hunger, disease, illiteracy, environmental degradation, and discrimination against women (see Exhibit 17-8 and Chapter 1). Among them was the goal to "halt, and begin to reverse, the spread of HIV/AIDS." Much of the global health focus of the next decade was on countries' progress in reaching those goals (see, for example, the 2010 UN report entitled *Keeping the Promise*).

Second, there were discussions on how to finance the attainment of the MDGs. With the new century

---

Exhibit 17-8   **The Eight Millennium Development Goals (MDGs)**

The MDGs were agreed upon in 2000 by 189 countries belonging to the United Nations, with the support of the International Monetary Fund and the World Bank, the Organization for Economic Cooperation and Development, and the G7 and G20 countries. There are eight goals:

- Eradicate extreme poverty and hunger
- Achieve universal primary education
- Promote gender equality and empower women
- Reduce child mortality
- Improve maternal health
- Combat HIV/AIDS, malaria, and other diseases
- Ensure environmental sustainability
- Develop a global partnership for development

Each goal has a number of targets and indicators. All of these goals are meant to be achieved by 2015, and have been monitored since their introduction.

Although the MDGs have been criticized (e.g., as neglecting noncommunicable diseases and injuries, both of which result in high levels of morbidity and mortality in many low- and middle-income countries), they do represent an unprecedented global agreement to address unacceptable inequalities between rich and poor countries. Nevertheless, achieving the goals by 2015 presents a major challenge. In a progress report, the UN Secretary General warned that with five years to go to the target date of 2015, "the prospect of falling short of achieving the Goals because of a lack of commitment is very real. This would be an unacceptable failure from both the moral and the practical standpoint. If we fail, the dangers in the world—instability, violence, epidemic diseases, environmental degradation, runaway population growth—will all be multiplied" (United Nations, 2010, p. 2).

While progress has been hampered by a global economic crisis, some advances were being seen by 2010. Under-five child mortality (MDG 4) declined to approximately 8.1 million deaths in 2009, down from 12.4 million deaths in 1990, and analysis of data for maternal mortality (MDG 5) from 1980 to 2008 for 181 countries showed a substantial decline in maternal deaths (World Health Statistics, 2011; United Nations, 2009).

---

came a realization that traditional aid—typically raised through taxation by donor governments and issued as grants to recipient governments and NGOs—had failed to generate sufficient funds to respond adequately to many of the world's most pressing health challenges. The International Conference on Financing for Development in Monterrey in 2002 resulted in a number of proposals being explored as a way to raise aid levels. One example was the establishment of UNITAID in 2006 (see Exhibit 17-9), which sought to raise additional funds through a levy on airline tickets for medicines and diagnostics to treat AIDS, tuberculosis, and malaria (and which later included maternal and child health). In 2007 the OECD reported that $22 billion was being raised annually for global health, although this represented just 0.05% of donors' gross domestic product (OECD, 2007).

In 2008, the High Level Taskforce on Innovative International Financing for Health Systems was established to develop new ways of raising funds to help strengthen health systems in the poorest countries in the world (Exhibit 17-10). This group calculated that an additional $10 billion per year by 2015 would be required to achieve its goal (Taskforce on Innovative International Financing for Health Systems, 2009). Innovation in this new global context meant finding new sources for raising revenues, usually outside the traditional tax revenue systems. In particular, the Taskforce drew attention to the potential of voluntary giving through initiatives such as Massive Good (Exhibit 17-9). These kinds of initiatives typically use social media and networks to encourage multiple, small donations from the general public, rather than relying on large, one-off donations from wealthy private benefactors.

Other new instruments were also created to raise investment for global health. Two examples are the Advanced Market Commitment (AMC) and the International Financing Facility for Immunization (IFFIm). AMCs encourage pharmaceutical companies to invest in research and development for neglected diseases because donors agree in advance to "buy out" newly developed medicines for an agreed

| Exhibit 17-9 | **UNITAID: Innovative Funding For Medicines** |

UNITAID is an international drug purchase facility focused on treatments for HIV, malaria, and tuberculosis. It was launched by the governments of Brazil, Chile, France, Norway, and the United Kingdom and the Bill and Melinda Gates Foundation in September 2006, in an effort to leverage price reductions for quality diagnostics and medicines and to accelerate the pace at which these items are made available. By 2010, UNITAID had committed more than $730 million to achieving its goal and was supporting 16 projects in 93 countries. In 2008, 29 countries supported the organization through financial contributions; 7 applied the airline tax, including Chile, France, Madagascar, Mauritius, Niger, and the Republic of Korea. Norway allocates part of its tax on carbon dioxide emissions from air travel to UNITAID. Jordan joined UNITAID in late 2008 and declared its intention of introducing the air tax. In addition, two African countries—Kenya and Burkina-Faso—pledged their intention of introducing the air tax in the near future to support UNITAID. Seventy percent of UNITAID's finances come from airline taxes (UNITAID, 2008).

In late 2009, a related initiative was launched. Entitled Massive Good, its intention was to invite travelers to make a $2, £2, or €2 voluntary "micro-contribution" toward major global health causes every time they buy a plane ticket, reserve a hotel room, or rent a car. By clicking on or saying "yes" to Massive Good, it is hoped that travelers will provide as much as $1 billion in additional funding for UNITAID (Massive Good, 2010).

| Exhibit 17-10 | **High Level Taskforce on Innovative International Financing for Health Systems** |

The Taskforce on Innovative International Financing for Health Systems was launched in September 2008 to help strengthen health systems in the 49 poorest countries in the world. The Taskforce was chaired by U.K. Prime Minister Gordon Brown and World Bank President Robert Zoellick. Two expert Working Groups were set up to produce detailed reports—one on the constraints to health systems strengthening and the costs of scaling-up essential health care, and the other on the sources of finance and the options for channeling such funding. The group's recommendations were presented to the UN General Assembly in New York City in September 2009 (Taskforce on Innovative International Financing for Health Systems, 2009).

The Taskforce took as a starting point the idea that expenditure on global health is an investment, not simply a cost. It recognized that raising additional resources at a time of global financial turmoil posed a challenge, but pointed out that the global recession made this task even more urgent. The Taskforce noted that 100 million of the world's poor had receded back into poverty because of the financial crisis.

Working Group 1 produced new estimates of the costs of strengthening health systems, which was difficult in the face of weak and conflicting data. Given a lack of consensus on the best approach to improving essential health care, group members presented two models—one proposed by WHO and its various technical partners, and the other proposed by UNICEF and the World Bank. Working Group 2 identified a menu of financing mechanisms to complement traditional aid and raise an additional $10 billion per year, which included, among other things:

- A $1 billion expansion of the International Finance Facility for Immunization (IFFIm). The IFFIm uses government guarantees to raise funds immediately by issuing bonds on the capital markets. The GAVI Alliance, in turn, uses these funds to purchase vaccines and provide support to strengthen national health systems. By 2010, the IFFIm had raised more than $2 billion for immunization programs.
- A new mechanism for making voluntary contributions when buying airline tickets, expected to raise as much as $3.2 billion by 2015 (see Exhibit 17-9 on UNITAID).
- Exploration of levies on tobacco and on currency transactions.
- Launch of a value-added tax (VAT) credit pilot scheme called De-Tax, expected to raise as much as $220 million per year in VAT resources (the scheme would earmark a share of VAT receipts from participating businesses that agree to add a share of their profits).

Among the commitments to the preceding recommendations was an undertaking by the GAVI Alliance, the Global Fund, the World Bank, and WHO to rationalize funding for health systems through a single funding stream to be in place in seven countries in 2010.

There were divergent views within the Taskforce and between Working Groups, largely regarding the potential role of the private sector (Fryatt, Mills, & Nordstrom, 2010). Some observers expressed disappointment in what were seen as the limitations of the new sources of finance. One said, "Although the endorsement of taxation as a legitimate source of global public finance for health and development is welcome, given the integrated and globalized nature of all economies, the actual recommendations put forward lack ambition and conviction. As the world enters a global economic recession on the back of unprecedented levels of inequality, and as climate change threatens to eclipse the health gains of the past 20 years, the opportunity to link taxes and revenue generation to a redistributive and environmental agenda has been ignored" (McCoy, 2009, p. 323).

amount comparable to revenues that the companies could expect to earn from affluent markets (GAVI Alliance, 2010). The IFFIm also relies on legally binding, future, financial commitments by donors. The aim of the IFFIm, however, is to fund rapid scale-up of immunization in poor countries. On the strength of a pledge by government donors (France, Italy, Spain, Sweden, Norway, and South Africa) to make total payments to the IFFIm of $5.3 billion over a 20-year period, the IFFIm issues AAA-rated bonds in the international capital markets. The first bond of $1 billion was issued in 2006, and any resources that accrue go to fund GAVI Alliance programs (IFFIm, 2010).

A third action that followed the UN Millennium Summit built on the experiment started by the GAVI Alliance in 1999 and the Global Fund in 2001 (see Exhibit 17-4), and established public–private partnerships between international organizations, governments, CSOs, and private, for-profit companies to deliver aid through performance-based support. Countries are expected to submit specific requests for aid (in the case of the GAVI Alliance, country applications have to demonstrate levels of immunization coverage, and explain how the country would increase these levels with provision of new-generation vaccines). Countries are then judged on their performance against their own stated goals. Grants are disbursed only in partial payments, and payouts can be moderated against performance—and even suspended if progress or remedial efforts are judged insufficient. GAVI also provides countries with a reward—$20 for each additional child immunized above an agreed-upon target level—and in so doing has supported increased immunization coverage (Lu, Michaud, Gakidou, Khan, & Murray, 2006).

The consequence of these changes has been a spectacular rise in additional funding for health: Annual development assistance for health increased from $2.5 billion in 1990 to approximately $16 billion in 2006—doubling between 2000 and 2009 (Taskforce, 2009). Sources of funding have also multiplied exponentially. In addition to traditional bilateral and multilateral development assistance for health, low-income countries typically receive funds from NGOs, global health partnerships, private foundations, the business/corporate sector, and individuals either indirectly through taxes or directly in the form of donations (Institute for Health Metrics and Evaluation [IHME], 2009; McCoy, Chand, & Sridhar, 2009). To give a sense of the rapid scale-up of funding, since 1989, the World Bank has committed approximately $4.2 billion in loans and credits to HIV/AIDS programs alone, disbursing approximately $3.1 bil-

lion; PEPFAR has donated approximately $26 billion since 2003 and authorized a further $48 billion in 2009 for 5 years; and since 2001 donors have pledged in excess of $21 billion to the Global Fund (Global Fund, 2010; PEPFAR, 2009; World Bank, 2010).

In the new millennium, there has also been an increasing emphasis on linking aid to notions of "good governance," democracy, and the growth of civil society. These attempts have included, for example, promoting increased accountability in the public sector, improving procedures and the rule of law, introducing transparency in financing and other systems, promoting human rights, and encouraging multiparty democratic systems—as well as emphasizing state stewardship of the sector as opposed to a service-delivery role. As Exhibit 17-4 shows, the Global Fund insisted that CSOs be involved in the development of proposals for funding through the establishment of Country Coordinating Mechanisms, and during the decade funds were frozen in several instances until alleged mismanagement of funds was resolved (Salaam-Blyther, 2008).

Vertical Representation to Horizontal Participation: The Implications for Health Policy

This chapter has suggested that states were once able to influence global health policy through their formal representation on the governing bodies or at meetings of the various organizations of the UN. In recent years, this channel of influence has diminished because global health policy is no longer largely decided through the UN or its specialized agency, WHO. Over the past three decades, cooperation on health has expanded to include a greater diversity of nonstate actors, which cooperate within partnerships that include the UN bodies but do not belong to them and do not necessarily act within their rules and regulations. This shift from representation to participation has some important implications for health policy cooperation in the new century, and it raises questions in five arenas: changes in the balance of power, mandates, competition and fragmentation, coordination, and governance. This final section of the chapter addresses those five areas of concern.

Shifts in Power

By the 2000s, the balance of power among the various organizations involved in global health had shifted significantly. The "shooting star" in the new millennium skies was the Bill and Melinda Gates Foundation, founded in 2000 with an initial investment of $1 billion. A further large injection of funds from Warren Buffet in 2007 made the Gates Foundation the most influential global investor in health. Its power is derived from its own grant-giving ability (for operational programs but also for research) as well as from its support for partnerships (e.g., funding for both the GAVI Alliance and the Global Fund). In 2008, the Gates Foundation paid out approximately $1.8 billion in grants related to global health (Gates Foundation, 2008). By comparison, the Global Fund disbursed $2.25 billion in 2008 (Global Fund, 2010); WHO's budget for 2008 was approximately $2 billion, only 22% of which came from member states' contributions (WHO, 2008), and the rest of which came from extrabudgetary sources earmarked for specific programs. To put the Gates Foundation contribution to global health financing into perspective, McCoy, Kembhavi, Patel, and Luintel (2009) noted, "The Foundation is now a bigger international health donor than all governments bar the United States and the United Kingdom" (p. 1645). As a partner and sponsor of many global initiatives, the Gates Foundation has significantly influenced the global policy agenda and broader discourses around health.

While most commentators have welcomed the additional funding for global health, praising the Gates Foundation for renewing the dynamism, credibility, and attractiveness of global health ("What Has the Gates Foundation Done for Global Health?," 2009), some questions have been raised about its tendency to support what are seen as technical fixes (e.g., vaccines) while paying insufficient attention to systems for delivery (Birn, 2005). Other critics have observed that the majority of the Gates Foundation's grants went to organizations in high-income countries, and that there was a large gap between what the Gates Foundation funded and the burden of disease of the poorest countries (Black, Bhan, Chopra, Rudan, & Victora, 2009). Nevertheless, such criticisms have been fairly muted.

Power has also been consolidated between global organizations. The G8—comprising the heads of state of eight nations (the United States, Canada, the United Kingdom, France, Russia, Japan, Germany, and Italy)—which meets annually, started to put health on its agenda regularly from 2001. In the wake of the HIV/AIDS pandemic, the terrorist attacks on September 11, 2001, and fears about bioterrorism, the G8 began to promote and support specific initiatives (for HIV vaccine development and polio eradication, for example). Some envisaged the G8 as evolving into a center for global health governance, replacing the UN and WHO. Others have been more circumspect,

given the broad political and economic agenda of the G8 members.

Another potentially powerful grouping is the H8, which was created in mid 2007. The informal group includes the heads of eight health-related organizations—WHO, UNICEF, UNFPA, UNAIDS, the Global Fund, the GAVI Alliance, the Gates Foundation, and the World Bank. It meets only once per year, and was established to stimulate a sense of urgency for achieving the health-related MDGs more quickly.

While both the G8 and the H8 meet infrequently, their continuity of membership and common interests in global health have combined to influence what goes onto the global health agenda. These groups also have the potential to improve collaboration between countries and agencies.

It is not only at the global level that the number of actors in health has diversified and power has shifted. Regional organizations such as the European Union (EU) have expanded their interests in health. In fact, by 2010 the EU accounted for 60% of all official development assistance globally. WHO's regional offices—particularly PAHO—act as relatively independent institutions in their own right. Bilateral organizations provide funds for health to regional organizations (approximately one-third of the United Kingdom's overseas development assistance is channeled through the EU) as well as continue to support WHO and have a significant presence at the country level. Indeed, many bilateral organizations expanded their activities to the country level by channeling funds through NGOs in the health field, leading to an explosion of NGO activity in the twenty-first century both at the country level and internationally. The percentage of overseas development aid channeled through NGOs by the U.S. government, for example, increased from 0.18% in 1980 to 6% in 2002 (OECD, 2005, quoted in McCoy, Chand, & Sridhar, 2009a). The entry of actors from the corporate sector (the pharmaceutical companies, for example) into health is further changing the landscape of health cooperation.

The power increasingly exercised by global health initiatives and partnerships has implications not only for the influence exercised by the traditional international organizations (such as WHO and the World Bank) over international health policy, but also for national governments, which have different relationships with these new entities than they did with international organizations (Buse & Harmer, 2004). These partnerships are often actively involved in setting technical norms and standards, and their support to countries often takes place within the confines of application criteria and performance results that may be far more restrictive than earlier conditions associated with bilateral support or loans from international finance institutions.

This pluralism of activity and partnership has raised the status of health on the world's policy agenda, and led to significantly increased expenditures on global health. At the same time, it has altered the balance of power and heightened concerns about overlapping mandates, competition and duplication of health activities, poor coordination, and other issues of governance.

Overlapping Mandates

As pointed out by Lee and associates (1996), many of the UN organizations' formal mandates (defined as an organization's statement of overall purpose) have evolved over time, and what the UN organizations are actually doing—their effective mandates—have changed considerably as well. For example, UNICEF's original mandate as "a temporary body to meet the emergency needs of children in postwar Europe" (Koivusalo & Ollila, 1997) graduated from temporary relief and emergency activities to development work with children, and later evolved to include the welfare of youth and women. UNFPA, which had a relatively clear formal mandate to promote population programs, did not stray far from activities concerning population issues, including family planning, until after the International Conference on Population and Development in 1994. It was at this conference that population activities were redefined as reproductive health activities, raising debates within UNFPA about its effective mandate. The World Bank, with a mandate to provide financial capital to assist with the reconstruction and development of member states, entered the health field through its support for population policies in the late 1960s, and in the 1990s led the way in establishing international health policy by focusing on financing reforms.

It is not clear whether the various global health partnerships will end up with a proliferation of arrangements that, far from filling gaps and strategic niches, actually lead to duplication and confusion. Concern has been expressed, for instance, at an attempt by the Centers for Disease Control and Prevention (CDC) to establish a global disease surveillance network that parallels WHO's surveillance network (Exhibit 17-11). Giving evidence to a U.K. government Select Committee in 2008, a WHO staff member, Dr. Heymann, made the following statement:

> CDC, which in the past was a very strong partner in the Global Outbreak Alert and Response Network, is now setting up its own bilateral Global Disease Detection Network. . . . It causes us very difficult problems, to the extent that many times there is difficulty knowing who is doing what in a country when there is an outbreak of disease. (U.K. Select Committee on Intergovernmental Organizations, 2008)

Exhibit 17-11   WHO and Surveillance: When to Declare a Pandemic?

One of WHO's functions is to help the global community protect itself against the spread of infectious diseases. To assist the organization in this task, the International Health Regulations (IHRs) are an international, legal agreement, binding on all governments, that outline obligations to prevent the spread of infectious diseases while minimizing disruption to international trade. In 2005, the IHRs were revised from covering only cholera, plague, and yellow fever, to include many other diseases, and to have a broader scope. The new IHRs cover the mandatory reporting of all public health events of international concern (PHEICs), which includes new types of communicable diseases such as severe acute respiratory syndrome (SARS) and avian influenza (H5N1).

To fulfill these obligations, governments must develop and maintain systems of surveillance, and link into WHO's Global Outbreak Alert and Response Network (GOARN). GOARN coordinates reports of and responses to outbreaks of infectious diseases, and receives reports from many different institutions in many countries, including CSOs.

While the revised IHRs are designed to strengthen member states' roles and responsibilities for preventing the spread of infectious diseases, their application has not been without problems. For example, some critics expressed concern that the 2005 IHR revisions would slow down governments' ability to mount a rapid response, by requiring WHO to first convene an emergency committee comprising technical experts before declaring a public health emergency (Kamradt-Scott, 2009). In 2009, there was criticism of WHO's declaration of the H1N1 virus as a pandemic (Watson, 2010). Questions were raised about the virulence of the disease, the definition of a "pandemic," and industry influence and conflicts of interest. Critics noted the fast-track approval given for vaccines whose impact on pregnant women had not been fully assessed. As a result, at least three separate inquiries were planned to investigate WHO's decision to declare the H1N1 virus a pandemic (Watson, 2010).

Competition and Duplication

A recurring concern in the governance of global health is the extent to which competition, fragmentation, and duplication of health activities occur because there are so many different actors, and the effect that this may have on domestic policy environments. MOHs, on the one hand, may experience negative cumulative effects, with multiple donors and partnerships making demands on officials' time, and each donor wanting its own project presentations, evaluations, accounting systems, and meetings. Governments, on the other hand, may sometimes use competition for attention to play donors off against one another.

For example, in a few countries where WHO had the lead role among UN agencies in negotiations with the MOH about healthcare reforms, the World Bank was perceived as a threat and a competitor because of its standing in the country and its access to policy elites beyond the MOH. Case studies of negotiations on healthcare reforms in Ecuador (Lucas et al., 1997) and the Dominican Republic (Glassman, Reich, Laserson, & Rojas, 1999) suggest that the World Bank was sometimes seen as competing not only with other international organizations, such as WHO, but also with certain institutions within the government.

In those low- and middle-income countries with weak administrative systems, the sheer number of international organizations, NGOs, and partnerships interacting with the host government can hide duplication of activities and programs. It is often difficult for the government to know who is doing what. In Vietnam in the mid-2000s, there were 25 bilateral aid donors, 19 multilateral organizations providing aid, 350 international NGOs, and 8,000 aid projects (Acharya, de Lima, & Moore, 2006)—and this proliferation was fairly typical for many low- and middle-income countries.

Poor Coordination

Poor coordination between organizations in health has long been recognized as a problem, especially at the country level. Global agreements through meetings, partnerships, and policy discussions of the G8 and H8 have attempted to secure greater policy cohesion at the global level. There have also been a number of attempts to achieve greater coherence at the country level. For example, the Paris Declaration on Aid Effectiveness was endorsed in 2005 by development officials and ministers from 91 countries, 26 donor organizations, the private sector, and CSOs. It committed participants to a series of measures that would help coordinate aid and make it more effective.

These principles have been adapted and adopted by the global health community. Exhibit 17-12 outlines the principles, indicators, and targets to be achieved.

Other attempts to coordinate have involved sector-wide approaches (SWAps), whereby donors agree to activities and support within a health plan designed by the recipient government (see Exhibit 17-13). SWAps were introduced in the late 1990s. The World Bank (2010) defines a SWAp as "an approach to a locally-owned program for a coherent sector in a comprehensive and coordinated manner, moving toward the use of country systems." These approaches have been perceived as being the answer to competition and duplication, as well as offering a more effective way of managing resources (Peters & Chao, 1998).

Although considerable support for this strategy has been observed, observers noted a number of obstacles to SWAps early on (Cassels, 1997; Walt, Pavignani, Gilson, & Buse, 1999), including weak institutional capacity to coordinate and manage, and continuing competition among donors. An evaluation in 2010 of health SWAps in six countries (Bangladesh, Ghana, Kyrgyzstan, Malawi, Nepal, and Tanzania) produced mixed results. On the one hand, the SWAps had been successful in putting in place tools and processes for improved sector coordination and oversight, and had made headway in improving the harmonization and alignment of development assistance. On the other hand, SWAps had been only modestly successful in achieving improvements in the efficiency of resource utilization, the ability to focus on results, and the enforcement of sector-wide accountabilities (of government and donors). The majority of completed programs of work had made only modest progress in achieving their nationally set development objectives (Vaillencourt, 2009).

As evidence accumulated that the global community was not on track to meet the MDG targets by 2015, and that weak health systems were undermining the achievement of these goals, two other initiatives were launched to coordinate action and accelerate joint efforts at global and national levels. Recognizing the need to strengthen poor countries' health systems, the International Health Partnership (IHP) was unveiled in London in 2007 (Exhibit 17-14). The IHP's goal was to encourage donors to work together more effectively to build strong and sustainable health systems.

Two years later, the GAVI Alliance, the World Bank, the Global Fund, and WHO were given a mandate by the High Level Task Force on Innovative Financing for Health Systems (Exhibit 17-10) to coordinate, mobilize, streamline, and channel resources to support

Exhibit 17-12	**Getting Donors and Countries to "Walk the Talk": The Paris Declaration**

Hosted by the French government in Paris in February 2005, the second High Level Forum (HLF) on aid effectiveness established five areas of reform (the "Paris Principles") in the delivery and management of donor aid necessary to achieve the Millennium Development Goals. Building on the first HLF held in Rome in 2003, the Paris Declaration included targets for 2010 and indicators against which progress could be measured.

	Principle	Indicator	Target for 2010
1	Ownership: partner countries exercise effective leadership over their development policies and strategies, and coordinate development actions.	Number of countries with national development strategies that have clear strategic priorities linked to a medium-term expenditure framework and reflected in annual budgets.	At least 75% of partner countries have operational development strategies.
2	Alignment: donors base their overall support on partner countries' national development strategies, institutions, and procedures.	Multiple indicators exist, including percentage of aid disbursements released according to agreed schedules in annual or multiyear frameworks.	Halve the gap—that is, halve the proportion of aid not disbursed within the fiscal year for which it was scheduled.
3	Harmonization: donors' actions are more harmonized, transparent, and collectively effective.	Multiple indicators exist, including percentage of aid provided as program-based approaches and percentage of joint field missions and analytic work.	Sixty-six percent of aid flow is provided in the context of program-based approaches; 40% of donor missions to the field are joint.
4	Managing for results: managing resources and improving decision-making for results.	Number of countries with transparent and monitorable performance assessment frameworks to assess progress against the national development strategies and sector programs.	Reduce the gap by one-third—that is, reduce the proportion of countries without transparent and monitorable performance assessment frameworks by one-third.
5	Mutual accountability: donors and partners enhance mutual accountability and transparency for development results and the use of resources.	Number of partner countries that undertake mutual assessments of progress in implementing agreed commitments on aid effectiveness, including those in the Paris Declaration.	All partner countries have mutual assessment reviews in place.

In September 2009, the third HLF was held in Accra, Ghana. Drawing on extensive consultation and country experiences, three areas of aid effectiveness were identified, where progress among both countries and donors remained slow and more needed to be done:

1. *Country ownership is key*. Low- and middle-income countries were encouraged to take stronger leadership roles in formulating their own development priorities; donors were encouraged to strengthen support for these country-led initiatives by investing in countries' human resources and institutions, and by using existing country systems rather than initiative-specific ones.
2. *Build more effective and inclusive partnerships*. Aid continued to be beset by problems of duplication and fragmentation. Good practice principles were required as well as country-led division of labor. Further untying of aid would increase aid's value for money. Development with all partners was emphasized, particularly with CSOs.
3. *Focus on achieving and accounting for development results*. The importance of transparency and accountability was stressed. Implementing mutual assessment reviews was declared a priority. Conditions for development support should be mutually agreed and mid-term predictability of aid improved.

Sources: Best Practice Principles for Global Health Partnership Activities at Country Level, Paris, November 14–15, 2005; Paris Declaration on Aid Effectiveness, 2nd High Level Forum on Aid Effectiveness, Paris, February 28–March 2, 2005; Accra Agenda for Action, 3rd High Level Forum on Aid Effectiveness, Accra, September 2–4, 2008; Overview of the Evaluation of the Implementation of the Paris Declaration, OECD. Retrieved from http://www.oecd.org/document/60/0,3343,en_21571361_34047972_38242748_1_1_1_1,00.html

Exhibit 17-13	What Is a SWAp?

Sector-wide approaches (SWAps), in the form of program aid, were promoted by the World Bank beginning in the late 1980s, although it was only in the mid-1990s that they were more generally accepted by bilateral agencies and some recipient governments. Derived from sector investment programs and sector expenditure programs, SWAps are instruments through which to deliver agreed-on health policies and to manage aid and domestic resources in a rational and optimal way. They embrace many of the principles of alignment and harmonization outlined in the Paris Declaration (see Exhibit 17-12). What makes SWAps attractive is that they are perceived as being able to strengthen governments' ability to oversee the entire health sector, develop policies and plans, and allocate and manage resources—including those provided by development partners.

In practice, health SWAps have been limited to a few countries and have not been supported by all donors. They have faced a number of difficulties over their two decades of existence:

- SWAps take time to be established. It took between three and five years to set up health SWAps in Uganda and Malawi, respectively.

- SWAps have to balance increased participation against unwieldy and large meetings.

- The need to agree on performance monitoring and indicators has proved challenging, with data collection to measure progress often being delayed.

- SWAps demand certain ways of working, and changes in aid instruments over the past decades have shifted the skills and competencies of those involved. For example, development partners need greater negotiation and facilitation skills than they did during the era of project design and management (Walford, 2007).

An evaluation in six countries in 2009 reported that in most of the countries, national health objectives were only modestly achieved under the SWAp (Vaillencourt, 2009). For example, the SWAps had largely succeeded in establishing new, country-led partnerships for the purposes of policy dialogue, joint annual planning and budgeting, and periodic reviews of sector performance. However, the accountabilities of development partners were weak, and guidance on conflict resolution was lacking. Another analysis of the long-established Bangladesh SWAp concluded that it was in poor shape, despite its undeniable achievements over the years. However, the author suggested that it was not the SWAp model that was at fault, but rather the way it was applied: Health sectors could not deliver more and better services if their basic health plans were badly conceived, whether or not a SWAp was in place (Martinez, 2008).

health systems and improve health-sector performance. As indicated by the slogan "More money for health, more health for the money," the aim of the Health Systems Funding Platform is to raise funds (as much as $5 billion) to help countries meet their national and MDG goals. It is not planned to be a finance mechanism in the sense of a global pool of funds with its own governance structure, but rather to be flexible and country focused; to reduce duplication of funding; to increase harmonization between the GAVI Alliance, the Global Fund, and the World Bank; and to align processes with country systems. All of these aims are similar to those found within the Paris Declaration (Exhibit 17-12) and IHP+ (Exhibit 17-14).

While these examples provide considerable justification for the view that the global health community is seriously concerned about the lack of health policy coherence, and is searching for ways of coordinating multiple actors and activities, it remains to be seen how well this concern is translated into practice at country level. Attempts to improve shortfalls in monitoring and evaluating health information

have led to the establishment of the Health Metrics Network (hosted by WHO) and to calls for improved health data by the H8 countries (Chan et. al., 2010). Nevertheless, some donors have failed to institutionalize the tools, incentives, and processes required to improve harmonization and alignment at the recipient country level, and the continuing complexity of the health arena at the country level raises doubts about recipient governments' ability to control "an unruly mélange" (Buse & Walt, 1997, p. 449) of actors. In one study, a senior government official was quoted as saying that managing aid was a "huge juggling act" (Brugha et al., 2004, p. 99). Another survey of donor practices in 11 recipient countries ranked the five highest burdens for countries as donor-driven priorities and systems, difficulties with donor procedures, uncoordinated donor practices, excessive demands on time, and delays in disbursements (OECD, 2003).

A study that looked at national and subnational coordination of HIV/AIDS programs in seven countries concluded that while global health initiatives such as the Global Fund had created opportunities for

---

Exhibit 17-14   IHP+: Strengthening Health Systems Through Coordination

The International Health Partnership plus related initiatives (IHP+) was launched in London in 2007. Recognizing the need for "urgent and collective action" to achieve the Millennium Development Goals, 10 donors, 8 low-income countries, and 8 international organizations signed a Global Compact that committed each partner to improve aid coordination, renew its commitment to the principles of aid effectiveness enshrined in the 2005 Paris Declaration, and leverage additional public funding for health care.

IHP+ is primarily a coordinating rather than a financing mechanism. It is not a formal institution such as the Global Fund, although it does have an administrative Core Team hosted by WHO and the World Bank.

IHP+ works by encouraging all partners to support one national health plan through a number of complementary actions:

- Supporting national sector planning processes. In January 2010, WHO launched a Country Planning Cycle Database to help coordinate and synchronize country health system planning.

- Encouraging joint assessment of national health plans by donors.

- Formalizing commitment to national plans through a Country Compact. As of March 2010, four countries had signed Compacts: Ethiopia, Mali, Mozambique and Nepal. Some, but not all, donors and international partners have signed these Compacts.

- Developing a results monitoring framework to track the implementation of national health plans and a Country Health Systems Surveillance (CheSS) system.

- Improving mutual accountability by monitoring progress against Country Compact commitments.

An additional feature of the IHP+ is the importance that it places on civil society participation. Two CSO representatives are members of the IHP+ executive board.

A short-term evaluation of the IHP+ reported that partners had made progress in reforming the ways they worked, but could do more to fully translate the principles of IHP+ into practice (Conway, Harmer, & Spicer, 2008). Despite some progress, there remained limited consensus not only about what constituted a Compact, but also—crucially—what role civil society should play in its development.

In 2010, a commentary in *The Lancet* by two members of the International Advisory Group to the team evaluating IHP+ lamented that the SuRG (the "Scaling-up Reference Group" that oversees IHP+) had decided to withhold the 2010 preliminary progress report from public release. According to these sources:

> There are some data to suggest that donors are aligning more with national plans, but most of the aid still reflects donor priorities. There is little evidence of health-systems strengthening. This lack of evidence does not mean the IHP+ is failing to deliver; it does mean that insufficient information to make this assessment was forthcoming. Difficulties with the reporting mechanism account for some of the reporting reluctance and a working group has since been established to create a new list of indicators. But disagreement over measures is not sufficient reason to withhold the first report from public discussion. (Labonte & Marriott, 2010, p.1506)

---

multisectoral participation, the quality of that participation was poor, and some global health initiatives bypassed coordination mechanisms, especially at the subnational level, thereby weakening their effectiveness (Spicer et. al., 2010). Some donors continue to finance programs that are off plan and off budget, and that are monitored through project-specific instruments.

The problems faced in coordination both among and between governments and donors arise for many reasons, including different interests, agendas, and cultures between the different actors; asymmetric power relations; and unique country contexts in

which institutional capacities and characteristics play a major role (Walt et al., 1999). Such barriers will continue to affect relationships in the shift from representation to participation, and their removal may require new tools, procedures, and incentives to support partnership processes.

Governance

Considerations about health governance arose during the 1980s, when aid was linked with "good governance," human rights, and multiparty democracy. The World Bank initially was concerned with governments that lacked accountability, transparency, and predictability, and countries where the rule of law was weak or absent. However, as Nelson and Eglinton (quoted in Killick et al., 1998) observe, these concerns led to broader issues:

> Transparency required not only open competition for public contracts, but adequate information on government projects and programs, and therefore the freedom of the media. Account-ability entails not only effective financial accounting and auditing, but penalties for corrupt or inept politicians. That in turn implies some form of elections and freedom of association and speech to make such elections meaningful. A predictable rule of law requires an independent and competent judiciary. (p. 95)

Although notions of governance have been applied largely to government, they are also applicable to global institutions and corporations. Are international organizations characterized by good governance? International organizations differ, but they are all accountable to their member states or governing bodies, which have clear mechanisms for challenging activities. Although budgets and expenditures are not always described as transparent, they are subject to annual audits and are accessible for perusal.

One of the most open of such organizations is the Global Fund. Its Office of Inspector General provides independent and objective assurance over the design and effectiveness of the Global Fund's programs and operations, and makes these publicly available on its website. There are clear rules governing the recruitment, selection, and behavior of those persons employed as international civil servants. In organizations such as WHO, representation of different interests is ensured through the WHA—although, in practice, the organization may be dominated by a smaller group of powerful members.

Through their ability to draw on worldwide policy communities to provide guidance on issues and reach consensus on policies and best practices, international organizations are vested with significant authority and legitimacy. Although the highest standards are not equally adhered to in all international agencies (UNESCO, for example, was criticized for nepotism, inefficiency, and corruption in the 1980s and again in 1999), the agencies are expected to be publicly accountable.

Since the late 1990s, global health partnerships and alliances have evolved alongside traditional intergovernmental relations between sovereign states and UN organizations, arguably establishing a new norm in relations among an increasingly diverse range of actors within the global health system (Szlezak, Bloom, Jamison, Keusch, Michaud, & Moon, 2010). The partnership model of global cooperation initially raised many questions and concerns about good governance (Buse, 2004; Buse & Walt, 2000): Would their actions be representative of the interests of multiple stakeholders? Would their actions be transparent? If partnerships were responsible to a myriad of constituencies (shareholders, governing boards, governments, beneficiaries, and consumers), would overall accountability fall between the cracks? These questions continue to elude attempts to provide definitive answers, but a clearer picture is emerging more than 10 years into the new century.

Representation in public–private partnerships remains a contentious and divisive issue at both national and global levels. At the global level, while many partnerships now recognize, and seek to profit from, synergy between multiple stakeholders (notably civil society and the private for-profit sector), board membership of partnerships remains skewed toward the private sector, with insufficient representation of the global South (Buse & Harmer, 2009). On the one hand, partnerships support (both financially and by capacity building) civil society and NGOs; on the other hand, many partnerships are perceived to embrace "private-sector thinking" that gives priority to expertise over representation when it comes to decision making (Adlide, Rowe, & Lob-Levyt, 2009).

Achieving the governance goal of transparency has also proved difficult. Differences in public and private ethos may create tensions or conflicts of interest for those involved. For example, sharing information may be difficult: Private industry or research groups may want to protect product leads or early data from trials. Practical limitations also impede monitoring progress, and a number of studies note that data systems are insufficiently developed to satisfy increasing demands for transparent reporting (Levine, 2006; Sridhar & Batniji, 2008). Independent evaluations of global health initiatives indicate that they, too, could do much more in the name of transparent best practice. In 2009, the Global Fund's Five Year Evaluation found that the Fund's support for transparency in reporting was not matched by its investment in data quality and availability (Macro International, 2009). A 2009 evaluation of the GAVI Alliance, however, applauded the organization for its transparent formula for allocation of funds—a formula that let countries know exactly how much they were entitled to request, thereby removing "a key element of uncertainty present, for example, in the Global Fund" (HLSP, 2009, p. 69)

Ensuring accountability is another continuing challenge. While governments are held accountable to their citizens through traditional political channels, it is less clear how multiple stakeholders can hold one another to account and be accountable to the countries in which they are working. Various attempts to address accountability have been initiated. In 2009, the One World Trust and Commonwealth Foundation piloted a Civil Society Accountability toolbox in four countries in an effort to strengthen the sector and reinforce its role in governance (One World Trust, 2010). Ten years after the UN established a Compact with the private sector, laying out the principles for public and private cooperation between the UN and private for-profit corporations, new guidelines were drafted in 2009 to reaffirm, among other things, the importance of social responsibility (UN, 2009). Ironically, one evaluation concluded that concerns about improving accountability in applications for funds—for example, GAVI Alliance applications for funding to strengthen country health systems—shifted attention away from efforts to ensure that funds secured were used effectively (HLSP, 2009).

Increasingly, good governance criteria are being applied not only to governments and international organizations, but also to corporations, NGOs, and global health initiatives. If Thomas Friedman (2008) is correct in asserting that in the current era of globalization "we are all partners now," then a strong case can be made that principles of governance "best practice" should apply to all who have a stake in ensuring better health for all.

Conclusion

The profile of international cooperation in health has changed considerably since the UN was established in the late 1940s as a putative means to bring peace and security to a world recovering from war. In the wake of its founding years of economic growth and relative security (with important exceptions in parts of the world), the UN facilitated the growth of overseas development assistance and led to considerable consensus in health cooperation. In the last few decades, however, economic growth has slowed—particularly in 2008–2009—and international insecurity has grown. The pace of globalization trends has changed perceptions and relationships among countries. As these changes have taken place, health cooperation has shifted from systems of formal, vertical representation to forms of horizontal partnership. The consequences of this transition are not clear, but three concluding points can be made.

First, increasing globalization will lead to different emphases in activities in health. Global health cooperation is likely to focus more on issues of governance and regulation at the global level, whether they involve environmental issues, which indirectly affect health, or transborder trade of health interventions and services, pharmaceuticals, and tobacco products. Nevertheless, much of the action relating to regulation and governance will likely center on the WTO in coming years, rather than on WHO. The global policy agenda will be influenced by the large investors in health, such as the Bill and Melinda Gates Foundation. Juxtaposed against this global-level activity, there is likely to be a continuation, or even growth, in international relief efforts at local levels if internal, ethnic, and secessionist conflicts continue as they have since the end of the Cold War.

Second, it is likely that public–private partnerships and alliances will be an increasing characteristic of cooperation in global health at the global, national, and local levels. Much remains to be learned about which sorts of partnerships work best, and under which conditions. Although there are clear advantages to this type of cooperation, ranging from the input of new ideas and energy to the harnessing of new financial resources, it is as yet unclear which sorts of problems will be generated through such partnerships. For example, how much will global health cooperation depend on focusing on narrow programs of disease control, which lend themselves to monitoring but neglect other important issues in health? How much will the calls for strengthening health systems help to develop good-quality and accessible health systems, given that outcomes and impact are more difficult to measure and take longer to demonstrate results? Partnerships may also raise issues of equity, by choosing to work in some countries with a particular disease rather than all countries. Also, if aid selectivity becomes a trend, such that aid is given only to those governments that demonstrate they have strong policy environments, what will happen to the people who live in countries considered to have weak policy environments?

Third, cooperation in health will no longer be dominated by the UN or its specialized agencies such as WHO, but rather will be represented by a much more diverse set of actors who form partnerships and networks. Included among them will be private-sector entities as well as a range of NGOs, including consumer and professional groups, large and small environmental groups, and other CSOs. The revolution in communications technology, which has made it so much easier to communicate electronically across borders, will allow a relatively fluid formation of informal networks and partnerships that may come together to campaign or demonstrate on specific issues.

For all these reasons, horizontal participation is likely to be the key feature of global health cooperation in the new millennium. Although the state will still play a role, it will not be primarily through formal vertical representation as it was in the twentieth century.

● ● ● Discussion Questions

1. List the most important actors in global health, differentiating between international organizations, bilateral organizations, NGOs, and public–private partnerships. For each organization, characterize its strengths in terms of financial resources or technical skills. Which other factors make organizations influential?

2. Give three reasons why states may cooperate, and identify the sorts of activities they might undertake together.

3. How has the role of WHO changed in the twenty-first century? Which factors have contributed most to this change?

4. What are the factors that have led to the shift from vertical to horizontal representation?

5. Name three benefits and three challenges facing global health partnerships.

• • • References

Abbasi, K. (1999). The World Bank on world health: Under fire. *British Medical Journal, 318,* 1003–1006.

Acharya, A., de Lima, A. T. F., & Moore, M. (2006). Proliferation and fragmentation: Transactions costs and the value of aid. *Journal of Development Studies, 42*(1), 1–21.

Adlide, G., Rowe, A., & Lob-Levyt, J. (2009). Public–private partnership to promote health: The GAVI Alliance experience. In A. Clapham & M. Robinson (Eds.), *Realizing the rights to health* (Vol. III, pp. 539–547). Geneva, Switzerland: Swiss Human Rights Books.

Basch, P. (1999). *Textbook of international health* (2nd ed.). Oxford, UK: Oxford University Press.

Biesma, R., Brugha, R., Harmer, A., Walsh, A., Spicer, N., & Walt, G. (2009). The effects of global health initiatives on country health systems: A review of the evidence from HIV/AIDS control. *Health Policy and Planning, 24*(4), 239–252.

Birn, E. (2005). Gates's grandest challenge: Transcending technology as public health ideology. *Lancet, 366* (9484), 514–519.

Black, E., Bhan, M., Chopra, M., Rudan, I., & Victora, C. (2009). Accelerating the health impact of the Global Fund. *Lancet, 373,* 1584–1585.

Brugha, R., Donoghue, M., Starling, M., Ndubani, P., Ssengoba, F., Fernandes, B., & Walt, G. (2004). The Global Fund: Managing great expectations. *Lancet, 364,* 95–100.

Budlanto, L. (2010, March 25) RI pushes for fair virus sharing scheme despite Obama visit. *Jakarta Post.* Retrieved from www.thejakartapost.com/news/2010/02/10/ri-pushes-fair-virus-sharing-scheme-despite-obama-visit.html

Buse, K. (2004). Governing public–private infectious disease partnerships. *Brown Journal of World Affairs, 10*(2), 225–242.

Buse, K., & Harmer, A. (2004). Power to the partners? The politics of public–private health partnerships. *Development, 47*(2), 43–48.

Buse, K., & Harmer, A. (2009). Global health partnerships: The mosh-pit of global health governance. In K. Buse, W. Hein, & N. Drager (Eds.), pp. 245–267. *Making sense of global health governance: The policy perspective.* London: Palgrave Macmillan.

Buse, K., & Walt, G. (1997). An unruly melange? Coordinating external resources to the health sector: A review. *Social Science and Medicine, 45,* 449–463.

Buse, K., & Walt, G. (2000). Global public–private partnerships: Part I—A new development in health? *Bulletin of the World Health Organization, 78*(4), 549–561.

Cassels, A. (1997). *A guide to sector-wide approaches to health development: Concepts, issues and working arrangements.* Geneva, Switzerland: World Health Organization.

Chan, M., Kazatchkine, M., Lob-Levyt, J., Obaid, T., Schwiezer, J., Sidibe, M., et al. (2010). Meeting the demand for results and accountability: A call for action on health data from eight global health agencies. *PLOS Medicine, 7*(1).doi:10.1371/journal.pmed.1000223

Childers, E., & Urquhart, B. (1994). *Renewing the United Nations system.* Uppsala, Sweden: Dag Hammarskjold Foundation.

Chowdury, Z., & Rowson, M. (2000). The people's health assembly. *British Medical Journal, 321,* 1361–1362.

Coker, R. (1999). Public health, civil liberties and tuberculosis. *British Medical Journal, 318,* 1434–1435.

Collin, J. (2004). Tobacco politics. *Development, 47,* 91–96.

Cometto, G., Ooms, G., Starrs, A., & Zeitz, P. (2009). A Global Fund for the health MDGs? *Lancet, 373,* 1500–1502.

Conway, S., Harmer, A., & Spicer, N. (2008). *External review of the International Health Partnership + related initiatives.* Johannesburg, South Africa: Responsible Action.

Fassin, D., & Schneider, H. (2003). The politics of AIDS in South Africa: Beyond the controversies. *British Medical Journal, 326*, 495–497.

Feldbaum, H., Patel, P., Sondorp, E., & Lee, K. (2004). *Global health and national security: The need for critical engagement*. Unpublished manuscript, Centre on Global Change and Health, London School of Hygiene and Tropical Medicine.

Ford, N., Wilson, D., Bunjumnong, O., & Van Schoen Angerer, T. (2004). The role of civil society in protecting public health over commercial interests: Lessons from Thailand. *Lancet, 363*, 560–563.

Forster, P. (2009). *The political economy of avian influenza in Indonesia*. STEPS Working Paper 17. Brighton, UK: STEPS Centre.

Friedman, T. L. (2008, October 18). The great Iceland meltdown. *New York Times*. Retrieved from www.nytimes.com/2008/10/19/opinion/19 friedman.html

Fryatt, B., Mills, A., & Nordstrum, A. (2010). Financing of health systems to achieve the health Millennium Development Goals in low-income countries. *Lancet, 375*, 419–426.

Gates Foundation. (2008). Annual report, p. 23. Retrieved April 20, 2010, from http://www .gatesfoundation.org/annualreport/2008/Docum ents/2008-annual-report.pdf

Gilmore, A., & Collin, J. (2002). The world's first international tobacco control treaty. *British Medical Journal, 325*, 846–847.

Glassman, A., Reich, M., Laserson, K., & Rojas, F. (1999). Applying political analysis to understand health reform: The case of the Dominican Republic. *Health Policy and Planning, 14*, 115–126.

Global Alliance for Vaccines and Immunization (GAVI) Alliance. (2010). Advanced market commitments. Retrieved from http://www.gavialliance .org/vision/policies/in_financing/amcs/index.php

Global Fund. (2010). Latest figures on pledges and contributions to the Global Fund. Retrieved from http://www.theglobalfund.org/documents/pledges_ contributions.xls

Godlee, F. (1994). The World Health Organization. *British Medical Journal, 309*, 1424–1428, 1491–1495, 1566–1570, 1636–1639.

Godlee, F. (1995). The World Health Organization. *British Medical Journal, 310*, 110–112, 178–182, 389–393, 583–586.

Greenough, P. (1995). Intimidation, coercion and resistance in the final stages of the South Asian smallpox eradication campaign, 1973–1975. *Social Science and Medicine, 41*, 633–645.

Haas, P. M. (1992). Introduction: Epistemic communities and international policy coordination. *International Organization, 46*, 1–35.

HLSP. (2009). *GAVI health systems strengthening support evaluation 2009, RFP-0006-08: Volume 2: Full evaluation report*. London: Author.

Hogan, M. C., Foreman, K. J., Naghavi, M., Ayn, S., Wang, M., Makela, S., et al. (2010, April 12). Maternal mortality for 181 countries, 1980–2008: A systematic analysis of progress towards Millennium Development Goal 5.

Howson, C., Fineberg, H., & Bloom, B. (1998). The pursuit of global health: The relevance of engagement for developed countries. *Lancet, 351*, 586–590.

Institute for Health Metrics and Evaluation (IHME). (2009). *Financing global health 2009: Tracking development assistance for health*. Seattle: Institute for Health Metrics and Evaluation.

International Financing Facility for Immunization (IFFIm). (2010) IFFIm: Supporting GAVI. Retrieved from http://www.iff-immunisation.org/index.html

Kamradt-Scott, A. (2009). *The evolving WHO: Implications for global health security*. Working paper. London: LSHTM.

Kanji, N., Hardon, A., Harnmeijer, J. W., Mamdani, M., & Walt, G. (1992). *Drugs policy in developing countries*. London: Zed Books.

Killick, T., Gunatillaka, R., & Marr, A. (1998). *Aid and the political economy of policy change*. London/New York: Routledge.

Koivusalo, M., & Ollila, E. (1997). *Making a healthy world: Agencies, actors, and policies in international health*. London: Zed Books.

Koplan, J., Bond, C., Merson, M., Reddy, K. S., Rodriguez, M. H., Sewankambo, N. K., & Wasserheit, J. N. (2009). Towards a common definition of global health. *Lancet, 373*, 1993–1995.

Labonte, R., & Marriot, A. (2010). The International Health Partnership+: Little progress in accountability, or just little progress? *Lancet, 375*, 1505–1507.

Lee, K. (1998). *Historical dictionary of the World Health Organization*. Lanham, MD: Scarecrow Press.

Lee, K., Collinson, S., Walt, G., & Gilson, L. (1996). Who should be doing what in international health: A confusion of mandates in the United Nations? *British Medical Journal, 312*, 302–307.

Levine, R. (2006). Following the money in global health. Centre for Global Development. Retrieved from http://www.cgdev.org/content/article/detail/1423555/

Lu, C., Michaud, C. M., Gakidou, E., Khan, K., & Murray, C. J. (2006). Effect of the Global Alliance for Vaccines and Immunisation on diphtheria, tetanus, and pertussis vaccine coverage: An independent assessment. *Lancet, 369*, 1088–1095.

Lucas, A., Mogedal, S., Walt, G., Hodne-Steen, S., Kruse, S. E., Lee, K., & Hawken, L. (1997). *Cooperation for development: The World Health Organization's support to programs at country level* [Report for the governments of Australia, Canada, Italy, Norway, Sweden, and United Kingdom]. London: London School of Hygiene and Tropical Medicine.

Macro International. (2009). *Global Fund five-year evaluation: Study area 3. The impact of collective efforts on the reduction of the disease burden of AIDS, tuberculosis and malaria*. Calverton, MD: Macro International Inc.

Mahler, H. (1983, May 3). *The full measure of the strategy for health for all*. Address to the World Health Assembly.

Martinez, J. (2008). *Sector wide approaches at critical times: The case of Bangladesh*. Technical approach paper. London: HSLP Institute.

Massive Good. (2010). Do "massive good": Fight AIDS, TB as you travel. Retrieved from http://travelplanning101.com/2010/03/do-massive-good-fight-aids-tb-as-you-travel/716

McCoy, D. (2009). The High Level Taskforce on Innovative International Financing for Health Systems. *Health Policy and Planning, 24*(5), 321–323.

McCoy, D., Chand, S., & Sridhar, D. (2009). Global health funding: How much, where it comes from, and where it goes. *Health Policy and Planning, 24*, 407–417.

McCoy, D., Kembhavi, G., Patel, J., & Luintel, A. (2009). The Bill and Melinda Gates Foundation's grant-making programme for global health. *Lancet, 373*, 1645–1653.

Nattrass, N. (2008). The (political) economy of antiretroviral treatment in developing countries. *Trends in Microbiology, 16*, 574–579.

One World Trust. (2010). Toolkits on CSO accountability. Retrieved from http://www.oneworldtrust.org/index.php?option=com_content&view=article&id=83&Itemid=70

Organization for Economic Cooperation and Development (OECD). (2003). *Harmonizing donor practices for effective aid delivery*. DAC Guidelines and Reference Series. Paris: Author.

Organization for Economic Cooperation and Development (OECD). (2007). *Financing development: Aid and beyond*. Paris: The Development Centre, OECD.

People's Health Movement. (2009). People's charter for health. Retrieved from http://www.phmovement.org/en/resources/charters/peopleshealth

Peters, C., & Chao, S. (1998). The sector-wide approach in health: What is it? Where is it leading? *International Journal of Health Planning and Management, 13*, 177–190.

Pollock, A. M., & Price, D. (2003). The public health implications of world trade negotiations on the general agreement on trade in services and public services. *Lancet, 363,* 1072–1075.

Pratley, N. (2004, April 14). Sisters who stirred the conscience of Coca-Cola. *The Guardian,* p. 26.

President's Emergency Plan for AIDS Relief (PEPFAR). (2009). Reauthorizing PEPFAR. Retrieved from http://www.pepfar.gov/press/107735.htm

Putnam, R., Leonari, R., & Nanetti, R. (1995). *Making democracy work.* Princeton, NJ: Princeton University Press.

Salaam-Blyther, T. (2008). *The Global Fund to Fight AIDS, Tuberculosis and Malaria: Progress report and issues for Congress.* CRS Report, RL33396.

Schneider, H. (2002). On the fault-line: The politics of AIDS policy in contemporary South Africa. *African Studies, 61*(1), 145–197.

Sedyaningsih, E. R., Isfandiri, S., Soendoro, T., & Supari, S. F. (2008). Towards mutual trust, transparency and equity in virus sharing mechanisms: The avian influenza case of Indonesia. *Annals of the Academy of Medicine of Singapore, 37,* 482–488.

Shiffman, J. (2008). Has donor prioritization of HIV/AIDS displaced aid for other health issues? *Health Policy and Planning, 23*(2), 95–100.

Smith, R. D., & MacKellar, L. (2007) Global public goods and the global health agenda: Problems, priorities and potential. *Globalization and Health, 3*(9), 1–17.

Spicer, N., Aleshkina, J., Biesma, R., Brugha, R., Caceres, C., Chilundo, B., et al. (2010). National and subnational HIV/AIDS coordination: Are global health initiatives closing the gap between intent and practice? *Globalization and Health, 6*(3). doi:10.1186/1744-8603-6-3

Sridhar, D., & Batniji, R. (2008). Misfinancing global health: A case for transparency in disbursements and decision making. *Lancet, 372,* 1185–1191.

Stiglitz, J. (2002). *Globalization and its discontents.* New York: W. W. Norton.

Szlezak, N., Bloom, B., Jamison, D., Keusch, G., Michaud, C., & Moon, S. (2010). The global health system: Actors, norms, and expectations in transition. *PLOS Med, 7*(1). doi:10.1371/journal.pmed.1000183

Taskforce on Innovative International Financing for Health Systems. (2009). *More money for health, and more health for the money.* Geneva, Switzerland: Author.

Taylor, P. (1993). *International organization in the modern world.* London: Pinter.

U.K. Select Committee on Intergovernmental Organizations, (2008). *Diseases know no frontiers: How effective are intergovernmental organizations in controlling their spread? Volume I: Report.* London: Stationery Office.

UNITAID. (2008). Annual report. Retrieved from http://www.unitaid.eu/images/news/annual_report_2008_en.pdf

United Nations (UN). (2009). Guidelines on cooperation between the United Nations and the private sector: Final draft. Retrieved from http://business.un.org/en/assets/fb72af6d-8ef0-48f7-82ff-38ebfc77787f.pdf

United Nations (UN). (2010). *Keeping the promise: Report of the Secretary-General to 64th General Assembly of the United Nations.* A/64/665

Vaillencourt, D. (2009). *Do health sector wide approaches achieve results?* Working paper, IEG. Washington, DC: World Bank.

Vaughan, J. P., Mogedal, S., Walt, G., Kruse, S. E., Lee, K., & de Wilde, K. (1996). WHO and the effects of extrabudgetary funds: Is the organization donor driven? *Health Policy and Planning, 11,* 253–264.

Walford, V. (2007). *A review of SWAps in Africa.* Technical paper. London: HLSP Institute.

Walt, G., & Gilson, L. (1994). Reforming the health sector in developing countries: The central role of policy analysis. *Health Policy and Planning, 4,* 353–370.

Walt, G., Pavignani, E., Gilson, L., & Buse, K. (1999). Managing external resources: Are there lessons for SWAps? *Health Policy and Planning, 14*(3), 273–284.

Watson, R. (2010). WHO is accused of "crying wolf" over its decision to declare the H1N1 virus a pandemic. *British Medical Journal, 340,* 783.

What has the Gates Foundation done for global health? [Editorial]. (2009). *Lancet, 373,* 1577.

World Bank. (2010). HIV/AIDS data. Retrieved from http://go.worldbank.org/SK5YQCIFT0

World Health Organization (WHO). (2004). *Financial report and audited financial statements presented to 57th World Health Assembly, April 2004.* Unpublished document A 57/20. Geneva, Switzerland: Author.

World Health Organization (WHO). (2008). Programme budget 2009–2009. Retrieved from apps.who.int/gb/ebwha/pdf_files/AMTSP-PPB/a-mtsp_4en.pdf

World Health Organization (WHO). (2009). *2009 summary report on global progress in implementation of the WHO Framework Convention on Tobacco Control.* Geneva, Switzerland: Author.

World Health Organization (WHO) Maximizing Positive Synergies Collaborative Group. (2009). An assessment of interactions between global health initiatives and country health systems. *Lancet, 373,* 2137–2169.

World Health Organization (WHO). (2011). *World Health Statistics 2011.* Geneva, Switzerland: Author.

Zarrilli, S., & Kinnon, C. (1998). *International trade in health services.* Geneva, Switzerland: UNCTAD/World Health Organization.

18

Globalization and Health

KELLEY LEE, DEREK YACH, AND ADAM KAMRADT-SCOTT

Widespread consensus now exists that fundamental changes to human societies around the world are presently under way, a trend broadly referred to as globalization. Although this evolution is historically rooted in how all societies have formed and adapted over millennia, there is a sense that the changes of recent decades are more intense and accelerated. The resultant impacts of globalization potentially affect every individual and community.

The changes arising from globalization can be understood to extend to the field of public health in three main ways. First, processes of global change are shaping the broad determinants of health. Along with individual lifestyle factors, globalization is influencing determinants of health such as employment, housing, education, water and sanitation, and agriculture and food production. Moreover, general socioeconomic, cultural, and environmental conditions are undergoing a transformation. Overall, globalization is restructuring human societies in diverse ways, and hence potentially influencing a broad range of factors that affect individual and population health.

Second, a growing body of evidence indicates that health status and outcomes are being variably influenced by globalization. Many argue that globalization is giving rise to new patterns of health and disease linked to the consequent restructuring of human societies. These patterns include the spread of new and re-emerging diseases, as well as the reconfiguration of existing health challenges, including health inequalities within and across countries. In short, contemporary forms of globalization are producing winners and losers, and health outcomes are one reflection of this separation.

Third, as a consequence of the factors mentioned previously, societies must adapt their collective responses to changing health determinants and outcomes. Within the broader context of global governance, and specifically global governance for health (see Chapter 17), globalization is influencing healthcare financing and service provision in a diverse range of countries, as well as the ways in which many products and services that affect health are regulated and marketed. The need to negotiate collective arrangements within and across countries, within the health sector and beyond, and across the public and private sectors has created new challenges.

This chapter provides an overview of how globalization is affecting health determinants, health status and outcomes, and the regulatory environment for public health, including healthcare financing and service provision. These impacts can be collectively understood as the effects of the transition from international to global public health. The chapter begins by defining the often-used term "globalization," its key drivers, and the precise changes it is creating. This explication is followed by a discussion of the links between globalization and shifting patterns of infectious and chronic diseases. Finally, the effects on collective responses to global health challenges are explored through consideration of the reform of healthcare financing and service provision, migration of health workers, and the restructuring of the pharmaceutical industry. The chapter concludes by outlining ways the public health community might potentially promote and protect health in an era of globalization, including the role of global health diplomacy.

What Is Globalization?

Globalization has undoubtedly caught the imagination of many, judging by the enthusiasm with which this term is so frequently used by scholars, policy makers, the business community, mass media, and the general public. Intuitively, the term articulates how the contemporary world is becoming more interconnected, with events in one part of the world having an impact elsewhere. If we are to understand the implications of globalization for public health, however, a more precise understanding of what it means is needed.

The Historical Context of Globalization

It is beyond the scope of this chapter to review the expansive literature on globalization. Moreover, the definition of this term remains highly contested, with ongoing debates about whether globalization is really happening, what its key drivers are, and, perhaps most controversially, whether it is having positive or negative impacts on human societies and the natural world. Nevertheless, beyond the rough-and-tumble of these debates, it is still possible to define globalization in more precise terms.

First, to assess whether a distinct phenomenon that can be called globalization is really happening, it is important to understand more recent developments in their historical context. Although many writers on globalization focus on changes taking place from the late twentieth century, it is helpful to see globalization as a longer process of social change occurring over the course of centuries, if not millennia (Berridge, Loughlin, & Herring, 2009). The early beginnings of globalization might be described as occurring when human species beginning with *Homo erectus* migrated out of Africa 1 million years ago, formed societies, and then interacted with one another across distant territories. This process accelerated and intensified with the development of long-distance modes of transportation (such as sea-going vessels) that enabled individuals to travel farther and in greater numbers. Major developments in social, political, and economic history marked the acceleration of globalization, such as the opening of the Silk Route between Asia and Europe, the arrival of Christopher Columbus in the Americas, the formation of the modern state system, European imperialism, the slave trade, and the Industrial Revolution. Characterizing all of these developments was an increased movement of people (voluntary or otherwise) and other life forms (plants and animals), capital, goods and services, and knowledge and ideas. Thus what many today refer to as globalization is simply the contemporary intensification of the long-established interaction of human societies across territorial space.

Changing patterns of health and disease have been integrally linked to this historical evolution of human societies. A familiar example is the spread of bubonic plague during the fourteenth century by travelers along trade routes between Asia and Europe. The disease killed millions, and eventually led to the introduction of quarantine practices that sought to regulate trade to prevent further importation of the disease. Similarly, the transition of cholera from an endemic disease of South Asia to a pandemic disease from the 1830s onward was caused in large part by the social, political, and economic upheavals inflicted on local communities, economies, and ecosystems by European imperialism (Lee & Dodgson, 2002). The resulting cholera pandemics of the nineteenth century led to the development of the International Sanitary Conventions (later renamed the International Health Regulations, discussed later in this chapter).

Yet, although globalization can be understood as a historical process linked to the evolution of human societies, it remains necessary to identify what is distinct about the term "globalization" per se. How is globalization different from internationalization, liberalization, universalization, and Westernization—terms that are so often used interchangeably? What is "global" about globalization? The work of Scholte (2000) is helpful in this respect. He defines each of these "redundant concepts of globalization" in the following ways:

- *Internationalization.* The most common usage of the term "globalization" is in reference to the increasing interaction and interdependence of people in different countries. Various measures, such as trade, communication, and migration, certainly confirm that there has been a substantial increase in cross-border exchanges. Historically, however, there have been many periods of intensified interconnections since the establishment of the modern system of sovereign states some 500 years ago—a system that still defines international relations today. Because these interactions refer to exchanges between nations, or "inter-national" interactions, the term "internationalization" is an accurate description.

- *Liberalization.* This term is used especially often by advocates of neoliberal ideas, and their critics, to signal a global world that is defined as "one without regulatory barriers to transfers of resources between countries." Historically, we can identify periods where statutory constraints on cross-border movements of capital, goods, and services have been reduced. For example, the second half of the twentieth century saw a significant expansion of international trade and commerce as a result of widespread liberalization. The rounds of negotiations under the General Agreement on Tariffs and Trade (GATT), which was later replaced by the World Trade Organization (WTO), from the end of World War II to 1995 also led to successive reductions in trade tariffs. The continuation of this process since the mid-1990s, under multilateral, regional, and bilateral trade agreements, has often been referred to as globalization. Scholte (2000) argues convincingly that, in this sense, the term "liberalization" is appropriate and there is "little need now to invent a new vocabulary for this old phenomenon." Distinguishing globalization from liberalization addresses criticisms that the former is nothing new.

- *Universalization.* Universalization generally refers to the spread of people and cultures to all corners of the world. Defined in this way, however, we can see that the human species has traveled intercontinentally for 1 million years or more. Similarly, several world religions have won followers worldwide, and trade has distributed goods and services on a worldwide scale for centuries. In this sense, the term "universalization" is deemed adequate and the new terminology of "globalization" unnecessary.

- *Westernization.* The term "Westernization" describes the belief that certain cultural values, aspirations, and behaviors characteristic of Western societies, and particularly U.S. society, are being adopted increasingly throughout the world. In this case, globalization is seen as a largely negative process of homogenization, a postindustrial form of colonization through Hollywood films, fast-food diets, and consumerism. Although it is undoubtedly the case that a certain degree of Westernization is taking place, Scholte (2000) argues that "intercontinental westernization, too, has unfolded since long before the recent emergence of globe-talk." He suggests that the concepts of modernization and imperialism readily capture ideas of Westernization and "[w]e do not need a new vocabulary of globalization to remake an old analysis."

Strictly speaking, Scholte casts aside these "redundant" terms, and reserves the term "globalization" to describe social interactions that not only cross national boundaries, but also transcend them. According to Scholte, only when territorial boundaries, based on physical geography, are circumvented or become irrelevant can we speak of globalization. Satellite communications, the Internet, illicit drug trafficking, and undocumented migration are examples of globalization in this strict sense. Thus it is important to be aware of how the term "globalization" is defined. A looser definition suggests that at least some aspects of what people call globalization today are not novel to the twenty-first century. A strict definition of globalization, as the transcendence of territorial boundaries, is more distinctive of the transition facing human societies in recent decades.

Key Drivers of Globalization

A second important definitional question is why globalization is occurring. In other words, what are the key drivers of globalization? McMichael (2001) usefully distinguishes between two types of global change.

The first type results from the interplay of natural forces (e.g., climatic dynamics, continental drift, evolution, and mass extinctions) that occurred during the history of the planet. For example, there have been five great natural extinctions since the advent of vertebrate life approximately 500 million years ago, the last of which marked the end of the dinosaurs 65 million years ago. This phenomenon was followed by a long period of cooling that eventually opened an evolutionary niche 6 million years ago "for an ape able to survive mostly out of the forest." Over the past million years, there have been eight major glaciations, during which *Homo erectus* began to spread throughout Eurasia. It was only during the final interglacial period that *Homo sapiens* began to move out of northeast Africa and migrate worldwide. More recently, the rapid post-glaciation temperature rise between 15,000 and 10,000 years ago, amounting to approximately 5°C, caused substantial environmental changes and the extinction of many species of plants and animals.

The second type of global change is human induced, or anthropomorphic. These changes to the world occur as a result of human actions, individually or collectively, intentional or otherwise. The classic work on this subject is *The Earth as Transformed by Human Action* by W. C. Clark and colleagues (1990), which focuses on anthropomorphic changes to the Earth and its atmosphere. For example, the bulk of existing scientific evidence shows that global warming of recent decades is the result of human activity such as the burning of fossil fuels and deforestation (United Nations Environment Program, 2001).

For the purposes of this chapter, the term "globalization" refers to human-induced rather than naturally occurring change. Globalization is driven, foremost, by the individual or collective actions of human beings—the formation of larger social groupings (e.g., megacities); the more frequent and farther-reaching mobility of populations; the adoption of larger-scale production and consumption patterns; the intensified use (and, increasingly overuse) of natural resources; the development and application of new technologies, knowledge, and ideas; and so on.

Some writers describe globalization as driven foremost by technology. It is assumed that communication and transportation technologies, in particular, are enabling people to travel the world more readily, interact with one another across vast distances, and carry out many forms of interaction that circumvent territorial boundaries. Hence, the advent of undersea cables, satellite communications, and the Internet, for instance, allows us to carry out financial transactions, information gathering and dissemination, and social interactions more quickly, cheaply and across greater distances (Hundley, Anderson, Bikson, & Neu, 2003). The availability of low-cost airlines, bullet trains, and automobiles allows millions of people to travel farther, faster, and more frequently. As Lawrence Summers, former Secretary of the U.S. Department of Treasury, stated, "Transportation is the industry that connects other industries . . . it is the key to globalization" (quoted in U.S. Department of Transportation, 2000).

Others argue that the key drivers of globalization are largely economic. Fukuyama (1992), for example, sees the emergence of a global economy as reflecting the ultimate triumph of capitalism over socialism. Liberal capitalism is described as "the final form of human government." Fukuyama believes that no viable alternative to capitalism is possible and that we have reached the "end of history" as far as ideological development is concerned. It is this assumed economic logic of globalization that lies behind arguments favoring the further unleashing of globalization forces in the form of policies favoring trade liberalization, privatization, deregulation, and foreign direct investment. This perspective argues that all countries must embrace the inevitable and progressive march of globalization, defined in this way, or be left on the economic sidelines (International Chamber of Commerce, 1997). The stark social and environmental effects of economic globalization, in part created by large-scale global financial crises, along with the dramatic shift in power to emerging economies such as China, India, and Brazil, suggest that global economic change continues apace.

Although technology and economics are certainly important drivers of globalization, it does not necessarily follow that globalization is somehow inevitable, singular, and rational in its current forms. Given that it comprises a set of change processes driven by human actions, it is vital to recognize that normative-based interests are embedded within current forms of globalization. Contemporary globalization is a manifestation of the vested interests of powerful individuals and groups who stand to benefit from it. This relationships suggests that not only is globalization within human capacity to shape and direct, but also that if the adverse social and environmental consequences resulting from globalization are to be minimized or at least shared fairly, it is imperative that these change processes be actively managed.

Effects of Globalization: Positive Versus Negative

This point brings us to the final issue of major debate on globalization—whether the resultant changes are having positive or negative impacts on human societies and the natural world. As described previously, globalization is having diverse effects on a wide range of social spheres, including the economic, political, cultural, technological, and environmental realms. These effects are creating both positive and negative impacts. Individually, each of us gains and loses from specific aspects of globalization. The Information Revolution has given us 24-hour access to news, entertainment, and personal messages, but at the expense of our ability to switch off and enjoy down time. The globalization of the food industry has potentially diversified our diets by, for example, offering access to fresh fruits and vegetables throughout the year. Yet the global spread of more intense farming methods, the transport of more and more products worldwide, and greater dependency on food imports are creating new risks.

It is also important to recognize that the distribution of these gains and losses varies considerably across population groups. For the relatively wealthy, educated, gainfully employed, literate (including computer literate), and mobile, globalization offers exciting opportunities for personal growth and material gain. The availability of an ever-expanding variety of goods and services, declining prices for many of these products due to economies of scale, the ability to retrieve information anytime from all corners of the globe, and the possibility of traveling abroad for business or pleasure are attractive benefits from globalization to which many aspire.

In contrast, for the relatively disadvantaged in terms of socioeconomic status, education, geographical location, race, and gender, the net balance between gains and losses from globalization can tip more toward the negative. As well as being less able to enjoy its benefits, they shoulder a relatively heavier burden of its costs. Lower wages, greater insecurity of employment, poorer housing and sanitation due to rapid urbanization, and greater vulnerability to environmental degradation define the experiences of globalization by the world's poor across all countries. As well as failing to realize the promised "trickle-down" effects of globalization, the globally disadvantaged may very likely remain so given how current forms of globalization may be stacked in favor of some at the expense of others.

A good example is the current cost of food. Between 2006 and 2008, the cost of food increased by 57%, prompting social unrest among the poor in approximately 33 low- and middle-income countries as people struggled to buy basic foods. Several factors have been identified as contributing to the sharp increase in food prices, including the devaluation of the U.S. dollar, higher oil prices, and new demand among wealthier citizens in emerging economies for grains, cereals, and meat. Another key factor has been growing demand for biofuels as an alternative energy source (Food and Agriculture Organization [FAO], 2009). This new industry, which comprises large corporations based primarily in the United States, Brazil, and the European Union, is supported by hefty government subsidies to produce ethanol. This development, in turn, is contributing to food shortages (and correspondingly higher prices) as surplus food crops are purchased for ethanol production and farmers are encouraged to convert their land from production of food crops to ethanol-producing crops (Tenenbaum, 2008).

Another structural inequity of contemporary globalization is the flow of development aid. Few countries have lived up to the agreed commitment to give 0.7% of their gross national income (GNI) as official development assistance (ODA). After a decade of declining aid levels, aid volume rose by 11% during 2002–2003 following the UN Financing for Development Summit held in Monterrey (Manning, 2004), which elicited widespread support for achieving the Millennium Development Goals (MDGs) by 2015 (see Chapter 17, Exhibit 17-8). Nonetheless, funding of the MDGs has been woefully inadequate

(Lee, Walt, & Haines, 2004). Although further commitments were made at the 2005 G8 Gleneagles Summit to increase aid (Fratianni, Kirton, & Savona, 2007), it is now estimated that a further 55 to 90 million more people will remain in extreme poverty (defined as people living on less than $1.25 per day) as a consequence of the 2008 global financial crisis and high-income countries attempting to reduce public expenditure (United Nations Development Program [UNDP], 2009).

The distribution of wealth through globalization has produced widening gaps not only between rich and poor countries, but also between rich and poor people within countries. Over the past two centuries, wealthier regions of the world led economic development, with massive inequalities emerging both between regions and between individual countries. By and large, however, income inequality within countries remained relatively stable, or was observed to decline as a middle class emerged. In the last 60 years, however, the situation has changed considerably, with countries such as China and India experiencing much more rapid economic growth than many Western countries historically. This trend, in turn, has changed the nature of global income inequality, with what appears to be a progressive equalization of wealth between regions and countries, but rising income inequality within countries (Firebaugh, 2003).

Alongside economic inequalities, health inequalities appear to be growing within and across countries as well. These trends are often more difficult to observe because of the aggregated nature of available data. Nonetheless, some evidence suggests that globalization is creating new patterns of health inequalities that do not conform to nationally defined populations. Many lower-income countries now have emerging upper and middle classes whose living conditions are increasingly similar to those in more affluent countries, yet who reside alongside large populations who remain deeply impoverished. Thus new patterns of winners and losers, in terms of the global distribution of health and ill health across countries, are emerging:

- Increased impoverishment among the globally disadvantaged has been accompanied by increased world hunger, with an estimated 1.02 billion people now undernourished. Most people suffering from hunger live in Asia (642 million) and sub-Saharan Africa (265 million). There are also 15 million undernourished people now living in high-income countries—a 50% increase since 2003 (FAO, 2009).

- A rising incidence of type 2 diabetes mellitus has been reported in children and adolescents in countries as diverse as the United States, Japan, Hong Kong, Singapore, Bangladesh, and Libya, among others. Until recently, most children with diabetes had type 1 disease. The rise in type 2 disease is associated with the increase in childhood obesity, which is linked in turn to the globalization of more sedentary lifestyles and diets containing a high fat, sugar, and salt content (O'Dea & Piers, 2002).

- The increased concentration of ownership in the tobacco industry, and the spread of the industry globally into so-called emerging markets, is expected to lead to a sharp rise in tobacco-related deaths. Today tobacco kills 5.4 million people annually, a figure expected to rise to 10 million by 2030, 70 percent of deaths to occur in the developing world (World Health Organization [WHO], 2008).

It is these sorts of global health inequalities, and a conviction that improved health conditions are a prerequisite for improved economic performance, that prompted the formation of the WHO Commission on Macroeconomics and Health in 2000 to investigate "how concrete health interventions can lead to economic growth and reduce inequity in developing countries." Among its tasks was to recommend "a set of measures designed to maximize the poverty reduction and economic benefits of health sector investment" (WHO, 2000).

Within the context just described, it is important to understand how globalization is affecting the broad determinants of health. As defined by Dahlgren and Whitehead (1991), health can be influenced by a broad range of factors (see Chapter 3, Figure 3-1). As discussed in this chapter, for example, a growing body of evidence indicates that human-induced changes to the world's climate (global warming) are affecting the distribution and epidemiology of diseases such as malaria and dengue fever. Similarly, the intensified competition for foreign direct investment within a globalizing economy is believed to be leading to pressures not to adopt necessary health and safety standards in the workplace. Liberalized trade in food and drink, as well as tobacco products, may be leading to lifestyle changes that will increase populations' risk of many chronic diseases. What will be critical for the public health community to understand better, if these practitioners are to address the existing health gaps and prevent globalization from widening them further, is how these diverse changes are influencing each type of determinant.

Globalization: A Summary

In summary, the shift from international to global health can be defined in the following ways:

- Globalization must be understood within a historical context over centuries, with contemporary forms of globalization distinguished by the intensity of cross-border (and in some cases transborder) activities taking place and the geographic extent of their reach.

- A strict definition of globalization focuses on the transcendence of geography, whereas looser definitions often use the term to describe related phenomena such as liberalization, Westernization, and universalization.

- Globalization is affecting a broad range of social spheres.

- Globalization is affecting different individuals and population groups in diverse ways.

- Contemporary forms of globalization appear to be worsening inequalities in health for certain individuals and population groups.

- The capacity to address these inequalities effectively requires that we understand globalization in relation to the broad determinants of health.

The Global Dimensions of Infectious Disease

The Risks from Infectious Diseases in a Globalizing World

Globalization has the potential to affect a broad range of biological, environmental, and social factors that influence human infections. Indeed, the implications of globalization on infectious diseases have received considerable attention in recent years. Most importantly, the interaction between human populations and pathogens must be seen in evolutionary terms, within a long history of the development, adaptation, and interaction of human societies. As human societies have formed and interacted with local environments and with other human societies, patterns of infection have evolved accordingly. Agrarian societies, for instance, where populations live in close proximity to domesticated animals, demonstrate a greater susceptibility to zoonotic infections. In contrast, urbanization, which is characterized by larger numbers of people living in relatively close proximity, demonstrates greater susceptibility to so-called crowd diseases, including infections spread by close human contact (e.g. plague, influenza). Greater mobility of individuals within and between societies raises the risk of infections spreading farther afield (e.g. SARS).

In this context, we can see how globalization might influence patterns of population mobility and, in turn, the susceptibility of specific populations to certain infections. A good example is the association of meningococcal disease with the centuries-old pilgrimage of Muslims to Mecca (in Saudi Arabia), known as the Hajj. Over the past 50 years, the scale of this annual event has grown markedly, with a 100% increase in numbers of pilgrims every decade since 1949. In 2009, an estimated 3 million people from more than 160 countries participated in the event, with the bulk of travelers coming from abroad. This growth has been supported by the expansion of facilities at the site, greater wealth among potential travelers, and increased accessibility of transportation (97% travel by air). Because the event brings ever larger numbers of people together from more widely dispersed communities, who then interact in close proximity and subsequently disburse again, the setting poses an opportunity for the global spread of infectious disease. The most well-known health consequence is regular epidemics of meningococcal disease that occur during and after the event. Cases linked to the pilgrimage have been reported in most parts of the world, with secondary epidemics occurring as long as 2 years later in destination countries (Saker, Lee, Cannito, Gilmore, & Campbell-Lendrum, 2004). Universal availability and mandatory use of quadrivalent conjugate meningococcal vaccine by all pilgrims appears to be successfully reducing the risk of such outbreaks (Borrow, 2009). In 2009, the Hajj took place during the H1N1 influenza pandemic which prompted Arab health officials to adopt travel warnings for high-risk groups and consider other restrictions (Al Jazeera, 2009).

Another association between globalization and infectious disease is the impact of global change (see Chapter 10) not only on the natural world, but also on built and social environments. The natural environment can be modified by local influences, such as pollution and growth of human settlements, as well as global-scale forces, such as changes in the world's biophysical systems that alter the climate. Environmental changes can either be natural or human induced, and all can play an important role in shaping human health (Saker et al., 2004).

A growing body of evidence has linked global climate change and the epidemiology of infectious diseases such as malaria, yellow fever, and dengue fever. Current concerns about climate change focus on rising global average land and sea surface temperatures (global warming) and the increasing frequency of extreme weather conditions in many parts of the world. There is now substantial evidence that average temperatures have risen by 0.6°C since the mid-nineteenth century, with most of this change occurring since 1976. The UN Intergovernmental Panel on Climate Change (IPCC) predicts that average global temperatures will rise by 1.8 to 4°C by 2100. Although the causes of this phenomenon remain the source of some controversy, the IPCC concludes that much of the global warming during the last 50 years can be attributed to human activity (IPCC, 2007).

Detecting the influence of observed and predicted changes in global climate on infectious disease transmission is not straightforward. An irrefutable case would require standardized monitoring of exposure (climate), the outcome (incidence of a particular infectious disease), and other determinants of disease (e.g., immunity, treatment, socioeconomic factors) over many years. Such data sets are rare. Nonetheless, best estimates of the likely current and future impacts of climate change come from theoretical consideration of the known effects of climate on disease transmission, and from indirect assessment based on the reported effects of climate on infectious diseases in the present or recent past. This information tells us that, in general, climate constrains the range of infectious disease, whereas weather affects the timing and intensity of outbreaks (Dobson & Carper, 1993). Higher ambient air temperatures, along with changes in precipitation and humidity, appear to affect the biology and ecology of certain disease vectors and intermediate hosts, the pathogens they transmit, and consequently the risk of transmission (Githeko, Lindsay, Confalonieri, & Patz, 2000).

Diseases carried by mosquitoes are especially sensitive to meteorological conditions because these insects have fastidious temperature thresholds for survival and are extremely vulnerable to changes in average ambient temperature (Epstein, 2001). Available evidence suggests that in parts of the United States, for example, small outbreaks of locally transmitted malaria have occurred during unseasonably hot weather spells. Malaria is now prevalent in elevated regions where it did not previously exist, such as in the rural highlands of Papua New Guinea (Githeko et al., 2000). Climate change may also be a factor contributing over the past 30 years to the dramatic advance of dengue fever, a disease of the tropics transmitted by the *Aedes aegypti* mosquito. In Mexico, higher median temperatures during the rainy season were found to be a strong predictor of dengue prevalence, while in the South Pacific region, outbreaks of dengue from 1970 to 1995 on the fringe of the endemic zone correlated with El Niño events (Hales, de Wet, Maindonald, & Woodward, 2002). Similarly, the first appearance of West Nile virus in the United States (which subsequently spread to Canada and, more recently, to southern Europe) is believed to be a consequence of mosquito proliferation following extreme summer drought conditions in the New York area (Githeko et al., 2000).

Although the increased risk from acute and "exotic" diseases and climate change are clearly worrying developments in terms of health impact, they are dwarfed by the challenge posed by the global spread of tuberculosis (TB). *Mycobacterium tuberculosis* has been present in the human population since antiquity, but it was not until 1944 that effective treatments (beginning with streptomycin) were developed. This discovery was followed by the development of a rapid succession of anti-TB drugs, leading public health experts to predict the long-awaited end to this ancient scourge.

In an age of globalization, however, we face a very different scenario. Today, one-third of the world's population is infected with TB, and the disease caused approximately 1.6 million deaths in 2005. Today the largest number of deaths occurs in Southeast Asia, but the highest mortality per capita is in Africa, where the HIV/AIDS pandemic has been associated with rapid increases in the incidence of TB. Transmission of TB across borders has increased as a result of population mobility, inadequate healthcare delivery, and ineffective coordination of control strategies. For example, between 1990 and 2008, TB cases reported in the United States declined from 25,701 to 12,904. However, the proportion of cases occurring among foreign-born persons rose from 24% to 59%, of which most originated from Mexico and Central America. In 2008, Mexico was the country of origin for 23% of all foreign-born persons with TB in the United States (Centers for Disease Control and Prevention [CDC], 2009).

Of particular concern is the spread of drug-resistant forms of TB, which have arisen from the incorrect or incomplete use of existing regimens (see Chapter 5). Drug-resistant TB is now found in all regions of the world. The prevalence of multidrug-resistant TB (MDR-TB) is especially high in the former Soviet Union, China, Ecuador, and Israel. As of 2009, India had the world's highest incidence of MDR-TB, with 25.7% of all TB cases in that country involving the drug-resistant pathogen (WHO, 2009c). As Mario Raviglione, director of WHO's Stop TB Department, states, "It is in the interest of

every country to support rapid scale-up of TB control if we are to overcome MDR-TB. Passport control will not halt drug resistance; investment in global TB prevention will" (quoted in WHO, 2004a).

Perhaps the most serious infectious disease threat of all, in an era of intensifying globalization, comes from "democratic" infections that are relatively indiscriminate in the populations they can infect. The common cold, for example, is probably the most widespread illness experienced by humans. Caused by more than 200 different viruses (notably rhinoviruses) and readily transmitted by air and close contact, colds affect adults with an average two to four episodes annually. Fortunately, colds are usually mild and rarely life threatening. The prospect of an infection emerging with the transmissibility of a cold but with more lethal consequences is the public health community's worst-case scenario. It was fears of this scenario that spurred the global response to the SARS outbreak of 2002–2003 (Exhibit 18-1).

Although the number of SARS cases and deaths was eventually less than feared, the experience focused attention on the likely capacity of public health systems to cope with the anticipated pandemic to come with the next major shift in the influenza A virus, which at the time of writing last occurred in April 2009 with the emergence of the H1N1 pandemic. Minor changes to the influenza virus (antigenic drift) happen continually over time, which explains its ability to reinfect populations. The change is usually so minimal that the previous year's influenza or vaccine offers some protection. Occasionally (every 10 to 12 years or so), there is an abrupt, major change in the virus (antigenic shift) against which most people have little or no protection. The H1N1 pandemic has, to date, been relatively mild, with fewer deaths on average compared to seasonal epidemics of influenza. By comparison, the Spanish influenza pandemic of 1918–1919 killed an estimated 40 million people worldwide. Influenza A viruses are found in many different animals, including ducks, chickens, pigs, whales, horses, and seals. Although it is unusual for people to contract influenza infections directly from animals, sporadic human infections and outbreaks caused by certain avian influenza A viruses have been reported.

The danger arising from an antigenic shift in the influenza virus is magnified by globalization. In East Asia, where new strains of influenza more frequently originate, population pressures combined with intense farming methods and close contact with domesticated animals may increase the likelihood of mutations emerging. Once the virus emerges, population mobility means that the outbreak is likely to

| Exhibit 18-1 | The Global Warning from Severe Acute Respiratory Syndrome |

The outbreak of severe acute respiratory syndrome (SARS) in 2002–2003 demonstrated how a globalizing world can be more vulnerable to infectious disease. SARS is a respiratory illness caused by a previously unknown type of coronavirus (SARS-CoV). Normally, coronaviruses cause mild to moderate upper respiratory symptoms. People with SARS develop a high fever (greater than 38°C), cough, shortness of breath, difficulty breathing, and other, more severe symptoms. Some develop severe pneumonia or respiratory failure that can be fatal. Between November 1, 2002, and July 31, 2003, there were 8,096 cumulative cases of SARS and 774 deaths in 27 countries (WHO, 2004b).

Although the eventual disease burden from SARS proved to be relatively low (by comparison, influenza causes 250,000 to 500,000 deaths each year worldwide), the outbreak was seen as an important lesson concerning the global management of such a public health emergency. The outbreak was described as unprecedented in the speed and extent of its global spread. Its airborne transmission, the lack of diagnostic technologies, the absence of an effective vaccine, and, perhaps most importantly, the disease's rapid spread via a globally mobile population made it "the first infectious disease epidemic since HIV/AIDS to pose a truly global threat" (Fidler, 2004). As described in a report by the University of Toronto, "In the Middle Ages, it took three years for the plague to spread from Asia to the western reaches of Europe. The SARS virus crossed from Hong Kong to Toronto in about 15 hours" (Joint Centre for Bioethics, 2003). It is believed that air travelers eventually spread SARS to 16 countries (Bonn, 2003).

The economic cost of the outbreak was estimated at between $30 billion and $100 billion (Smith & Sommers, 2003). These costs were distributed across a wide range of countries, illustrating the vulnerability of a globalizing economy to public health emergencies of international concern. Had the outbreak been more serious, or another outbreak occurs, the economic impact on the global economy would likely be even more substantial. As described in a report by the U.S. National Intelligence Council, "an outbreak of SARS in major trade centers again would be likely to have significant economic and political implications. . . . global trade and investment flows could seize up if quarantines shut down factories and shipments" (Monaghan, 2003). As such, the outbreak demonstrates the shared interest by all countries in ensuring effective management of such emergencies.

SARS served as an important opportunity to test existing systems of international health cooperation. The initial refusal by the Chinese government to report cases confirmed inherent weaknesses in the International Health Regulations, which required member states to report on only three diseases (yellow fever, plague, and cholera). WHO thus lacks the formal authority to command information that is potentially vital to the world's health, and action comes down to the willingness of the Director-General to challenge the mettle of sovereign states.

Once the outbreak was confirmed, the international community began to mobilize. Within two weeks of the Hong Kong outbreak, on March 12, 2003, WHO declared SARS to be a global health emergency. On March 17, the WHO collaborative multicenter research project on SARS diagnosis was established to identify the causative agent and develop a diagnostic test.

For many public health practitioners, WHO's handling of the SARS outbreak reaffirmed the organization's vital and unique role in global health. No other organization had the legitimacy to pull together the international health community. At the same time, the outbreak highlighted the inherent weaknesses in the International Health Regulations as well as the national public health systems of affected countries. SARS also demonstrated how infectious diseases can provoke public fears, fueled both by the unknown nature of the disease and by the mass media. Fortunately, SARS proved less serious than anticipated, providing a timely opportunity for the global public health community to prepare itself for the next emergency outbreak.

spread worldwide with great speed. After World War I, influenza spread globally within a month, facilitated by large-scale movements of civilians and armed forces. With the advent of modern transport systems, a new strain of influenza can reach anywhere in the world in a matter of hours, as the 2009 H1N1 pandemic demonstrated.

Enhancing Global Governance for Communicable Disease Prevention, Control, and Treatment

Of foremost importance to enabling the public health community to detect and respond to a communicable disease outbreak are epidemiologic and clinical data.

The challenges posed by globalization have reinvigorated efforts to strengthen how the global public health community might respond to infectious disease outbreaks. The historical underpinning for international cooperation on infectious disease control is the International Health Regulations (IHR). As mentioned earlier, this legislative framework has its origins in the International Sanitary Conferences of the nineteenth century, but the more formal version of the treaty was first ratified in 1951 by the 4th World Health Assembly (WHA). Between 1951 and 1981, the guidelines underwent a series of revisions, not only resulting in a name change (from "International Sanitary Regulations" to "IHR"), but also reducing their scope to cover only three diseases—cholera, plague, and yellow fever. Yet while countries were obliged to report outbreaks of these diseases, compliance remained poor due to the economic consequences that often accompanied notification of disease outbreaks. In short, the framework lacked both the means and the incentives to encourage greater collaboration (WHO, 2002).

In 1995, the WHA authorized the WHO Director-General to substantially revise and update the IHR in the wake of concerns about the impact of globalization on human health. A series of disease outbreaks ranging from cholera in Latin America (1991), to plague in India (1994), to Ebola virus in Zaire (1995) added to new concerns following the discovery of the former Soviet Union's biological weapons program (1991) and a bioterrorist attack on a Tokyo subway (1994). At the time of the 2003 SARS outbreak, the IHR revision process remained incomplete, and the event served as a catalyst, lending much needed political impetus to develop a new framework. In 2004, an intergovernmental working group was convened to finalize the revision process. The revised IHR was subsequently completed and endorsed by the WHA in 2005, and the new treaty entered into force in June 2007.

Under the revised IHR, countries are obligated to report any adverse health event that has the potential to spread beyond their borders (referred to as a "public health emergency of international concern" [PHEIC]). This requirement includes not only infectious disease outbreaks, but other threats to human health as well. To avoid replicating the compliance problems in reporting, the revised IHR permits WHO to be notified about PHEICs from both government and nongovernmental sources (Table 18-1). In addition, whereas the previous framework mainly emphasized the need to bolster border surveillance (to prevent the importation of disease), the new framework requires countries to strengthen their health systems so that they can detect, verify, and respond to health events before they threaten other countries.

Yet while the scope of the revised IHR has been expanded considerably, and the new version represents a marked improvement over the former regulations, weaknesses within the system persist, some of which were highlighted by the 2009 H1N1 pandemic. For example, one of the core problems under the former system was the ability of member states to impose trade and travel restrictions against countries experiencing disease outbreaks to an extent that might be excessive and even adversely harmful to affected economies. Although the revised IHR was ideally meant to address this challenge, in practice countries still can, and do, take such measures. In 2009, for instance, several countries banned live pig and pork

Table 18-1	Broadening Data Sources for Communicable Disease Surveillance
National	U.S. Centers for Disease Control and Prevention Pasteur Institutes, Sentiweb UK Public Health Laboratory Service Health Canada WHO country offices
Regional	WHO regional offices European Community (EC) Rapid Alert System for Non-food Products (RAPEX) European Network for Diagnostics of "Imported" Viral Diseases (ENIVD) Pacific Public Health Surveillance Network (PACNET)
International	WHO UN Global Program on HIV/AIDS UN High Commissioner for Refugees UN Development Program UN Children's Fund
Global	Global Public Health Intelligence Network (GPHIN–Health Canada) PROMED (Federation of American Scientists) TravelMed Red Cross/Red Crescent Médicins Sans Frontières (MSF) Merlin International Rescue Committee

meat imports despite the absence of scientific evidence that humans could contract the H1N1 ("swine flu") virus from eating or working with pigs (WHO, 2009b). As such, no system of governance currently exists to regulate the economic impact on countries of disease outbreaks, and countries continue to suffer losses disproportionate to the actual health risk posed.

To summarize, human populations and infectious diseases have historically coexisted and coevolved over time, and it may be tempting to overplay the threat from infectious diseases being created by globalization. This unwarranted suspicion can result in the stigmatization of certain population groups (e.g., migrant populations, ethnic minorities) and the skewing of resources and policy priorities. Nonetheless, changes in global patterns of human settlement and interaction among human societies have led to corresponding changes in infectious disease susceptibility. It is necessary, in this context, to ask how contemporary forms of globalization are changing the epidemiology of some infectious diseases, and how corresponding adaptation by human societies is needed to protect and promote human health.

The Globalization of Chronic Diseases

Chapter 7 highlights the impact of chronic diseases and risks on health and economies. As mentioned in that chapter, important processes of globalization—trade, foreign investment, marketing, and technological change—have implications for the spread and alleviation of chronic diseases. These issues are expanded upon in this section.

Trade Liberalization and Chronic Diseases

Tobacco, alcohol, and food products are being produced and marketed on an unprecedented scale by transnational corporations (TNCs) seeking to increase their economies of scale and, therefore, their profits through expansion into new markets across the world. In the case of tobacco, trade liberalization has facilitated a shift in market share, from traditional markets to emerging markets in Asia, Latin America, the Middle East, and the former Soviet Union. Most overtly, the United States used bilateral trade relations in the late 1980s to exert pressure on countries such as Thailand, Taiwan, and South Korea to open up their domestic markets to cigarette imports. The Uruguay Round of the GATT, which concluded in 1994, liberalized trade in unmanufactured tobacco.

Since 1995, multilateral trade agreements under the WTO have significantly reduced tariff and nontariff barriers to tobacco trade (Bettcher et al., 2003). In addition, pressure has been exerted by tobacco manufacturers' home countries to include tobacco in negotiations to liberalize the agricultural sector, and industry objections have squelched stronger tobacco control measures under the terms of trade agreements (Peterson, 2010). This has resulted in increased and more competitive tobacco trade between countries, leading to increased supply, more extensive marketing, and lower prices.

More research is needed to understand the implications of changing trends in food production for chronic diseases. For example, the trade of oilseeds and corn for livestock feed may be associated with the dramatic increase of livestock production in many low- and middle-income countries and associated rise in meat consumption. Another trend that may have implications for dietary patterns is the increased trade of high-value processed agricultural products (e.g., meats, dairy products, frozen foods). Exports of these products from the United States are growing faster than any other category of agricultural exports (Bolling, 1998; Whitton, 2004). The global health implications of increased marketing of processed and fast foods are discussed later in this chapter.

The Impact of Foreign Direct Investment

Foreign direct investment (FDI) has played an unprecedented role in recent decades as a source of capital for economic growth and development. FDI is an investment by an enterprise from one country into an entity or affiliate in another, in which the parent firm owns a substantial but not necessarily majority interest. The foreign enterprise becomes an affiliate of the parent company, thereby creating or joining a TNC. FDI is one of the mechanisms through which TNCs enter new markets, and it reflects an intention to remain invested over the long term.

Over the past 25 years FDI has risen dramatically, largely among high-income countries. Since the 1990s, however, emerging markets in low and middle-income countries have attracted substantial FDI. In 2002, $162 billion of foreign money flowed into the low- and middle-income world, mainly from TNCs based in high-income countries (United Nations Conference on Trade and Development, 2003). The global economic and financial crisis of the late 2000s saw a sharp decline in FDI worldwide, from more than $2 trillion in 2007 to less than $1 trillion in 2009. Importantly, this decline has been less marked in emerging economies, which, for the first time, have attracted more FDI than high-income countries (UN Conference on Trade and Development, 2009).

These trends in FDI can have important implications for the globalization of chronic diseases where it represents a strong investment in tobacco, unhealthy food, and alcohol products, especially in emerging markets where there is the most potential for growth in consumption. The privatization of national industries can offer further opportunities for FDI, notably where such products can be more expensive to produce abroad and transport, which in turn encourages their local production by subsidiaries or licensed manufacturers (Bolling, 2002; Walkenhorst, 2001). Finally, regional trade agreements can create incentives for TNCs to relocate within trade-partner areas to take advantage of more favorable tariff rates.

Evidence suggests several trends in FDI warrant closer scrutiny in relation to chronic diseases (Exhibit 18-2). For example, 10 of the 100 largest TNCs (ranked by foreign assets) manufacture tobacco, food, or alcohol, as do a high proportion of the largest affiliates of foreign TNCs in emerging economies. The substantial FDI by these companies can bring much-needed capital, skills, technology, and goods and services to the local market, encouraging host countries to liberalize investment rules and other incentives to attract FDI (Organization for Economic Cooperation and Development [OECD], 2000). At the same time, such regimes can preclude the introduction of regulations or standards intended to protect public health interests. For example, the desire to attract FDI may bring with it pressures for lower tax rates, thereby re-

---

Exhibit 18-2	The Food Industry, Foreign Direct Investment, and Chronic Disease Risks

Foreign direct investment has so far been overlooked as an important driver of the diet transition. FDI into food processing, service, and retail has become particularly significant since the mid-1980s. Food companies, based mainly (but not exclusively) in Western Europe and the United States, have a significant international presence.* By 2001, 12 transnational food companies (TFCs) were among the top 100 holders of foreign assets globally, double the number in 1990. The foreign assets of these companies amounted to $257.7 billion in 2002, an enormous increase (658%) from $34 billion in 1990. During the same period, foreign sales increased from $88.8 trillion to $234.1 billion (164%) (Hawkes, 2004b). By 2007, global sales in packaged foods were estimated to have reached $1.3 trillion, and the top 10 companies accounted for 35% of the revenue (ETC Group, 2008). A high proportion of foreign assets and sales are in high-income countries, but foreign affiliates of TFCs are frequently among the largest companies in the tertiary sector in the low- and middle-income world. This factor has contributed to a "nutrition transition" in terms of food availability and consumption patterns, as diets based on local staples have given way to nutritional regimes that contain higher levels of fats, animal products, and sweeteners (Thow & Hawkes, 2009).

Globally, food processing is the most important recipient of FDI relative to other parts of the food system, including the farm sector. American FDI into foreign food processing companies grew from $9 billion in 1980 to $36 billion in 2000, and between 2000 and 2006 U.S. FDI in food processing virtually doubled to $67 billion (Hawkes & Murphy, 2010). As FDI has increased, the allocation of investment has shifted toward highly processed foods for sale in the host market, and away from products for export to the home market and those produced by primary processing (although these items may remain important in certain cases). The tendency to allocate investment into highly processed foods is illustrated by the economies of Central and Eastern Europe, and the Baltic states, which attracted soaring rates of FDI in the food sector in the 1990s. Such investment largely concentrated on soft drinks and confectionery. The confectionery sector in Poland, for example, attracted FDI of $963 million between 1990 and 1999—more than the FDI in meat, fish, flour, pasta, bread, sugar, potato products, fruits, vegetables, vegetable oils, and fats put together (Hawkes, 2004b). By 2003, FDI in Poland's food processing industry had reached around $3.4 billion and by 2006 it had almost doubled to $6.6 billion (Jansik, 2009). On a global scale, this trend has led to the dominance of foreign investors in the highly processed food sector. In China and Mexico, foreign investors dominate packaged foods, such as instant noodles, soft drinks, snacks, sweet biscuits, and fast foods.

Processed food sales in low- and middle-income countries are lower than those in high-income countries (one-fourth or less of all food expenditures compared with almost half). Yet wider availability, lower prices, and new purchasing channels are driving rapid sales growth. The annual sales growth for processed foods is approximately 29% in low-middle-income countries, compared with 7% in upper-middle-income countries. The market for highly processed foods is expanding fast, and TFCs clearly perceive that their best chances for sales growth lie in low- and middle-income countries. Vietnam, China, and Indonesia are expected to be the fastest-growing markets for packaged food retail sales over the coming years, with growth rates forecasted at 11%, 10%, and 8%, respectively. Korea, Thailand, India, and the Philippines rank among the top 10 fastest-growing markets, with total packaged food retail sales expected to grow 5% to 7% annually (Hawkes, 2004b). It is still not clear how the consumption of highly processed foods has affected the diets and nutrition of different households and individuals, but it is likely to fuel increases in diet-related chronic diseases unless effective policies are implemented.

Two potential approaches to influence FDI and redirect the diet transition toward better health have been proposed. One would be to impose health-oriented conditions on FDI by TFCs. These policy options (and others) are contained in the

continues

Exhibit 18-2	continued

WHO Global Strategy on Diet, Physical Activity and Health, and many countries have the structures in place to implement them. Through its position upstream, FDI would be a single entry point at which to implement a multiple range of public health policies.

A second option would be to look directly to TFCs for a solution. An alternative to the regulatory option might be to encourage TFCs to invest in healthier products, such as less salty snacks and baked goods and more low-fat products, nutrient-rich foods, or even foods with functional benefits. At the same time, this approach would ensure that TFCs do not market unhealthy products and lifestyles to children.

These two different approaches reflect one of the fundamental tensions in policy development today: how to balance the role of government and transnational corporations. A mixed approach will probably evolve over time.

*Here the term "food company" refers to a company that is involved in the processing, service, or sale of highly processed food. It includes diversified companies that manufacture, serve, or sell products other than food, such as personal care products or tobacco. It excludes companies concerned solely with agricultural production, processing, or research.

moving a significant barrier in discouraging tobacco consumption. In the food sector, TNCs may exert pressure on government agencies to minimize labeling requirements or nutritional standards, or to soften restrictions on marketing and advertising such as to children. Such negotiations are often conducted between TNCs and ministries of trade and finance with minimal public health input, despite the fact that they have obvious public health consequences.

Gilmore and McKee (2004) offer a case study of how British American Tobacco and Philip Morris—the world's two largest transnational tobacco companies—are among the largest foreign investors in Russia and Moldova. Given their importance as source of new investment, these companies have been able to negotiate advantageous conditions that benefit their businesses, such as tax breaks, exemption from monopoly regulation, and even a role in drafting health legislation. The International Monetary Fund (IMF) has traditionally supported the privatization of state-owned enterprises in emerging markets, including the tobacco industry. Although this position may make sense from a macroeconomic perspective, it ignores the impact that privatization without appropriate government regulation and tax policies can have on a major risk factor in health. Importantly, if the IMF were to draw on the World Bank's more recent policy prescriptions for tobacco control, and support governments prior to privatization, macroeconomic and health goals could be met together.

The Globalization of Marketing, Advertising, and Promotion

The increasingly global pattern of consumption for certain goods and services has been facilitated, in large part, by marketing, advertising, and promotion campaigns. These activities, in the form of brand names, imagery, logos, and messages, seek to influence consumer behavior.

TNCs invest heavily in marketing, advertising, and promotion of their products, in the process creating a growing number of regional and global brands to be sold in diverse local settings. From a public health perspective, evidence suggests such activities have been effectively used to increase the consumption of tobacco, alcohol, and unhealthy food products (Babor, 2003; Jackson, Hastings, Wheeler, Eadie, & Mackintosh, 2002). In low- and middle-income countries, regulation of such activities can often be relatively weak, enabling TNCs to target selected population groups, such as the poorly educated, children, women, or young adults, who represent promising targets for market growth but can be particularly vulnerable to commercial claims (Hawkes, 2002, 2004a). In Asian countries, for example, tobacco companies use glamorous images to advertise "light" and "mild" cigarettes specifically to young adults—notably, girls and women (Lee, Carpenter, Challa, Lee, Connelly, & Koh, 2009; Mackay & Eriksen, 2002). Similarly, some food companies attempt to increase "stomach share" in the low- and middle-income world through campaigns aimed at children. Where high-calorie products are involved, such efforts are believed to be contributing to rising levels of obesity by adversely influencing the "human energy equation" (Witkowski, 2007).

Globalization, Politics, and Chronic Disease Prevention

In recent years, greater efforts have been made to address global influences on chronic diseases through collective action across countries. The experiences of developing the Framework Convention on Tobacco Control (FCTC) and the Global Strategy on Diet and Physical Activity and Health provide valuable lessons for public health.

From an economic perspective, both tobacco and sugar have been regarded as highly valuable export commodities. Both have been highly subsidized and protected, and seen as a source of export earnings. When evidence that they could be of harm to health first appeared, the response by producers and manufacturers was similar: consistent denial of the evidence, creation of front groups to oppose public health action, and intense and sustained lobbying of policy makers to thwart stronger regulation at the national and international levels.

As evidence of the public health harms of tobacco use and poor diet accumulated, two different approaches were taken by governments, in large part influenced by the intensity of industry pressure and the degree of acceptance by the public of the need for government intervention. Nordic countries, supported by Canada, have argued that for "healthy choices to be the easy choices," social, environmental, and commercial influences on health need to be addressed through government regulation, fiscal policy, and intersectoral action, combined with health education. In contrast, the United States has given primacy to the importance of individual responsibility and, therefore, health education. Generally, industry has supported the U.S. approach, whereas many nongovernmental organizations (NGOs) have supported the Nordic approach. These approaches have also been debated at every WHO session that addresses public health and behavioral change.

Enhancing Global Governance for Chronic Disease Prevention and Control

As the factors influencing chronic diseases have become increasingly global, collective action to prevent and control them has also been forced to adapt accordingly. This governance has proved difficult to achieve on a global level, however, for several reasons.

First, among the many global health players influencing the broad determinants of chronic diseases, some have yet to become fully engaged in such activities. These entities include the World Bank, IMF, CDC, World Heart Federation, International Union Against Cancer (UICC), World Medical Association, representatives of the WHO collaborating centers, International Federation of Pharmaceutical Manufacturers Association (IFPMA), UNICEF, and FAO. Some of these organizations do not see themselves as playing a major role in public health. The mission of the FAO, for example, is to raise nutrition levels, promote food security, improve agricultural productivity, better the lives of rural populations, and contribute to the growth of the world economy. These goals can bring the FAO into conflict with WHO's efforts to re-

duce tobacco and sugar production and consumption. The importance of promoting intersectoral action for chronic disease control requires a more sustained and rigorous effort that should include deeper involvement with those responsible for agriculture, transport, urban design, and education policy.

The experience of the ad hoc Task Force on Tobacco Control, as an example of efforts to strengthen policy coherence on tobacco control during negotiation of the FCTC (see Exhibit 18-3), suggests that considerable progress can be made by having the FAO, World Bank, IMF, and others develop a shared approach to a public health problem, and use their different channels of influence to affect change at the country level. The establishment of similar interagency bodies on chronic diseases could improve policy coherence among different institutions, identify institutional strengths and weaknesses, lead to development of actions based on comparative advantages, and define potential partnerships and collaborations. Comparable models of governance could be developed at the country level.

Second, fuller consideration might be given to which incentives are needed to encourage global industries whose goods or services influence chronic disease risks and outcomes, as well as members of the investment community, to act in ways that are both profitable and beneficial to public health goals. This approach would require, among other things, careful consideration of the regulatory environment and financial mechanisms in place for goods and services that contribute positively to health. Agreement on global standards concerning production, manufacture, and marketing is needed, as is enforcement of such standards at the national level. In the absence of binding global agreement, "soft" measures to encourage compliance may be effective. Metrics related to desired corporate behaviors and actions, for example, might be developed to provide consumers and investors with indices of compliance with agreed-upon public health standards. Such metrics are already used to report on ethical business practices and environmental sustainability (e.g., Dow Jones Sustainability Index, Global Reporting System). In addition, more critical analysis of the potential to develop reporting systems for public health, which could reward progressive companies that are supportive of health goals, is needed.

Third, there is a need for enhanced capacity building for tackling chronic diseases, notably in the low- and middle-income world (see Chapter 7). Without significant investment in capacity building, global progress in chronic disease prevention and control

Exhibit 18-3	Building Policy Coherence for Global Tobacco Control

Policy coherence on tobacco control was strengthened among UN organizations in the following ways:

- The Policy Strategy Advisory Committee (PSAC) was established by WHO to improve policy coherence on tobacco control, solidify support for WHO activities, and expand the base of advocacy and action. The PSAC includes representatives from the World Bank, United Nations Children's Fund (UNICEF), World Self-Medication Industry (WSMI), International Nongovernmental Coalition Against Tobacco (INGCAT), Campaign for Tobacco-Free Kids, and U.S. Centers for Disease Control and Prevention (CDC).
- WHO was asked by the UN Secretary-General to convene the Ad Hoc Inter-Agency Task Force on Tobacco Control. The Task Force replaced the former UN tobacco focal point, which had been situated within the UN Conference on Trade and Development (UNCTAD). This move shifted the tobacco debate within the UN from one of addressing issues relating to supply of tobacco as a first-order priority (i.e., protection of tobacco farming) to one of putting the protection and promotion of health first. Fifteen UN organizations, as well as the World Bank, the IMF, and the WTO, participate in the work of the Task Force.

Among nongovernmental organizations, policy coherence was improved in the following ways:

- In 1999, WHO obtained funding from the UN Foundation to develop partnerships with civil society organizations (CSOs) to raise awareness and counter the global marketing practices of the tobacco industry. Based on the successful California counter-advertising campaign, which had pioneered the strategy of exposing the tobacco industry's behavior, the "Don't Be Duped" campaign sought a new language, a new idiom, and a new sense of purpose and direction for tobacco control. One particularly effective campaign, aimed at countering the rise of the Marlboro man as the twentieth century's most successful global advertising icon, was to replace the traditional "No Smoking" sign with an image of two Marlboro cowboys riding into the sunset with one confiding to the other that he has cancer. The campaign engaged and supported nationally based tobacco control champions and became an important avenue for accessing nongovernmental partners to support and advocate for the FCTC.
- WHO ensured early civil society participation in the FCTC process when it held its first-ever public hearings in October 2000. All interested parties, including representatives of the tobacco industry, were invited to present their views on the FCTC. During 2 days of testimony, more than 90 public heath groups took the floor, along with representatives from all 4 leading tobacco companies (Philip Morris, British American Tobacco, Japan Tobacco International, and Imperial Tobacco). The hearings were widely reported on by the world's media, and the publicity helped to intensify the emerging global tobacco control debate. Although some tobacco industry representatives challenged the evidence base linking passive smoking to disease, the public hearings did provide the first truly global forum in which tobacco companies admitted the addictive and deadly effects of active smoking.

will be limited and unsustained. Considerable expertise is already available within academic centers in high-income countries and could, with modest increased support, be made more widely available. Twinning arrangements between researchers in high- and low-income countries, such as those supported by the U.S. National Institutes of Health's Fogarty Interna-tional Center, could be pursued with urgency. "South–south" cooperation among low- and middle-income countries should be particularly encouraged. A mixture of short-course and longer degree programs in chronic disease control for low- and middle-income countries could be stimulated though exchanges with major donor agencies.

Finally, there is need for active support for the implementation of agreed-upon global norms and standards to enhance health promotion. The Bangkok Charter on Health Promotion in a Globalized World, which was ratified in 2005, identifies actions, commitments, and pledges required to address the broad determinants of health in a globalized world. Unfortunately, it remains a statement without clear mechanisms or authority to enforce its provisions. More progress has been achieved through the FCTC, which, as of May 2011, had been ratified or acceded to by 172 countries. As a binding treaty, the FCTC represents a milestone for the promotion of public health by requiring each party to submit to the Conference of the Parties (COP) periodic reports on its implementation of the Convention. The objective of reporting is to enable parties to learn from one another's experience in implementing the FCTC; the reporting also serves as a compliance mechanism to ensure fulfillment of obligations. Importantly, additional protocols and guidelines can be adopted to support implementation of specific articles. For example, four sessions of the Intergovernmental Negotiating Body for the elaboration of a Protocol on Illicit Trade in Tobacco Products had been held as of March 2010, with a fifth and final session scheduled for 2012.

Unfortunately, resources to enable implementation of these requirements at the national level remain woefully inadequate despite the clear public health benefits to be gained. In general, global norms and standards for health promotion remain in their infancy and will require much greater political and economic support to be truly effective.

Impacts on Healthcare Financing and Service Provision

In addition to having varied impacts on health status and outcomes, globalization is believed to be leading to changes in healthcare provision and financing (Smith, 2004). In providing an introduction to some of these changes, this section examines three areas: the migration of health workers, the globalization of the pharmaceutical industry, and the global spread of health-sector reform.

Migration of Health Workers

Population mobility is a core feature of contemporary globalization, encompassing many types of migration, including temporary visitors (e.g., tourists, students), permanent settlers, documented and undocumented migrant laborers, asylum seekers, refugees, and internally displaced persons (International Organization for Migration, 2010). An estimated 214 million people (3.1% of the world's population) lived outside their country of birth in 2009, an increase from 100 million (1.8% of the world's population) in 1995, and a more than doubling since 1965. Data on the various types of population movement are notoriously incomplete across countries. Nonetheless, it is clear that globalization has been contributing to a marked increase in the number of people moving across national borders, the frequency of such movements, and the distances traveled. As Martin (2001, p. 41) writes,

> Few countries remain untouched by migration. Nations as varied as Haiti, India, and the former Yugoslavia feed international flows. The United States receives by far the most international migrants, but migrants also pour into Germany,

France, Canada, Saudi Arabia, and Iran. Some countries, such as Mexico, send emigrants to other lands, but also receive immigrants—both those planning to settle and those on their way elsewhere.

Given the intensified scale and global reach of migration, countries have sought to improve the means of regulating and managing population flows. These efforts have been aimed at easing the movement of selected populations (e.g., skilled workers to fill labor shortages) through such measures as harmonizing accreditation and licensing requirements, or reciprocal agreements between countries on workforce migration. Conversely, migration policies have sought to restrict certain populations whom governments wish to deter from greater mobility (e.g., human trafficking, criminals, economic migrants).

Trends in the migration of healthcare workers suggest an emerging global marketplace for such labor. In the past, health workers have represented only a small proportion of highly skilled workers who migrate, given national licensing, language, and other requirements. Nonetheless, there has been a clear trend toward the increased migration of doctors and nurses, along with pharmacists, physiotherapists, dentists, laboratory technicians, and other health-related workers. Historically, health workers have long migrated to greener pastures, enticed by differentials in wages, training opportunities, and working conditions.

The so-called brain drain of health workers from poorer to richer countries has raised considerable concern. During the 1960s and 1970s, a large number of doctors and nurses from other parts of the British Commonwealth migrated to the United Kingdom to meet staffing shortages. By the 1980s, it was estimated that 35% of all hospital physicians in the United Kingdom were trained overseas, 60% of these in low-income countries (Abel-Smith, 1986, cited in Martineau, Decker, & Bundred, 2002). Worldwide, at least 140,000 physicians (6% of the world total, excluding China) were based outside their country of birth or training in 1971. Similarly, approximately 135,000 nurses (4% of the world total) worked outside their country of birth or training during the 1970s (Mejia, 1978).

From the 1990s onward, a marked increase in the number of health workers migrating from the low- and middle-income world was noted, with a wider range of countries involved in these outflows and inflows. One of the drivers of this change, according to Martineau, Decker, and Bundred (2002), was "the globalization of markets and the development of free trade agreements." According to these authors, this factor "facilitated international migration and reduced barriers to trade and mobility of services, products and people, including the skills of health professionals." Harmonization of qualifications within the European Union, for example, enabled a greater flow among member states. Another driving force was growing demand on healthcare systems owing to aging populations, which put pressure on high-income countries to fill labor gaps. Furthermore, worsened economic conditions in many low- and middle-income countries encouraged health workers to seek better job prospects elsewhere. For example, the Philippines has been a historically important source of migrant health workers to the world. Given the value of overseas remittances to the national economy, the government has even supported a policy of intentionally training health workers for export. An estimated 85% of Filipino nurses (more than 150,000) worked overseas by 2003, even though there were more than 30,000 unfilled nursing posts in their home country (Aitken, Buchan, Sochalski, Nichols, & Powell, 2004). Data on why health workers migrate are limited, but clearly complex push and pull factors are at play. Nonetheless, the opportunity to secure better working conditions, salaries, and quality of life has been important.

The brain drain out of Africa has been especially worrisome because of the shortage of staff and the impact of the HIV/AIDS epidemic on health worker numbers. At a time when additional external funds were made available to provide antiretroviral therapy, there was declining availability of qualified staff to provide this treatment (Padarath, Chamberlain, McCoy, Ntuli, Rowson, & Loewenson, 2003). In Zimbabwe, for example, approximately 340 nurses graduated each year between 1998 and 2000, while the annual number of Zimbabwean nurses registering in the United Kingdom in 2000 totaled 382 (Stilwell, Diallo, Zurn, Dal Poz, Adams, & Buchan, 2003). Similarly, more than 500 nurses left Ghana in 2000—more than twice the number graduating from nursing programs that year (Buchan & Sochalski, 2004). Between 2000 and 2004, more nurses left Malawi to work abroad than the 330 who remained to care for the country's 11.6 million people (Dugger, 2004). In contrast to high-income countries, which have ratios of more than 1,000 doctors/nurses per 100,000 people (Chen, 2010), in 2010 it was estimated that there were only 17 nurses for every 100,000 people in Malawi (Senior, 2010).

The United Kingdom has been a key destination for migrating health workers from Commonwealth countries. Between 1999 and 2002, the number of foreign-trained nurses based in the United Kingdom and eligible to practice doubled to around 42,000 (Buchan, 2003). By 2008, this number had grown a further 16% to 48,782 (Nursing and Midwifery Council, 2008). In the future, the collective demand for health workers by the United States, Canada, Ireland, Australia, New Zealand, and the United Kingdom is predicted to be "large enough to deplete the supply of qualified nurses throughout the developing world" (Aitken et al., 2004). For example, by 2020 it is projected that the shortfall of nurses in the United States will reach 800,000 (Dugger, 2004).

While the issue of health worker migration must be considered within the context of the wider need to improve the global governance of migration, the majority of action to date has been pursued on a country-by-country basis. For example, in November 1999 the U.K. Department of Health introduced voluntary guidelines to limit the recruitment of health workers from low- and middle-income countries. However, these guidelines excluded private recruitment agencies and employers (Stilwell et al., 2003). While they initially seemed to result in a decline in new registrants from South Africa and the West Indies, the effect was transitory: It was soon followed by a doubling of registrants from low-income countries in 2001–2002 (Buchan and Dovlo, 2004).

In 2004, the World Health Assembly passed a resolution (WHA 57.19) that acknowledged the problems associated with health worker migration, and tasked the WHO Secretariat with developing a new international code of conduct on health worker recruitment that member states would be encouraged to voluntarily adhere to (Buchan, 2010). In 2009, a WHO expert committee also set out a strategy to improve retention of health workers in remote areas, by focusing on three main categories of intervention: education and regulation, financial incentives, and management environment and social support (WHO, 2009a). Reaching international consensus on the necessary measures to implement, along with the adoption of appropriate and effective legislative frameworks and the designation of clear organizational responsibilities, remain major challenges (Martin, 2001).

Globalization and the Pharmaceutical Industry

In recent decades, the pharmaceutical industry has grown in total size, as have the sizes of the largest companies within it. In 2003, the industry earned $492 billion in sales worldwide. By 2009, worldwide

Table 18-2	World's Ten Largest Pharmaceutical Companies, 2008			
Rank (2007 Rank)	Company and Headquarters (website)	2008 Global Pharmaceutical Sales (change from 2007)	R&D Spend	2008 Top-Selling Drugs (2008 sales)
1 (1)	Pfizer; New York, NY (pfizer.com)	$44.2 billion (−0.5%)	$7.9 billion	Lipitor ($12.4 billion), Lyrica ($2.6 billion), Celebrex ($2.5 billion)
2 (2)	GlaxoSmithKline; Brentford, England (gsk.com)	$43.0 billion (11.2%)	$5.2 billion	Seretide/Advair ($6.0 billion), Valtrex ($1.7 billion), Lamictal ($1.4 billion)
3 (3)	Sanofi-Aventis; Paris, France (sanofi-aventis.com)	$38.7 billion (4.8%)	$6.5 billioh	Lovenox ($3.9 billion), Plavix ($3.7 billion), Lantus ($3.5 billion)
4 (4)	Novartis; Basel, Switzerland (novartis.com)	$36.0 billion (10.7%)	$7.2 billion	Diovan/Co-Diovan ($5.7 billion), Gleevec/Glivec ($3.7 billion), Zometa ($1.4 billion)
5 (5)	AstraZeneca; London, England (astrazeneca.com)	$31.6 billion (10.1%)	$5.1 billion	Nexium ($5.2 billion), Seroquel ($4.5 billion), Crestor ($3.6 billion)
6 (6)	Johnson & Johnson; New Brunswick, NJ (jnj.com)	$24.6 billion (−1.2%)	$5.1 billion	Remicade ($3.7 billion), Topamax ($2.7 billion), Procrit ($2.5 billion)
7 (7)	Merck; Whitehouse Station, NJ (merck.com)	$23.6 billion (−2.4%)	$4.8 billion	Singulair ($4.4 billion), Cozaar/Hyzaar ($3.6 billion), Fosamax ($1.6 billion)
8 (8)	Roche; Basel, Switzerland (roche.com)	$21.0 billion (3.4%)	$7.2 billion	MabThera/Rituxan ($5.6 billion), Avastin ($4.9 billion), Herceptin ($4.8 billion)
9 (10)	Eli Lilly; Indianapolis, IN (lilly.com)	$19.3 billion (9.6%)	$3.8 billion	Zyprexa ($4.7 billion), Cymbalta ($2.7 billion), Gemzar ($1.6 billion)
10 (9)	Wyeth; Madison, NJ (wyeth.com)	$19.0 billion (2.3%)	$3.4 billion	Effexor ($3.9 billion), Prevnar ($2.7 billion), Enbrel ($2.6 billion)

Source: Reprinted with permission from *Pharmaceutical Executive*, 29(5), 70, May 2009, New York. *Pharmaceutical Executive* is a copyrighted publication of Advanstar Communications Inc. All rights reserved.

sales had almost doubled to $750 billion (Trombetta, 2009). Perhaps not surprisingly, the pharmaceutical industry is dominated by large MNCs. In 2008, the 10 largest companies earned almost half of the total revenues ($301 billion) garnered by the world pharmaceuticals market (Table 18-2). Together they marketed 30 products that earned more than $1 billion each in sales. Importantly, emerging markets such as Brazil, China, and India are rapidly becoming global players in the pharmaceutical industry, as both producers and consumers (Deutsch Bank Research, 2008).

Analysis by Taribusi and Vickery (1998) found that the pharmaceutical industry has been indeed undergoing major restructuring. This transition has been the result of a flurry of mergers and acquisitions as companies have sought to increase economies of scale (and with it cost savings, market access, and portfolios of products).

More recently, Busfield (2003) looked more carefully at the extent to which the term "globalization"

can be strictly applied to describe the pharmaceutical industry. She confirms that the consolidation of the industry has continued into the early twenty-first century, with no signs of abatement. The percentage of the world market held by the top 10 companies has continued to increase and now sits at almost half of the total market, up from approximately one-third in 1995.

Although it is clear that the pharmaceutical industry has become larger in scale and more concentrated in ownership, the extent to which production has become globalized remains subject to debate. Busfield (2003) concludes that it is more accurate to describe the industry as becoming highly internationalized and perhaps globalizing, but not yet globalized. She notes that the industry as yet does not have companies without clear national identities, nor do those companies demonstrate internationalized management or willingness to relocate across the world. So far production and consumption remains concentrated in high-income countries, though signs suggest that richer low- and middle-income countries have begun playing a more prominent role in recent years.

Setting aside these debates, the increased economic might and reach of the industry do raise important policy issues. Pharmaceutical companies, and notably the industry leaders, argue that there is an economic logic to expanding their size because of the increasing need to compete in the global marketplace. According to this perspective, it is their size, in turn, that enables them to access sufficient resources needed to develop and market new products. As private-sector (profit-seeking) companies, global pharmaceutical companies insist that the demands of the marketplace must invariably drive product development. This practice means ensuring that pricing and ultimately profits give a sufficient return to shareholders and investment in research and development (R&D).

Public health advocates, however, have raised concerns about the dominance of the industry by a small number of large firms and, more specifically, their ability to determine the products and prices available to consumers. One important issue is which products are produced and for what purposes. Critics argue that the market-driven approach of drug companies means that they compete for the lucrative customers of the rich world or focus almost exclusively on conditions where there are sufficient buyers, at the expense of those consumers who are less able to pay for drugs or who have rarer conditions without a sufficient "customer base." This phenomenon explains, for example, the proliferation of "me-too" drugs and the huge investments in drugs to treat obesity and impotence, while investment in conditions more common to the low- and middle-income world is less forthcoming.

Another key issue that has gained increasing prominence in recent years is the drive to improve access to medicines. In 1977, WHO published its first Model List of Essential Drugs, which identified some 220 essential drugs that a country could use to meet the majority of its people's health problems calling for drug solutions. The list, both then and now, serves as a model for countries in developing their own national lists. Since 1977, the WHO list has been updated to include the most effective and cost-effective drugs. If a pharmaceutical company successfully brings a new product to market, which typically requires spending an average of $500 million on R&D, the firm will rely on patent protection under intellectual property rights (IPR) to recoup its development costs and earn profits. For the world's poor, this practice means higher drug prices that often put important medicines beyond their reach.

This clear tension between meeting important public health needs and the practical workings of the market came into intense focus in 2001 with the dispute over access to antiretroviral treatment for HIV/AIDS (Exhibit 18-4). The case highlighted the challenge of reconciling the interests of two very different communities, increasingly brought together by globalization. As a follow-up to the dispute, the British government initiated a Commission on Intellectual Property Rights in 2001 to look at how IPR might work better for poor people and low- and middle-income countries. The commission was asked to consider the following issues:

Exhibit 18-4   The Implications of the TRIPS Agreement for Pharmaceuticals

The Agreement on Trade Related Property Rights (TRIPS) was adopted at the end of the Uruguay Round of international trade negotiations in 1994. The agreement establishes minimum standards for protecting and enforcing nearly all forms of intellectual property rights (i.e., patents, trademarks, and copyrights) for WTO member states, with standards derived from legislation in high-income countries. All member states must comply with these standards, where necessary modifying their national legislation. Importantly, the agreement explicitly acknowledges in Article 8 that, in framing national laws, members "may   .   .   .
adopt measures necessary to protect public health and nutrition, and to promote the public interest."

In an important departure from previous conventions, pharmaceutical products are accorded full intellectual property rights under TRIPS. Pharmaceutical companies are granted the legal means, as patent owners of new drug products, to prevent others from making, using, or selling the new invention for a limited period of time. This provision led to concerns within the public health community over its potential implications for access to medicines. TRIPS specifies that patents must be available for all discoveries that "are new, involve an inventive step and are capable of industrial application" (Article 27). Thus patent protection can be obtained for new drug products, which enables the patent holder to have exclusive rights to produce and sell the product. Pharmaceutical companies argue that such rights, and the consequent ability to charge a higher price for a drug under patent, are necessary to recoup the many millions of dollars spent to research and develop a drug and bring it to market. Without the prospect of earning such prices, the incentive to invest in research and development would

continues

| Exhibit 18-4 | continued |

is made possible—viable—by two important features of our economic system: one is market-based pricing . . . the other is intellectual property protection."

Within the public health community, however, the increased prices charged for drugs under patent protection raise concerns about access to medicines. For drugs unprotected by patent rights—because such rights were not granted, are not asserted, or have expired—other producers can manufacture generic versions that can be sold at more competitive prices. This process leads to lower drug prices for consumers, which is an especially important consideration in low-income communities and countries. Where a drug is needed for an important public health condition, the high cost of patented drugs becomes a particularly acute issue.

The tension between market economics and public health need came to a head in 2001 when the South African government sought an amendment to the South African Medicines and Related Substances Control Amendment Act that would allow the import and use of cheaper generic versions of prescription drugs. The key clause stated that the government could find and "parallel import" the cheapest drug available and grant "compulsory licensing" to other companies allowing them to make copies of patented drugs. It was argued that the prevalence of HIV/AIDS in the country warranted such measures. Thirty-nine pharmaceutical companies, including GlaxoSmithKline, Merck, and Roche, launched legal action against the amendment as a direct violation of their patent rights. Supported by the campaigning of NGOs such as Health Action International and Médicins sans Frontières, the case generated huge public pressure. Faced with negative publicity and strong criticism, the pharmaceutical companies ultimately withdrew the case in April 2001.

Attempts to address continued concerns related to public health protections available under TRIPS led to the Declaration on the TRIPS Agreement and Public Health (known as the Doha Declaration). This agreement affirmed the right of WTO member states to interpret and implement TRIPS in a manner supporting the protection of public health and, in particular, access to medicines. While the TRIPS agreement was initially well received, consternation soon arose over the interpretation of Article 31(f), which states that a compulsory license can be issued only for primarily domestic use. This paragraph precluded generic drug production for export to countries without their own domestic capabilities, leaving the poorest countries still without access to generic medicines. After a further two years of deliberation, the WTO's decision on the interpretation of Paragraph 6 was announced in 2003: It waived this requirement, thereby allowing a country to issue a compulsory license for either domestic use or export, on the basis of public health need. Following the decision, countries remained reluctant to use available flexibilities for fear that pharmaceutical companies would withdraw access to other drugs. The negotiation of reduced prices directly from patent holders became an alternative option. Since the mid- to late-2000s, Thailand, Brazil, and other countries have issued compulsory licenses to produce or import patented drugs despite industry pressure.

Today, three key problems continue to hinder access to medicines. The first is the inability of many very poor countries to implement the flexibilities given their stark resource constraints. Even at reduced cost, increased and innovative financing remains needed. The second is the undermining of TRIPS flexibilities by provisions adopted under bilateral and regional trade agreements. Known as "TRIPS plus" or "WTO plus" measures, the standard of IPRs being negotiated and adopted under subsequent trade agreements can be more restrictive of public health protections. Third, achievement of an appropriate balance between ensuring access to medicines and creating incentives for drug development and innovation has remained elusive. Since 2004, an Independent Commission, Intergovernmental Working Group, and Global Strategy and Plan of Action on Public Health, Innovation and Intellectual Property have been tasked with finding a regulatory framework that reconciles the interests of industry and public health and can gain consensus among the WTO members.

Sources: World Health Organization. (2001). *Globalization, TRIPS and access to pharmaceuticals: WHO policy perspectives on medicine no. 3.* Geneva, Switzerland: Author; World Trade Organization. (2003). *TRIPS and pharmaceutical patents.* Geneva, Switzerland: Author; and World Health Organization. (2008). *The global strategy and plan of action on public health, innovation and intellectual property (GSPOA).* Geneva, Switzerland: Author.

- How national IPR regimes could best be designed to benefit low- and middle-income countries within the context of international agreements, including the Agreement on Trade Related Property Rights (TRIPS)

- How the international framework of rules and agreements might be improved and developed (for instance, in the area of traditional knowledge) and what the relationship between IPR rules and regimes covering access to genetic resources should be

- The broader policy framework needed to complement intellectual property regimes

In its final report published in 2002, the Commission put forth a series of recommendations to integrate development objectives into the protection of IPR in low- and middle-income countries (Commission on Intellectual Property Rights, 2002).

Internationally, the need to balance the creation of new medicines and access to medicines led to the Doha Declaration on TRIPS and Public Health in November 2001. The declaration stated that WTO members had the right to grant compulsory licenses and engage in parallel importing where "public health crises" made this necessary. The declaration also extended exemptions on pharmaceutical patent protection for the poorest countries until 2016.

The key dilemma—that is, the tradeoff between access to medicines and innovation—led WHO to create the Commission on Intellectual Property Rights, Innovation and Public Health in 2004. While its final report provides an important review of the existing evidence and proposals for improving current incentive and funding regimes so as to stimulate the creation of new medicines and other products, disagreement has persisted regarding the effectiveness of the flexibilities available under TRIPS for increasing access to medicines in countries without manufacturing capacity. The impact of data exclusivity laws and of intellectual property provisions in bilateral trade agreements have also raised major concerns (WHO, 2006). Policy debates since the late 2000s have largely focused on the potential contributions of patent pools, advance purchasing agreements, and innovative financing mechanisms.

In conclusion, it is more accurate to describe the pharmaceutical industry as a globalizing, rather than globalized, sector. Efforts to standardize products, regulation, and intellectual property rights worldwide can be seen as steps toward the creation of a global market for pharmaceuticals. However, concerns about access to medicines and product development, for example, have led to debates about the costs and benefits to public health of such trends. The term "internationalization," rather than "globalization," perhaps more accurately describes the sector so far given the continued concentration of ownership, staff, R&D, and markets in high-income countries. Globalization would evolve the industry so that production and consumption become distributed more broadly across the world, and companies no longer have clear national identities but truly internationalized management.

Globalization and Health-Sector Reform

One of the key aspects of globalization concerns changes to how we see ourselves and the world around us. Globalization is affecting a wide range of thought processes, including values and beliefs, cultural identities and products, scientific research, and policy decisions (Lee, 2003). Health sector reform over the past two decades is an example of the global power of ideas. Around the world, countries have grappled with the challenge of improving the financing and provision of health care. At the root of this en-

deavor are shifts in thinking about health care—for example, how better health can best be achieved, how health systems should be restructured, whose needs should get priority, and who should pay for it. The reforms put forth to address these questions have been underpinned by values, beliefs, ideologies, research, and other cognitive processes about what needs to be changed.

The thinking that has driven health-sector reform over the past three decades can be described as globalizing, in the sense that ideas about reform have flowed across a diverse range of countries, involving both public- and private-sector actors. In the United States, this effort was brought into sharp focus in 2009 with the healthcare reform debates that compared the U.S. system to the British National Health Service (Clark, 2009). The origins of this wave of reform are complex, but stem foremost from pressures on governments to address rising health costs and improve the quality of health services. As Dixon and Preker (1999, p.1449) describe,

> [I]t would be too easy to blame ideology and economic crises alone for exposing public services to competitive market forces and increasing private sector participation. In reality, the welfare state approach has not always met the health needs of populations. Although state involvement is clearly needed, it has been dogged with the failure of the public sector to provide the services well.

Although there has been considerable debate about how best to meet these challenges, a clear set of ideas emerged from the early 1980s focused on rethinking (and in many cases reducing) the role of the state and introducing market mechanisms to manage and deliver health services. Initially introduced in the United States and United Kingdom, where enthusiasm for health reforms was perhaps most pronounced, these ideas began to be taken up in a wide variety of settings, including many parts of the low- and middle-income world.

The publication of *World Development Report 1993: Investing in Health* by the World Bank (1993) marked an important point in the emerging discourse of health-sector reform. Based on the innovative, yet controversial findings of the Global Burden of Disease project, which was carried out by the Harvard School of Public Health, the report ignited fierce debates about setting priorities and financing health care in the low- and middle-income world. *World Development Report 1993* set out a new approach to priority setting that sought to target those conditions inflicting the heaviest disease or disability burden (measured by DALYs) for which cost-effective interventions are available. In addition, a new language of reform known broadly as the "new public management" began to permeate health policy at the national and global levels—internal markets, contracting out, public–private mix, decentralization, cost-effectiveness, rationing, autonomous hospitals, managed care—all bent on making health systems worldwide leaner and meaner.

The content of these reforms, and assessments of their relative merits and demerits at achieving their declared intentions, has been dealt with extensively elsewhere (see, for example, Berman & Bossert, 2000; Mills, 2001). What is interesting here, in the context of globalization, is the way in which such policy ideas flowed across territorial boundaries more readily than ever before. This phenomenon might be explained by the inherent "rightness" of the policies themselves, which claim to offer proven and effective measures to deal with practical problems in public-sector management common across countries. However, the adoption of reforms in so many countries prior to the availability of supporting evidence of their effec-

tiveness directly challenges this view. So do the sometimes heated debates surrounding specific reforms—the appropriateness of reforms to local settings, the inequitable effects imposed on certain population groups (especially the poor), the quality of the evidence base and methodology, and the underlying assumptions and values. The debate over WHO's efforts in 2001 to comparatively assess the world's health systems is a good example (Exhibit 18-5).

The sometimes controversial response suggests that the flow of ideas about health-sector reform over the past decade or so cannot be solely explained by the quality of their content. Rather, it is important to recognize that the messengers have been as important as the messages themselves. At the national level, successive conservative-thinking governments favored the adoption of policies based on neoliberal economic principles such as downsizing of the state, deregulation and privatization, and strengthening the market. At the global level, organizations such as the World Bank, IMF, and U.S. Agency for International Development (USAID) advocated similar policies, including structural adjustment programs, which became known as the "Washington consensus." Given

---

Exhibit 18-5 | **The Global Debate over *World Health Report 2000***

In 2001, WHO published its *World Health Report 2000: Health Systems—Improving Performance* (WHO, 2001c) as "the first ever analysis of the world's health systems." Using five performance indicators (overall level of population health, health inequalities within the population, health system responsiveness, distribution of responsiveness, and distribution of the health system's financial burden within the population) to measure health systems in 191 member states, the report was intended "to stimulate a vigorous debate about better ways of measuring health system performance and thus finding a successful new direction for health systems to follow." The report stated that "[b]y shedding new light on what makes health systems behave in certain ways, WHO also hopes to help policy-makers weigh the many complex issues involved, examine their options, and make wise choices." The results found France to be providing the best overall health care, followed by Italy, Spain, Oman, Austria, and Japan. The U.S. health system, which consumes a higher portion of gross domestic product than any other country's health system, ranked 37th (WHO, 2001b).

The analysis immediately met with strong criticism on methodological grounds. Many public health practitioners objected to countries being ranked on the basis of untested methods that they felt were also based on ethically unacceptable assumptions. For example, Almeida and associates (2001, p. 1692) wrote that the "measures of health inequalities and fair financing do not seem conceptually sound or useful to guide policy; of particular concern are some ethical aspects of the methodology for both these measures, whose implications for social policy are cause for concern." Similarly, Nolte and McKee (2003) challenged the report's assessment of overall performance of health systems as a composite measure and, in particular, the attribution of health attainment to health systems. Many determinants of health lie outside of health care, and the method used by the *World Health Report* has been criticized for inadequately allowing for them. Applying a measure known as "avoidable mortality" to 19 countries, Nolte and McKee (2003) found that "no country retained the same rank with both methods." Even the editor-in-chief of the report subsequently called the data "spurious" and "of no use for judging how well a health system performs" (Musgrove, 2003).

Although a second report with methodological refinements and new rankings never appeared, and criticisms continue to question WHO's political judgment in undertaking such an exercise, the report was successful in drawing attention to the importance of better understanding health systems. The exercise spurred efforts to develop better methods and then to use them to unravel the "black box" of health systems' performance.

these factors, together with the increased opportunities for policy makers to interact with their counterparts across the world, it is perhaps unsurprising that a considerable degree of policy convergence has occurred. Much more needs to be understood about how this evolution takes place, which key individuals and institutions are involved, and which policy issues have been most affected. New areas of research such as policy transfer, policy learning, and network analysis seek to grapple with these questions.

In short, health-sector reforms in recent decades illustrate well how transborder flows of thought processes are a key aspect of globalization. Ideas today move across national borders in a variety of forms via the mass media, the advertising industry, research institutions, consultancy firms, governments, civil society, corporations, international organizations, and individuals (e.g., via the Internet). The health sector is an arena in which ever-changing knowledge and ideas are at the core of practice. As a consequence, we can speak of health-sector reforms as being "globalized" to the extent that these ideas driving reform have become universally debated and, in many cases, adopted by diverse health systems around the world.

Although knowledge and ideas have flowed across societies throughout history, the technological advances that characterize contemporary forms of globalization have intensified this intellectual exchange to an unprecedented degree. Global policy networks of influential individuals and institutions, in turn, shape which ideas are put into practice in healthcare financing and service delivery.

The Growing Importance of Global Health Diplomacy

The changing nature of health determinants and outcomes as a result of globalization has prompted concerted reflection on the need for more effective global health governance. As a part of this reflection, growing attention has been paid to global health diplomacy as a means of facilitating consensus on collective action. Global health diplomacy can be defined as "policy shaping processes through which States, intergovernmental organizations, and non-State actors negotiate responses to health challenges or utilize health concepts or mechanisms in policy-shaping and negotiation strategies to achieve other political, economic, or social objectives" (Smith, Fidler, & Lee, 2009, p. 1). Such processes recognize that the changing roles and responsibilities of the increasingly diverse

public and private actors concerned with global health require a range of approaches to collective action. Of significance is the absence of an overarching authority to adopt and enforce legally binding measures. Yet the world's experiences with SARS and H1N1 influenza, for example, have reemphasized the shared nature of global health challenges. To date, the focus has largely centered on negotiating global governance mechanisms to deal with acute public health threats—notably, infectious diseases outbreaks. However, greater attention needs to be given to how state and nonstate actors at different policy levels can work more effectively together to address other global health issues such as strengthening health systems, health worker migration, access to medicines, and preventing and controlling the rapid increase in chronic diseases.

Over the past six decades, WHO has been at the forefront of global health diplomacy as the UN specialized agency for health. The World Health Assembly has served as a valued forum for debating issues and encouraging consensus among member states. The post–Cold War era, however, has seen the rise of the Group of Eight (G8) countries as a core influence in international relations. More recently, the rapidly growing economies of China, India, and Brazil have ensured growing prominence for the Group of Twenty (G20) countries. Both the G8 and G20, along with major forums within which they participate, such as the World Economic Forum (WEF) and the Organization for Economic Cooperation and Development (OECD), will remain key players in foreign policy.

Moreover, as discussed earlier in this chapter, global health actors embrace a broad range of nonstate actors—notably, private companies and civil society organizations, and the public–private partnerships that bring them together with state actors. This interweaving of organizations directed at global health is complicated further by the influence of other sectors, including trade, security, environment, migration and agriculture. The greater complexity of issues, and the diverse actors that need to be engaged to address them, means that global health diplomacy has assumed even greater importance. WHO has sought to diversify its engagement activities by hosting issue-specific meetings, convening working groups, and disseminating best-practice guidelines and recommendations (Kickbusch, Silberschmidt, & Buss, 2007). Yet, far greater understanding is required regarding how diplomatic negotiations should be conducted, which skills are needed for effective negotiation, and which ends global health diplomacy should seek to achieve.

Conclusions: Health Protection and Promotion Amid Globalization

This chapter has presented an introduction to the subject of globalization and health. Globalization is a wide-ranging subject that is plagued by definitional ambiguity, heated debate, and a limited, albeit steadily growing, evidence base. Despite the sometimes muddy waters surrounding this issue, it is clear that the public health community is faced with fundamentally critical and, in some cases, unprecedented challenges. It is increasingly accepted that a transition from international to global public health is taking place, as evident in shifting patterns of health and disease within and across countries. More complex is the need to better understand, and respond effectively to, the causes of these health impacts. Coming to terms with globalization requires tackling its implications for the broad determinants of health, which quickly takes the public health community beyond its usual comfort zone. Such issues as foreign policy, trade and finance, agricultural subsidies, corporate restructuring, and international law are unavoidably bumping up against more familiar public health agendas. Dealing with the overlap necessitates the acquisition of new sets of knowledge, new skills to deploy them, and seats at unfamiliar decision-making tables to voice public health concerns.

On some issues, signs indicate that the public health community is rising to the challenge. High-profile efforts to globalize tobacco control and to strengthen global responses to infectious disease outbreaks have received deserved attention. Away from the spotlight, there have been efforts to globalize many essential public health functions. For example, the tenth revision of the International Classification of Diseases is part of the ongoing development of common definitions of diseases and deaths carried out since 1893. Such initiatives represent an important example of how globalization of standards has led to better decision making and improved prospects for global surveillance of major risks and diseases, and smoothed the way toward standardized approaches to prevent and treat conditions. Similarly, common standards for surveillance have been developed for infectious diseases and for chronic disease risks and outcomes.

More controversial outcomes have resulted when public health advocates have sought to tackle the broader determinants of health, such as poverty and inequality, which are embedded within the structures of contemporary globalization. As a starting point, there remains acute variation in health systems capacity among countries. The International Classification of Diseases, for example, must be underpinned by national systems for surveillance, diagnostics, and reporting. The value of global standards, in other words, is determined by the ability to implement them meaningfully. Drawing much-needed attention to unacceptable weaknesses in health systems, along with persistent inequities in health status and outcomes, amidst a world of rapid globalization, requires political courage to point fingers at inadequate regulation, weak political will, and the dominance of vested interests. It has meant making deeper forays into new territories for the public health community, but such incursions are critical if the health of the public is to be appropriately protected and promoted in an increasingly globalized world.

● ● ● Discussion Questions

1. Identify at least two positive and two negative examples of how globalization is affecting the broad determinants of health.

2. Name some goods and services that could benefit or harm health if traded more readily worldwide.

3. How do you think your own specific field of work or interest within public health is being influenced by globalization? Which regulatory measures or incentive systems might be needed to tackle the issues raised?

• • • References

Abel-Smith, B. (1986). The patterns of medical practice in England and the Third World. In S. J. Kingma (Ed.), *The principles and practice of primary health care*. Geneva, Switzerland: Christian Medical Commission and World Council of Churches.

Aitken, L., Buchan, J., Sochalski, J., Nichols, B., & Powell, M. (2004). Trends in international nurse migration. *Health Affairs, 23*(3), 69–77.

Al Jazeera. (2009, July 23). H1N1 prompts Hajj restrictions. Retrieved March 30, 2010, from http://english.aljazeera.net/news/middleeast/2009/07/200972311236123448.html

Almeida, C., Braveman, P., Gold, M., Szwarcwald, C., Ribeiro, J., Miglionico, A. et al. (2001). Methodological concerns and recommendations on policy consequences of the *World Health Report 2000*. *Lancet, 357*, 1692–1697.

Babor, T. (2003). *Alcohol: No ordinary commodity. Research and public policy*. Oxford, UK: Oxford University Press.

Berman, P., & Bossert, T. (2000). *A decade of health sector reform in developing countries: What have we learned?* Cambridge, MA: Harvard School of Public Health.

Berridge, V., Loughlin, K., & Herring, R. (2009). Historical dimensions of global health governance. In K. Buse, W. Hein, & N. Drager, *Making sense of global health governance: a policy perspective* (pp. 28–46). Hampshire, UK: Palgrave Macmillan.

Bettcher, D., Subramaniam, C., Guindon, E., Perucic, A.-M., Soll, L., Grabman, G., et al. (2003). *Confronting the tobacco epidemic in an era of trade liberalization*. Geneva, Switzerland: World Health Organization.

Bolling, C. (1998). Appendix 4: U.S. foreign direct investment in the global processed food industries. In M. E. Burfisher & E. A. Jones, *Regional trade agreements and U.S. agriculture* (pp. 84–86). Washington, DC: U.S. Department of Agriculture.

Bolling, C. (2002). Globalization of the soft drink industry. *Agricultural Outlook, 297*, 25–27.

Bonn, D. (2003). Closing in on the cause of SARS. *Lancet Infectious Diseases, 3*(5), 268.

Borrow, R. (2009). Meningococcal disease and prevention at the Hajj. *Travel Medicine and Infectious Disease, 7*(4), 219–225.

Buchan, J. (2003). *Here to stay? International nurses in the UK*. London: Royal College of Nursing.

Buchan, J. (2010). Can the WHO code on international recruitment succeed? *British Medical Journal, 340*(7750), 791–793.

Buchan, J., & Dovlo, D. (2004). *International recruitment of health workers to the UK: A report for DFID*. London: DFID Health Systems Resource Centre.

Buchan, J., & Sochalski, J. (2004). The migration of nurses: Trends and policies. *Bulletin of the World Health Organization, 82*(8), 587–594.

Busfield, J. (2003). Globalization and the pharmaceutical industry revisited. *International Journal of Health Services, 33*(3), 581–605.

Centers for Disease Control and Prevention (CDC). (2009). *Reported tuberculosis in the United States, 2008*. Atlanta: U.S. Department of Health and Human Services.

Chen, L. C. (2010). Striking the right balance: Health workforce retention in remote and rural areas. *Bulletin of the World Health Organization, 88*(5), 323–324.

Clark, A. (2009, August 11). "Evil and Orwellian": America's right turns its fire on NHS. *The Guardian*. Retrieved from http://www.guardian.co.uk/world/2009/aug/11/nhs-united-states-republican-health

Clark, W. C., Kates, R. W., Richards, J. F., Mathews, J. T., Meyer, W. B., & Turner, B. L. (Eds.). (1990). *The Earth as transformed by human action*. Cambridge, UK: Cambridge University Press.

Commission on Intellectual Property Rights. (2002, September). *Integrating intellectual property rights and development policy*. London: Author.

Dahlgren, G., & Whitehead, M. (1991). *Policies and strategies to promote social equity in health.* Stockholm, Sweden: Institute for Futures Studies.

Deutsch Bank Research. (2008). India's pharmaceutical industry on course for globalisation. Retrieved from http://www.dbresearch.com/PROD/ DBR_INTERNET_EN-PROD/PROD0000000000 224095.pdf

Dixon, J., & Preker, A. (1999). Learning from the NHS. *British Medical Journal, 319,* 1449–1450.

Dobson, A., & Carper, R. (1993). Biodiversity. *Lancet, 342,* 1096–1099.

Dugger, C. (2004, July 12). An exodus of African nurses puts infants and the ill in peril. *New York Times.* Retrieved from http://www.nytimes.com/ 2004/07/12/world/an-exodus-of-african-nurses-puts-infants-and-the-ill-in-peril.html

Epstein, P. (2001). Climate change and emerging infectious diseases. *Microbes and Infection, 3,* 747–754.

ETC Group. (2008). *Who owns nature? Corporate power and the final frontier in the commodification of life.* Ottawa: ETC Group.

Fidler, D. (2004). *SARS, governance, and the globalization of disease.* London: Palgrave Macmillan.

Firebaugh, G. (2003). *The new geography of global income inequality.* Cambridge, MA: Harvard University Press.

Food and Agriculture Organization (FAO). (2009). *The state of agricultural commodity markets: High food prices and the food crisis—experiences and lessons learned.* Rome: Author.

Fratianni, M., Kirton, J., & Savona, P. (2007). *Financing development: The G8 and UN contribution.* Hampshire, UK: Ashgate.

Fukuyama, F. (1992). *The end of history and the last man.* New York: Free Press.

Gilmore, A. B., & McKee, M. (2004). Moving east: How the transnational tobacco industry gained entry to the emerging markets of the former Soviet

Union. Part I: Establishing cigarette imports. *Tobacco Control, 13,* 143–150.

Githeko, A., Lindsay, S., Confalonieri, U., & Patz, J. (2000). Climate change and vector-borne diseases: A regional analysis. *Bulletin of the World Health Organization, 78*(9), 1136–1147.

Hales, S., de Wet, N., Maindonald, J., & Woodward, A. (2002). Potential effect of population and climate changes on global distribution of dengue fever: An empirical model. *Lancet, 360,* 830–834.

Hawkes, C. (2002). Marketing activities of global soft drink and fast food companies in emerging markets: A review. Retrieved from http://whqlibdoc.who.int/publications/9241590 416.pdf. In World Health Organization, *Globalization, diets and noncommunicable diseases.* Geneva, Switzerland: Author.

Hawkes, C. (2004a). *The global regulatory environment around marketing food to children.* Geneva, Switzerland: World Health Organization.

Hawkes, C. (2004b). *The global regulatory environment around nutrition labels and health claims.* Geneva, Switzerland: World Health Organization.

Hawkes, C. & Murphy, S. (2010). An overview of global food trade. In C. Hawkes, C. Blouin, S. Henson, & N. Drager (Eds.), *Trade, food, diet and health: Perspectives and policy options* (pp. 16–33). London: Wiley-Blackwell.

Hundley, R. O., Anderson, R. H., Bikson, T. K., & Neu, C. R. (2003). *The global course of the information revolution, recurring themes and regional variations.* Washington, DC: RAND Corporation.

International Chamber of Commerce. (1997, May 23). Business and the global economy. Statement on behalf of world business to the heads of state and government attending the Denver summit, 20–22 June 1997, Paris. Retrieved from http://www.iccwbo .org/home/shared_pages/gloecon.asp

International Organization for Migration. (2010). Global estimates and trends. Retrieved from http://www.iom.int/jahia/Jahia/about-migration/

facts-and-figures/global-estimates-and-trends#1

Jackson, M. C., Hastings, G., Wheeler, C., Eadie, D., & Mackintosh, A. M. (2002). Marketing alcohol to young people: Implications for industry regulation and research policy. *Addiction, 95*(suppl 4), S597–S608.

Jansik, C. (2009). Geographical aspects of food industry FDI in CEE countries. *EuroChoices, 8*(1), 46–51.

Joint Centre for Bioethics. (2003, August 13). *Ethics and SARS: Learning lessons from the Toronto experience.* Working paper, University of Toronto. Retrieved from http://www.utoronto.ca/jcb/SARS_workingpaper.asp

Kickbusch, I., Silberschmidt, G., & Buss, P. (2007). Global health diplomacy: The need for new perspectives, strategic approaches and skills in global health. *Bulletin of the World Health Organization, 85*(3), 230–232.

Lee, K. (2003). *Globalization and health: An introduction.* London: Palgrave Macmillan.

Lee, K., Carpenter, C., Challa, C., Lee, S. Y. Connelly, G. N., & Koh, H. (2009). The strategic targeting of females by transnational tobacco companies in South Korea following trade liberalisation. *Globalization and Health, 5*(2), 1–10.

Lee, K., & Dodgson, R. (2002). Globalization and cholera: Implications for global governance. In K. Lee (Ed.), *Health impacts of globalization: Towards global governance* (pp. 123–143). London: Palgrave Macmillan.

Lee, K., Walt, G., & Haines, A. (2004). The challenge to improve global health: Financing the Millennium Development Goals. *Journal of the American Medical Association, 291*(21), 2636–2638.

Mackay, J., & Eriksen, M. (2002). *The tobacco atlas.* Geneva, Switzerland: World Health Organization.

Manning, R. (2004). Development challenge. *OECD Observer, 243,* 36–37.

Martin, S. (2001). Heavy traffic: International migration in an era of globalization. *Brookings Review, 19*(4), 41–44.

Martineau, T., Decker, K., & Bundred, P. (2002). *Briefing note on international migration of health professionals: Levelling the playing field for developing country health systems.* Briefing paper, Liverpool School of Tropical Medicine, Liverpool, UK.

McMichael, A. J. (2001). *Human frontiers, environments and disease.* Cambridge, UK: Cambridge University Press.

Mejia, A. (1978). Migration of physicians and nurses: A world wide picture. *International Journal of Epidemiology, 7*(3), 207–215.

Mills, A. (2001). *The challenge of health sector reform: What must governments do?* London: Palgrave Macmillan.

Monaghan, K. (2003). *SARS Down But Still a Threat, Intelligence Community Assessment.* Retrieved from http://www.dni.gov/nic/special_sarsthreat.html. Washington, DC: U.S. National Intelligence Council.

Musgrove, P. (2003). Judging health systems: Reflections on WHO's methods. *Lancet, 361,* 1817–1820.

Nolte, E., & McKee, M. (2003). Measuring the health of nations: Analysis of mortality amenable to health care. *British Medical Journal, 327,* 1129–1133.

Nursing and Midwifery Council. (2008). Statistical analysis of the register 1 April 2007 to 31 March 2008. Retrieved from http://www.nmc-uk.org/aDisplayDocument.aspx?DocumentID=5730

O'Dea, K., & Piers, L. S. (2002). Diabetes. In B. Caballero & B. M. Popkin (Eds.), *The nutrition transition: Diet and disease in the developing world* (pp. 165–190). London: Academic Press.

Organization for Economic Cooperation and Development (OECD). (2000). *Foreign direct investment, development and corporate responsibility.* Paris: Author.

Padarath, A., Chamberlain, C., McCoy, D., Ntuli, A., Rowson, M., & Loewenson, R. (2003). *Health personnel in southern Africa: Confronting maldistribution and brain drain* (EQUINET Discussion Paper No. 3). Harari, South Africa: Health Systems Trust and Medact.

Peterson, L. E. (2010, March 10). Big Tobacco tests anti-smoking rules. *Embassy*. Retrieved March 30, 2010, from http://www.embassymag.ca/page/view/bigtobacco-03-10-2010

Saker, L., Lee, K., Cannito, B., Gilmore, A., & Campbell-Lendrum, D. (2004). *Globalization and infectious diseases: A review of the linkages.* Geneva, Switzerland: UNICEF/UNDP/World Bank/WHO Special Programme for Research and Training in Tropical Diseases.

Scholte, J. A. (2000). *Globalization: A critical introduction.* London: Macmillan.

Senior, K. (2010). Wanted: 2.4 million nurses, and that's just in India. *Bulletin of the World Health Organization, 88*(5), 327–328.

Smith, R. (2004). Foreign direct investment and trade in health services: A review of the literature. *Social Science and Medicine, 59,* 2313–2323.

Smith, R., Fidler, D. F., & Lee, K. (2009). *Global health diplomacy research.* Geneva, Switzerland: WHO Trade, Foreign Policy, Diplomacy and Health Working Paper Series.

Smith, R., & Sommers, T. (2003, July). *Assessing the economic impact of communicable disease outbreaks: The case of SARS.* Report prepared for the Strategy Unit, World Health Organization, Geneva, Switzerland.

Stilwell, B., Diallo, K., Zurn, P., Dal Poz, M, Adams, O., & Buchan, J. (2003). Developing evidence-based ethical policies on the migration of health workers: Conceptual and practical challenges. *Human Resources for Health, 1*(8). Retrieved from http://www.human-resources-health.com/content/1/1/8

Taribusi, C., & Vickery, G. (1998). Globalization in the pharmaceutical industry, part 1. *International Journal of Health Services, 28*(1), 67–105.

Taurel, S. (2003, November 4). *Where drugs come from: The facts of life about pharmaceutical innovation.* Remarks to Hudson Institute Forum, National Press Club, Washington, DC.

Tenenbaum, D. J. (2008). Food vs. fuel: Diversion of crops could cause more hunger. *Environmental Health Perspectives, 116*(6), A254–A257.

Thow, A. M. & Hawkes, C. (2009). The implications of trade liberalization for diet and health: A case study from Central America. *Globalization and Health, 5*(5). Retrieved from http://www.globalizationandhealth.com/content/5/1/5

Trombetta, B. (2009). Industry audit 2009. Retrieved from http://pharmexec.findpharma.com/pharmexec/Strategy/Industry-Audit-2009/ArticleStandard/Article/detail/625744

United Nations Conference on Trade and Development. (2003). *World investment report 2003. FDI policies for development: National and international perspectives.* Geneva, Switzerland: Author.

United Nations Conference on Trade and Development. (2009). *World investment report 2009. Transnational corporations, agricultural production and development.* Geneva, Switzerland: Author.

United Nations Development Program (UNDP). (2009). *The Millennium Development Goals report 2009.* New York: United Nations.

United Nations Environment Program. (2001). *IPCC third assessment report. Climate change 2001: The scientific basis.* New York: UN Environment Program, Intergovernmental Panel on Climate Change.

United Nations Intergovernmental Panel on Climate Change (IPCC). (2007). *Climate change 2007, fourth assessment report: Working Group I report, the physical science basis.* Geneva, Switzerland: Author. Retrieved from http://www1.ipcc.ch/ipccreports/ar4-wg1.htm

U.S. Department of Transportation. (2000). *The changing face of transportation.* Washington, DC: Bureau of Transportation Statistics.

Walkenhorst, P. (2001). The geography of foreign direct investment in Poland's food industry. *Journal of Agricultural Economics, 52,* 71–86.

Whitton, C. (2004). *Processed agricultural exports led gains in U.S. agricultural exports between 1976 and 2002* (Electronic Output Report FAU-85-01). Washington, DC: U.S. Department of Agriculture, Economic Research Service.

Witkowski, T. H. (2007). Food Marketing and obesity in developing countries: Analysis, ethics, and public policy. *Journal of Macromarketing, 27*(2), 126–137.

World Bank. (1993). *World development report 1993: Investing in health.* Washington, DC: International Bank for Reconstruction and Development.

World Health Organization. (2000, January 18). WHO, internationally-renowned economists launch commission on macroeconomics and health [Press release].

World Health Organization (WHO). (2001b, July 21). World Health Organization assesses the world's health systems [Press release].

World Health Organization (WHO). (2001c). *World health report 2000: Health systems—Improving performance.* Geneva, Switzerland: Author.

World Health Organization (WHO). (2002). *Global crises—global solutions: Managing public health emergencies of international concern through the revised International Health Regulations.* Geneva, Switzerland: International Health Regulations Revision Project.

World Health Organization (WHO). (2004a, March 16). Drug resistant tuberculosis levels ten times higher in eastern Europe and Central Asia [Press release].

World Health Organization (WHO). (2004b). Summary of probable SARS cases with onset of illness between 1 November 2002 to 31 July 2003. Retrieved from http://www.who.int/csr/sars/country/table2004_04_21/en.

World Health Organization (WHO). (2006). *Public health, innovation and intellectual property rights: Report of the Commission on Intellectual Property Rights, Innovation and Public Health.* Geneva, Switzerland: Author.

World Health Organization (WHO). (2008). *The global tobacco epidemic 2008.* Geneva, Switzerland: Tobacco Free Initiative.

World Health Organization (WHO). (2009a). *Report on the first core group expert consultation on increasing access to health workers in remote and rural areas through improved retention.* Geneva, Switzerland: Author.

World Health Organization (WHO). (2009b). Transcript of virtual press conference with Gregory Hartl, WHO Spokesperson for Epidemic and Pandemic Diseases, and Dr Peter Ben Embarek, WHO Food Safety Scientist, World Health Organization, 3 May 2009. Retrieved from http://www.who.int/mediacentre/swineflu_presstranscript_2009_05_03.pdf

Acronyms

ACC/SCN Administrative Committee on Coordination/Subcommittee on Nutrition (United Nations)

ACF Action Contre la Faim

ACT artemisinin-based combination therapy

AIDS acquired immunodeficiency syndrome

ALRI acute lower respiratory infection

AMC advanced market commitment

ANC antenatal care

ARI acute respiratory infection

ARV antiretroviral therapy

ASEAN Association of Southeast Asian Nations

AZT zidovudine

BBC British Broadcasting Corporation

BCG bacillus Calmette-Guérin (vaccine)

BMI body mass index

CBH community-based health

CBHI community-based health insurance

CCM country coordination mechanism

CCMD Chinese Classification of Mental Disorders

CDC Centers for Disease Control and Prevention

CDR case disability ratio

CE complex emergency

CFR case fatality ratio

CHD coronary artery disease

CHE complex humanitarian emergency

CHeSS Country Health Systems Surveillance

CHW community health worker

CMD common mental disorder

CMR crude mortality rate

COPD chronic obstructive pulmonary disease

CRA comparative risk assessment

CSO civil society organization

CSR corporate social responsibility

CVD cardiovascular disease

CVI Childhood Vaccine Initiative

DALE disability-adjusted life expectancy

DALY disability-adjusted life year

DDT dichlorodiphenyltrichloroethane

DFID Department for International Development (United Kingdom)

DFLE disability-free life expectancy

DHS demographic and health survey

DOTS directly observed treatment, short course

DPSEEA driving force-pressure-state-exposure-effect-action

DPT diptheria, pertussis, tetanus vaccine

DRC Democratic Republic of Congo

DSM-IV *Diagnostic Statistical Manual of the American Psychiatric Association, Fourth Edition*

DSS Demographic Surveillance Site

ECOSOC Economic and Social Council

EHRA environmental health risk assessment

EIA environmental impact assessment

EMRO Eastern Mediterranean Regional Office (WHO)

EPI Expanded Program on Immunization

EPIDOS European Patent Information and Documentation Systems

ERA environmental risk assessment

ERAP Epilepsy Rapid Assessment Procedures

ERHI employment-related health insurance

ERR economic rate of return

ETEC enterotoxigenic *Escherichia coli*

ETS environmental tobacco smoke

EU European Union

FAO Food and Agriculture Organization

FCTC Framework Convention on Tobacco Control

FDA U.S. Food and Drug Administration

FDI foreign direct investment

G20 Group of 20

G8 Group of Eight

GAVI Global Alliance for Vaccines and Immunizations

GBD Global Burden of Disease

GBS Global Burden of Disease Studies

GDP gross domestic product

GFATM Global Fund to Fight AIDS, Tuberculosis and Malaria (Global Fund)

GHI global health initiative

GNI gross national income

GNP gross national product

GOARN Global Outbreak Alert and Response Network

GOBI growth monitoring, oral rehydration, breastfeeding, and immunization

GYTS Global Youth Tobacco Survey

HALE health-adjusted life expectancy

HeaLY healthy life years

HIA Health Impact Assessment

HIV human immunodeficiency virus

HIV/AIDS human immunodeficiency virus/acquired immunodeficiency syndrome

HMO health maintenance organization

HPV human papillomavirus

HR human resources

IARC International Agency for Research on Cancer

IAVI International AIDS Vaccine Initiative

ICCC Innovative Care for Chronic Conditions

ICD *International Classification of Diseases*

ICD-10 *International Classification of Diseases-Tenth Revision*

ICF International Classification of Functioning, Disability and Health

ICIDH International Classification of Impairments, Disabilities, and Handicaps

ICPD International Conference on Population Development

ICRC International Committee of the Red Cross

IDD iodine deficiency disorders

IDP internally displaced person

IFI international financial institutions

IFPMA International Federation of Pharmaceutical Manufacturers Association

IGO international governmental organization

IHP International Health Partnership

IHR International Health Regulations

ILO International Labour Organization

IMCI Integrated Management of Childhood Illness

IMF International Monetary Fund

IMR infant mortality rates

INCAP Instituto Nutricional de Central America y Panama

INGCAT International Nongovernmental Coalition Against Tobacco

INTERFET International Force in East Timor

IPCC United Nations Intergovernmental Panel on Climate Change

IPR intellectual property rights

IPV injectable polio vaccine

ITN insecticide-treated nets

IVACG International Vitamin A Consultative Group

LFA local fund agent

LMIC low- and middle-income countries

MAC *Mycobacterium avium* complex

MDGs Millennium Development Goals

MDR-TB multi-drug resistant tuberculosis

MISP minimum initial service package

MMV Medicines for Malaria Venture

MNCH maternal, newborn, and child health

MOH Ministry of Health

MSAs medical savings accounts

MSF Médecins sans Frontières

MUAC middle upper arm circumference

NCD noncommunicable disease

NGO nongovernmental organization

NID National Immunization Day

NIH National Institutes of Health

NPV net present value

OCHA Office for the Coordination of Humanitarian Affairs

OCP Onchocerciasis Control Program

OECD Organization for Economic Cooperation and Development

OPV oral polio vaccine

ORS oral rehydration solution

ORT oral rehydration therapy

PAHO Pan American Health Organization

PCBs polychlorinated biphenyls

PEM protein-energy malnutrition

PEPFAR President's Emergency Plan for AIDS Relief

PEV Expanded Program on Immigration (French)

PHC primary health care

PHEIC public health emergency of international concern

PPI Private Participation in Infrastructure

PPP purchasing power parity

PPYL productive years of life lost

PR Principal Recipient

PSAC Policy Strategy Advisory Committee

PSR pressure-state-response

QALY quality-adjusted life year

QWB quality of well-being

RAP Rapid Assessment Procedures

RARE Rapid Assessment, Response and Evaluation

RBM Roll Back Malaria Partnership

RCT randomized controlled trial

RDA Recommended Dietary Allowance

RENAMO Resistência Nacional Moçambicana

RHU refugee health unit

R&D research and development

SARS severe acute respiratory syndrome

SDR social discount rate

SFP supplementary feeding program

SIDA Swedish International Development Agency

SIPs sector investment programs

STEPS STEPwise approach to Surveillance

SWAp sector wide approach

SWOT strengths, weaknesses, opportunities, and threats

TAC Treatment Action Campaign

TB tuberculosis

TDR WHO-based Special Programme for Research and Training in Tropical Diseases

TEA total exposure assessment

TFC transnational food companies

TFP therapeutic feeding programs

TFR total fertility rate

TGR total goiter rate

TNCs transnational corporations

TRIPS Trade Related Aspects of Intellectual Property Rights

TRL Transport Research Laboratory

TT tetanus toxoid

UCHA United Nations Office for Coordination of Humanitarian Affairs

UICC International Union Against Cancer (French)

UN United Nations

UNAIDS United Nations Programme on HIV/AIDS

UNCHR United Nations Commission on Human Rights

UNCTAD United Nations Conference on Trade and Development

UNDP United Nations Development Program

UNESCO United Nations Educational, Scientific and Cultural Organization

UNFPA United Nations Population Fund

UNHCR United Nations High Commissioner for Refugees

UNICEF United Nations Children's Fund

USAID United States Agency for International Development

USI universal salt iodization

UVR ultraviolet radiation

VAC vitamin A capsule

VAT value-added tax

WCH women's and children's health

WDR *World Development Report*

WEF World Economic Forum

WFP World Food Program

WHA World Health Assembly

WHO World Health Organization

WHR *World Health Report*

WPRO Western Pacific Regional Office (WHO)

WSMI World Self Medication Industry

WTO World Trade Organization

YLD years lived with disability

YLL years of life lost

Index

Exhibits, figures and tables are indicated by e, f, and t following page numbers.